OPERATIVE PLASTIC SURGERY

OPERATIVE PLASTIC SURGERY

SECOND EDITION

EDITED BY

Gregory R. D. Evans, MD, FACS

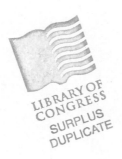

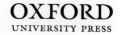
OXFORD
UNIVERSITY PRESS

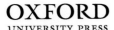

UNIVERSITY PRESS

Oxford University Press is a department of the University of Oxford. It furthers
the University's objective of excellence in research, scholarship, and education
by publishing worldwide. Oxford is a registered trade mark of Oxford University
Press in the UK and certain other countries.

Published in the United States of America by Oxford University Press
198 Madison Avenue, New York, NY 10016, United States of America.

First Edition published in 2000
Second Edition published in 2019

CIP data is on file at the Library of Congress
ISBN 978-0-19-049907-5

9 8 7 6 5 4 3 2 1

Printed by Sheridan Books, Inc., United States of America

CONTENTS

CONTRIBUTORS

Omotinuwe Adepoju, MD
Department of Plastic and Hand Surgery
Regions Hospital
St. Paul, Minnesota

Joshua M. Adkinson, MD
Assistant Professor of Surgery
Department of Surgery
Division of Plastic Surgery
Indiana University School of Medicine
Indianapolis, Indiana

Husain T. AlQattan, MD
General Surgery Resident
Dewitt Daughtry Department of Surgery
Division of Plastic Aesthetic and Reconstructive Surgery
Miller School of Medicine
University of Miami
Miami, Florida

Al Aly, MD
Consultant Plastic Surgeon—Professor of Plastic Surgery
Cleveland Clinic Abu Dhabi
Abu Dhabi, United Arab Emirates

Dalit Amar, MD
Attending Plastic Surgeon, Clinical Lecturer
Director, Body Contouring Service
Department of Plastic, Reconstructive and Aesthetic Surgery
Hadassah Hebrew University Medical Center
Jerusalem, Israel

William B. Armstrong, MD
Professor of Clinical Otolaryngology—Head and Neck Surgery
Department of Otolaryngology—Head and Neck Surgery
University of California, Irvine
Orange, California

Alfonso Barrera, MD, FACS
Diplomate, American Board of Plastic Surgery & American Board of Otolaryngology Head and Neck Surgery
Clinical Assistant Professor of Plastic Surgery
Baylor College of Medicine
Houston, Texas

Ruth J. Barta, MD
Adjunct Clinical Assistant Professor
Regions Hospital Department of Plastic and Hand Surgery
St. Paul, Minnesota

Erica L. Bartlett, MD
Resident Physician
Baylor College of Medicine
Division of Plastic Surgery
Houston, Texas

Natalie Barton, MD, MS
Resident Physician
Department of Plastic Surgery
University of California, Irvine
Orange, California

Joseph Baylan, MD
Resident Physician
Stanford University School of Medicine
Palo Alto, California

Bradley P. Bengtson, MD, FACS
Founder, Bengtson Center for Aesthetics and Plastic Surgery
Assistant Professor of Plastic Surgery
Michigan State University Department of Surgery
Grand Rapids, Michigan

Michael L. Bentz, MD, FAAP, FACS
Chair, Division of Plastic and Reconstructive Surgery
Vice Chair of Clinical Affairs
Department of Surgery

Layton F. Rikkers MD
Chair of Surgical Leadership
Professor of Surgery, Pediatrics, and Neurosurgery
University of Wisconsin School of Medicine and Public Health
Madison, Wisconsin

Nishant Bhatt, MD
Assistant Professor
Division of Plastic Surgery
University of North Carolina
Chapel Hill, North Carolina

James Martin Bourgeois, MD
Plastic Surgeon
Baton Rouge, Louisiana

Keith E. Brandt, MD
Executive Director, American Board of Plastic Surgery
William G. Hamm Professor of Surgery
Division of Plastic Surgery
Washington University School of Medicine
Saint Louis, Missouri

Richard E. Brown, MD
Private Practice
Springfield, IL

Steven R. Buchman, MD, FACS
M. Haskell Newman Professor in Plastic Surgery
Professor of Neurosurgery
Program Director, Craniofacial Surgery Fellowship
University of Michigan Medical School
Chief, Pediatric Plastic Surgery
CS Mott Children's Hospital
Director, Craniofacial Anomalies Program
University of Michigan Medical Center
Ann Arbor, Michigan

Michael Budd, MD
Plastic Surgeon (Partner)
Southern California Permanente Medical Group (SCPMG)
Downey, California

Bernard W. Chang, MD
Chief of Plastic Surgery
Mercy Medical Center
Baltimore, Maryland

David W. Chang, MD, FACS
Chief of Plastic Reconstructive Surgery
Director of Microsurgery Fellowship
Professor of Surgery
The University of Chicago Medicine & Biological Sciences
Chicago, Illinois

Elaina Y. Chen, MD
Assistant Professor of Surgery
Division of Plastic Surgery, Department of Surgery
University of Rochester Medical Center
Rochester, New York

Ming-Huei Cheng, MD, MBA, FACS
Professor
Department of Plastic Surgery
Chang Gung Memorial Hospital, Taiwan
Taoyuan, Taiwan

Brian M. Christie, MD, MPH
Resident
Plastic and Reconstructive Surgery
University of Wisconsin Hospital and Clinics
Madison, Wisconsin

Kevin C. Chung, MS, MD
Chief of Hand Surgery, Michigan Medicine
Charles B. G. de Nancrede Professor of Surgery
Professor of Plastic Surgery and Orthopaedic Surgery
Assistant Dean for Faculty Affairs
Associate Director of Global REACH
University of Michigan Medical School
Ann Arbor, Michigan

Michael E. Ciaravino, MD
Plastic Surgeon
Ciaravino Total Beauty
Houston, Texas

Mark W. Clemens, MD
Associate Professor
University of Texas MD Anderson Cancer Center
Houston, Texas

Benjamin E. Cohen, MD
Clinical Professor of Surgery
Weill Cornell Medical College
New York, New York

Mimis N. Cohen, MD, FACS, FAAP
Professor and Chief
Division of Plastic, Reconstructive and Cosmetic Surgery
Director, Craniofacial Center
University of Illinois
Chicago, Illinois

Bruce Cunningham, MD, MSc
Professor Emeritus and Past Chief of Plastic Surgery
University of Minnesota
Minneapolis, Minnesota

Alessandro G. Cusano, DDS, MD
Plastic Surgery Fellow
Department of Surgery, Division of Plastic Surgery
University of California Davis
Sacramento, California

Gehaan D'Souza, MD
CEO, Iconic Plastic Surgery
Carlsbad, California

David A. Daar, MD, MBA
Resident, Plastic Surgery
Hansjorg Wyss Department of Plastic Surgery
NYU Langone Health
New York, New York

Joseph J. Disa, MD, FACS
Attending Surgeon
Vice Chair of Clinical Activities
Plastic and Reconstructive Surgery Service
Department of Surgery
Memorial Sloan Kettering Cancer Center
Professor of Surgery
Weill Cornell Medical College
New York, New York

Marek K. Dobke, MD, PhD
Professor of Plastic Surgery
Department of Surgery
University of California San Diego
San Diego, California

Marco F. Ellis, MD, FACS
Assistant Professor
Division of Plastic Surgery
Department of Neurological Sciences
Feinberg School of Medicine, Northwestern University
Chicago, Illinois

Christopher L. Ellstrom, MD
Private Practice
Newport Beach, California

Russell E. Ettinger, MD
Chief Resident
Section of Plastic & Reconstructive Surgery
University of Michigan
Ann Arbor, Michigan

Maristella S. Evangelista, MD, MBA
Physician, Plastic Surgery
Veteran Affairs Palo Alto Health Care System
Palo Alto, California

Brogan G. A. Evans, MD Candidate (MS-III)
Texas A&M Health Science Center
College of Medicine
Bryan, Texas

Gregory R. D. Evans, MD, FACS
Professor of Plastic Surgery and Biomedical Engineering
Founding Chair, Department of Plastic Surgery
The University of California, Irvine
Orange, California

Jeffrey D. Friedman, MD
Associate Professor of Plastic Surgery
Institute for Reconstructive Surgery
Houston Methodist Hospital
Weill Cornell Medical College
Houston, Texas

David W. Furnas, MD
Professor Emeritus
Department of Plastic Surgery
University of California, Irvine
Orange, California

Shaili Gal, MD
Plastic and Reconstructive Surgery Fellow
Division of Plastic Surgery
Department of Surgery
University of California, Davis
Sacramento, California

Catharine B. Garland, MD
Assistant Professor, Plastic and Reconstructive Surgery
University of Wisconsin School of Medicine and Public Health
Madison, Wisconsin

Patrick B. Garvey, MD
Associate Professor of Plastic Surgery
University of Texas MD Anderson Cancer Center
Houston, Texas

Guilio Gheradini, MD
Private Practice
Rome, Italy

Daniel Goldberg, MD
Assistant Professor
Case Western Reserve University
Cleveland, Ohio

Arun K. Gosain, MD
Professor and Chief
Division of Pediatric Plastic Surgery
Lurie Children's Hospital
Northwestern University Feinberg School of Medicine
Chicago, Illinois

Amanda Gosman, MD
Professor and Interim Chief of Plastic Surgery Director of
    Craniofacial and Pediatric Plastic Surgery Plastic Surgery
    Program Director, Craniofacial Fellowship Director
University of California, San Diego Chief of Plastic
    Surgery, Rady Children's Hospital San Diego
San Diego, California

Lawrence J. Gottlieb, MD, FACS
Professor of Surgery
Section of Plastic and Reconstructive Surgery
The University of Chicago Medicine & Biological
    Sciences
Chicago, Illinois

Thomas Griffin Jr., MD
Dermatology Associates of Plymouth Meeting
Plymouth Meeting, Pennsylvania

Seanna R. Grob, MD
ASOPRS Fellow
University of California, Irvine
Orange, California

Ronald P. Gruber, MD
Clinical Associate Professor
University of California, San Francisco
San Francisco, California
Stanford University
Stanford, California

Kristy L. Hamilton, MD
Resident Physician
Division of Plastic Surgery
Baylor College of Medicine
Houston, Texas

Brett C. Hartman, DO
Assistant Professor of Plastic Surgery
Department of Surgery
Division of Plastic Surgery
Indiana University School of Medicine
Indianapolis, Indiana

Antony Hazel, MD
Clinical Instructor
Department of Orthopaedic Surgery
University of Louisville
Louisville, Kentucky

Matthew T. Houdek, MD
Assistant Professor of Orthopedic Surgery
Mayo Clinic College of Medicine and Science
Rochester, Minnesota

Keith A. Hurvitz, MD, FACS
Chief of Plastic Surgery
Long Beach Memorial Medical Center
Long Beach, California

Dana N. Johns, MD
Assistant Professor, Division of Plastic Surgery
University of Utah Hospital
Salt Lake City, Utah

Shepard P. Johnson, MBBS
Resident Physician
Department of Plastic Surgery
Vanderbilt University
Nashville, Tennessee

Neil F. Jones, MD, FRCS
Chief of Hand Surgery
Professor of Plastic and Reconstructive Surgery
Professor of Orthopedic Surgery
University of California, Irvine
Orange, California
Consultant
Hand Surgery and Microsurgery,
Shriners Hospital for Children
Los Angeles, California
Children's Hospital of Orange County
Orange, California

Melissa Kanack, MD
Resident Physician
University of California, Irvine
Orange, California

Jordan Kaplan, MD
Resident, Division of Plastic Surgery
Baylor College of Medicine
Houston, Texas

Raffy Karamanoukian, MD, FACS
Kare Plastic Surgery + Skin Health Center
Santa Monica, California

Rahul Kasukurthi, MD
Plastic Surgeon
Division of Plastic Surgery
Kaiser Permanente Northwest
Portland, Oregon

Ibrahim Khansa, MD
Fellow in Craniofacial Surgery
Children's Hospital Los Angeles
Los Angeles, California

Don O. Kikkawa, MD, FACS
Professor of Clinical Ophthalmology
Vice-Chairman, Department of Ophthalmology
Chief, Division of Oculofacial Plastic and Reconstructive
    Surgery
University of California, San Diego
San Diego, California

Elizabeth Killion, MD
Chief Resident
Baylor College of Medicine
Division of Plastic and Reconstructive Surgery
Houston, Texas

Brian M. Kinney, MD, FACS, MSME
Clinical Associate Professor of Plastic Surgery
University of Southern California (USC)
Plastic and Reconstructive Surgery
Beverly Hills, California

W. John Kitzmiller, MD, FACS
Henry W. and Margaret C. Neale Endowed Professor of
    Plastic Surgery
Chief, Section of Plastics/Burn Surgery
Medical Director of Ambulatory Surgery
University of Cincinnati Medical Center
Cincinnati, Ohio

Michael Klebuc, MD
Associate Professor of Clinical Plastic & Reconstructive
    Surgery
Houston Methodist Hospital—Weill Cornell Medical College
Houston, Texas

Grant M. Kleiber, MD
Assistant Professor of Surgery
Georgetown University
Washington, District of Columbia

Jason H. Ko, MD
Associate Professor
Division of Plastic and Reconstructive Surgery
Department of Orthopedic Surgery
Northwestern University Feinberg School of Medicine
Chicago, Illinois

Aaron M. Kosins, MD
Assistant Professor
University of California, Irvine
Private Practice
Newport Beach, California

Stephen S. Kroll, MD
Professor of Plastic Surgery
Anderson Cancer Center

Mark E. Krugman, MD
Assistant Clinical Professor of Plastic Surgery
University of California, Irvine, School of Medicine
Orange, California

Shadi Lalezari, MD, MBA
Physician
University of California, Irvine
Orange, California

Val Lambros, MD
Clinical Professor
Department of Plastic Surgery
University of California, Irvine
Orange, California

Samuel Lance, MD
Assistant Professor of Plastic Surgery
Associate Residency Program Director
University of California, San Diego
Division of Plastic Surgery, Rady Children's Hospital
    San Diego
San Diego, California

Karen T. Lane, MD, FACS
Clinical Director
Breast Health Center, Surgery School of Medicine
University of California, Irvine
Orange, California

Howard N. Langstein, MD
Professor of Surgery
Chief, Division of Plastic Surgery
Department of Surgery
University of Rochester Medical Center
Rochester, New York

Vincent G. Laurence, MD
Clinical Instructor
University of Pittsburgh Medical Center (UPMC)
    Orthopedic Specialists
Pittsburgh, Pennsylvania

Christine J. Lee, MD
Physician
Department of Plastic Surgery
University of California, Irvine
Orange, California

Michael Lee, MD
Private Practice
Dallas, TX

Amber R. Leis, MD
Director of Hand Surgery
Assistant Program Director
University of California at Irvine
Orange, California

Benjamin T. Lemelman, MD
PGY-6
Department of Surgery
The University of Chicago
Chicago, Illinois

Vivian V. Le-Tran, DO
Private Practice
CA, USA

Erin Lin, DO, FACOS, FACS
Assistant Clinical Professor
Department of Surgery
University of California, Irvine Health
Orange, California

Kant Y. Lin, MD, FACS
Professor and Chief
Division of Plastic Surgery
University of Kentucky College of Medicine
Lexington, Kentucky

H. Peter Lorenz, MD
Professor of Plastic Surgery
Director, Craniofacial Surgery Fellowship
Service Chief, Pediatric Plastic Surgery
Stanford University
Stanford, California

Joseph E. Losee, MD, FACS, FAAP
Ross H. Musgrave Professor of Pediatric
    Plastic Surgery
Children's Hospital of Pittsburgh of UPMC
Pittsburgh, Pennsylvania

Edward A. Luce, MD
Professor of Plastic Surgery
University of Tennessee
Memphis, Tennessee

Gina A. Mackert, MD
Resident of Plastic Surgery
Department of Hand-, Plastic and Reconstructive Surgery
Burn Center
Affiliated Department of Plastic Surgery of the University
    of Heidelberg
BG Trauma Center City
Ludwigshafen, Germany

Alan Matarasso, MD
Clinical Professor of Surgery
Hofstra University
Northwell School of Medicine
President-Elect, American Society of Plastic Surgeons,
    Executive Committee & Board of Directors
Past President, the Rhinoplasty Society & Chair Board of
    Trustees
Past President, New York Regional Society of Plastic
    Surgeons & Chair Board of Trustees
New York, New York

Evan Matros, MD, MMSc, MPH
Associate Professor, Weill Cornell Medical College
Associate Attending, Memorial Sloan Kettering
    Cancer Center
New York, New York

Gennaya L. Mattison, MD
Plastic Surgery Resident
University of California at Irvine
Orange, California

Jennifer L. McGrath, MD
Resident
Division of Plastic Surgery
Northwestern University Feinberg School of Medicine
Chicago, Illinois

Jillian M. McLaughlin, MD
Resident, PGY-4
Department of Surgery
University of Texas Medical Branch
Galveston, Texas

Heather A. McMahon, MD
Resident
University of Virginia School of Medicine

Alexander F. Mericli, MD
Assistant Professor of Plastic Surgery
University of Texas MD Anderson Cancer Center
Houston, Texas

Paul Mittermiller, MD
Plastic Surgery Resident Physician
Stanford University
Stanford, California

M. Mark Mofid, MD, FACS
Diplomate, American Board of Plastic Surgery
Diplomate, American Board of Facial Plastic and
    Reconstructive Surgery
Associate Clinical Professor of Plastic Surgery (Voluntary)
University of California, San Diego
La Jolla, California

Amy M. Moore, MD
Department of Surgery
Washington University School of Medicine
Saint Louis, Missouri

Ryan M. Moore, MD
Resident, Department of Plastic Surgery
University of California, Irvine
Orange, California

Steven L. Moran, MD
Professor of Plastic Surgery and Orthopedic Surgery
Mayo Clinic College of Medicine and Science
Rochester, Minnesota

Scott W. Mosser, MD
Plastic Surgeon
Scott W. Mosser Plastic Surgery
San Francisco, California

Donald S. Mowlds, MD, MBA
Resident Physician
Department of Plastic Surgery
University of California, Irvine
Orange, California

Melissa Mueller, MD
University of California, Irvine
Department of Plastic Surgery
Orange, California

Daniel Murariu, MD, MPH
Private Practice
Pittsburgh, PA

Maurice Y. Nahabedian, MD, FACS
Professor of Plastic Surgery
Virginia Commonwealth University—Inova Branch
National Center for Plastic Surgery
McLean, Virginia

Peter C. Neligan, MB, FRCS(I), FRCSC, FACS
Professor of Surgery
Division of Plastic Surgery
University of Washington Medical Center
Seattle, Washington

David T. Netscher, MD
Professor
Department of Orthopedic Surgery
Houston, Texas

Michael W. Neumeister, MD, FRCSC, FACS
Chief, Microsurgery & Research, SIUSOM
Director, Wound Care Center, Memorial Medical
    Center, Springfield, IL
Department of Surgery—Vice Chairman of
    Research, SIUSOM
Professor, SIUSOM
Chairman of Plastic Surgery, SIUSOM
Program Director—Hand/Micro Surgery Fellowship,
    SIUSOM
Director, Regional Burn Center, Memorial
    Medical Center
Medical Director—Baylis Outpatient Surgery Center
Chairman of Surgery, SIUSOM Microsurgery
Springfield, Illinois

Wendy Kar Yee Ng, MD, FRCSC
Assistant Clinical Professor of Plastic Surgery
University of California Irvine
Orange, California

Dananh Nguyen, BS
Private Practice
Pittsburgh, PA

Ajani Nugent, MD
Assistant Professor
Dewitt Daughtry Department of Surgery
Division of Plastic Aesthetic and Reconstructive
    Surgery
Miller School of Medicine
University of Miami
Miami, Florida

Scott D. Oates, MD
Professor
Department of Plastic Surgery
University of Texas MD Anderson Cancer Center
Houston, Texas

Windy A. Olaya, BS, MD
St. Joseph Hospital, Orange, California
Children's Hospital of Orange County
Orange, California

D. J. John Park, MD, FACS
Plastic Surgeon and Oculoplastic Surgeon
Newport Beach, California
Assistant Clinical Professor in Plastic Surgery
ASOPRS Associate Fellowship Preceptor
University of California, Irvine
Orange, California

Lauren D. Patty, MD, MS
Resident Physician, PGY 2
Department of Plastic Surgery
University of California, Irvine
Orange, California

Malcolm D. Paul, MD, FACS
Clinical Professor of Surgery
Department of Plastic Surgery
University of California, Irvine
Orange, California

Linda G. Phillips, MD, FACS
The Truman G. Blocker Jr., MD, Distinguished Professor
    and Chief
Division of Plastic Surgery
Department of Surgery
University of Texas Medical Branch
Galveston, Texas

Julian J. Pribaz, MD, FRCS (Edin), FRACS
Professor of Surgery Morsani College of Medicine
Department of Plastic Surgery
University of Florida
Tampa, Florida

Lee L. Q. Pu, MD
Professor of Surgery
Department of Surgery, Division of Plastic Surgery
University of California Davis
Sacramento, California

Gregory Rafijah, MD
Associate Professor
Department of Orthopaedic Surgery
University of California, Irvine
Orange, California

Edward Ray, MD, FACS
Assistant Professor of Surgery
Cedars-Sinai Medical Center
Los Angeles, California

Greg P. Reece, BS, MD
Professor of Plastic Surgery
University of Texas MD Anderson Cancer Center
Houston, Texas

J. Peter Rubin, MD
UPMC Endowed Professor and Chair of Plastic Surgery
Director, Life After Weight Loss Body Contouring
    Program
University of Pittsburgh
Pittsburgh, Pennsylvania

Eric S. Ruff, BS
Medical Student
Texas A&M Medical School
College Station, Texas

Nazanin Saedi, MD
Associate Professor
Thomas Jefferson University
Philadelphia, Pennsylvania

Ali Sajjadian, MD
Private Practice
Newport Beach, CA

Arthur Salibian, MD
Clinical Professor
Aesthetic and Plastic Surgery Institute
UC Irvine Medical Center, Orange, California
St. Joseph Hospital
Orange, California

**Mark V. Schaverien, MBChB, MSc, Med, MD, FRCS
    (Plast)**
Assistant Professor of Plastic Surgery
University of Texas MD Anderson Cancer Center
Houston, Texas

Warren Schubert, MD, FACS
Professor, University of Minnesota
Chair, Department of Plastic & Hand Surgery, Regions
    Hospital
St. Paul, Minnesota

Hisham Seify, MD, PhD
Assistant Clinical Professor
University of California, Los Angeles
Los Angeles, California

Jesse Selber, MD
Associate Professor of Plastic and Reconstructive Surgery
University of Texas MD Anderson Cancer Center
Houston, Texas

Ashkaun Shaterian, MD
Plastic Surgery Resident, Post Graduate Year 5
Department of Plastic Surgery
University of California, Irvine
Orange, California

Deana S. Shenaq, MD
Section of Plastic and Reconstructive Surgery
The University of Chicago Medicine & Biological
    Sciences
Chicago, Illinois

Kenneth C. Shestak, MD
Department of Plastic Surgery
University of Pittsburgh
Pittsburgh, Pennsylvania

Erica L. Sivak, MD
Department of Anesthesiology
Division of Pediatric Anesthesia
University of Pittsburgh
Pittsburgh, Pennsylvania

Wesley N. Sivak, MD, PhD
Fellow, Department of Plastic Surgery
Department of Plastic Surgery
University of Pittsburgh
Pittsburgh, Pennsylvania

Sheri Slezak, MD
Chief, Division of Plastic Surgery
Professor, University of Maryland School
    of Medicine
Baltimore, Maryland

Darren M. Smith, MD
Aesthetic and Craniofacial Plastic Surgeon
Private Practice
New York, New York

4000**Jesse Smith, MD**
Private Practice
Fort Worth & Colleyville, TX

David H. Song, MD, FACS
Physician Executive Director
MedStar Health Plastic & Reconstructive Surgery
Professor and Chairman
Department of Plastic Surgery
Georgetown University School of Medicine
Washington, District of Columbia

Rajiv Sood, MD
Chief of Plastic Surgery
Department of Surgery
Division of Plastic Surgery
Indiana University School of Medicine
Indianapolis, Indiana

Darlene M. Sparkman, MD
Director of Plastic Surgery at Hillcrest
Division of Plastic and Reconstructive Surgery
Baylor Scott & White Health
Waco, Texas

Aldona J. Spiegel, MD
Associate Professor
Weill Cornell Medicine
Institute for Reconstructive Surgery
Houston Methodist Hospital
Houston, Texas

Ahmed Suliman, MD
Associate Professor
Department of Surgery
University of California, San Diego
La Jolla, California

Chad M. Teven, MD
PGY-6
Department of Surgery
The University of Chicago
Chicago, Illinois

Seth Thaller, DMD, MD
Professor
Dewitt Daughtry Department of Surgery
Division of Plastic Aesthetic and Reconstructive Surgery
Miller School of Medicine
University of Miami
Miami, Florida

Yeshaswini Thelekkat, MDS
Senior Lecturer, Oral & Maxillofacial Surgeon
Oral Diagnostics and Surgical Sciences
International Medical University
Kuala Lumpur, Malaysia

Tjoson Tjoa, MD
Assistant Clinical Professor
Head and Neck Surgical Oncology
Microvascular Reconstruction
Department of Otolaryngology
University of California at Irvine
Orange, California

Catherine Tsai, MD
Resident Physician
University of California, San Diego
San Diego, California

Jonathan T. Unkart, MD, MS
Resident
Department of Surgery
University of California, San Diego
La Jolla, California

Mark M. Urata, MD, DDS, FACS, FAAP
Audrey Skirball Kenis Endowed Chair and
    Chief, Division of Plastic and Reconstructive
    Surgery
Keck School of Medicine, University of Southern
    California
Chair, Division of Oral and Maxillofacial Surgery
Ostrow School of Dentistry, University of Southern
    California
Division Head, Division of Plastic and Maxillofacial
    Surgery
Children's Hospital Los Angeles
Los Angeles, California

Leo J. Urbinelli, MD, MA
Assistant Professor of Plastic Surgery
Oregon Health & Science University
Portland, Oregon

Nicholas B. Vedder, MD
Professor of Surgery and Orthopaedics
Chief of Plastic Surgery
University of Washington
Seattle, Washington

Raj M. Vyas, MD
Associate Professor
Department of Plastic Surgery
University of California, Irvine, School of Medicine
Orange, California

Anne M. Wallace, MD
Professor of Surgery
Director, Comprehensive Breast Health Center
Department of Surgery
University of California, San Diego
La Jolla, California

Derrick Wan, MD
Associate Professor, Department of Surgery
Stanford University School of Medicine
Stanford, California

Nicholas A. Wingate, MD
Resident, Plastic Surgery
Division of Plastic Surgery, Department of Surgery
University of Rochester Medical Center
Rochester, New York

Michael S. Wong, MD
Professor of Surgery
Department of Surgery, Division of Plastic Surgery
University of California Davis
Sacramento, California

Peirong Yu, MD, MS
Professor
Department of Plastic Surgery
University of Texas MD Anderson Cancer Center
Houston, Texas

Christopher B. Zachary, FRCP
Professor and Chair
University of California, Irvine
Orange, California

Sanam Zahedi, MD
Resident, PGY-4
Department of Surgery
University of Texas Medical Branch
Galveston, Texas

Jonathan A. Zelken, MD
Plastic Surgeon
Zelken Institute for Aesthetic Medicine
Newport Beach, California

PART I.

PRINCIPLES

1.

INTRODUCTION

Gregory R. D. Evans

The art of plastic surgery is the restoration of form and function with the resultant improvement not only in aesthetic outcomes but also in the quality of life. The word "plastic" is derived from the Greek *plastikos* ("fit for molding"). While the term "plastique" was used by Desault in 1798, it was the publication of Zeis's *Handbuch der plastischen Chirurgie* in 1838 that popularized the term.

> The longer you look back, the further you can look forward.
>
> —*Churchill*

Tissue restoration has its heritage in ancient Egypt with the first well-documented manuscript written in 1600 BC on a 12-inch-wide, 25-yard-long scroll, the Ebers Papyrus. This document described multiple operations to restore missing structures of facial expression, such as the nose and ears, in an attempt to restore socially acceptable features.

Civil and penal responsibility of the physician developed during the Assyrian period with the code of Hammurabi. The threat of hand amputation was great incentive for success in the restoration of form and function. Current litigants are much less of a treat than the former physical punishment, and the "above all, do no harm" philosophy has been maintained through today's current medical practice.

The *Sushruta Samhita* (circa 600 BC) from ancient India described 15 operations for restoring split or mutilated ears. Records further indicate the earliest rhinoplasty and the repair of nasal defects from cheek tissue. It was against the religious principles of the Hindu priests to contaminate themselves by contact with injured or diseased flesh. Thus, reparative surgery was relegated to the members of the lower caste.

The transformation from the Bronze to the Iron Age is exemplified by Homer's *Iliad* and *Odyssey*. This coincided with the transformation of the practice of medicine from priests or members of the lower caste to more formalized training. Hippocrates (460 to 370 BC) believed that war was the only proper school for a surgeon. He discussed in the *Corpus Hippocraticum* (400 BC) the pathology and treatment of scars (burns) in an attempt to prevent deformities and mold tissue to more acceptable results.

Celsus (25 BC to 50 AD) described in detail plastic surgery on the nose, lips, eyelids, and ears. He was probably the originator of the island flap, and his techniques included molding tissue by the use of sliding grafts to cover quadrilateral and triangular defects.

After the barbarian invasions, the vestiges of Greek and Roman medicine and plastic surgery remained in the Islamic schools. The Middle Ages (1096–1438 AD) were devoid of innovation, and the medieval church opposed surgeons. Not until the fifteenth century did the invention of the printing press make possible books on tissue restoration that included medical illustrations.

The fourteenth through sixteenth centuries marked a rebirth in medicine and plastic surgery. The Renaissance produced many gifted surgeons, including Guido Lanfranchi, Guy de Chauliac, and the Brancas family. However, it was left to Gaspare Tagliacozzi (1545–1599) to lay the cornerstone of modern plastic surgery. A professor at the University of Bologna and chief surgeon to the Grand Duke of Tuscany, he provided the first record of plastic surgery in his 1597 treatise, *De curtorum chirurgia per insitionem*: "We restore, repair and make whole, those parts of the face which nature has given but which fortune has taken away. . . ."

With Tagliacozzi's treatises, plastic surgery was thrust into the modern era. Over the next few centuries, surgeons continued to restore form and function. In 1794, a letter describing the traditional Indian nasal reconstruction of Cowasjee, a bullock driver with the English army in the war of 1792, was written to Mr. Urban, the editor of *Gentleman's* magazine. The transfer of the forehead flap on an axial pattern blood supply brought the concepts of tissue transfer into the Western world.

With Morton's use of ether in 1846, surgery was thrust into the contemporary age. More reliable methods for wound closure were advanced. Local pedicle flaps were slowly replaced by more reliable tissue transfers. One such method was the development of microvascular free tissue transfer, and the first clinical series was performed in 1964 by Nakayama, who transferred intestinal segments into the cervical esophagus of 21 patients. Another flurry of clinical reports occurred in 1971, with Antia and Buch, McLean and Buncke, Daniel, Taylor, and O'Brien. Bowel, skin, muscle, and bone were now available for one-stage, immediate reconstruction.

These time-honored techniques, developed over the preceding 5,000 years, have allowed us to approach patients systematically. This systematic approach, along with patient considerations, has been used to outline the chapters in this second edition of the original book. In the approach to the patient, the surgeon must first consider the assessment of the defect. What are the important preoperative factors in addressing the problem at hand? How does the influence of medical or adjuvant therapy affect efforts to address the defect? What is the pathology of the defect? What role does trauma play in operative repair? What is the correct marriage of donor to recipient tissue?

The second consideration is the operative indications. When would the operative technique be indicated, and when would alternative techniques be used? The third consideration is contraindications. What are the contraindications to the operative procedure? What defects would not lend themselves to operative closure or repair?

The operative room setup must also be considered. What is required to proceed with the operative plan? What are the tricks one employs to make the procedure run smoothly? How should the patient be positioned? When these considerations have been assessed, patient markings for operative intervention must be performed. How should the patient be marked to proceed with the operative plan? Are the patient markings position-dependent? Do alterations in muscular tone, initiated by anesthesia, affect the operative outline? The sixth consideration is the operative technique. What are the step-by-step procedures that must be followed to correct the defect or deformity?

Finally, postoperative care and details of pertinent dressings to be used must be reviewed. Should an occlusive dressing be used? Are stints, tape, or sutures necessary? What is the standard of care following these surgical closures? What type of rehabilitation is necessary? Are splints required? If flap monitoring is required, what type should be used? What is the time frame for the removal of packing or drains? How should hardware be managed? Is occupational or physical therapy required? In addition, we must learn from the procedure. If complications occur, how can we change our operative technique to avoid potential difficulties? Was the timing of the operation appropriate?

"Not for self, not for the fulfillment of any earthly desire or gain but solely for the salvage of suffering humanity," says the *Sushruta Samhita*. Three thousand years later, the same philosophy holds. We have come from the transfer of local, pedicle, and free flaps to the understanding of the requirements for angiogenesis and the physiology of tissue molding. Despite our efforts, our ability to modify tissues remains somewhat primitive and still requires the use of autogenous donor tissue. What lies ahead? Ahead lies a future bright with ideas and concepts that we are just beginning to explore, such as translational research, fat grafting, stem cells, and tissue engineering.

SELECTED READINGS

Absolon KB, Rogers W, Aust JB. Some historical developments of the surgical therapy of tongue cancer from the seventeenth to the nineteenth century. *Am J Surg* 1962;104:686.

Antia NH, Buch VI. Transfer of an abdominal dermo-fat graft by direct anastomosis of blood vessels. *Br J Plast Surg* 1971;24:15.

Ariyan S. The pectoralis major myocutaneous flap: a versatile flap for reconstruction in the head and neck. *Plast Reconstr Surg* 1979;63:73.

Ariyan S. The pectoralis major for single-stage reconstruction of the difficult wounds of the orbit and pharyngoesophagus. *Plast Reconstr Surg* 1983;72:468.

Ariyan S, Chicarill ZN. Cancer of the upper aerodigestive system. In: McCarthy JG, ed. *Plastic Surgery*. Philadelphia: WB Saunders Co., 1990:3412–3478.

Ariyan S, Krizek TJ. Reconstruction after resection of head and neck cancer. Cline clinics. Clinical Congress of the American College of Surgeons, Dallas, October 1977.

Bakamjian VY. A two-stage method for pharyngoesophageal reconstruction with a primary pectoral skin flap. *Plast Reconstr Surg* 1965;36:173.

Bhishagratna KK. *An English Translation of the Sushruta Samhita Based on Original Sanskrit Text.* 3 vols. Calcutta: Bose, 1916.

Daniel RK, Taylor GI. Distant transfer of an island flap by microvascular anastomoses. *Plast Reconstr Surg* 1973;52:111.

Desault PJ. *Oeuvres chirurgicales ou exposé de la doctrine et de la plastique.* Vol. 2. Paris: Megegnon, 1798.

Erol ÖO, Spira M. Utilization of a composite island flap employing omentum in organ reconstruction: an experimental investigation. *Plast Reconstr Surg* 1981;68:561–570.

Hirase Y, Valauri FA, Buncke HJ. Prefabricated sensate myocutaneous and osteomyocutaneous free flaps: an experimental model. Preliminary report. *Plast Reconstr Surg* 1988;82:440–445.

Hussl H., Russell RC, Zook EG, Eriksson E. Experimental evaluation of tissue: revascularization using a transferred muscular-vascular pedicle. *Ann Plast Surg* 1986;17:299–305.

Hyakusoku H, Okubo M, Umeda Ta, Fumiiri M. A prefabricated hair-bearing island flap for lip reconstruction. *Br J Plast Surg* 1987;40:37–39.

Itoh Y. An experimental study of prefabricated flaps using silicone sheets, with reference to the vascular patternization process. *Ann Plast Surg* 1992;28:140–146.

Jurkiewica MJ. Vascularized intestinal graft for reconstruction of the cervical esophagus and pharynx. *Plast Reconstr Surg* 1965;36:509.

Khouri RK, Koudsi B, Reddi H. Tissue transformation into bone in vivo. *JAMA* 1991;266:1953–1955.

Khouri RK, Tark KC, Shaw WW. Prefabrication of flaps using an arteriovenous bundle and angiogenesis factors. *Surg Forum* 1992;15:597–2599.

Khouri RK, Upton J, Shaw WW. Prefabrication of composite free flaps through staged microvascular transfer: an experimental and clinical study. *Plast Reconstr Surg* 1991;87:108–115.

Kim WS, Vacanti CA, Upton J, Vacanti JP. Bone defect repair with tissue-engineered cartilage. *Plast Reconstr Surg* 1994;94:580–584.

Langer R, Vancanti CA. Tissue engineering. *Science* 1993;260:920–926. Review.

McLean DH, Bunke HJ. Auto transplant of omentum to a large scalp defect with microsurgical revascularization. *Plast Reconstr Surg* 1972;49:268.

Mulliken JB, Glowacki J. Induced osteogenesis for repair and construction in the craniofacial region. *Plast Reconstr Surg* 1980;65:553–560.

Nakayama K, Yamamoto K, Tamiya T, et al. Experience with free autografts of the bowel with a new venous anastomosis apparatus. *Surgery* 1964;55:796–802.

O'Brien BM, MacLeod AM, Milly GD, et al. Successful transfer of a large island flap from the groin to the foot by microvascular anastomoses. *Plast Reconstr Surg* 1973;52:271.

Özgentaş, HE, Shenaq S, Spira M. Prefabrication of a secondary TRAM flap. *Plast Reconstr Surg* 1995;95:441–449.

Serafin D, Rios AV, Georgiade N. Fourteen free groin flap transfers. *Plast Reconstr Surg* 1976;57:707–715.

Stark GB, Hong C, Futrell JW. Enhanced neovascularization of rat tubed pedicle flaps with low perfusion of the wound margin. *Plast Reconstr Surg* 1987;80:814–824.

Talgliacozzi G. *De curtorum chirurgia per insitionem*. Venice: Gaspare Bindoni, 1597.

Tzuyao S. Experimental study of tissue graft vascularization by means of vascular implantation and subcutaneous burying. *Plast Reconstr Surg* 1984;73:403–410.

Upton J, Ferraro N, Healy G, et al. The use of prefabricated fascial flaps for lining of the oral and nasal cavities. *Plast Reconstr Surg* 1994;94:573–579.

Vacanti CA, Langer R, Schloo B, Vacanti JP. Synthetic polymers seeded with chondrocytes provide a template for new cartilage formation. *Plast Reconstr Surg* 1991;88:753–759.

Zeis E. *Handbuch der plastichen Chirurgie (Nebsteiner Vorrede von J. F. Dieffenbach)*. Berlin: Reimer, 1838.

2.

ANESTHESIA
LOCAL NERVE BLOCKS

Wesley N. Sivak, Erica L. Sivak, and Kenneth C. Shestak

INTRODUCTION

Regional anesthesia refers to the use of local anesthetics to block nerve signals emanating from discrete anatomic areas of the body. It allows surgical procedures to be performed on anesthetized regions of the body without necessarily rendering a patient unconscious. As such, it has many advantages over general anesthesia, as there are less interferences and disturbances of normal homeostasis. This is particularly important for patients with significant medical comorbidities involving the cardiovascular, respiratory, or renal systems. Additionally, regional anesthesia can be performed quickly and is useful in emergency situations without delaying care, such as when a patient may have recently eaten and is at increased risk for general anesthesia due to aspiration. Furthermore, postoperative morbidity, including pulmonary edema, atelectasis, and other respiratory complications related to general anesthesia, can be markedly reduced with the use of regional anesthesia techniques. There can also be a significant benefit from a nursing and medical standpoint corresponding to decreases in after-care requirements when techniques are planned and implemented appropriately.

Regional anesthesia encompasses a broad range of techniques. In its simplest form, infiltration of local tissues with anesthetic agents can provide a small field under which to perform minor surgical procedures. Peripheral nerves of all sizes can also be targeted to render discrete anatomic areas and even entire limbs insensate. In its most complex form, regional anesthesia can be delivered to the central nervous system, blocking entire regions of the body encompassing multiple dermatomal distributions. Regional techniques have even allowed patients to remain awake during major surgery, as evidenced by a recent trend toward "wide awake surgery" being utilized for many plastic surgery procedures.

Local anesthetic agents are essential to create and maintain regional blockades. These drugs fall into two main classifications: esters and amides, with the latter by far the most frequently used. A list of commonly used local anesthetic agents is presented in Table 2.1. Local anesthetic agents are delivered to the target tissues, where they produce a temporary block of nerve conduction by interfering with action potential propagation via their effects on sodium channels. After being taken up by bodily tissues, esters are eliminated locally by plasma pseudocholinesterase, but amides must be absorbed into the systemic circulation to be metabolized by the liver. Use of epinephrine, typically at concentrations of 1:200,000 (or 5 μg/mL), can prolong the expected duration of regional anesthetic blockade. Other techniques employing controlled-release formulations or placement of catheters for continuous infusion of local anesthetics have been described and have further expanded the clinical indications for regional anesthesia.

Local anesthetics, when used in dosages within the normal clinical range, have minimal noxious effects on target tissues. There is negligible neurotoxicity, as exemplified by complete recovery of neural function after regional blocks have been performed. The local adverse effects of anesthetic agents can include manifestations such as prolonged anesthesia (i.e., numbness) and paresthesia (i.e., tingling, feeling of "pins and needles," or strange sensations). These symptoms can be related to damage, usually caused by intraneural injection or expansion of fluid into a closed anatomic space, including untoward sequela such as hematoma. Systemic adverse effects are directly related to circulating plasma levels. Symptoms follow a predictable pattern affecting first peripheral nerves, then the central nervous system, and finally the heart. Side effects on the central nervous system and the heart may be severe and potentially fatal. However, toxicity occurs only at plasma levels that are

TABLE 2.1 LOCAL ANESTHETIC AGENTS

Esters	Amides
Cocaine	Lidocaine (Xylocaine)
Procaine (Novocaine)	Mepivacaine (Carbocaine)
Tetracaine (Pontocaine)	Prilocaine (Citanest)
Chloroprocaine (Nesacaine)	Bupivacaine (Marcaine, Sensorcaine)
Benzocaine (Americaine)	Etidocaine (Duranest)

rarely reached if proper technique is followed. Epinephrine, in addition to prolonging the anesthetic effect via vasoconstriction, can also shift the timeframe for occurrence of peak plasma levels. A detailed discussion of local anesthetic pharmacokinetics is beyond the scope of this chapter, but the characteristics of the commonly used anesthetic agents, including normal dosages, are listed in Table 2.2.

Adverse reactions to local anesthetics are not uncommon, but true allergic reaction remains rare. Allergic reactions occur only with the esters; are usually due to sensitivity to their metabolite, para-aminobenzoic acid (PABA); and do not result in cross-allergy to amide agents. Also, cases of allergy to paraben derivatives occur, which are often added as preservatives to local anesthetic solutions. Methemoglobinemia, a process in which the oxygen-carrying ability of iron in hemoglobin is altered, produces cyanosis and symptoms of hypoxia. Benzocaine, lidocaine, and prilocaine can all produce this effect, especially benzocaine. Thus, a careful medical history should be obtained from every patient, highlighting any previous adverse effect involving local anesthetic agents prior to considering regional anesthesia.

ASSESSMENT OF THE DEFECT

Regional anesthesia is ideal for any surgical procedure being performed on an anatomic site with a pattern of nervous innervation emerging from a point that is accessible for local anesthetic blockade.

INDICATIONS

Regional anesthesia can be used as the sole anesthetic (with or without sedation) or as a supplement to general anesthesia to improve postoperative analgesia. General considerations include (1) suitability for the type of surgery being performed, (2) surgeon's preferences, (3) institutional experience in performing the technique, (4) physiologic and psychologic state of the patient, and (5) patient acceptance of temporary loss of motor/sensory function. Benefits of regional anesthesia can include (1) improved patient satisfaction, (2) less immunosuppression relative to general anesthesia, (3) decreased incidence of postoperative nausea and vomiting, (4) alternative for patients with a history of malignant hyperthermia, (5) alternative for patients who are hemodynamically unstable or too ill to tolerate general anesthesia, (6) superior pain control in the immediate postoperative period, (7) decreased alteration of the patient's cardiopulmonary physiological status, and (8) less postoperative cognitive impairment (especially in the elderly). General risks of regional anesthesia include (1) toxicity of local anesthetics (especially with indwelling catheters), (2) transient or chronic paresthesia, (3) potential nerve damage, (4) intraarterial injection, (5) seizure, (6) cardiac

TABLE 2.2 CHARACTERISTICS OF COMMONLY USED ANESTHETIC DRUGS

Generic Name (Proprietary Name)	Concentrations (mg %)		Maximum Dose[a] (mg/kg)	Approximate Duration (hr)
	Infiltration	Nerve Block		
Procaine (Novocaine)	0.75	1.5–3.0	10–14	0.75–1.50
Chloroprocaine (Nesacaine)	0.75	1.5–3.0	12.15	Short-acting
Lidocaine (Xylocaine)	0.50	1.0–2.0	8–11	1.5–3.0
Mepivacaine (Carbocaine)	0.50	1.0–2.0	8–11	Medium duration
Tetracaine (Pontocaine)	0.05	0.15–0.20	2	
Bupivacaine (Marcaine)	0.25	0.25–0.50	2.5–3.5	3.0–10.0
Etidocaine (Duranest)	0.50	0.5–1.0	4.0–5.5	Long-acting
Ropivacaine (Naropin)	0.25	0.25–0.50	2.5–3.5	

[a] Higher dose with the use of 1:200 000 epinephrine.

arrest, (7) block failure and need to supplement and/or convert to general anesthesia, and (8) infection.

Regional anesthesia remains the procedure of choice in most patients undergoing upper extremity surgery. Anesthetics can be employed at the level of the brachial plexus, but blocks that anesthetize the entire limb are most commonly carried out in the form of an axillary block. Additionally, blocks can be performed around the elbow or in the forearm, including blocks of the ulnar nerve, medial nerve, radial nerve, and medial and lateral antebrachial cutaneous nerves. Another commonly administered regional block is the wrist block. Wrist blocks are very helpful in producing anesthesia of the palm and in median nerve distribution for carpal tunnel release and release of Guyon's canal. Finally, the most commonly used block in the hand is the digital block, which provides anesthesia to a single digit. This invaluable method of anesthesia for emergency hand surgery is the most common type employed in the management of emergency surgical procedures on the hand.

CONTRAINDICATIONS

There are several factors to consider when choosing anesthetic techniques. Examine the patient for surgical scars, scoliosis, skin lesions, and anatomy that may interfere with nerve blockade. There are no routine preoperative tests for healthy patients undergoing regional anesthesia. However, patients with a history of medications/medical conditions that may increase the risk of bleeding should have coagulation studies and platelet counts drawn. Every patient should be assessed for thrombocytopenia prior to the initiation of spinal anesthesia. The following signs and symptom may indicate bleeding tendencies: (1) blood in the urine, (2) bleeding around the gums, and (3) diffuse petechiae. In addition, the patient should be carefully questioned about tendency to bruise easily and any difficulty forming blood clots or prolonged bleeding.

Contraindications for regional anesthesia can be either relative or absolute. Absolute contraindications include (1) patient refusal, (2) infection at the injection site, (3) a true allergy to local anesthetics, (4) inability to guarantee sterile equipment, and (5) high risk of local anesthetic toxicity (i.e., bilateral axillary block). Relative contraindications include (1) pediatric, combative, and/or demented patients; (2) bleeding disorder, either medication induced (i.e., Coumadin) or genetic (i.e., hemophilia) or acquired (i.e., disseminated intravascular coagulation [DIC]); (3) existing peripheral nerve neuropathies that

may increase the risk for permanent nerve damage; (4) severe hypovolemia; (5) anemia; and (6) stenotic heart valve lesions. Careful documentation of any existing sensory and/or motor deficits should occur prior to the initiation of any regional approach. Bleeding disorders are an absolute contraindication for any spinal anesthetic due to the risk of hematoma and subsequent cord compression.

ROOM SETUP AND MARKINGS

The room setup and markings will be specific for each case and the type of regional anesthesia being utilized. Regional anesthetic techniques will most often be employed by the plastic surgeon during upper extremity cases. In such instances, the room should include an operating room table with a hand or arm board coming off at a 90-degree angle for arm positioning, overhead operating room lighting, an arm pneumatic tourniquet, and movable stools around both sides of the arm board. There must also be a place to store the anesthetic agents and sterile supplies, such as gloves, towels, syringes, needles, and tubing. The commonly used needles are 1.5- and 3.8-cm long and either 22 or 25 gauge. The syringes necessary are 5 cc, 10 cc, 30 cc, and 50 cc capacity syringes.

SPECIFIC BLOCKS

AXILLARY BLOCK

The most common technique for providing regional anesthesia of the upper extremity is the axillary block, which blocks the major nerves at the level of the third part of the axillary artery. The artery and major nerves are superficial, permitting consistent anesthesia of the extremity with infiltration of the anesthetic agent.

Anatomy

At the level of the third part of the axillary artery, the brachial plexus cords form three major nerves. Using the axillary artery as a point of reference in the area immediately below the shoulder crease on the medial side of the humerus, the median nerve lies anterior and superficial, the ulnar nerve lies posterior and superficial, and the radial nerve lies deep (Figure 2.1). The artery and vein are enclosed in their own subdivision of the fascial sheath, which envelops the entire brachial plexus. The axillary and musculocutaneous nerves egress from the plexus at the level of the coracoid process

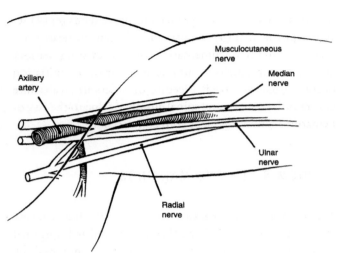

Figure 2.1. Axillary block. Median, ulnar, and radial nerves may be located using axillary artery as point of reference in area immediately below shoulder crease on medial side of humerus.

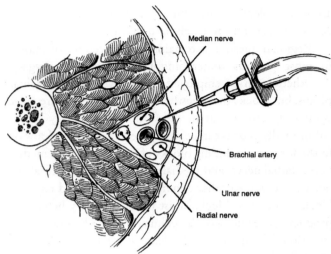

Figure 2.2. Axillary block technique: perivascular approach. Injecting anesthetic agent into sheath above and then below axillary artery.

and are not routinely anesthetized during the performance of an axillary block.

Technique

The original description of the axillary block technique was by Hirshel in 1911. Subsequent to this, all techniques were performed with the arm abducted 90 degrees, with the humerus placed in a position of slight external rotation. Historically, the most common techniques were the arterial puncture and the paresthesia techniques. More recently, the perivascular technique, which is the technique of infiltrating above and below the artery without puncturing the artery or producing paresthesias, has been employed and utilizes ultrasound guidance for delivery of local anesthetic to the axillary sheath.

Since the nerves to be anesthetized surround the axillary artery, the technique of deliberately puncturing the artery with a 22-gauge needle while aspirating blood through the syringe was developed. The needle is advanced through the artery, and an injection is performed only when no further blood can be aspirated. At this point, 40–50 mL of lidocaine or bupivacaine is injected into the sheath surrounding the plexus. It is imperative to hold digital pressure on the area of arterial puncture to prevent hematoma formation, which, if present, may interfere with the production of a satisfactory block.

With the paresthesia technique, the needle is used to explore the region just anterior and just posterior to the axillary artery. It is relatively easy to elicit paresthesias from the median and ulnar nerves since they are superficial, but more difficult to evoke paresthesias from the radial nerve. After paresthesias are noted, approximately 10 mL of local anesthetic agent is injected around each nerve.

Currently, the most popular technique of achieving an axillary block is the perivascular approach (Figure 2.2). In this method, the penetration of the axillary sheath by the injecting needle is noted when a "click" is felt just above and just below the artery. Approximately 40 mL of anesthetic agent is injected into the sheath, and again digital pressure is applied after completion of the injection. The arm is then adducted, and this maneuver, along with the digital pressure, promotes central and proximal migration of the anesthetic solution. This block is relatively simple and is consistently attainable with experience; ultrasound guidance is routinely used to enhance accuracy of this technique.

Precautions

The technique cannot be used when it is not possible to abduct the arm. When using the paresthesia technique, there has been some concern regarding neuritis following injection, especially when epinephrine is added to the local anesthetic. With these concerns in mind, the axillary block remains the technique of choice for regional anesthesia of the upper extremity.

BLOCKS AROUND THE ELBOW

Blocks around the elbow are not frequently performed since there is significant overlap of the distribution of the ulnar, median, and radial nerves, and the variation of this distribution necessitates multiple blocks. Therefore, instead of performing the necessary multiple blocks at the elbow level, it is easier to achieve whole-arm anesthesia with an axillary block. Individual nerve blocks at the elbow are most often used to supplement an axillary block. However, diagnostic nerve blocks at the elbow are useful in the evaluation of pathologic nerve lesions, such as neuromas, or to investigate pain syndromes of the forearm, wrist, and hand.

ULNAR NERVE BLOCK

Technique

The ulnar nerve passes from the posterior aspect of the upper arm to the anterior aspect of the forearm at the elbow, running through the groove between the olecranon and the medial epicondyle. It can be palpated at this level and is anesthetized by the placement of 5 mL of 2% lidocaine solution administered through a 1.5-cm, 25-gauge needle.

Precautions

It is imperative to avoid injection of the local anesthetic directly into the ulnar nerve, which is quite superficial.

RADIAL NERVE BLOCK

Technique

The radial nerve travels on the lateral aspect of the upper arm in the interval between the brachialis and brachioradialis muscles. The nerve is blocked two fingerbreadths above this landmark in the interval between the two muscle bellies, using a 3- to 8-cm, 25-gauge needle. Paresthesias should be sought, and once obtained, 5–10 mL of 2% lidocaine solution is infused.

The medial and lateral antebrachial cutaneous (MAC and LAC) nerves can be blocked distal to the elbow. The MAC runs just lateral to the medial basilic vein, and the LAC runs just medial to the cephalic vein. Approximately 3–5 mL of local anesthetic can be placed into this location, or, alternatively, a subcutaneous ring of local anesthetic can be injected just distal to the elbow flexion crease.

WRIST BLOCKS

Wrist blocks are very valuable and used often in hand surgery. They are safe, well tolerated by the patient, and simple to perform.

MEDIAN NERVE BLOCK

Anatomy

Anesthesia of the median nerve is critical in the performance of carpal tunnel release. This nerve is readily accessible to the infiltration of local anesthetic in the form of either lidocaine or bupivacaine.

The nerve is derived from the medial cord of the brachial plexus. It runs on the anterior aspect of the upper arm and then in the plane between the flexor digitorum superficialis and flexor digitorum profundus in the upper forearm. At approximately the distal third of the forearm, the nerve becomes relatively superficial. Just above the wrist flexion crease, it lies in a position between the flexor carpi radialis (FCR) and the palmaris longus (PL). At this level, it can be anesthetized by the infiltration of local anesthesia.

Technique

Routinely, the patient is asked to oppose the tip of the ring finger to the tip of the thumb. This allows careful and precise location of the PL tendon. The PL lies on the ulnar side of the median nerve. Local anesthetic can then be injected radial to this landmark along the nerve (Figure 2.3). An injection of the nerve in the carpal tunnel

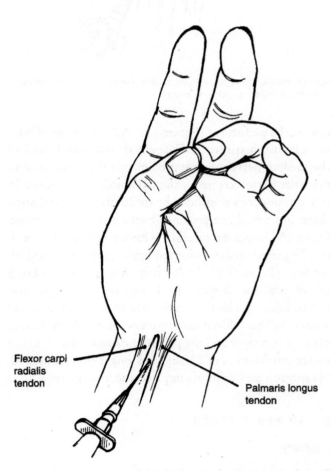

Flexor carpi radialis tendon

Palmaris longus tendon

Figure 2.3. Median nerve block. Injecting local anesthetic radial to palmaris longus along nerve.

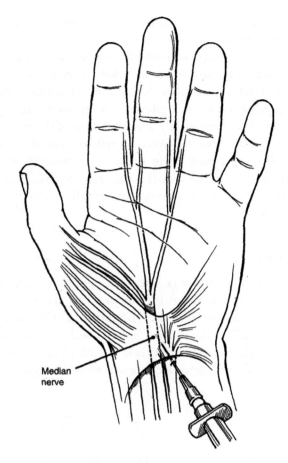

Figure 2.4. Median nerve block. Injecting local anesthetic in carpal tunnel with entrance ulnar to palmaris longus.

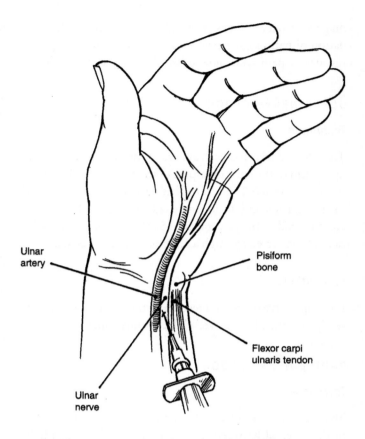

Figure 2.5. Ulnar nerve block. Injection proximal to wrist flexion crease and just radial to flexor carpi ulnaris tendon.

can also be performed (Figure 2.4). A 2% solution of lidocaine is customarily used. The palmar cutaneous branch of the median nerve arises approximately 6 cm proximal to the wrist flexion crease on the radial side of the nerve. It, too, can undergo anesthesia by infiltrating the local anesthetic in a wheal just proximal to the wrist flexion crease. Using 2% lidocaine solution without epinephrine, a 4-cm, 25-gauge needle is inserted between the FCR and PL tendons (Figure 2.3). At the first sign of paresthesias, 5 mL of local anesthetic is slowly injected. It is imperative not to inject the local directly into the nerve, but rather around it. This infiltration produces anesthesia in the median nerve proper and the palmar cutaneous bands with a maximum duration of 2 hours. If a longer effect is desired, the surgeon may infiltrate bupivacaine into the region.

ULNAR NERVE BLOCK

Anatomy

The ulnar nerve is also superficial in its position: it lies radial to the flexor carpi ulnaris tendon, which inserts into the pisiform bone (Figure 2.5). This pisiform bone is readily palpated at the wrist. The ulnar artery lies radial to the ulnar nerve (Figure 2.5), and the surgeon must not inject local anesthesia into the artery. The dorsal sensory branch of the ulnar nerve exits 6 cm proximal to the wrist, passing over the ulnar aspect of the forearm.

Technique

The pisiform bone is palpated on the palmar aspect of the wrist, and the patient is asked to flex and deviate the wrist toward the ulna, allowing precise identification of the flexor carpi ulnaris (FCU) tendon. Next, a 4- cm, 25-gauge needle, which is attached to a syringe containing 2% lidocaine solution, is passed just radial to the FCU tendon until paresthesias are sensed. At this point, the needle is slightly withdrawn so as to not directly inject the nerve, and 5 mL of the lidocaine is injected slowly (Figure 2.5). To obtain a block of the dorsal sensory branch of the ulnar nerve, an additional 5 mL of lidocaine is injected 6 cm proximal to the wrist flexion crease on the ulnar and dorsal aspect of the forearm in the subcutaneous tissue.

RADIAL NERVE BLOCK

Anatomy

The radial nerve is a pure sensory nerve after giving rise to the posterior interosseous nerve in the proximal forearm. It runs on the volar aspect of the forearm deep to the brachioradialis muscle and emerges through this muscle 8–10 cm proximal to the wrist. It then passes radial and dorsal at a point 6 cm proximal to the wrist flexion crease (Figure 2.6) to supply sensory innervation to the dorsoradial aspect of the hand and radial digits (thumb through ring finger).

Technique

The radial nerve is readily blocked at the level of the wrist by placing 5–8 mL of 2% lidocaine solution in the subcutaneous tissues 6 cm proximal to the wrist flexion crease on the radial and dorsoradial aspect of the forearm.

DIGITAL NERVE BLOCK

Perhaps the most frequently used nerve block for surgery on the hand is the digital nerve block. It is easy to administer, well tolerated by the patient, and invaluable for many of the outpatient emergency procedures performed on the digit. Historically, it has been taught to never inject local anesthetic agents containing epinephrine when performing this block.

Anatomy

Each digit is supplied by four nerve branches. Two of these run on the palmar aspect of the finger and are commonly

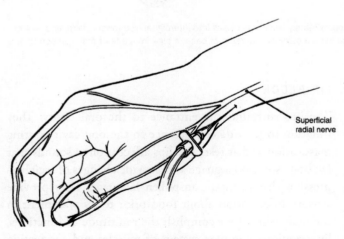

Figure 2.6. Radial nerve block. Subcutaneous injection along radial side of forearm 5 cm proximal to wrist flexion crease.

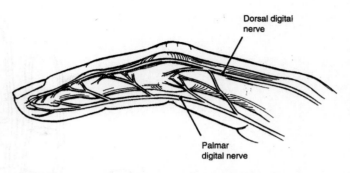

Figure 2.7. Digital nerve block. Dorsal and palmar digital nerve anatomy.

referred to as the digital nerves. They arise from either the median nerve (thumb, index, and middle fingers and radial aspect of the ring finger) or the ulnar nerve (ulnar side of ring and small finger in the proximal portion of the palm). The two corresponding dorsal sensory branches to the digits arise from either the dorsal radial nerve or the dorsal ulnar nerve (Figure 2.7).

Technique

Either of two techniques is used to achieve anesthesia in the distribution of the proper digital nerves from either the main median or ulnar nerve. The preferred method starts with the dorsal skin surface as a reference, where a 25-gauge needle is inserted into the interdigital web two-thirds of the way toward the palm. The needle is inserted approximately 2 cm deep, and 3–4 mL of 2% lidocaine solution is injected (Figure 2.8A). The same maneuver is performed on the opposite side of the digit. Next, additional local anesthetic is injected subcutaneously over the dorsum of the base of the digit from the site of the first injection to the site of the second injection (Figure 2.8B).

An alternative to injecting the interdigital web space to achieve a block of the proper digital nerves is to begin the injection on the dorsum of the hand in the distal hand at a level corresponding to the distal palmar crease on either side of the metacarpal ray. A 4-cm, 25-gauge needle is introduced through the dorsal skin of hand. A small amount of 2% lidocaine solution is injected into the subcutaneous tissue, and the needle is further inserted toward the palmar skin. Contact with the dermis on the palm side will produce discomfort: at this time the needle is withdrawn slightly, and 3 mL of the lidocaine solution is injected on one side of the metacarpal ray; then the procedure is repeated on the other side of this metacarpal. Again, it is also necessary to inject local anesthesia into the subcutaneous tissues over

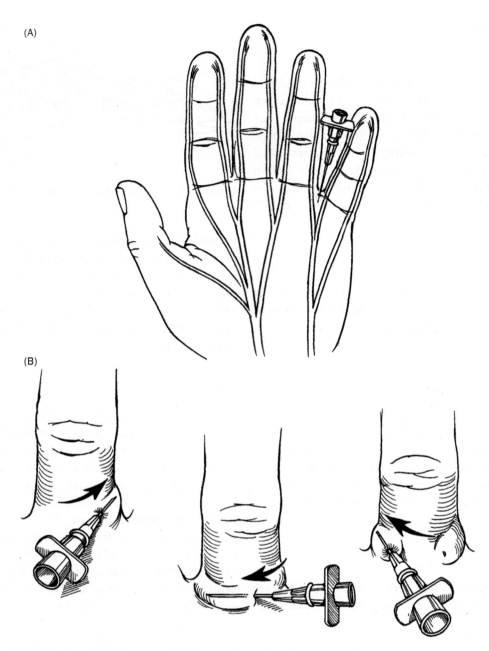

(A)

(B)

Figure 2.8. Digital nerve block technique. (A) A 25-gauge needle is inserted approximately two-thirds of way into interdigital web toward palm, and 3–4 mL of lidocaine solution is injected. (B) Additional local anesthetic is injected subcutaneously over dorsum of base of digit from site of first injection to site of second injection.

the entire dorsum of the digit to block the dorsal sensory nerves.

FACIAL BLOCKS

Facial blocks are very valuable and used often in plastic surgery to facilitate simple office procedures or allow for emergent repair of injuries. They are safe, well tolerated by the patient, and simple to perform.

LIP BLOCK

The lips surround the entrance to the oral cavity. They function to provide competence to the oral cavity during mastication and at rest. The lips affect uttered sounds that facilitate spoken language and provide changes of facial expression that facilitate unspoken language. They provide sensory information about food prior to its placement in the oral cavity. To accomplish the multitude of functions, lips require a complex system of muscles and supporting structures.

Anatomy

The sensory innervation to the perioral region is from the maxillary and mandibular branches of the fifth cranial nerve. The infraorbital nerve, which is a terminal branch of the maxillary nerve, innervates the upper lip. This nerve exits the infraorbital foramen 4–7 mm below the inferior orbital rim on a vertical line that descends from the medial limbus of the iris. The nerve runs beneath the levator labii superioris and superficial to the levator anguli oris to supply the lateral nasal sidewall, ala, columella, medial cheek, and upper lip.

The lower lip and chin receive sensory innervation from branches of the mandibular nerve. The inferior alveolar nerve, a branch of the mandibular nerve, forms the nerve to the mylohyoid just proximal to entering the lingula of the mandible. The inferior alveolar nerve travels through the body of the mandible to exit from the mental foramen. The mental foramen is located below the apex of the second mandibular bicuspid with 6–10 mm of lateral variability. The mental nerve ramifies to supply the lower lip skin down to the labiomental fold and, occasionally, down the chin as well. The nerve is located in the submucosa as it exits the foramen and frequently is visible in its location.

Technique

Either an intraoral or extraoral approach can be used to block the infraorbital nerve, while the mental nerve is routinely blocked from within the oral cavity at its location within the lower gingival buccal sulcus (Figure 2.9). When blocking the infraorbital nerve via an intraoral approach,

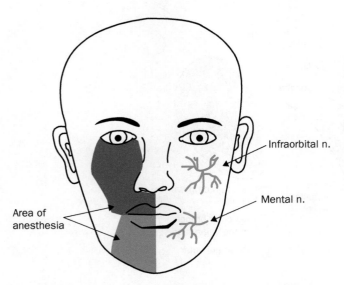

Figure 2.9. Sensory innervation to the periorbital region arises from the infraorbital and mental nerves.

a finger should be placed over the infraorbital rim to protect the globe from accidental puncture. The cheek is retracted on the desired side and a 4-cm, 25-gauge needle is introduced into the mucosa comprising the upper gingival buccal sulcus above the second premolar. The needle is kept parallel with the long axis of the second premolar until it is palpated through the skin near the foramen lying approximately 2.5 cm cephalad. If the needle is extended too far superiorly and posteriorly, the orbit may be entered. Once the needle is positioned properly, aspirate to ensure that the needle is not within a vessel and inject 2.3 mL of anesthetic solution adjacent to the foramen. For the extraoral approach to the infraorbital nerve, a finger is again placed on the infraorbital rim to protect the globe. The skin is pierced with a 4-cm, 25-gauge needle perpendicular to the skin surface one fingerbreadth below the infraorbital rim in a position directly below the later corneal limbus. Again, 2.3 mL of local anesthetic solution is injected around the foramen.

For blocking the mental nerve, the cheek is retracted laterally. The mental nerve foramen is located approximately 2 cm below the alveolar ridge in line with the second premolar in adults. The needle is inserted into the lower gingival buccal sulcus directly under the second premolar and 2–3 mL of local anesthetic solution is injected around the foramen.

NASAL BLOCK

Nasal anesthesia is required for the management of common routine and emergency procedures including management of nasal and facial trauma. General anesthesia may not be an option because of the emergent need for intervention, medical risk factors, or operating room availability.

Anatomy

The understanding of nasal innervation can be simplified by dividing it into the internal and external aspects of the nose. The external nose is innervated by the ophthalmic (V1) and maxillary (V2) nerves, which are the first two divisions of the trigeminal nerve (cranial nerve V). The anterior-superior aspect of the nose, including the tip, is supplied by the infratrochlear nerve (V1), the supratrochlear nerve (V1), and the external nasal branch of the anterior ethmoid nerve (V1). The infraorbital nerve (V2) supplies the inferior and lateral aspects of the nose, extending to the lower eyelids.

The internal nasal cavity may be subdivided into the nasal septum, the lateral walls, and the cribriform plate. The superior inner aspect of the lateral nasal wall is supplied by the anterior and posterior ethmoid nerves (V1). The sphenopalatine ganglion (V2) is located at the posterior end of the middle turbinate and innervates the posterior nasal cavity. The anterior and posterior ethmoid nerves (V1) and the sphenopalatine ganglion (through the nasopalatine nerve) provide sensation to most of the septum. The cribriform plate contains the special sensory branches of the olfactory nerve.

Technique

For a comprehensive nerve block, a series of injections is performed. The practitioner must attempt to limit the number of times the needle is inserted into the skin by performing a series of sequential injections. First, block the external nasal nerve with an intercartilaginous injection of the nasal dorsum from the region of the rhinion to the supratip region. Next, block the nasopalatine nerve with an injection at the base of the columella and nasal tip. Inject the other side in a similar fashion. Next, pass the needle through the vestibule into the facial soft tissue to a point just below the mid-orbital rim to anesthetize the infraorbital nerve.

EAR BLOCK

Anesthesia of the ear is useful for repair of lacerations, hematoma incision and drainage, and other painful procedures of the ear.

Anatomy

Four sensory nerves supply the external ear: (1) greater auricular nerve, (2) lesser occipital nerve, (3) auricular branch of the vagus nerve (i.e., Arnold's nerve), and (4) auriculotemporal nerve. The greater auricular nerve is a branch of the cervical plexus. It innervates the posteromedial, posterolateral, and inferior auricle (lower two-thirds both anteriorly and posteriorly). The lesser occipital nerve innervates a small portion of the helix. The auricular branch of the vagus nerve innervates the concha and most of the area around the auditory meatus. The auriculotemporal nerve originates from the mandibular branch of the trigeminal nerve. It innervates the anterosuperior and anteromedial aspects of the auricle.

Technique

The choice of technique depends on the area of the ear that requires anesthesia. The ring block around the entire ear can anesthetize the entire ear, excluding the concha and external auditory canal. To perform this technique, insert a 4-cm, 25-gauge needle into the skin just inferior to the attachment of the earlobe caudally. Advance the needle just anterior to the tragus, aspirating as the needle advances. Aspirate and then inject 2.3 mL of anesthetic while withdrawing the needle slowly back toward the puncture site without removing it from the skin. Once back at the puncture site, redirect and advance the needle posteriorly along the inferior posterior auricular sulcus, again aspirating as it is advanced. Then inject 2.3 mL of anesthetic while withdrawing the needle Figure 2.10.

The needle is then removed and reinserted just superior to the attachment of the helix to the scalp. Direct and advance the needle just anterior to the tragus, aspirating as it is advanced. Aspirate and inject 2.3 mL of anesthetic

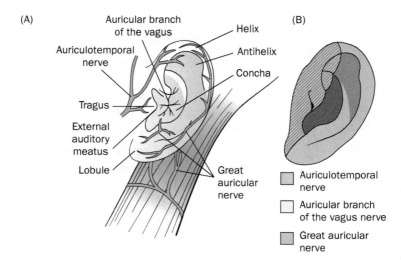

Figure 2.10. Sensory innervation to the ear arises from four distinct sources: (1) greater auricular nerve, (2) lesser occipital nerve, (3) auricular branch of the vagus nerve (i.e., Arnold's nerve), and (4) auriculotemporal nerve.

while withdrawing the needle toward the skin puncture site without removing it. Be cognizant to inject the subcutaneous tissue, not the ear cartilage. Once just under the skin at the needle puncture site, redirect and advance the needle posteriorly along the superior posterior auricular sulcus, aspirating as it is advanced. Again aspirate and inject 2.3 mL of anesthetic while withdrawing the needle. Be mindful of the superficial temporal artery, located anterior to the ear as it crosses over the zygomatic arch. The concha and ear canal can be difficult to anesthetize due to the sensation arising from the auricular branch of the vagus nerve.

INTRAVENOUS REGIONAL ANESTHESIA

Intravenous regional anesthesia, also known as a Bier block, is a very simple technique that is increasingly being used for hand surgery procedures and for fracture reduction procedures in the upper extremity.

TECHNIQUE

A double tourniquet is placed on the upper arm and each of the dual compartments is carefully checked. An intravenous line is started in the arm to be anesthetized, using a 20- or 22-gauge venous cannula, and it is taped securely. The arm is elevated and exsanguinated with an Esmarch bandage from the digital tips to the tourniquet; this exsanguination must be thorough. After this maneuver, the proximal tourniquet is inflated. Next, the intravenous infusion of lidocaine without epinephrine is begun using 0.5% lidocaine solution. A dose of 3 mg/kg is administered through the intravenous line. Anesthesia in the extremity is noted approximately 4 minutes after the infusion. The proximal tourniquet is left up until the patient senses discomfort (usually 20–30 minutes) and then the distal cuff of the tourniquet is inflated. The proximal cuff is deflated when it is ascertained that the distal cuff is stable. The distal cuff can remain inflated for up to 40 minutes without producing significant discomfort.

At the completion of the procedure, the tourniquet is released for short intervals of approximately 15 seconds and then reinflated. This procedure is repeated four times if the procedure was less than 10 minutes in duration, three times if it was less than 20 minutes in duration, and two times if it was less than 40 minutes in duration. This prevents a bolus of lidocaine from entering the circulation. Fifty percent of the local anesthetic is still bound to the tissues for 30 minutes. If additional anesthesia is needed within 30 minutes after deflation of the tourniquet, additional lidocaine can be administered in half of the original dose.

The advantages of this procedure are that it is very easy to perform, and it is safe and effective for outpatient surgery. Rapid return of motor function occurs after tourniquet release, allowing the surgeon to evaluate tendon and joint motion in cases of tenolysis. Disadvantages of this technique include the potential for tourniquet pain, especially if the procedure lasts longer than 1 hour. Other potential problems include lack of anesthesia after cuff deflation, lack of muscle relaxation, equipment problems, and problems with tourniquet release.

FIELD BLOCK ANESTHESIA

This type of anesthesia has limited application in hand surgery, but it is valuable for certain procedures, including carpal tunnel release, trigger finger release, and release of the second extensor compartment for de Quervain's tenosynovitis. For surgery on the preceding three conditions, a field block-type anesthesia is effective and facilitates rapid recovery when these surgical procedures are performed under sedative anesthesia.

ANATOMY

Carpal tunnel release is performed using an incision ulnar to and parallel with the thenar flexion crease. The transverse carpal ligament is released from the superficial palmar arch to the volar carpal ligament. The characteristic incision varies from 3–5 cm in length.

Technique

Using 1% lidocaine solution without epinephrine, 2 mL is injected proximal in the wrist flexion crease after intravenous sedation has been administered. Next, an additional 8 mL of 1% lidocaine solution is injected into the subcutaneous tissues, both immediately below the dermis and immediately above the palmar fascia in the line of intended incision. This provides excellent anesthesia in the hand, and the operation can be performed with the assistance of either a forearm or upper arm tourniquet.

For trigger finger release operations or for release of the first extensor compartments to treat de Quervain's disease, the local anesthetic is instilled into the intended line of incision, and, again, either a forearm or upper arm tourniquet is used.

STELLATE GANGLION BLOCK

This is a special block designed to interrupt the sympathetic innervation of the extremity, which is used to treat the early phases of a reflex pain syndrome. It can be very useful in the treatment of reflex sympathetic dystrophy. If the initial block is successful, repeated blocks are also likely to be successful.

TECHNIQUE

The most commonly used technique is the paratracheal approach, for which the patient is placed in the supine position. The sternoclavicular junction is palpated and the sternocleidomastoid muscle is displaced laterally. A 4-cm, 22-gauge needle is inserted two fingerbreadths above and lateral to the sternoclavicular junction until the seventh transverse process is contacted (Figure 2.11). After aspiration, the needle is withdrawn 2 mm and 10–15 mL of 1% lidocaine solution is injected. The development of Horner's syndrome is observed within a few minutes. Increased skin temperature and the absence of swelling are evidence that the sympathetic input has been blocked.

INTERCOSTAL NERVE BLOCK

Intercostal block produces discrete band-like segmental anesthesia in the chosen levels. The intercostal block is an excellent analgesic option for a variety of surgical procedures. The beneficial effect of intercostal blockade on respiratory function following thoracic or upper abdominal surgery, or following chest wall trauma, is well documented. Although similar in many ways to the paravertebral block, intercostal blocks are generally simpler to perform because the osseous landmarks are more readily palpable. However, the risks of pneumothorax and local anesthetic systemic toxicity are present, and care must be taken to prevent these potentially serious complications.

ANATOMY

After emerging from their respective intervertebral foramina, the thoracic nerve roots divide into dorsal and ventral rami. The dorsal ramus provides innervation to the skin and muscle of the paravertebral region; the ventral ramus continues laterally as the intercostal nerve. This nerve then pierces the posterior intercostal membrane

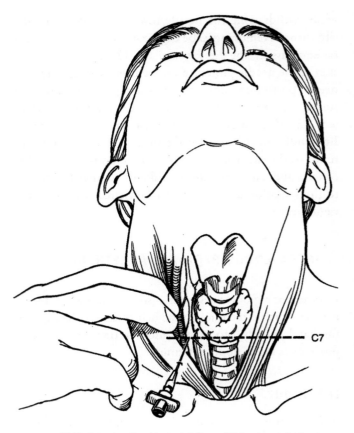

Figure 2.11. (A) Stellate ganglion block. A 3.8 cm, 22-gauge needle is inserted two fingers' breadth above and lateral to sternoclavicular junction until the seventh transverse process is contacted; needle is withdrawn 2 mm and 10–15 mL of 1% lidocaine solution is injected. Disadvantages of this technique include the potential for tourniquet pain, especially if the procedure lasts longer than 1 hour. Other potential problems include lack of anesthesia after cuff deflation, lack of muscle relaxation, equipment problems, and problems with tourniquet release.

approximately 3 cm lateral to the intervertebral foramen and enters the subcostal groove of the rib, where it travels inferiorly to the intercostal artery and vein. Initially, the nerve lies between the parietal pleura and the inner most intercostal muscle. Immediately proximal to the angle of the rib, it passes into the space between the innermost and internal intercostal muscles, where it remains for much of the remainder of its course. At the midaxillary line, the intercostal nerve gives rise to the lateral cutaneous branch, which pierces the internal and external intercostal muscles and supplies the muscles and skin of the lateral trunk. The continuation of the intercostal nerve terminates as the anterior cutaneous branch, which supplies the skin and muscles of the anterior trunk, including the skin overlying the sternum and rectus abdominis.

Intercostal blocks can be more challenging to perform above the level of T7 because the scapula prevents access to the ribs. Although an intercostal block is an excellent choice for analgesic purposes, it is often inadequate as a complete surgical anesthesia. For this application, supplementation with another anesthesia technique usually is required.

TECHNIQUE

After cleaning the skin with an antiseptic solution, 1–2 mL of dilute local anesthetic is infiltrated subcutaneously at each planned level injection site. The fingers of the palpating hand should straddle the insertion site at the inferior border of the rib and fix the skin to avoid unwanted skin movement. A 2-cm, 22-gauge needle is introduced through the skin and contact with the rib should be made. While maintaining the same angle of insertion, the needle is walked off the inferior border of the rib. Then the needle is advanced 3 mm below the inferior margin of the rib, with the goal of placing the tip in the space containing the neurovascular bundle between the internal and innermost intercostal muscles. The end point for advancement should be the predetermined distance (3 mm). Following negative aspiration for blood or air, 3–5 mL of local anesthetic is injected. The process is repeated for the remaining levels of blockade.

TRANSVERSUS ABDOMINIS PLANE BLOCK

The transverse abdominis plane (TAP) block is a peripheral nerve block designed to anesthetize the nerves supplying the anterior abdominal wall (T6–L1). It was first described in 2001 by Rafi as a traditional blind landmark technique using the lumbar triangle of Petit. In recent studies, the TAP block was shown to reduce the need for postoperative opioid use, increase the time to first request for further analgesia, and provide more effective pain relief while decreasing opioid-related side effects such as sedation and postoperative nausea and vomiting. The introduction of ultrasound has allowed providers to identify the appropriate tissue plane and perform this block with greater accuracy under direct visualization. Often, the plastic surgeon will have direct access to the abdominal wall through a lower abdominal incision.

ANATOMY

The abdominal wall is composed of five paired muscles: two midline vertical muscles (the rectus abdominis and the pyramidalis) and three lateral layered flat muscles (external abdominal oblique, the internal abdominal oblique, and the transversus abdominis muscles). The internal oblique muscle is the intermediate layer of the three lateral abdominal muscles. It originates broadly from the anterior portion of the iliac crest, lateral half of the inguinal ligament, and thoracolumbar fascia. The internal oblique inserts on the inferior border of the 10th–12th ribs, the linea alba, and the pubic crest via the conjoint tendon. The muscle fibers of the internal abdominal oblique course upward in a superomedial orientation, perpendicular to the muscle fibers of the external abdominal oblique.

The transversus abdominis muscle is the deepest of the three paired, flat abdominal muscles. It originates on the internal surfaces of the 7th–12th costal cartilages, thoracolumbar fascia, anterior three-fourths of the iliac crest, and lateral third of the inguinal ligament. As with the other flat muscles, the transversus abdominis forms a broad aponeurosis that helps make up the rectus sheath before it fuses in the midline to the linea alba. Above the arcuate line, the transversus abdominis aponeurosis contributes to the posterior rectus sheath. Below the arcuate line, it is fused with the other flat muscles as the anterior rectus sheath.

TECHNIQUE

In the traditional blind approach, the lumbar triangle of Petit is identified. The triangle of Petit is formed by the iliac crest as the base, the external oblique muscle as the anterior border, and the latissimus dorsi muscle as the posterior border. The floor of the triangle is made up of the fascia from both the external and internal oblique muscles. A needle is inserted perpendicular to the skin just cephalad to the iliac crest near the mid-axillary line. The TAP is identified using a "two-pop" sensation or loss of resistance. The first pop indicates penetration of the fascia of the external oblique muscle, and the second indicates penetration of the fascia of the internal oblique muscle. Local anesthetic is then injected with multiple aspirations. Recently, ultrasound has eliminated the blind approach and has greatly enhanced both the safety and efficacy of the TAP block.

PERTINENT DRESSINGS

There are no special dressings required. However, sterile gauze should be available to hold pressure on the site of infiltration or local anesthetic infusion.

UNIQUE ASPECTS OF POSTOPERATIVE CARE

The performance of surgery under regional anesthesia routinely results in a rapid return of motor and sensory function dependent upon the type of local anesthesia used. Sometimes the goal of regional anesthesia is not only to provide surgical anesthesia, but to provide pain control for many hours after surgery. This type of anesthesia does not interfere in any way with the application of the desired dressing or splint, with the necessary arm and hand positioning, or with subsequent therapy.

CAVEATS

Consistency with regional anesthesia requires a thorough knowledge of anatomy and experience in administering the respective blocks.

SELECTED READINGS

Adams JP, Dealy EJ, Kenmore PI. Intravenous regional anesthesia in hand surgery. *J Bone Joint Surg* 1964;46A:811–816.

Adrani J. *Nerve Blocks: A Manual of Regional Anesthesia for Practitioners of Medicine*. Springfield, IL: Charles C Thomas, 1954.

Bier A. Uber einen leg local Anesthetie in den Gleidmassen zu erzeugen. *Arch Klin Chir* 1908;86:1007–1016.

Graham WP III. Intravenous regional anesthesia for outpatient operations on the upper extremity. *Industrial Med* 1970;39:213–214.

Hadzic A. *Textbook of Regional Anesthesia and Acute Pain Management*. McGraw-Hill Education, 2016.

Malamed SF. *Handbook of Local Anesthesia*. Elsevier Health Sciences, 2014.

Mustoe TA, Buck DW, Lalonde DH. The safe management of anesthesia, sedation, and pain in plastic surgery. *Plast Reconstruct Surg* 2010;126(4): 165e–176e.

Ramamurthy S, Hickey R. Anesthesia. In: Green DP, ed. *Operative Hand Surgery*. New York: Churchill Livingstone, 1993.

Winnie AP, Ramamurthy S, Durrani Z. Diagnostic and therapeutic nerve blocks: recent advances in techniques. In: Bonica JJ, ed. *Advances in Neurology*. Vol 4. New York: Raven Press, 1974.

Winnie AP, Tay CH, Patel KP, et al. Pharmacokinetics of local anesthetics during plexus blocks. *Anesth Analg* 1977;56:852–861.

3.

WOUND CLOSURE

David A. Daar and Maristella S. Evangelista

The main duty of plastic surgeons is to restore form and function to their patients. Wound closure is the principal means of accomplishing this task. In order to successfully allow for healing, proper wound assessment and planning are of paramount importance. Successful closure of a wound cannot be achieved with a simple algorithm; rather, it involves a decision made after consideration of wound characteristics, patient characteristics, and reconstructive options.

ASSESSMENT OF THE DEFECT

A thorough history is always the first step in the assessment of a wound. Understanding of the mechanism of injury, chronicity of the wound, and associated symptoms can signal important considerations such as the potential for contamination, infection, or other disease processes. Patient factors such as age, medical history, family history, and social history will also be important in the management of their wounds and will be discussed in more detail in subsequent sections.

On physical exam, assess the location and characteristics of the defect, including size, shape, depth, and color. Is there active drainage or discharge? Does the area have good blood flow? One should consider the anatomy in the area and look for damage to or exposure of surrounding structures, including vessels, nerves, tendons, joints, muscle, or bone.[1] If structures are not visible, their function should still be evaluated as this may indicate a concealed or ongoing process.

Healthy tissue will appear red or pink and may have punctate bleeding. Devitalized tissue may appear gray, purple, or black. Infected wounds may be malodorous or have purulent drainage. Other nonhealing wounds may show hardened fibrotic tissue or yellow debris. Chronic nonhealing wounds should heighten suspicion for chronic patient factors and potentially even malignancy. In traumatic injuries, consider the potential for contamination or retained foreign bodies. Sharp lacerations tend to be confined to the area of the wound, whereas avulsion injuries and blast injuries will create zones of injury beyond initial assessment.

INDICATIONS FOR SURGICAL CLOSURE

In traumatic injuries, the urgency of closure is something to quickly evaluate. Leaving wounds open may increase the risk of infection. Are critical structures exposed or damaged? Is there active bleeding? Is the wound contaminated? Closure performed in the emergency room may be easier and faster but will require good local anesthetic and patient cooperation. Going to the operating room is a more involved process but offers better light, specialized instruments, and greater ability to manipulate, repair, and debride tissue. In times of uncontrolled bleeding, damage to critical structures, evidence of joint or bone involvement, high contamination, high complexity, and/or uncooperative or high-risk patients, the operating room is indicated. Patient safety and comfort is the primary concern—if there is any doubt, manage the patient in the operating room.

Barring contraindications, traumatic wounds should be closed within 6 hours to minimize infection.[2] Open fractures should undergo thorough irrigation and debridement within 8 hours to decrease infection risk.[3,4] Closure may be delayed if further debridement of ischemic or contaminated tissue is needed. The advent of negative pressure wound therapy (NWPT) has revolutionized management of open fractures and allowed for safe delay of closure in these settings. NWPT will be discussed further in the "Operative Technique" section.

In the closure of other surgical defects, the same principles apply. Immediate closure may be preferred if there are exposed critical structures or hardware. Final closure should be delayed when there is concern for continued infection, contamination, devitalized tissue, or residual malignancy. Careful preoperative planning, coordination with referring physicians, and consideration of several intrinsic and extrinsic factors are necessary in the decision to perform closure. These are further detailed in the next section.

CONTRAINDICATIONS TO SURGICAL WOUND CLOSURE

There are few absolute contraindications to wound closure. However, factors that impair healing should be considered as relative contraindications in order to ensure patient safety and successful wound closure. Possible risks for wound healing can be divided into wound factors as well as intrinsic and extrinsic patient factors. In each case, use of NPWT and/or dressing changes can provide temporary coverage and promote a clean, healthy wound bed until the closure is appropriate.

INFECTION

When the bacterial load within the wound reaches greater than 10^5 organisms per gram of tissue, there is an increased risk of wound infection.[5] Inadequate debridement is often the cause for persistent infection. Exposed bone or hardware is presumed infected and should be debrided or removed if possible. Antibiotic regimens should initially cover a broad spectrum of organism and be de-escalated as soon as possible based on culture and sensitivity results. Because bacteria will colonize all exposed areas, aim to obtain cultures from deep, nonexposed areas or after superficial debridement has taken place.

FOREIGN BODY

Presence of a foreign body may impede wound healing, particularly if infected or contaminated. In trauma situations, an x-ray may be indicated in order to identify the possible presence of a foreign body.[1] Exposed hardware should be presumed contaminated and should be removed if possible prior to final closure.

AGE

Aging has shown to delay wound healing in healthy adults without actually impairing the healing quality.[6] Aging delays each stage of the wound healing process, including inflammatory response, angiogenesis, re-epithelialization, and collagen turnover. Hormonal changes in aging patients also affect rate of wound healing. In particular, estrogen has shown to improve age-related wound healing and may explain the gender discrepancy in which aged males heal more slowly than aged females.

NUTRITION

Malnutrition delays wound healing and alters immune system function, thus increasing the risk of infection.[7] Protein malnutrition affects all stages of wound healing. Recommended range of protein intake is between 1.25 and 1.5 g/kg/day in chronic wounds, and adequate intake can be gauged by testing serum prealbumin (PAB) and albumin levels.[7] C-reactive protein (CRP) should be checked alongside prealbumin as elevated levels may indicate unreliable PAB. Arginine and glutamine are two amino acids integral to wound healing, yet their supplementation has shown mixed results.[7,8]

Vitamins C and A are involved in collagen synthesis and the inflammatory phase of wound healing, respectively.[7,8] Recommended supplementation for vitamin C is 60 mg/day for deficient patients. Magnesium, copper, and zinc are micronutrients essential to wound healing due to their role as cofactors for various enzymes, yet benefits of supplementation are unproved.[8,9] Beware of zinc deficiency in patients with diarrhea, malabsorption, or hypermetabolic states (e.g., sepsis, burns, serious injury, etc.).

STEROIDS

Corticosteroid use affects wound healing by impairing inflammation and collagen production as well as inhibiting epithelialization.[8] Their use should be discontinued prior to surgery if possible. Patients taking corticosteroids can be offered vitamin A supplementation to mitigate delayed wound healing, although risk of wound contraction and infection still remain.[7,9]

SMOKING

Nicotine impairs wound healing through its vasoconstrictive effects and increased risk of thrombus formation.[10] Studies show a two- to threefold increased risk of tissue necrosis, delayed healing, dehiscence, and infectious complications with cigarette smoking.[11] Digital blood flow velocity can decrease by roughly 42% after smoking a single cigarette.[12] It is recommended that patients quit smoking for at least 4 weeks prior to surgery, with progressive risk reduction out to 6 weeks.[11]Nicotine products, such as nicotine gum, nicotine patches, and electronic cigarettes, will also affect the wound healing process and should be addressed similarly.

DIABETES

Diabetes is a well-known risk factor for wound complications due to hyperglycemia and vascular impairment.[8] Poor control, both long-term and perioperatively, is associated with increased risk of infectious and noninfectious wound complications.[13] Plastic surgery literature suggests cutoffs for adequate control as a hemoglobin A1c level of 6.5% and perioperative glucose level of 200 mg/dL for patients undergoing primary wound closure.[14] Delay closure, if possible, in poorly controlled patients.

CANCER

Cancer patients are at significant risk for impaired wound healing due to both the nature of disease as well as the multimodal treatment they undergo. Approximately 40–80% of patients are malnourished, due to various reasons, and impacts of chemoradiation and corticosteroid use can be additive.[15]

CHEMOTHERAPY

Multiple animal studies have demonstrated decreased wound strength after neoadjuvant or adjuvant chemotherapy, especially in the early postsurgical period.[16] While clinical evidence regarding the risk of postsurgical wound complications in the setting of chemotherapy remains inconclusive, estimates suggest an interval of at least 5–8 weeks between chemotherapy and surgery.[8,17–19]

RADIATION

Ionizing radiation causes DNA damage and acute microvascular occlusion and stasis that predisposes tissue to edema, thrombosis, and poor healing.[20] Wounds involving irradiated skin are at increased risk for dehiscence and infection, and, if possible, irradiated skin should be excised and then sutured to a well-vascularized flap.[8,21] Studies show enhanced equilibrium of tissues at 6 months post-radiation and one should consider delaying reconstruction until that time.

ROOM SETUP

Whether performing closure in the emergency room or operating room, preparation of proper instrumentation, medications, and devices is essential. A surgeon should consider all the steps of the proposed operation from beginning to end and communicate his or her plan to any support staff, assistants, or collaborating teams (anesthesia, consulting services, etc.). It is often helpful to have this plan in writing, both for the surgeon's preparation and for his or her team. Considerations of room setup include:

- *Anesthesia*: Local versus sedation versus general anesthesia
- *Patient positioning*: Longer cords and tubing needed if turning table
- *Pressure ulcer prevention*: Pad bony prominences
- *Nerve damage prevention*: Facilitate natural position of extremities and spine
- *Deep vein thrombosis (DVT) prophylaxis*: Sequential compression devices, heparin, enoxaparin
- *Fluid management*: Foley catheter placement if anticipated time for procedure is more than 3 hours
- *Antibiotics*: Preoperative antibiotics and/or antibiotic irrigation
- *Lighting*: Room lights, headlights, lighted retractors
- *Sterile prep and drape*: Chlorhexidine gluconate, povidone-iodine
- *Debridement instruments*: Curettes, rongeurs, pulse lavage, cystoscopy tubing
- *Cultures and specimens*: Culture swabs and specimen cups
- *Instruments for dissection, retraction, mobilization, and hemostasis*: Instrument trays, Bovie or handheld cautery, hemoclips or suture ties, gauze sponges or laps
- *Special implants*: Hardware or mesh
- *Imaging*: Obtained and available for display

- *Sutures*: Deep tissue and skin closure
- *Drains*: Jackson-Pratt, Blake, Penrose
- *Dressings*: Steri-Strips, Xeroform, bacitracin, gauze, tape, Dermabond

Though the name of this section may imply otherwise, part of setup should always include patient counseling. Patients should understand the potential risks, benefits, alternatives, and indications of your procedure (i.e., informed consent). They should understand the likely outcome and recovery as well as possible scars, deformities, donor site morbidities, postoperative restrictions, and other potential complications that may occur. One should estimate how long the procedure will take and prepare patients for the possibility of multiple stages if indicated. Thorough patient preparation is the best way to gain patients' trust and to keep patients and their families at ease.

PATIENT MARKINGS

The defect should be measured and nearby anatomy adequately assessed. Patient markings will depend on the specific reconstructive option chosen, which will be discussed in subsequent chapters. In the case of local and distant flaps, ensure patient markings provide sufficient pedicle length and the ability to transpose the flap. When possible, use relaxed skin tension lines (RSTLs) and junctions of aesthetic subunits to identify incision sites and flap design that will minimize scar visibility.[22] This will be discussed further in future chapters.

OPERATIVE TECHNIQUES

Techniques of wound closure in plastic surgery include everything from primary closure to free tissue transfer. The traditional reconstructive ladder (Figure 3.1), developed in 1982 by Mathes and Nahai, implied approaching closure options from simple to complex.[23] However, many now refer to the traditional ladder as a reconstructive elevator, where a surgeon may skip rungs to higher complexity surgeries when appropriate. Recent advances, namely NPWT and dermal regenerative substitutes, have affected the approach and management of many wounds. For the purposes of this chapter, we will discuss closure techniques of primary closure, secondary intention, tissue expansion, NPWT, and dermal regenerative substitutes. Future chapters will cover more complex closure techniques such as local flaps, skin grafts, regional flaps, and distant flaps.

PRIMARY CLOSURE

Primary closure is often the preferred method of closure if there is minimal tissue loss and/or appropriate skin laxity. Principles of primary closure include good eversion of the tissue, precise alignment of skin edges, adequate achievement of hemostasis, and minimization of wound tension while using atraumatic technique.[24,25] Choice of technique, suture material, and needle depend on location and intrinsic aspects of the wound and will be covered in more detail in the subsequent chapter, "Suture Material." Undermining surrounding tissues, scoring of fascia or galea, and utilizing mechanical creep are techniques that can help to minimize tension and allow for primary closure. Suturing techniques (Figure 3.2) to consider in primary closure include:

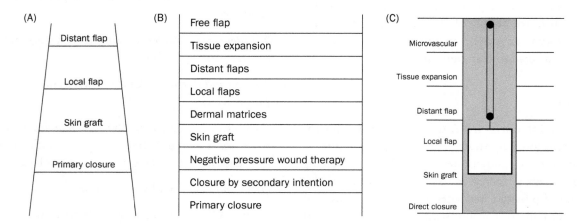

Figure 3.1. (A) The traditional reconstructive ladder as compared to the (B) new reconstructive ladder and the (C) reconstructive elevator.

- *Simple interrupted sutures*: The most common suture technique that involves piercing through skin and dermis on one side of the wound and then exiting the wound on the other side. One should aim to enter and exit at a 90-degree angle and then supinate the wrist to allow the curve of the needle to guide the suture. The deep portion of the throw should be farther from the wound edge than the superficial portion which allows for good eversion of the skin edges when the knots are tied.[25–27]

- *Simple running suture (baseball stitch)*: This suture involves the same technique as the simple interrupted but is continuous, only requiring knots at the beginning and the end. It is faster to complete but has less precise ability to achieve good alignment and eversion and thus requires good prior skin alignment and/or deep sutures to have a good aesthetic result.

- *Deep dermal or buried sutures*: These sutures are kept under the surface of the skin and start deep in the dermis and exit superficial at the dermal-epidermal junction. It takes the reverse course on the opposite side of the wound. By exaggerating a 90-degree angle of entry and exit, the wound edges will achieve good eversion. Grabbing a healthy bite of dermis will enhance strength. Burying the suture ends deep will prevent exposure or "spitting" of the suture knots.[25]

- *Vertical mattress sutures*: These sutures are used when you require more eversion than is possible with simple interrupted sutures. They also help distribute tension and can be helpful in higher tension areas, such as joints, hands, or feet. Sutures are placed in a "far-far near-near" fashion in relation to wound edges. Hatch-mark scars are imminent if sutures are left in place for too long.[25,27]

- *Horizontal mattress sutures* (Figure 3.3): Similar to a vertical mattress, these sutures will enhance eversion and help distribute tension and may be preferred in high tension areas. The suture is started like a simple

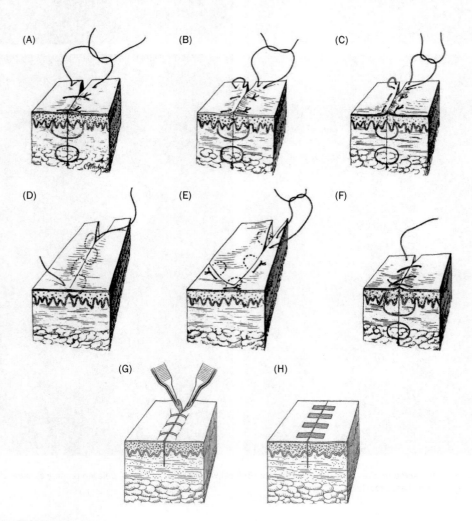

Figure 3.2. Various suture techniques.

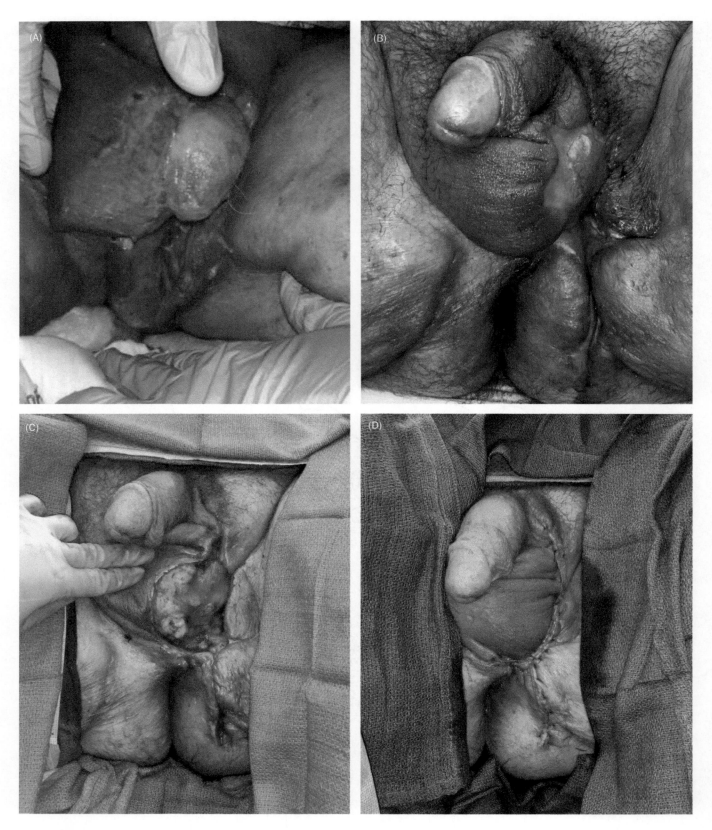

Figure 3.3. Fournier's gangrene of the scrotum after (A) initial debridement (B) local wound care, and (C–D) delayed primary closure after infection control, smoking cessation, and control of diabetes mellitus.

interrupted but instead of tying the suture after the first throw, the suture is passed from the exit side to the entry side after moving a distance down the wound. This cannot be tied too tightly as there is a risk for tissue necrosis in between the suture throws.

- *Half-buried horizontal mattress sutures*: When closing V-shaped wounds, or when hiding one side of suture knots is desired (e.g., hair-bearing areas adjacent to non–hair-bearing areas, a half-buried horizontal mattress suture is placed. Flap edges/corners can benefit from this suture because it minimizes ischemia of the skin on the buried side. Suture is similar to a horizontal mattress but there is no exit on the opposing side. Instead, the opposing side is addressed by a horizontal throw deep to the skin surface prior to exiting back out the original side several millimeters down from its origin.

- *Running subcuticular suture*: This suture is thrown horizontally under the surface of the skin and is used to reapproximate the superficial layer of skin. It is often used after a deep dermal or other deeper stitch to provide a final, more precise layer of skin closure.

- *Staples*: This is the most expedient way to close a wound, and it is still possible to get good alignment and eversion. These are ideal for the scalp because sutures have higher tendency to cause alopecia. They are easy to remove and should be removed early to prevent track marks.

- *Tapes*: Surgical tapes and glue are not commonly used for primary closure alone but can be used in superficial wounds or in wounds that are approximated by deep stitches. They are often used as an adjunct overlying a closed wound.

CLOSURE BY SECONDARY INTENTION

Secondary intention (Figure 3.4) is a good option to employ when wounds are not able to be closed primarily.

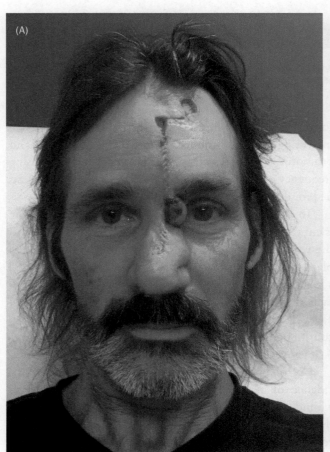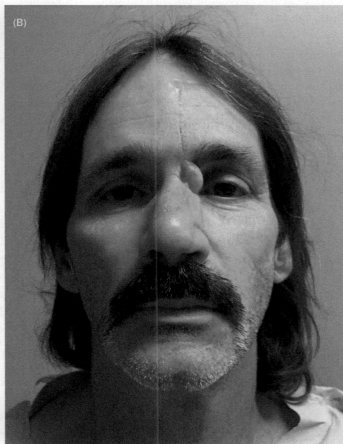

Figure 3.4. Forehead flap defect (A) 1 week after closure with combination of primary closure and secondary intention. (B) At 9 weeks, there is minimal deformity at the donor site.

This may occur in areas without good laxity or in tissue that is too friable to be sutured. It is also useful in highly specialized areas such as the fingertips where regrowth of specialized function can be beneficial. Generally, this technique involves local dressings such as a "wet-to-moist" dressing, where moistened saline gauze is covered by dry gauze and changed 1–3 times daily. This will optimize the wound bed while the wound re-epithelializes from the sides in. In some areas, this can yield closure that almost resembles the native skin in both appearance and function. In larger areas, it can lead to depressed scars and visible scar deformity. It will not be ideal in areas of exposed bone, cartilage, or other critical structures. It also takes more time to heal than other closure techniques and requires patient compliance with wound care.

TISSUE EXPANSION

Tissue expansion can be performed by internal or external means. Internal tissue expanders can be placed under the skin and fascia adjacent to a wound and serially filled with saline to provide stretch of the adjacent tissue. The gradual filling process allows expanded tissue to have improved vascularity, so tissue may be advanced and primary closure achieved.[28,29] The amount of advancement achieved is calculated by adding the lengths of the sides and top of the expander and subtracting the base of the expander. The expander is filled every week after a 2- to 3-week resting period, and removal and advancement is performed 4 weeks after final expansion. Large areas can be covered; however, multiple procedures are required and unsightly deformities may occur during the expansion process. In addition, tissue expanders are a foreign body that can be prone to extrusion and infection.

External tissue expanders (Figure 3.5) are devices that are affixed to skin surrounding wound using sutures, tapes, or tacks/staples. They utilize mechanical creep over time and can promote stretch of tissues without inserting an internal foreign body. The DermaClose device is one such option, where 85% of maximal stretch is achieved by 5 days and thus final closure can be performed 5–10 days after application of the device. External devices are more limited than internal devices in the amount of expansion they can provide. In addition, traction on the epidermis can yield visible scars that may be suboptimal for patients.

NEGATIVE PRESSURE WOUND THERAPY

Since its development in the 1990s, NPWT (Figure 3.6) has revolutionized the management of wounds. It is thought

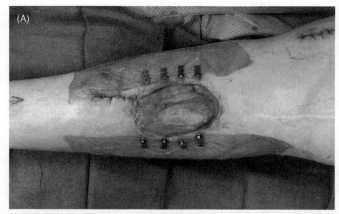

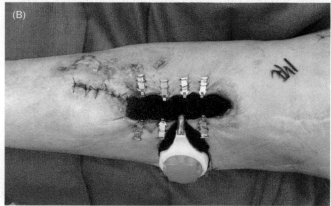

Figure 3.5. Leg wound, 5 × 8 cm (A) before and (B) 1 week after application of DermaClose external tissue expander.

to promote wound healing by reducing fluid and edema, increasing tissue perfusion, clearing bacteria and debris, and promoting granulation tissue.[30,31] It can assist in decreasing frequency of dressing changes as well as prepare the wound bed for definitive surgical closure.[31–33]

To apply NPWT to an open wound, a foam dressing is cut to fit the shape of the wound and placed gently onto the wound bed. Next, a polyacrylate adhesive dressing is placed over the foam to create a pneumatic seal. Finally, a hole is cut in the dressing and track pad with tubing attached to the dressing and is connected to the machine. Negative pressure therapy is typically set at 125 mm Hg continuous pressure. Standard dressing changes occur 3 times weekly.

Use of a single sponge is ideal to minimize the incidence of retained sponge, which can interfere with wound healing. Circumferential dressing application should be avoided as this may increase risk of vascular compromise.[34] Adjacent wounds can be bridged with sponge to create a single NPWT dressing. Alternatively, a Y-connector can connect two dressings to one machine. In wounds over bony prominences or weight-bearing

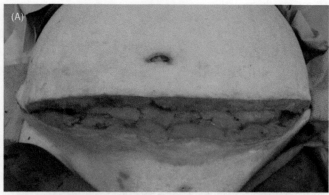

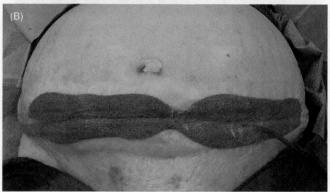

Figure 3.6. Infected abdominal wound (A) before and (B) after application of negative-pressure wound therapy, silver sponge.

areas, off-loading is advised; track pad can also be bridged to a non–weight-bearing surface. Direct placement over vessels, nerves, or tendons is not recommended. Other contraindications to NPWT include malignancy in the wound, untreated osteomyelitis, nonenteric and unexplored fistulas, necrotic tissue with eschar present, and sensitivity to silver (silver dressing only).[34,35]

Variations to standard therapy are now available to enhance customized wound characteristics. Ten percent silver polyurethane foam can be use and serves as an added barrier to bacteria. White polyvinyl alcohol foam reduces adherence and can thus be used over critical structures or in wounds with significant tunneling. Pressure settings can be set to as lower as 50 mm Hg in areas of sensitivity or by critical structures. When used over grafts, dressing changes are not employed as often and usually occur every 1–3 weeks.

Newer innovations in NPWT include NPWT with instillation and dwell time (NPWTi), which offers the ability to irrigate the wound with saline or other antiseptic/antimicrobial solution to potentially decrease bioburden.[36] Recent studies promote its use in complex wounds involving severe trauma, diabetic foot infections, and invasive infection or widespread biofilm.

DERMAL SUBSTITUTES

Dermal substitutes are another area of significant advancement in wound closure in the past decade. These biologic scaffold materials promote cellular invasion and capillary growth. The result is a "neodermis" or enhanced granulation bed over which wounds can then be skin grafted or allowed to heal by secondary intention. Wounds that would generally not take skin grafts (exposed bone, tendon, even exposed hardware in some reports) can be treated with these materials. Dermal substitutes thereby offer a less invasive treatment modality than a local, regional, or distant flap. For patients with significant comorbidities or who simply do not desire a more invasive procedure, they are an excellent option.

Integra Dermal Regeneration Template is a popular dermal substitute that has two layers: a thin outer layer of silicone and a thick inner matrix layer of pure bovine collagen and glycosaminoglycan (GAG) from shark cartilage. Graft is placed in a clean wound bed with silicone side up and is affixed to the wound with a bolster. The graft will act as an extracellular matrix, promoting cellular growth and collagen synthesis. It biodegrades while being replaced by autologous dermal tissue. Outer dressing can be changed once a week or as needed. Three to four weeks later, the graft is expected to have fully incorporated. The silicone layer is removed and the wound can be grafted.

ACell (Figure 3.7) is a similar dermal substitute that comes in sheet and powder form. Grafts are derived porcine urinary bladder extracellular matrix. The wound should be debrided and clean prior to graft placement. The graft is hydrated in room temperature sterile saline (0.9%) or sterile lactated Ringer's solution. There is a triangular notch in the top right of all sheet grafts to indicate the correct side up. The graft is cut and placed in the wound and affixed with a nonadherent bolster dressing. In dry wounds, it is recommended to apply hydrogel to keep the wound moist. In wet wounds, an absorptive dressing may be needed. The outer dressing should be changed weekly, and the wound will be ready for grafting and/or start to re-epithelialize in 3–6 weeks. The powder form is a moralized version of the graft that can be layered over time to promote further granulation tissue. It is noted that this graft does have a yellow fibrinous appearance and mild odor as part of the normal incorporation process, and this should not be debrided.

POSTOPERATIVE CONSIDERATIONS

The stages of wound healing include an inflammatory phase (4–6 days), a proliferative phase (4–14 days), and

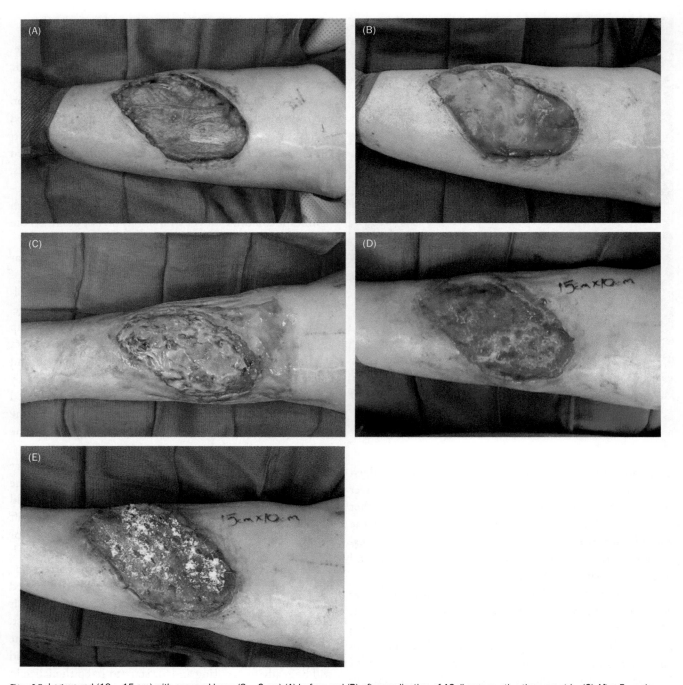

Figure 3.7. Leg wound (10 × 15 cm) with exposed bone (3 × 6 cm) (A) before and (B) after application of ACell regenerative tissue matrix. (C) After 5 weeks of incorporation, you can see an elevated wound bed and no exposed bone. The yellow fibrinous material on the surface graft will continue to incorporate and need not be debrided. Wound bed (D) before and (E) after skin grafting. ACell powder is applied to the skin graft bed to enhance skin graft incorporation.

a remodeling phase (14 days–1 year). Tensile strength is only 3% of normal skin at 1 week and about 30% of normal skin at 3 weeks. At 12 weeks, the wound approaches maximum tensile strength at approximately 80% of normal skin.

Just as important as placing sutures is the timing of removal of permanent sutures, which varies with wound location. Sutures on the face should be removed in 3–5 days; scalp and arms in 7–10 days; trunk, legs, and hands/feet in 10–14 days; and palms or soles in 14–21 days. Areas of considerable tension (e.g., joints) require longer suture implantation.[26,37]

The principles of scar optimization following wound closure include (1) minimizing sun/ultraviolet radiation exposure; (2) reducing tension and forces of mechanical stress; (2) hydrating, taping, or occluding the surgical site; and (4) using pressure garments.[38,39] Because the wound healing process extends over several weeks and months, it is important to guide postoperative restrictions and to manage patient expectations.

CAVEATS

Timing and technique of wound closure is an individualized process which depends on wound factors, patient factors, and surgeon factors. While the reconstructive ladder is a useful tool for considering options from simple to complex, sometimes an elevator approach is indicated.

SELECTED READINGS

1. Bullocks J, Hsu P, Izaddoost S, Hollier L, Stal S. *Plastic Surgery Emergencies: Principles and Techniques.* 1st ed. New York: Thieme; 2008.
2. Eliya-Masamba MC, Banda GW. Primary closure versus delayed closure for non bite traumatic wounds within 24 hours post injury. *Cochrane Database Syst Rev* 2013(10):CD008574.
3. Lenarz CJ, Watson JT, Moed BR, Israel H, Mullen JD, Macdonald JB. Timing of wound closure in open fractures based on cultures obtained after debridement. *J Bone Joint Surg Am* 2010;92(10):1921–1926.
4. Malhotra AK, Goldberg S, Graham J, et al. Open extremity fractures: impact of delay in operative debridement and irrigation. *J Trauma Acute Care Surg* 2014;76(5):1201–1207.
5. Bowler PG. The 10(5) bacterial growth guideline: reassessing its clinical relevance in wound healing. *Ostomy Wound Manage* 2003;49(1):44–53.
6. Guo S, Dipietro LA. Factors affecting wound healing. *J Dent Res* 2010;89(3):219–229.
7. Stechmiller J. Understanding the role of nutrition and wound healing. *Nutr Clin Pract* 2010;25(1):61–68.
8. Janis JE, Harrison B. Wound healing: part I. Basic science. *Plast Reconstr Surg* 2014;133(2):199e–207e.
9. Anstead G. Steroids, retinoids, and wound healing. *Adv Wound Care* 1998;11:277–285.
10. Rinker B. The evils of nicotine: an evidence-based guide to smoking and plastic surgery. *Ann Plast Surg* 2013;70(5):599–605.
11. Sorensen L. Wound healing and infection in surgery. The clinical impact of smoking and smoking cessation: a systematic review and meta-analysis. *Arch Surg* 2012;147(4):373–383.
12. Sarin C, Austin J, Nickel W. Effects of smoking on digital blood-flow velocity. *JAMA* 1974;229(10):1327–1328.
13. Myers TG, Lowery NJ, Frykberg RG, Wukich DK. Ankle and hindfoot fusions: comparison of outcomes in patients with and without diabetes. *Foot Ankle Int* 2012;33(1):20–28.
14. Endara M, Masden D, Goldstein J, Gondek S, Steinberg J, Attinger C. The role of chronic and perioperative glucose management in high-risk surgical closures: a case for tighter glycemic control. *Plast Reconstr Surg* 2013;132(4):996–1004.
15. Payne WG, Naidu DK, Wheeler CK, et al. Wound healing in patients with cancer. *Eplasty* 2008;8:e9.
16. Warren Peled A, Itakura K, Foster RD, et al. Impact of chemotherapy on postoperative complications after mastectomy and immediate breast reconstruction. *Arch Surg* 2010;145(9):880–885.
17. Erinjeri JP, Fong AJ, Kemeny NE, Brown KT, Getrajdman GI, Solomon SB. Timing of administration of bevacizumab chemotherapy affects wound healing after chest wall port placement. *Cancer* 2011;117(6):1296–1301.
18. Kapalschinski N, Goertz O, Harati K, et al. Plastic surgery in the multimodal treatment concept of soft tissue sarcoma: influence of radiation, chemotherapy, and isolated limb perfusion on plastic surgery techniques. *Front Oncol* 2015;5:268.
19. Sanniec KJ, Swanson S, Casey WJ, 3rd, Schwartz A, Bryant L, Rebecca AM. Predictive factors of wound complications after sarcoma resection requiring plastic surgeon involvement. *Ann Plast Surg* 2013;71(3):283–285.
20. Olascoaga A, Vilar-Compte D, Poitevin-Chacon A, Contreras-Ruiz J. Wound healing in radiated skin: pathophysiology and treatment options. *Int Wound J* 2008;5(2):246–257.
21. Janis JE, Kwon RK, Lalonde DH. A practical guide to wound healing. *Plast Reconstr Surg* 2010;125(6):230e–244e.
22. Maciel-Miranda A, Morris SF, Hallock GG. Local flaps, including pedicled perforator flaps: anatomy, technique, and applications. *Plast Reconstr Surg* 2013;131(6):896e–911e.
23. Mathes SJ, Nahai F. *Reconstructive Surgery: Principles, Anatomy & Technique.* Vol 2. New York: Churchill Livingstone; St. Louis: Quality Medical; 1997.
24. Regula CG, Yag-Howard C. Suture products and techniques: what to use, where, and why. *Dermatol Surg* 2015;41 Suppl 10:S187–S200.
25. Thorne C, Chung KC, Gosain A, et al. *Grabb and Smith's Plastic Surgery.* 7th ed. Philadelphia: Wolters Kluwer/Lippincott Williams & Wilkins; 2014.
26. Singer A, Hollander J, Quinn J. Evaluation and management of traumatic lacerations. *N Engl J Med* 1997;337(16):1142–1148.
27. Hochberg J, Meyer KM, Marion MD. Suture choice and other methods of skin closure. *Surg Clin North Am* 2009;89(3):627–641.
28. Baker SR. Fundamentals of expanded tissue. *Head Neck* 1991;13(4):327–333.
29. Cherry GW, Austad E, Pasyk K, McClatchey K, Rohrich RJ. Increased survival and vascularity of random-pattern skin flaps elevated in controlled, expanded skin. *Plast Reconstr Surg* 1983;72(5):680–687.
30. Orgill DP, Bayer LR. Update on negative-pressure wound therapy. *Plast Reconstr Surg* 2011;127 Suppl 1:105S–115S.
31. Buchanan PJ, Kung TA, Cederna PS. Evidence-based medicine: wound closure. *Plast Reconstr Surg.* 2014;134(6):1391–1404.
32. Webster J, Scuffham P, Stankiewicz M, Chaboyer WP. Negative pressure wound therapy for skin grafts and surgical wounds healing by primary intention. *Cochrane Database Syst Rev* 2014(10):CD009261.
33. Dumville JC, Owens GL, Crosbie EJ, Peinemann F, Liu Z. Negative pressure wound therapy for treating surgical wounds healing by secondary intention. *Cochrane Database Syst Rev* 2015(6):CD011278.
34. Orgill DP, Bayer LR. Negative pressure wound therapy: past, present and future. *Int Wound J* 2013;10(Suppl 1):15–19.
35. V.A.C. *Therapy Clinical Guidelines: A Reference Source for Clinicians.* San Antonio, TX: Acelity; 2015.
36. Kim PJ, Attinger CE, Olawoye O, et al. Negative pressure wound therapy with instillation: review of evidence and recommendations. *Wounds* 2015;27(12):S2–S19.
37. Mirastschijski U, Jokuszies A, Vogt P. Skin wound healing: repair biology, wound, and scar treatment. In: Neligan P, ed. *Plastic Surgery.* vol 1. 3rd ed. London: Elsevier; 2013:267–296.
38. Monstrey S, Middelkoop E, Vranckx JJ, et al. Updated scar management practical guidelines: non-invasive and invasive measures. *J Plast Reconstr Aesthet Surg* 2014;67(8):1017–1025.
39. Gurtner GC, Dauskardt RH, Wong VW, et al. Improving cutaneous scar formation by controlling the mechanical environment: large animal and phase I studies. *Ann Surg* 2011;254(2):217–225.

4.

MATERIAL

Jeffrey D. Friedman, Scott W. Mosser, and Eric Ruff

Choosing the type of closure for a specific occasion demands a complete working knowledge of the materials available. Having this appreciation for the particular strengths and weaknesses of the various suture materials also complements the particular task at hand. The use of suture materials to close various wounds extends as far back as 5000 BC with reports of crude wound closures with natural materials. The arrival of synthetic suture materials in the 1940s and synthetic absorbable materials beginning in 1970 has offered an expanding wealth of options to the wound closure expert. The surgeon must be well acquainted with these materials to take full advantage of their specific differences, since the type of closure chosen is now as integral a part of the procedure as any other. This is even more true in the field of plastic and reconstructive surgery, in which the visual result of the wound closure can have equal importance with the functional result.

ASSESSMENT OF SUTURE MATERIALS

Various suture materials are often described in terms of how they relate to the hypothetical ideal suture. This refers to a suture that, when broken down into each of its qualities, exemplifies the epitome of that quality. The ideal suture would have superior tensile strength and knot security, be easy to handle, evoke a minimal inflammatory response, be resistant to infection, and eventually reabsorb once the wound strength compensated for the operative injury.[6] Unfortunately, some of the factors contributing to each of these characteristics can be mutually exclusive so that a particular suture material may only exhibit a few of these ideal characteristics. Each of these qualities is described

separately, but the final determination of an appropriate suture material lies in a careful assessment of the special needs of each individual closure (Table 4.1).

TENSILE STRENGTH

The tensile strength of a suture is the amount of weight required to break a suture divided by the cross-sectional area. For each compound, this number is a constant (Table 4.2).[1] From this value, the strengths of sutures are determined based on the United States Pharmacopoeia (USP) rating, given in #-0 values. Since the USP rating refers to breaking strength, two 3-0 sutures of different materials can have very different diameters. Steel, for example, which is the material with the highest tensile strength, would have the smallest diameter of all sutures, rated 2-0, and would be much thinner than a 2-0 silk suture.[9] After the metals, the synthetic materials have the next highest tensile strength, and, finally, the natural fibers (i.e., silk, catgut) have the least tensile strength of all materials.

The concept of an "ideal tensile strength" is largely subjective. While a suture of high tensile strength is desirable to ensure adequate wound closure, the diameter of the material being used should also be considered. Under certain circumstances, a thicker suture than necessary might leave a larger, more noticeable scar, while under different conditions, a thinner suture might cut through swollen tissue instead of holding it together. All things considered, for cutaneous sutures under the normal low tension of final closure, using a smaller diameter suture is much more important cosmetically than using a thicker suture with a higher breaking threshold. Under these conditions of minimal skin tension, thinner sutures are

TABLE 4.1 NONABSORBABLE SUTURE QUALITIES

Material	Configuration	Tensile Strength	Reactivity	Handling	Knot Security
Cotton	Twisted	Good	High	Good	Low
Silk	Braided	Good	High	Good	Low
Nylon					
Monofilament	Monofilament	High	Low	Poor	High
Ethilon					
Dermalon					
Surgamid					
Braided	Braided	High	Medium	Good	Fair
Nurolon					
Polypropylene	Monofilament	Fair	Low	Poor	High
Prolene					
Surgilene					
Dermalene					
Polybutester	Monofilament	High	Low	Fair	Low
Novafil					
Polyester					
Uncoated	Braided	High	Medium	Good	Fair
Mersilene					
Dacron					
Polyviolene					
Coated	Braided	High	Medium	Good	Fair
Ethibond					
Poydek					
Tri-Cron	Braided	High	Medium	Poor	Fair
Tevdek					
Stainless steel	Monofilament	High	Low	Poor	Poor

usually adequate. Placing a wound under greater tension with a thicker stitch may cause significant trauma and ultimate tissue necrosis.

CONFIGURATION

A suture material can have a configuration of either monofilament or multifilament. Multifilament suture can be further classified as either twisted or braided. Since monofilament sutures have a smooth surface that passes easily through tissue, they cause the least amount of tissue trauma and are believed to be more resistant to the adhesion of bacteria. Although braided materials are easiest to handle, simplest to tie, and have significantly enhanced knot strength, they have the ability to harbor debris and bacteria through a process of capillary uptake. This may predispose to local wound contamination and possibly wound infection. Braided sutures, such as polyglactin 910 (Vicryl), polyglycolic acid (Dexon), and silk, should generally be avoided in heavily contaminated areas.

KNOT SECURITY

A number of factors define the characteristic of knot security for a given suture. This is best thought of as a measurement of the force necessary to cause a knot to slip, which is proportional to the coefficient of friction and the ability of the suture to stretch. The braided sutures score highest

TABLE 4.2 RELATIVE STRENGTHS OF SUTURE MATERIALS

Increasing Strength	Nonabsorbable	Absorbable
	Steel	
	Polyester	Polyglycolic acid
	Nylon (monofilament)	Polyglactin 910
	Nylon (braided)	
	Polypropylene	
	Silk, cotton	
		Catgut, collagen

Adapted with permission from Bennett RG. Selection of wound closure materials. *Amer Acad Derm*. 1988;18(4):619.

in this area since they tend to have a remarkably higher co-efficient of friction than monofilament or multifilament sutures. Silk, for example, has among the highest rating for knot security, while nylon and polypropylene have remarkably lower knot security and require more throws to ensure a secure tie.[5]

ELASTICITY

The tendency of a suture to return to its original length after stretching is the elasticity of the material. This quality is desirable because elastic sutures will stretch in edematous wounds. As the local edema subsides, these sutures return to normal size while maintaining tension on the wound. Nonelastic sutures, on the other hand, will tend to cut through edematous tissues instead of forgiving the added tension. This can result in wound dehiscence if swelling is severe. Nylon is one of the more elastic synthetic compounds, while the metals, such as steel, are quite inelastic.

MEMORY

It can be difficult to understand the difference between elasticity and memory. Memory is the tendency of a suture material to return to its original shape and is similar to the stiffness of the material. Sutures with more memory tend to be less pliable and are generally more difficult to handle. Because materials with high memory ratings may tend to relax over time and knots unravel more easily, knot strength is inversely proportional to the memory of the suture material. Most of the monofilament synthetic materials (i.e., polypropylene) have a high degree of memory.

REACTIVITY

With the development of synthetic suture material, the availability of nonreactive materials for wound closure has greatly increased. Reactivity, simply stated, is the degree to which the inflammatory response is activated as a result of the presence of the suture material. Usually, this is measured after the inflammatory phase of wound healing subsides, normally 2–7 days. Typically, after 2 days, the inflammation present in the local wound environment is predominantly the result of the type of foreign body present. The relative tissue reactivity of different absorbable suture materials can be seen in Table 4.3. Overall, naturally occurring materials are more reactive than synthetic materials.

FLUID ABSORPTION AND CAPILLARITY

Fluid absorption and capillarity are similar qualities. Fluid absorption is literally the amount of fluid retained by a suture per unit of weight, while capillarity is a measure of the tendency of fluid to travel along a suture. While fluid absorption might reveal little more than the tendency of a suture material to remain dry, capillarity is thought to correlate well with adhesion and harboring of bacteria, should the suture become contaminated. This is because capillarity implies the existence of crevices within which bacteria may be harbored away from the immune system. Multifilament sutures have the highest capillarity by far and demonstrate a greater incidence of contamination than monofilament sutures.

TABLE 4.3 RELATIVE TISSUE REACTIVITY TO SUTURES

Increasing Reactivity	Nonabsorbable	Absorbable
		Catgut
	Silk, cotton	
	Polyester (coated)	Polyglactin 910
	Polyester (uncoated)	Polyglycolic acid
	Nylon	
	Polypropylene	

Adapted with permission from Bennett RG. Selection of wound closure materials. *Amer Acad Derm*. 1988;18(4):619.

COST

Although synthetic sutures cost more than natural materials as a whole, the cost consideration of a suture is largely based on the price of the needle used. This is particularly true in the case where the sharpest needles (so-called *precision needles*) are desired. These needles are made of a stronger alloy and honed an additional two dozen times. Sutures bearing these needles are about twice as costly as the same-sized sutures with nonprecision needles.

VISIBILITY

Finally, the visibility of the suture can be of importance, both intraoperatively and postoperatively. Many sutures are darkly colored to aid either in intraoperative visibility or to aid in removal (i.e., purple scalp sutures in a patient with dark hair). Other sutures are either monofilament clear (used in skin closure to be less noticeable) or braided. Braided sutures are usually visible even if undyed since they can become saturated with blood intraoperatively and can therefore become darkly colored over time. There have been reports of colored absorbable suture "tattooing" the dermis of a subcuticular closure. In addition, as scars may thin out over time, dyed permanent suture may become increasingly visible beneath the skin. For this reason, we recommend only undyed suture for absorbable subcuticular and dermal closures.

INDICATIONS AND CONTRAINDICATIONS FOR SUTURE TYPE AND ABSORPTION

The role of sutures varies in the different phases of wound healing. Wound healing is divided into three phases. In the *substrate phase*, initial inflammation is associated with wound induration and swelling. During this 4- to 5-day period, the surgical wound depends exclusively on the sutures to maintain tissue edge opposition and security of the closure. During the *proliferative phase* (days 5–42), fibroblasts begin to produce collagen, which contributes to the rapid gain in wound tensile strength. In spite of the increasing strength of the wound, the suture that is in place still has an important role in preventing wound edge retraction. Loss of suture integrity during the early period of this phase (through dissolution, for example) can result in widening of the suture line in areas of higher tension. This is particularly true of the back, knee, and shoulder region. Finally, during the *remodeling (or maturation) phase*, which lasts from about postoperative day 42 until approximately 1 year later, the wound continues to gain strength as the collagen fibers become further cross-linked. In this phase, most absorbable suture has already dissolved and is of little consequence to healing or scarring.

The idea of a suture being "absorbable" can actually be somewhat arbitrary depending on the time allotted for this process to take place. Although there is significant evidence that both nylon and silk slowly dissolve over a number of years, it is generally accepted that an absorbable suture is one that has lost more than half its tensile strength within 60 days. Some suture materials have a much faster rate of absorption. For example, catgut loses half its tensile strength within 7 days and, after 2 weeks. contributes very little to wound integrity. Such sutures might be useful when the task at hand calls for a short-term opposition of edges that are under minimal tension.[8] These sutures are particularly useful when their removal is not desirable (i.e., patient noncompliance to follow-up, patient reluctance, or children with wounds in inconspicuous areas). A summary of the various rates of dissolution of absorbable suture materials can be found in Table 4.4.

In some cases, an absorbable suture with tensile strength that lasts several weeks is desirable. This is because the loss of suture tension should be equivalent to or slower than the gain in wound strength through collagen deposition and cross-linking. The choice of this type of material is often dependent on the inherent tension on the wound edges. After a procedure, skin strength can be expected to regain 5% of its original strength within a week, nearly 50% within 4 weeks, and 80% within 6 weeks of skin closure. Even after collagen maturation is complete (6 months to 1 year postoperatively), the wound regains only 80% of its original strength. Therefore, this rate of self-repair should be kept in mind when choosing an absorbable compound that is placed under a significant amount of tension.

Enzymatic degradation of sutures occurs through either proteolytic or hydrolytic mechanisms. All natural suture materials are absorbed through a proteolytic process, which, as noted earlier, is associated with a greater inflammatory response. This is because proteolytic degradation results in a significant amount of suture debris that must be processed and digested by phagocytic cells. Synthetic materials, such as polyglycolic acid and polyglactin 910, are degraded by the process of hydrolysis, which does not appear to stimulate mononuclear phagocytes and therefore results in less inflammation.

TABLE 4.4 PROPERTIES OF ABSORBABLE SUTURE MATERIALS

Material	Source	Approximate Half-life	Reactivity	Knot Security	Memory	Absorption
Plain catgut	Intestinal submucosa (sheep) or serosa (cattle)	5–6 d	High	Poor	Low	Unpredictable (12 wk)
Treated (chromic) catgut	Intestinal submucosa (sheep) or serosa (cattle)	14 d	Medium	Fair	Low	Unpredictable (14–80 d)
Polyglactin 910 (Vicryl)[3]	Synthetic	2–3 wk	Low	Fair	Low	Predictable (80 d)
Poliglecaprone 25 (Monocryl)	Synthetic	7–14 d	Low	Fair	High	Predictable (91–119 d)
Polyglycolic acid (Dexon)[3]	Synthetic	2–3 wk	Low	Good	Low	Predictable (90 d)
Polyglyconate (Maxon)	Synthetic	4 wk	Low			
Polydioxanone (PDS)[7]	Synthetic	4 wk	Low	Poor	High	Predictable (180 d)
Barbed (V-loc Unidirectional) (Quill Bidirectional)	Synthetic	4 wk	Low	High	High	Predictable (90–180 d)

EPITHELIAL TRACKING AND CYST FORMATION

Epithelial cells that abut a skin suture form a cylindrical cuff as they grow downward along the suture from the skin borders. If these epithelial progenitor cells are established along the suture lines, they will continue to develop after the suture is removed, thus keratinizing the length of the suture track. This keratinization results in inflammation and punctate scar formation. Tract formation may be especially problematic for full-thickness sutures left in place in the eyelid for longer than 2–3 days. In these cases, early track formation may form a tunnel that remains patent after suture removal, necessitating operative intervention for correction. Although epithelial tracking begins within 48 hours, most sutures can generally be removed up until the eighth postoperative day with resultant regression of the epithelium and no noticeable tracks. Because most absorbable suture materials remain in the skin for more than 8 days, absorbable sutures have a high risk of epithelial tracking if not removed. Therefore, the plastic surgeon should be aware of this or plan to remove the final skin sutures that were not placed as a subcuticular closure. General guidelines for the timing of suture removal are listed in Table 4.5.

A "railroad track" scar implies the formation of punctate scars from epithelial tracking and parallel rows of scarring from beneath each suture strand. This results from pressure necrosis of the skin and subcutaneous tissue beneath the external suture. Generally, this can be prevented by tying

TABLE 4.5 OPTIMAL TIMING OF SUTURE REMOVAL BY BODY SITE

Bodily Area	Days to Removal
Eyelid	3–5
Face	5–7
Lip	5–7
Hands/feet	10–14
Trunk	7–10
Breast	7–10

sutures loose enough to allow for edematous change and removing the sutures within a reasonable time period.

Close postoperative follow-up should be attempted so that, in the event of a complication of wound closure, the problem can be promptly addressed. This may reduce the probability of the need for further corrective procedures. Suture cysts can be unroofed and allowed to heal, while any infected suture must be removed to affect prompt resolution of the infection.

NEEDLES

At this time, there is no standard nomenclature for the different needle types. Each suture company has its own set of model numbers to describe its product. It is more useful, then, to understand the major variables between various needle types and become familiar with their usefulness in specific situations.[1]

Needles are attached to sutures through a process of *swaging*, whereby the cylinder of metal at the rear of the needle is swaged around the suture material. This method of needle production has resulted in less tissue trauma compared with previous methods (i.e., using a threaded needle through which a suture was placed). Although a swaged needle has a slightly larger diameter than the suture material itself, the effect is still superior to pulling two threads of suture through tissue on an eyed needle. However, one must be cognizant of this difference in diameters and take care to choose both an appropriately sized suture and needle to avoid undesirable microtrauma.

Needles are classified based on the qualities of strength and ductility. Strength is the ability to withstand outward bending, while ductility is the ability to withstand breaking on bending. More expensive needles are made of alloys, which are superior in both respects and, though more costly, may actually save money over a repeated dulling or breaking of inferior needles.

Although there are numerous variations, needles can basically be configured in one of three ways. Tapered needles are conical in shape, with very little tendency for the suture to cut through the tissue postoperatively. Cutting and reverse-cutting needles have a pyramidal cross-section, the flat base of the pyramid being either outside (cutting) or inside (reverse-cutting) the curve of the needle, as seen in

Figure 4.1. Reverse-cutting needles are used far more often in skin closures than are cutting needles since the flat surface on the inner side of the curve creates a tract that makes it less likely that the suture will tear through the tissue. However, only tapered needles should be used in suturing cartilage because cutting needles tend to tear the cartilage, increasing the likelihood of fracture at this point and the possibility of sutures pulling through the cartilage.

TECHNIQUE AND SPECIFIC CONSIDERATIONS

The concept of an ideal wound closure follows a number of basic principles to achieve an optimal result. Precise wound approximation may require skin marking with perpendicular hatchmarks before the procedure is begun or, in the case of a large flap, temporarily securing the closure with staples or towel clips to ensure proper alignment. For smaller closures, in which the operative site is not marked, a single hook can be used to stretch the margins of the skin and plan the alignment of the skin edges.

Since the reticular dermis is one particular region where collagen deposition contributes significantly to the final appearance of the scar, the tension on this skin layer should be reduced as much as possible. Sutures should be placed so that the tension is on the deeper layers. If an absorbable suture is used under tension, it should be chosen to

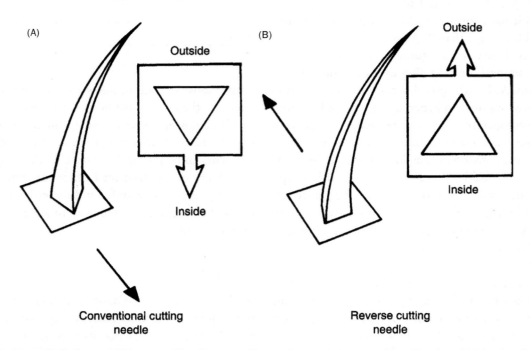

Figure 4.1. Needles in use. (A) Cutting and (B) reverse-cutting. Reverse-cutting needles create tract away from skin edge, which lessens likelihood of sutures pulling through skin margin.

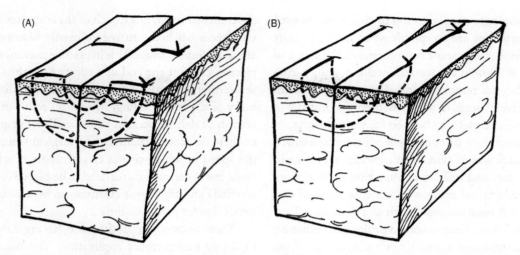

Figure 4.2. Mattress stitch. (A) vertical and (B) horizontal mattress sutures. Though both methods allow for eversion of skin edges, horizontal mattress technique produces greater eversion and is used in areas where inversion of the skin edges is particularly problematic (hands, feet).

maintain this tension throughout the initial healing period. Otherwise, the collagen deposition might cause the wound edges to migrate farther apart, resulting in a wider scar. An ideal final skin closure should provide coaptation of the skin edges with slight eversion of the margins, indicating minimal tension on the most superficial layer.[2]

Wound edges must be maximally everted. Without initial eversion, a remodeling scar will contract downward, leaving a depression in the site of closure. Eversion of the skin edges is easily accomplished with both vertical and horizontal mattress sutures (Figure 4.2). This becomes especially problematic in hand closures, where a palmar depression can be a site of excessive moisture collection and discomfort.

Postoperative discomfort can also be derived from surface irregularities beneath a scar. This typically occurs as a result of not inverting absorbable suture knots deeply enough in a dermal closure. All knots not tied to remain outside the skin should be inverted. Running sutures can save time and

are an acceptable means of closure provided that the sutures are well secured at the ends. We prefer to avoid knots at the end of subcuticular closures, but instead the ends of the suture are brought through the skin and held down with adhesive tape (e.g., Steri-Strips) or skin glue.

In the past, the subcuticular closure was a perpendicular stitch, with the exiting stitch on one end entering at the same point on the other skin edge. We find that the closure is most secure if, instead of entering the dermis directly across from the exiting bite on the opposite side, the entrance is chosen slightly upstream (Figure 4.3). In our experience, direct perpendicular bites do not hold the wound edges as well as this backtracking pattern.

OTHER WOUND CLOSURE METHODS

In addition to suturing wounds, both staples and wound taping have become useful for effecting a closure.[4] Although

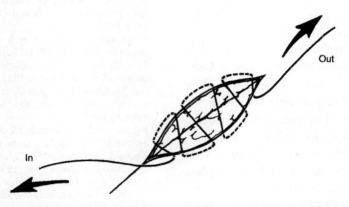

Figure 4.3. Optimal subcuticular closure method. Method demonstrates need to overlap each suture as one progresses. Suture may be tied at each end with buried knots or placed as pullout sutures securing either end with adhesive tape.

staples are a seemingly crude method of closure when used in plastic surgery, they are acceptable when used to ensure skin-edge eversion, when some room between the skin and the staple bar is allowed for wound swelling, and, particularly, when they are removed early. There are two widths of staples available: regular width is used for most skin closures, and wide staples may be used for scalp closures.

Taping wounds with strips of sterile adhesive tape can be a useful and quick way to close simple excisions. Normally, however, they are used only in conjunction with sutures, to offer some additional support in the first week or two postoperatively. A local adhesive, such as a tincture of benzoin, or Mastisol is an effective way to prolong the adhesive property of the tape and is usually safe if kept out of the wound. On occasion, patients can demonstrate tape allergy from the adhesive, with resultant local skin irritation and inflammation. More frequently, however, skin lesions from tape are in the form of blisters, which occur as a result of swelling in the area where the tape is applied. If significant swelling is expected over the next several days, taping is done loosely or not at all.

Recently, various cyanoacrylate skin glues have been adopted to replace the need for external taping of skin closures in order to provide greater wound edge support (e.g., Dermabond). We have found these materials to be quite effective in maintaining the integrity of skin closures. Their use may allow for the earlier removal of external sutures or provide greater wound stability and therefore reduce the number of dermal sutures required for a suitable subcuticular closure. In some cases, these external adhesives may obviate the need for external sutures, particularly simple lacerations located in tension-free anatomic areas. One must, however, be cognizant of the fact that some patients may develop significant skin reactions to these adhesives and thus necessitate the early removal of the glue in the postoperative period.

BARBED SUTURE

The advent of barbed suture technology has been widely adopted by surgical practitioners over the past decade. These devices were approved by the US Food and Drug Administration (FDA) in 2004 and were touted as the first commercially available knotless wound closure suture devices (Quill, Angiotech Pharmaceuticals, Vancouver, BC).[10] Since that time, several other manufacturers have introduced similar barbed devices to the marketplace that avoid the use of knots in order to secure tension on wound closures (V-Loc, STRATAFIX). Despite the minor difference in technology, each of these sutures utilizes small unidirectional barbs to secure evenly distributed tension along a wound closure. This in essence prevents the need for placing knots at the end of a suture line, thus maintaining the tensile strength of the suture and avoiding the possibility of the knots failing, which can result in wound separation or dehiscence. An additional advantage for the use of these devices, particularly for surgical wound closure, is the speed at which tissues can be approximated. In most cases, fewer dermal sutures need to be placed (or completely avoided) and thus most closures can be accomplished in a much shorter period of time.

These sutures are produced as having either unidirectional or bidirectional application. The use of unidirectional materials requires that the suture is passed through a loop at one end of the wound in order to secure the suture at this point, and closure the proceeds along the length of the wound until the wound is closed. By contrast, the bidirectional suture is double-armed, and closure begins in the middle of the wound. Approximation of the wound edges is carried out by approximating the tissues in either direction, typically in a subcuticular fashion. A variety of absorbable and nonabsorbable materials are used in the production of these devices. Selection of these suture materials is based on the particular characteristics of the wound and the tensile strength requirements of the tissues being approximated.

SELECTED READINGS

1. Bennett RG. Selection of wound closure materials. *Amer Acad Derm* 1988;18:619.
2. Cohen M. *Mastery of Plastic and Reconstructive Surgery.* New York: Little, Brown, 1994:7.
3. Craig PH, Williams JA, Davis KW, et al. A biologic comparison of polyglactin 910 and polyglycolic acid synthetic absorbable sutures. *Surg Gynecol Obstet* 1975;141:1.
4. Edlich RF, Becker DG, Thacker JG, Rodeheaver GT. Scientific basis for selecting staple and tape skin closures. *Clin Plast Surg* 1990;17:571.
5. Herrmann JB. Tensile strength and knot security of surgical suture materials. *Amer Surg* 1971;37:209.
6. Moy RL, Lee A, Zalka A. Commonly used suture materials in skin surgery. *Am Fam Physician* 1991;44:2123.
7. Ray JA, Doddi N, Regula D, et al. Polydioxanone (PDS), a novel monofilament synthetic absorbable suture. *Surg Gynecol Obstet* 1981;153:497.
8. Swanson NA, Tromovitch TA. Suture materials, 1980s: properties, uses, and abuses. *Int J Dermatol* 1982;21:373.
9. *United States Pharmacopeia.* 22nd ed. Rockville, MD: United States Pharmacopeial Convention, 1990.
10. Greenberg JA, Goldman RH. Barbed suture: a review of the technology and clinical uses in obstetrics and gynecology. *Rev Obstet Gynecol* 2013;6(3–4):107.

5.

LOCAL RANDOM PATTERN FLAPS

Brian M. Christie and Michael L. Bentz

The local random pattern flap may be considered an apt representation of the distillation of plastic surgery. Requiring creativity, planning, and a fundamental grasp of both geometry and tissue dynamics, the local flap is a versatile technique that can be utilized for both prevention of and as a solution to difficult wounds. Local flaps are utilized across the body following tumor extirpation or for closure of traumatic defects and must be individualized based on anatomic defect location, available and desired tissue characteristics, and patient clinical factors. They are used commonly in hand reconstruction following trauma, pressure sore reconstruction, following skin cancer removal on the face, and in burn reconstruction. In this chapter, an approach to utilization of the local random pattern flap will be discussed, including assessment of the defect, indications/contraindications for use of a local flap, practicalities of design and technique, and postoperative care. Various specific local flaps and examples of their use will be reviewed.

ASSESSMENT OF THE DEFECT

The plastic surgeon performing local flap reconstruction of a defect may be presented with an existing defect or may be performing tumor extirpation. In either situation, but especially the former, the plastic surgeon must be of two minds. The surgeon performing cancer resection must prioritize margin clearance without consideration for the size or location of the defect created. Any attempt to limit margins will compromise both the primary goal of the operation (to achieve a cancer-free wound) and secondary efforts of definitive reconstruction. It is essential that the reconstructive component of the procedure not be planned until margins are confirmed cancer-free.

Once the defect is created, it should be fully assessed. The initial evaluation must include assessment of all missing tissues, including skin, subcutaneous tissue, and mucosal lining, as well as structural tissue such as bone or cartilage. Second, any exposed structures must be noted, including bone without periosteum and tendon denuded of paratenon, as well as exposed nerves and arteries. Third, the physical characteristics of the defect must be considered. These include the contour of the defect (concave, flat, or convex), the skin quality (thick, thin, and color), and the presence or absence of hair. Last, one must consider the function of the reconstructed tissue—whether the ultimate goal is a closed wound, a minimally visible scar (in the setting of facial reconstruction), or a durable construct (pressure sores and palmar hand tissues). In the situation where a local flap is selected, multiple potential incisions should be evaluated in order to optimize the donor and recipient sites. In facial flap reconstruction, incisions are made along lines of minimal tension and designed to lie in creases and concave surfaces. In the setting of pressure sore reconstruction, this often involves planning incisions so that they do not ultimately lie directly over the reconstructed area or any future pressure points.

INDICATIONS

Once the defect has been adequately assessed, available options must then be inventoried and organized according to their relative location on the reconstructive ladder. The reconstructive surgeon should feel totally comfortable, however, skipping "rungs" on the ladder when the optimal solution is not the simplest one. While primary closure is often the initial goal, in some settings it can result in excessive tension which can threaten a closure or lead to unfavorable scarring or, in the setting of pressure sore reconstruction, can result in an incision placed directly over the offending pressure point, thus dramatically increasing the risk of failure When primary closure is suboptimal or not possible, secondary closure, split and full thickness skin grafts, and axial pattern flaps should all be considered (in addition to local random pattern flaps). Second-intention healing can result in scar contracture, which can distort surrounding tissue. Skin grafts may not be able to be used if other grafts, such as mucosa or cartilage, are to be used and are generally not as durable as local flap options. Additionally, both full- and split-thickness skin grafts can result in donor/recipient site characteristic mismatch and are prone to hyperpigmentation. Assessment of utilized and surrounding tissue quality and laxity is essential if a local flap is to be considered. Local flaps are often an ideal choice for reconstruction in that the adjacent tissue is of similar quality to the original defect tissue. Incisions, dissection, and operative time are often also considerably less than utilization of a regional or axial pattern flap. Consideration of the desired characteristics of the reconstructed tissue, as well as the goals and physical characteristics of the patient, will often lead to the most appropriate choice.

CONTRAINDICATIONS

If local flap options are limited, whether due to the size of the defect or the availability of appropriate local tissue, then they should be avoided. In situations where local tissue may have considerably different characteristics, such as in the hair-bearing scalp or the alar rim, other options such as tissue expansion, composite grafting, or axial pattern flaps may be more appropriate. Great caution should be used when considering the use of radiated tissue for local flap reconstruction due to the permanently diminished and unpredictable blood supply. In this setting, regional flaps are often a more suitable and reliable choice.

OPERATING ROOM LOGISTICS

Excellent exposure is paramount in the evaluation and design of local flaps. In facial reconstruction, the entire face and neck should be prepped to allow for comparison of the defect to the intact contralateral side and to allow consideration of multiple options with room for back-cuts or wide undermining. Similarly, the entire scalp or extremity should be exposed as well. In the setting of pressure sore reconstruction, the patient is positioned prone and the extremity on the involved side is prepped down to the level of the knee, again to allow for consideration of all options to and ensure room for mobilization of necessary tissue.

PATIENT MARKING

In surgical planning, use of a marking pen and rough measurement of distance and angles can greatly assist in determining the feasibility of a proposed local flap and resulting final incision lines. Often, this is not practical until the patient is positioned on the operating room table.

FLAP TYPES

ROTATION FLAPS

Rotation flaps involve tissue moved around the circumference of a circle. One side of the wound becomes the leading edge of the flap, which is rotated to cover the opposite aspect of the wound. A major advantage of rotation flaps is their typically broad-based and robust blood supply. A disadvantage can be the amount of tissue undermining required for donor defect coverage. Rotation flaps typically require significant undermining, including a consideration of flap size to defect size ratio of at least 4:1. Crucially, the surgeon must grasp the concept of the point of rotation about which the tissue will rotate, which is defined as the center of the theoretical circle around which the flap will rotate. If the flap is not designed so that the base of the rotation flap is also the point of rotation, then the flap may not rotate far enough to fully close the defect. This rotation can be approximated using a piece of stretched gauze or suture, with one end placed at the point of rotation and the other at the leading edge of the flap to approximate the rotated tissue. While some tissues may have enough laxity to allow for rotation of the flap using only a circular cut, other flaps may require a back cut in the flap to permit adequate advancement with rotation of the tissue to cover the defect. The back cut should be made thoughtfully because it can jeopardize the blood supply to the flap and may require skin grafting for donor site closure.

Examples of commonly used rotation flaps include coverage of hair-bearing scalp defects (especially those involving the crown) and cheek defects, as well as sacral pressure sores (Figures 5.1–5.3).

TRANSPOSITION FLAPS

Transposition flaps involve rotation of tissue to cover a defect that occurs over an intervening area of intact skin. An advantage is that the tissue for the flap can be designed to match that of the defect, whether circular, rectangular, or asymmetrically shaped, and can be taken from an area of

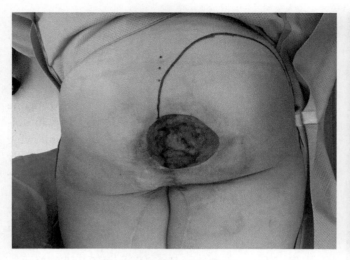

Figure 5.1. Design of rotational flap for coverage of a squamous cell carcinoma. The flap is designed to be large and wide to allow for distribution of tension over a large area, maintenance of robust vascular supply, and the potential of re-rotation in the future should the neoplasm recur.

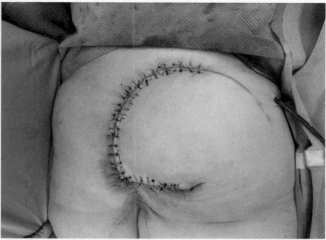

Figure 5.3. Inset of the rotational flap. Note that the suture line is located off midline to minimize the chance of dehiscence when pressure is reapplied over the sacral area.

maximum laxity. Careful planning is required to ensure that the flap donor defect can be primarily closed. The concept of the arc of rotation must be followed in the setting of transposition flaps as well to ensure that the transposed tissue will adequately rotate to fill the defect.

A commonly used transposition flap in facial reconstruction is the *bilobe flap*. The bilobe flap is often used in reconstruction of the nasal dorsum and lateral nasal walls. It consists of two transposition flaps, one to close the defect and another to close the secondary donor site. The flap is designed using tissue from the nasal sidewall and ingeniously allows for coverage of a larger defect (up to 1.5 cm in

diameter) by ultimately borrowing from the more lax tissue of the nasal sidewall.

Another extremely common use of transposition involves the design of a *z-plasty*, which involves two opposing transposition flaps designed most often to lengthen and redirect scarred or contracted tissue. The transposition flaps in a z-plasty are designed so that each shares a side with the scarred tissue or area to be transposed. The flaps are then designed with identical angles that can be adjusted depending on the amount of lengthening needed, although 60 degrees is commonly used as it will yield a maximal 75% length increase. The flaps are then transposed over each other and sutured in place, thus redirecting and lengthening the central scar or local tissue. It is often used in oncologic reconstruction (Figures 5.4–5.7), secondary

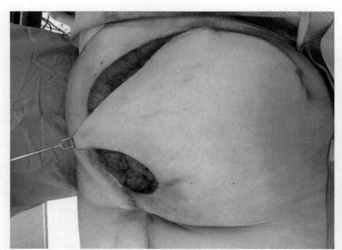

Figure 5.2. Rotation of the flap. While the incision is drawn and designed to allow for a large amount of potential tissue dissection and advancement, the amount of tissue laxity and flap advancement is assessed intraoperatively, and often the entire designed flap length is not required.

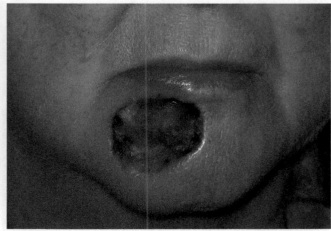

Figure 5.4. Large defect following Mohs excision of a squamous cell carcinoma.

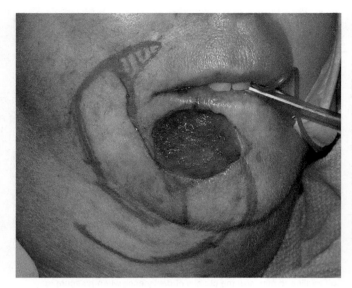

Figure 5.5. Design of two flaps for coverage of the defect: an inferiorly based transposition flap for coverage of the superolateral defect and advancement of the inferior wound edge utilizing the laxity of the anterior neck for coverage of the inferior aspect of the defect.

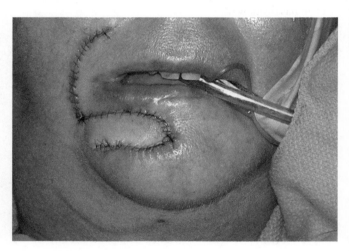

Figure 5.6. Inset of the transposition flap with advancement of the inferior aspect of the wound.

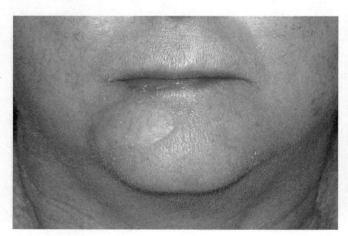

Figure 5.7. Patient at 2 years.

burn reconstruction, flexor contracture release of the volatile/palmar upper extremity, and in cleft palate repair.

ADVANCEMENT FLAPS

Advancement flaps involve advancement of tissue from one edge of the wound, with undermining of the flap and bilateral incisions to allow for adequate mobility. Following advancement, burrows triangles may be excised bilaterally to allow for closure without dog ears. A common type of advancement flap is the V-Y advancement flap, which involves an initial V-shaped incision to permit mobility with direct closure of the donor defect, resulting in a Y-shaped incision line. Advancement flaps are commonly used for Mohs reconstruction (Figures 5.8–5.11), coverage of ischial and sacral pressure sores, and for coverage of distal thumb defects (Moberg flap).

RHOMBOID FLAPS

Rhomboid flaps are a specific type of transposition flap that are geometrically designed to match a specifically created defect. The defect is fashioned into a rhomboid with angles of 60 and 120 degrees. From this design, four different flap variations are possible that the surgeon may choose from, based on donor site tissue laxity and resultant incision location. A line is extended laterally from the 120-degree angle in identical length to the rhomboid, and an additional line is made parallel to the defect rhomboid line (depending on which flap variation is chosen). The flap is undermined and transposed into the defect. The donor defect can typically be closed primarily.

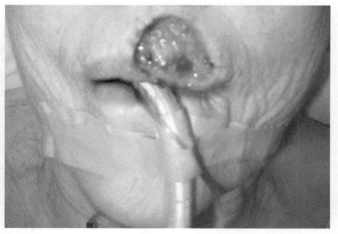

Figure 5.8. A complex defect of the upper lip following Mohs excision of a basal cell carcinoma with involvement of the dry vermillion.

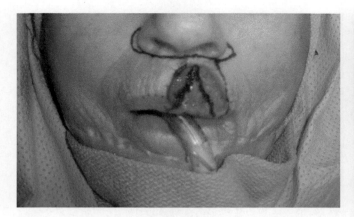

Figure 5.9. Design of bilateral advancement flaps for coverage of this approximately one-third defect of the upper lip. The defect must be recut pentagonally to allow for appropriate alignment of the vermillion border, maintenance of vermillion height, to prevent excess tissue (i.e., dog ear formation) of the subcolumnellar upper lip, and to protect against linear contraction.

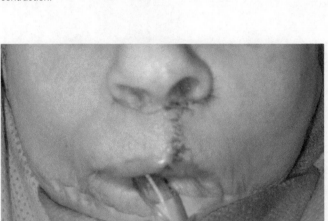

Figure 5.10. Following inset of a unilateral left advancement flap, with attention focused on precise alignment of the vermillion border (white line).

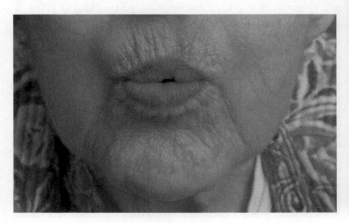

Figure 5.11. One-year follow-up with excellent continuity of the vermillion border and preservation of orbicularis function.

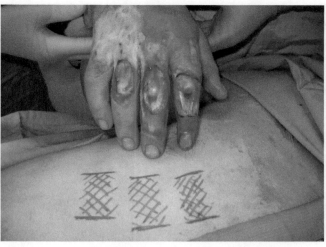

Figure 5.12. A 38-year-old man following motor vehicle accident with full thickness tissue loss of dorsal soft tissue and tendon/joint exposure over the index, long, and ring finger proximal phalanges of the right hand.

Rhomboid flaps can be used throughout the body but are particularly useful on the lower midface (Figures 5.12–5.14), upper extremity, and back. Variations of the rhomboid flap include double and triple rhomboids, which divide defects into multiple individual rhomboid defects which are then closed in a similar manner as described.

ISLAND FLAPS

Island flaps are another type of transposition flap in which the blood supply, based on random subcutaneous vessels, is transposed under intact skin to the donor defect. This results in a donor site that is remote from the defect and does not share an incision line. Island flaps rely on the principle of a point of rotation in order to ensure adequate

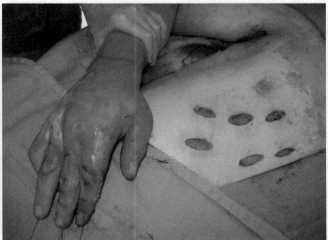

Figure 5.13. Bipedicled thoracoepigastric flaps designed as pockets for coverage of the exposed proximal interphalangeal (PIP) joints.

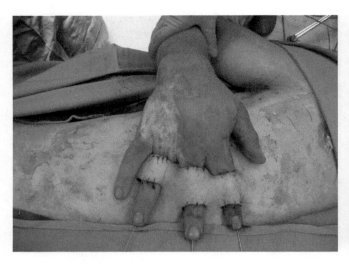

Figure 5.14. The bipedicled flaps are inset into the fingers, which traverse the "pocket" created to allow for vascular ingrowth via inosculation.

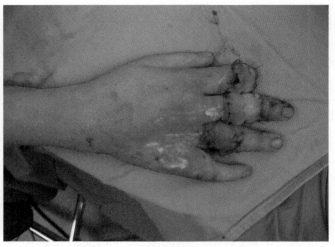

Figure 5.15. Division and inset at 3 weeks.

rotation and coverage of the defect. Care should be taken to assure that the undermined subcutaneous tunnel is not too tight, which can threaten compression of the island's blood supply. Additionally, as a random pattern flap, it is crucial to ensure that the flap blood supply is not too long and does not exceed a 3:1 length to width ratio.

BIPEDICLE FLAPS

Bipedicle flaps are an excellent technique for safe coverage of a defect when a random pattern local flap is indicated in a setting where blood supply is less predictable. By creating two parallel incisions, one along the edge of the defect and one remote from it, the flap maintains blood supply from two separate sources. Along with increased reliability, this also allows for flap dimensions beyond the usual 3:1 ratio, although at the potential cost of flap mobility. The donor site may have to be back-grafted. Bipedicle flaps may be used in multiple settings throughout the body (Figures 5.15–5.18) and are especially helpful in the distal lower extremity.

DELAY TECHNIQUES

Use of random pattern flaps necessitate careful consideration of the vascularity of the designed flap. In certain settings, such as that of previous irradiated tissue or in the lower third of the lower extremity, the use of delay techniques may help to improve the reliability of a random pattern flap. Partial division of the flap prior to definitive mobilization and inset may stress the tissue, encouraging dilation of choke vessels and potentially also promoting angiogenesis. Specific techniques include bipedicle dissection of the flap initially, with division of the distal aspect of the flap 2–3 weeks later (Figures 5.19–5.22). Another technique involves complete division of the flap

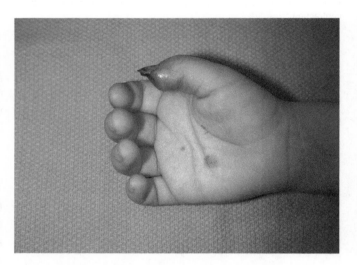

Figure 5.16. A 14-year-old man who sustained a tablesaw injury to the right volar thumb. Exposure of the distal phalanx at the wound base and loss of nail plate support necessitate durable soft tissue coverage in order to preserve length.

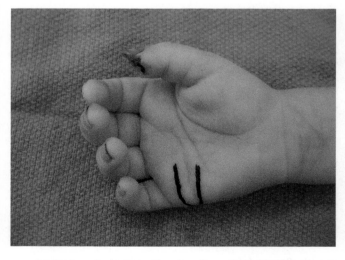

Figure 5.17. Design of a random-pattern hypothenar flap. While the flap will provide the durable soft tissue cover required, it must be delayed in order to allow adequate vascular ingrowth into the recipient bed.

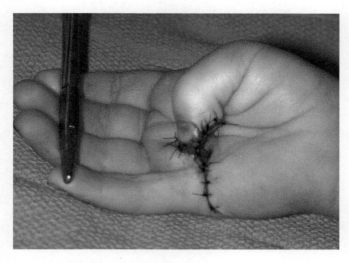

Figure 5.18. Thenar flap inset into defect.

without rotation/advancement/transposition, replacement of the flap in its donor bed, and reelevation with movement to the defect 2–3 weeks later. Often, inert materials such as silicone sheeting are inserted under the flap to prevent the flap from readhering and inosculating its donor bed.

DRESSINGS

Large, bulky dressings are often unnecessary with use of local flaps. Furthermore, they can often hinder the frequent

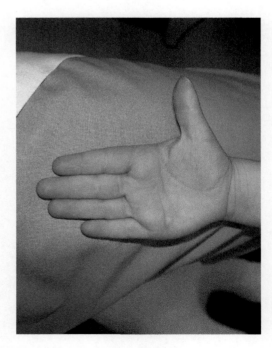

Figure 5.19. One year after division and inset of the thenar flap.

assessment of vascularity and shroud a compromised flap that could potentially be salvaged with interventions such as the use of nitroglycerin paste, removal of tight sutures, drainage of a hematoma, or treatment of a cellulitis that could benefit from antibiotics. Most often, use of a petroleum ointment over incision lines is adequate.

DRAINS

The use of drains depends on the defect being reconstructed and the amount of tissue undermined. In facial reconstruction, drains are rarely helpful or indicated. In pressure sore reconstruction, however, suction drains function to reduce the large amount of dead space created by the defect and the flap used to fill the defect. These are typically maintained for a significant amount of time, until the patient has completed a wedging protocol and output has decreased. In scalp reconstruction, Penrose drains may be helpful to facilitate dead space reduction and allow for drainage of interstitial fluid. These are typically removed after a few days.

POSTOPERATIVE CARE

Following inset of the flap and completion of the operation, the patient is advised to elevate the flap site as much as possible for the first postoperative week. Instructions are given to minimize the risk of bleeding by prevention of elevation of heart rate or blood pressure through lifting or exercise. Showering is permitted, and keeping the surgical site open to air without a dressing is encouraged.

CAVEATS

The majority of complications can be avoided with careful planning and flap design and good technique. Consideration of the 3:1 length-to-width ratio of reliable vascularity in random pattern flaps is essential. Close attention to optimal points of rotation, flap dimensions, and angles will prevent the avoidable circumstance of a flap that will not cover the wound. When a flap does not appear to reach the defect, additional undermining of the defect can sometimes permit closure. In the case that the flap appears congested, indicative of limited venous outflow, release of sutures may relieve compression, and prudent use of leech therapy may be of benefit.

CONCLUSION

The local random pattern flap is an essential tool in the plastic surgeon's armamentarium, providing versatility when faced with daunting wounds that might otherwise require much more extensive reconstructive options. The ability to provide vascularized, adjacent tissue can deliver superior results compared with selections "from rungs above or below" on the reconstructive ladder. By adhering to basic principles of geometry and respecting flap vascularity, the local random pattern flap can offer uniquely advantageous reconstructive opportunities to both surgeon and patient.

6.

PRINCIPLES OF MICROSURGERY

Gregory R. D. Evans and Jordan Kaplan

ASSESSMENT OF THE DEFECT

Proper flap selection requires a careful defect assessment. The surgeon must initially formulate a list of tissues that are needed for the most efficient and durable reconstruction. The defect usually involves some combination of skin, subcutaneous tissue, mucosa, muscle, fascia, tendon, or bone. Neurosensory flaps should be considered when reconstructing the hand, plantar surface of the foot, and potential defects around the mouth. Defects involving the oral cavity may require either soft tissue bulk to facilitate swallowing and speech or mucosal replacement to protect the underlying vital structures in the neck. Reconstruction of muscles may be required if important function has been sacrificed. Fascial reconstruction may be needed for structural integrity or to facilitate tendon gliding over exposed surfaces. Finally, bony defects that result in significant functional impairment should be restored.

Several factors influence the reconstructive plan. Both systemic and local wound healing must be considered. Radiated wounds and wounds in patients undergoing chemotherapy are notoriously difficult to heal. Peripheral vascular disease, cigarette smoking, and diabetes also adversely effect wound healing. In these high-risk patients, aggressive reconstructive efforts, often involving free tissue transfer, are often the best option. While it is true that free tissue transfer is less tolerant of surgical error than many of the more traditional pedicled flaps, the complication rate is frequently higher in pedicle flaps, owing their complications to a less tolerant and less reliable vascular supply. Wound complications can lead to delayed adjuvant therapy and prolonged hospitalization. Thus, free tissue transfer for wound closure in these high-risk patients offers highly reliable, single-stage reconstruction. Because complications and delayed wound healing are minimized, patients are able to return to valuable family time.

Before proceeding, details of the operation should be explained to the patient at a suitable level of detail. Information concerning the donor site, donor site morbidity, intraoperative and postoperative course, and surgical complications, as well as discomfort and scarring should all be discussed with the patient as well as his or her immediate support group.

INDICATIONS

Flap selection can occur only after the defect is cataloged, factors influencing wound healing are considered, and the available tissue is assessed. Tissue available for reconstruction may be local, regional, or distant. Local flaps may be adequate for many smaller defects or those requiring only skin, but these are rarely adequate for more complex defects. Local and regional flaps are frequently unreliable owing to scarring, previous irradiation, trauma, infection, and insufficient surface area or volume. When local and regional tissue is unsatisfactory, distant free tissue transfer must be considered.

We consider free tissue transfer the method of choice in many reconstructive situations. The use of free flaps for breast reconstruction allows aggressive shaping of the tissue, the ability to vary chest wall position, and the ability to sculpture the flap to achieve symmetry. After head and neck resection, free flaps allow for simultaneous composite reconstruction of skin, mucosa, and bone with good to excellent functional outcomes. Complicated wounds involving fistulae and osteoradionecrosis mandate the use of free tissue transfer. The cervical esophagus can also be replaced immediately after resection, leading to early swallowing and minimal weight loss. Large extremity wounds, which involve blood vessels, nerves, and bone, can also be restored with microsurgical techniques, allowing good to excellent functional outcomes. As a result, limb salvage is now the standard in all but a few situations. The use of free tissue transfer has expanded the horizons of ablative surgery. Currently, tumors can be resected without compromising margins for fear of creating a wound "too large" to close.

Free tissue transfer should not remain at the apex of the reconstructive ladder or be used only when local or regional tissue is unavailable. It should be considered whenever the wound is complex and requires multiple composite tissues or when variation in geometric design is necessary. Free tissue transfer is indicated whenever reliable wound healing is mandated in the presence of risk factors for healing.

CONTRAINDICATIONS

Microsurgical reconstruction of a given defect may be contraindicated for reasons related to the surgeon or the patient. The surgeon and the support staff providing operative and postoperative care should be experienced with free tissue transfer. Rather than undertake a case under difficult circumstances, it may be prudent to postpone the reconstruction until these problems can be addressed.

Neither extreme youth nor age are contraindications to microvascular surgery; however, medical optimization may be required in chronically ill patients. Well-controlled coronary artery disease and diabetes do not adversely effect patency. However, delayed wound healing may be expected. Atherosclerosis is more prevalent in these patients, and preoperative angiography may be indicated. Buerger's disease, Raynaud's syndrome, scleroderma, and other collagen vascular diseases increase the risk of potential thrombosis and flap failure. Venous ulcers or superficial varicosities should alert the surgeon to potential outflow difficulties, which could compromise flap survival.

Nicotine, from cigarettes, patches, or gum, is a potent vasoconstrictor and leads to an increased rate of flap failure. However, free flap failure in chronic smokers who have stopped smoking preoperatively is not increased when compared with nonsmokers. Delayed wound healing at both the donor and recipient sites should, however, be expected. Random skin paddle extensions are less reliable in smokers, and this should be considered in any type of flap reconstruction.

Free tissue transfer is challenging in patients with sickle cell anemia. To optimize patency, we recommend (1) preoperative and postoperative exchange transfusions, (2) liberal use of anticoagulants, and (3) maintenance of adequate blood volume and oxygenation. Preoperative consultation with a hematologist can be valuable.

Elective free flaps are contraindicated in pregnancy. Pregnancy results in an increased red blood cell mass, decreased plasma volume, increased clotting factor activity, and lower limb venous stasis, resulting from mass effect exerted by the uterus. All of these factors combine to make the risk of flap loss unacceptably high.

Corticosteroids, cyclosporine, and cancer chemotherapy do not effect anastomotic patency; however, wound healing will be delayed. Free tissue transfer should be postponed until the absolute neutrophil count is above 1, usually 3–4 weeks after chemotherapy administration. Postoperative chemotherapy may begin about 2 weeks after free tissue transfer, provided wound healing is proceeding.

Irradiation causes progressive subendothelial proliferation, reduced compliance, and atherosclerotic changes in blood vessels. Although most authors report no increase in flap loss when irradiated recipient vessels are used, rigid technique must be employed. Hydration of the head and neck patient in the postoperative period is required. Collapse of the internal jugular vein due to fluid loss creates a thrombogenic potential that is less tolerated in the irradiated patient. A good rule of thumb is to delay surgery following radiotherapy 1 week for every week of irradiation treatment. Postoperative radiotherapy may begin approximately 2 weeks after free tissue transfer, provided wound healing is progressing. Flap edema and acute radiation changes are well tolerated by free flaps, but the long-term late effects of irradiation are currently unknown.

As a result of advances in anesthesia and perioperative care, free tissue transfer is now routine in seriously ill patients; however, selection remains important. In the elective setting, patients who are able to withstand major resections will generally tolerate microsurgical reconstruction. Emergency free tissue transfer should be used with caution until the patient is adequately resuscitated. Although some advocate "minimal" operations for elderly, chronically ill, or severely injured patients, well-executed microvascular tissue transfer may actually reduce postoperative complications and accelerate recovery of these patients. Consequently, we are not of the philosophy that a lesser form of reconstruction is always better. The correct solution for a given situation requires the compatible marriage of donor tissue to the defect while minimizing both complications and the number of operations.

CHOOSING A FLAP

Detailed planning of the reconstruction must take place before surgery. There are many different factors that go into deciding what tissue type is best for achieving the surgeon's reconstructive goals. First, the surgeon must determine what components of the tissue are missing from the defect. Is only skin and subcutaneous fat missing, or is muscle and bone missing as well? Next, the surgeon must determine the necessary thickness of the flap, the required dimensions, and volume. A decision of what tissue will be used to reconstruct the defect can only be made once these questions have been answered. A discussion of what anatomical flaps are used to correct specific defects is beyond the scope of this text.

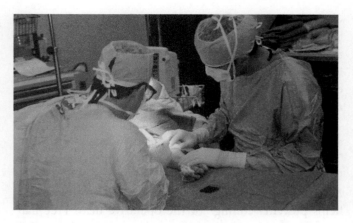

Figure 6.1. Operating table with surgeon and assistant seated.

ROOM SETUP

It is imperative that the patient be kept warm during microvascular surgery. Forced-air warming systems (e.g., Bair Hugger) are ideal and maintain the patient's temperature, while the ambient temperature in the operating room can be adjusted. Exposed surface area causes rapid cooling, which may lead to vasospasm, a reduction in peripheral capillary function, and flap failure. If possible, the patient should be positioned to allow for simultaneous harvest of the flap and preparation of the defect. Foam and gel pads are used liberally for skin protection. An uninvolved arm or leg should always be available for potential vein or skin grafts.

Optical magnification allows the surgeon to more clearly see structures that are not visible to the naked eye. As magnification increases, the depth of focus and the field size concurrently decrease, and more light is required for clear visualization. Both floor- and ceiling-mounted microscopes are available, and either is suitable for most cases. Upper extremity and hand surgery is traditionally performed with the surgeon seated and the limb positioned on a table. The table should allow for the operator's wrists and elbows to rest on a solid surface while the back and neck are straight (Figure 6.1). Microsurgery on the foot can usually be carried out while seated; however, breast, head, neck, and most other types of reconstruction are technically easier with the surgeon standing. In these situations, a seated surgeon has difficulty bracing his or her wrists and elbows on the table (Figure 6.2). The microscope in either situation should be positioned to allow the assistant easy access to the patient.

The microscope consists of a light source, a head that contains the objective lens, and the eyepieces. Most commonly, eyepieces with a magnification of 10× are used. A positive and negative diopter scale is provided on the eyepieces for individual adjustment up to 3.0 diopters. Eyeglasses should be worn while working under the microscope if correction of more than 2 or 3 diopters is required.

The eyepieces frequently become maladjusted when the microscope is moved or cleaned. If difficulty in focusing the microscope is encountered, check to see that both eyepieces are properly seated on the head of the microscope.

The objective lens determines the focal length of the microscope. Standard focal lengths range from 150 to 400 mm. A 200 mm lens is suitable in most instances.

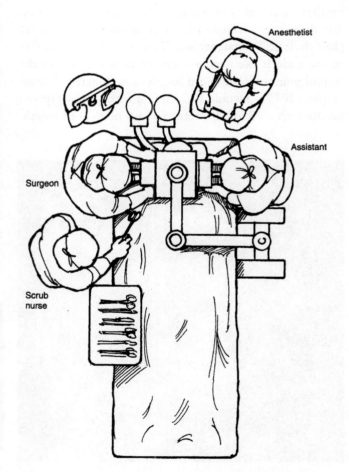

Figure 6.2. Surgeon and assistant standing on either side of operative microscope while performing head and neck reconstruction.

Controls to adjust focus and magnification and to position the objective lens in the X and Y axes are located on the floor or on a sterile hand apparatus. Initially, the focus is adjusted with the microscope set at high power. This ensures that the field will remain in focus with all levels of magnification.

Loupes generally provide magnification of 2.5× to 8× and are useful for structures that are 2–3 mm in diameter. The focal length is fixed (most often 19 inches), and focus is maintained by the surgeon adjusting his or her head. Most loupes are available with wide-field optics, which helps prevent "coning" of the operative field. Free flap operations and most nerve reconstruction can be carried out effectively under loupe magnification. However, this technique requires considerable experience, and, when available, the microscope usually provides better optics and lighting and can be a better tool for teaching (Figure 6.3).

Microsurgical sutures range from 8-0 (45-µm diameter) to 11-0 (14-µm diameter). Needle diameters range from 30 to 150 µm. The body of the needle is flat to improve stability while held in the needle holder. Ethicon needles are coded as to shape, diameter, and chord length. The shape codes include BV (three-quarters circle), BVH (half circle), ST (straight), and V (taper). The first number in the code is the needle diameter in microns, and the second number is the chord length in millimeters. For example, a BV 75-3 would be a three-quarters circle tapered needle with a 75 µm diameter and a 3 mm chord length.

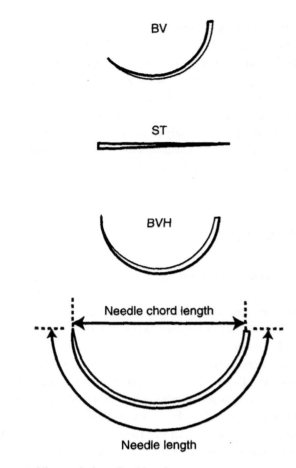

Figure 6.4. Microsurgical needle with codes.

The Sharpoint suture is labeled with the needle diameter, and its arc is described in degrees (Figure 6.4).

Papaverine solution (60 mg/30 mL of injectable normal saline) is commonly used for its local vasodilator effect. For general irrigating and to assist with intraluminal clot removal, we use heparin solution (I prefer 10,000 units in a liter of saline; however, other physicians may only use 1,000 units). The heparin is filled in 10 cc syringes with an ophthalmology needle for easy intraluminal irrigation (Figure 6.5).

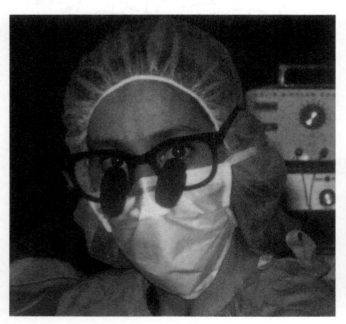

Figure 6.3. Surgeon with operative loupes.

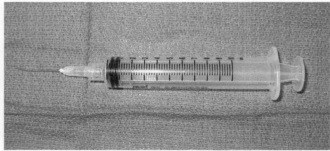

Figure 6.5. The heparin is filled in 10 cc syringes with an ophthalmology needle for easy intraluminal irrigation.

Incisions should be planned and marked both for flap harvest and over the recipient vessels. For head and neck reconstruction, we prefer to use the external carotid artery and internal jugular vein or their branches as recipient vessels. If these are not readily visible, an incision is usually planned along the anterior border of the sternocleidomastoid muscle. The donor vessels can be routed to the defect through a tunnel, or, if a skin bridge exists between the neck incision and the defect, this can be opened. Stumps of the sacrificed branches from the external carotid artery or the facial artery can also be used.

For immediate breast reconstruction, the thoracodorsal vessels are usually visible in the axilla. An end-to-end anastomosis can be performed just proximal to the serratus branch, allowing further use of the latissimus dorsi for salvage procedures. For delayed breast reconstruction, the thoracodorsal vessels can be explored using the axillary portion of the mastectomy incision. An alternative approach is to use the internal mammary vessels, which can be found by making a transverse incision in the second or third interspace, just lateral to the sternum, and the cartilage of the rib is removed for easier access. Unlike the thoracodorsal vessels, the internal mammary vessels are generally free of scarring in the delayed procedure and following irradiation. These vessels, however, especially the vein, can be small and friable, especially on the right.

For upper limb reconstruction, the more common recipient vessels are the radial or ulnar artery or its corresponding branches. These should be exposed through longitudinal incisions directly over the appropriate vessels. In the lower extremity, the popliteal vessels are approached through a Z incision at the popliteal fossa that extends just medial to the midline of the calf. An incision between the tibialis anterior and the extensor digitorum longus allows exposure of the anterior tibial artery, and, for distal leg or foot defects, the posterior tibial artery can be exposed at the medial malleolus. Recipient vessels can be selected either proximal or distal to the zone of injury. Vessels in the field of irradiation and trauma should be avoided when possible, with consideration of the use of vein grafts from distant nonirradiated vessels.

OPERATIVE TECHNIQUES

ARTERIAL ANASTOMOSIS

Preparation begins with trimming the donor artery with sharp scissors. If the vessel is damaged or plaque is present

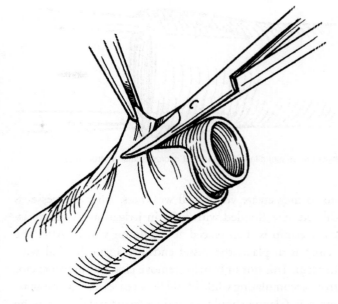

Figure 6.6. Trimming of microvascular vessels in preparation for anastomosis.

at the end of the vessel, it should be trimmed back to an area that is healthy. The adventitia and periadventitial tissues should be excised sharply while the vessel is held steady by an assistant (Figure 6.6). This prevents strands of adventitia from becoming interposed between the donor and recipient vessels, which is highly thrombogenic. All side branches should be sealed with bipolar cautery or vessel hemoclips. Intraluminal clots are removed by irrigation with heparinized saline solution (Figure 6.7). The artery is dilated by inserting either blunt microneedle holders or vessel dilators parallel to the long axis of the vessel (Figure 6.8). Care is required to avoid repeatedly dilating the vessel at exactly the same point. Instead, the dilator or needle driver should be rotated a few degrees. Failure to

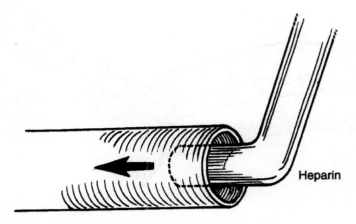

Figure 6.7. Vessel irrigated with Heparin and ophthalmology needle.

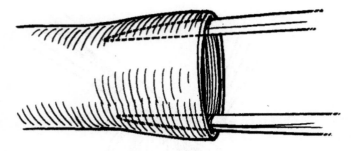

Figure 6.8. Vessel dilation with use of microvascular instruments.

do so may create vessel wall weakness. After the vessel is dilated, it is flooded with heparin irrigation. A microvascular clamp is then placed at the donor vessels. After the clamp is in place, the vessel ends are again flooded with heparin. This not only helps remove clot, but prevents clot from accumulating while blood flow ceases during the anastomosis. Clamps should not induce structural defects in the vessel (clamp pressure must be less than 30 mm Hg).

The recipient vessels are prepared in a similar fashion. If recipient vessels have been subjected to previous irradiation, preparation requires extreme care. Radiated vessels are fragile, atherosclerotic, and fibrotic. It can be difficult to recognize the junction between the adventitia and media. If the media is damaged during preparation, the vessel will be weakened and prone to leakage and thrombosis. The intima of irradiated vessels may fracture during preparation, allowing sections to separate and lift away from the underlying media, which is highly thrombogenic (Figure 6.9).

When possible, end-to-side arterial anastomoses are preferred. The principal advantage of this technique is that distal blood flow is preserved. If an end-to-side anastomosis is planned, the arteriotomy in the recipient vessel can be made with either microscissor or an aortic punch. We prefer to make a small incision in the artery with the Beaver blade

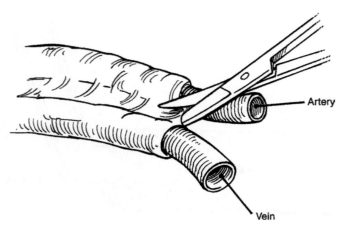

Figure 6.9. Preparation of recipient vessels by dissection of adventitia.

and then insert a 2.4–2.7 mm aortic punch to complete the arteriotomy (Figure 6.10). This creates a consistent round defect. If larger or smaller arteriotomies are required, or if the geometry must be tailored, microscissors may be more appropriate or the use of alternative size aortic punches. Size discrepancies between donor and recipient vessels are of little importance with the end-to-side technique. Blood flow is stopped within the recipient vessels with the use of vessel loops. A clamp on the donor vessel may or may not be necessary in this instance (Figure 6.11). In contrast, an end-to-end anastomosis is intolerant to size discrepancies. Size discrepancies up to 1.5:1 can be equalized by selectively dilating only the smaller vessel, whereas size discrepancies up to 3:1 can be overcome by spatulation, which involves a longitudinal cut on the smaller vessel, effectively increasing the circumference. Greater discrepancies require interposition vein grafting or excision of a longitudinal wedge of the arterial wall to cone down the larger vessel (Figure 6.12). Patency rates for end-to-side and end-to-end anastomoses are equivalent. End-to-side anastomoses are performed by placing the suture at both the head and toe of the vessels. The sutures may be run and tied at the opposite end. Alternatively, the suture may be interrupted. Care must be taken to ensure that the continuous sutures are tight.

An end-to-end anastomosis is easiest to perform with the vessel ends in a double-bar approximating clamp. Running or interrupted suture techniques can be used and result in equivalent patency rates (Figure 6.13). If running sutures are used, two 9-0 or 10-0 nylon sutures are initially placed 180 degrees apart at the opposite ends of the anastomosis. The posterior wall is usually more difficult to suture and is completed first. Once completed, the clamp is rotated, allowing the anterior wall to come into view, which is then sutured. Any gaps between the arteries will lead to suture line bleeding and thrombosis. Care is required to avoid narrowing the anastomosis with this technique, and spatulating the vessels may be required. Alternatively, an interrupted technique may be used. Gaps between the sutures are closed as needed. The last two sutures are not tied until both are in place, which allows for a final inspection of the back wall intima before anastomosis closure. The interrupted technique may be more prudent for small and irradiated vessels.

Regardless of which technique is used, each suture must enter the vessel perpendicular to its axis and include all three wall layers. Poor technique raises intimal flaps, weakening and potentiating the development of pseudoaneurysms. The needles should be placed equidistant from each other and from the vessel end. Too few sutures leads to bleeding and thrombus formation, whereas too many may result in

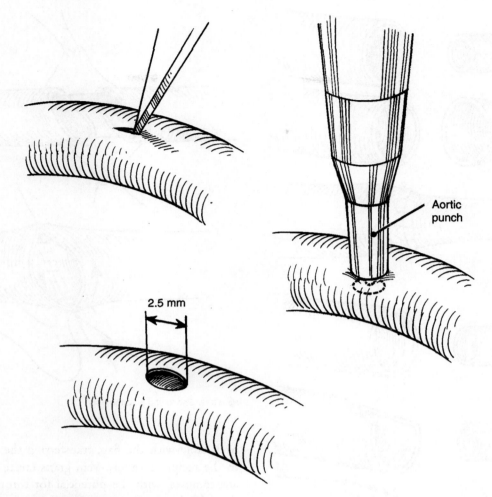

Figure 6.10. End-to-side arteriotomy with 2.4–2.7-mm aortic punch.

2.5 mm

Aortic
punch

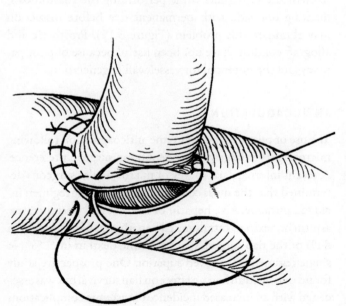

Figure 6.11. End-to-side anastomosis.

increased damage to the endothelium. The optimal number of sutures needed for the anastomosis in the clinical setting is enough to "get the job done" without bleeding from the vessel.

VENOUS ANASTOMOSIS

Despite its reputation for difficulty, the venous anastomosis is often more forgiving than the arterial side. Usually, multiple large veins are present and an end-to-end anastomosis can be done without regard for reducing distal venous drainage. Technical approaches to the venous anastomosis are essentially the same as for the artery.

COUPLING

For 1.5–2.0 mm vessels, patency rates are equivalent for hand-sewn and stapled anastomoses. The vessel ends must be everted onto the device, which shortens available length.

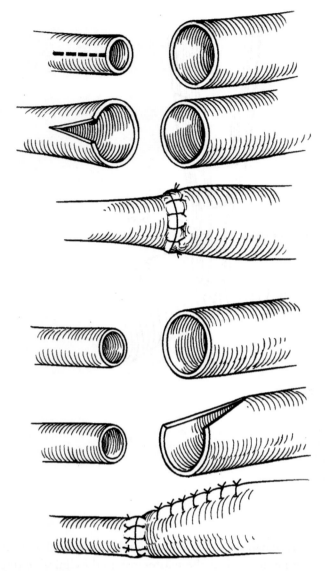

Figure 6.12. Addressing vessel size discrepancies with use of spatulation or longitudinal wedge resection.

Flexibility is minimized to correct size discrepancies, and the stapling device occasionally is too bulky to fit in tight spaces. We have found that the coupler fits nicely in the axilla and chest wall during breast reconstruction and that its use may be more applicable for veins as it tends to stent the anastomosis open. The stapler has not generally been employed for arteries and is not appropriate for irradiated vessels (Figure 6.14).

VEIN GRAFTS

When pedicle length is inadequate, vein grafts are needed. Loops can be created between the arterial and venous systems and are allowed to perfuse and mature before anastomosing the donor vessels to the cut ends of the vein. Alternatively, the vein grafts may be anastomosed on the

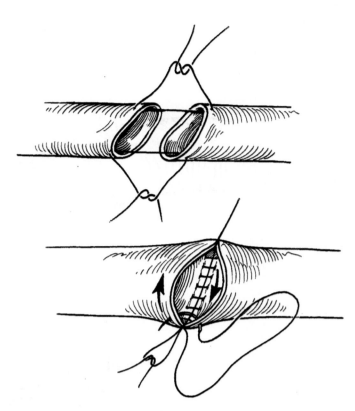

Figure 6.13. End-to-end anastomosis.

back table with the flap, transferring the entire complex to the recipient vessels. Vein grafts create two additional anastomoses, with the potential for thrombosis. Despite this added complexity, patency does not appear to be altered with the use of vein grafts. Care must be taken not to twist the vein grafts while performing the anastomosis; marking one side with permanent dye before dissection may eliminate this problem (Figure 6.15). Prosthetic and allograft conduits have not been useful because of poor patency and the potential for vessel wall degeneration.

ANTICOAGULATION

The use of postoperative systemic anticoagulation following microsurgery is largely dependent upon surgeon preference. A recent international survey of microvascular surgeons determined that the most common anticoagulant regimen included intraoperative heparin or dextran and postoperative aspirin or dextran. Intraluminal heparin was administered in 84% of the flap surgeries and systemic dextran in 60%. No single regimen was proved superior. One prospective study found that dextran had no effect on flap survival but was associated with an increased incidence of systemic complications when compared with aspirin. Animal studies have shown that the use of topical heparin improves patency of the

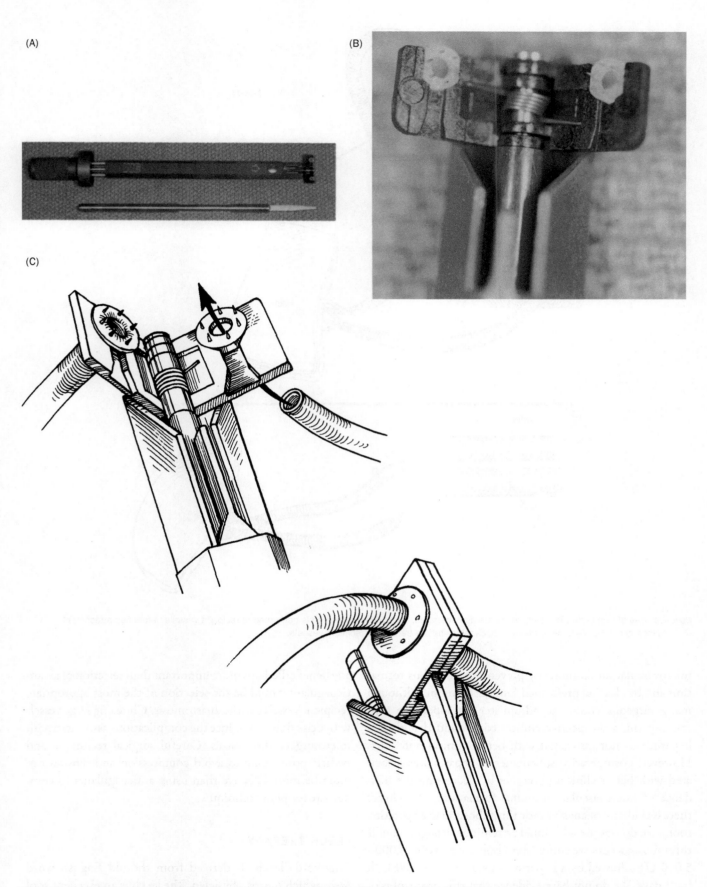

Figure 6.14. (A–C). 3M coupling device used for end-to-end anastomosis. Vessel is everted and device closed, securing anastomosis.

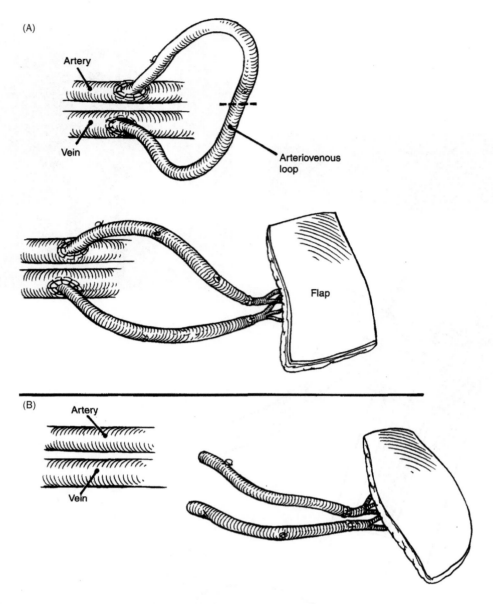

Figure 6.15. Use of vein grafts. Two techniques are demonstrated. (A) Arteriovenous loop is performed to recipient vessels before flap attachment. (B) Vein loop anastomosis is performed on "back table" before transfer to recipient vessels.

microvascular anastomosis by preventing thrombus formation and by clearing preformed luminal thrombi. Although many surgeons choose to administer intraoperative topical heparin, a prospective clinical trial found that topical heparin was not associated with better clinical outcomes. However, postoperative subcutaneous heparin was associated with better clinical outcomes by decreasing the incidence of microvascular thrombus formation.[10,18,20] Unless there is evidence of anastomotic thrombosis in the operating room, we do not use additional systemic anticoagulation. If thrombosis occurs, we administer a bolus of heparin (3,000–5,000 U) followed by a heparin infusion at 100–300 U/h for 5 days. We do not have evidence that this protocol is of

any benefit. Perhaps more important than selection of an anticoagulant would be the selection of the most appropriate recipient vessels for the anastomosis. Choosing large vessels with brisk flow can reduce the complications associated with microsurgery thrombosis. Careful surgical technique and pedicle positioning to avoid compression and tension can often be more effective than using anticoagulants to compensate for poor technique.

LEECH THERAPY

The word "leech" is derived from the old English word *laece*, which means physician. The leech is an excellent tool for venous congestion and is indicated for flaps with adequate inflow but limited drainage despite a *patent* venous anastomosis. The leech can consume up to 6 mL of blood at one meal and decompress the congested flap until capillary ingrowth occurs and venous drainage improves. The bacteria *Aeromonas (Pseudomonas) hydrophila* is present in the leech's digestive system; thus, patients should be treated with prophylactic antibiotics (an aminoglycoside or a second- or third-generation cephalosporin). After satiety, the leech usually falls off; if not, a solution of 70% alcohol can be applied. Leeches should not be avulsed from the patient because their teeth may remain in the wound. Leech application *should not replace re-exploration* of the venous anastomosis if patency is in question.

DRESSINGS

We prefer to minimize dressings after free tissue transfer so that the entire flap is easily visible for inspection. Frequent clinical inspection should be encouraged and made as easy as possible for the nursing staff. There is no particular advantage to large, bulky dressings, which may obscure portions of the flap and, as a result, delay detection of wound complications or prevent detection of a change in the flap's color, which may be indicative of an anastomotic problem.

After breast reconstruction with large transverse rectus abdominis myocutaneous (TRAM) flaps, surgical or sports bras can be worn beginning at discharge from the hospital. This allows easier ambulation and prevents the weight of the reconstructed breast from stressing the incisions or possibly stretching the vascular pedicle. We typically do not apply dressings to flaps used for head and neck reconstruction. For flaps on the extremity, splints are employed for 5–7 days, followed by progressive, supervised range-of-motion exercises. The extremity should be elevated in the postoperative period to help with the management of edema. Splints should be designed to allow easy inspection of the flap while avoiding flap compression.

POSTOPERATIVE CARE

Vascular thrombosis leading to flap loss is rare, occurring in 1–3% of cases. Complications related to flap thrombosis usually occur within the first 24–48 hours, although flap loss can occur several days or weeks after surgery. Early failure is often related to anastomotic imperfections (e.g., leaks, intimal flaps), hematoma near the pedicle, or problems with the pedicle position (e.g., twists, kinks, compression). A plethora of monitoring techniques has been developed to predict initial flap ischemia and detect flap failure. These techniques are helpful but do not replace clinical observation, which is the gold standard for postoperative flap evaluation. If occlusion of arterial inflow or venous outflow occurs, a free flap can still be salvaged by exploration and revision of the microanastomoses. The success rate of flap salvage surgery approaches 80% but is inversely related to the time interval between the onset of flap ischemia and its clinical recognition. If circulation cannot be reestablished within 8–12 hours, salvage of a free flap is usually impossible. Therefore, if flap viability is at all questionable, prompt operative exploration is in order. It is preferable to explore a patent anastomosis than to wait for total flap loss that will require alternative reconstruction.

At the University of California Irvine, we usually monitor free flaps by clinical inspection and a handheld Doppler probe. After completion of the anastomosis, a cutaneous perforator is identified with the Doppler probe and marked with a fine suture. Alternatively, these can frequently be Dopplered and marked prior to surgery, especially on the abdomen. Once the patient arrives in the recovery room, the surgeon and the nurses listen to the Doppler signal together, so there is no confusion as to signal interpretation or location. The flap is monitored every hour for the first days by the nursing staff. The character of the Doppler pulse, color, duration of capillary refill, and subjective temperature of the flap are recorded. If there is any change in the character of the pulse or color or temperature of the flap, or if the capillary refill becomes rapid (<1.5–2.0 seconds) or slow (<3–4 seconds), the surgeon is notified. Rapid capillary refill and flap congestion are especially important because these are the most sensitive predictors of venous thrombosis. A strong arterial pulse will persist for hours after venous occlusion.

If an adequate Doppler signal cannot be detected from the skin paddle in the operating room despite adequate perfusion, if the flap is covered by a skin graft, or if the flap is completely buried and inspection is impossible, an alternative is the use of the implantable Doppler device (Cook-Swartz). A small transducer mounted in a Gore-Tex cuff is sutured around the draining vein just proximal to the anastomosis. The Doppler pulse character is monitored continuously, and the transducer can be connected to a computer to calculate total flow within the flap. Occasionally, spurious signals are heard from adjacent vessels, but the range of the transducer can be adjusted to correct for this. The cutaneous wires connecting the Gore-Tex cuff to the Doppler machine can be removed by gentle traction after 2–3 weeks.

ALTERNATIVE TECHNIQUES IN FLAP MONITORING

As discussed earlier, clinical observation is the gold standard for postoperative flap monitoring. In addition to clinical observation, free flaps are usually monitored by handheld Doppler unless characteristics of the flap require an implantable Doppler to be used. While the majority of flaps are monitored by these methods, other techniques are utilized to evaluate flaps postoperatively.[10,19,20]

Near-Infrared Spectroscopy

Near-infrared spectroscopy (NIRS) is a noninvasive technique that utilizes optical spectrometry to evaluate flap oxygenation and perfusion. A probe is attached to the skin which delivers calibrated wavelengths of near-infrared light that is absorbed by chromophores in hemoglobin. By measuring the amount of light absorbed, this technique is able to quantify both oxygenated and deoxygenated hemoglobin concentrations within the flap. This technique allows surgeons to monitor a greater depth of tissue than other methods and allows for flap failure to be detected before clinical signs arise. One of the potential downsides to using NIRS is the burden of additional cost. However, a study conducted by Pelletier et al. concluded that the use of NIRS plus standard hospital nursing care showed a mean cost reduction of $1,937 per patient when compared to patients who were monitored in an intensive care unit (ICU) setting. This number does not account for the additional revenue that would be generated by opening an ICU bed for a different patient.[13,19]

Color Duplex Sonography

Color duplex sonography records both blood flow velocity and direction to asses anastomotic patency and flap viability. Its main strengths are its ability to quantitatively measure inflow and outflow of buried flaps that could not otherwise be monitored by conventional techniques.[19]

Laser Doppler Flowmetry

Laser Doppler flowmetry is a continuous means of measuring tissue perfusion. It utilizes backscattered laser light to determine blood flow and velocity. When analyzing results of laser Doppler flowmetry it is more important to asses trends rather than absolute values because this can help differentiate between venous and arterial occlusion. Often it is used in conjunction with tissue spectrometry to help make this distinction.[19]

Microdialysis

Microdialysis is a sensitive monitoring technique that can be utilized when flaps are difficult to monitor by clinical observation due to depth or location. It evaluates flap metabolism by measuring glucose, lactate, pyruvate, and glycerol concentrations in the interstitial fluid surrounding the flap. Falling glucose levels combined with an increased lactate to pyruvate ratio indicates anaerobic metabolism and arterial insufficiency, whereas rising glycerol levels indicate cell membrane damage that results from both venous and arterial insufficiency.[19]

MICROSURGERY TRAINING TECHNIQUES

A wide variety of training techniques have been used to teach surgeons the skills needed to preform the complex anastomoses used in free flap reconstructive surgery. Classically, ex vivo prosthetic models have been used to teach microsurgery suturing techniques. Materials include latex gloves as well as silicon sheets and tubing. Many training programs also utilize nonliving animal models such as chicken or turkey legs. While these methods allow for the individual to practice microvascular anastomosis, they do not improve anatomical knowledge. In vivo training models offer a more realistic training environment by simulating normal clotting processes that often complicate free flap reconstruction. While this is advantageous to the learner, cost, tight regulation on animal experimentation, and constant scrutiny of the ethical use of laboratory animals limits the use of in vivo animal models.

A new method of training that is currently being evaluated uses human cadaver models. While certain conditions cannot be mimicked with this model, this pedagogic method allows trainees to practice flap harvesting thereby improving their knowledge of the anatomic basis of the flap. In addition, training surgeons are able to prepare recipient vessels.[20]

CAVEATS

There is little to be lost in exploring a well-perfused flap, but much can be lost if a failing flap remains unexplored. Therefore, the threshold for returning to the operating room to evaluate the microvascular anastomosis should be low. If there is any concern at all that either anastomosis is not functioning, operative exploration is indicated.

The best flap monitoring technique is clinical observation. Any flap that appears congested or cool or to have altered capillary refill on clinical inspection should be evaluated in the operating room. Exploration should be carried out even in the face of strong or unchanged Doppler signals.

It is easiest to be a successful microsurgeon if one avoids true *micro*surgery. Flaps should be designed to take advantage of the largest recipient and donor vessels available. The importance of this principle cannot be overemphasized.

SELECTED READINGS

1. Belker AM. Principles of microsurgery. *Urol Clin North Am* 1994; 21:487–504.
2. Bengtson BP, Schusterman MA, Baldwin BJ, et al. Influence of prior radiotherapy on the development of postoperative complications and success of free tissue transfers in head and neck cancer reconstruction. *Am J Surg* Oct 1993;166:326–330.
3. Colen LB, Gonzales FP, Buncke JH. The relationship between the number of sutures and the strength of microvascular anastomoses. *Plast Reconstr Surg* 1979;64:325.
4. Khouri R. *Practice Patterns and Outcome Data in a Prospective Survey of 495 Microvascular Free Flaps.* Abstract, January 12, 1996; Tucson, AZ: American Society of Reconstructive Microsurgery. Abstract.
5. Krizek TJ, Tani T, Desprez JD, Kiehn CL. Experimental transplantation of composite grafts by microsurgical vascular anastomoses. *Plast Reconstr Surg* 1965;36:538–546.
6. Kroll SS, ed. *Reconstructive Plastic Surgery for Cancer.* St Louis: Mosby CV, 1996.
7. Mackinnon SE, Dellon AL. *Surgery of the Peripheral Nerve.* New York: Thieme, 1988.
8. Manktelow RT. Functioning microsurgical muscle transfer. *Hand Clin* 1988;4:289.
9. Miller MJ, Schusterman MA, Reece GP, Kroll SS. Interposition vein grafting in head and neck reconstructive surgery. *J Reconstr Microsurg* 1993;9:245–252.
10. Motakef S, Mountziaris P, Ismail I, et al. Emerging paradigms in perioperative management for microsurgical free tissue transfer: review of the literature and evidence-based guidelines. *Plast Reconstr Surg* 2015;131:290–299.
11. Nakayama K, Yamamoto K, Tamiya T, et al. Experience with free autografts of the bowel with a new venous anastomosis apparatus. *Surgery* 1964;55:796–802.
12. Neligan PC. Monitoring techniques for the detection of flow failure in the postoperative period. *Microsurgery* 1993;14:162–164.
13. Pelletier A, Tseng C, Agarwall S, Park J, Song D. Cost analysis of near-infrared spectroscopy tissue Oximetry for monitoring autologous free tissue breast reconstruction. *J Reconstr Microsurg* 2011;27:487–494.
14. Reus WF, Colen LB, Straker DJ. Tobacco smoking and complications in elective microsurgery. *Plast Reconstr Surg* 1992;89:490–493.
15. Schusterman MA, Horndeski G. Analysis of the morbidity associated with immediate microvascular reconstruction in head and neck cancer patients. *Head Neck* 1991;13:51–55.
16. Shaw WM, Ahn CY. Microvascular free flaps in breast reconstruction. *Clin Plast Surg* 1992;19:917–926.
17. Shestak K, Myer EN, Ramasastry SS, et al. Vascularized free-tissue transfer in head and neck surgery. *Am J Otolaryngol* 1993;14:148–154.
18. Siemionow M, Eisenmann-Klein M, eds. *Plastic and Reconstructive Surgery.* London/New York: Springer, 2010.
19. Smit JM, Zeebregts CJ, Acosta R, Werker P. Advancements in free flap monitoring in the last decade: a critical review. *Plast Reconstr Surg* 2010;125:177–185.
20. Thorne C, Chung K, Gosain A, et al., eds. *Grabb and Smith's Plastic Surgery.* Seventh ed. Philadelphia: Lippincott Williams & Wilkins, 2014.
21. Wells MD, Manktelow RT, Boyd JB, Bowen V. The medical leech: an old treatment revisited. *Microsurgery* 1993;14:183–186.
22. Yajima H, Tamai S, Mizumoto S, et al. Vascular complications of vascularized composite tissue transfer: outcome and salvage techniques. *Microsurgery* 1993;14:473–478.

PART II.

TISSUE HARVEST

7.

SKIN GRAFTING

Stephen M. Milner

Skin grafting is a process whereby skin is detached from its blood supply and incorporated into a host bed. It is a means of replacing skin loss, most commonly due to infection, burns, excised cutaneous lesions and scars, non-healing ulcers or following surgical loss (e.g., to cover open areas created when raising flaps). Skin grafts can be classified as split-thickness, consisting of varying quantities of dermis, or full-thickness, containing the entire dermis. The procedure demands maintenance of contact between the apposed raw surfaces of the graft and a vascular bed and relies on a dynamic and intricate array of coordinated physiological events.[1] Initially bound to the wound bed by fibrin, the graft is nourished by osmotic diffusion in a process termed *serum imbibition* for 24–48 hours.[2,3] There follows an *inosculatory phase*, in which a new circulation is established within the graft, so that by the fifth or sixth day the graft is pink and adherent to the defect, with further remodeling continuing in succeeding months.[4] Disruption of any of these steps will prevent graft survival ("take"). Successful grafting therefore depends on the condition of the recipient site, the general health of the patient, and the operative technique.

ASSESSMENT OF THE DEFECT AND DONOR SITE

Each defect is assessed according to its size, anatomical site, and aesthetic importance. Successful grafting necessitates a vascular recipient bed, which includes muscle, fascia, blood vessels, nerves, and granulation tissue.[5] The bed should also be as clean as possible. Necrotic tissue must be thoroughly debrided. Hypertrophic granulation tissue usually harbors bacteria and should be re-excised prior to surgery. Signs of infection, such as surrounding erythema, drainage, or discolored granulation tissue, warrant a biopsy for quantitative

bacteriology. Grafting is delayed should there be counts greater than 10^5 organisms per gram of tissue.[6]

Consideration is also given to the compatibility of color, texture, and hair density of the donor site with that of the defect. All split-thickness skin graft donor sites heal by re-epithelialization with scar and pigmentary changes. Thus, in general, the thighs and buttocks are preferential sites because they can be concealed by clothing. The scalp is also an excellent donor site when resurfacing large facial defects since grafts taken from above the clavicle provide a superior color match, and the donor scar is imperceptible following hair growth.[7]

INDICATIONS

The choice of graft depends on the size and location of the defect. Split-thickness skin grafts are most often used to close large wounds. They readily "take," and the donor sites heal by re-epithelialization from the skin appendages left in the dermis. This is especially important in large burns where donor sites may be limited and where, once healed, the procedure can be repeated. Since dermis never regenerates, the number of times a site can be harvested will depend on the thickness of the donor site and the depth at which the graft is harvested.

As soon as a skin graft is removed from its donor site it undergoes primary contraction, believed to be due to recoil of its elastic fibers. Although a split-thickness graft loses only about 10% of its original length, its secondary contraction, which occurs as the graft heals, is considerable. Thus thin skin grafts have a lack of durability and texture, and there is a tendency for contraction of the grafted wound. Sometimes the secondary contraction can be used to advantage, with the resulting smaller wound allowing excision of the defect as a secondary procedure.

Full-thickness grafts are best suited to resurface small defects such as on the face or hands, where it is important that texture, good color match, and mobility occur without distortion. Larger donor defects may be closed by a split-thickness skin graft. Full-thickness grafts contain all the epithelial appendages, and so the implication of transferring hair follicles to the recipient site should not be overlooked. Although a full-thickness graft immediately loses about 40% of its original length, secondary contraction is minimal.[8] Thus the size of full-thickness grafts remains stable, and they are ideal for use in sites where contraction would impair function, such as in the eyelids, web spaces, or neck.[9,10] Full-thickness grafts are also more durable and may be used where split-thickness grafts would be likely to break down. Compared to split-thickness grafts, they retain sweat and sebaceous gland function, thus requiring less lubrication; sensory return is greater because of a greater availability of neurilemmal sheaths; and they are less likely to become hyperpigmented.[11,12] Another advantage is that the donor site can be closed primarily, leaving only a linear scar, which may be inconspicuous.

PREOPERATIVE PREPARATION

The operation is usually performed under general anesthesia; however, long-acting local anesthetic infiltration (0.25% Marcaine, with epinephrine) or regional nerve blocks may be used in selected patients. Although calibrated hand-driven instruments such as a Humby or Goulian knives (Weck blades) may be used to harvest split-thickness skin grafts, power-driven dermatomes (e.g., Zimmer dermatome) are more commonly chosen in the United States, and the use of a power-driven dermatome will be described in this chapter (Figure 7.1). Convex surfaces of the body are best chosen, in particular the thighs, especially when large sheets of skin are required. For smaller defects, however, it is preferable to select a less noticeable area such as the buttocks since the donor site scar may be visible years later.

Before harvesting the graft, the donor area is shaved, and, if the thigh is selected, it should be prepped and draped circumferentially so that the limb is freely mobile. The dermatome and blade are assembled on the back table and an appropriate guard chosen for the correct width. The screws are tightened with fingertip pressure only, and the dermatome set for the depth of harvesting, which will usually be 0012–0014 inch. The length of the required graft is then marked on the donor site.

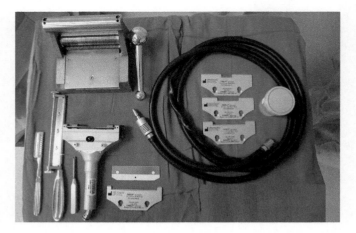

Figure 7.1. Instrument setup. Zimmer dermatome with blade, guards and screwdriver, power cord, Humby knife, Goulian knife, mineral oil, and Brennen skin graft mesher.

SURGICAL TECHNIQUE

SPLIT-THICKNESS GRAFTS

The assistant stretches the skin to produce as flat a surface as possible. It may also be necessary for the assistant to place a hand beneath the limb to press the thigh upward. The dermatome is switched on and abruptly contacts the skin at an angle of 30–45 degrees. It is guided forward, exerting a steady downward pressure against the assistant's countertraction (Figure 7.2). We prefer to allow the cut graft to accumulate in the pocket of the handpiece although some surgeons prefer to use tissue forceps to gently lift the graft as it emerges. When an adequate amount of skin has been cut, the leading edge is severed from the donor site by

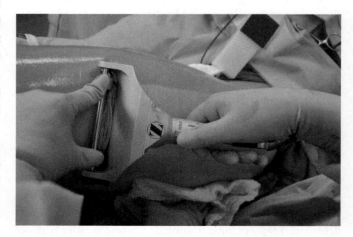

Figure 7.2. Harvesting split-thickness skin graft with a dermatome. The instrument is steadied with the index finger and thumb to give total control of the instrument. The graft accumulates in the pocket of the handpiece.

an upward movement with the dermatome still running. If the graft remains stuck to the blade it can be trimmed off with a scissor. The dermatome is released and the skin graft retrieved. Between successive harvests, the blade should be thoroughly cleaned, and our practice is to change the blade after every three passes.

Modifications of the technique include infiltration of saline over the ribs, spine, or iliac crest to facilitate harvesting over bony prominences.

The graft is then placed in a bowl of normal saline while Telfa soaked in 1:100,000 epinephrine solution is used to secure hemostasis of the donor site.

Thin split-thickness skin grafts can be easily expanded by meshing, a process whereby slits are cut into the graft to allow it to be stretched.[13] This allows egress of blood through the interstices and decreases the likelihood of hematoma formation. A disadvantage is a less than ideal "cobblestone" appearance making it unsuitable for use on the face and hands. We prefer the Brennen Skin Graft Mesher, which is available in a variety of ratios and does not require a carrier (Figure 7.3). It should be noted that the actual expansion of skin is less than that anticipated from the meshing ratio. Widely expanded meshed (4:1) autologous split-thickness skin grafts, used in large wounds, are best overlaid with unexpanded (2:1) meshed allograft split skin to prevent desiccation of the interstices. This "sandwich technique" promotes rapid epithelialization of the interstices of the autograft and shedding of the allograft before inducing acute rejection.[14]

There is currently no ideal way to dress the donor site. In most cases, we use Xeroform and bacitracin covered with burn dressings. We also advise placing a nonadherent

dressing (Telfa) over the Xeroform to facilitate removal of the outer dressing on the first postoperative day. For smaller areas bio-occlusive dressings, such as OpSite, have been favored since they are said to reduce pain; however, the weeping of large amounts of fluid from the wound during the first 24 hours can distress some patients.[15]

The skin graft is then applied to the defect in one or more strips. In cosmetically sensitive areas, we prefer to leave the graft a millimeter short of the edge to prevent a step deformity, which can be difficult to correct postoperatively. Sufficient graft should be used to avoid tenting over concave areas of the wound. The graft can be easily secured to these areas using staples or sutures (4.0/5.0 chromic catgut) (Figures 7.4 and 7.5).

In total resurfacing of the face it is important to place the sheet graft in the regional aesthetic units[16] (Figure 7.6).

All shearing forces must be limited. Hands are carefully splinted where grafts are placed across joints to achieve maximal stretch of the graft for 5 days. Vacuum-assisted closure has proved helpful for postoperative management.[17]

FULL-THICKNESS GRAFTS

Prior to creating the full-thickness defect, donor sites are chosen where direct closure can be achieved. Since full-thickness skin grafts grow hair, nonhirsute donor areas should be chosen. Ideal sites include postauricular and supraclavicular skin, which gives excellent color match for the eyelids and small nasal defects. The groin and lower abdomen provide a larger area, and this area is commonly used where color match is not so essential. It is sometimes more convenient to remove smaller pieces of skin from

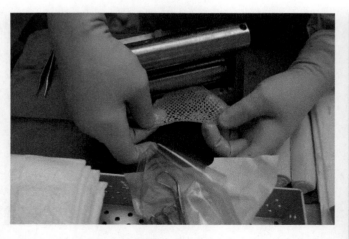

Figure 7.3. Skin grafts are expanded with the Brennen skin graft mesher. The skin is fed into the mesher dermis side up and meshed by turning the hand crank. It is important that the instrument is not hot after sterilization.

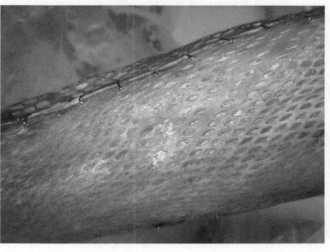

Figure 7.4. A 2:1 meshed skin graft placed on the bed of an excised burn and stapled into position.

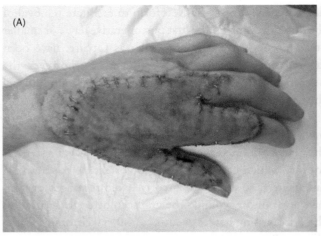
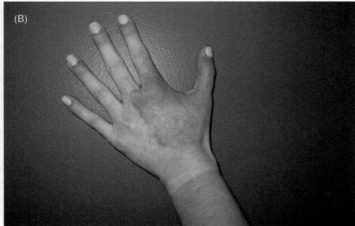

Figure 7.5. (A) Sheet graft placed on hand. (B) Appearance at 6 months.

an extremity where this falls within the operative site, for example, the medial aspect of the arm.

Because of the pronounced primary contracture associated with harvesting full-thickness grafts, an exact pattern is first drawn on a suitable template such as glove paper, and orientation marks are added. If necessary, the pattern can be extended into an ellipse for ease of closure. The template is then transferred to the donor site, and the graft is harvested using a scalpel (Figure 7.7).

The corner of the graft is picked up with forceps, and the graft is separated with a scalpel at the junction of the dermis and subcutaneous fat. Care is taken not to create any button-holes. Any fat remaining is later trimmed using curved scissors, with the graft supported by the convex surface of a finger while keeping the tissue moist. Once perfect hemostasis of the bed is achieved, the graft is meticulously inset with interrupted sutures of 3-0–5-0 silk. A Xeroform and cotton and mineral oil bolster dressing is held in place with the tie-over sutures to protect the graft from shearing forces that may disrupt neovascularization. The donor site is closed in a layered

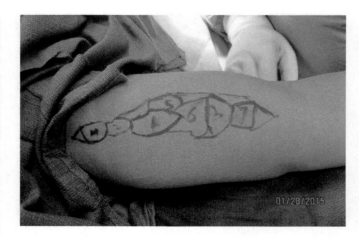

Figure 7.7. Pattern of grafts from several templates marked on medial aspect of arm used for resurfacing multiple defects on hands. The periphery is incised full-thickness, whereas the intermediate lines are scored and separated by sharp scissors once the graft is removed.

Figure 7.6. Total resurfacing of face with split-thickness skin grafts applied in the aesthetic units of the face and sutured with 5.0 chromic catgut.

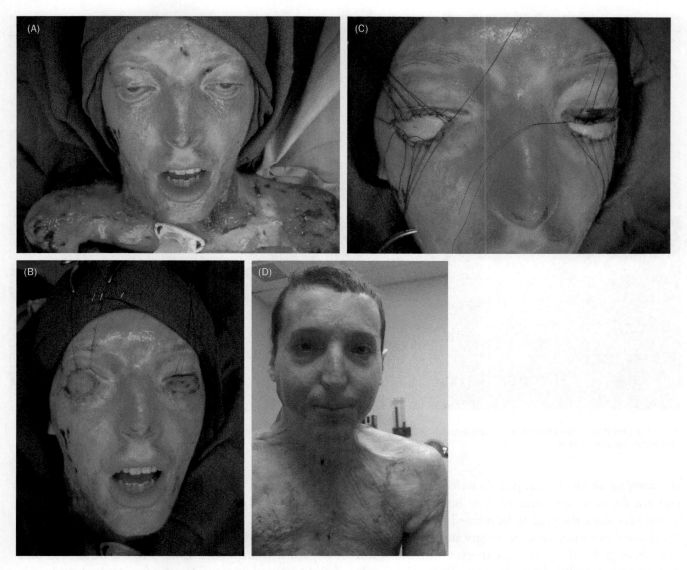

Figure 7.8. (A) Ectropion of lower eyelids. (B) Release of lower lid ectropions. (C) Full-thickness skin grafts. (D) One year after surgery.

fashion with buried dermal and subcuticular sutures (Figure 7.8).

HARVESTING OF SCALP DONOR SITE

The head is shaved on the morning of surgery. It is important that the frontal hairline is marked with a pen or by leaving a rim of frontal area to avoid accidentally harvesting from the forehead. The scalp is infiltrated with 1:500,000 solution of epinephrine in the subgaleal plane to facilitate taking as wide a graft as possible and to reduce bleeding. An appropriate Zimmer dermatome guard is held against the scalp to enable the width of each harvest to be determined and the order of the operation planned (Figure 7.9A, B). The thickness of the graft is set for patients older than 7 years between 0.0012 and 0.0016 inch. The Zimmer dermatome

is used with even pressure while an assistant supports the head. The handle of the handpiece is elevated as the instrument is moved over the scalp, keeping the blade of the dermatome at 45 degrees to the skin. Hemostasis is achieved by application of Telfa and epinephrine soaks. The graft is rinsed gently in normal saline to remove any hairs and is applied and secured to the donor site (Figure 7.9C, D). The donor scalp is dressed with Xeroform, which separates spontaneously over the next 2 weeks as the scalp regenerates and hair regrows.

POSTOPERATIVE CONSIDERATIONS

Views vary regarding the timing of dressing removal for split-thickness skin grafts. Our practice is to take down

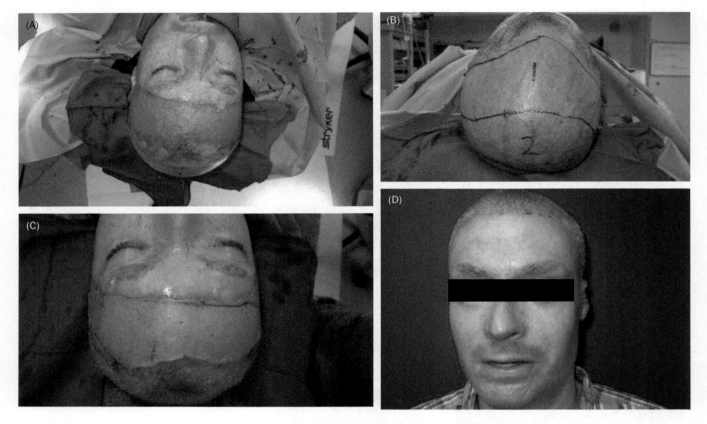

Figure 7.9. (A) Forehead wound bed following burn excision. (B) Skin harvest planned. (C) Split-thickness skin graft fixed to forehead with fibrin glue.[18] (D) Appearance at 6 months.

the dressing on the fourth postoperative day. If there is concern for hematoma formation or infection, early removal may allow the graft to be rescued. The donor sites are exposed to air the day after surgery and allowed to dry out. Sheet grafts of the face are dressed with Xeroform and protected with a burn dressing. They are initially inspected hourly. Any hematomas can be milked with a cotton swab through an incision over the fluid collection. Grafts on the lower extremities are supported by double elastic (Ace) wraps for a few weeks, and the patients can be mobilized early. The bolsters on full-thickness grafts are removed at 7 days.

CAVEATS

Successful skin grafting requires accurate approximation of a skin graft to an adequately vascularized recipient bed. Exposed bone, tendon, or cartilage will not support a graft. Hemostasis is paramount since any barrier between the graft and recipient sites will prevent revascularization. Immobilization is necessary to prevent shearing in the early postoperative period. The wound bed should be

bacteriologically clean and free of dead tissue to avoid destruction of the graft by infection. The donor site should be selected with care since every patient is left with a visible scar. Meshed skin grafts should be avoided in cosmetically sensitive areas, such as the face and hands. The ideal full-thickness donor site for the face is the hairless skin behind the ear and the supraclavicular area. These are best immobilized with a soft bolster and tie-over stent.

SELECTED READINGS

1. Billingham RE, Medawar PB. The Technique of Free Skin Grafting in Mammals. *J Exp Biol* 1951;28:385–402.
2. Hinshaw JT, Miller ER. Histology of healing split-thickness, full-thickness autogenous skin grafts and donor sites. *Arch Surg* 1965;91:658–670.
3. Rudolph R, Klein L. Healing processes in skin grafts. *Surg Gynecol Obstet* 1973;136:641–654.
4. Haller JA, Billingham RE. Studies of the origin of the vasculature in free skin grafts. *Ann Surg* 1967;166:896–901.
5. Gingrass P, Grabb WC, Gingrass RP. Skin graft survival on avascular defects. *Plast Reconstr Surg* 1975;55:65–70.
6. Robson MC, Heggers JP. Delayed wound closure based on bacterial counts. *J Surg Oncol* 1970;2:379–383.
7. Valencia JC, Falabella AF, Eaglstein. Skin grafting. *Dermatol Clin* 2000;18:521–532.

8. Kamran A, Mohammad FJ, Sahram F, Jaber MS. A comparison of survival and secondary contraction in expanded versus conventional full-thickness skin grafts: an experimental study in rats. *Eplasty* 2012;12:e20.

9. Milner SM, Fauerbach JA, Hahn A, et al. Cody. *Eplasty* 2015;15:e35.

10. Iwuagwu F, Wilson, D, Bailie F. The use of skin grafts in postburn contracture release: a 10-year review. *Plast Reconstr Surg* 1999;103: 1198–1204.

11. Waris T, Astrand K, Hämäläinen H, Piironen J, Valtimo J, Järvilehto T. Regeneration of cold, warmth and heat-pain sensibility in human skin grafts. Br *J Plast Surg* 1989;42:576–580.

12. Smahel J. The healing of skin grafts. *Clin Plast Surg* 1977;4:409–424

13. Knight SL, Moorghen M. Configurational changes within the dermis of meshed split skin grafts: a histological study. *Br J Plast Surg* 1987;40:420–422.

14. Alexander JW, Macmillan BG, Law E, et al. Treatment of severe burns with widely meshed skin autograft and meshed skin allograft overlay. *J Trauma* 1981;21:433–438.

15. Masella PC, Balent EM, Carlson TL, Lee KW, Pierce LM. Evaluation of six split-thickness skin graft donor-site dressing materials in a swine model. *Plast Reconstr Surg Glob Open* 2014 Jan 6;1:e84.

16. Gonzalex-Ulloa. Restoration of the face covering by means of selected skin in regional aesthetic units. *Br J Plast Surg* 1956;9:212–221.

17. Blackburn JH, Boemi L, Hall WW, Jeffors K et al. Negative-pressure dressings as a bolster for skin grafts. *Ann Plast Surg* 1998;40:453–457.

18. Currie LJ, Sharpe JR, Martin R. The use of fibrin glue in skin grafts and tissue-engineered skin replacements: a review. *Plast Reconstr Surg* 2001;108:1713–1726.

8.

CRANIAL BONE GRAFTING

Raj M. Vyas

INDICATIONS

Calvarial bone grafts are utilized to fill osseous defects and augment the craniofacial skeleton. Augmentations may be done for minimal hypoplasia, such as malar or mandibular gonial angle flatness, or moderate hypoplasia, such as perinasal maxillary retrusion secondary to cleft lip or palate. For most moderate to severe defects, however, distraction osteogenesis is the method of choice. For minor defects or in patients who decline distraction osteogenesis, calvarial bone grafting is an option for reconstruction.

Osseous defects requiring grafting may be congenital in origin, such as the alveolar clefting that occurs in cleft lip and palate (see the "Alveolar Bone Grafting" chapter 12 for more information) or the aplastic zygoma of Treacher Collins syndrome. They can also be acquired from head trauma or ablative surgery. The needs of the recipient site dominate decision-making regarding the calvarial graft. These needs include structural integrity, size, shape, and fixation of the graft.

ANATOMY

The mature calvaria is a trilamellar structure consisting of two cortical lamella, the inner and outer tables, and an interposed medullary cavity, the diploe. The macroanatomy allows for delamination of the two tables through the diploe, yielding up to double the surface area of the original amount of cortical bone harvested.

ASSESSMENT OF THE DEFECT

Autogenous calvarial grafting is a valuable technique for any surgeon working in craniofacial surgery. With proper consideration of recipient site needs and harvest technique, autogenous calvarial grafting is a useful procedure with benefits outweighing the inherent surgical risks. Several key components are taken into account when evaluating and deciding graft type to utilize.

STRUCTURAL INTEGRITY

The structural integrity of the calvarial graft required at the recipient site determines whether to utilize a full- or split-thickness graft. A full-thickness calvarial graft provides a relatively thin, solid, and rigid piece of bone. This can be useful for support of hypoplastic or contracted soft tissues, such as in nasal or malar reconstruction. Full-thickness calvarial grafts are, however, by nature curved. They can be difficult to shape due the brittle nature of the graft. If a more malleable and thinner graft is desired, the unique anatomy of the calvaria allows for split-thickness harvest. These grafts are useful for superficial contour augmentation such as in the forehead, orbital rim, or orbital wall reconstruction. The structural integrity of a split-thickness calvarial graft depends on the method of harvest. Split-thickness grafts harvested in situ often have microfractures that can facilitate bending, an asset for onlay grafts, but one that limits structural integrity and is a liability for cantilever grafts.

SIZE

To a certain degree, the size of the desired graft determines the means of graft harvest and choice of graft thickness. A full-thickness graft is harvested as a craniectomy, its size limited by concern for the endocranial attachments of the sagittal and transverse sinuses as well as the dura at calvarial sutures. Split-thickness grafts are restricted to the confines of discrete calvarial bones because calvaria does not split well across sutures. A split-thickness graft can be harvested in situ or as a full-thickness craniectomy that is split on the back table.

Small grafts, less than 4 by 4 cm, and narrow rectangular grafts, with a maximum width of about 4 cm, can often be harvested in situ. If a larger, split-thickness calvarial graft with structural integrity is desired, the authors prefer full-thickness harvest with back table splitting to minimize microfractures and perforations as well as to improve the safety of harvest. The outer table is then replaced with miniplate fixation.

SHAPE

The shape of the desired graft contributes to decision-making regarding the site of graft harvest, means of harvest, and the choice of graft thickness. If a full-thickness calvarial graft of a specific shape is desired, then the surface curvature of the site from which the graft is harvested becomes critical. A semirigid metallic template can transfer size and special shape information from the recipient to the donor sites. When split-thickness calvaria is harvested, post-harvest mechanical bone deformation becomes more feasible to produce a desired spatial configuration.

DEGREE OF FIXATION

The degree of fixation needed at the recipient site may affect the choice of calvarial graft. If the graft is to be an onlay without probability of displacement after short-term wound healing is completed, a wide range of fixation techniques will suffice. These can include a constraining soft tissue pocket, suture, wire, screw, or plate with screws. Such grafts can be thin split-thickness or even full-thickness calvaria. If the graft is in a motion area, such as on the dura or mandible, or if the graft must support a tight soft tissue envelope, such as a nasal dorsum cantilever, rigid fixation with screws alone or combined with plates is preferred. Grafts that are exposed to active forces tend to survive better if they are full-thickness calvaria as opposed to split-thickness grafts.

PROCEDURE

ROOM SETUP

For calvarial bone harvesting, no specific room setup is required. You will need to have the patient positioned supine or prone, depending on the site to be harvested, and on a Mayfield horseshoe headrest. The operating room is otherwise arranged for the planned reconstructive procedure, with a back table available for ex vivo splitting of the calvarial graft as needed.

MARKINGS

Calvarial graft harvest access depends on associated procedures. If the patient requires scalp elevation for cranioplasty or access to the facial skeleton, the primary scalp incision suffices for cranial bone harvest with additional scalp mobilization. If the primary procedure does not require a scalp incision, a linear T or H incision is made for direct exposure of the harvest site. The pattern and size of the incisions depend on the size of the calvarial graft harvest. Once the reconstructive defect size is determined, a template of the defect can be drawn and transferred or measurements taken and utilized for design of the donor site area to harvest.

SURGICAL TECHNIQUE

Harvest and Delamination

There are two available methods of calvarial harvest, full-thickness calvarectomy and in situ harvest. Full-thickness calvarial harvest, or craniectomy, has been practiced for more than a century by neurosurgeons to gain access to the intracranial contents. In the same manner, a full-thickness portion of calvarium can be raised and then delaminated. In situ harvest is also possible with removal of the outer table from the inner, without disruption of the inner table during harvest.

If the graft is harvested full-thickness (i.e., craniectomy), the method of demalination bears no patient morbidity. Narrow grafts up to 4 cm in width can be split with a chisel or osteotome. For larger grafts, the diploe can be split around the entire perimeter with a long sagittal saw followed by use of an osteotome to complete the central portion inaccessible to a saw blade. This method minimizes microfractures, fenestrations, and fragmentation. Calvarium can be split in infants as young as 3 months of age. In this pediatric population, we prefer to use a 15 blade and/or a fine linear pencil-like drill bit to separate the cortices.

If the graft is to be harvested in situ for split thickness, the outer table is disrupted around the perimeter of the graft and the diploid space entered to permit separation of the outer from the inner table. The perimeter to be harvested can be etched with a saw, sagittal or reciprocating, or a burr. The diploic space can then be entered with a saw, chisel, or osteotome parallel to the surface of the outer table. The author's preference is to utilize an olive-tip shaped burr to remove 3–5 mm of the outer table around the marked perimeter of the desired graft, exposing the diploe. A 5–10 m chisel or osteotome with the blade oriented slightly outward is utilized to minimize the chance of inner table penetration. It is introduced with a series of gentle mallet taps, and care is taken to minimize the chance of inner table penetration. Even with careful in situ harvesting, it is not unusual to have a small portion of full-thickness harvest in the central portion of the graft due to disruption of the inner table from the mechanical action of the chisel or osteotome. In situ harvest often results in a graft with micro- or macro-fractures. During split thickness in situ harvest, one must be careful to guard against the potential for indirect central nervous system damage with percussion because sharp instruments can penetrate the dura, vessels, or even the brain itself. Harvest of in situ grafts is not suitable in children due to their thin calvaria. Additionally, they are almost always contraindicated in individuals with craniosynostoses due to the frequent obliteration of diploe, converting the calvaria to a thin monolayer of cortical bone without inner and outer table delineation. Due to the risks, if a split-thickness in situ graft is to be obtained, it should be done preferably over the calvaria overlying the nondominant cerebral hemisphere. The major indication for in situ harvesting is the need for a small graft requiring curvature shaping, such as for orbital fractures. Otherwise, when possible, the graft is harvested full-thickness and split on the back table as described earlier.

DONOR SITE DEFECT

Management of the donor site defect depends on the method of harvest as well as the size and location of the defect. If a split thickness in situ harvest is performed successfully, no specific donor site management is indicated. Bleeding is addressed with focally placed bone wax prior to closure, and a drain is placed as indicated. Harvest of the graft by calvarectomy, the generally utilized method of harvest at our institution, requires reconstruction of the donor defect by either replacement of the outer table in the case of splitting the graft or by autogenous or alloplastic material. The preferred autogenous material is a split-thickness calvarial graft, generally obtained by harvesting a second piece of full-thickness calvarium. This is usually obtained by harvesting a second piece of full-thickness calvaria adjacent to the initial donor defect that is the same size as the defect. The second piece is delaminated on the back table and then the outer table replaced in the most visible area of the defect with the inner table placed in the less visible area.

Some surgeons advocate use of split rib to reconstruct such defect. Other options for reconstruction include alloplastic materials such titanium mesh or one of the various "bone cements" available today.

The theoretical amount of bone that can be harvested from the calvaria without leaving a donor defect exceeds 50% of the calvaria itself assuming all donor calvaria can be split into two solid lamina. In actual practice, the presence of sutures prevents perfect delamination of an entire hemicalvaria.

POSTOPERATIVE CARE

Postoperatively, drains utilized are removed once the drainage is less than 15 cc/day. The patient is advised to take care to avoid any head trauma or activity that could result in trauma to the head for 6 weeks postoperatively. If the patient is unable to follow directions well, such as with very young children, and more than one-eighth the calvaria is compromised, a postoperative protective helmet can be utilized during waking hours. Patients are allowed to return to regular activity after approximately 6 weeks if healing is uneventful and uncomplicated.

CONTRAINDICATIONS

There are relative and absolute contraindications to calvarial bone harvest. Any patient who is an acceptable anesthesia risk for some sort of craniofacial surgery is generally a candidate for full-thickness calvarial harvest, with or without back table split. Contraindications related to in situ split harvest include prior neurologic injury or deficit or insufficient or obliterated diploe.

FUTURE

In recent years, virtual surgical planning (VSP) has contributed an additional option for calvarial defect reconstruction by broadening the treatment options to include custom three-dimensional printed polyether ether ketone (PEEK) inlays. With continued advancements in technology and industry, more defects can potentially be treated in this fashion, thus diminishing the need for calvarial grafting and donor site morbidity.

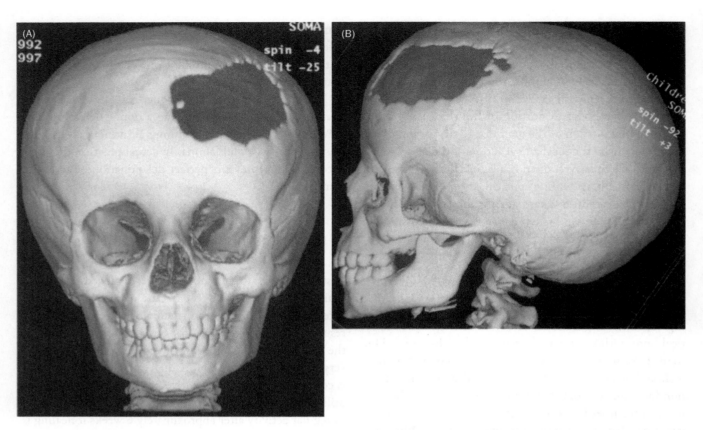

Figure 8.1. Osseous surface three-dimensional computer topographic scan reformations frontal (A) and left lateral (B) of the skull of a five year old female one year after traumatic partial loss of frontal bone. The defect was covered acutely with a full thickness scalp rotation flap with split-thicknsss skin grafting of the donor site

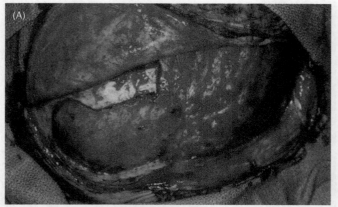

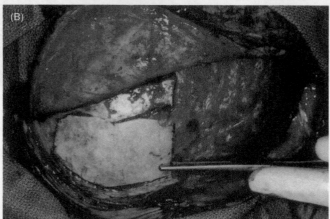

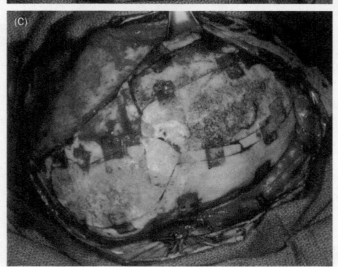

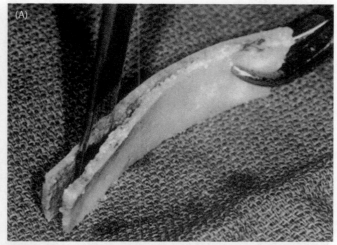

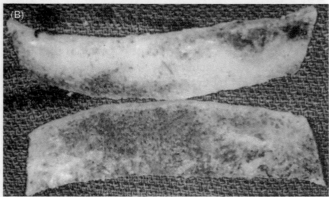

Figure 8.3. Technique of back table split. Full thickness calvaria graft has been scored with a sagittal saw. A, split is completed with an osteotome. B, two solid grafts, without microfracture or lacunae, result.

Figure 8.2. Intraoperative photographs of autogenous split-thickness calvarial cranioplasty. A, preexisting incision along interior edge of scalp rotation flap was opened, exposing posttraumatic defect. Dura was freed from the defect, bone edges freshened to bleeding bone, and template draw. The template was then placed adjacent to the posterior margin of the defect and the donor calvectomy marked and harvested. B, full-thickness bone graft was split on the back table using a combination of a sagittal saw and osteotome. The outer table was contoured with bone-bending forceps to match the recipient site. C, the inner table was returned to the donor site and an additional strip of calvaria was harvested and split to complete the reconstruction. Grafts were fixed to the recipient and donor sites with biodegradable plates.

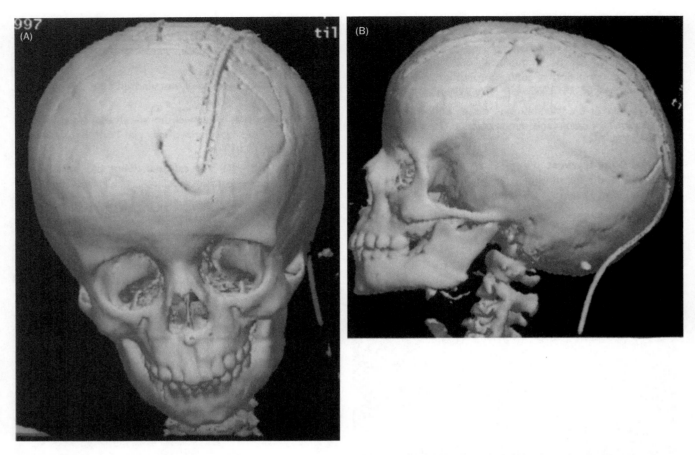

Figure 8.4. Osseous surface three-dimensional computed tomographic scan reformations, frontal (A) and left lateral (B) immediately after autogenous splits thickness calvarial reconstruction.

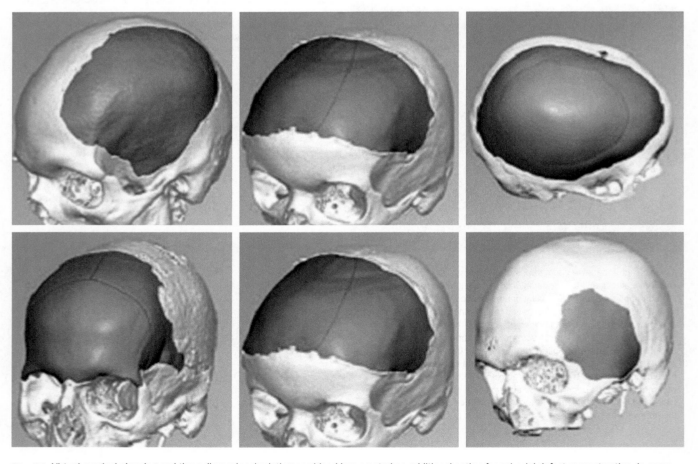

Figure 8.5. Virtual surgical planning and three-dimensional printing combined has created an additional option for calvarial defect reconstruction, in some cases eliminating the need for donor site defects.

9.

ILIAC CREST AND RIB BONE GRAFTS

Paul Mittermiller, Joseph Baylan, Dana N. Johns, Derrick Wan, and H. Peter Lorenz

The most frequent donor sites for autologous bone in reconstructive surgery are the cranium, iliac crest, and ribs. The purpose of this chapter is to detail the use and harvesting of iliac crest and rib bone grafts.

ILIAC CREST: OPEN APPROACH

The iliac crest is an excellent donor site for large amounts of both cortical and cancellous bone. Both anterior and posterior crests are used for bone grafts. The anterior approach is the technique most commonly used by plastic surgeons and is highlighted in this chapter.

INDICATIONS

Autologous bone from the iliac crest is used for reconstruction of small defects of the mandible (i.e., <2.5 cm) and in locations where primarily cancellous bone is needed, such as alveolar clefts. Iliac bone can also be used when a significant amount of bone is required around the orbit or the maxilla, typically when calvarial bone is not available.

TECHNIQUE

Initially, the type and size of desired bone graft must be determined. The patient is placed in the recumbent position and the anterior superior iliac spine (ASIS) is marked. An incision is marked along the inferior edge of the crest (Figure 9.1). The incision is usually 2–3 cm in length, although this varies depending on the size and type of bone required.

The skin is stretched superiorly to allow the incision to ultimately lie underneath the iliac crest to prevent irritation and wound breakdown. The site is incised using a scalpel, and electrocautery dissection is carried down through subcutaneous fat to the iliac crest. The aponeurosis of the external oblique and tensor fascia lata is incised along the ridge of the iliac crest over its lateral edge.

Care is taken during the dissection to avoid the peripheral nerves in the area. The lateral cutaneous branch of the T12 subcostal nerve, the anterior cutaneous branch of the iliohypogastric nerve, and the lateral femoral cutaneous nerve are the most likely to be encountered or injured during the operation.[1] The lateral cutaneous branch of the subcostal nerve runs diagonally across the midpoint of the anterior iliac crest, while the anterior cutaneous branch of the iliohypogastric area crosses immediately behind the ASIS.[2,3] The lateral femoral cutaneous nerve normally courses anterior to the ASIS underneath the inguinal ligament, but anatomical variants have demonstrated the nerve crossing over the iliac crest within 3 cm of the ASIS.[1]

In cases where only cancellous bone is required, an oscillating saw or osteotome is used to make a tricortical bone cap out of the superior portion of the iliac crest (Figure 9.2). The bone cap is reflected medially, hinging on the periosteum that is still attached on the medial surface of the ilium. Bone gouges or curettes are used to harvest the cancellous bone. Gel foam soaked in 0.25% bupivacaine can be packed into the donor site for postoperative analgesia, and the bone plate is placed back into its natural position.

In cases where cortical and cancellous bone are needed, a wide subcutaneous pocket is dissected and the muscular insertions are incised. The lateral cortical bone is then marked with methylene blue and cut with an oscillating saw. Heavy osteotomes are used to remove the bone. Bone gouges are used to harvest any additional cancellous bone. Gel foam soaked in 0.25% bupivacaine can be packed into the donor site.

A closed suction drain can be placed in the subperiosteal pocket after cortical bone harvest, although for smaller bone graft harvests this may not be necessary. The aponeurosis is closed tightly to contain bleeding with large resorbable suture, and the remainder of the wound is closed in layers.

79

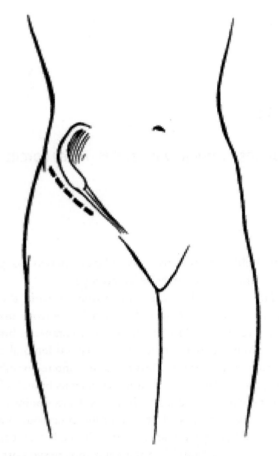

Figure 9.1. Incision in iliac crest is made 2 cm below crest.

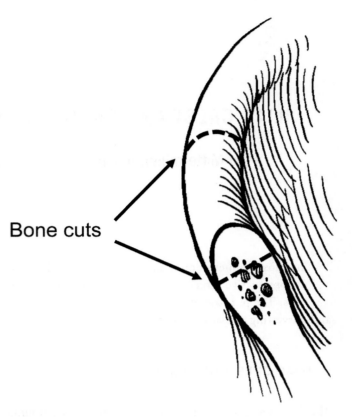

Bone cuts

Figure 9.2. Iliac crest is split below crest to create a bone cap that can be reflected medially for access to cancellous bone as well as lateral wall cortical bone.

An adhesive bandage is applied. The suction drain is removed after 2 days of less than 20 –30 mL of drainage per day.

CAVEATS AND COMPLICATIONS

The complications associated with iliac bone graft harvest include pain, infection, hematoma formation, palpable defects of the ilium, fractures of the ilium, herniation of abdominal contents through the bony defect, neuralgias, and paresthesias.[4] Controversy exists as to which nerve is the most commonly injured as a result of the operation.[1] Nerves at risk include branches of the iliohypogastric and the lateral femoral cutaneous nerves (Figure 9.3). Despite these possible complications, iliac bone is still the donor site of choice for cases in which significant quantities of cancellous and cortical bone are required.

ILIAC CREST: PERCUTANEOUS APPROACH

Iliac crest bone has historically been harvested through an open approach. However, a percutaneous approach can also be used when only cancellous bone is needed.

INDICATIONS

Percutaneously harvested iliac crest cancellous bone can be used for the same indications as that harvested using an open approach.[5] Harvesting iliac crest cancellous bone through a percutaneous approach is thought to result in decreased postoperative pain, duration of hospital stay, and rate of gait disturbanes.[6, 7] It uses a smaller incision, is thought to decrease rates of infection, does not disturb the growth plate in children, and does not require dissection of the cartilage cap in the pediatric population.

Technique

The location of the anterior superior iliac spine is palpated and an insertion site is marked two finger breadths posterior to the ASIS on the superior surface of the iliac crest. A scalpel is used to make a stab incision through the skin.

There are a variety of percutaneous bone graft harvesting instruments. The senior author currently uses the Imbibe bone marrow aspiration needle by Stryker. This disposable instrument has a cannula with a sharp trocar. With the trocar seated in the cannula, the instrument is placed through the incision and the tip is pushed through the

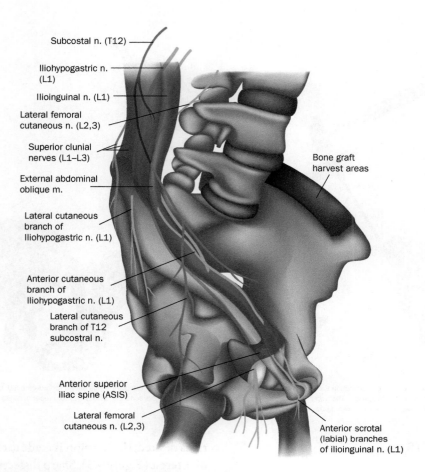

Subcostal n. (T12)

Iliohypogastric n. (L1)

Ilioinguinal n. (L1)

Lateral femoral cutaneous n. (L2,3)

Superior clunial nerves (L1–L3)

External abdominal oblique m.

Lateral cutaneous branch of Iliohypogastric n. (L1)

Anterior cutaneous branch of Iliohypogastric n. (L1)

Lateral cutaneous branch of T12 subcostral n.

Anterior superior iliac spine (ASIS)

Lateral femoral cutaneous n. (L2,3)

Bone graft harvest areas

Anterior scrotal (labial) branches of ilioinguinal n. (L1)

Figure 9.3. Iliac crest harvest area (*purple*) and nearby sensory nerves at risk for injury during graft harvest.

soft tissue to the iliac crest. The center of the iliac crest is identified, and a mallet is used to seat the instrument into the cortical bone. The surgeon then palpates the shape of the iliac wing and aligns the instrument parallel to the wing, as shown in Figure 9.4. With multiple mallet taps, the surgeon penetrates the cortical bone and guides the instrument into the cancellous bone. Care should be taken to avoid an approach that aims too medially as this can theoretically penetrate the medial plate of the ilium and cause intraabdominal injuries. An approach that aims too laterally can cause the surgeon to miss the cancellous space.

Once the surgeon has the tip of the instrument located within the cancellous bone, the trocar is exchanged for a rounded stylet. This allows advancement of the instrument in the cancellous bone without penetrating the cortical bone. The stylet allows the instrument to glide along the inner surface of the cortex, as shown in Figure 9.4. The instrument should be advanced roughly 2–3 cm to position the fenestrations of the instrument within the cortical space. The stylet should then be removed and the surgeon can aspirate marrow into a syringe.

In order to obtain a sufficient amount of bone, the stylet needs to be replaced to further advance the instrument. Once readvanced, aspiration can be repeated. The instrument can also be fanned anteriorly and posteriorly to create new tracts for marrow aspiration. Once a sufficient amount of bone is obtained, it is minced with straight Mayo scissors to facilitate placement in the graft site.

The instrument is removed, and the incision is closed using a combination of deep dermal and simple interrupted sutures. The incision is covered with a small piece of gauze and held in place with a transparent film dressing.

CAVEATS AND COMPLICATIONS

The most feared complication from percutaneous gone graft harvest is penetration of the medial cortex of the iliac wing and visceral perforation. There are currently no reported cases of this complication in the literature. Additional complications include pain, infection, and neuralgias. The general consensus is that morbidity with this approach is lower than that with an open approach.

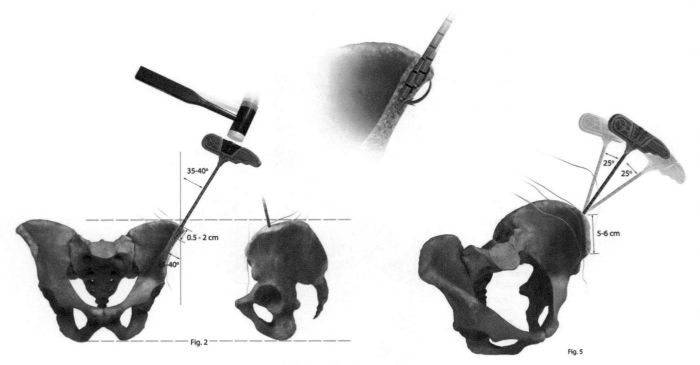

Figure 9.4. Proper placement of percutaneous bone collection tool is shown in the bottom left image. Placement of the blunt stylus allows for movement through the cancellous bone without penetrating the cortical bone, as shown in the top image. The trocar has approximately 25 degrees of movement around the central axis for proper cancellous bone harvest as shown in the bottom right image. Copyright Adam Questell, A KYU Design, LLC.

RIB BONE GRAFTS

INDICATIONS

Rib bone grafts are used for a variety of purposes in facial reconstruction, including replacing bone defects of the mandible, maxilla, zygoma, and calvarium.[8, 9] The approach to the donor site varies according to the material needed and the sex of the patient. This chapter focuses on the approach for harvesting rib bone grafts.

TECHNIQUE

The anatomy of the bony thorax reveals that cartilages of the paired upper seven ribs articulate directly with the sternum, while the eighth rib may or may not be part of the chondrosynctium. The eighth, ninth, and tenth ribs usually articulate with each other through fibrous unions. The floating ribs (eleven and twelve) are not attached to the rib cage (Figure 9.5).

The patient is placed in the supine position and the sixth, seventh, and eighth ribs are identified. The location of the inframammary fold or crease is noted and an incision is made within this natural crease. In young children, the future location of the inframammary fold is estimated and used. This is less important in males. If a more inferior rib is desired, the incision is made directly overlying the rib of interest (Figure 9.5). Sharp dissection is carried through the skin, and electrocautery dissection is used to dissect through the subcutaneous tissue and the external oblique muscle. Mobility of the chest wall skin allows for retraction of the incision 8-10 cm in all directions. The incision is retracted over the rib of interest, and the periosteum on the anterior surface is incised longitudinally. Transverse incisions in the periosteum are created at the medial and lateral aspects to facilitate reflection of the periosteum and exposure of the rib. The periosteum is lifted off the anterior surface of the rib, and subperiosteal dissection is continued around the superior, inferior, and posterior surfaces. Care should be taken to ensure circumferential dissection of the bone graft while avoiding posterior tears of the periosteum and parietal pleura. The medial aspect of the bone is incised at the costochondral junction using a scalpel while protecting the soft tissue posteriorly with a malleable retractor or Doyen elevator. Dissection in the subperiosteal plane is carried laterally and the bone is cut laterally using rib shears.

After hemostasis is obtained, the patient is checked for a pleural tear. The wound is filled with saline, and the anesthesiologist inflates the patient's lungs. A pleural tear is identified if a positive Valsalva maneuver causes air bubbles to emanate from the wound. If a pleural tear is identified,

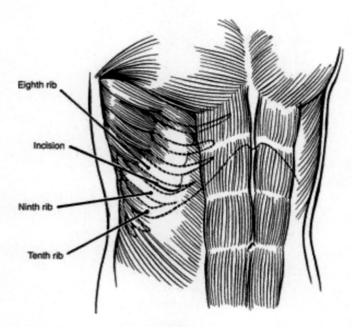

Figure 9.5. Location of the ribs in relation to surface landmarks. An incision is made within the inframammary fold or directly overlying the rib of interest.

Eighth rib

Incision

Ninth rib

Tenth rib

a red rubber No. 19 catheter is inserted into the pleural cavity. The overlying soft tissue is closed around the catheter in a purse string fashion. The catheter is connected to suction and removed while the purse string suture is tied. If there is an ongoing air leak from injury to the visceral pleura, a chest tube is inserted.

The external oblique and subcutaneous tissues are closed in layers over the periosteal sheath. Before closing the wound, a 0.25% bupivacaine solution is injected. The skin is then closed. An adhesive bandage is placed over the wound. If a large pleural tear was identified and treated intraoperatively, a postoperative chest x-ray film is obtained in the recovery room.

CAVEATS AND COMPLICATIONS

Complications of rib graft harvest include pleural tear with or without pneumothorax, scarring, and pain.[10]

ACKNOWLEDGMENTS

We thank Dr. John F. Teichgraeber for his contributions to this chapter in a prior edition.

SUGGESTED READINGS

1. Zouhary KJ. Bone graft harvesting from distant sites: concepts and techniques. *Oral Maxillofacial Surg Clin NA* 2010;22:301–316.
2. Chou D, Storm PB, Campbell JN. Vulnerability of the subcostal nerve to injury during bone graft harvesting from the iliac crest. *J Neurosurg Spine* 2004;1:87–89.
3. Maigne JY, Maigne R, Guérin-Surville H. Anatomic study of the lateral cutaneous rami of the subcostal and iliohypogastric nerves. *Surg Radiologic Anat* 1986;8:251–256.
4. Arrington ED, Smith WJ, Chambers HG, et al. Complications of iliac crest bone graft harvesting. *Clin Orthopaed Related Res* 1996:300–309.
5. Shepard GH, Dierberg WJ. Use of the cylinder osteotome for cancellous bone grafting. *Plast Reconstr Surg* 1987;80:129–132.
6. Hardy SP, Wilke RC, Doyle JF. Advantages of percutaneous hollow needle technique for iliac bone harvest in alveolar cleft grafting. *Cleft Palate-Craniofacial J* 1999;36:252–255.
7. Bartels RHMA. Single-blinded prospective randomized study comparing open versus needle technique for obtaining autologous cancellous bone from the iliac crest. *Eur Spine J* 2005;14:649–653.
8. Abdel-Haleem AK, Nouby R, Taghian M. The use of the rib grafts in head and neck reconstruction. *Egypt J Ear, Nose, Throat Allied Sci* 2011;12:89–98.
9. James DR, Irvine GH. Autogenous rib grafts in maxillofacial surgery. *J Maxillofacial Surg* 1983;11:201–203.
10. Laurie SW, Kaban LB, Mulliken JB, et al. Donor-site morbidity after harvesting rib and iliac bone. *Plast Reconstr Surg* 1984;73:933–938.

10.

COSTAL CARTILAGE GRAFTS

Guilio Gheradini and Ronald P. Gruber

ASSESSMENT OF THE DEFECT

Cartilage is a specialized form of connective tissue with unique properties that make it an ideal source of grafting material for nasal and facial defects. Cartilage is avascular and relies on the neighboring tissue for nutritional support; it has a very slow metabolic rate, equal to 0.2– 1% of the metabolic rate of other human tissues; it is generally accepted to be an immunologically privileged tissue. In general, cartilage grafts are used for many purposes. In assessing the defect to be filled with costal cartilage, some factors must be taken into account. The length of the defect can extend up to 6–7 cm; a larger defect would require multiple grafts or bone grafts (usually vascularized). Large costal cartilage grafts are also difficult to harvest and have increased morbidity at the donor and recipient sites. The rigidity and firmness of costal cartilage can be used for structural augmentation (i.e., correction of saddle-nose deformities or to provide structural rigidity to the trachea and eyelid). However, costal cartilage cannot be considered a substitute for bone grafts when significant structural support is needed. Costal cartilage grafts can be used as onlay-type grafts to correct traumatic, congenital, or surgically induced facial deformities and as spacers to maintain mobility of the temporomandibular joint.

INDICATIONS

Costal cartilage grafts are the best choice when large amounts of material are needed. Cases such as major nasal reconstruction, total ear reconstruction, contour restoration, and maxillary hypoplasia augmentation lend themselves to the use of costal cartilage. Costal cartilage is also the material of choice when semi-rigid support is necessary. Patients with bilateral cleft lip frequently have depressed nasal tips with absence of the nasal spine and caudal septum. After soft tissue columella lengthening, costal cartilage can be used to extend the septum and support the tip. Rib cartilage may be used as an onlay graft for malar or maxillary contour in locations where bone grafts would normally suffer from significant resorption. Rib cartilage is of the hyaline type, and, as with all cartilage, it retains its original characteristics when transplanted. Functional stress is not necessary for survival of the bulk of cartilaginous rib grafts, although care should be taken to appropriately shape the graft. Appropriate rib selection helps facilitate graft carving and success. For example, the seventh costal cartilage is relatively straight and lends itself well to nasal dorsal augmentation, while the eighth is more suited for malar maxillary onlay.

Osseous rib grafts can be included with the cartilage transplant when a bony graft is also needed. This site is especially useful for patients in whom other sources have already been exhausted or in children whose septal cartilage should not be harvested. The site of harvesting is chosen according to patient and surgeon preferences, the presence of previous incisions or scars that can be used, and the type of reconstruction to be performed. For nasal reconstruction, the majority of surgeons prefer the right side to harvest cartilage; for other reconstruction, either side is used.

Cartilage has a variety of differences with free-bone graft, although they can both serve overlapping functions. In general, cartilaginous grafts are easy to shape and do not require functional stress for retention of bulk. The receiving vascular supply of a cartilage graft does not need to be as developed as that for a corresponding bone graft, and cartilage has a lower resorption rate. Cartilage donor sites frequently cause less morbidity than bone donor sites. Cartilage grafts, however, do have a tendency to warpage, less inherent strength and support, possible migration, and possible rapid absorption if exposed to pressure or infection. In general, cranial or rib bone grafts are preferred for cases of severe hypoplasia or saddle-nose deformity (more than 3–4 cm needed) or in total nose reconstruction, when a rigid structural support of the nose is needed. In this case, the bone grafts can be fixed to the proximal nasal bone with interosseous wires. Cartilaginous grafts are preferred to augment tip projection and create supratip concavity and a contoured double break.

CONTRAINDICATIONS

Donor site complications, specifically chest wall deformities and thoracic scoliosis, are described in the literature as occurring after harvest of costal cartilage grafts. Preexistent bony deformities of the chest wall constitute a relative contraindication to the use of this graft. Recently, attention has been focused on the patient's age at the time of cartilage harvest. Thoracic deformities seem to be less frequent if cartilage is harvested from patients older than 10 years of age, probably because the seventh rib possesses the strongest growth capacity. However, young age is not a contraindication to the harvest of costal cartilage grafts. Advanced age (>60 years) is accompanied by various degrees of calcification of the costal cartilages. This condition is a relative contraindication to the use of this donor site because the structural characteristics of the cartilage graft (e.g., strength, low resorption rate) become similar to those of bone grafts, and there is an increased risk of postoperative morbidity. Other contraindications to rib cartilage graft include the general contraindications to surgery.

PATIENT POSITION AND ROOM SETUP

The patient lies in a supine position on the operating table with a rolled towel or a shoulder support under the middle back to provide chest extension. A 15-degree rotation of the chest opposite to the donor side is preferred. The surgeon is positioned at the right side of the patient, and the assistant is positioned at the opposite side. General preoperative measures are observed: no solid food is allowed for at least 6 hours before the operation. Endotracheal anesthesia is preferred.

OPERATIVE TECHNIQUE

The optimal site for harvesting rib cartilage is in the lower chest wall, specifically the anterior medial synchondrosis of ribs seven, eight, and nine (Figure 10.1). The lower

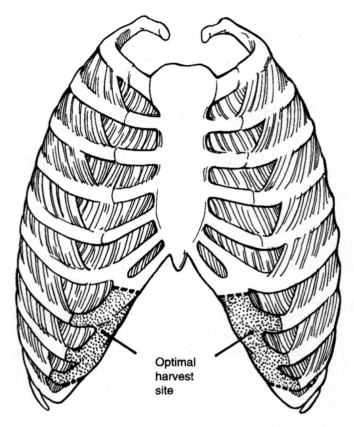

Figure 10.1. Cartilaginous portion of seventh, eighth, and ninth ribs can be used as donor site for cartilage harvesting.

ribs are marked on the chest wall after palpation, 5–7 mL of lidocaine (0.5% solution) with 1:200,000 epinephrine is injected in the area to minimize blood loss, and a 2- to 3-cm incision is made anterior laterally (6 cm from the midline), depending on the cartilage chosen (usually rib eight). Alternatively, the incision can be placed at the level of the inframammary fold, especially if the operation is performed on an adult female. Since the chest wall skin is very mobile, a large amount of cartilage can be exposed by moving the retractors. Usually, a self-retaining retractor is used (Figure 10.2). The incision is deepened to the level of the perichondrium, and total or subtotal removal of the rib cartilage is accomplished. For the subtotal excision, a no. 66 Beaver blade, or a no. 11 blade can be used to create a right-angle incision to dissect the outer 75% of the cartilage (Figure 10.3). Another possibility is to use a dental elevator altered into a Joseph elevator to dissect out the perichondrium before totally resecting the cartilage. The appropriate amount of cartilage is removed, and the wound is closed anatomically in three layers without a drain. A light pressure dressing is helpful.

The anterior portion of the cartilage is excised with a no. 11 blade, and the middle portion is used as needed.

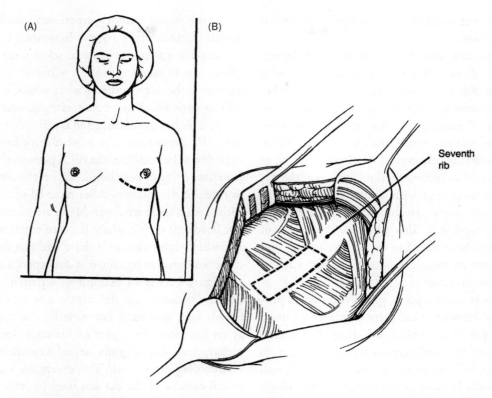

Seventh rib

Figure 10.2. (A) Cartilage is exposed through incision along long axis of rib. (B) Self-retaining retractor assists with exposure and rib harvest.

The shavings of the cartilage should be saved since they can be used as onlay grafts for alar cartilage. When crushed in a Cottle cartilage crusher, these shavings also make excellent camouflage overlay in static areas. We have experienced the most difficulty when rib cartilage is used for large defects on the nasal dorsum. Warping of these grafts

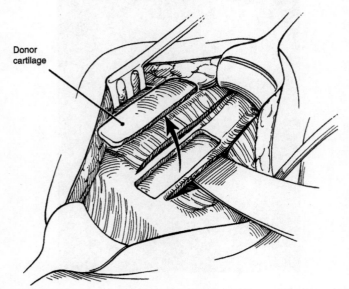

Donor cartilage

Figure 10.3. Dissection is completed with no. 11 blade. Approximately 75% of cartilage can be removed.

occurs frequently even after appropriate cross-sectional carving. This subtotal approach to rib harvesting takes 20–25 minutes from start to finish. A second surgeon should create the recipient soft tissue pocket in the face while harvesting is in process.

RIB GRAFTS FOR RHINOPLASTY

Rib grafts have become an essential part of rhinoplasty, particularly in secondary rhinoplasty. The typical situation is when there is not enough donor material for reconstruction because the septum was harvested previously. Perhaps the ear was harvested as well, which is a favorite of many surgeons. However, a number of surgeons by-pass ear cartilage as donor material because it tends to be weak and curved and prefer rib cartilage in all circumstances—despite the fact that cartilage stiffness and straightness has been improved with suture techniques in recent years.

In the past, the problems with rib grafts for dorsal augmentation have been (1) warping, (2) technical difficulty of carving a piece for the dorsum that is just right in terms of the size, (3) technical difficulties in removing the rib cartilage, and (4) morbidity (pain) to the patient. However, most of these issues have been largely resolved or at least much improved. Warping has largely been overcome by using the interior portion of the rib cartilage, as described by Toriumi and others.

A simpler approach is to slice the resected rib (much like a salami) into slices that are approximately the width of septal cartilage. Rib removal should be done at the beginning of the operation, with the specimens placed in saline for at least 30 minutes to allow any early warping to take place. The straight specimens can be used where needed, and even the slightly curved specimens may be of value for certain types of reconstruction, such as at the tip. Straightening the specimens with mattress sutures, as is done for septoplasty, lateral crus bulbosity, and ear donor cartilage, does not work well. This is because these slices of rib cartilage tend to be stiffer than ear or rib cartilage and often brittle. However, there are usually enough straight specimens for reconstruction of any kind.

When one has an abundance of grafts, it is easy to proceed comfortably knowing that there is plenty of good material for the job of biological sculpting. This means replacing all parts of the cartilaginous framework. The rib specimens are typically cut into segments that are 3 mm long and 6 mm wide. Because of the slicing just described, the segments are usually 1 mm wide. These segments make good lateral crus grafts (described by Gunter), spreader grafts, dorsal grafts, batten grafts of the lateral wall, columellar struts, and tip grafts. Of all the grafts, however, the rib tip graft is probably surpassed by concha of the ear or septum because thin rib grafts are very stiff. They need to be scored to provide a gentle curvature and the edges carefully beveled. By working with these sized units, it is much easier to rebuild any part of the nasal framework. This mimics the way many artists who work with clay create a face, by adding or subtracting small pieces until the result seems favorable.

This approach is predicated on the notion that it is not necessary to perform the traditional large dorsal augmentation with a large single graft. It is the senior author's opinion that multiple single layer grafts or even diced cartilage, as Daniel has described, is better than trying to carve a single large dorsal cartilaginous implant. One other advantage of using the multiple thin (salami) slices approach is that there is no obligation to resect the entire thickness of rib. Resecting the anterior (superficial) half or two-thirds of the rib with a septal knife or other such semi-sharp instrument works well and minimizes the risk of pneumothorax. Partial superficial resection is also helpful when one only needs a small amount of donor material and there are no septal or ear donor possibilities. Furthermore, it can be done under local anesthesia if one proceeds slowly with the injection of the local.

In the senior author's experience, the best site is the medial inframammary region. In women it is easy to hide the scar. No attempt is made to select a rib ahead of time. Dissection is taken down to whatever cartilaginous rib happens to be deep to the incision, which is commonly the fifth or sixth rib. A generously size incision is made (commonly 2 inches), and dissection is taken down to the periosteum. The periosteum is somewhat thick here and is incised right down the middle of the rib. A periosteal elevator is used to elevate a flap of perichondrium on the superior and inferior side of the incision. After removal of the cartilage, the entire area is infiltrated with Marcaine, particularly the inferior border of the rib where the intercostal nerve is located. A multiple-layer closure is done without drains. If a dead space is allowed to remain, one can expect a seroma postop.

Figure 10.4 is an example of a patient who exhibited dorsal deficiency, tip deficiency, a somewhat short nose for his face, and weak lateral walls. He required thin rib grafts for most every part of his nose, including a columellar strut, dorsal grafts, septal extension graft, and an intercartilaginous graft. The exception was the tip, for which concha of the ear was used because of the reasons mentioned earlier. Postop results indicated considerable improvement, in large part due to augmentation rhinoplasty with costal (rib) grafts.

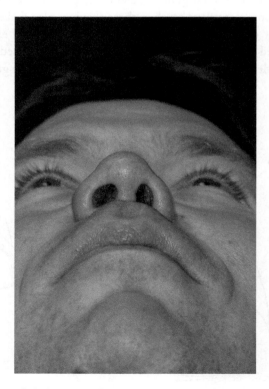

Figure 10.4. Typical example of short columella with relatively tick skin and short nose. These features largely benefit from costal cartilage rib graft in most parts of the nose.

POSTOPERATIVE CARE AND FOLLOW-UP EVALUATION

Postoperative morbidity is generally minimal. Patients receive intravenous antibiotics at the time of surgery, and oral antibiotics are continued for 1 week. Postoperative pain may be controlled with morphine immediately after surgery, and an analgesic containing codeine is prescribed for 2–3 days. Usually, the patient is discharged to home the same day or kept in the hospital for 1 day. Full activity is allowed after 4 weeks.

CAVEATS

The technique for rib cartilage harvesting described here is relatively easy to perform, provides outstanding material for facial aesthetic and reconstructive surgery, and causes little donor site morbidity. The only serious complication is pneumothorax. This risk is particularly high when a near-total removal of the rib chondral cartilage is necessary, such as for an ear reconstruction. Atelectasis is sometimes observed, owing to postoperative pain or splinting. Some authors suggest the infiltration of 0.25% bupivacaine solution at the end of the procedure to minimize the pain. It is advisable to harvest a larger segment of cartilage than needed since it must be carved, and equal amounts are removed from both sides (balanced cross-section) to prevent warping and bending.

SELECTED READINGS

Abrahams M, Duggan TC. The mechanical characteristics of costal cartilage. In: Kenedi RM, ed. *Biomechanics and Related Bioengineering Topics*. Proceedings of Science and Plastic Surgery Symposium held in Glasgow, Scotland, June 1963. London: Pergamon Press, 1965:285.

Adamson PA, Warner J, Becker D, Rom TJ 3rd, Toriumi DM. Revision rhinoplasty: *panel discussion, controversies, and techniques. Facial Plast Surg Clinics NA* 2014;22:57–96.

Bujia J, Alsalameh S, Naumann A, et al. Humoral immune response against minor collagens type IX and XI in patients with cartilage graft resorption after reconstructive surgery. *Ann Rheum Dis* 1994;53:229.

Constantian MB. Distant effects of dorsal and tip grafting in rhinoplasty. *Plast Reconstr Surg* 1992;90:405–418.

Calvert JW, Patel AC, Daniel RK. Reconstructive rhinoplasty: operative revision of patients with previous autologous costal cartilage grafts. *Plast Reconstr Surg* 2014;133:1087–1096.

Converse JM. The absorption and shrinkage of maternal ear cartilage used as living homografts: follow-up report of 21 of Gillies' patients. In: Converse JM, ed. *Reconstructive Plastic Surgery*. 2nd ed. Philadelphia: WB Saunders, 1997:308.

Daniel RK. Rhinoplasty and rib grafts: evolving a flexible operative technique. *Plast Reconstr Surg* 1994;94:597–609.

Gibson T, Davis WB. The distortion of autogenous cartilage grafts: its cause and prevention. *Br J Plast Surg* 1957;10:257.

Gibson T, Davis WB, Curran RC. The long-term survival of cartilage homografts in man. *Br J Plast Surg* 1958;11:177.

Herdon CH, Chase SW. Experimental studies in the transplantation of whole joints. *J Bone Joint Surg* 1952;34:564–578.

Horton CE, Matthews MS. Nasal reconstruction with autologous rib cartilage: a 43-year follow-up. *Plast Reconstr Surg* 1992;89:131.

Kruger E. Absorption of human rib cartilage grafts transplanted to rabbits after preservation by different methods. *Br J Plast Surg* 1964;17:254.

Kim DW, Shah AR, Toriumi DM. Concentric and eccentric carved costal cartilage. *Arch Facial Plast Surg* 2006; 8:42.

Lester CW. Tissue replacement after subperichondrial resection of costal cartilage: two case reports. *Plast Recontr Surg* 1959;23:49.

Lopez MA, Shah AR, Westine JG, O'Grady K, Toriumi DM. Analysis of the physical properties of costal cartilage in a porcine model. *Arch Facial Plast Surg.* 2007;9:35–39.

Muhlbauer WD, Schmidt-Tintemann U, Glaser M. Long-term behavior of preserved homologous rib cartilage in the correction of saddle nose deformity. *Br J Plast Surg* 1971;24:325.

Ohara K, Nakamura K, Ohta EO. Chest wall deformities and thoracic scoliosis after costal cartilage graft harvesting. *Plast Reconstr Surg* 1997;93:1030.

Ortiz-Monasterio F, Olmedo A, Oscoy LO. The use of cartilage grafts in primary aesthetic rhinoplasty. *Plast Reconstr Surg* 1981;67:597.

Peck GC. The onlay graft for nasal tip projection. *Plast Reconstr Surg* 1983;71:27.

Schuller DE, Baradach J, Krause CJ. Irradiated homologous costal cartilage for facial contour restoration. *Arch Otolaryngol* 1977; 103:12.

Sheen JH, Sheen AP. *Aesthetic Rhinoplasty*. Vol 1. St. Louis: CV Mosby, 1987:514.

Skouteris CA, Sotereanos GC. Donor site morbidity following harvesting of autogenous rib grafts. *J Oral Maxillofac Surg* 1989;47:808.

Stal S, Netscher D, Spira M. Cartilage grafting. In: Russell R, ed. *Instructional Courses*. St. Louis: Mosby-Year Book, 1991:43–60.

11.

AURICULAR CARTILAGE

Ali Sajjadian

INDICATIONS AND CONTRAINDICATIONS

The ear is generally not a first choice as a cartilage graft donor site for several reasons, none of which is valid. One reason is the scar at the donor site. Even when the graft is harvested anteriorly, the scar is well-concealed as long as the incision is placed within the rim of the conchal bowl, which make it imperceptible as it falls at the border of a light and shadow region. Another reason is the volume of cartilage available. Although no site can provide as much cartilage as the rib, the auricle can provide a surprisingly large amount of graft material (Figure 11.1). Additionally, its shape is well suited to assist in several aspects of nasal reconstruction, including reconstituting the lower lateral cartilages, nonanatomic rim strips, and tip grafts. There is also characteristically minimal morbidity with the harvest of auricular cartilage. This distinguishes it from rib cartilage harvest, which may be accompanied by significant postoperative pain and occasionally pneumothorax. In addition, septal harvest may cause bleeding, saddling of the nose symptomatic of septal perforation, and other airflow disturbances. The most important and major problem with ear cartilage is the flaccidity inherent in its structure. This makes it a poor choice when significant structural support is mandatory.

LANDMARKS, PATIENT MARKINGS, AND OPERATIVE METHOD

Both anterior and posterior approaches can be used to harvest auricular cartilage. If a graft for reconstruction of the lower lateral cartilage or an isolated tip graft is needed, an anterior approach may be the preferred method. The skin is first infiltrated with 1% lidocaine solution with 1:100,000 epinephrine. This provides hemostasis and partially hydrodissects the proper plane of dissection.

The incision is made at the light–shadow region to help conceal the final scar. Several 15-gauge needles can be used to mark the proposed area. The incision is typically made 3–4 mm inside of the conchal bowl (Figure 11.2). This helps to preserve the rim of the conchal bowl for support. A fine scissor is then used to elevate the anterior skin off the cartilage. The cartilage to be used is then incised full-thickness with a scalpel, and the posterior skin is dissected completely free from the conchal bowl (Figure 11.3). The graft harvesting process is completed

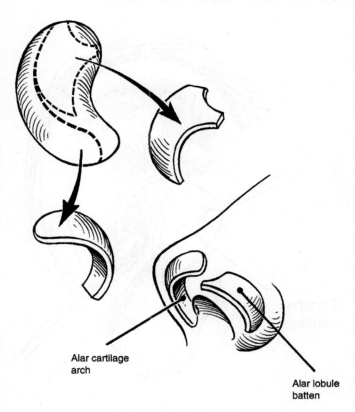

Alar cartilage arch

Alar lobule batten

Figure 11.1. Conchal cartilage can provide large batten volume of graft material for nasal reconstruction.

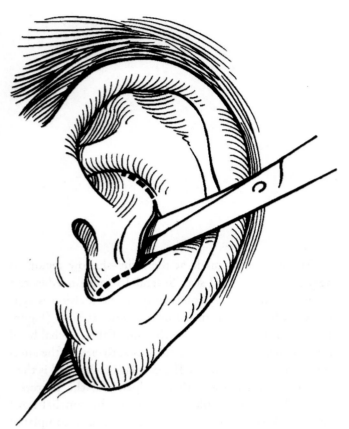

Figure 11.2. Anterior incision is placed just inside of conchal bowl rim.

by incising the cartilage medially. Hemostasis is achieved, and the incision is closed in two layers with interrupted deep 5-0 Vicryl sutures and running 5-0 fast absorbing catgut suture. When a larger graft is needed, such as for dorsal augmentation of the nose, a posterior approach is preferred (Figure 11.4). This medial access facilitates visualization of the entire conchal bowl. Again, the posterior skin is infiltrated with 1% lidocaine solution with 1:100,000 epinephrine. To preserve the conchal rim and at least 3 mm of bowl cartilage, it is helpful to mark the proposed cartilage incision. Typically, multiple 25-gauge needles are used to mark the proposed area, with a marking pen connecting the exit sites of the needle. Alternatively, a 25-gauge needle placed on a tuberculin syringe filled with methylene blue can be used to mark the areas of the cartilage to be dissected.

From a point 3 mm inside the conchal bowl, the needle is passed full-thickness through the cartilage from anterior to posterior, releasing a small amount of dye (Figure 11.5). The posterior skin incision is then made along the concho-cephalicl angle, and the skin is dissected free of

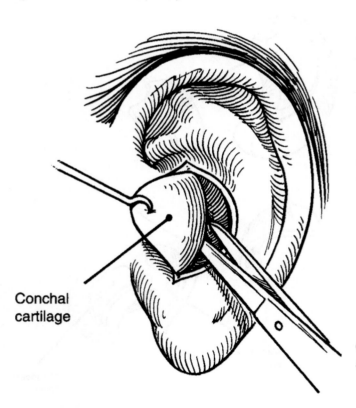

Conchal cartilage

Figure 11.3. Using hook on conchal cartilage for traction, posterior auricular skin is dissected free.

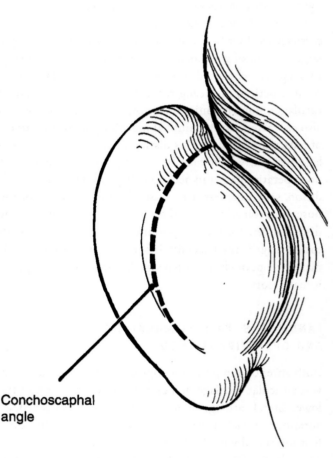

Conchoscaphal angle

Figure 11.4. Incision for posterior approach is placed at conchoscaphal angle.

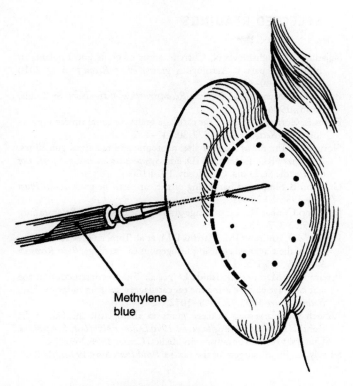

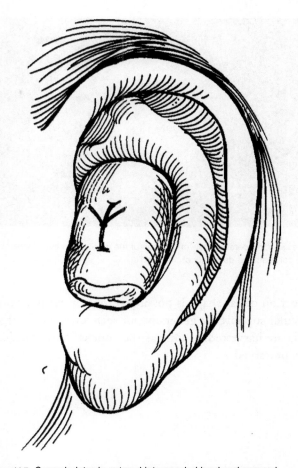

Figure 11.5. A 25-gauge needle is passed from anterior to posterior to mark line of proposed incision maintaining rim of conchal bowl.

the cartilage down to the auriculo-cephalic attachment. It is important to note that the posterior dissection can be more tedious as the perichondrium is closely adherent to the cartilage. Using the markings previously placed, a full-thickness cartilage cut is made (Figure 11.6). The anterior dissection is then completed with a scissor. The harvest

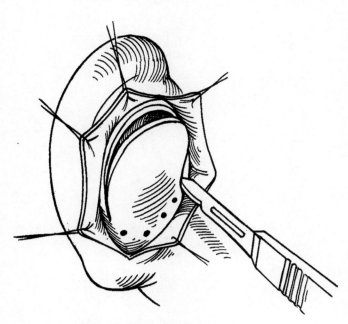

Figure 11.6. Conchal cartilage is incised along dotted line.

Figure 11.7. Gauze bolster is sutured into conchal bowl and secured with sutures through anterior and posterior auricular skin to obliterate dead space.

is completed by incising the cartilage medially, taking great care not to perforate the anterior skin (Figure 11.8). Hemostasis is achieved, and the incision is closed in two layers with interrupted deep 5-0 Vicryl sutures and running 5-0 fast-absorbing catgut suture. In all cases in which ear cartilage is harvested, a tie-over bolster of Xeroform or cotton within a fine mesh gauze is used to close the dead space created and to prevent hematoma formation. This is secured with a 4-0 Prolene suture placed through the anterior and posterior skin (Figure 11.7). The bolster dressing is removed in 5 days.

POSTOPERATIVE CONSIDERATIONS

Very little postoperative care is necessary for the harvest site. The only potential significant risk is hematoma within the dead space created, but this should be prevented by the bolster dressing. If hematoma is noticed in the early postoperative period, it should be gently expressed or aspirated and pressure applied. If this is not done, resorption and deformity of surrounding cartilage and

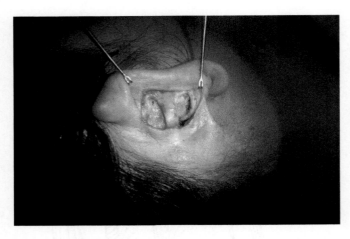

Figure 11.8. Intraoperative view of excision of the cartilage in two pieces to avoid collapse and deformity of the auricle.

distortion of ear shape is possible. Problems with lack of auricular support are generally not seen, even when large grafts are harvested, as long as the conchal bowl rim has been preserved.

SELECTED READINGS

Sajjadian A, Naghshineh N. Current status of grafts and implants in rhinoplasty: part I. Autologous grafts. *Plast Reconstr Surg* 2010 Feb;125(2):40–49.

Burget GC, Menick FJ. *Aesthetic Reconstruction of the Nose.* St. Louis: Mosby, 1994.

Falces E, Gorney M. Use of ear cartilage grafts for nasal tip reconstruction. *Plast Reconstr Surg* 1972;50:147–152.

Gorney M. The ear as a donor site: anatomic and technical guidelines. In: Tanzer RD, Edgerton MD, eds. *Symposium on Reconstruction of the Auricle.* St. Louis: CV Mosby, 1974:106.

Guyuron B. Simplified harvesting of the ear cartilage graft. *Aesth Plast Surg* 1986;10:29–41.

Juri J, Juri C, Elias JC. Ear cartilage grafts to the nose. *Plast Reconstr Surg* 1979;63:377–382.

Pereira MD, Andrews JM, Martins DM, et al. Total en bloc reconstruction of the alar cartilage using autogenous ear cartilage. *Plast Reconstr Surg* 1995;95:168–172.

Pereira MD, Marques AF, Ishida LC, et al. Total reconstruction of the alar cartilage en bloc using the ear cartilage: a study in cadavers. *Plast Reconstr Surg* 1995;96:1045–1052.

Rohrich RJ. Harvesting cartilage grafts in rhinoplasty. In: Gunter JP, Rohrich RJ, eds. *Course Syllabus for 1996 Dallas Rhinoplasty Symposium.* University of Texas Southwestern Medical Center, 1996:369–374.

Snively SL. Plastic surgery of the ear. *Sel Read Plast Surg* 1994;7:1–22.

12.

ALVEOLAR BONE GRAFTING

Raj M. Vyas and Gennaya L. Mattison

INDICATIONS

Alveolar bone grafting plays a crucial role in cleft reconstruction. In orofacial clefting, approximately 75% of patients require bony augmentation of the alveolar ridge. When neonatal presurgical orthodontia is successful in aligning the cleft segments, alveolar reconstruction can be initiated as a gingivoperiosteoplasty during primary cleft lip repair. Later in childhood, bone graft is required for alveolar reconstruction. The reconstruction is critical for normal dental eruption and subsequent orthodontic adjustments and therefore must be appropriately timed. Excessively early reconstruction has been associated with midface hypoplasia while late reconstruction can result in loss of canine eruption. In children with cleft palate, alveolar bone grafting is usually done after transverse maxillary expansion with a palatal expander. Exact timing of bone grafting is controversial; most centers initiate orthodontic evaluation/expansion between ages 7 and 8 years (beginning of mixed dentition) with an aim to bone graft before age 10 in order to allow osteogenic incorporation prior to eruption of the permanent canine.

ANATOMY AND EMBRYOLOGY

The face forms from the frontonasal prominence, bilateral maxillary prominences, and bilateral mandibular prominences. The maxillary prominences result in the bilateral sides of the mouth, while the frontonasal prominence result in the forehead, nose, and top of the mouth. Cleft lip occurs with failure of fusion of the maxillary prominences with the medial nasal process from the frontonasal prominence (Figure 12.1) during weeks 4–7 of gestation. The resulting cleft can be present from the lip

to the incisive foramen, passing between the cuspid and lateral incisor. It can result in defect of bone in the alveolar ridge requiring eventual grafting as the child ages and enters mixed dentition.

ASSESSMENT

Following orthodontic expansion (when needed), preoperative assessment of the alveolar bone defect is accomplished with a cone beam computed tomography (CBCT) scan to minimize radiation exposure. This defines the three-dimensional volume of the alveolar cleft, allowing the surgeon to plan appropriately for bone harvest. CBCT imaging also evaluates stages of dental eruption and provides a baseline to compare post-grafting results when needed. Additionally, in the case of syndromic patients, a full preoperative workup should be performed to evaluate the safety of undergoing operative intervention and anesthesia. Palatal expanders are removed 1–2 days prior to scheduled surgery.

PROCEDURE

ROOM SETUP

The room should be set up to turn the patient 180 degrees after oral intubation. The endotracheal tube is secured to the lower lip midline. The patient is positioned on a Mayfield horseshoe headrest. If bone harvest is to be performed concurrently with intraoral exposure, two Mayo stands should be prepared to keep the intraoral instruments separate from the sterile bone graft harvest setup.

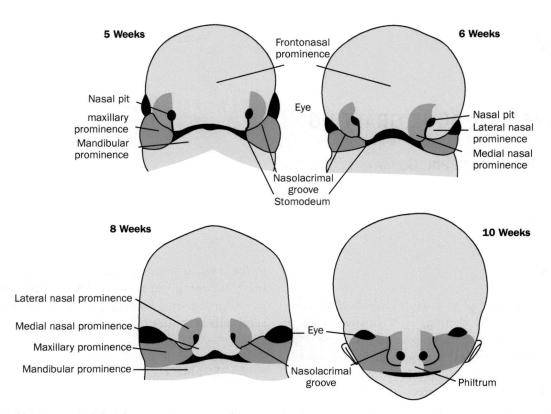

Figure 12.1. Embryologic development and fusion of the maxillary prominence with the medial nasal prominence in lip formation.

SURGICAL TECHNIQUE

The patient is brought to the operating room and placed supine on the operating table. The airway is secured and the patient appropriately positioned. The hip is cleaned grossly with alcohol pads, and the anterior superior iliac crest is marked on the patient's nondominant side. While marking the proposed surgical incision site, the skin is pulled from inferolateral to superomedial so that the eventual scar is hidden in the normal underwear line. With this skin displacement, a 2 cm surgical incision is marked 2 cm behind the anterior superior iliac spine. The surgical field is infiltrated down to bone with 0.25% Marcaine containing 1:100,000 epinephrine. Chlorhexidine is used for surgical preparation of the hip.

The intraoral surgical site is cleaned next with Peridex and a soft toothbrush to debride any gross contaminate. Again, 0.25% Marcaine with 1:100,000 epinephrine is injected into the gingiva, gingivobuccal sulci, bilateral infraorbital nerves, the anterior palatal mucosa, and around any existing nasolabial fistulas. A throat pack is placed and accounted for. Betadine is used for surgical preparation of the mouth and face. The patient is then draped in the typical sterile fashion. Antibiotic prophylaxis with Unasyn is given, and the surgical "time out" is executed. There are two options for proceeding from this point: two surgical teams can start simultaneously with separate instruments,

or the procedure is performed sequentially with attention first given to harvesting the iliac bone graft. Both of these methods help prevent the contamination of the iliac bone graft donor site with instruments utilized intraorally.

To harvest the iliac bone graft, an assistant displaces the skin as previously described while the surgeon makes the marked incision (2 cm above the anterior superior iliac spine), and dissection is carried down to the perichondrium/periosteum. The perichondrium and cartilage are scored with electrocautery such that they can be elevated as a medially hinged trap door flap that can be later restored. The cancellous bone is then harvested. Our preferred technique is to use a trephine drill system. Regardless of method utilized, the cancellous bone is transferred to a sterile container and kept in saline solution. Once an adequate graft is obtained, the donor site is packed with Marcaine-soaked gel foam for hemostasis and postoperative analgesia. Attention is then turned to closure. The cartilage cap and perichondrium are closed with 3-0 Vicryl suture. The deep facial layer is also closed with interrupted 3-0 Vicryl. 3-0 Monocryl is used to close the dermis with buried interrupted sutures, and a running 4-0 Monocryl is used for intracuticular closure. Surgical glue (Dermabond) is placed and the incision can be covered with a heart-shaped nonadherent dressing (Telfa) and then a semi-occlusive transparent film dressing (Tegaderm).

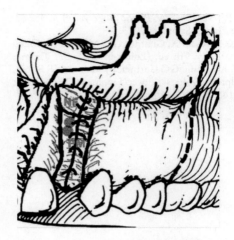

Closure of nasal floor
mucosa superiorly (NF)
and palatal mucosa (PM)
posteriorly

Figure 12.2. Elevation of the flap with demonstration of the nasal floor mucosa superiorly and the palatal mucosa posteriorly.

For the intraoral component of the surgery, an incision is made along the alveolar cleft margins that extends superiorly around any nasolabial fistula. The attached gingival is sharply elevated off the maxilla such that a gingival apron flap is elevated from the non-cleft lateral incisor to the first molar on the cleft side. The periosteum is scored to allow for medial movement of the apron flap and tension free closure (Figure 12.2). A back-cut can be made at the level of the first molar of the lesser maxillary segment; if needed this can remain open and allowed to heal by secondary intention (Figure 12.3). If there is a nasolabial fistula, methylene

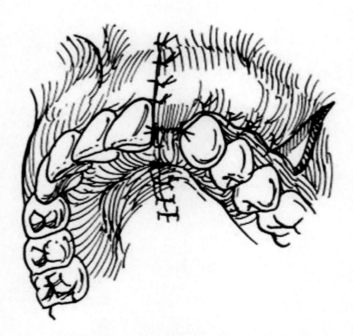

Figure 12.3. Illustration of the dissection of the flap with closure occasionally warranting a back cut for advancement of the gingival over the newly grafted site.

blue is placed in the cleft nostril to help delineate and dissect it rostrally; the fistula is then imbricated and closed with interrupted 4-0 Vicryl suture. Methylene blue is again used to confirm the fistula is sealed prior to placement of graft material. The medial alveolar cleft margins are reflected palatally to form a posterior wall to the alveolar gap. 4-0 Vicryl sutures unite these flaps, with knots tied on the palatal side.

With the deficient alveolar gap exposed, bone edges are mildly scraped to encourage bone graft take and the area copiously irrigated. Iliac crest bone is then carefully placed into the cleft site, being sure to pack thoroughly and include the deficiency in the nasal floor and pyriform margin. Care should be taken to transfer bone such that it is not contaminated by exposure to oral bacteria.

After completion of bone grafting, attention is turned to closure. The gingival apron flap is brought down over the bone graft and sewn back to the palatal mucosa with interrupted through-and-through interdental 4-0 Vicryl sutures. The mouth is then irrigated and the throat pack is removed. The stomach and oropharynx are suctioned, the face is cleansed, and the patient turned 180 degrees for safe extubation.

ALTERNATIVE TECHNIQUES

In patients who have completed eruption of adult dentition, an alternative to autogenous bone grafting is alloplastic grafting with BMP. This reduces operative time and eliminates donor site morbidity. It is our experience that recombinant human BMP with demineralized bone matrix placed prior to eruption of the canines can result in blocked eruption because the tooth cannot advance through the alloplast.

POSTOPERATIVE CARE

Postoperatively, the patient is started on a clear liquid diet for the first 24 hours, advanced to full liquids the subsequent 48–72 hours, and then maintained on a soft diet for 6 weeks. Strict instructions are given to maintain oral hygiene with chlorhexidine mouthwash and gentle tooth brushing. Augmentin is given for five days. Dental and orthodontic work (including expander replacement) is held for 2 months until the bone graft is mostly incorporated. Patients are seen at 2 and 6 weeks postoperatively. Bone graft incorporation is analyzed with a CBCT at approximately 3 months after surgery; results are provided to the patient's orthodontist.

SUGGESTED READINGS

1. Brown DL, Borschel GH, Levi B. *Michigan Manual of Plastic Surgery*. 2nd ed. Philadelphia: Lippincott Williams & Wilkins/ Wolters Kluwer, 2014.
2. Janis JE. *Essentials of Plastic Surgery*. 2nd ed. St. Louis, MO/Boca Raton, FL: Quality Medical Publishing/CRC Press/Taylor & Francis Group, 2014.
3. Neligan P, Warren RJ, Van Beek A. *Plastic Surgery*. Vol 3. 3rd ed. London/New York: Elsevier Saunders, 2013.
4. Thorne C, Chung KC, Gosain A, Guntner GC, Mehrara BJ. *Grabb and Smith's Plastic Surgery*. 7th ed. (Editor-in-chief, *CH* Thorne; editors, KC Chung, A Gosain, GC Gurtner, BJ Mehrara, JP Rubin, SL Spear.) Philadelphia: Wolters Kluwer/Lippincott Williams & Wilkins Health, 2014.

13

BASIC TECHNIQUES IN SEPTORHINOPLASTY

Aaron M. Kosins, Rollin Daniel, and Dananh Nguyen

INDICATIONS

Indications for septorhinoplasty include both cosmetic and/or functional issues. Common cosmetic complaints include a hump, bulbous tip, wide dorsum and/or base, plunging tip, and asymmetry. Functional issues can be due to the nasal septum and turbinates, as well as to the internal and external nasal valves.

During the initial assessment, it is very important to discuss your patient's individual wishes and concerns. Realistic expectations are paramount.

CONTRAINDICATIONS

General contraindications to surgery are likewise contraindications to rhinoplasty. Specific contraindications include smoking, nasal steroid use, chronic substance abuse (particularly of cocaine), and septorhinoplasty within the past year. Unrealistic expectations are a contraindication if the goals, expectations, and/or motivations are not fully understood by the patient as well as the surgeon.

OPEN SEPTORHINOPLASTY

The authors prefer an external or open approach for primary septorhinoplasty. The open approach allows for accurate diagnosis and treatment as the structures of the nose can be visualized. The extended open approach that has been introduced with piezosurgery has extended the advantages to the bony vault as well. The most important advantage for the average surgeon regards tip surgery. In the authors' opinions, the closed approach increases the risk of asymmetry, contour irregularities, and external valve/vestibular collapse.

Disadvantages of the open approach include the presence of the transcolumellar scar. Swelling does not appear to be increased with the open approach. Likewise, the nose can be "opened" in less than 5 minutes by an experienced surgeon.

PATIENT PREPARATION

All patients undergoing septorhinoplasty are started on Mupirocin ointment 5 days before surgery to be used twice daily around the nostrils. Smoking must be stopped 3 weeks in advance. A complete blood count is required.

PATIENT POSITIONING AND ROOM SETUP

In the preoperative holding area, markings are made by marking the desired profile and tip-defining point. After induction of general anesthesia using an oral ray tube and throat pack, the bed is turned 90 degrees away from the anesthesiologist and the head is elevated approximately 15 degrees. A foam donut is placed under the head to allow movement.

Lighting is paramount. One light illuminates the face from above, and a second light is directed to the base of the nose from below. A fiberoptic headlight is recommended as are loupe magnification.

The nasal vestibule hair is trimmed and the external nares are cleaned with Betadine, as is the nasal airway. The nose is then injected with 10–15 mL of lidocaine (1.0% solution) with 1:100,000 epinephrine using a 25-gauge needle at the level of the dorsum, the piriform aperture, the base, the septum, and the tip. The septum is injected in a subperichondrial plane all the way back to the perpendicular plate of the ethmoid. Nu-form gauze is moistened with 4% cocaine solution and placed along the floor of the nose and nasal septum. The purpose of this packing is vasoconstriction and local anesthesia. It is not removed until the septum is approached.

OPERATIVE TECHNIQUE (OPEN)

OPENING THE NOSE

The incisions for the open rhinoplasty approach should be marked and incised precisely. First, an infracartilaginous incision is placed bilaterally following the caudal margin of the lower lateral cartilage. An inverted V transcolumellar incision is made and extends posterior to the medial crura (see Figure 13.1). This incision is then turned 90 degrees and connected to the infracartilaginous incisions. An angled Converse scissor is advanced across the columella between the skin and the anterior edge of the medial crura. A three-point retraction is used with two double hooks and a single hook for ease of exposure (see Figure 13.1). One double hook is placed at the level of the transcolumellar incision and the other in the soft triangle to retract the columellar flap. The single hook is used as countertraction on the ipsilateral footplate. Soft tissue is incised superficial to the lower lateral cartilages, making sure to leave as much tissue as possible on the nasal flap. This plane of dissection can be adjusted for patients with thin skin (subperichondrial) and thick skin (subcutaneous). Once over the domes, the hooks are retracted inferiorly using a 10-mm double hook to complete undermining.

At the anterior septal angle, care is taken to enter a subsuperficial musculoapaneurotic system plane all the way up to the caudal portion of the nasal bones. Once the bones are reached, they are incised on the right and left sides and dissected in a subperiosteal plane. These planes are connected in the midline and dissection is done cephalically to the nasal radix.

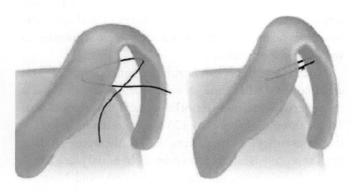

Figure 13.1. An inverted V or W incision is made at the narrowest point in the columella and connected to bilateral infracartilaginous incisions. It is important to make the incision perfectly perpendicular, and we prefer the use of a no. 11 blade scalpel.

EXPOSING THE SEPTUM

Most commonly, a unilateral, right transfixion incision is made and a subperichondrial plane is entered. Dissection is carried back to the perpendicular plate of the ethmoid. The incision is made at the caudal border of the septum, and each side is exposed. The cartilage is incised in a criss-cross fashion with a no. 15 blade and then scraped with a dental amalgam. Once the cartilage is exposed, a Cottle elevator is used to enter the subperichondrial plane. Dissection carries back along the anterior portion of the septum, and then the surgeon sweeps down to expose cephalically. Last, the anteroinferior perichondrium is lifted by sweeping toward the nares from the back.

DORSAL REDUCTION

Setting the nasal profile is the first step in performing a septorhinoplasty. Dorsal reduction is done as planned preoperatively by first taking the bony cap off of the cartilaginous dorsum. Either a pull rasp or Piezo scraper is used to remove this cap. An osteotome is not used so that cartilage can be spared. The upper lateral cartilages are then split from the dorsal septum, and then the dorsal septum is reduced using a straight scissors. Upper lateral cartilage is spared as much as possible and only trimmed as necessary.

CAUDAL REDUCTION

Caudal septal reduction (Figure 13.2) as well as anterior nasal spine reduction, is then carried out if necessary to shorten the nose and/or to make room for a columellar strut. This is done with a no. 15 blade.

SEPTOPLASTY

When it comes to doing septal work, the authors agree that if you are not willing to operate on the septum, then you should not operate on the nose. Resection of the septal body is always done to harvest cartilage for grafting. A 10–12 mm L-shaped strut is always left in place to prevent collapse and saddle nose deformity. Submucous resection of the septal body will help to alleviate most deviations.

A hemitransfixion incision is made through the mucosa of the caudal septum to minimize loss of tip projection. The septum is score with a no. 15 blade and a dental amalgam is used to scratch through the perichondrium and expose the septum. A Cottle elevator is used to lift the mucoperichondrium all the way back to the perpendicular plate of the ethmoid and down to the nasal spine

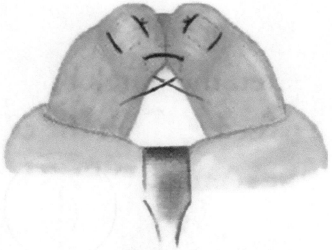

Figure 13.2. Caudal septal reduction is done in more than 90% of septorhinoplasties to both shorten the long nose and also to make room for insertion of a columellar strut. Reductions of 2–4 mm are common. Posterior septal reductions shorten the nose, while anterior septal reductions help with tip rotation.

and vomer. Using a no. 15 blade, a full-thickness incision is made 1 cm behind the caudal septum and back to the ethmoid. The cartilage is then disarticulated out of the vomer and ethmoid bones and removed with forceps (see Figure 13.3).

RELOCATION OF CAUDAL SEPTUM

Issues such as weakness and deviations of the caudal septum can be simplified with three maneuvers: relocation, reinforcement, or replacement. *Relocation* refers to a caudal septum that is deviated off the nasal spine and must be relocated centrally or to the other side. This is done via a drill hole in the anterior nasal spine and using a figure-of-eight suture with a 4-0 PDS. Reinforcement is done with septal cartilage or perpendicular placement of ethmoid bone to strengthen a weak or floppy caudal septum. *Replacement* is done when the caudal septum is unusually weak, deviated, or collapsed.

OSTEOTOMIES

All osteotomies are now done with Piezo saws as osteotomes have proven to be less accurate and are no longer used (see Figure 13.4). Medial oblique osteotomies are used to narrow the dorsum, and lateral osteotomies are used to narrow the nasal bony width. Convexities are rasped down using ultrasonic rhinosculpture using Piezo scrapers and rasps.

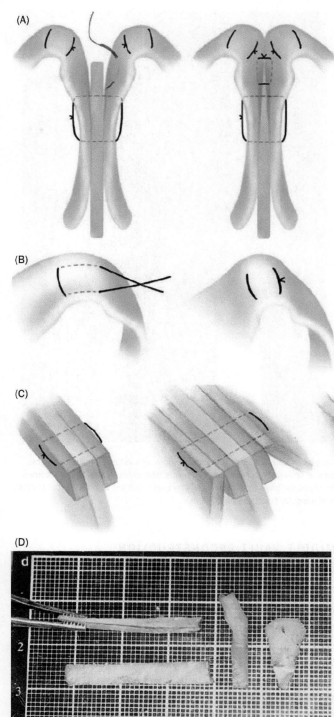

Figure 13.3. (A) A Cottle elevator is used to develop submucoperichondrial leaflets off the cartilaginous septum all the way down to the vomer and back to the perpendicular plate of the ethmoid. (B) The first cut in a submucosal resection of the septal body is at least 10 mm parallel to the dorsal septum *post-reduction*. The second cut is at least 10 mm parallel to the caudal septum *post-reduction*. (C) A Cottle elevator is used to push the septum out of the vomer and finally off the perpendicular plate of the ethmoid. (D) The last maneuver is a septal body resection in gaining access to the septal tail by pushing out of the vomerine ridge.

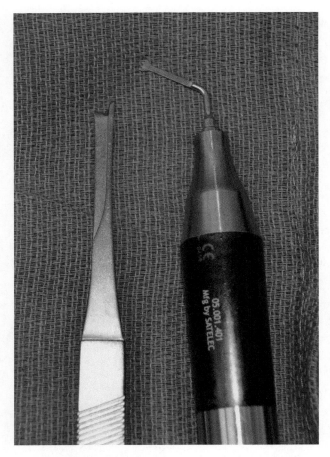

Figure 13.4. Both a conventional osteotome as well as a Piezo ultrasonic saw is shown. We prefer Piezo osteotomies to conventional osteotomes because we have found them to be precise, cutting without mucosal injury and irregular fracture lines.

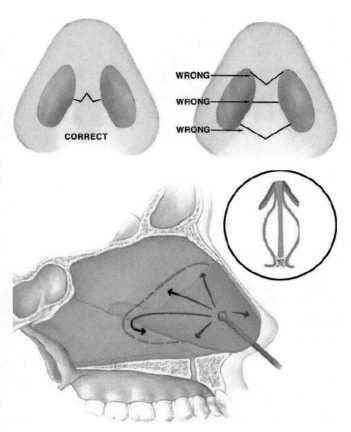

Figure 13.5. Spreader grafts are an integral part of middle vault reconstruction in septorhinoplasty. They are usually made from septal cartilage and help to open the internal valve, smooth the osseocartilaginous junction, and account for any dorsal asymmetries. They are placed on one or both sides of the septum and secured with polydioxanone (PDS) suture.

MIDDLE VAULT RECONSTRUCTION (SPREADER GRAFTS VERSUS FLAPS)

The middle vault is *always* reconstructed if the dorsal reduction is more than 1 mm to avoid internal valve collapse, asymmetries, and inverted-V deformities. Almost all secondary rhinoplasty performed by the authors are in some way connected to a failure of middle vault reconstruction.

Spreader grafts are thin pieces of cartilage that are placed on either side of the septum (Figure 13.5). They help to straighten the septum, mask asymmetries, and open the internal valve. Spreader flaps "turn in" the upper lateral cartilages and also help to stent open the internal valve.

TIP SURGERY

If the external rhinoplasty approach is utilized, a columellar strut of the strong septal cartilage is *always* used. This acts a jig to help build the tip. Cephalic trim is used to decrease the bulk of the nasal tip, and 6–7 mm should always be left behind to prevent alar collapse. Tip suturing can be broken down to four basic sutures (see Figure 13.6). Domal creation or cranial tip sutures are used to create definition of the nasal tip. Intradomal sutures are used to narrow the tip. A domal equalization suture is used to bring symmetry to the domes. Finally, a tip position suture is used for rotation and projection. Concealer grafts of cephalic trim cartilage are often used to camouflage asymmetries.

SUPPORT OF THE ALAR RIMS

If there is felt to be weakness at the alar rims, alar rim grafts can be used to strengthen the rim. These are 12 × 2 mm pieces of cartilage placed through a stab incision in the nasal vestibule. They are nonanatomic in nature and run along the alar rim. Alar rim support grafts are similar but are sewn into the closure along a rim incision. They are more powerful and can also be used to shape the nostrils. Finally, lateral crural strut grafts are placed underneath the lateral crura and are used to strengthen the lateral crura,

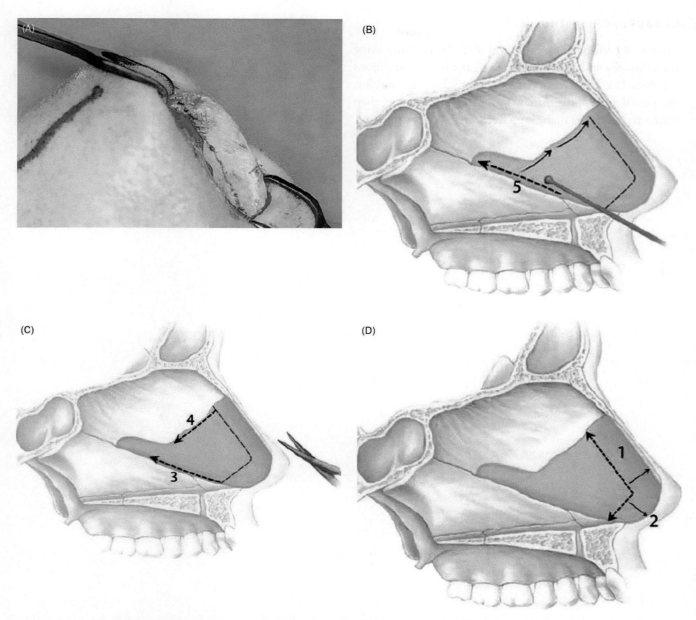

Figure 13.6. The standard tip suturing sequence can be used in more than 85% of septorhinoplasties to create an aesthetic tip. (A) A domal creation suture is a horizontal mattress suture placed at the existing dome to create domal definition in the middle crura and concavity in the lateral crura of the lower lateral cartilages. (B) A interdomal suture is used to narrow the nasal tip and is done by suturing the together above the columellar strut. This can be tied incrementally depending on the amount of narrowing desired. (C) A domal equalization suture is done to bring symmetry to the domes and to narrow the supratip. (D) A tip position suture is done to increase projection and rotation by reattaching Pitanguy's ligament to the anterior septal angle. Not all sutures need to be done for every tip. They can be used as needed.

to straighten the lateral crura, and to support the alar rim. Their use is more valuable in secondary surgery but also necessary in certain primary cases.

ALAR BASE SURGERY

Alar base surgery is used to either narrow the nostril width or nostril flare. Nostril width is determined by measuring the distance between each alar crease. If this is greater than the distance between the medial canthi, a nostril sill excision is often warranted via a trapezoidal excision of the nostril sill. Nostril flare occurs when the widest point of the nostril extends beyond the alar crease. An alar wedge, or Weir excision is warranted to reduce the flare. These can also be combined, and this is often done in certain ethnic populations (i.e., Asian patients).

CLOSURE/SPLINTING

Closure is performed carefully with 6-0 Vicryl suture along the columella and 5-0 Chromic along the infracartilaginous incisions. Doyle splints as well as an external Aquaplast splint are placed for approximately 1 week. The patient is then instructed to tape at night for 3 weeks to decrease swelling.

Intravenous antibiotics are given at the time of surgery, and oral antibiotics are continued for 1 weeks. Patients are discharged home the same day and kept on a soft diet for several days. Blowing the nose is discouraged until the second postoperative week. The final result may be appreciated in 12–18 months, depending on the quality of the skin.

PART III.

BODY CONTOURING

14.

LIPOSUCTION OF THE HIPS AND THIGHS

Hisham Seify

INTRODUCTION AND HISTORICAL BACKGROUND

Liposuction of the hips and thighs constitute a valuable tool in the armamentarium used for body contouring. Whether used as an isolated procedure or in conjunction with excisional procedures (thigh lift, body lift), the suction-assisted lipectomy (the Illouz technique) is here to stay.

The popularity of liposuction attests to its safety and efficacy in the hands of a well-trained specialist. The simple and straightforward concept of vacuum aspiration of fat using a hollow, blunt-tip cannula represents a great achievement in body contouring surgery. Different types of liposuction techniques (laser-assisted; ultrasound-assisted; power-assisted [PAL], Separation, aspiration, and fat equalization [SAFE], etc.) emerged from the original technique, while the original concept is still the same.

As originally conceived and performed, liposuction resulted in significant blood loss. Vigorous perioperative resuscitation, including autologous blood transfusion, was frequently necessary. Guidelines suggested administration of a parenteral intravenous fluid that was three times the volume of the aspirate to treat third-spacing and fluid shifts! For every 1.5 L of fat removal, 1 U of autologous blood was administered. As the volume of fat removal increased, so did the need for additional blood replacement (e.g., 2–2.5 L of fat removal required 2 U of autologous blood; 3 L of fat removal required 3 U of autologous blood). Liposuction, as originally performed using the "dry technique," represented a physiologic trauma to the patient and was associated with significant blood loss and prolonged postoperative convalescence. There was an absolute limit to the amount of fat that could be removed because of the concurrent blood loss. The absolute limit of fat removal was approximately 3 or 4 L, even with a 3-U autologous blood transfusion.

Significant innovations have subsequently occurred, lessening the blood loss associated with liposuction. The dry technique gave way to the "wet technique." The wet (Hetter) technique evolved via the process of "hydrotomy" (Illouz technique), where *hypotonic* epinephrine-containing solutions were used. The wet technique is the infiltration of the dilute solutions containing epinephrine into the subcutaneous fat that is to be suctioned. When an appropriate volume of this fluid is infiltrated, significantly less blood loss occurs during liposuction. As the advantages of the wet technique became readily apparent, the infiltration volumes of epinephrine-containing solutions were increased. As infiltration volumes of these "wetting solutions" continued to increase, the process evolved into the "superwet technique" (Fodor technique).

Finally, as greater volumes of increasingly diluted wetting solutions were infiltrated, creating a firm, turgid feel to the tissue (the *tumesced state*), the "tumescent technique" came to be. The advantage of this evolution in wetting solution volume is apparent by examining blood loss. For the dry technique, 200–400 mL of whole blood is lost per liter of liposuction aspirate. When the wet technique is used, blood loss decreases to approximately 100-300 mL/L. When the tumescent technique is used, a dramatic reduction in blood loss is noted; specifically, 6 or 7 mL of whole blood is lost per liter of aspirate. When this is extrapolated, only 11 mL of whole blood is lost per liter of pure fat removal (Figure 14.1).

The tumescent technique uses the infiltration of large volumes of diluted lidocaine- and epinephrine-containing solutions. The infiltrated fluid is pressurized to achieve a firm, turgid, or hard feel of the tissue. To achieve the maximum benefits of tumescent liposuction, it is strongly suggested that the tumesced state be produced.

The standard infiltration fluid contains between 250 and 1000 mg of lidocaine per liter. In all cases, the standard

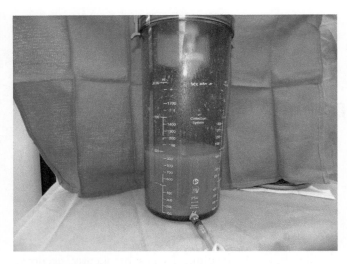

Figure 14.1. Blood loss associated with tumescent liposuction.

tumescent infiltration of lidocaine at 35 mg/kg provides a significant level of safety with a maximum plasma lidocaine level never exceeding 2 μg/mL, which is significantly below the 3–5 μg/mL level at which the first signs of lidocaine toxicity occur. Some studies demonstrated Lidocaine safety using up to 55 mg/kg, but it is better not to exceed the traditional levels due to variation in lidocaine metabolism by the liver.

PREOPERATIVE ASSESSMENT

MEDICAL HISTORY

When considering contouring of the hips and thighs, the primary indication for the procedure is an otherwise healthy patient with localized lipodystrophy of these areas.

Women aged 25–50 most commonly request liposuction of the hips and thighs. However, the procedure can be appropriate for both male and female patients in their late teens to mid-60s and beyond.

A patient history must be taken to determine allergies to drugs (especially when prescribing postoperative medications), previous experiences and concerns regarding anesthesia, current medications (particularly those with anticoagulant properties, e.g., aspirin), and general health, with specific emphasis on the cardiopulmonary system. Although smoking is not an absolute contraindication to liposuction surgery, physicians should stress the negative effects of carbon monoxide and nicotine on blood supply and wound healing and offer their services to help patients with smoking cessation. A general lab panel (complete blood count [CBC], Chem 7 panel, prothrombin

time [PT], partial thromboplastin time [PTT], and pregnancy test) is ordered to address any underlying medical conditions. Electrocardiogram (EKG) and chest x-ray are ordered for patients older than 50 years or as needed.

EXAMINATION OF THE DEFORMITY

A determination of the amount to be removed and the defect that results from subcutaneous fat removal is very important. In patients whose muscle and skeletal structures contribute significantly to these deformities, liposuction can offer only limited benefit. However, for most patients, liposuction can offer significant improvement because the fullness in these areas is largely attributable to excess subcutaneous fat. A physical examination should be conducted to evaluate the thickness of the subcutaneous fat layer in body areas that concern the patient. The skin's tone must also be taken into account because when the volume of the fat is reduced, skin elasticity and retraction is necessary to help lessen contour irregularities and noticeable skin laxity.

Proposed openings (entry sites) for tumescent infiltration and liposuction should be described to the patient before surgery so that he or she will have agreed to having a permanent scar in these locations.

The pinch test is useful in the hip rolls and thighs in determining the amount of excess adiposity that is present and estimating the amount of fat that can be removed. It is important to demonstrate to the patient what can and cannot be achieved. Showing the patient the amount of fat to be left in place gives him or her an idea of the final outcome. When the thighs and hips are evaluated, they should be examined circumferentially; evaluation includes the prepatellar fat, medial knee, inner thigh, anterior thigh, lateral thigh (commonly referred to as the saddlebag), the infragluteal fullness (commonly referred to as the banana fold), the posterior inner thigh, and posterior thigh. These areas should be carefully evaluated and reviewed because they are all amenable to suction.

Suctioning in the banana fold area should be performed only *superficially*. If deep suction with a large cannula is performed here, the supportive structures of the gluteus itself will be weakened and the buttock will develop ptosis, which is often unilateral and difficult to correct.

The posterior and anterior thigh have traditionally been taboo areas for liposuction. However, using tumescent infiltration and small-diameter cannulae, these areas can be effectively suctioned, with minimal complications of waviness and irregularity, to achieve an improved result by circumferential suctioning.

A patient who demonstrates significant cellulite (i.e., skin dimpling from musculocutaneous bands and excess intervening adiposity) must be warned that liposuction is not specifically designed to treat cellulite. However, by thoroughly performing liposuction with small cannulae facilitated by tumescent infiltration, some improvement may be achieved in these patients.

Inner-thigh skin tone should be reviewed with all patients. If a large-diameter (>4 mm) cannula is used, the skin laxity in this tenuous region may be worsened after liposuction, and patients may be concerned with postoperative skin redundancy. Patients with poor skin elasticity must be warned before surgery that inner-thigh lifting procedures may be necessary to truly achieve a tightened skin envelope. The procedure specifics, including cost and postoperative recovery, should be reviewed.

Anesthetic considerations should also be discussed with the patient. The tumescent technique itself is a method of anesthesia and may be used as the sole means of anesthesia (particularly for small areas or touch-ups). Tumescent infiltration combined with intravenous sedation can be useful in virtually all types of liposuction. Our current preference is tumescent infiltration performed in conjunction with local anesthesia.

CONTRAINDICATIONS

Contraindications for tumescent liposuction of the hips and thighs include an objection to the necessary entry site scars for the procedure. Some modification to these entry site locations can usually be performed to allay patient concerns. With the use of small-diameter cannulae, the openings can be as small as 3 mm, which is inconspicuous. If ultrasonic liposuction is being considered, the entry sites become significantly larger (approximately 8–12 mm) because skin protection devices are required.

Patients who are taking anticoagulant medicines that interfere with hemostasis (e.g., aspirin, nonsteroidal anti-inflammatory agents) should discontinue these for a minimum of 10 days (preferably, 2 weeks) before surgery. For patients with a history of deep venous thrombosis, heart valve disorders, or other conditions requiring continual anticoagulation, liposuction is probably contraindicated. Tumescent liposuction is usually reserved for patients who are ASA class I or II, a designation by the American Society of Anesthesiology. For patients in class III or above, consultation between the anesthesiologist and the patient's primary care physician is suggested.

Patients having sedation or general anesthesia require someone to be with them after surgery. They must be picked up, taken home, and cared for by a responsible adult for at least 24 hours after surgery, and they must not operate a car or any machinery for at least 24 hours after surgery. Patients must accept and be willing to abide by these conditions for their safety. Overnight care for the patient in the office, outpatient surgery facility, or hospital setting can be useful, particularly when large-volume liposuction is performed and the patient lives out of town.

Patients must be made aware of and agree with the postoperative convalescence requirements. It will certainly be a number of days or weeks before the patient returns to a relative degree of normalcy. They must be willing to endure this postoperative convalescence period and be realistic about returning to a normal lifestyle.

PATIENT MARKINGS

Patient markings are performed in the immediate preoperative period, with the patient standing. Without careful preoperative markings, the postoperative result for the patient is unpredictable and may result in a high revision rate. The patient should review his or her own markings in a mirror. When the patient agrees with the markings and the location of the entry sites, he or she becomes an active participant in the decision-making process—committed to the procedure. By being an involved partner in the operation, the patient assumes a greater degree of responsibility for the final outcome and experiences a greater degree of satisfaction in the overall result.

The medial aspect of the knee is used as an entry site to access the medial superior and inferior knee regions, but it can also be used to suction the inner thigh. The inner thigh entry site is designed to be hidden within swimwear and can be used for access to the inner thigh and the anterior thigh. The entry site at the trochanteric "zone of adherence," although used less frequently, is best suited to treat the fullness of the hip rolls, saddlebags, and inferior gluteal region. The gluteal crease entry site is best suited to access the posterior inner thigh, the infragluteal "banana fold," the saddlebag, and fullness in the inferior posterior thigh. A frank discussion with the patient about these entry sites accompanied by anatomic drawings is very helpful and will lessen postoperative patient concerns. It is not unusual to use a preexisting scar to access these areas. The criss-crossing method is utilized in all areas to achieve the most symmetric results.

We like to start the patient's drawing by identifying the anatomical landmarks and the patient specific deformity in a 360-degree manner.

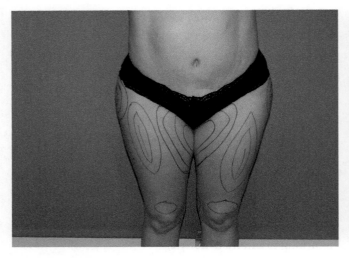

Figure 14.2. Marking of the anterior and inner thigh areas.

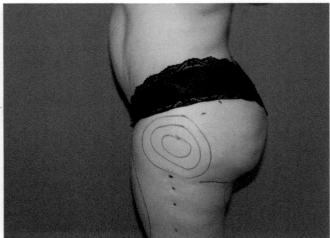

Figure 14.4. Marking of the left zone of adherence, the left lateral hip roll, and the left saddlebag area.

Anteriorly, the groin crease, the medial thigh bulge, the knee bulge, and the junction between the medical bulge and the knee area are marked bilaterally while the patient is standing (Figure 14.2).

Posteriorly, we identify the buttock crease, the zone of adherence, the post thigh lipodystrophy, and the medial thigh excess (Figure 14.3).

Laterally, the zone of adherence, the lateral hip roll, and the saddlebag region are marked (Figures 14.4 and 14.5).

The "zone of adherence" is a landmark at the level of the greater trochanter that separates the hip roll and saddlebag regions on the lateral thigh. This is a condensation of superficial fascia that becomes adherent to the underlying trochanter and defines a very distinct border between the hip roll fat and the saddlebag fat: it is a key point to

be marked and can be used also as an effective entry site to address both of these areas. With the patient standing and the surgeon sitting, the patient is then marked topographically, delineating the relative areas of maximum fullness of the hip roll and saddlebags and then marking the residual area of this fullness anteriorly.

The best entry site in the gluteal crease to address the posterior medial thigh, banana fold, and saddlebag region is selected. If excess fullness is identified in the posterior thigh, this is marked as well. The patient is then returned to the forward facing position and the entry sites in the medial aspect of the knee and pubic area are marked. The pubic thigh crease and the point of maximum fullness of the inner thigh are marked. The medial knee bulge is carefully marked, along with any bulge superior and inferior to the patella. The area of

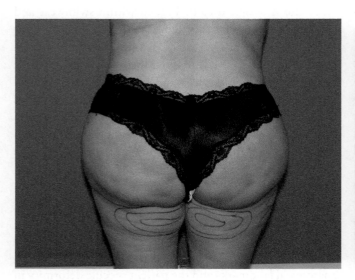

Figure 14.3. Marking of the posterior thigh, the buttock crease, and the zone of adherence.

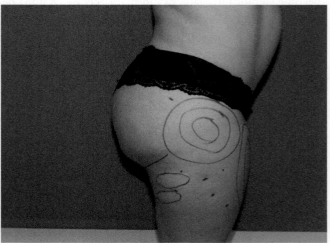

Figure 14.5. Marking of the right zone of adherence, the right lateral hip roll and the right saddlebag area.

BODY CONTOURING

minimal fullness, superior to the patellar bulge and inferior to the fullness of the anterior thigh, must be treated with care. Without careful attention to this area of relative fat deficiency, a postoperative physical depression can result after surgery.

Medial knee fullness should be checked with the patient in the sitting position, which reveals what should and should not be removed. The medial knee should be reviewed in this position, because if only a standing position is evaluated, overresection is possible. If these areas are aggressively suctioned, a postoperative depression can be created, particularly in the area immediately superior to the patella. The fullness of the anterior thigh is then marked, completing the anterior markings. The patient is then turned around with the legs spread apart so that the remainder of the medial thigh marking can be done. Two-thirds of the fullness in the medial thigh is posterior, and this must be carefully identified.

Any points of cellulite, depression, or contour irregularity should be marked and identified for the patient. After completion of the markings, the patient is asked to carefully examine them to be sure that all areas to be suctioned are marked and that the patient agrees with the markings. After the patient has agreed, anterior and posterior photographs can be taken to further document the mutually accepted markings.

The patient should now be weighed. Just as with preoperative photographs, there is only one opportunity to obtain this measurement. Postoperatively, if a patient believes that inadequate fat was removed, weighing the patient often reveals weight gain that is responsible for hip or thigh fullness, which can help address the patient concern.

ROOM SETUP

The operating room table should be centered in the operating room with the anesthesia staff at the patient's head. There should be ample space on the sides of the patient and at the foot of the table so that the surgeon and assistant can freely navigate around the patient. The back table should have the necessary instrumentation, including various diameters and lengths of liposuction cannulae, handles, and tubing. A basic instrument setup to suture the entry sites is required. The liposuction machine is placed inside the operating room. If the syringe technique is used, 60-cc Toomey syringes and Hub locks and syringe cannulae are necessary. If ultrasonic- or laser-assisted liposuction is to be used, the ultrasonic machine, electrical cables, transducer, handle, cannulae, and skin protectors are required. In most cases, one ergonomic cart could host the suction machine, laser, or PAL. This is a great space saver.

TUMESCENT FLUID FORMULATION

The original formula described for the tumescent technique (after Klein) is a normal saline-based solution (Table 14.1). Normal saline is inherently acidic (pH about 5), and sodium bicarbonate was added to neutralize this fluid. Changing the carrier fluid from normal saline to lactated Ringer's solution (average pH about 6.5) obviated the need to add sodium bicarbonate. Another advantage of lactated Ringer's solution is that, per liter, it contains 45 mEq sodium less than normal saline, which is important for postoperative fluid management. Lactated Ringer's solution is considered more "physiologic" for fat cells, which is important when performing fat grafting. It is to be noted that the amount of Lidocaine per liter is 75–100 mL/L in cases performed under local anesthesia. The total amount of Lidocaine delivered should still be 35 mg/kg to avoid Lidocaine toxicity.

Warming the fluid to 38°C, has proved effective in minimizing core body temperature loss and improving patient comfort during and after surgery (Table 14.1).

TABLE 14.1 COMPARISON BETWEEN ORIGINAL (KLEIN) AND RECOMMENDED (HUNSTAD) INFILTRATION FORMULAS FOR TUMESCENT LIPOSUCTION

Tumescent Formula (Klein)		Modified Tumescent Formula (Hunstad)[b]	
Normal saline solution[a]	1,000 mL	Lactated Ringer's solution[c]	1000 mL
1% lidocaine	50 mL	1% lidocaine	25–50 mL
0.1% epinephrine (1:1,000)	1 mL	0.1% epinephrine (1:1,000)	1 mL
8.4% sodium bicarbonate	8.4 mL		

Final concentrations for both formulas: lidocaine, 0.05%; epinephrine, 1:1,000,000.

[a] 0.9% sodium chloride

[b] Warmed to 38°C–40°C

[c] Lactated Ringer's solution is recommended because it is more physiologic, has a neutral pH (6.5), contains 45 mEq/L less sodium than normal saline (pH 5), and the solution is warmed to maintain core body temperature.

OPERATIVE TECHNIQUE

Preparing and draping the field can be done with the patient either in the supine position on the operating room table or standing (Figure 14.6). We use povidone iodine (Betadine) solution, but other solutions can be used as deemed appropriate. After the solution is applied (warmed), it usually dries before surgery begins, thus achieving maximum antiseptic capability. If the patient is prepared standing, he or she sits on sterile towels and is maneuvered into a lying position, and the feet are covered with stockinettes.

Having the patient circumferentially prepared facilitates any position change during surgery without repeating preparation and draping. Sterile drapes are placed so that the areas to be suctioned are completely in view and can be evaluated during the procedure.

INFILTRATION TECHNIQUE

Instrumentation for tumescent infiltration includes a device for fluid infiltration, large-diameter tubing, a handle for fluid control, and several lengths of blunt tip infiltration needles. Creating the entry site can be done with a sharp no. 11 knife blade or by using a punch or an awl device (Figure 14.7).

Tumescent infiltration is performed beginning with the anterior thigh through the medial patellar entry site. Variable lengths of cannula are used, depending on the need, to infiltrate from the knees; throughout the entire anterior thigh, a relatively long cannula is used. Longitudinal strokes allow a uniform dispersion of tumescent fluid to be achieved, which provides a thorough infiltration. Using the pubic entry sites, the remainder of the medial thigh

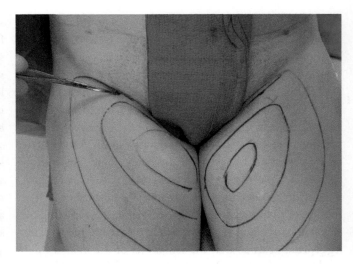

Figure 14.7. Patient set up and access for anterior thigh liposuction.

and anterior thigh is infiltrated. The pubic site is the most common entry site for infiltration and suction; however, when used in conjunction with the medial knee site, it may be less important to the overall contouring and shape (Figure 14.8).

When ultrasonic-assisted liposuction (UAL) or laser-assisted lipo is performed, patients are routinely in the prone position. This is because UAL cannulae are not flexible; they must remain straight, and thus the position is necessary to eliminate any chance of "end hits" or burns. However, the knee-chest, frog-legged, and cross-legged positions (after Mladick) are very useful when performing circumferential thigh liposuction in the supine-only position.

A trochanteric entry site can be used for this technique, but it is usually avoided for UAL. When the patient is turned in the prone position, the gluteal entry site is used

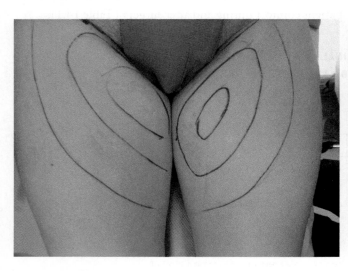

Figure 14.6. Patient set up and access for anterior thigh liposuction.

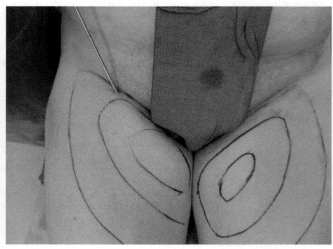

Figure 14.8. Medial thigh access incision and positioning.

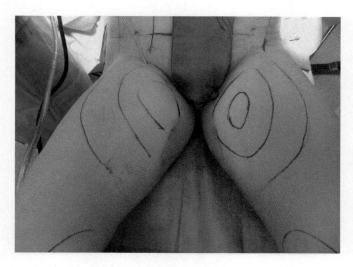

Figure 14.9. Medial thigh access incision and positioning.

to completely suction the saddlebag region, which avoids using the trochanter entry site and creating a visible scar.

In the supine cross-legged and knee-chest positions, the trochanteric entry site is used to uniformly infiltrate the saddlebags and the inferior buttocks, although the major site of entry for the latter region is the infragluteal site. The lateral thigh, cross-legged position is often used when performing circumferential thigh liposuction in the supine position because this position facilitates not only infiltration, but also suctioning of the hip rolls, saddlebags, and inferior buttocks (Figure 14.9). Care must be taken not to oversuction, particularly over the trochanteric area, to avoid a depression.

In the knee-chest position, the hip is flexed and the thigh is brought up so that the anterior thigh literally touches the abdomen. The gluteal crease or infragluteal entry site is used for infiltration and suctioning. The areas that are treated include the posterior medial thigh (where two-thirds of the inner thigh fat resides), the posterior thigh, the infragluteal fullness (banana fold), inferior buttocks, and posterior lateral saddlebag.

Profound vasoconstriction is achieved with proper tumescent infiltration. Although the epinephrine ratio is only 1:100000 we believe that the pressurized infiltration of fluid to the point of achieving tissue turgor does produce a profound vasoconstriction by "internal exsanguination" of the tissue, allowing the epinephrine to be most effective on compressed and elongated vessels. Fluid should be infiltrated until the tissue is firm and turgid, but also until a clinical sign, known as the "fountain sign," that demonstrates adequate tumescence can be elicited: when interstitial pressure changes from −2 cm H_2O to perhaps 100 mm Hg or more, a jet or fountain of fluid from the entry site is noted when

the infiltration cannula is removed. This demonstrates adequate infiltration and is a desirable clinical finding.

Once properly infiltrated, the areas treated should show profound vasoconstriction, blanching, and turgor. The vasoconstriction spreads across the area treated, demonstrating adequate infiltration. We prefer to wait for 20 minutes between the start of infiltration and liposuction. If laser-assisted liposuction is used, the laser is introduced to the field and approximately 5,000 j delivered to each area. It is important to use universal laser precautions (using goggles, avoiding direct exposure to the laser beam, constant gentle movement to avoid overheating of any specific area, care when withdrawing the laser fiber to avoid burn at the entry site).

Liposuction of the knees is performed first through the medial patella entry site. Liposuction of the medial knees and anterior knee bulges is done with, usually, a small-diameter (3 mm) cannula, which allows a great degree of precision and minimizes the chance of waviness and irregularity. A uniform, thin layer of subcutaneous fat is left, which allows for the desired contour and does not create a depression or irregularity. This is done by a thorough suctioning of these areas, creating multiple tunnels without creating any cavity or space. Repeated passes are made throughout this region, slowly and incrementally achieving the final desired contour.

The anterior thigh is next suctioned, again through the medial patellar and inguinal entry sites (Figure 14.10). A long cannula, usually 3 mm or possibly 4 mm in diameter, is used to suction the anterior thigh, treating the entire area of fullness. Longitudinal strokes achieve a uniform final contour and lessen the chance of overresection or demarcation that can occur from using only an inguinal entry

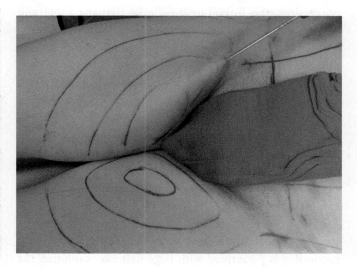

Figure 14.10. Medial thigh access incision and positioning.

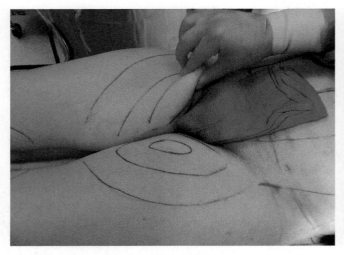

Figure 14.11. Skin pinch test to insure symmetry and appropriate thickness.

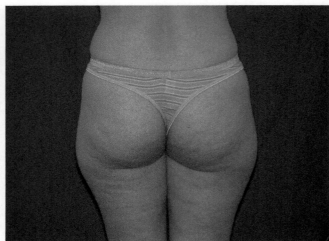

Figure 14.12. Thigh liposuction, preoperative.

site. The medial thigh suctioning is performed through the medial patellar entry site and also through the inguinal entry site. Continual evaluation and inspection is necessary to prevent overresection. As the desired final outcome is reached, this side should continually be compared to the opposite side to achieve symmetry. This must be done throughout the entire procedure, again using all methods for end point determination that are available. These clinical determinations include inspection, palpation, side-by-side two-point tests, and volume comparisons of the aspirate (Figure 14.11).

Hip-roll liposuctioning can be performed through the trochanteric entry site or, preferably, with UAL and other techniques through a buttock entry site in the prone position. If the trochanteric entry site is chosen, this can be used to successfully treat the saddlebag and hip rolls. Through the trochanteric and gluteal crease entry sites, the infragluteal fullness (banana fold) and posterior thigh again are suctioned.

Although the posterior thigh has been traditionally considered taboo, thorough tumescence achieves a magnified deformity that can be successfully treated with small-diameter cannulae (e.g., 3 or 4 mm), achieving a significant improvement in contour, allowing for circumferential suctioning with its intended advantages of circumferential contour improvement, and yet minimizing chances of waviness and irregularity that occur without tumescence and with the use of large cannulae (Figure 14.13).

The infragluteal fullness of the banana fold *must* be treated superficially. If deep suctioning is performed, or if suctioning is performed with large-diameter cannulae, the supportive structures that maintain buttock position will

be weakened. Should this be the case, buttock ptosis, which is often unilateral and very difficult to correct, will result. Correction requires creation of a higher gluteal crease on the affected side, which is difficult to achieve. Attention to detail and avoidance is preferable to attempting a revision in this area.

We prefer not to use drains, and, in patients undergoing large-volume liposuction, we leave a few of the incisions open to drain. In our experience this does not lead to any problems in the healing due to the small size of these access wounds.

The final outcome should be restoring a natural anatomy by removing the excess undesired fat while keeping a uniform layer of subcutaneous fat and avoiding dents and irregularities (Figures 14.12 and 14.13).

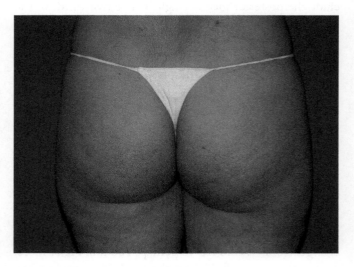

Figure 14.13. Thigh liposuction, postoperative.

PERTINENT DRESSINGS AND TECHNIQUES OF APPLICATION

There are many choices for postoperative tumescent liposuction dressings. Some surgeons use no dressings whatsoever. Most patients, however, find some sort of dressing helpful, particularly in the early postoperative phase. Because much of the infiltrated fluid remains in the subcutaneous tissue, there is a high likelihood that it will drain from one or more of the entry sites postoperatively. This usually subsides in 24 hours. The patient *must* be informed of this eventuality and be prepared. Impervious drapes covered by absorbent cloths are necessary on the car seat on the way home and in the patient's recliner or bed and along the pathway from the bed to the bathroom. Patients *must* be informed that fluid will drain or pour down their legs for 24–30 hours after surgery.

Absorbent dressings around the knees and in the pubic area, such as adult diapers, can be helpful. Other methods of attaching absorbent washcloths or other absorbent dressings around the most dependent areas (knees) may be necessary.

We find it useful to apply the dressings with the patient standing after the early recovery period. When the patient is standing, the dressings can be applied with less difficulty, and body compression garments can be much more easily placed. They can also be placed immediately after surgery, when the patient wakes up.

Patients like to be clean and to begin their normal routine as soon as possible. We allow all of our patients to take a brief, warm shower the day *after* surgery. They must, however, remove their compression garments while sitting. When garments are removed too quickly or if patient is standing, blood will pool, and he or she may become dizzy and pass out. Patients should be warned of this possibility and advised to sit and undress with the help of their caregiver. When the patient can stand without any difficulty, a warm shower can be taken.

The shower should be brief, and all of the patient's entry sites (covered with tape) should be patted dry. The original compression garment is frequently soiled at this point; it should be laundered and left to hang dry. A second garment can be immediately applied, or the patient can rest supine until the original garment is dry. The skin can then be lightly coated with body powder to facilitate sliding on the compressive garment.

The garment should be worn for approximately 3–6 weeks after surgery. If swelling is resolving rapidly, these garments can be replaced with bicycle or workout clothing made with spandex (Lycra). If the patient feels secure with the garments, they may be worn for longer than 3 weeks. The tapes applied over the entry sites should be changed after the first day to a dry adhesive bandage (e.g., Band-Aid) to minimize skin maceration. Postoperative bruising after tumescent liposuction is usually minimal and resolves rapidly.

POSTOPERATIVE CARE

Postoperative care following tumescent liposuction is straightforward. Patients are allowed to begin walking the day after surgery and advance to their normal level of activity as soon as they feel comfortable. A conservative approach must be stressed, however. When the patient is not walking, he or she should remain supine with the feet and legs elevated to facilitate the reabsorption of fluid and lessen edema in the calves, ankles, and feet. If patients are experiencing edema around the feet and ankles, they should elevate their legs and, if necessary, use elastic wraps to gently compress these swollen areas. Postoperative ultrasound, massage therapy, or Endermologie have proved helpful. These techniques are thought useful by many surgeons to decrease the need for revision and to speed recovery. The subcutaneous fat in the immediate postoperative period is somewhat "malleable." If an area is felt to be slightly full in this time period, massage, Endermologie, or other treatments can help mobilize the tissue and distribute it more evenly, creating a smoother overall contour.

Minimal restrictions are placed on patients during this phase, and they are actually encouraged to move to a level of activity that is comfortable for them. Many are eager to resume their preoperative exercise activities; this should be encouraged.

Patients are seen within a few days following surgery (possibly the first day), and then usually at 1, 3, 6, and 12 weeks after surgery. It takes at least 3 months for the edema to resolve; this should be stressed preoperatively. At 3 months, if the patient is doing well, he or she can be released for follow-up either at 6 months, 1 year, or on an as-needed basis, depending on surgeon and patient preference.

CAVEATS

The tumescent technique has dramatically changed, if not revolutionized, liposuction for most plastic surgeons by virtually eliminating blood loss during surgery and the need for autologous transfusion in most patients. Recovery is significantly enhanced and morbidity decreased. In addition to the marked decrease in blood loss during surgery, the tumescent technique magnifies all areas of deformity, which facilitates their correction. By enlarging an area of fullness, tumescent infiltration makes a satisfactory final result easier to obtain, just as magnification of a small vessel or nerve when performing microsurgery enhances accuracy.

Lidocaine-containing infiltration fluid may allow tumescent liposuction to be performed without any additional anesthesia or with sedation alone. When general anesthesia is chosen, the tumescent technique is used in exactly the same way. The lidocaine in the infiltration fluid lessens the level of general anesthesia required, allowing for a much more rapid awakening following surgery and, in addition, prolonged postoperative comfort for patients. The lidocaine remains within the subcutaneous tissue for at least 40 hours following surgery, significantly lessening discomfort and pain medication requirements.

SUGGESTED READINGS

Cárdenas-Camarena L, Andino-Ulloa R, Mora RC, Fajardo-Barajas D. Laboratory and histopathologic comparative study of internal ultrasound-assisted lipoplasty and tumescent lipoplasty. *Plast Reconstr Surg* 2002;110:1158–1164, discussion 1165.

Coleman WP III, Badame A, Phillips JH III. A new technique for injection of tumescent anesthetic mixtures. *J Dermatol Surg Oncol* 1991;17:535.

Courtiss EH. Suction lipectomy: a retrospective analysis of 100 patients. *Plast Reconstr Surg* 1984;73:780–794.

Fodor PB. Wetting solutions in aspirative lipoplasty: a plea for safety in liposuction. *Aesth Plast Surg* 1995;19:379.

Gasparotti M, Lewis CM, Toledo LS. *Superficial Liposculpture Manual of Technique*. New York: Springer-Verlag, 1993.

Gilliland MD. *Mega-volume pressurized liposuction. Presented at the 12th Biennial Congress of the International Society of Aesthetic Plastic Surgery*; September 1995, New York.

Grazer FM. Suction-assisted lipectomy, suction lipectomy, lipolysis, and lipexeresis. *Plast Reconstr Surg* 1983;72:620.

Hetter GP. Guidelines: blood and fluid replacement of lipoplasty procedures. *Clin Plast Surg* 1989;16:245.

Hunstad JP. Addressing difficult areas in body contouring with emphasis on combined tumescent and syringe techniques. *Clin Plast Surg* 1996;23:57.

Hunstad JP. Body contouring in the obese patient. *Clin Plast Surg* 1996;23:647.

Hunstad JP. Tumescent and syringe liposculpture: a logical partnership. *Aesth Plast Surg* 1995;19:321.

Illouz YG. Body contouring by lipolysis: a 5-year experience with over 3000 cases. *Plast Reconstr Surg* 1983;72:591–597.

Klein JA. The tumescent technique: anesthesia and modified liposuction technique. *Dermatol Clin* 1990;8:425.

Klein JA. Tumescent technique for regional anesthesia permits lidocaine doses of 35 mg/kg for liposuction. *J Dermatol Surg Oncol* 1990;16:248.

Lillis PJ. Liposuction surgery under local anesthesia: limited blood loss and minimal lidocaine absorption. *J Dermatol Surg Oncol* 1988;14:1145.

Mladick RA. Circumferential "intermediate" lipoplasty of the legs. *Aesth Plast Surg* 1994;18:165.

Pitman GH. Liposuction: refinement in technique for improved cosmetic results and increased safety. *Aesthet Surg J* 1998;18:455–457.

Rohrich RJ, Leedy JE, Swamy R, et al. Fluid resuscitation in liposuction: a retrospective review of 89 consecutive patients. *Plast Reconstr Surg* 2006;117:431–435.

Scuderi N, Paolini G, Grippaudo FR, Tenna S. Comparative evaluation of traditional, ultrasonic, and pneumatic assisted lipoplasty: analysis of local and systemic effects, efficacy, and costs of these methods. *Aesthetic Plast Surg* 2000;24:395–400.

Wall SH Jr, Lee MR. Separation, aspiration, and fat equalization: SAFE liposuction concepts for comprehensive body contouring. *Plast Reconstr Surg* 138(6):1192–1201, December 2016.

15.

ABDOMINOPLASTY

Malcolm D. Paul

Operative procedures used to change the shape and form of the abdomen include suction lipectomy; abdominoplasty, or the classic dermolipectomy; the modified or "mini-abdominoplasty"; circumferential, or "belt," abdominoplasty; and panniculectomy. The first recorded abdominoplasty procedure was performed by Demars and Marx in 1890. Kelly, in 1899, described an abdominal lipectomy. These procedures have evolved over the course of the twentieth century from operations directed at the correction of functional problems (e.g., hernia repair, which was done with long, often vertical, incisions placed directly over the defect with little or no undermining) to an approach with transverse, more concealed lower abdominal incisions marked by extensive undermining of the skin and adipose layer, as described by Pitanguy with a bikini line incision and by Grazer with a "smile line incision." The introduction of liposuction by Illouz in 1982 allowed the gradual evolution of abdominal contouring into much more than muscle aponeurotic plication and skin and fat removal. Illouz in 1982 described liposuction-assisted abdominoplasty. This technique was further modified by Avelar in 1985 and in 2006, and by Saldanha et al. in 2010, describing a technique named *lipoabdominoplasty* with a more limited area of abdominal wall undermining combined with liposuction. These techniques led to the ability to treat the most pronounced forms of skin and fat excess and muscle laxity. Importantly, a comprehensive understanding of the blood supply of the abdominal wall favored a more limited, inverted V dissection combined with liposuction to allow better contouring while ensuring satisfactory blood flow to the abdominal flap.

In an effort to reduce the incidence of seroma formation, basting sutures were first described by Baroudi and later validated with a large clinical series by Pollack and Pollack. To allow for more definition of the abdominal wall and to minimize tension at the incision line, progressive tension sutures were also described by Pollack and Pollack and others. The most recent addition to the history of abdominoplasty was the development of "high-definition abdominoplasty," described by Hoyos. His technique includes some of the classic steps in a full abdominoplasty along with utilizing ultrasonic energy for fat emulsification, fascial plications frequently performed in multiple areas for better definition, and fat grafting for a well-defined contour.

As patients presented with less pronounced deformities, modifications of the classic abdominoplasty were used to shorten the incisions and decrease operative morbidity. A modified abdominoplasty technique, designed to treat mainly postpartum lower abdominal wall deformities, was described by Greminger in 1987 and by Wilkinson in 1988. The incorporation of the endoscope has expanded the "reach," allowing muscle plication at a higher level through smaller incisions.

In addition to surgical options in abdominal wall aesthetic improvement, multiple energy-based systems have been described to allow improvement in contour with selective reduction of subcutaneous fat. Energy-based options can be performed as minimally invasive or noninvasive techniques and include laser liposuction, ultrasonic emulsion of fat, freezing of fat, and radiofrequency energy-based fat reduction.

The use of fat-dissolving injectables containing desoxycholic acid have limited use because a large volume of injectable agent would be required to obtain a noticeable difference in the appearance of the abdominal wall.

ASSESSMENT OF THE DEFECT

Selection of a particular procedure must be individualized on the basis of presenting complaints, aesthetic goals, and the specific abdominal deformity of each patient.

TABLE 15.1 **FIVE TYPES OF ABDOMINAL DEFORMITIES**

Type	Clinical findings	Treatment
1	Fat deposit, normal musculoaponeurotic layer, no excess skin	Suction-assisted lipectomy
2	Mild skin excess, normal musculoaponeurotic layer, fat may or may not be in excess	Elliptical skin resection; suction-assisted lipectomy
3	Mild skin excess, laxity of the infraumbilical area of the musculoaponeurotic layer, mild to moderate excess of fat	Elliptical skin resection; suture of the rectus abdominis sheath from the pubis to the umbilicus; suction-assisted lipectomy or defatting
4	Mild skin excess, laxity of the overall musculoaponeurotic layer, fat may or may not be in excess	Elliptical skin resection; transection of the umbilical stalk; suture of the rectus abdominis sheath from the pubis to the xiphoid; suction-assisted lipectomy or plicative defatting when needed
5	Large skin excess, laxity of the musculoaponeurotic layer with or without hernias, fat may or may not be in excess	Traditional abdominoplasty; resection of skin from the pubis to the umbilicus; suture of the rectus abdominis sheath from the pubis to the xiphoid; suction-assisted lipectomy when needed

From Bozola AR, Psillakis JM. Abdominoplasty: a new concept and classification for treatment. *Plast Reconstr Surg* 1988;82:983. Reprinted with permission.

A careful analysis of the patient's anatomy, breaking down each deformity into its significant components (e.g., skin and fat excess, muscle laxity) helps to select the best procedure for each individual situation. Analysis includes a classification of the deformity; our schema for classification is similar to that proposed by Bozola and Psillakis (Table 15.1).

INDICATIONS

The selection of the particular technique for abdominal wall contouring depends on the deformity exhibited by the patient. The classification proposed by Psillakis has been helpful to us in selecting the appropriate procedure (Table 15.1).

It is essential to carefully listen to the patient's chief complaint. This may be related to excess skin, excess adipose tissue, protuberance of the abdomen, lack of definition in the waist, or other specific concerns. As part of the history, it is imperative to find out whether the patient suffers from constipation or difficulty in passing urine. Inquiries as to the patient's clothing preference, especially preference for bathing suit style, is important. In addition, dietary habits, exercise, and general level of activity should be discussed before surgery. The patient's height and weight should be recorded as part of the preoperative history and physical examination. Dress size, waist measurement, and pant size are also recorded.

In focusing on the abdomen, the general length of the abdomen and the relationship of the costal margin to the iliac crest region should be noted. In the frontal view, note the spatial relationships between the costal margins,

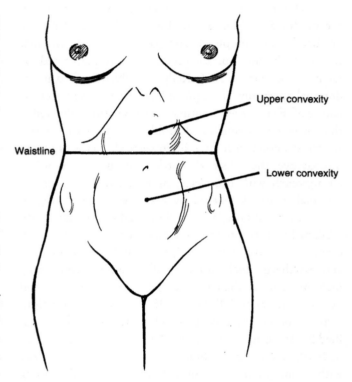

Figure 15.1. Surface anatomy of abdomen. Note relation of xiphoid to umbilicus and pubic area. Waist is narrowest just above umbilicus. Note gentle supraumbilical and infraumbilical convex contours.

xiphoid, umbilicus, pubis, and iliac crests (Figure 15.1). The contours of the abdomen in the lateral view should be considered, keeping in mind the normal gentle curves in the upper and lower abdomen (Figure 15.1). The relationship of the lowest point of the costal margin to the iliac crests determines the waist configuration and potential for increasing definition at the waist. Patients are classified as being either short-waisted or long-waisted (Figure 15.2).

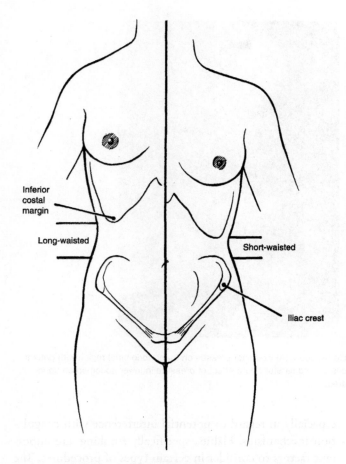

Figure 15.2. In patients who are "short-waisted," note distance between costal margin and iliac crest (R, 5–6 cm in short-waisted persons; L, 10–11 cm in long-waisted persons).

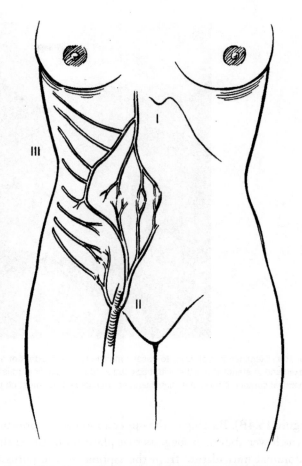

Figure 15.3. Abdominal wall vascular supply. I, from superior epigastric system; II, from inferior epigastric system; III, from segmental perforators from intercostal vessels.

Finally, as procedures are selected, it is crucial to keep in mind the blood supply to the abdominal wall, which has been outlined by Huger (Figure 15.3). The presence and orientation of existing abdominal incisions may affect this blood supply.

The physical examination must be systematic and complete. Previous incisions should be carefully assessed. Examine each patient both in the standing, or upright, position and in the supine position. The supine examination is done to disclose signs of abdominal mass or organomegaly and to determine whether or not incisional hernias are present, if the patient has undergone previous surgery. Carefully palpate the umbilical region to rule out umbilical hernias. Having the patient lift his or her head off of the examining table is helpful in disclosing such hernias. The patient is asked to do a sit-up without using the hands to ascertain the general strength of the abdominal musculature.

Examination in the upright position is probably more important than in the supine position. In this position, the surgeon must note the abdominal contour as well as the skin quality and tone. The presence of any discoloration or striae is noted, along with the degree of skin laxity. The amount and distribution of abdominal fat is also determined in the standing position. The patient is asked to relax, and the contour of the abdomen is examined. The patient is then asked to tighten, or "tense," the abdominal musculature, and any change in the abdominal contour is noted. If laxity is present, decipher whether this is generalized abdominal muscle laxity or laxity located predominately in the lower abdominal region. Absence of the posterior rectus sheath below the arcuate line predisposes to a laxity in the lower abdomen, especially after pregnancy. If laxity is present in the lower abdominal or infraumbilical area alone, the patient is asked to stand against a wall or door that supports the back. In this position, the examiner presses on the lower abdomen to simulate the effect of lower abdominal rectus muscle plication. Enough pressure is exerted to alter the contour of the lower abdomen (Figure 15.4A). While performing this maneuver, the examiner looks at the upper abdominal region to carefully assess any tendency for bulging

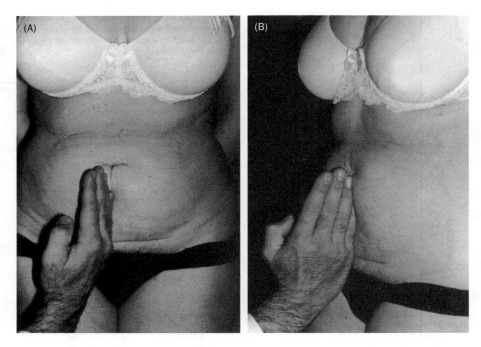

Figure 15.4. Examination maneuver to assess muscle tone and extent of muscle plication. (A) Examiner presses on lower abdominal region with patient relaxed and in standing position with back supported. (B) Examiner must focus on and carefully note effect of pressure in lower abdomen on upper abdominal contour. If bulging is significant, entire muscle layer must be plicated.

(Figure 15.4B). Bulging in the upper abdomen on pressure in the lower abdomen suggests that plication of the entire abdominal musculature from the xiphoid to the pubis is necessary to improve abdominal contour. If, on the other hand, the protuberance in the lower abdomen is corrected by externally applied pressure without causing a significant bulge in the upper abdomen, then infraumbilical muscle plication is all that is necessary to achieve correction.

After careful consideration of the patient's chief complaint, along with an analysis of the abdominal region, the surgeon suggests the appropriate procedure to treat the problem.

CONTRAINDICATIONS

The surgeon must know whether the patient has undergone previous abdominal surgery and for what conditions. Physical examination discloses the particular orientation of any previous incision. The plastic surgeon should also inquire about how the incision healed and whether there was any difficulty with the surgery.

Medical comorbidity should be investigated, including conditions such as lung disease or chronic cough, difficulties with bleeding (as suggested by heavy menses or bleeding after dental work), and any history of previous deep vein thrombophlebitis (DVT). A medication inventory is critical, especially in regard to potential interference with coagulation mechanisms. Habits, specifically smoking, are important factors to consider in certain types of procedures. The development of the Caprini scale has provided a grading system that will indicate the level of risk a given patient may be at for developing DVT. As the Caprini score increases, indicating a higher risk for developing a DVT, the suggestion is made to utilize chemoprophylaxis that would decrease the risk for unwanted blood clotting and the most dreaded complication of an abdominoplasty, a fatal pulmonary embolus. In addition, the surgeon should consider having the patient perform a bowel prep similar to that required for a colonoscopy. This is particularly relevant in patients who have a body mass index (BMI) of higher than 30 and in those patients who will have concomitant liposuction. Decreasing the abdominal fullness by emptying the colon will prevent a heavy colon from exerting pressure on the iliac veins, potentially setting the stage for a pulmonary embolus. This is also important as general anesthesia and the use of narcotics slows bowel motility. When the Valsalva maneuver is utilized to force evacuation of the colon, a clot can be dislodged and become a potentially fatal pulmonary embolus. Patients are not too pleased with this requirement, but they are much more comfortable when they understand why it is being recommended. They also are typically more comfortable postoperatively when they are not suffering from constipation.

TYPE 1 DEFORMITY

ROOM SETUP AND PATIENT MARKINGS

Type 1 deformity is marked by excess adipose tissue in the abdominal region with normal skin quantity, good skin tone, and good muscle tone. This clinical situation is normally seen in young patients. Such patients are excellent candidates for suction lipectomy alone, without the need for abdominal incisional procedures. It is important to carefully analyze the skin tone, including any tendency toward skin laxity, irregularities of surface contour (cellulite), and striae. Additionally, carefully note the distribution and quality of the adipose tissue. Asymmetries of the fatty layer are common. These must be identified and elucidated for the patient preoperatively.

As described by Markman and Barton, adipose tissue throughout the body is arranged in two layers, including a septated superficial layer and a more loosely arranged deeper layer, and separated by the superficial fascial system.

Suction lipectomy can generally be performed as outpatient surgery under local anesthesia with intravenous sedation. This operation has been markedly facilitated by the tumescent technique, which uses the infusion of large volumes of fluid containing epinephrine and lidocaine (see Chapter 13). The procedure can be performed with traditional machine-controlled aspiration technology or syringe aspiration technology. Ultrasound-assisted lipoplasty is also very helpful in many situations, including revisional surgery treatment of areas in which there is significant fibrosis in the fatty tissue, such as the back.

The postoperative routine is explained to the patient before surgery, including the need for postoperative compression garments and activity restrictions. Drains are rarely required after abdominal liposuction, but this remote possibility is usually mentioned to the patient before surgery in case drains are needed.

All patients undergoing body contouring procedures of the abdomen, including liposuction, are carefully evaluated in the standing position. Areas to be treated are outlined directly on the skin, using a skin-marking pen. Areas to be intensely treated are emphasized, and, similarly, areas that are not to be treated are also marked. The placement of incisions is also determined at this point. Our preference is to use multiple small, round incisions, which heal as small "dots" or pock marks. As many incisions as necessary are used since they heal with an almost inconspicuous scar.

SURGICAL TECHNIQUE

The patient is placed on the operating table and an intravenous line is started. General anesthesia or, preferably, intravenous sedation is begun. All patients wear support hose and have intermittent compression devices attached to both calves throughout the procedure as well as during the recovery period. If the patient will remain in the surgery center or hospital overnight, the compression devices are continued until discharge. The patient is customarily placed in the supine position. If the flanks, or "love handles," are to be treated, this is done first, with the patient in the prone position. Prophylactic antibiotics are administered, most often a broad-spectrum antibiotic, such as cefazolin sodium (Ancef), in a dose of 1 g intravenously. Intravenous corticosteroids are not given for liposuction. The surgical preparation includes all the areas to be treated.

The areas of adipose tissue that will be liposuctioned are prepared by infiltrating epinephrine and lidocaine in lactated Ringer's solution to facilitate homeostasis and to allow the procedure to be done in a painless fashion. This is customarily made by mixing 1 L of lactated Ringer's solution with 1 mg of epinephrine and either 12.5 or 25 mL of 1% lidocaine solution. The tissues are infused until they are turgid, or achieve a state of tumescence, which is reached when fluid begins to emanate from the small entrance incisions used for infiltration.

During the suction procedure, the deep fat layer is treated first. Fat in this layer is less well septated and is easily aspirated. The superficial layer is treated next. A consistent and methodical approach to suction lipectomy is required. The surgeon should avoid getting too superficial or performing repeated suctioning in the same tunnel. Cannula sizes ranging from 3.0 mm to 4.6 mm are used for abdominal wall liposuction.

Tumescence allows a relatively bloodless fat aspirate. This improves the precision of the procedure and also facilitates the aggressiveness with which this operation can be performed.

PERTINENT DRESSINGS

At the conclusion of the procedure, the entrance incisions are closed with rapid-absorbing sutures. We characteristically use topically applied nonadherent foam to minimize bruising. This is placed directly against the skin. The patient is immediately placed in a compression garment. Drains are rarely needed following suction lipectomy, but, in the event that they are, a drain may be inserted by attaching it to a cannula to insert it through the incision site.

UNIQUE ASPECTS OF POSTOPERATIVE CARE

When indicated, chemoprophylaxis begins one hour after surgery has been completed and daily at the same time for 6 or 7 days. The patient is left in the compression garment for 2 weeks (day and night) and for an additional 4 weeks for as many hours per day as can be tolerated. Patients are allowed to shower on the third postoperative day and replace the nonadherent foam pads and binder. They are instructed to wash the treated area gently over the first week and more vigorously thereafter, with the idea of massaging the tissues by milking the skin toward the regional lymph nodal basin (i.e., in the direction of the groin or the axillary region).

CAVEATS

Untoward sequelae include waviness of the skin, contour asymmetry, numbness or annoying dysesthesias and paresthesias in the skin, pigmentation changes in the skin, and contour deformities that cause indentations. Extremely rare conditions include injuries to the abdominal musculature or abdominal viscera and injury to the ribs and chest. There is always the potential for pulmonary embolism syndrome, but this is an exceedingly rare condition, and chemoprophylaxis will diminish the incidence of this adverse event. Nevertheless, we mention these potential complications to patients before surgery.

TYPE 2 DEFORMITY

PATIENT MARKINGS

Patients with type 2 deformity have a mild to moderate degree of excess skin in the lower abdomen and an excess of adipose tissue. There is no evidence of musculoaponeurotic laxity. Such patients are candidates for a combination of suction lipectomy and excision of skin excess. The procedure performed to correct this deformity is called "mini-abdominoplasty," which can be performed under local anesthesia with sedation. The use of fluid infiltration to produce tumescence facilitates both the suction lipectomy and the skin excision.

The areas to be treated by suction lipectomy are marked preoperatively in the standing position, using a marking pencil on the skin. Again, areas to be avoided are similarly marked, usually with a different color of marking pen (Figure 15.5).

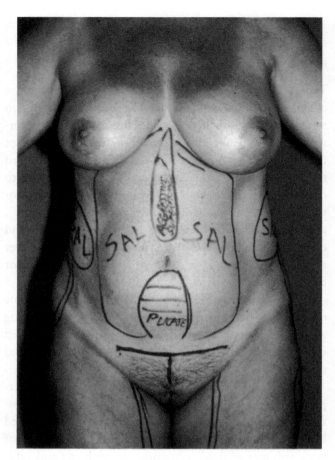

Figure 15.5. Markings for mini-abdominoplasty.

It is possible to estimate how much skin needs to be removed before surgery. With the patient in the standing position, the "pinch test" is performed by the examiner placing his or her finger on the lower abdominal tissue and advancing the tissue in the infraumbilical area toward the pubic region. This provides a fairly accurate estimate of how much skin is to be removed. The length of the incision necessary to remove this tissue depends on the amount of tissue to be removed and whether or not skin folds are present. The incision must be long enough to remove skin folds (Figure 15.5).

SURGICAL TECHNIQUE

The suction lipectomy is done first in a manner similar to the procedure for patients with type 1 deformity. After completion of liposuction, the incision is made along the upper and lower aspect of the inscribed ellipse that was devised from the pinch test. The skin flap in the lower abdomen is then elevated off the musculature toward the umbilicus. Undermining is maintained in the midline as much as possible. This limits the transection of sensory nerves that run with the perforating blood vessels from the underlying rectus abdominis muscles. In some patients, it is necessary to undermine more laterally to achieve adequate tissue drape of this flap. After skin excision, the wound is temporarily approximated with staples. We routinely use a single suction drain introduced through a small incision in the pubic area. This is maintained until it is draining less than 30 mL/day. The wound is closed in layers, with care being taken to close the superficial fascial system (Scarpa's fascia), which is performed with a running 2-0 bidirectional absorbable barbed suture. The skin is closed with an intradermal running 3-0 bidirectional absorbable polyglycolic acid suture. Topical nonadherent foam is again used, and a compression garment is given to the patient with instructions identical to those for type 1 patients. Activity restrictions include a 6-week abstinence from vigorous exercise.

TYPE 3 DEFORMITY

Patients with type 3 deformities exhibit a mild to moderate excess of skin, a moderate to mild excess of subcutaneous adipose tissue, and infraumbilical muscle laxity. Such laxity is more commonly seen in women after pregnancy. Again, careful preoperative evaluation in the standing position, including the effect of tightening of the muscle girdle and simulating the plication maneuver by pressing in the midline of the abdomen between the pubis and the umbilicus, helps to evaluate and predict the effect of infraumbilical muscle plication.

PATIENT MARKINGS

Marking is performed preoperatively for contour adjustment with suction lipectomy (Figure 15.5). The skin to be removed is estimated with the pinch test. The effect of muscle plication and whether laxity exists only in the lower abdomen or throughout the entire abdomen must be determined before surgery.

The maneuver to make this determination involves having the patient totally relaxed and in the standing position with his or her back supported. The examiner exerts pressure in the abdominal region to simulate the correction that will be achieved by infraumbilical rectus abdominis plication (Figure 15.4A). As this maneuver is carried out, the examiner's gaze is focused on the upper abdomen (Figure 15.4B). Significant bulging in the upper abdomen is evidence that plication will be needed in the upper abdomen as well as the lower abdomen. If only a small amount of bulging occurs and if there is a significant adipose layer in the upper abdomen, it is often possible to plicate just the infraumbilical abdominal musculature and perform an aggressive suction lipectomy in the upper abdomen to compensate for the slight bulging there.

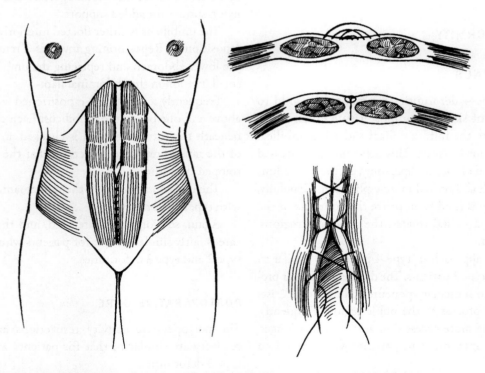

Figure 15.6. Outline for rectus abdominis plication inferior to umbilicus. Note plication suture placement and technique.

The operative sequence is similar to that for a type 2 procedure. The suction lipectomy is done first after fluid infiltration for tumescence. Once again, local anesthesia with intravenous sedation is adequate.

This procedure requires a short lower abdominal incision. Suction lipectomy is done first, using tumescent technique. Next, the abdominal skin flap is elevated off the musculoaponeurotic layer to the umbilicus. The area to be plicated is carefully marked intraoperatively with methylene blue. This marking is important because the tendency is to overplicate when done without marking. Plication is done with an absorbable, 0 or no. 1 bidirectional barbed suture, reinforced with a few 3-0 nylon sutures. The muscle is plicated from the umbilicus to the pubic area (Figure 15.6).

After this procedure, the wound is closed by advancing the tissues and closing the superficial fascial system (Scarpa's fascia) and closing the rest of the wound, all performed with barbed sutures. A drain is placed before completing the wound and superficial fascial system closure, and it is brought out through a small wound in the pubic area. The postoperative care is as noted for previously described procedures.

Representative case examples, illustrating the effect of combining aggressive suction lipectomy with this mini-abdominoplasty, are shown in Figure 15.7A through 7F.

TYPE 4 DEFORMITY

PATIENT MARKINGS

Patients with type 4 deformities are marked by mild to moderate excess of skin and adipose tissue excess along with laxity of both the infraumbilical and supraumbilical rectus abdominis musculature. This deformity is addressed with a combination of suction lipectomy, excision of redundant skin, and full abdominal muscle plication. Generally, suction lipectomy is used to improve the contours of the upper midline abdominal tissues, the subcostal regions, and the waist area.

The operative approach in type 4 patients is similar to that in type 2 and type 3 patients. The difference in their presentation relates to muscular aponeurotic laxity that exists from the xiphoid process to the pubic region. Frequently, these patients have more excess skin and require a longer, lower abdominal incision than patients with types 1 to 3 deformities.

The procedure is again begun by performing the suction lipectomy after fluid infiltration to attain tumescence.

Next, undermining is carried out after making the abdominal incision above the pubic area as inscribed on the skin preoperatively. The skin flap is elevated at the muscular aponeurotic level, and undermining is carried out to the umbilical region. At this point, the surgeon must decide whether to "float" the umbilicus by transecting the stalk or to dissect around it. Dissecting around it and above it requires long instruments, a head light or lighted retractors, and an optional use of the endoscope. If the amount of skin to be removed is minimal, the umbilicus may be floated and repositioned so that the new umbilical position is aesthetic in its relationship to the xiphoid and the suprapubic region.

In these patients, plication is indicated from the xiphoid to the pubic area. This is done in the upper abdomen with a running 0 or no. 1 absorbable bidirectional barbed suture. The suture begins at the umbilical area. One half of the suture runs to the xiphoid and the other half from the umbilicus to the pubic area. A running suture is necessitated by the long "tunnel" created by undermining the upper abdominal area through a short incision in the lower abdomen. Using the endoscope requires some practice, but this instrument greatly facilitates the placement of sutures and the plication maneuver in the upper abdomen when the incision in the lower abdomen is very short. The absorbable barbed suture line repair is reinforced with a few 3-0 nylon sutures for added support.

The umbilicus is either floated inferiorly or it is slightly repositioned. Repositioning involves a removal of skin in the lower abdomen and replacing the umbilicus through a small incision in the abdominal flap.

Frequently, a pain pump is positioned with one catheter above and one below the umbilicus. Each catheter lies just beneath the suture line and is checked at the conclusion of the muscle repair to be certain that the needle has not trapped the catheter.

The incision is closed in the same manner as in patient with type 2 deformity.

Again, suction drains are used, and the postoperative care is fairly similar to that for patients who are treated for type 2 and type 3 deformities.

POSTOPERATIVE CARE

The postoperative activity restrictions and anticipated recovery are similar to that for patients with type 2 and type 3 deformities.

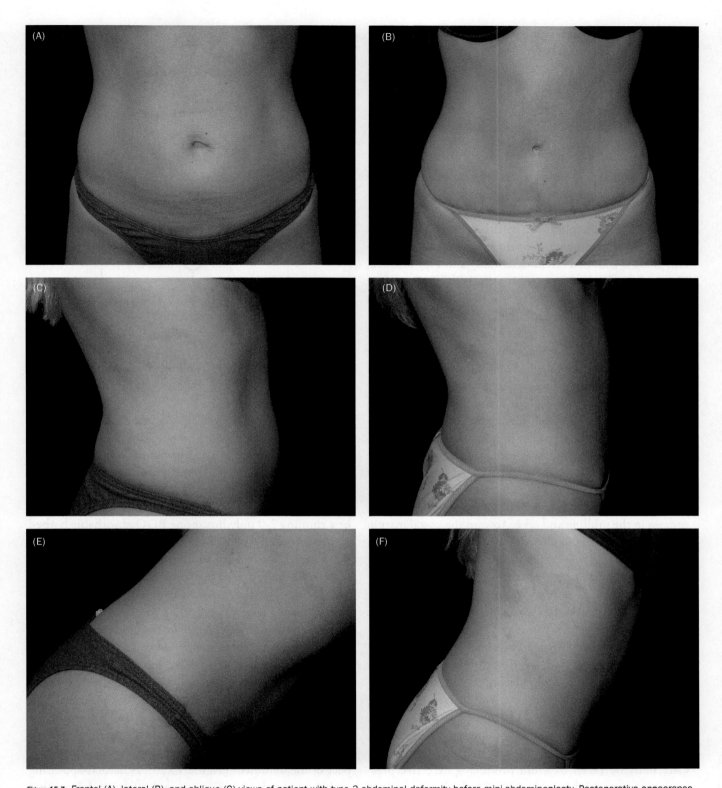

Figure 15.7. Frontal (A), lateral (B), and oblique (C) views of patient with type 3 abdominal deformity before mini-abdominoplasty. Postoperative appearance of patient in frontal (D), lateral (E), and oblique (F) views. Patient also lost 15 pounds.

CAVEATS

Risks and complications include widened scar, sensitive scar, abdominal asymmetry, wrinkling of the skin, seroma formation, hematoma, injury to the umbilicus, injury to the abdominal musculature or abdominal viscera, injury to chest structure (if liposuction is done in the chest region), and pulmonary embolism syndrome. The latter complications are exceedingly rare.

TYPE 5 DEFORMITY

SURGICAL TECHNIQUE

Patients with type 5 deformities require more extensive skin and fat excision, more significant undermining (especially laterally toward the costal margins), and more significant muscle plication, which is best done with full exposure through an open approach. The umbilicus is always incised circumferentially and repositioned. The umbilical stalk is sutured with 3-0 polydioxanone (PDS) sutures to the rectus fascia at the 3, 6, and 9 o'clock positions. This will prevent anterior traction on the umbilicus which can jeopardize its blood supply. An added cosmetic benefit is that the small abdominal flaps have to be sutured down to the hidden umbilicus, which will invaginate the closure. The skin to be excised is normally that from the area just above the umbilicus down to the pubic region. It is possible to make the upper incision first, but many surgeons prefer to make the lower incision first. Tumescent anesthesia is infiltrated throughout the area to be undermined as well as over the costal margins and laterally into the flanks. Undermining is performed at the level of the muscular aponeurotic layer to the xiphoid process in the midline and taken toward the costal margin laterally, but it is limited to an inverted V-shaped pattern to preserve the blood supply to the flap. The extremes of the lateral undermining over the oblique muscles is limited to just what is needed to obtain a nice skin drape and to achieve closure of the lateral skin tissues without a "dog ear."

After complete undermining is accomplished, hemostasis is meticulously achieved with the electrocautery device. Plication of the musculature can be done in a vertical orientation (most common), transverse orientation, or oblique orientation, especially in the area of the waist, or vertically along the linea semilunaris (Figure 15.8). Plication technique is the same as in type 4 deformity. Care must be taken to avoid producing excessive pressure on the intraabdominal contents, which can produce a compartment syndrome with pulmonary sequelae. Pain pump catheters are routinely placed within, but not below the fascial repair. Power-assisted liposuction is then performed of the entire flap (except in smokers), preserving the perforators to the flap, which

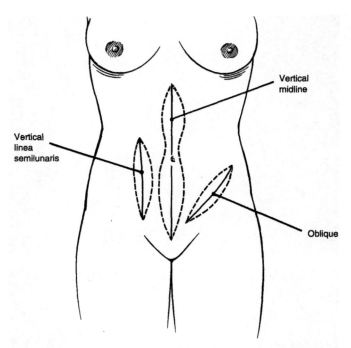

Figure 15.8. Plication patterns for full abdominoplasty, including vertical midline plication, oblique plication, and vertical linea semilunaris plication.

is an inherent component of the inverted V dissection. Then the amount of skin to be excised is determined. This is usually done by flexing the patient on the operating table and advancing the skin distally. The excess skin is marked and excised (Figure 15.9). At this point, multiple basting sutures with interrupted 2 or 3-0 PDS or a running 2-0 polydioxanone PDO absorbable barbed suture is are used to eliminate the dead space, but these same sutures are placed under tension between Scarpa's fascia and the fascia of the rectus, external, and internal oblique muscle fascias to further define the abdominal wall contour.

The umbilicus is replaced in the midline by making a small incision, either ovoid or round, depending on the umbilical appearance before surgery or developing a V-shaped flap and inserting it into a V-shaped recipient area in the umbilicus at its 12 o'clock position. One can also use a technique in which the lateral and inferior aspects of the umbilicus are tacked to the underlying fascia to produce an appearance of "hooding" in the superior aspect of the umbilicus (Figure 15.10). A natural-appearing umbilicus avoids the operative look of an umbilicus that has a circular visible scar. Therefore, invaginating the small abdominal skin flaps to the hidden umbilicus provides a natural appearance. Two suction drains are placed through small incisions in the pubic area (Figure 15.9). Wounds are closed in layers, with careful attention being given to

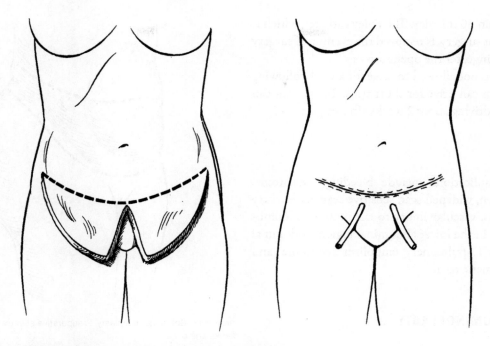

Figure 15.9. Excess tissue from abdomen resected and completed closure with drain placement.

closing the superficial fascia system (Scarpa's fascia), especially laterally. We use absorbable barbed sutures for repair of all of the skin wounds. Interestingly, the use of bidirectional barbed sutures has an accordion-like effect on the closure, decreasing the horizontal length of the wound as an added benefit to the reduced operative time required for wound closure.

UNIQUE ASPECTS OF POSTOPERATIVE CARE

Postoperatively, the patient is maintained in a position with the hips and knees flexed and the back elevated. Patients get out of bed the night of surgery and may resume normal activity quickly. Customary postoperative hospital stays are 24–48 hours. Drains are maintained until they are

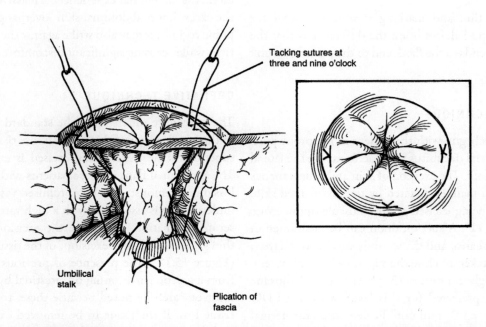

Figure 15.10. Technique for umbilicoplasty with tacking of umbilicus to fascia at three, six, and nine o'clock positions to produce "hooding." (Six o'clock position not shown on left side of figure.)

draining less than 30 mL/day. The Foley catheter, which is used throughout surgery, is removed the evening of surgery or on the morning after the operation.

The patient is not allowed to drive for a week following surgery and then can drive for short trips. The patient can resume normal driving about 2 weeks after surgery.

CAVEATS

Risks and complications include bleeding, hematoma, seroma, infection, widened scar, sensitive scar, eccentricity of the umbilicus, vascular injury to the umbilicus, numbness of the skin in the lower abdominal region, abdominal asymmetry, DVT, pulmonary embolism syndrome, and suboptimal cosmetic result.

BELT ABDOMINOPLASTY

INDICATIONS

Belt abdominoplasty is a variation of the classic abdominal dermolipectomy that incorporates a circumferential excision of excess skin and subcutaneous tissue by extending the lateral aspect of the incisions on each side around to the midline of the back. Suitable patients usually have a large girth and a circumferential excess of tissue.

PATIENT MARKINGS

Patient examination and marking is similar to that for patients with type 5 deformities; the difference is that the skin excision extends to the flank and to the posterior trunk (Figure 15.11).

OPERATIVE TECHNIQUE

The procedure is begun with the patient in the prone position or in the lateral decubitus position to expose the lateral and posterior trunk. The excision of skin and subcutaneous fat proceeds in a manner dictated by the pre-marked skin, with the tissue being excised at the musculo-aponeurotic level (Figure 15.11). A suction drain can be positioned in the posterolateral area, and the wounds are closed in layers, with care being taken to close the superficial fascial system. Absorbable polyglactin sutures (3-0 Vicryl) or polydioxane (3-0 PDO) are preferred for this layer, with 3-0 PDO (Monoderm) or a 3-0 "pull-out" Prolene used for dermal closure and for careful coaptation of the wound edges.

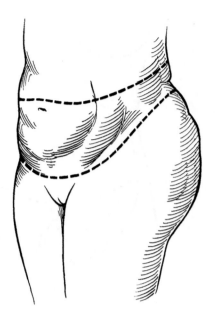

Figure 15.11. Belt abdominoplasty. Preoperative skin excision as outlined on flanks and back.

PANNICULECTOMY

INDICATIONS

This is a modification of a standard abdominoplasty that is used to treat patients with a large overhanging abdominal skin apron, or "pannus," that has caused a problem with skin breakdown or rash in the groin or pubic area. Most often, the patient has experienced a massive weight loss and the excess lower abdominal skin "overhangs" the groin and pubic regions. It may also strike against the thighs as the patient walks, causing significant discomfort.

OPERATIVE TECHNIQUE

The procedure differs from the standard abdominoplasty in that the amount of skin and adipose tissue undermining superior to the tissue being excised is *extremely* limited. The abdominal flaps in these patients with massive weight loss often demonstrate a compromised vascular status, and undermining is associated with a high rate of skin loss and seroma formation. Therefore, the excision can almost be thought of as a "wedge excision" of the tissue to be removed (Figure 15.12). The presence of previous incisions (often from a gastric partitioning or intestinal bypass procedure) must be carefully noted because these, too, predispose to tissue loss. If the tissue to be removed extends above the umbilicus, an umbilectomy is discussed with the patient

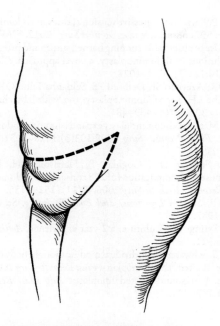

Figure 15.12. Panniculectomy planning. Note that tissue between superior and inferior lines is removed by "wedge" excision with minimal undermining above superior line.

preoperatively and is often performed at the time of the panniculectomy.

The excision of the redundant abdominal skin and subcutaneous tissue is performed from inferior to superior, with the dissection proceeding at the musculoaponeurotic level. Closure proceeds in a manner similar to an abdominoplasty, again with careful attention being paid to closing

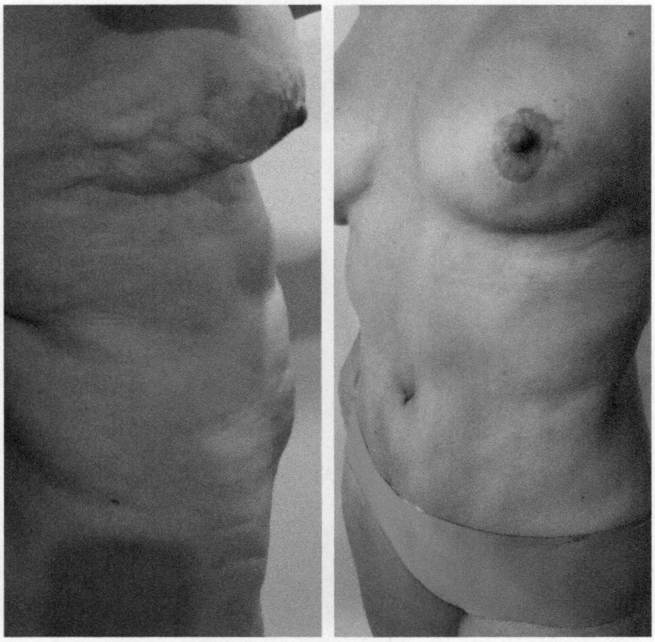

the superficial fascial system, deep dermis, and intradermal layers. Suction drains are always used; they are brought out through small incisions in the pubic region and left in place until they drain less than 30 mL/day. Patients get out of bed the night of surgery and then at least three times daily. The normal duration of hospital stay is between 3 and 5 days.

CAVEATS

Possible complications following these procedures include altered skin sensation, contour asymmetry, induration or lumpiness in the abdominal fat, thickening or hypertrophy of the scar, sensitivity of the scar, bleeding with potential hematoma formation, seroma formation, infection, and the remote possibilities of injuries to abdominal viscera, DVT, pulmonary embolism, and fat embolism. Careful patient selection and preoperative planning, along with consistent surgical technique, can keep these untoward sequelae to a minimum and keep patient satisfaction high.

SELECTED READINGS

Avelar J. Fat suction versus abdominoplasty. *Aesthetic Plast Surg* 1985;9(4):265–275.

Avelar JM. Abdominoplasty combined with lipoplasty without panniculus undermining: abdominolipoplasty–a safe technique. *Clin Plast Surg* 2006;33:79–90

Baroudi R, Ferreira CAA. Seroma: how to avoid it and how to treat it. *Aesthet Surg J* 1998;18;439–441.

Bozola AR, Psillakis JM. Abdominoplasty: a new concept and classification for treatment. *Plast Reconstr Surg* 1988;82:983.

Cimino WW. Physics of soft tissue fragmentation using ultrasonic frequency vibration of metal probes. *Clin Plast Surg* 1999;26:447–461.

Cooper MA. Mini-abdominoplasty. *Plast Reconstr Surg* 1988;81(3):473–475.

Demars, Marx. In: Voloir P., ed. *Operations plastiques aus-aponevrotiques sur la paroiabdominale anterieure.* Vol. 1. Paris: These; 1960:25.

Ferraro GA, Rossano F, Miccoli A, Contaldo L, D'Andrea F. Modified mini-abdominoplasty: navel transposition and horizontal residual scar. *Aesthetic Plast Surg* 2007;31(6):663–665.

Grazer FM, Goldwyn RM. Abdominoplasty assessed by survey with emphasis on complications. *Plast Reconstr Surg* 1977;59:513.

Gremminger RF. The mini-abdominoplasty. *Plast Reconstr Surg* 1987;79:365.

Hetter GP. *Lipolysis: The Theory and Practice of Suction Lipectomy.* Boston: Little, Brown, 1984.

Hoyos AE, Millard JA. Vaser-assisted high definition lipoplasty. *Aesthetic Surg J* 2007;27:594–604.

Huger WE Jr. The anatomic rationale for abdominal lipectomy. *Amer Surg* 1979;45:612.

Illouz YG. A new safe and aesthetic approach to suction abdominoplasty. *Aesthetic Plast Surg* 1992;16(3):237–245

Isaac KV, Lista F, McIsaac MP, Ahmad J. Drainless abdominoplasty using barbed progressive tension sutures. *Aesthetic Surg J* 2017; 37 (4):428–439.

Figure 15.13. 62 y.o female pre and post-op full abdominoplasty for correction of post liposuction and fat grafting deformities of the abdomen and breast.

Jewell MI, Fodor PB, de Souza Pinto EB, Al Shammari MA. Clinical application of VASER-assisted lipoplasty: a pilot clinical study. *Aesthetic Surg J* 2002;22:131–146.

Kelly HA. Report of gynecological cases. *Johns Hopkins Med J* 1899;10:197.

Klein JA. Tumescent technique for local anesthesia improves safety in large-volume liposuction. *Plast Reconstr Surg* 1983;92:1085.

Klein, JA. Tumescent technique for regional anesthesia permits lidocaine doses of 35mg/kg for liposuction. *J Dermatol Surg Oncol*1990;16(3)248–263.

Lee MJ, Mustoe TA. Simplified technique for creating a youthful umbilicus in abdominoplasty. *Plast Reconstr Surg* 2002;109(6): 2136–2140.

Lockwood TE. Superficial fascial system (SFS) of the trunk and extremities: a new concept. *Plast Reconstr Surg* 1991;87:1009.

Markman B, Barton FE. Anatomy of the subcutaneous tissue of the trunk and lower extremity. *Plast Reconstr Surg* 1987;80:248.

Matarasso A. Liposuction as an adjunct to a full abdominoplasty revisited. *Plast Reconstr Surg* 2000;106(5)1197–1202; discussion 1203–1205.

Pitman J, Holzer R. Safe suctions: fluid replacement and blood loss parameters. *Perspect Plast Surg* 1991;5:79.

Pollock TA, Pollack H. Progressive tension sutures in abdominoplasty: a review of 597 consecutive cases. *Aesthet Surg J* 2012; 32(6):729–742.

Rosen AD. Use of absorbable running barbed suture and progressive tension technique in abdominoplasty: a novel approach. *Plast Reconstr Surg* 2010;125(3):1024–1027.

Saldanha, OR, Azevedo SF, Delboni PS, Saldanha Filho OR, Saldanha CB, Uribe LH. Lipoabdominoplasty: the Saldnha technique. *Clin Plast Surg* 2010;37(3):469–481.

Shestak KC. Marriage abdominoplasty expands the mini-abdominoplasty concept. *Plast Reconstr Surg* 1999;103(3):1020–1031; discussion 1032–1035

Stewart KJ, Stewart DA, Coghlan B, Harrison DH, Jones BM, Waterhouse N. Complications of 278 consecutive abdominoplasties. *J Plast Reconstr Aesthetic Surg* 2006;59(11)1152–1155.

Teimourian B. *Suction Lipectomy and Body Sculpting*. St. Louis: CV Mosby, 1987.

Toledo LD. Syringe liposculpture: a 2-year experience. *Aesth Plast Surg* 1991;15:321.

Wilkinson TS, Schwartz BE. Individual modifications in body contour surgery: the "limited" abdominoplasty. *Plast Reconstr Surg* 1986;77:779.

Zocchi, ML. Ultrasound-assisted lipoplasty. *Adv Plast Reconstr Surg* 1995;11:197–221.

16.

BASIC TECHNIQUES OF FAT GRAFTING

Shaili Gal and Lee L. Q. Pu

INTRODUCTION

Fat grafting has been utilized for more than 100 years. Illouz reported the transfer of liposuction aspirate fat in 1984 and in 1986; Ellenbogen reported the use of free pearl fat autografts in a variety of atrophic and posttraumatic facial deficits.[1] Due to its abundance and biocompatibility, as well as being readily available, autologous fat transfer has become a popular method for soft tissue augmentation. While fat grafting has become more mainstream, the overall fat graft survival rate still remains about 50% in most reports, continuing to perplex clinicians as well as scientists.[2] Therefore, fat grafting technique has been refined and studied in order to achieve higher graft survival or "take" in a recipient site.

While there is much interest in fat grafting for different applications, there is still a lack of standardization to the technique.[3,4] Furthermore, different recipient sites require different methods of grafting technique. In this chapter, we describe a more rationalized approach to fat grafting that could be applied to diverse purposes and potentially yield the best results in terms of fat graft viability for each patient's specific needs.

ASSESSMENT OF THE DEFECT: CLASSIFICATIONS FOR FAT GRAFTING

Each fat grafting candidate should be approached on an individual basis and the basic technique tailored to the specific patient's needs and his or her specific deformity or cosmetic goal.

Fat grafting can be classified into three categories based on the volume needed: small-volume fat grafting (<100 mL), large-volume fat grafting (100–200 mL), and mega-volume fat grafting (>300 mL) are the three main categories. The fat grafting technique utilized should be based on the patient's unique requirements. For example, small-volume fat grafting is mainly used for facial rejuvenation, large-volume grafting primarily for breast and body contouring, and mega-volume grafting for buttock or breast augmentation as well as for reconstruction.[5]

INDICATIONS

After a full history and physical exam, fat grafting can be undertaken for soft tissue augmentation in various areas of the body. In addition, it has also been used as a regenerative approach for improvement of burn scars as well as irradiated tissue and chronic wounds. It is used to improve tissue atrophy from aging as well as for cosmetic enhancement.

CONTRAINDICATIONS

Most contraindications are relative, not absolute, and maintain that the patient doesn't have any major comorbidities withholding him or her from undergoing general anesthesia or disease processes that impede wound healing. Another relative contraindication is patients who are too thin and don't have enough adipose tissue available for fat grafting. It is important to realize that some reconstruction patients may not want to have another procedure performed on an additional part of their body in order to harvest fat grafts. In addition, it is still controversial to utilize autologous fat grafting augmentation in a breast that has a prior history of partial mastectomy for cancer.

SURGICAL TECHNIQUE

The basic fat grafting procedure can be arbitrarily divided into four parts: donor site selection, harvesting, processing, and placement.

ROOM SETUP AND PATIENT MARKINGS

Each patient will be marked on an individual basis based on location of donor site and recipient site to be grafted. The patient should be evaluated in the standing position preoperatively

In general, the donor area is outlined directly on the skin using a skin marking pen, as is the area to be grafted. Placement of incisions for cannula insertion can also be determined at this point to assure ease of tunneling (Figure 16.1A, B).

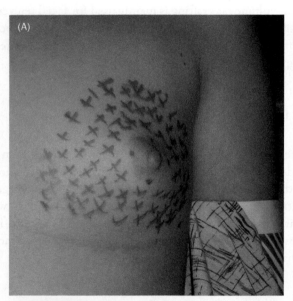

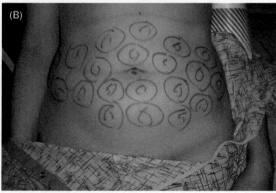

Figure 16.1. (A) Preoperative marking for fat grafting recipient site of the breast shows areas for fat graft placement and periareolar and lateral inframammary entrance sites for fat graft injection. (B) Preoperative marking for fat grafting donor site of the abdomen shows areas for fat graft donor sites and periumbilical entrance sites for fat graft harvest.

The room should be able to facilitate general anesthesia as well as have all equipment available for the fat grafting procedure.

BASIC CONSIDERATIONS FOR FAT GRAFTING

Anesthesia

Fat graft harvesting can be performed under general, epidural, or local anesthesia with or without sedation. Intravenous sedation is routinely used along with regional or local anesthesia if requested by the patient. As far as the tumescent solution used for the donor site fat graft harvesting, the lowest concentration of lidocaine should be used because in high concentration it may have a detrimental effect on adipocyte function and viability.

The author prefers 0.03% of lidocaine in lactated Ringer's if the procedure is performed under general anesthesia. Otherwise, 0.04% if the procedure is to be performed under local anesthesia with or without sedation.[2] Again, a higher concentration of lidocaine may have toxic effects on adipocytes and thus should be avoided.[6] The tumescent solution also contains epinephrine with a concentration of 1:1,000,000.

Donor Site Selection

Donor sites are usually selected based on ease of accessibility from a supine position and contour enhancement. While fat graft viability is considered equal from all sites, it was shown in one study that the number of adipose-derived stem cells (ADSCs) is highest in the lower abdomen and inner thighs.[7,8] These are therefore good choices for donor fat graft sites. Both of these locations are easily accessible from the supine position and are scientifically sound, as long as enough adipose tissue is located there. For mega-volume harvesting, the patient can be placed in prone position in order to gain access to the posterior medial thigh, lateral thigh, and flank. The palm and pinch test should be utilized to assess how much fat can be harvested and to decide if there is adequate fat reserve in a particular location. A palm is roughly measured as 200 cm², and the pinch test estimates the layer of thickness that can be harvested from a site.[9]

Fat Graft Harvesting

Syringe aspiration should be considered the method of choice for harvesting fat grafts since it is relatively less traumatic. However, this method can be time-consuming.

Small-Volume Harvesting

Placement of incisions can be made with a no. 11 blade in a location where the scar will be easily concealed. Inducing tumescence and harvesting can be done via the same incisions. The incision is typically 2–3 mm and should be dilated using a tenotomy scissor. The tumescence solution is then infiltrated about 10–15 minutes before fat harvesting commences to allow for adequate vasoconstriction and greater fat harvesting ease. The ratio of tumescent to lipoaspirate should be 1:1.

We recommend a 10 mL Luer-Lok syringe connected to a harvesting cannula. This is less cumbersome in hand. The harvesting cannula should be a 15-cm-long blunt-tip cannula with dual openings in the shape of a bucket handle. The plunger should be gently pulled back to create negative pressure in the syringe (Figure 16.2). Fluid that collects within the syringe can be pushed out from the syringe by placing it in a vertical position. Once harvesting is complete, all incision sites are closed with 6-0 interrupted suture.[2]

Large- or Mega-Volume Harvesting

Lower aspiration pressure (<250 mm Hg) is preferred for large-volume or mega-volume harvesting since it may yield more viable adipocytes according to one study.[10] Khouri et al. designed a constant low-pressure vacuum (300 mm Hg) liposuction with a specially designed device to harvest the fat graft at a constant low pressure through rolled ribbon springs. The fat can then be centrifuged at low G forces (15 G for 2–3 minutes) using a hand-cranked centrifuge for mega-volume fat graft harvest and processing.[9] Additionally, the newly designed harvesting cannula by Khouri may be more efficient to use and cause less trauma to adipocytes with its 12-gauge, 12-hole design (Figure 16.3).

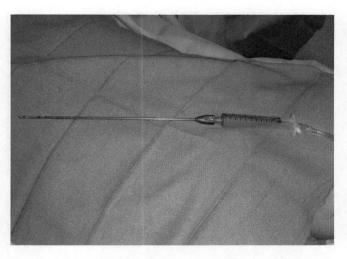

Figure 16.3. A newly designed Khouri cannula with multiple side holes for large- or mega-volume fat graft harvest.

Fat Graft Processing

Many methods exist for fat graft processing, and this may be the most controversial part of the fat grafting procedure. Some of the more common techniques include centrifugation, filtration, or gravity sedimentation. The authors' preferred method is centrifugation, as proposed by Coleman.[11] Studies show that centrifugation with a force of 50 g for 2 minutes will yield more viable adipocytes at the bottom of the middle layer, leading to easier manipulation of the fat grafts for use.[12,13] Recent studies have shown that centrifugation can concentrate ADSCs as well as several angiogenic growth factors.[14,15] Since both of these factors correlate with improved fat graft survival, centrifugation at 3,000 rpm (about 1,200 G) for 3 minutes should be the method of choice for fat graft processing, more so for small-volume fat grafting.[12]

Centrifugation

At the completion of fat harvesting, the Luer-Lok aperture of the 10 mL syringe is locked with a plug. After removal of the plunger, all lipoaspirate-filled syringes are placed in a centrifuge at 3,000 rpm (about 1,200 G) for 3 minutes. During this process, it is important to avoid fat graft exposure to air and bacterial contamination. After centrifugation, the lipoaspirate is divided into three layers: the oil content in the upper layer, fatty tissue in the middle layer, and a fluid portion at the bottom (Figure 16.4). The oil should be decanted from the Luer-Lok syringe. The fluid at the bottom will be easily drained once the plug is removed. The concentrated fat can thus be placed in a 1 mL syringe (the authors' preferred size) with an adapter. Air bubbles from within the syringe should be removed so the amount injected can be quantified and correctly recorded.

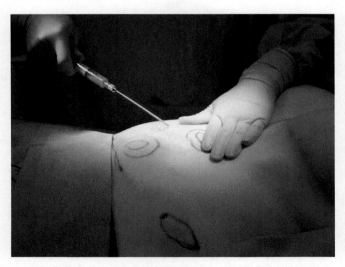

Figure 16.2. An intraoperative view shows fat graft harvesting technique: back- and-forth movement with a 10 mL syringe and a 2 mL space vacuum of negative pressure, and fat grafts are aspirated into the syringe.

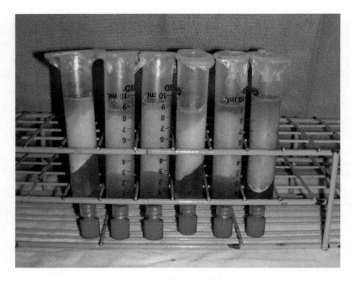

Figure 16.4. Syringes are placed after centrifugation at 3,000 rpm for 3 minutes. Three layers are formed: the upper layer, oil; middle layer, fat grafts; and the lower layer, liquid.

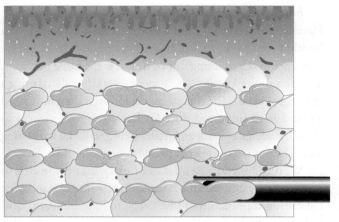

Figure 16.5. A schematic diagram shows proper technique of fat graft injection. Placement of minuscule amounts of fat grafts with each pass as the cannula is withdrawn. Fat grafts should be placed with multiple passes but in multiple tissue planes and tunnels.

Filtration or Gravity Sedimentation

Several studies failed to prove the superiority of filtration or gravity sedimentation in fat graft processing as compared to centrifugation. Fat grafts processed with filtration or sedimentation may contain many inflammatory mediators in comparison to processing with proper centrifugation.[2,16,17] Thus, centrifugation should be utilized even for large- or mega-volume fat grafting, as advocated by Khouri, utilizing a hand-held cranked centrifuge at 15 G for 2–3 minutes.[9]

Placement of Fat Grafts

Fat graft survival depends on maximal contact with the recipient site in order to achieve imbibition and neovascularization; hence, it is important to evenly distribute the fat grafts upon placement. Since grafting a small amount per pass will not only lead to a better aesthetic outcome but also result in less complications including fibrosis, oil cyst formation, calcification, and even infection, this is preferred to large bolus grafting. Thus, a small volume (no more than 0.1 mL) should be injected with each pass at a slow rate of 0.5–1.0 mL/s during the withdrawal phase to lessen trauma to the adipocytes. Furthermore, the fat grafts should be placed with multiple passes in multiple tissue planes and tunnels in multiple directions (Figure 16.5). Inject gently to avoid possible injury to vessels or nerves.

Injection cannulas range from 20- to 12-gauge in diameter and vary in length and shape according to the volume of the area to be grafted. The tip of the cannula is usually blunt and has one opening on the side. For facial procedures, cannula length is usually between 5 and 9 cm, while a length of 9 to 15 cm is used for body procedures. Additionally, cannulas may be curved or straight or have a blunt or a forked tip that can cut through more fibrotic tissues. It is important to remain conscientious of where the cannula tip is throughout the entire injection process so as not to inadvertently cause injury to the patient.

For large- or mega-volume grafting, the principles remain the same, but a larger volume (1 mL of fat grafts) can be injected with each pass since the recipient site is much larger. Fat boluses, especially with larger injected volumes, should be carefully avoided to assure better outcome and prevent fat necrosis (Figure 16.6).

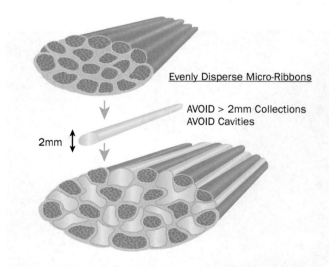

Figure 16.6. A schematic diagram shows proper technique of fat graft placement within the tissue. No more than 2 mm placement in each pass should be performed, and placement of fat grafts into cavities should also be avoided.

POSTOPERATIVE CARE AND PERTINENT DRESSINGS

Patients should be informed that swelling in the recipient site is normal and may last for 1–2 weeks postoperatively and that these areas can become firm and hard during these first few weeks. In the face, swelling may last up to 6 weeks. During recovery, ice packs, tight compression garments, or massage of the grafted area should be avoided because this may compromise viability and ultimate outcome. Otherwise, dressing over grafted areas may provide some relief to these areas and prevent patients from pressing or touching these areas (Figure 16.7A, B). Direct trauma and shear force should be avoided as well in order to improve fat graft survival.

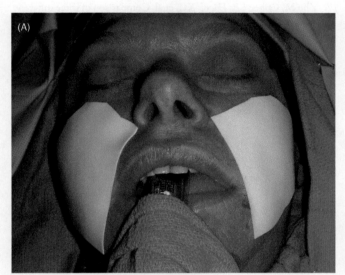

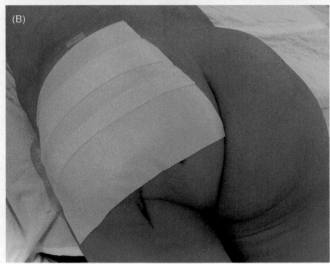

Figure 16.7. Taping the injected area for immediate postoperative care after fat grafting to avoid shear force on the placed fat grafts. (A) After small-volume facial fat grafting. (B) After large-volume fat grafting for buttock augmentation.

Abdominal binders and compressive dressings should be applied to the donor sites.

SUBSEQUENT PROCEDURES

Assessment of results can usually be done at 4–6 weeks post fat grafting procedure. This time frame allows for the swelling to go down and is also dependent upon the volume grafted. Since overall fat graft "take" ranges from 50% to 90% in even the most experienced of hands, additional procedures are most likely necessary to achieve the desired result. There is no specific study that has addressed the timing of these procedures; rather, only expert opinion exists within the literature regarding this topic. The authors have observed that it usually takes 3 months for the transplanted fat to stabilize postoperatively. Thus the timing for subsequent fat grafting procedures should be deferred at least 3–6 months from the initial fat grafting procedure. This also allows time to minimize the effect of the inflammatory response in the grafted area.

CAVEATS

Risks and complications include all possible untoward sequelae related to lipoaspirate harvesting as well as grafting. These include bleeding, infection, scarring, asymmetry, loss of fat volume over time, increase of fat volume due to weight gain, possible need for future treatments to achieve desired effect, firmness or lumpiness, contour deformity of donor site, loss of skin or tissue in the treated area, fat embolism, accidental intravascular injection causing arterial embolism, formation of cysts, deep vein thrombosis, pulmonary embolism, and even death. While the latter complications are exceedingly rare, they should all be included in the consent the patient will sign preoperatively.

DISCLOSURE

The authors have no financial interests in any of the drugs, products, or devices mentioned in this article.

REFERENCES

1. Rinker BD, Vyas KS. Do stem cells have an effect when we fat graft? Fat versus fiction. *Ann Plast Surg* 2015.

2. Lin JY, Wang C, Pu LL. Can we standardize the techniques for fat grafting? *Clin Plastic Surg* 2015;42:199–208.
3. Kaufman MR, Bradley JP, Dickinson B, et al. Autologous fat transfer national consensus survey: trends in techniques for harvest, preparation, and application, and perception of short- and long-term results. *Plast Reconstr Surg* 2007;119:323–331.
4. Kaufman MR, Miller TA, Huang C, et al. Autologous fat transfer for facial recontouring: is there science behind the art? *Plast Reconstr Surg* 2007;119:2287–2296.
5. Del Vecchio D, Rohrich RJ. A classification of clinical fat grafting: different problems, different solutions. *Plast Reconstr Surg* 2012;130:511–522.
6. Keck M, Zeyda M, Gollinger K, et al. Local anesthetics have a major impact on the viability of preadipocytes and their differentiation into adipocytes. *Plast Reconstr Surg* 2010;123:1500–1505.
7. Padoin AV, Braga-Silva J, Martins P, et al. Sources of processed lipoaspirate cells: influence on donor site on cell concentration. *Plast Reconstr Surg* 2008;122:614–618.
8. Geissler PJ, Davis K, Roostaeian J, et al. Improving fat transfer viability: the role of aging, body mass index and harvest site. *Plast Reconstr Surg* 2014;134:227–232.
9. Khouri RK, Rigotti G, Cardoso E, et al. Megavolume autologous transfer: part II. Practice and techniques. *Plast Reconstr Surg* 2014;133:1369–1377.
10. Cheriyan T, Kao HK, Qiao X, et al. Low harvest pressure enhances autologous fat graft viability. *Plast Reconstr Surg* 2014;133:1365–1368.
11. Pu LL, Coleman SR, Cui X, et al. Autologous fat grafts harvested and refined by the Coleman technique: a comparative study. *Plast Reconstr Surg* 2008;122:932–937.
12. Boscher MT, BeeCKert BW, Puckett CL, et al. Analysis of lipocyte viability after liposuction. *Plast Reconstr Surg* 2002;109:761–765.
13. Pu LL, Cui X, Fink BF, et al. The viability of fatty tissue within adipose aspirates after conventional liposuction: a comprehensive study. *Ann Plast Surg* 2005;54:288–292.
14. Kurita M, Matsumoto D, Shigeura T, et al. Influences of centrifugation on cells and tissues in liposuction aspirates: optimized centrifugation for lipotransfer and cell isolation. *Plast Reconstr Surg* 2008;121:1033–1041.
15. Pallua N, Pulsfort AK, Suschek C, et al. Content of the growth factors bFGF, IGF-1, VEGF, and PDGF-BB in freshly harvested lipoaspirate after centrifugation and incubation. *Plast Reconstr Surg* 2009;123:826–833.
16. Ansorge H, Garza JR, McCormack MC, et al. Autologous fat processing via Revolve system: quality and quantity of fat retention evaluated in an animal model. *Aesthet Surg J* 2014;34:438–447.
17. Zhu M, Cohen SR, Hicok KC, et al. Comparison of three different fat graft preparation methods: gravity separation, centrifugation, and simultaneous washing and filtration in a closed system. *Plast Reconstr Surg* 2013;131:873–880.

17.

BODY CONTOURING AFTER WEIGHT LOSS

Dalit Amar and J. Peter Rubin

INTRODUCTION

Body contouring following massive weight loss (MWL) is a constantly evolving subspecialty of plastic surgery, fueled by the obesity epidemic and successful outcomes from bariatric surgery. MWL patients represent a unique population that differs from typical aesthetic body contouring patients. Preoperative evaluation of this unique cohort must take into account complex medical and psychosocial issues associated with obesity, and operative planning requires unique strategies.

The goal of this chapter is to provide a comprehensive approach to management of MWL patients. The topics covered include the medical impact of obesity and the rise in bariatric surgical procedures that has increased the demand for plastic surgical reconstruction after MWL, critical factors for consideration in the preoperative evaluation of the MWL patient presenting for body contouring surgery, essential elements of intraoperative patient management, and a framework for deciding when to combine multiple procedures and when to perform them in separate stages.

OBESITY AND IMPACT OF BARIATRIC SURGERY

Overweight and *obesity* refer to ranges of weight that are greater than what is generally considered healthy for a given height. The key measurement for categorizing obesity is the body mass index (BMI).[1] According to the World Health Organization (WHO), overweight is defined as a BMI between 25 and 29.99 kg/m²; obesity is further categorized to obese class I (BMI between 30 and 34.99 kg/m²), obese class II (BMI between 35 and 39.99 kg/m², formerly known as severe obesity), and obese class III (BMI >40 kg/m²,

formerly known as morbid obesity)[2]. Modifications to the classification have been added, including the categories of super obese (50–60 kg/m²) and super, super obese (>60 kg/m²).[3] According to the 2015 data from the Centers for Disease Control and Prevention (CDC), more than one-third (34.9% or 78.6 million) of US adults are obese.[4] Worldwide, the World Obesity Federation estimates that overweight and obesity prevalence is 27.5% among men, 35.8% among women, 32.1% among boys, and 33.7% among girls.[5]

Obesity is an independent risk factor not only for all-cause mortality but also for major diseases including coronary heart disease, type 2 diabetes mellitus, hypertension, hyperlipidemia, obstructive sleep apnea (OSA), gastroesophageal reflux disease (GERD), certain malignancies, and musculoskeletal disorders such as osteoarthritis.[6] One cannot ignore the significant psychosocial impact of obesity. Obesity is predicted to overtake smoking as the leading cause of death in the United States.[7] The most effective treatment for morbid obesity is bariatric surgery. Bariatric surgeries have been shown to provide cost-effective, durable, long-term weight control in the severe to morbid obese population.[8–9] Improvements in safety as well as decreases in morbidity associated with bariatric surgery have led to a concomitant rise in bariatric surgical procedures, with more than 200,000 people undergoing various weight loss procedures annually.[10] The improvement of obesity-related medical disorders following bariatric surgery has been a major health benefit.[11]

The striking rise in the post bariatric population results in growing numbers of patients seeking removal of the excess skin and fat remaining following their weight loss. Nearly every region of the body can be affected, resulting in redundant, loose, hanging rolls of skin and fat.[12] These deformities lead to intertriginous rashes, chronic fungal infections, skin breakdown, and social embarrassment. Patients frequently seek consultation with a plastic surgeon to address these deformities and often consider body contouring as the final phase of their weight loss journey. With the increased number of bariatric procedures, body contouring has been a tremendous area of growth in plastic surgery, and the majority of plastic surgeons worldwide are now exposed to the weight loss population in their training and practices.[13]

INDICATIONS AND PREOPERATIVE PATIENT EVALUATION

Body contouring procedures are purely elective surgeries performed on complex patients, therefore deferring surgery to modify risk factors is always reasonable and acceptable.

Seven key assessment points in a comprehensive preoperative evaluation of the MWL patient were identified and include (1) method of weight reduction, (2) timing of body contouring surgery relative to bariatric surgery or other method of weight reduction, (3) BMI at presentation, (4) nutritional assessment, (5) evaluation for medical comorbidities of obesity, (6) psychosocial evaluation, and (7) assessment of the physical deformities.

The approach of the surgeon and the office staff to the MWL patient must be supportive, empathic, and compassionate, recognizing the major transformation these patients have undergone through great dedication and constant struggling to accomplish their goals.

TIMING OF BODY CONTOURING SURGERY RELATIVE TO BARIATRIC SURGERY OR OTHER METHOD OF WEIGHT REDUCTION

Patient evaluation includes a complete medical history with special emphasis on weight loss history. A history of the age of onset of obesity, family history of obesity, and course of obesity over the patient's life leading up to bariatric surgery is obtained. A detailed history of the type of bariatric procedure performed includes the type of procedure, date of procedure, any postoperative complications and/or additional procedures, and course of weight loss since the procedure. An accurate weight is obtained in the office, including the patient's goal weight and changes in weight status during the previous 3 months prior to presentation. The highest BMI prior to bariatric surgery, the lowest BMI since bariatric surgery, and the current BMI at the time of presentation are calculated and recorded. Eligibility to

body contouring surgery requires weight stability, defined by not more than 5 lb of weight change per month in the previous 3 months.

Timing of plastic surgery following MWL is an important factor, and patients must be at a stable weight before undergoing body contouring procedures. In general, a minimum of 12 months should elapse following weight loss surgery to enable the patient to reach a plateau, and often a plateau is not observed until 18 months postop. A patient still undergoing rapid weight loss may not have achieved metabolic and nutritional homeostasis and could be at risk for suboptimal wound healing and compromised aesthetic results, especially if still losing a significant amount of weight after body contouring surgery. Therefore, patients still actively losing weight are deferred and reassessed in 3 months.

BMI AT PRESENTATION

There is no absolute threshold for BMI prior to surgery, but the best candidates for extensive body contouring surgery typically have a BMI of less than 30 kg/m² and can be considered for multiple procedures and a wide range of procedures if their medical and psychological conditions are favorable.[7] Many successful bariatric patients will present in the BMI range of 25–30 kg/m². At higher BMIs, between 30 and 35 kg/m², one must be more selective and evaluate individual patterns of body fat distribution to guide surgical planning. Patients with a BMI between 35 and 40 kg/m² tend to have findings that limit effective aesthetic contouring, including a thicker subcutaneous adipose layer and a large intraabdominal fat compartment. In this patient group, one has to focus on single-procedure, functional operations to relieve symptoms and encourage further weight loss. For example, an initial panniculectomy or breast reduction can greatly improve comfort and ability to exercise as the patient strives for further weight loss. Surgery is usually deferred for patients with a BMI of greater than 40 kg/m² until they achieve further weight loss unless symptoms are unusually severe (i.e., severe or acute panniculitis).

NUTRITIONAL ASSESSMENT

Screening for nutritional status is important. Protein intake by history is considered adequate if 70–100 g of protein per day is reported. Serum protein measurement is also indicated before post-bariatric body contouring. Following bariatric surgery, protein is one of the major nutrients affected and may be reflected as hypoalbuminemia, anemia, and edema. Protein intake is essential for wound healing, especially if multiple contouring procedures are performed. Serum prealbumin and albumin levels elucidate issues with protein intake and absorption. Protein supplementation may be required preoperatively.

Deficiencies in nutrients and vitamins, such as thiamine, calcium, folate, vitamin B_{12}, and iron are common.[14,15] A history of current or past supplementation may screen for this.

Anemia is also common in the MWL population and may be related to generalized or specific nutrient deficiencies. Although iron deficiency is most common and may be seen in association with any gastric bypass procedure, micronutrients such as B_{12}, folate, copper, fat-soluble vitamins A and E, and zinc may be deficient and contribute to anemia. In some cases, iron deficiencies may be refractory to oral supplemental therapy and require more aggressive treatment with parenteral iron, blood transfusions, or surgical interventions.[14]

EVALUATION FOR MEDICAL COMORBIDITIES OF OBESITY AND CONTRAINDICATIONS FOR BODY CONTOURING SURGERY

Weight loss induced by bariatric surgery improves health and alleviates or resolves active diseases. These benefits commonly occur within 2–5 months following bariatric surgery.[16] However, the plastic surgeon must actively inquire about the most common comorbidities of obesity and search for unresolved issues.

While Pories et al.[8] demonstrated that 82% of obese patients with type 2 diabetes mellitus had resolution of their disease following weight loss, patients with persistent insulin resistance will still present to the plastic surgeon when seeking for body contouring. Hemoglobin A1C is checked as an indicator of glucose control. Oral hypoglycemic agents are held on the morning of surgery, and insulin dose is reduced on the morning of surgery consistent with the fasting state. For all diabetic patients, glucose is monitored every 4 hours postoperatively and treated with an insulin sliding scale for tight glycemic control. Endocrinology consult may be required in complex cases.

Obstructive sleep apnea (OSA) is another common comorbidity of obesity and may still be present in patients presenting for plastic surgery. Risks and complications associated with OSA include myocardial infarction, stroke, arrhythmia, and sudden death. Patients should be questioned about recent sleep studies and recommendations for perioperative management

obtained from their treating pulmonologist or internist. If patients use continuous positive airway pressure (CPAP) devices at home, they should be instructed to bring their own CPAP machine and mask for use after surgery as their device will be well tolerated and will increase compliance during the inpatient stay.

It is imperative to question the patient about symptoms of active cardiovascular disease, including exertional dyspnea and chest pain. Exercise tolerance is a useful measure as patients who routinely tolerate 45 minutes of vigorous exercise are likely to tolerate the stress of surgery. Given the magnitude of major body contouring procedures, the plastic surgeon should not hesitate to refer patients for a preoperative stress test and other appropriate cardiovascular studies.

Risk factors for venous thromboembolism (VTE) are assessed, including current obesity state, immobility, age, and venous varicosities.[17] The potential for hereditary coagulopathies is considered as well. A history of multiple spontaneous abortions should arouse suspicion of an underlying thrombophilia.[18] All patients with a documented history of VTE are tested for hypercoagulable disorders and referred where indicated to a hematologist for perioperative risk assessment and recommendations. For particularly high-risk patients, placement of a temporary inferior vena cava filter is considered. Shermak et al. investigated the incidence of VTE in the post-bariatric body contouring population. They showed an overall risk of 2.9% for VTE for all patients undergoing body contouring surgery. This rate increased to 8.9% for patients with a BMI of 35 kg/m² or greater.[19] While clear evidence-based guidelines for the use of chemoprophylaxis have not been established for plastic surgery, all patients should have sequential pneumatic compression devices applied prior to the induction of general anesthesia. Early ambulation is critical and must be stressed during hospitalization and at the time of discharge.

Risk of platelet dysfunction from medications, including aspirin and nonsteroidal anti-inflammatory agents (NSAIDs), is considered and these medications are discontinued for at least 2 weeks before surgery. Herbal medications and certain vitamins and foods that are found to increase the risk of bleeding are also held 2 weeks preoperatively.

Tobacco use is another modifiable risk factor for postoperative complications. An aggressive approach should be adopted for this issue, and patient education for smoking cessation for at least 6 weeks prior to surgery and 6 weeks after surgery is addressed. Often, a surgery is not scheduled until the patient has stopped tobacco use.

PSYCHOSOCIAL EVALUATION

Body image issues and low self-esteem are prevalent in the bariatric population even after successful weight loss, and abundant, excess, loose-hanging skin may be one cause.[20] The psychological issues are complex, and the risk of major depression is nearly five times higher in individuals with a BMI of greater than 40 kg/m^2 when compared with individuals of average weight.[21] Unlike diabetes and hypertension, which often resolve after weight loss, the mood and personality disorders, destructive eating patterns, and poor body image issues seen in obese patients often do not resolve.[22] The common finding of controlled depression in the MWL patient is not, in itself, a contraindication to body contouring surgery. However, patients with a diagnosis of a bipolar disorder or schizophrenia require an evaluation and clearance from their mental health provider before body contouring surgery.[23] A supportive social network is vital during the recovery period from major body contouring procedures. Before undertaking major procedures, the plastic surgeon should make sure adequate support systems are in place.

Setting expectations begins with an understanding of motivations and priorities. Patients must verbalize an understanding that they will accept the scars and significant recovery period and accept the concept that they will be significantly improved but not "perfect." When patients are scar-averse and use terms such as "normal" for the expected outcome, the surgeon is wise to defer intervention. In such circumstances, it is nearly impossible to meet expectations no matter how skillfully the surgery is performed.

Even with a good outcome, patients tend to forget their preoperative appearance. Occasional review of the preoperative photos during postoperative visits helps remind the patients how far they have progressed and keeps them motivated.[24]

Despite the fact that MWL patients have significant deformities, they can still have body dysmorphic disorder or similar severe body image derangements that preclude satisfactory outcome. During the consultation, it is vital to observe the patient's affect and mood while they describe their lifestyle and the impact of the hanging skin on it. Patients who are overly preoccupied with their deformities and spend a substantial amount of time thinking about their loose skin are likely poor candidates for body contouring surgery. Importantly, patients who attribute problems with job performance, career advancement, relationships, and general self-esteem to their loose skin are to be avoided. With proper screening, this is a very happy patient population.

ASSESSMENT OF THE PHYSICAL DEFORMITIES

The MWL patient is unique in that nearly every part of the body can be affected. A thorough evaluation considers the areas of loose skin, the relative body type (android vs. gynoid), overall body fat distribution, skin tone in different regions, number and location of skin rolls, and regional adiposity. Zones of adherence, which are tight, nonyielding areas of fascial attachment to the underlying muscular system act as tethering points from which skin laxity will hang. These areas of restriction are located in the midline of the anterior and posterior trunk and around the pelvic rim. Areas of skin and soft tissue that are farthest in distance from the zones of adherence descend the most following MWL, which in most patients includes the lateral truncal tissues. Characteristically, patients will present with predictable patterns of tissue descent around the body. The Pittsburgh Rating Scale is a point-based rating system for severity of deformities in the MWL patient by anatomic region[12] and correlates severity to the type of treatment. Challenging cases require that both loose skin and excess adipose deposits are addressed, and this may entail a combination of excisional surgery and liposuction. Additionally, an important surgical concept is that not all excess adipose tissue is best treated by excision; some adipose tissue can be transposed to a new location, for example, adding volume and shape to the breast or buttock region.

During physical examination, scars from prior surgeries are important to document as a reduction in blood supply may require technical modifications during surgery. Commonly, rectus diastasis may be discovered. Ventral hernias should be identified when present, A breast examination should be performed, noting masses, position of the nipple areola complex, and skin envelope quality. Asymmetries are pointed out to the patient. Lateral thoracic skin rolls are noted. Standardized photographs are taken.

PREOPERATIVE INVESTIGATIONS, PATIENT COUNSELING, AND EDUCATION

A proper preoperative medical workup is essential. Preoperative clearance from internists, psychiatrists, and other physicians that care for the patient should be strongly considered. Preoperative testing is selected based on age and medical profile, and may include chest x-ray, electrocardiogram, complete blood count (CBC), coagulation profile, prealbumin, albumin, pregnancy screen in females of child-bearing age, and a mammogram if breast surgery is considered.[25] Abdominal computed tomography (CT) scan is done in cases of suspected hernias and will aid surgical planning.

Preoperative counseling exploring the patient's goals, expectations, and areas of greatest concern aids in patient selection. Patients are questioned on areas of the body of greatest priority requiring correction, especially when multiple procedures are performed. Discussion on the appropriate staging of procedures is also undertaken. Patients must be aware of the lengthy scars that occur with large skin resections and must be willing to trade a better contour with the resultant scar.

Abstinence from aspirin, NSAIDs, and herbal medications that predispose to bleeding is important. Smoking cessation will reduce risk of complications, and we ask all our patients to cease tobacco use prior to surgery. Informed consent is a key element of preoperative counseling. Patients must understand that body contouring after MWL may require multiple stages and possible revisionary surgeries. In general, MWL patients experience mild to moderate amounts of skin relaxation postoperatively, resulting in the need for further skin resections. There is also the possibility of contour irregularities and postoperative dog-ears at the ends of the scar.

SURGICAL TECHNIQUES BY ANATOMIC REGIONS

ABDOMINAL CONTOURING

Patient Evaluation

The abdominal area is the most common reason patients seek plastic surgical consultation after MWL. Apart of aesthetic concerns, a hanging abdominal pannus may be symptomatic and cause functional disabilities, such as recurrent intertrigo, infections in the skin fold, limited ambulation, intimacy problems, and the like. Performing panniculectomy or abdominoplasty on MWL patients may consistently improve their body image and quality of life.[26]

Evaluation of the patient presenting for abdominal contouring includes complete history and physical examination and all the following issues:

- Presence of multiple skin rolls
- Quality of abdominal skin
- Degree and location of adiposity
- Prior surgical scars

- Presence or absence of diastasis rectus
- Presence or absence of ventral hernias and/or umbilical hernias
- Extent of lateral and circumferential excess skin
- Coexisting genital deformities (i.e., mons ptosis, buried penis)

Operative Planning and Technique

A panniculectomy is primarily a reconstructive procedure aiming to remove skin and fat from the anterior abdominal area, thereby relieving symptoms related to the overhanging pannus. It is performed for patients with higher BMIs who are not at their optimal weight or for patients with more severe medical comorbidities. During panniculectomy, skin flap undermining is limited, and no muscular plication is performed. The umbilicus may or may not be sacrificed. Unlike panniculectomy, abdominoplasty is primarily an aesthetic procedure involving the removal of abdominal skin and fat, along with selective plication of rectus muscles and umbilical repositioning. In the MWL patient, there are often components of both procedures applied.

Evaluation of the presence or absence of ventral hernias and/or umbilical hernias is key. Abdominal wall reconstruction for ventral or umbilical hernias may be accessed through the low transverse abdominal incision. Small to moderate ventral hernia repairs may easily be combined with other body contouring procedures. However, more extensive hernias require wider dissection and lysis of intraabdominal adhesions. In these cases, the amount of concomitant procedures is decreased for patient safety reasons.[25] The decision whether to use prosthetic materials for the reconstruction of the abdominal wall should be carefully judged since these patient are at higher risk of wound dehiscence and infection. Components separation of the abdominal wall is an excellent technique for repair of ventral hernias and may avoid the use of mesh prosthetics.[27] Care must be taken to ensure that the abdominal cavity will accommodate the reduction of intraabdominal contents without causing excessive tension on the abdominal wall reconstruction. If not, the patient is counseled to lose further weight prior to reconstruction. Final scar placement must be considered. The inferior margin of the transverse resection is planned 6 cm superior to the anterior labial commissure in females and from the base of the penis in males. This position allows the final scar to be hidden in the patient's underwear.

Special Considerations

Special consideration is made for the giant pannus (*panniculus morbidus*). Associated with a high BMI, a giant pannus causes significant morbidity. Hygiene issues including recurrent intertrigo and rashes, interference with ambulation, and chronic pannus lymphedema may be alleviated with resection.[28,29] Since a large mass of tissue is present, special lifts provide access to incision sites. Steinman pins may be placed superficially into the edge of the pannus. One must always bear in mind that an incisional or umbilical hernia may be present. These pins may be connected to a Hoyer hydraulic lift.[30] Elevation is essential since it allows venous drainage from the pannus, hence better control of large blood vessels. Meticulous hemostasis should be addressed in these cases. In most cases, umbilical excision is necessary.

In patients with significant epigastric laxity, a vertical trunk excision may be combined with the low transverse excision, creating a fleur-de-lis (FDL) type abdominoplasty.[31] Care must be taken to minimize undermining at the edges of the vertical excision to preserve as many local perforators as possible and to avoid excessive triple-point tension to preserve flap viability.[32] Umbilical inset is made within the vertical incision; creating a cut-out for the inset will create an unaesthetic widened umbilicus over time. The resultant dog-ear at the cephalad limit of the vertical excision may be reduced by defatting superior to it. Advantages of the FDL abdominoplasty include the ability to enhance waist definition and contour the epigastrium. Disadvantages include the potential for overtightening at the waist in males, creating a feminine-appearing torso and the additional vertical abdominal scar. In the setting of a prior subcostal scar, an FDL abdominoplasty should be considered because it will correct the contour with minimal direct undermining in the epigastric region.

Ptosis of the mons area is frequently seen in the MWL patient. Subscarpal defatting of the pubic area may be required to match abdominal flap thickness. Resuspension of the mons is performed with nonabsorbable sutures from the anterior abdominal fascia to the superficial fascial system of the pubic area at three to five points.

Extreme cases of pubic ptosis accompanied by excess pubic fat in males results in a buried penis syndrome, in which the shaft and glans penis are concealed from view. Buried penis is a debilitating condition, interfering with normal urination, sexual activity, and proper hygiene. In buried penis syndrome, the penis is tethered by the suspensory ligament, while the abdominal fat is not.[33,34]

With recurrent episodes of infection, superficial skin breakdown and persistent moisture, cicatricial changes occur, trapping the penis. Correction of such a deformity is complex and includes escutcheonectomy, penile degloving and coverage with a split-thickness skin graft, scrotoplasty, and a panniculectomy.[35–37] These surgeries are often combined with a urology team. Prolonged urethral catheterization is necessary.

Complications and Caveats

Early local postoperative complications include hematoma, seroma, wound infection, and wound dehiscence. Late local postoperative complications include asymmetries involving scar position, contour irregularities, lateral dog-ears (avoided if care is taken in surgical planning or choice of procedure), and over- or underresection. Recurrence of tissue laxity and relapse of the pannus may require further skin tightening procedures. Resuspension of the mons pubis may cause temporary alteration in the angle of urine stream. Systemic postoperative complications include deep vein thrombosis and pulmonary embolism, hence prophylactic measures and early postoperative ambulation are advised.

LOWER BODY LIFT

In many MWL patients, the success of abdominal contouring alone is limited by circumferential excess skin and fat. A lower body lift, belt lipectomy, or circumferential torsoplasty will provide a more aesthetic results in these patients. In the MWL population, ptotic buttocks with loose skin and adiposity in the lateral thighs accompany a hanging pannus, therefore, lower body lift procedures should achieve circumferential trunk contouring. The buttocks, abdomen, and thighs must be treated as a single unit.[38,39] Some advanced surgical developments such as superficial fascial system (SFS) suspension by Lockwood[40] and buttock auto-augmentation using local de-epithelialized gluteal flaps[41] have improved results.

Patient Evaluation

In addition to the patient evaluation described in the abdominal section, one should assess the lateral thighs and buttocks region. This assessment includes the quality, elasticity, and quantity of skin in these areas; the translation of pull, which is determined by the pinch test; the volume and location of fat deposits; and buttocks volume and projection.

Preoperatively, the patient must be counseled on the extent of scarring and postoperative expectations. In many cases, staging of the procedures in the MWL patient is advised such as in patients undergoing both lower body circumferential contouring procedures and medial thigh lift procedures. The authors prefer to perform the lower body lift in a first stage, followed by the medial thigh lift in a second stage.

Operative Planning and Technique

Markings for circumferential lower body procedures may be placed inferiorly or superiorly:

1. *Placing the resection superiorly.* This allows more control over the excision of flank rolls, provides some elevation force on the lateral thighs, and accentuates the waist. However, buttock reshaping with auto-augmentation is more difficult with this higher positioning.

2. *Placing the resection inferiorly.* This allows greater elevation force on the lateral thighs, and buttock reshaping is easier with this approach. Waist definition may be enhanced by rectus plication and an FDL abdominoplasty.

Choice of resection depends on individual body type and surgical goals. When possible, the authors prefer to keep the resection low (inferior) to add control to lateral thigh contour, to prevent gluteal flattening, and to keep the final scar position covered by undergarments. In the supine position, a distance of 6 cm is marked from the superior aspect of the anterior vulvar commissure in females and from the base of the penis in males. Posterior markings are made with the patient standing and facing away from the surgeon. The superior anchor line posteriorly is determined in the midline and extended bilaterally to the mid-axillary line. Vertical reference marks are spaced 6 cm apart. Laterally, the amount of resected tissue is estimated with a pinch test and marked with the patient's legs slightly abducted. This creates the lateral margins of the inferior resection line. The inferior resection line is drawn. A transition zone between the posterior and anterior resections is usually marked in the mid-axillary line. The areas within the resection lines that are to be preserved for buttock auto-augmentation are marked. With the patient facing the surgeon and holding the abdominal skin on vertical stretch, the points marking the lower lateral margin of resection bilaterally are connected to the point 6 cm superior to the anterior vulvar commissure in the midline. This is the inferior margin of resection of the abdominal contouring portion of the procedure. Areas of adjunct liposuction are marked as well.

The surgery is a two-position procedure, beginning with the patient in the prone position and then supine. Routine Foley catheter, warming blankets, and sequential compression devices are used. Beginning in the prone position, the gluteal flaps to be preserved for buttock auto-augmentation are de-epithelialized. Then, the superior anchor line is incised and an inferiorly based flap is elevated, avoiding the de-epithelialized gluteal flaps. The inferior line is checked during the procedure and adjusted to ensure reasonable closure and the resection is then completed. Laterally, the buttock flaps are undermined and shaped with absorbable sutures for increased buttock projection and auto-augmentation. Inferior to the gluteal flaps, moderate undermining is performed in order to accommodate the flaps volume. The lateral thigh region is mobilized with the Lockwood discontinuous undermining device passed into the subcutaneous tissue. The patient's legs are abducted to decrease lateral tension and towel clamps are used to hold the wound together. Wound closure is performed over drains. The lateral dog-ears are temporarily stapled closed. In the supine position, the procedure continues as a traditional abdominoplasty. Attention should be paid when flexing the waist during abdominal closure as it may lead to greater tension on the back wound. Coaptation of the SFS in the lateral aspect of the wound with absorbable sutures is essential. The abdominal wound is closed over drains as in the usual fashion (see Figure 17.1 for representative case).

Postoperative Care

The patient is kept in a flexed waist position. Perioperative antibiotics and chemoprophylaxis for VTE are administered. Sequential compression devices are maintained. The Foley catheter is removed on postoperative day 1, and ambulation and mobilization with assistance are encouraged at this time. The expected duration of hospitalization is 2 nights. Drains are removed when output is less than 30 mL in a 24-hour period.

VERTICAL MEDIAL THIGH LIFT

Patient Evaluation

The thigh must be conceptually divided into lateral and medial areas. No single procedure can address changes in both medial and lateral thighs in MWL patients. Procedures such as lower body lift and lateral thigh lift may contour the lateral thighs but leave the medial thighs minimally affected. Conversely, a vertical medial thigh lift will only tighten the medial thigh, leaving the lateral thigh unaffected. There are several characteristic changes in the medial thighs in the MWL population. These include inferior descent of the

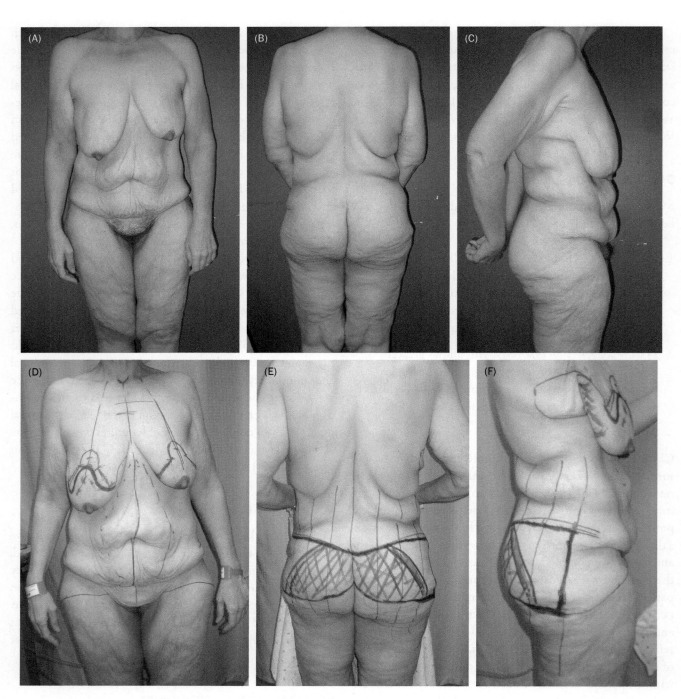

Figure 17.1. A 49-year-old woman following massive weight loss, shown preoperatively (A, B, C). Markings were designed for a circumferential lower body lift with preservation of gluteal fat pads and transposition of a flap for volume enhancement and shaping. Note the fairly low position of the posterior resection to enable buttock shaping. The patient is also marked for a concurrent mastopexy (D, E, F). In the operating room, gluteal shape is enhanced by lateral undermining of the gluteal fat pad and medial rotation (G). This use of gluteal flaps for buttock shaping is used selectively and can increase projection, as noted on the intraoperative photograph (H). The patient is shown 6 months after mastopexy and body lift. While not performed in the same setting as the lower body lift, the patient subsequently underwent posterior upper body lift 3 months after the lower body lift. These procedures are staged because of the opposing vectors of pull (I, J, K).

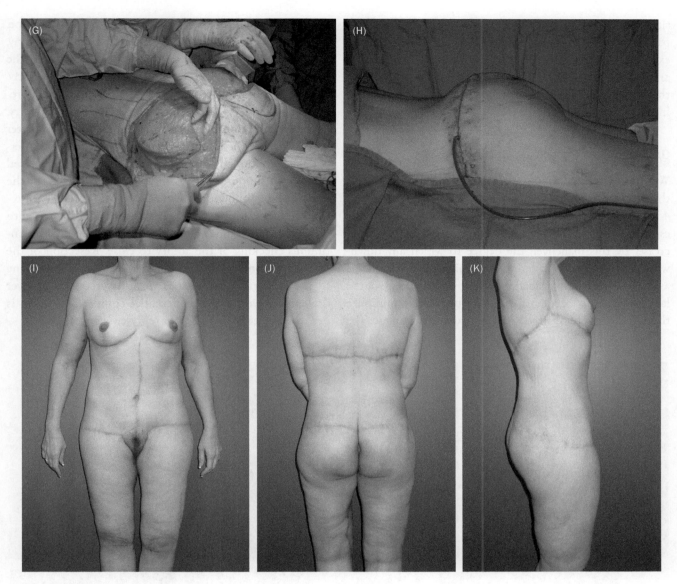

Figure 17.1. Continued

soft tissues, significant deflation, and decreased adherence of the skin–fat envelope of the medial thigh compared to the lateral thigh. These changes contribute to a significant horizontal tissue excess that needs to be addressed.[42] Minor medial thigh laxity can be treated with a vertical vector of pull toward the groin and a crescentic resection of excess skin, placing the scar in the groin and perineal crease. This transverse medial thigh lift addresses only the upper third of the thigh.[43] Further modifications were made in this procedure, including anchoring the inner thigh to Colles's fascia. This modification helped in minimizing scar widening, vulvar deformity, and recurrence of upper medial thigh ptosis. Even with its advantages, the transverse medial thigh lift does not address laxity of the distal third of the medial thigh, with which most MWL patients present. To address

the laxity of the distal third of the medial thigh, a vertical medial thigh lift is performed. The aim of vertical medial thigh lift is to primarily correct horizontal laxity with the resection of a vertical component. The widest aspect of the thigh is located 2–3 cm below the perineal crease. The only transverse component of excision in a vertical medial thigh lift is at the superior aspect of the incision, used to remove the resultant dog-ear in the proximal thigh. Depending on the distal extent of skin laxity and the patient's preference and acceptance of the length of the scar, the scar may be shortened or lengthened toward the medial knee. A history of lymphedema or significant varicosities is important to document preoperatively. Physical examination should include the degree and distal extent of skin laxity and quality and the amount of lipodystrophy. The amount of possible skin resection is demonstrated by a pinch test. In the MWL patient with residual thigh non-deflated adiposity and skin excess, either further weight reduction is recommended or an initial debulking liposuction procedure of the medial thigh area is performed, followed by a second-stage vertical medial thigh lift.

Operative Planning and Technique

With the patient in the supine position with legs abducted, the line of incision in the groin crease is marked beginning 4 cm lateral to the midline of the mons pubis. A pinch test estimates the transverse crescentic resection in the groin crease. By this maneuver, the degree to which any downward traction is transmitted to the genital area in females is assessed. Postoperative labial spreading with exposure of the labia minora may occur and care must be taken to minimize this risk. Next, the vertical resection markings are made. The

proposed scar position is marked on the anterior anchor line. This line is marked by pulling the thigh tissues posteriorly, thereby simulating the lift of the anterior thigh tissues. The posterior mark is made with a similar traction anteriorly. Reference lines are placed every 6 cm perpendicular to the resection. Bilateral thigh markings are compared for symmetry.

After induction of general anesthesia, a Foley catheter is inserted and the legs are prepped and draped circumferentially. Additionally, an extra set of arm boards are placed laterally to support the legs in abduction. Incision of the anterior line, followed by flap elevation toward the posterior line, is performed. Plane of dissection is superficial to the saphenous vein. The excess skin is resected, with continuous checking of the ability to close. Resection of the horizontal component is performed in a superficial plane to preserve groin lymphatics. Multilayered closure over drains, followed by circumferential compressive wraps is performed (see Figure 17.2 for representative case).

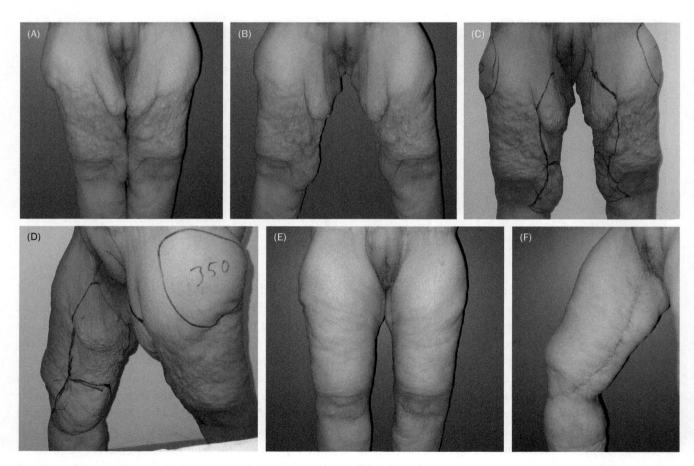

Figure 17.2. A 59-year-old woman following massive weight loss with lax skin in the medial thighs and festoons in the proximal thighs bilaterally (A, B). Markings for a vertical medial thigh lift are shown (C, D) along with lateral thigh liposuction. Vertical medial thigh lift markings curve under the patella to capture redundant skin and fat in the medial knee region. The proximal termination of the pattern can be a simple vertical incision running into the groin crease, an "L" pattern running posteriorly or anteriorly, or a "T" pattern. A "T" pattern is used only when necessary because a fresh triple-point in the groin region can be prone to wound healing problems. Results are shown are at 4 months (E, F) with significant reduction of the redundant skin and a longitudinal scar crossing the knee joint in the mid-axial position.

During the immediate postoperative period, the legs remain elevated. Ambulation is encouraged on the evening of surgery. Foley catheter is removed on postoperative day 1. Compressive stockings should be applied for 4 weeks. Drains are removed when the output is less than 30 mL in a 24-hour period.

Complications and Caveats

Common complications such as hematoma, seroma, poor scarring, and asymmetries are possible and encountered after medial thigh lift procedures. Temporary lower extremity edema develops in virtually all patients undergoing medial thigh lift procedures. Leg elevation and compression garments may aid in minimizing edema in the early postoperative period. In most cases, the edema resolves within months. The lymphatic structures of the leg are primarily concentrated medially and deep to the plane of the saphenous vein until the vessels begin to converge in the femoral triangle. Inadvertent injury to the lymphatics during thigh lift procedures may result in lymphedema of the lower extremity. This complication can lead to significant disability. Careful flap elevation and superficial dissection in the femoral triangle may help avoid this feared complication. Labial spreading with exposure of the labia minora may occur when including any horizontal skin resection adjacent to the groin. This is a leading cause of medicolegal action in thigh lift procedures.

UPPER BODY LIFT

Patient Evaluation

Upper body lift includes contouring of rolls of excess skin and lipodystrophy in the back area. Upper body lift may be combined with breast procedures (reduction mammaplasty or mastopexy) in females or with excisional gynecomastia procedures in males. These combined procedures enable medial rotation of the lateral breast skin and subcutaneous flap to restore volume to a deflated breast based on the lateral intercostal perforators. As with any elective body contouring procedure, the patient is assessed for medical comorbidities. A complete weight history (minimum, maximum, and current weights; calculation of BMI; fluctuations in weight in the past 3 months) is recorded. Patients are counseled about smoking cessation if they actively smoke and about the lengthy scars that are produced with large skin and soft tissue resections. In upper body lift of the trunk, the transverse excision may be hidden within the bra line, therefore trading scarring of the back with improvement in body contour.

Physical examination should include assessment of the back and adjacent areas that may require contouring (arms, breasts, abdomen). The predominance of excess skin versus fat is an important consideration for adequate surgical planning. Back rolls may range in number from one to four on either side of the midline.[50] Documentation of the number of rolls and their level of descent is important, along with the position of the inframammary crease. The highest of the back rolls that may be present is the posterolateral extension of the breast roll. Other possible rolls in descending order include the scapular, lower thoracic, and hip rolls. These rolls tend to be tethered at zones of adherence in the midlines of the chest and back, producing maximum tissue descent laterally (inverted-V deformity).

Choice of procedure for back contouring depends on the relative excesses of skin and fat along with the patient's skin elasticity. In patients with lipodystrophy and only mild amounts of skin excess, back rolls may be treated with liposuction alone. If moderate to severe amounts of skin redundancy are present, excisional procedures are necessary. There are three main excisional options: (1) transverse excision that extends from the mid-axillary line to the midline of the back, (2) vertical excision in the mid-axillary line that extends from the axilla to the iliac crest, and (3) extension from an excisional brachioplasty down through the lateral chest to the inframammary crease.

The patient should be informed about staging procedures (i.e., full transverse body lifts should not be performed concurrently with a lower body lift because there may be significant concurrent opposing vectors of pull).

Operative Planning and Technique

If transverse excisional upper body lift is executed, the patient is marked standing. If concomitant breast procedures are to be performed, the anterior chest markings are made first. In female patients, the patient is asked to bring in a bra of her choice to enable hiding the final scar position in the outline of her bra line. The proposed final scar position is marked. The superior margin of resection is made within the bra line, extending the mid-axillary line. The inferior tissues are pinched upward to stimulate resection. Using this maneuver, the inferior resection is marked to the mid-axillary line, where it merges with anterior chest markings. Vertical reference lines are made every 6 cm. Eventually, symmetry is assessed.

The procedure begins in the prone position. If concomitant chest or abdominal procedures are planned, they are performed after the upper body lift procedure. The superior mark is incised and dissection carried to the deep fascia, after encountering the strong SFS layer. An inferiorly based flap is elevated superficial to the muscle fascia to the proposed inferior resection line and continued laterally to the mid-axillary line. Towel clamps are used to estimate the safety of resection. Laterally, the vertical mark in the mid-axillary line that is the merge point with the chest procedure is incised to complete the resection. The wound is closed in layers: SFS is approximated with 2-0 braided absorbable sutures, followed by closure of deep dermal and subcuticular layers with 3-0 monofilament absorbable sutures. Skin glue is applied topically. The resultant lateral dog-ears are temporarily closed with staples and will be resected with the anterior chest procedures with the patient in the supine position. Drains usually come anteriorly from the chest. The patient is then flipped to the supine position for further anterior procedures, as needed (see Figure 17.3).

Postoperative Care, Complications, and Caveats

A compressive wrap (Ace wrap) is placed in the immediate postoperative period. Drains are removed when outputs are less than 30 mL over a 24-hr period. If combined with brachioplasty or breast surgeries, postoperative care for these procedures is also initiated.

Complications in back contouring include hematoma, poor scarring, wound dehiscence, asymmetry, and seroma. Most seromas are managed conservatively with serial aspirations in the office.

MASTOPEXY AND BREAST RESHAPING IN THE MWL PATIENT

Patient Evaluation

In the MWL population, the breast deformity is complex. Traditional mastopexy techniques do not offer a

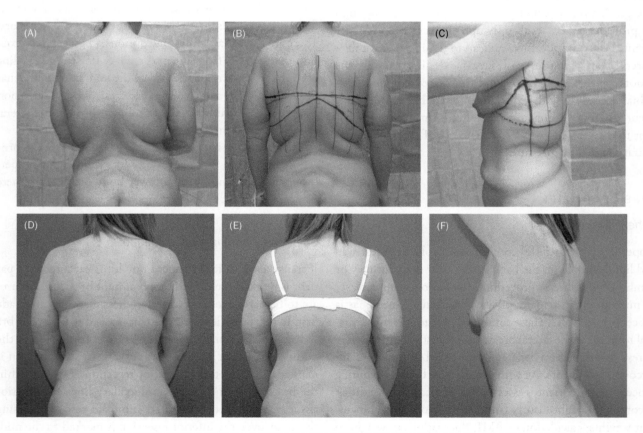

Figure 17.3. A 32-year-old woman presented with complaints of upper back rolls following massive weight loss (A). The patient was marked for a transverse upper body lift. Note that more tissue is excised in the lateral aspect of the pattern. Vertical reference marks aid in reapproximation of the wound edges after excision (B). The lateral view of the markings demonstrates that the anterior dog-ear is simply run into the inframammary fold (C). This procedure can be performed concurrently with a breast shaping procedure or independently. If performed concurrently with a breast shaping procedure, the posterior resection is still performed first, and a dog-ear is stapled temporarily at the lateral margin. The patient is then turned to the supine position and the breast shaping procedure performed. The dog-ear is then merged with the inframammary fold in a similar fashion. In this case, the patient is shown postoperatively at 3 months with the posterior transverse incision lying beneath the brassiere (D, E). On the posterior three-quarter view, the scar can be observed terminating into the inframammary fold.

long-standing result, therefore the surgeon is forced to adopt newer techniques for this challenging deformity. Characteristic changes in the breast following MWL include volume deflation, resulting in a stretched, thin, and inelastic skin envelope; significant ptosis; flattening of the overall breast shape; medialization of the nipple-areolar complex (NAC); and the development of a lateral chest wall roll. Moreover, breast asymmetry may coexist, along with significant skin excess, deficient parenchymal volume; and attenuated internal support structures of the breast. Traditional mastopexy techniques are usually inadequate for these deformities. To better describe breast deformities following MWL, the Pittsburgh Rating Scale was developed to classify contour deformities in this unique group of patients.[12] It takes into account the degree of breast ptosis, volume loss, loose skin, and the presence or absence of lateral chest wall skin rolls.

Goals in mastopexy after MWL include:

- Breast reshaping and tightening of the skin envelope

- Elevation and repositioning of the NAC to the breast meridian

- Restoration of superior pole fullness

- Development of a natural and aesthetic curve of the lateral breast

- Recruitment of volume from the lateral chest roll

- Minimization of scars and proper scar placement

- Creating a long-standing result

As in any breast procedure, a complete breast and medical history is collected and includes weight history, bra size (largest, current, ideal), personal and family history of breast cancer, genetic predisposition to breast cancer, history of ovarian/colon cancer, prior breast masses, prior breast surgeries or biopsies, previous mammographic history, breast-feeding history, future plans for breast-feeding, and smoking status. Physical examination should include distances (suprasternal notch to nipple, nipple to inframammary fold [IMF], breast meridian at clavicle to nipple), position of the NAC, asymmetries, presence of masses and/or irregularities, presence of lateral chest wall roll, scars, quality of skin envelope, parenchymal volume, and mobility of the IMF.

According to the American Cancer Society, screening guidelines are as follows: women aged 40–44 should have the choice to start annual breast cancer screening with mammograms if they wish to do so; women aged 45–54

should get mammograms every year. Women aged 55 and older should switch to mammograms every 2 years or can continue yearly screening.

Women with a positive family history of breast cancer or a genetic predisposition should be screened with magnetic resonance imaging (MRI) along with mammograms.[51]

After MWL, the breasts are usually lacking in upper pole fullness. Traditional breast reduction techniques (Wise pattern or vertical), augmentation mammoplasty with implants and augmentation mastopexy, may not produce a long-standing result in the MWL patient. Some methods to reshape the breast include dermal suspension techniques and/or the use of local tissues for auto-augmentation. One should not ignore deformities of structures adjacent to the breast in the MWL patient (axillary fold, lateral chest wall roll); these tissues are to be addressed during breast reshaping surgery and might be used for auto-augmentation. The addition of a lateral thoracic flap based on intercostal perforators allows the recruitment of soft tissue to augment insufficient breast volume along with simultaneous removal of commonly found lateral thoracic soft tissue excess. These intercostal perforators are located along the anterior axillary line, parallel to the lateral border of the breast. Parenchymal tissues may be either suspended to stable chest wall structures (pectoralis fascia, rib periosteum) or by a loop of pectoralis muscle.[52] Plication of parenchymal or de-epithelialized dermis allows for increased projection and reshaping of the underlying glandular structure.[53] If implants are to be considered for augmentation of breast volume, larger sizes may further stretch a poorly elastic skin envelope and the implant is prone to descent. Smaller sized implants or the use of additional support such as a cadaveric dermis sling may prevent this recurrent ptosis and worsening implant descent.

The authors present their technique and management. For further elaboration, the reader may refer to the other mastopexy chapter 63 in this book.

We describe a technique developed by the senior author, based on the Wise pattern, that achieves all of the goals of mastopexy following MWL.[54,55] This technique is called *dermal suspension and total parenchymal reshaping* (DSPR) mastopexy. The main principles of this technique include elevation of the NAC, tightening of the breast skin envelope, reshaping the breast mound, auto-augmentation by recruiting a laterally based dermoglandular flap, and simultaneous ablation of the lateral chest wall roll. This technique establishes a long-lasting, stable result.

Dermal Suspension and Total Parenchymal Reshaping Mastopexy: Operative Planning and Technique

With the patient in the standing position, the suprasternal notch and breast meridians are marked. The new nipple position is in the height of the IMF, and it is lateralized (because of medialization of the NAC in many MWL patients). A standard Wise pattern is drawn with a lateral extension to encompass the lateral thoracic roll. The keyhole pattern is placed 2 cm above the proposed new nipple position, with 5 cm vertical limbs and a 42 mm diameter areola. Back rolls may be treated with horizontal upper body lift excision, thus merging with the lateral extent of the mastopexy. If rolls are oriented more vertically, a vertical excision in the mid-axillary line may be performed, merging with brachioplasty incisions.

After induction of general anesthesia, de-epithelialization is carried out over the entire Wise pattern marking. An infero-centrally based pedicle is raised down to pectoralis fascia by completely degloving the breast parenchyma with 1–1.5 cm thick flaps overlying the breast capsule. The width of the base of the pedicle is maintained at 10 cm. The lateral and medial extensions of the Wise pattern are raised off the chest wall. The lateral wing is supplied by intercostal perforators. Once the chest wall is reached, dissection continues cephalad to the level of the clavicles. Suspension of the central keyhole dermoglandular extension to the second or third rib periosteum along the breast meridian is performed utilizing nonabsorbable braided nylon sutures. This suspension should raise the nipple to its intended position and allow stable elevation

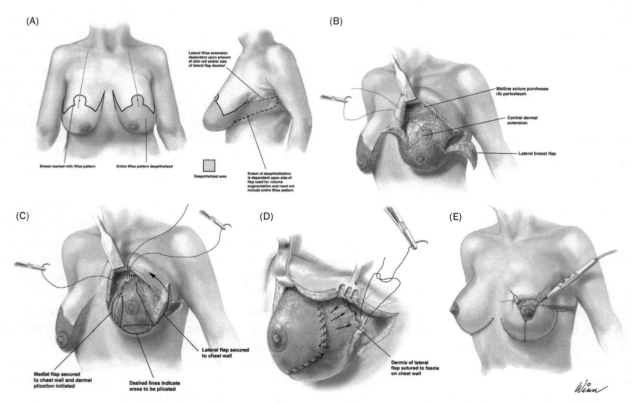

Figure 17.4. The design of the dermal suspension mastopexy is shown in (A). This procedure is based on an extended Wise pattern with the lateral extension extending as far as the posterior axillary line. The lateral extension of the Wise pattern will be elevated as a fasciocutaneous flap and transposed into the mastopexy to both enhance volume and establish the shape of the lateral curve. The entire shaded area will be stripped of epidermis to expose the dermal layer. Note that this illustration highlights the fact that many patients after weight loss have a medial nipple position that must be corrected and placed on a more lateral breast meridian. Once the epidermis is removed from the entire area within the Wise pattern, the medial and lateral wings of the Wise pattern are elevated as fasciocutaneous flaps (B). A tissue flap measuring 1–1.5 cm thick is elevated off the breast parenchyma, and the dissection continued along the pectoralis muscle to the level of the clavicle to create a generous subcutaneous pocket. The edge of the dermis on the top of the keyhole pattern is then secured to rib periosteum using 1-0 permanent braided nylon suture. Next (C), the medial and lateral wings are secured by their dermal edges to rib periosteum with the braided nylon suture. Two sutures are placed at each of the three points of fixation between dermis and periosteum. Once those points of fixation are secure, 2-0 braided absorbable suture is used to plicate the broad dermal surface area to shape the breast. This shaping is done to the satisfaction of the surgeon rather than adhering to a specific pattern. Following the plication, the lateral curve of the breast is shaped (D). This is done by securing the lateral dermal edge to deep fascia using a series of interrupted braided nylon sutures. This adds additional suspension to the breast complex and shapes the lateral curve of the breast. As a final step (E), any tethering of the nipple is gently released by scoring the dermas adjacent to the areola with the electric cautery. This is done selectively and is a safe maneuver because of the central pedicle blood supply.

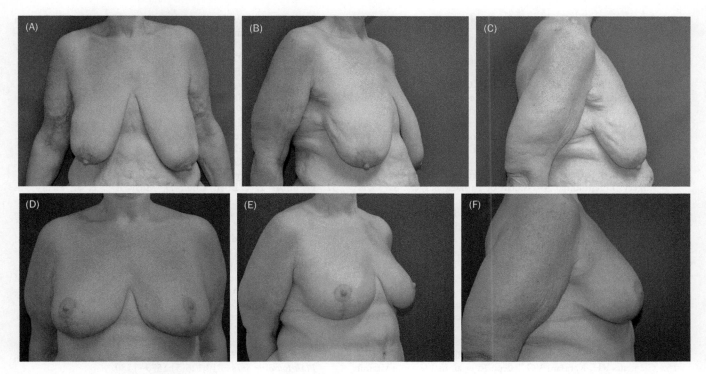

Figure 17.5. A 62-year-old woman presented with breast ptosis following massive weigh loss (A, B, C). She is shown 1 year postoperatively after a dermal suspension mastopexy (D, E, F).

with long-lasting fullness. The lateral breast flap is rotated medially to auto-augment breast volume. It is suspended to a position one rib lower than the initial suture. This reestablishes a natural lateral breast curvature. The medial breast flap is also suspended. Total parenchymal reshaping with plication of dermal elements is performed with absorbable sutures. The lateral and medial flaps are sutured to the central extension to enhance projection. Laterally, the breast flap is sutured to the serratus fascia to emphasize the lateral breast curve. If necessary, the inferior pole of the breast is plicated to shorten the distance from the nipple to the IMF. The remaining skin–parenchymal envelope is redraped over the new breast scaffold. Symmetry is assessed by sitting the patient up during surgery. Release of the dermis adjacent to a portion of the NAC may be necessary to allow better inset if tethered. Multilayered closure over drains is performed.

The DSPR mastopexy technique is safe and reliable. It may be performed in conjunction with other body contouring procedures. Disadvantages of this technique include longer operative time, creation of lengthy scars, and a great deal of intraoperative tailoring. Figure 17.4 shows illustrations of the markings and key steps of the operation, and Figure 17.5 shows a representative case.

Postoperative Care, Complications, and Caveats

A lightly compressive dressing is applied at the end of surgery and maintained until the first postoperative visit. After that, patients are instructed to wear a supportive bra and avoid underwire bras for 4 weeks. Drains are removed once output is less than 30 mL over a 24-hour period. Heavy lifting of items of more than 10 lb for 4–6 weeks postoperatively is discouraged.

The common complications related to DSPR include hematoma, seroma, minor wound dehiscence primarily at the "triple-point," changes in nipple sensation, dog-ears at the ends of resection, asymmetry, scarring, and fat necrosis.

SUGGESTED READINGS

1. CDC. Overweight and obesity. April 27, 2012. Available at: http://www.cdc.gov/obesity/defining.html
2. World Health Organization, Global Database on Body Mass Index. BMI Classification. 2004. Available at: http://apps.who.int/bmi/index.jsp?introPage= intro_3.html
3. Renquist K. Obesity classification. *Obes Surg* 1998;8(4):480.
4. CDC US Obesity Trends. September 21, 2015. Available at: http://www.cdc.gov/obesity/data/adult.html
5. World Obesity Federation. 2015. Available at: http://www.worldobesity.org/resources/trend-maps/?map=trend-maps

6. PiSunyer FX. Medical hazards of obesity. *Ann Intern Med* 1993;119(7 Pt 2):655–660.
7. Allison DB, Fontaine KR, Manson JE, et al. Annual deaths attributable to obesity in the United States. *JAMA* 1999;282(16):1530–1538.
8. Pories WJ, Swanson MS, MacDonald KG, et al. Who would have thought it? An operation proves to be the most effective therapy for adult-onset diabetes mellitus. *Ann Surg* 1995;222(3):339–352.
9. Picot J, Jones J, Colquitt JL, et al. The clinical effectiveness and cost-effectiveness of bariatric (weight loss) surgery for obesity: a systematic review and economic evaluation. *Health Technol Assess* 2009;13(41):1–190, 215–357, iii–iv.
10. Belle S, Berk P, Courcoulas A, et al. Safety and efficacy of bariatric surgery: Longitudinal Assessment of Bariatric Surgery. *Surg Obes Relat Dis* 2007 Mar–Apr;3(2):116–126.
11. Sjöström L, Lindroos A, Peltonen M, et al. Lifestyle, diabetes, and cardiovascular risk factors 10 years after bariatric surgery. *N Engl J Med* 2004 Dec 23;351(26):2683–2693.
12. Song A, Jean R, Hurwitz D, et al. A classification of contour deformities after bariatric weight loss: the Pittsburgh Rating Scale. *Plast Reconstr Surg* 2005 Oct;116(5):1535–1544.
13. American Society of Plastic Surgeons. Cosmetic surgery trends. Available at: http://www.plasticsurgery.org/Documents/news-resources/statistics/2014-statistics/cosmetic-procedure-trends-2014.pdf
14. Love AL, Billett HH. Obesity, bariatric surgery, and iron deficiency: true, true, true and related. *Am J Hematol* 2008;83(5):403–409.
15. Clements RH, Katasani VG, Palepu R, et al. Incidence of vitamin deficiency after laparoscopic RouxenY gastric bypass in a university hospital setting. *Am Surg* 2006;72(12):1196–1204.
16. Buchwald H. Consensus conference statement bariatric surgery for morbid obesity: health implications for patients, health professionals, and third-party payers. *Surg Obes Relat Dis* 2005;1(3):371–381.
17. Geerts W, Pineo G, Heit J, et al. Prevention of venous thromboembolism. *Chest* 2004; 126:338S.
18. Friedman T, Coon D, Michaels J, et al. Hereditary coagulopathies: practical diagnosis and management for the plastic surgeon. *Plast Reconstr Surg* 2010;125(5):1545–1552.
19. Shermak M, Chang D, Heller J. Factors impacting thromboembolism after bariatric body contouring surgery. *Plast Reconstr Surg* 2007;119:1590–1596.
20. Song A, Fernstrom MH. Nutritional and psychological considerations after bariatric surgery. *Aesthet Surg J* 2008;28(2):195–199.
21. Onyike C, Crum R, Lee H, et al. Is obesity associated with major depression? Results from the Third National Health and Nutrition Examination Survey. *Am J Epidemiol* 2003;158(12):1139–1147.
22. Sarwer D, Fabricatore A. Psychiatric considerations of the massive weight loss patient. *Clin Plastic Surg* 2008;35:1–10.
23. Rubin JP, O'Toole JP. Evaluation of the massive weight loss patient who presents for body contouring surgery. In: Rubin JP, Matarasso A, eds. *Aesthetic Surgery After Massive Weight Loss*. London: Elsevier; 2007;13–20.
24. Song AY, Rubin JP, Thomas V, et al. Body image and quality of life in post massive weight loss body contouring patients. *Obesity* 2006;14:1626–1636.
25. Rubin JP, Nguyen V, Schwentker A. Perioperative management of the post-gastric bypass patient presenting for body contour surgery. *Clin Plast Surg* 2004;31(4):601–610, vi.
26. Stuerz K, Piza H, Niermann K, et al. Psychosocial impact of abdominoplasty. *Obes Surg* 2008;18(1):34–38.
27. Borud LJ, Grunwaldt L, Janz B, et al. Components separation combined with abdominal wall plication for repair of large abdominal wall hernias following bariatric surgery. *Plast Reconstr Surg* 2007;119(6):1792–1798.
28. Petty P, Manson PN, Black R, et al. Panniculus morbidus. *Ann Plast Surg* 1992;28(5):442–452.
29. Manahan MA, Shermak MA. Massive panniculectomy after massive weight loss. *Plast Reconstr Surg* 2006;117(7):2191–2199.
30. Jensen PL, Sanger JR, Matloub HS, et al. Use of a portable floor crane as an aid to resection of the massive panniculus. *Ann Plast Surg* 1990;25(3):234–235.
31. RamseyStewart G. Radical "fleur-de-lis" abdominal after bariatric surgery. *Obes Surg* 1993;3(4):410–414.
32. Friedman T, O'Brien Coon D, Michaels J, et al. Fleur-de-lis abdominoplasty: a safe alternative to traditional abdominoplasty for the massive weight loss patient. *Plast Reconstr Surg* 2010;125(5):1525–1535.
33. Warren AG, Peled ZM, Borud LJ. Surgical correction of a buried penis focusing on the mons as an anatomic unit. *J Plast Reconstr Aesthet Surg* 2009;62(3):388–392.
34. Pestana IA, Greenfield JM, Walsh M, et al. Management of "buried" penis in adulthood: an overview. *Plast Reconstr Surg* 2009;124(4):1186–1195.
35. Donatucci CF, Ritter EF. Management of the buried penis in adults. *J Urol* 1998;159(2):420–424.
36. Blanton MW, Pestana IA, Donatucci CF, et al. A unique abdominoplasty approach in management of "buried" penis in adulthood. *Plast Reconstr Surg* 2010;125(5):1579–1580.
37. Alter GJ. Surgical techniques: surgery to correct hidden penis. *J Sex Med* 2006;3(5):939–942.
38. Van Geertruyden JP, Vandeweyer E, de Fontaine S, et al. Circumferential torsoplasty. *Br J Plast Surg* 1999;52(8):623–628.
39. Carwell GR, Horton Sr CE. Circumferential torsoplasty. *Ann Plast Surg* 1997;38(3):213–216.
40. Lockwood TE. Superficial fascial system (SFS) of the trunk and extremities: a new concept. *Plast Reconstr Surg* 1991;87(6): 1009–1018.
41. Centeno RF. Autologous gluteal augmentation with circumferential body lift in the massive weight loss and aesthetic patient. *Clin Plast Surg* 2006;33(3):479–496.
42. Cram A, Aly A. Thigh reduction in the massive weight loss patient. *Clin Plast Surg* 2008;35(1):165–172.
43. Le Louarn C, Pascal JF. The concentric medial thigh lift. *Aesthetic Plast Surg* 2004;28(1):20–23.
44. Strauch B, Rohde C, Patel MK, et al. Back contouring in weight loss patients. *Plast Reconstr Surg* 2007;120(6):1692–1696.
45. CRI. Detailed guide: breast cancer 2016. Available at: www.cancer.org/healthy/findcancerearly/cancerscreeningguidelines/american-cancer-society-guidelines-for-the-early-detection-of-cancer
46. Graf RM, Mansur AE, Tenius FP, et al. Mastopexy after massive weight loss: extended chest wall-based flap associated with a loop of pectoralis muscle. *Aesthetic Plast Surg* 2008;32(2):371–374.
47. Rubin JP, Khachi G. Mastopexy after massive weight loss: dermal suspension and selective auto-augmentation. *Clin Plast Surg* 2008;35(1):123–129.
48. Rubin JP. Mastopexy after massive weight loss: dermal suspension and total parenchymal reshaping. *Aesthet Surg J* 2006;26(2):214–222.
49. Rubin JP, Gusenoff JA, Coon D. Dermal suspension and parenchymal reshaping mastopexy after massive weight loss: statistical analysis with concomitant procedures from a prospective registry. *Plast Reconstr Surg* 2009;123(3):782–789.

18

BRACHIOPLASTY

Al Aly

INTRODUCTION

Brachioplasty procedures have become considerably more popular since the emergence of bariatric surgery with its resultant massive weight loss (MWL) patients. Upper arm excess can present on a spectrum of deformities, and although there are many classification systems in the literature, the author does not feel that they are very helpful in clinical decision-making. The technique described in this chapter is geared toward patients who present with a significant amount of upper arm skin excess with varying degrees of lipodystrophy.

ASSESSMENT OF THE DEFECT

As a basic principle of plastic surgery, it is imperative that the presenting deformity is defined accurately. One of the major contributions that the author feels he has made to brachioplasty surgery is the delineation of the posterior axillary fold and its extension onto the upper arm as the deformity encountered in all patients (Figure 18.1).

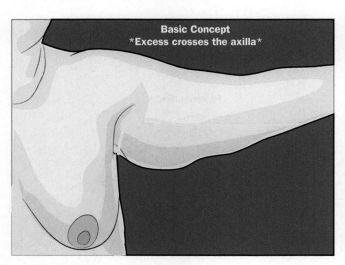

Basic Concept
Excess crosses the axilla

Figure 18.1. Excess crosses the axilla.

By definition, then, the posterior axillary fold traverses from the upper arm to the lateral chest wall; thus the deformity crosses the axilla onto the lateral chest wall. This is a very important concept because, as another basic principle of plastic surgery, once the deformity is accurately delineated, a logical operation can be created to treat it.

INDICATIONS AND CONTRAINDICATIONS

As in all body contouring procedures, especially MWL body contouring, the patient's weight should be stable for at least 3–6 months. The patient should be medically and psychiatrically stable, and the author prefers not to perform this surgery on smokers or diabetics. A complete set of nutritional lab values should be obtained and be within normal limits.

The ideal patient to undergo brachioplasty utilizing a "posterior scar Aly technique" is one who has a deflated upper arm with a significant amount of excess skin. Patients who present with a significant amount of lipodystrophy of the upper arms despite their weight loss are best treated with a preliminary liposuction procedure to deflate the arm. Three to six months after the liposuction procedure, when all the induration has resolved, the procedure described in this chapter is undertaken.

If the patient presents with an intermediate level of lipodystrophy, a decision has to be made by the patient and surgeon to determine the level of improvement that the patient is interested in since the results will not be at the level of a deflated arm.

Brachioplasty maybe performed by itself or in combination with an upper body lift, which includes breast, upper back, and upper arm surgery combined into one surgery.

ROOM SETUP

If brachioplasty is to be performed by itself, then the patient can be placed in the supine position with an arm board on either side to allow for full manipulation of the arms during the procedure. Usually the operating room bed is pushed away from anesthesia to allow an assistant to stand above the arm. When brachioplasty is combined with an upper body lift, the arm portion of the procedure in some cases is performed in the supine position while in others in a lateral decubitus position.

MARKINGS

Brachioplasty is a fairly unforgiving procedure that can easily lead to either an inability to close the arm at the end of the procedure or underresection. The anatomy of the arm can be likened to a cylinder, with a hard inner core made up of the musculoskeletal system that takes up the majority of the volume of the cylinder. The skin–fat envelope makes up a relatively small percentage of the cylinder's volume. Since the musculoskeletal core is largely noncompressible, the skin–fat envelope cannot tolerate much swelling before the arm cannot be closed after a fairly aggressive resection (Figure 18.2).

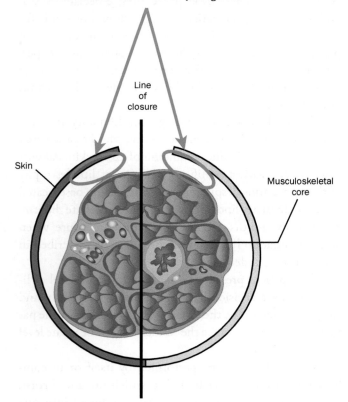

Figure 18.2. Minor edema.

Unlike other areas of the body, such as the face or abdomen, it is not possible to undermine tissues in the arm to decrease tension or help close an overresected arm. Thus, the author's marking methodology and surgical technique are designed to avoid these issues.

Overall, the markings can be thought of as creating an ellipse of tissue based on the posterior axillary fold and its extension onto the lateral chest wall medially and the upper arm distally. The author prefers to mark patients 1–2 days prior to surgery, after which they are photographed so that the surgeon can gain insight over time on how to improve by comparing the postoperative results with the marking photographs. The patient's arms are abducted to 90 degrees at the axilla and elbows for the marking process.

THE DOUBLE ELLIPSE MARKING TECHNIQUE

The meridian of the ellipse to be resected is marked on the inferior border of the posterior axillary fold, with its extension onto the lateral chest wall proximally and the upper arm distally.

The tissues are pinched and marked, equally on both sides of the meridian every few centimeters, just under the muscle mass. This is done with the intent to match the final contour to the underlying anatomy (Figures 18.3–18.6).

The dots are then connected to create the first ellipse by tapering on either end.

A second, inner ellipse is marked within the first ellipse based on repinching every few centimeters of the first ellipse and noting the distance between the fingers during the pinch. So, if the pinch in any particular point has a distance of 2 cm between the fingers, then this second set of

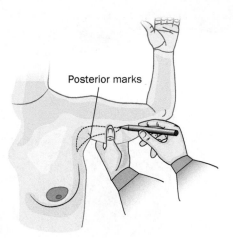

Figure 18.3. Marking technique I.

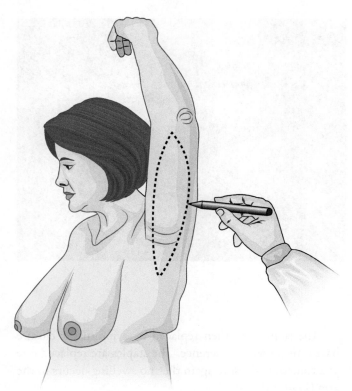

Figure 18.4. Marking technique II.

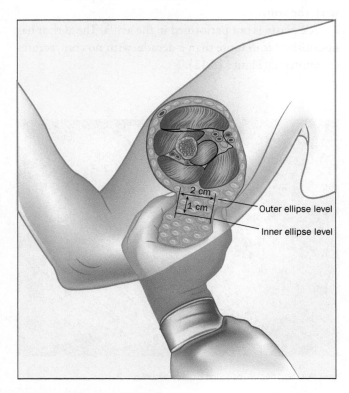

Figure 18.5. Marking technique III.

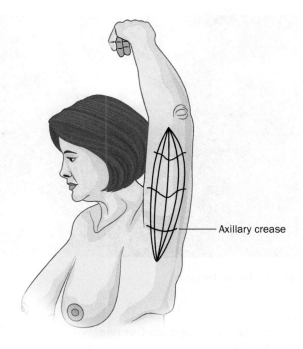

Axillary crease

Figure 18.6. Marking technique IV.

marks is moved in 1 cm on either side of the first ellipse. This maneuver is performed to make sure there is enough skin left behind to account for the distance between the pinched fingers.

Connecting this second set of anterior and posterior dots marks the inner ellipse. This is the ellipse that will be used as the resection edges.

Horizontal cross-hash marks are placed every 10–15 cm to help with alignment after resection.

SURGICAL TECHNIQUE

After the patient is anesthetized, the horizontal hash marks are tattooed with methylene blue and the inner ellipse is injected with epinephrine-containing solution to reduce bleeding during the resection.

The patient is prepped and draped, and the entire inner ellipse is then tailor tacked, starting distal and moving proximal, to simulate an actual closure. The reason for starting distally is that pinched tissues are pushed proximally, leading to less aggressive resection proximally. This will ultimately cause the arm shape to better reflect a normal upper arm—narrower at the elbow and larger at the axilla (Figure 18.7).

The resection is performed in what has been coined by the author as the "segmental resection-closure technique," which was designed to avoid swelling.

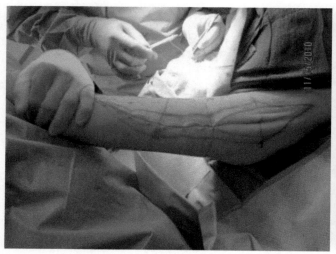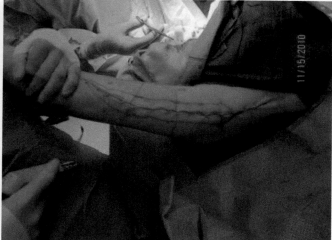

Figure 18.7. Surgical technique.

The tailor tacking staples are removed and the markings are adjusted.

Starting distally, the inner ellipse marks are incised, both anteriorly and posteriorly, up to the first horizontal hash mark. The incision is deepened to the level of the underlying muscle fascia. The skin and subcutaneous fat are elevated off the muscle fascia up to the hash mark (Figure 18.8).

The wound edges are then reapproximated with staples to simulate the final closure and to prevent any more swelling from occurring in this area of resection (Figure 18.9).

This same process is repeated from one hash mark to the next until the entire elliptical resection is completed.

The staples are then replaced by a multilayer closure based on surgeon preference. The staples are replaced one at a time to make sure again that no swelling occurs in the arm (Figure 18.10).

The author prefers the final layer to be a subcuticular layer with no external skin sutures and uses external skin staples on either side of the axillary crease to help reduce the risk of dehiscence in the axilla.

No drains are utilized, and the author prefers not to wrap the arm.

A z-plasty is not performed in the axilla. The author has not utilized it in more than a decade, with no contractures encountered (Figure 18.11).

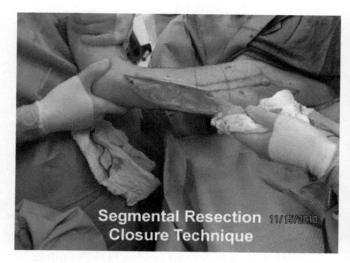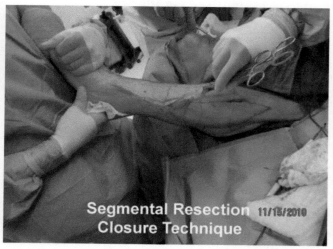

Figure 18.8. Segmental resection closure technique I.

Figure 18.9. Segmental resection closure technique II.

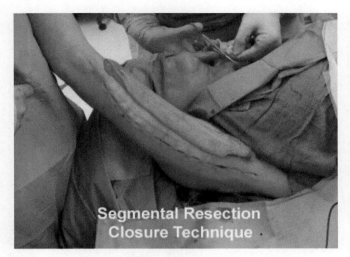

Figure 18.10. Segmental resection closure technique III.

POSTOPERATIVE CARE AND USUAL COURSE

Patients are asked to keep their arms above heart level with the elbow in neutral position for 2 weeks except for meals and going to the bathroom. The staples located in the axilla are removed 2 weeks after surgery. Some patients will experience swelling and scalloping for months after surgery. The scar matures over a longer period of time than most scars created elsewhere in the body, usually over a 2-year period.

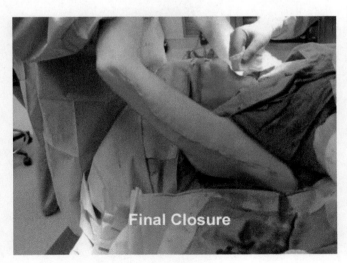

Figure 18.11. Final closure.

COMPLICATIONS

Infection and hematoma are possible complications. Dehiscence or separation of the wound is most likely to occur in the axilla and is most often treated conservatively.

Seromas tend to occur 4–5 weeks out from surgery and most likely in the distal third of the upper arm. The author has never had to operate on a seroma of the arm. Treatment usually involves the following steps, which are performed in the order listed if the previous step is not effective:

- Aspirate and apply compression every 2–3 days.

- Inject the seroma pocket with an astringent such as doxycycline and then aspirate, along with compression, every 2–3 days.

- Open the incision for 1 cm over the seroma pocket and insert a Penrose drain that is sutured in place and left in place until the pocket closes around it, which may take weeks to completely resolve.

- The patient is placed on a low dose diuretic such as hydrochlorothiazide, 25 mg/day, for 30 days whether a seroma is encountered or not.

An inability to close the arm defect should be avoided by using the technique described in this chapter.

CAVEATS

The excess in the upper arm is the posterior axillary roll with its extensions onto the lateral chest wall and the upper arm.

The excision must cross from the upper arm, through the axilla, and onto the lateral chest wall to allow for the large amount of excess skin that is usually associated with MWL.

The arm is a cylinder with a hard inner musculoskeletal core that does not compress, which makes the resection potentially dangerous.

During the marking process, the distance between the pinching fingers must be accounted for.

During the surgical procedure it is important not to allow swelling to occur in the unclosed arm.

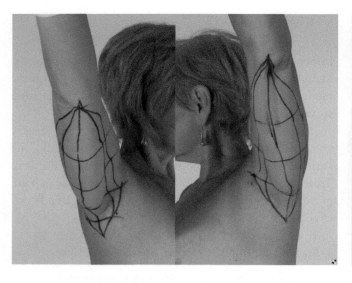

Figure 18.12. Shows the markings of a typical patient.

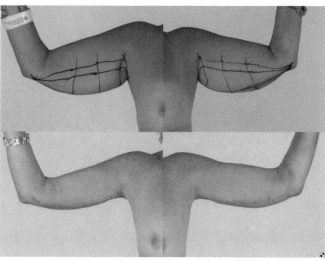

Figure 18.13. Shows the markings next to the final result, which is what should be compared in order for the surgeon to improve their technique technique

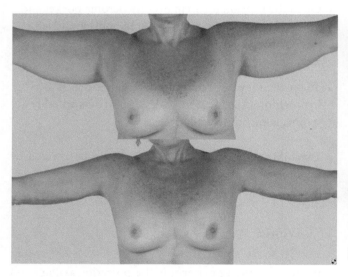

Figure 18.14. Show the arms before and after surgery anteriorly and posteriorly.

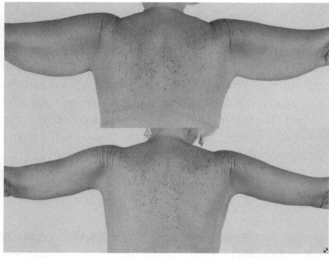

Figure 18.15. Show the arms before and after surgery anteriorly and posteriorly.

SELECTED READINGS

Aly AS, ed. *Body Contouring After Massive Weight Loss*. St Louis, MO: Quality Medical Publishing; 2006.

Aly, A, Soliman, S, Cram, A. Brachioplasty in the massive weight loss patient. In A. Aly, ed., *Clinics in Plastic Surgery. Body Contouring After Massive Weight Loss*. 2008 Jan;35(1).

Aly A, Tolazzi A, Soliman S, Cram A. Quantitative analysis of aesthetic results: introducing a new paradigm. *Aesthet Surg J* 2012 Jan;32(1):120–124.

Soliman S, Rotemberg SC, Pace D, Bark A, Mansur A, Cram A, Aly A. Upper body lift. In A. Aly, ed., *Clinics in Plastic Surgery. Body Contouring After Massive Weight Loss*. 2008 Jan;35(1).

PART IV.

NONINVASIVE TECHNIQUES

19.

PRINCIPLES OF INJECTABLE FACIAL FILLING

Donald S. Mowlds and Val Lambros

In the past decade, the use of fillers to correct wrinkles and creases as well as to restore volume to the aged face has grown rapidly, marking the most significant contribution to rehabilitation of the face since the introduction of the facelift. Because these substances are relatively easy to use, they have broadened the base of clinicians and others offering rejuvenation services, for better and worse.

ASSESSMENT OF THE PATIENT

The aging face develops excesses, creases, demarcations, hollows, and wrinkles. These changes have been part of the human condition since primitive times; our generation is certainly not the first to notice them. The interested reader can thumb through Shakespeare's sonnets and find many lamenting references to the passage of time on the human face. From the late 1890s to the 1920s, clinicians used injectable soft tissue fillers to counteract age-related changes and deformities, much as is done today. Unfortunately, the substances used were petroleum-based, like Vaseline and paraffin, and had an inordinate complication rate.

For the next 70 years, the aesthetic care of the face was primarily in the hands of surgeons, resulting in a natural shift in focus from volume addition to more subtractive procedures aimed at "tightening" tissue planes of the face and removal of fat. These procedures proved to be enduring and a commercial success, largely benefiting patients who fit the operation and when not repeated in excess. However, older faces were made to look thin and overly defined with tight and sometimes visibly pulled cheek skin. The orbits were routinely hollowed by fat removal, resulting in a rounder, shorter orbit with exposure of the underlying bony structures, all of which are attributes of aged eyes (Figure 19.1A,B). The limitations of surgery as the sole instrument for facial rejuvenation is evident in the untoward distortion of a face subjected to multiple procedures.

For many decades, there was nothing available to address facial volume disproportion or loss. When volume concepts were "rediscovered" in the late 1980s, after the emergence of liposuction and fat grafting, they were met with resistance because surgeons were conditioned by decades of surgical teaching and practice with opposite goals.

Although fat grafting of the face has some issues which make it difficult to use, its emergence did encourage

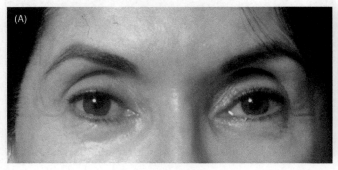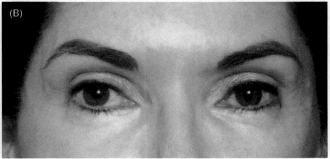

Figure 19.1. (A) A 68-year-old woman who has previously undergone a blepharoplasty. She was treated with 1 cc of hyaluronic acid (HA) filler and then another the year following. The post-injection image (B) is 3 years after the first injection.

practitioners to analyze and treat the face as a three-dimensional entity, a challenge to the dogma of surgeons from generations ago.

INDICATIONS AND CONTRAINDICATIONS

In the face, curves have meaning and are intimately tied to the emotional projection of the face. The difference between an agreeable appearance and a dour face may be the presence of marionette lines ("bitterness lines" in French) or a large tear trough shadow, which causes faces to appear tired. High cheekbones and hollow cheeks may be acceptable in a young person but are signs of age and ill health in the older patient. Similarly, hollow temples can look gaunt and detract from the appearance of a youthful, healthy state.

At present, the term "fillers" typically refers to injectable off-the-shelf products used to treat skin irregularities and volume deficiencies, a nebulous art where the basic proportions of the face are changed in an attempt to impart youthfulness or approximate an aesthetic ideal.

Commercially available fillers are priced as wrinkle treatments and are quite expensive. As volume deficits of the aged face may exceed 20 cc, the use of off-the-shelf fillers for full restoration may be financially impractical. Clinical judgment must be used, therefore, in order to maximize the visual gains while minimizing the amount of filler used.

The deep subcutaneous space should be avoided at the superior-most extent of the nasolabial crease where the nasal artery lies, as well as at the medial glabellar frown lines, which are directly superficial to the supratrochlear artery. Injections performed here carry an increased risk of vascular penetration and material embolization.

TECHNIQUES

NEEDLES VERSUS CANNULAS

Fillers have traditionally been injected using sharp hypodermic needles. In the past several years, disposable cannulas (22–30 gauge) have been promoted for the injection of filler and have proved invaluable. The cannulas are blunt and have a side port, resulting in less pain and bruising when compared to sharp-tipped needles. Furthermore, the cannulas are typically longer than needles, facilitating greater reach from a single injection site and allowing the use of both the bolus and threading techniques. Additionally, there is a theoretical increase in safety as blunt cannulas are thought to be less likely to result in vessel perforation and its ensuing complications. The authors prefer cannulas for most facial injections.

DISTRIBUTION OF FILLERS, TECHNIQUES, AND VOLUME CORRECTIONS

Ritual and habit play a significant role in any human endeavor, and, though beyond the scope of this discussion, their role in cosmetic facial treatments cannot be minimized. The tendency of clinicians to bias their treatment to particular areas of the face likely results from a lack of vision and unwillingness to treat outside areas of familiarity.

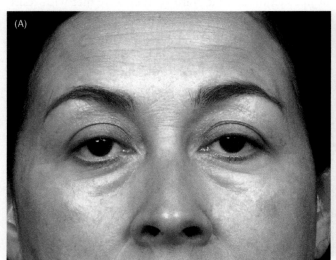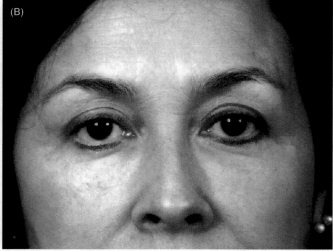

Figure 19.2. (A,B) This patient underwent injection of her tear troughs and brow; the pictures are 4 years apart and illustrate the extreme longevity of hyaluronic acid (HA) fillers in this location. Similar longevity can be seen in the brows and temples. She also exhibits a mild Tyndall effect in the lower lid where the site of injection is slightly bluish.

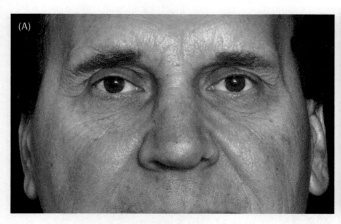
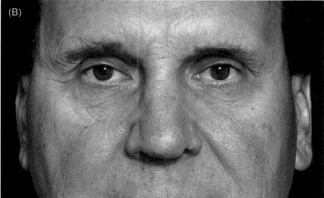

Figure 19.3. (A) A 62-year-old male with hollow temples. (B) His face assumes a more youthful shape after injection of 2 cc of hyaluronic acid (HA) filler into each temple.

A craftsman-like vision and technical expertise are necessary to achieve the desired aesthetic goals.

The technical aspects of filler injection are basic but nonetheless important. One must be able to fill lines and creases evenly as well as create three-dimensional shapes in the subcutaneous space. Basic techniques for filling surface lines and wrinkles include radial injections from a single insertion point or cross-hatching via orthogonal approaches.

Correction of facial contour irregularities such as the marionette line or tear trough (Figure 19.2A,B) may be partially addressed by subcutaneous injection of filler material, but three-dimensional consideration must be given to certain treatment areas. For example, submalar hollowing is counterbalanced by an injection volume that resembles a teardrop, while the temple is best addressed with one that is

pancake-shaped (Figures 19.3 and 19.4). The anterior jawline is managed using a bean-shaped volume. We now inject lips with a cannula in a simple threading maneuver at the vermilion border or submucosal body of the lips after suitable anesthesia (Figure 19.5A,B).

Free-form linear injection techniques, where the speed of the needle or cannula is varied in accordance with the desired treatment, can be used. Alternatively, we have come to prefer a depot technique where the treatment area is marked with dots spaced according to the severity of the indentation. A cannula or a needle is then used to bolus beneath each dot. As most contour injections are made at the deep subcutaneous or preperiosteal level, a bolus of 0.1 cc or less is not visible individually. Creating a three-dimensional object with a two-dimensional instrument, like a needle or

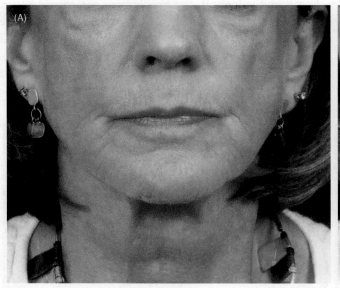
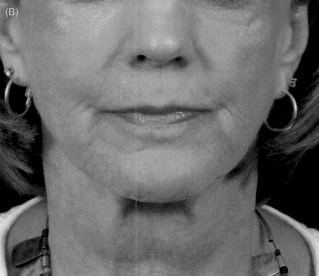

Figure 19.4. (A) This patient was diagnosed with scleroderma in her 60s, which is believed to be responsible for the hollowing of her cheekbone. (B) The follow-up image was taken 1 year after injection of 3 cc of hyaluronic acid (HA) filler into each cheek.

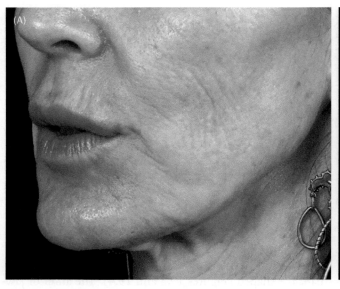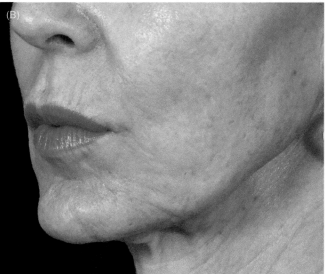

Figure 19.5. (A,B) A 22-year-old female patient 2 weeks after injection of 1 cc of hyaluronic acid (HA) filler into her upper lip.

cannula, is difficult and not always intuitive, but, with practice, the focused clinician can successfully master these basic shapes and ultimately improve their outcomes.

FILLERS FOR WRINKLES

Treatment of age-related wrinkles and creases is an obvious target for filler use. When patients are asked to describe the appearance they would like to achieve, they invariably pull the cheeks backward, erasing wrinkles and flattening creases. Though considered pedestrian and artless by some, wrinkle filling provides great benefit to the older face and has technical subtleties. If one examines a forehead or nasolabial crease by pinching it at a right angle to its long axis, one will feel what one sees, an indentation distinct from the dermis itself. In other words, the deficiency is in the subcutaneous space. Therefore, nasolabial, forehead, and marionette creases need to be filled primarily in the subcutaneous space with extension into the actual dermis if necessary.

To treat true dermal wrinkles, a topical anesthetic is applied following meticulous marking of the creases to be addressed. Fillers marketed for intradermal use or dilute hyaluronic acid (HA) fillers are used with excellent results. Once the skin is anesthetized, the injections are performed with magnification and 30–33 gauge needles. Both depot and linear threading techniques are useful depending on the clinical indication. These injections are technically demanding as great precision is required to thread the needle into the intradermal plane while remaining directly beneath the wrinkle to be filled. Failure to place the filler material beneath the wrinkle will result in accentuation. When one can see the bluish shaft of the needle through the overlying dermis and epidermis, the needle is in the correct plane. Attention to this is critical, as most cosmetic injections are subdermal despite clinicians' best intention. Concatenated pores, which do not fill well, are distinct from true wrinkles and ought to be avoided. Figure 19.6A and B demonstrates the effect of superficial injections to treat dermal wrinkles.

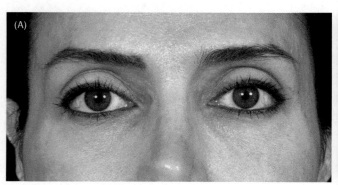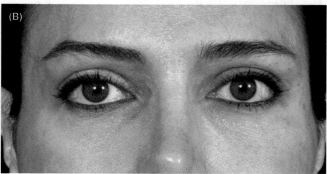

Figure 19.6. (A,B) These figures demonstrate the effect of superficial injections to treat dermal wrinkles.

NONINVASIVE TECHNIQUES

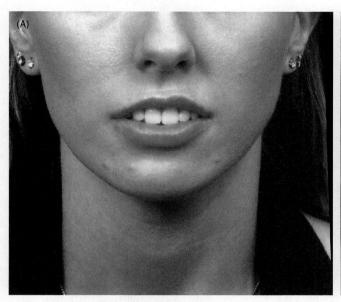 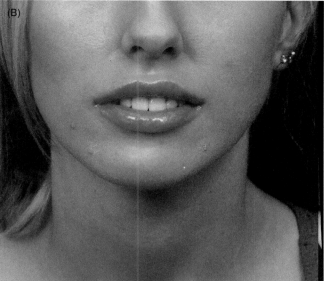

Figure 19.7. (A,B) These images illustrate the power of previsualizing an injection using local anesthetic. It is very difficult, if not impossible, to explain the outcome of an intended treatment verbally because it is a visual concept. If the patient is satisfied with the preview, we proceed with the injection immediately as the area is now numb and vasoconstricted.

Some clinicians offer patients topical and/or injectable anesthetic. In the latter group, the volume of the local anesthetic can be used to demonstrate the intended result of the final injection. We find this technique to be invaluable, especially when treating the brows, temples, and anterior jawline where "previewing" the intended result allows the clinician and client to make adjustments with impunity (Figure 19.7A,B).

POSTPROCEDURAL CARE

Injections of HA fillers beneath the skin can result in a bluish discoloration which is popularly ascribed to the Tyndall effect. Commonly seen in the lower lids and nasolabial folds, it results from having a lake or accumulation of filler beneath the skin. It is thought that short wavelength blue light is backscattered through the skin, imparting the bluish blush, which disappears after dissolving with hyaluronidase or draining the product with a needle stick (Figure 19.2B).[12–15] Interestingly, it is not seen with extremely superficial injections.

CAVEATS

The judgment required to achieve the most visible gain from facial injections is an acquired skill. Nevertheless, the following are suggested:

1. In general, dermal wrinkles are treated with true dermal injections. Creases, like the nasolabial crease and marionette line, are treated in the subcutaneous space, and volumization is accomplished in the deep subcutaneous space or adjacent to the periosteum.

2. Volume treatments of the face work best in an environment of tight skin. In general, heavy faces with skin excess do not respond well to filling because the treatments are small relative to the mass and extra skin, requiring large volumes to achieve facial smoothness. As in almost all cosmetic treatments of the face, the patient who needs them the most does the least well.

3. Treat one area well rather than undertreating multiple areas. Treating nasolabial folds, cheekbones, and marionette lines all together with one syringe of filler will result in a patient who sees no change in any of these locations. Unfortunately, perceptible change requires a certain minimum volume, which may be outside of the patient's financial means. Set realistic expectations with the patient.

4. As a general rule, older faces benefit the most from filling hollows while younger faces benefit from expanding prominences. For example, expanding the malar prominences in younger patients makes the cheekbones more defined. Filling the malar

prominence on an older patient with a submalar hollow makes the hollow more pronounced and increases gauntness. Instead, bringing the submalar hollow to the level of the nasojugal fold restores balance.

5. The temples are corrected by filling the subcutaneous space near or above the deep temporal fascia. Alternatively, injections may pierce the temporalis muscle to fill the space directly above the periosteum. The deep temporal fascia is difficult to expand, making the latter technique inefficient.

Most filler complications are aesthetic and related to lumps, overinjection, or persistent treatment of areas previously injected.

Granulomas are unusual with HA fillers and seem to be more common with calcium and poly-l-lactic acid (PLLA) fillers. Although rare, the most severe complication is intravascular injection. Skin slough of the nose, lips, cheeks, and forehead as well as blindness and even stroke and death have been described following intraarterial injection and embolization. Blunt cannulas in constant motion with slow product delivery are recommended. Aspirating before injecting may signal impending intravascular placement; however, this technique becomes unreliable when fine needles are used due to product viscosity. In scarred areas, vessels are not easily displaced by a passing cannula, and channels created within the tissue may funnel material into a perforated vessel.

Although these suggestions appear to be intuitively obvious, there is no evidence that implementing them has prevented arterial injuries.

SELECTED READINGS

American Society for Aesthetic Plastic Surgery. Cosmetic Surgery National Data Bank Statistics. *The American Society for Aesthetic Plastic Surgery's Cosmetic Surgery Statistics*. Web. 15 May 2016. https://www.surgery.org/sites/default/files/ASAPS-Stats2016.pdf

American Society of Plastic Surgeons. 2015 Plastic Surgery Statistics Report. *Plastic Surgery Procedural Statistics*. Web. 15 May 2016. https://www.google.com/url?sa=t&rct=j&q=&esrc=s&source=web&cd=11&cad=rja&uact=8&ved=2ahUKEwj2ip6n0aHdAhUDQK0KHfl4BAM4ChAWMAB6BAgKEAI&url=https%3A%2F%2Fd2wirczt3b6wjm.cloudfront.net%2FNews%2FStatistics%2F2015%2Fcosmetic-procedure-trends-2015.pdf&usg=AOvVaw0vVBnhXs-L5m46QerlZ7Az

Bailey SH, Cohen JL, Kenkel JM. Etiology, prevention, and treatment of dermal filler complications. *Aesthetic Surg J* 2011;31(1):110–121.

Carruthers JDA, Fagien S, Rohrich RJ, Weinkle, Carruthers A. Blindness caused by cosmetic filler injection: a review of cause and therapy. *Plast Reconstr Surg* 2014;134(6):1197–1201.

Carruthers JDA, Fagien S, Rohrich RJ, Weinkle S, Carruthers A. Blindness caused by cosmetic filler injection: a review of cause and therapy. *Plast Reconstr Surg* 2014;134(6):1197–1201.

Coleman SR. Facial reconstruction with lipostructure. *Clin Plast Surg* 1997;24:347–367.

Coleman, SR. Avoidance of arterial occlusion from injection of soft tissue fillers. *Aesthetic Surg J* 2002;22:555–557.

DeLorenzi C. Complications of injectable fillers, part I. *Aesthetic Surg J* 2013;33(4):561–575.

Douse-Dean T, Jacob CI. Fast and easy treatment for reduction of the Tyndall effect secondary to cosmetic use of hyaluronic acid. *J Drugs Dermatol* 2008;7:281–283.

Fagien S, Cassuto, D. Reconstituted injectable hyaluronic acid: expanded applications in facial aesthetics and additional thoughts on the mechanism of action in cosmetic medicine. *Plast Reconstr Surg* 2012;130: 208–217.

Goldwyn R, The paraffin story. *Plast Reconstr Surg* 1980;65(4):517–524.

Hirsch RJ, Narurkar V, Carruthers J. Management of injected hyaluronic acid induced Tyndall effects. *Lasers Surg Med* 2006;38:202–204.

Lam S, Glasgold R, Galsgold M. Analysis of facial aesthetics as applied to injectables. *Plast Reconstr Surg* 2015;136(5 suppl):11S–21S.

Lambros V. A technique for filling the temples with highly diluted hyaluronic acid: the "dilution solution." *Aesthetic Surg J* 2011;31(1):89–94.

Lambros V. The use of hyaluronidase to reverse the effects of hyaluronic acid filler. *Plast Reconstr Surg* 2004;114(1):277.

Lambros V. Volumizing the brow with hyaluronic acid fillers. *Aesthetic Surg J* 2009;29(3):174–179.

Lemperle G, Rullan PP, Gauthier-Hazan N. Avoiding and treating dermal filler complications. *Plast Reconstr Surg* 2006;118(3S):92S–107S.

Ozturk CN, Li Y, Tung R, Parker L, Piliang MP, Zins JE. Complications following injection of soft-tissue fillers. *Aesthetic Surg J* 2013;33(6): 862–877.

Rzany B, DeLorenzi C. Understanding, avoiding, and managing severe filler complications. *Plast Reconstr Surg* 2015;136(5 suppl):196S–203S.

Sykes JM, Cotofana S, Trevidic P, et al. Upper face: clinical anatomy and regional approaches with injectable fillers. *Plast Reconstr Surg* 2015;136(5 suppl):204S–218S.

20

BOTULINUM TOXINS AND RADIO FREQUENCY FOR FACIAL REJUVENATION

Brian M. Kinney

INTRODUCTION

According to the American Society of Plastic Surgeons Statistics Report, more than 7 million botulinum toxin injections were performed by its members in 2016. This represents a 4% increase over 2015.[1] Less than 4 million procedures were performed in 2005, less than 1 million in 2000, and data show a 797% increase in the 16-year interval.

Its use has become such a part of popular culture, reported in the news and magazines and spoken in common parlance, that the term "Botox" is listed in Merriam-Webster's dictionary as a verb.[2] Cosmetic minimally invasive procedures outnumber surgical almost 10 to 1 (15,411,829 vs. 1,780,987).

Most patients have a full response to toxin injection for 3–4 months, but residual weakness and effects are evident up to double than time. Due to this short duration and the need for repeated injections to achieve the desired effect, an alternative approach has emerged in the past 5 years: *radiofrequency (RF) ablation* for long-term (i.e., 1-year) duration.[3] There are clinical reports of even "permanent" duration at 4–5 years.[4] This mechanism of action is a heat-induced nerve injury. The therapeutic goal is at least a third-degree injury where the axon and endoneurium are disrupted with mild to moderate reduction in function for months or a fourth-degree injury where the axon and endo- and perineurium are injured with a moderate to severe reduction in function but recovery is possible, sometimes taking up to a year or more. Permanent injury is achieved with a fifth-degree lesion, with complete destruction of the nerve leading to irreversible nerve damage and, thus, muscle denervation.

ASSESSMENT AND INDICATIONS

Desired aesthetic results with treatment are not entirely related to facial aging and, in fact, most patients present for aesthetic improvement related to expressive, dynamic complaints even at a young age. Branches of the facial nerve innervate the muscles of facial expression through the temporal, zygomatic, buccal, and marginal mandibular branches. The cervical branch of the facial nerve innervates the platysma muscle and is a prime focus of rejuvenation as well. Some portion of facial expression is almost involuntary as the emotional state of the patient influences muscular contraction during speech, concentration, athletic competition, activities of daily living, and even at rest. Many patients come to treatment to improve hyperactive muscles; some to improve resting, baseline tone; some to "balance" the anatomy influenced by complementary muscles (e.g., eyebrow); and some to treat disease states or congenital conditions (e.g., congenital blepharophimosis, stroke or posttraumatic defects).

GENERAL ASSESSMENT AND APPROACH

There are a number of components in the evaluation of the patient presenting for aesthetic modification of facial muscles:

1. Ascertain patient goals.

2. Perform a history and physical.

3. Evaluate the patient's face when animated and resting; use photography and video as needed.

4. Perform a symmetry assessment.

5. Look for muscle action more than presence of lines.

6. Think of shape and balance of the face versus smoothing and paralyzing muscles.

7. Avoid the "porcelain doll" frozen look; instead think "natural."

To aesthetically improve the face, balance complementary muscles, smooth lines, and shrink bulky muscles, understanding the anatomy in detail is key, both its form and function. While it is easy to "inject the dots" or "push the plunger" in a standard pattern, this will provide a technically approximate result, but not an aesthetically superior one. In fact, some patient will be made worse by following this as a standard protocol. There are many variations in anatomy, and standard anatomy textbook depictions are inadequate for aesthetic excellence. There can be no underestimating how important it is to appreciate the myriad individual variations in facial anatomy and the patient's desire to be treated individually. Understanding the details of the functional anatomy of the face as elucidated by Rubin may be considered a gold standard.[5]

The assessment for toxin and RF patients is essentially the same; however, the therapeutic goals are somewhat different. The toxin patients can expect a shorter duration effect and a more focal response immediately in the area of the injection, usually within 1 cm. RF patients can expect anywhere from double the duration up to a permanent effect. The area of response is much larger, anywhere an innervated muscle is downstream of the point of the neural lesion. RF patients can experience a therapeutic effect even if immunized for botulism or naturally resistant to the effects of a toxin. RF has been cleared for creating lesions in nerves[6]; therefore, the aesthetic consequences of this, even though RF is not specifically cleared as an aesthetic procedure, are within the regulatory clearance because creating the lesion may result in an aesthetic effect.

INDICATIONS

Indications for on-label toxin use include:

1. Moderate to severe glabellar rhytids associated with corrugator and/or procerus muscle activity in adult patients.

2. Moderate to severe lateral canthal lines associated with orbicularis oculi activity in adult patients (crow's feet).

Indications for on-label RF use include:

1. Creating lesions in nerves (note that this means any nerve, in any location and not just specifically for aesthetics, spasm, or pain).

Indications for toxin off-label use and RF on-label effects are:

1. Eyebrow position and asymmetry

2. Transverse forehead lines

3. Lower eyelid lines

4. Nasal lines

5. Perioral lines (smoker's and oral commissure lines)

6. Chin dimpling

7. Platysmal bands

8. Any area where modulating muscle function will improve aesthetics (e.g., asymmetry, complications of aesthetic procedures)

CONTRAINDICATIONS

In the use of toxins, there are a number of contraindications due to conflicting concomitant chemical effects or neurological conditions. In the use of RF, the action is strictly local or limited to the distribution of the nerve under treatment, so systemic effects are relatively less concerning. Local considerations remain.

TOXIN CONTRAINDICATIONS

1. Use of aminoglycoside antibiotics

2. Use of anticholinergic drugs

3. Other botulinum toxin products

4. Muscle relaxants

5. Neuromuscular diseases (e.g., myasthenia gravis, amyotrophic lateral sclerosis, Lambert-Eaton syndrome)

6. Known allergy to botulinum toxin

7. Known hypersensitivity

8. Dysphagia and breathing difficulties

9. Under treatment for urinary tract infection

10. Injection of toxin in the previous two weeks

11. Prophylactic immunization for botulism

TOXIN AND RF CONTRAINDICATIONS

1. Active Bell's palsy, recent stroke, or another acute neurological event

2. Preexisting conditions at the site of treatment

3. Active infection at the site of injection

4. Pregnancy and breast-feeding

Disruption of the nerve, chemically or thermally, leads to dose-dependent muscular paresis or paralysis, sympathetic blockade of the skin, and concomitant effects such as hypohidrosis and smoothing of skin pores. Therefore, clinical techniques are focused generally on smoothing facial rhytids, balancing complementary muscle functions, and elevating or depressing facial muscles.

ROOM SETUP

Very little equipment is required. It is simply the equipment required for an injection. The list includes the following for toxin injection:

1. Sterile gloves

2. 1 cc Luer lock syringe with 30-gauge 1-inch needle for injection

3. 3 cc Luer lock syringe with 18-gauge needle for mixing

4. Sterile saline solution

5. Alcohol swab

6. Botulinum toxin bottle (onabotulinum vs. abobotulinum vs. incobotulinum)

7. Sterile saline (dilute 4 vs. 2.5)

8. Hand-held mirror for patient

9. Head of bed set at 45–90 degrees

The clinical effects of toxins are dose-related and dilution-dependent,[7] and the release of the 150 kDa neurotoxin is pH- and time-dependent.[8] Complexing proteins may be associated with nonresponse caused by neutralizing antibodies. Multiple small doses are more precise in predicting outcome, and the effects balance between agonist and antagonist muscles.[7] The effects diminish after regeneration of the nerve terminals, and, in general, comparable patient satisfaction can be achieved with understanding of dosing, preparation, storage, and immune characteristics.[9] See Table 20.1 for a

TABLE 20.1 COMPARISON OF BOTULINUM TOXIN A CHARACTERISTICS

	Onabotulinum	Abobotulinum	Incobotulinum
Vial Size	50 U, 100 U	300 U	50 U, 100 U
Stabilization	Vacuum-dried	Lyophilized	Lyophilized
Composition	C botulinum toxin type A ATCC 3502 (Hall strain) hemagglutinin complex	C botulinum toxin type A ATCC 3502 (Hall strain) hemagglutinin complex	C botulinum toxin type A ATCC 3502 (Hall strain)
	0.25 mg HSA, 0.5 mg HSA	0.125 mg HSA	1.0 mg HSA (both vial sizes)
	0.45 mg NaCl, 0.9 mg NaCl	2.5 mg lactose	4.7 mg sucrose (both vial sizes)
Molecular weight	900 kDa	500–900 kDa	150 kDa
Clostridial protein per 100 U	0.73 ng[4]	0.65 ng[4]	0.44 ng[4]
Specific biologic activity	60 MU-E/ng[5]	100 MU-E/ng[5]	167 MU-E/ng[5]
Storage (packaged product)	36°F–46°F for 36 mo.	36°F–46°F until vial expiration	68°F–77°F for 36 mo.
Storage (once reconstituted)	36°F–46°F, use within 24 h	36°F–46°F, use within 4 h	36°F–46°F, use within 24 h

HSA - Human Serum Albumin
MU-E - Mouse Units Equivalence

[1] BOTOX Cosmetic [package insert]. Irvine, CA: Allergan, Inc.; 2011.
[2] DYSPORT Cosmetic [package insert]. Scottsdale, AZ: Medicis Aesthetics Inc.; 2010.
[3] XEOMIN [package insert]. Greensboro, NC. Merz Pharmaceuticals, LLC; 2011.
[4] Frevert J. *Drugs R D*. 2010;10(2):67–73.
[5] Dressler D et al. *Disabil Rehabil*. 2007;29(23):1761–1768.

comparison of Botulinum Toxins A and their relative biological activities, stabilization, and other attributes.

Commonly used human serum albumin (HAS) in equivalence mouse units (MU-E).

In general, I prefer 2.5 u/0.1 mL solution (4 mL/100 u bottle) for injection for ona- and incobotulinum, whereas for abototulinum the 2.5 mL dilution yields a preparation with three times the number of units. Nonetheless, in a practical clinical situation, generally the injections are about 0.1 mL in each area via the serial puncture method as the abobotulinum toxin preparation is not as potent unit for unit. The ratio is generally about 3:1 compared to the other two preparations. Table 20.2 shows highlights from the US Food and Drug Administration (FDA) package inserts on the preparation of the solutions.

RF SETUP DETAILS

A small amount of equipment is required for an RF procedure compared to a surgical procedure, but more than a simple injection.

1. Cutaneous nerve stimulator and custom grounding pad for nerve mapping

2. Forward looking infrared (FLiR) camera with tripod or boom at 90-degree angle to skin

3. RF generator and computer monitor

4. 18-gauge hypodermic needle to create access point

5. 22-gauge active RF probe with outer sheath and three-way side injection port

TABLE 20.2 ON-LABEL PREPARATION AND USE OF BOTULINUM TOXINS-A

BOTOX Cosmetic[1] (100 U vial)	DYSPORT[2] (300 U vial)	XEOMIN[3] (100 U vial)
Preservative-free saline	Preservative-free saline	Preservative-free saline
2.5 mL diluent volume	2.5 mL or 1.5 mL diluent volume	0.5 mL–8.0 mL diluent volume
Use within 24 h	Use within 4 h	Use within 24 h
Single patient use vial	Single patient use vial	Single patient use vial

[1] BOTOX Cosmetic [package insert]. Irvine, CA: Allergan, Inc.; 2011.
[2] DYSPORT Cosmetic [package insert]. Scottsdale, AZ: Medicis Aesthetics Inc.; 2010.
[3] XEOMIN [package insert]. Greensboro, NC. Merz Pharmaceuticals, LLC; 2011.

6. Grounding pad

7. Betadine topical antiseptic

8. 4% lidocaine glass vial (~4 cc)

9. Sterile gloves and drapes

10. Basin with room-temperature sterile saline for topical cooling as needed

11. 4 × 4 gauze

12. Nonsterile marking pen

13. Head of bed set to 20–30 degrees

14. Porous paper tape for dressing

15. Compressive bandage

PATIENT MARKINGS

Initial evaluation of the patient is similar for both the toxin and RF approach. For the most detailed preparation and documentation, as in a learning or teaching setting, use animated and resting photos, as well as short videos. However, in a busy, practical clinical setting, a facial injection anatomy sheet is used and not much else. This should provide adequate details of the muscles injected and pinpoint the areas of the face with precision. Ink marks are rarely used. Instead, the injection points are keyed toward the bulk of the muscle targeted for diminishment and not the lines themselves. Always have the patient voluntarily animate multiple times, weakly and strongly. I use a routine that takes about 7 seconds to completely evaluate the upper face. It goes like this: (1) raise your eyebrows high, (2) relax, (3) squeeze your eyebrows together, (4) relax, (5) scrunch your nose, (6) relax, (7) gently close your eyes like you are dozing off, (8) open and relax, (9) squeeze your eyelids tightly like "soap in your eyes," (10) open and relax, (11) open your eyes wide like "you saw a ghost," and finally (12) relax. This allows me to see the muscles in multiple configurations, with gentle and forceful contractions, full and partial excursion. Subtleties in anatomy are almost always highlighted.

For the RF patient, the approach is supplemented with additional maneuvers. In this setting, the nerve is mapped cutaneously with an external nerve stimulator (Stimpod). This demonstrates in real-time the contraction of the muscle and the variations in the anatomy. An electrocardiogram (EKG)-style grounding pad is placed on the neck, and a pencil probe is placed over the proximal innervation of the target muscles. For example, in mapping the corrugator function, the supraorbital branch of the temporal facial nerve is found at the lateral eyebrow just superior to the bony orbital rim. For the procerus muscle, the angular branch is found inferior and lateral to the vertical line of the medial canthus and superior to the nasal alar rim. These branches are marked with ink dots from proximal to medial over a distance of at least 10–20 mm. A single lesion in the nerve is insufficient to achieve a clinical effect beyond a short time. My clinical experience with hundreds of lesions shows that a treated length along the nerve of 2 cm will result in 9–12 months of clinical effect, sometimes more. A permanent effect may be achieved with a few millimeters more. The animation sequence used in the toxin patients is also performed in this setting.

A good clinical axiom is "if you can map it, you can treat it." However, if the nerve cannot be mapped successfully, randomly heating in the area is *not* indicated due to increased risk of untoward thermal injury to other tissues. All branches of the facial nerve can be targeted and mapped. Inability to map can be due to previous toxin injection within the last 4–6 months, heavy fatty layer overlying the nerve acting as an electrical insulator, and other factors. The clinical versatility and power of the RF method is undeniable; however, great care and respect must be held for Rubin's functional anatomy and the numerous and subtle variations in the face from patient to patient.

PROCEDURE TECHNIQUE

GLABELLA

Toxin

Dosing depends on the desired effect and the bulk of the muscle. For the "paralyzed" look, up to 20–25 units of ona- or incobotulinum may be used in the male and 15–17 units in the female. For a minimally mobile or softened look without complete paralysis, the doses may be 12–15 units and 9–12 units, respectively.

The lateral corrugator almost always can be identified in a transitional "bump" medial to the vertical line of the pupil superior to the orbital rim. Serial puncture injection in the corrugator is performed lateral to medial in aliquots of 0.05–0.1 mL or less. Spacing can be as close as 3–4 mm or as far apart as 5–7 mm depending on muscle bulk and length. Some practitioners prefer a linear threading

technique, but this is less precise in my hands. Care must be taken not to allow injection to descend into the upper eyelid and orbicularis.

In many patients, the medial corrugators contribute almost all the lines and contours. Many patients will call these vertical paramedian lines the "elevens."

Results are highly reliable and generally excellent. See Figures 20.1 through 20.4 for preprocedure status and representative four month post-procedure results. Interestingly, Figures 20.5 through 20.18 demonstrate 13 consecutive months after injections in the glabella at months 0, 4, and 8 months. The effect at 5 months following the third injection is comparable with a 4-month post-injection in cycle two injection.

Radiofrequency

After the ink marks have been created, 0.05–0.1 mL of 1% lidocaine with 1:100,000 epinephrine is injected 5 mm lateral to the most lateral mark superior to the brow. An 18-gauge needle is used to create an access point for the 22-gauge RF probe. The patient is grounded on the high back or anterior trunk. Both the probe and grounding pad are connected to the RF generator and the temperature is set to 85°C with the time set to 1 minute.

The 22-gauge probe is advanced under the skin from the access point to the most proximal ink mark at the lateral orbital rim and the device is set to stimulate the motor nerve at 0.3 v, 2 Hz, and 1 ms pulse duration. Stimulate internally and increase the voltage only as necessary until the weakest contraction can be visualized.

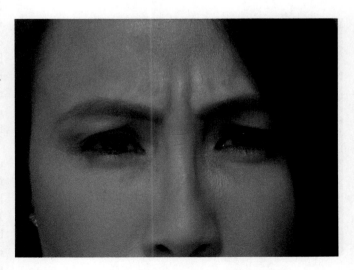

Figure 20.1. Preoperative view of contracted corrugators (note the "11's").

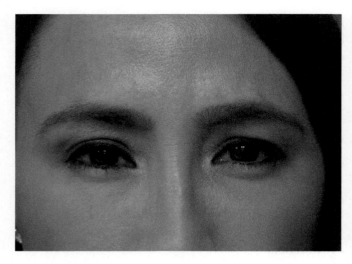

Figure 20.2. Postoperative view at 2 months of "contracted" corrugators (note the lack of "11's").

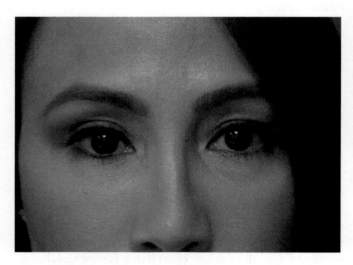

Figure 20.3. Preoperative view of relaxed upper face (note faint presence of "11's").

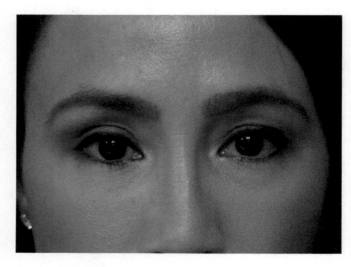

Figure 20.4. Postoperative view at 2 months of relaxed upper face (note smoother skin, in addition to loss of "11's").

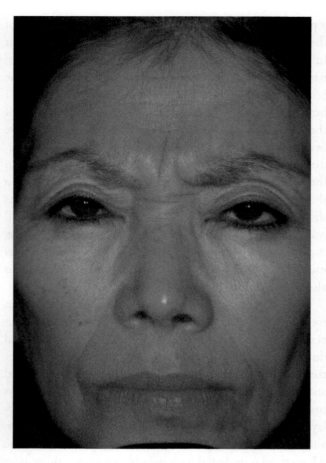

Figure 20.5. Thirteen consecutive months, preoperative view of contracted corrugators (notice procerus lines in addition to the "11's").

This means the probe is as close to the nerve as possible. Higher voltages may cause stimulation of the muscle directly or of adjacent nerves.

Once the nerve is located, 0.05–0.1 mL of 4% lidocaine is injected very slowly in a "microdroplet" technique to minimize diffusion. The idea is to bathe the epi-, peri-, and endoneurium but not anesthetize the axon and completely block the motor function of the nerve. The nerve is then treated at 85°C for 1 minute. The active, heated portion of the tip is 5 mm, and the effect of 1 minute of heating is immediate on the muscle. The lateral portion of the corrugator is rendered noncontractile.

The sequence from here is to advance (the probe), stimulate (the muscle to visualize the next treatment sequence), inject (to anesthetize the nerve), and treat (to immobilize the muscle). That is, advance, stimulate, inject, treat. In real time, the nerve can be disabled and the muscle can be shaped, denervated, or paralyzed. Generally, 5 minutes of heating in a zone of 2 cm or slightly larger achieves optimal results. One of the benefits of RF is the ability to treat asymmetries "live" and to achieve long-term or even

NONINVASIVE TECHNIQUES

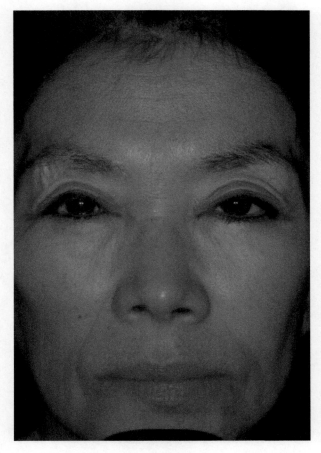

Figure 20.6. Thirteen consecutive months, postoperative view at 1 month of "contracted" corrugators (notice mild persistence of procerus lines in addition to the "11's" and lower forehead completely treated).

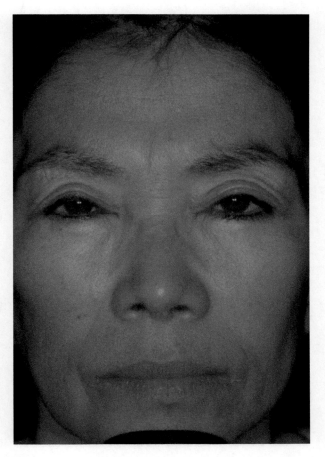

Figure 20.7. Thirteen consecutive months, postoperative view at 2 months of "contracted" corrugators (notice mild recurrence of procerus lines and the "11's" and minimal recurrence of lower forehead).

permanent results. In addition, the skin and subcutaneous tissue can be tightened, lifted, or shaped clinically.

Generally, creating two to three lesions is associated with a 6- to 9-month effect. See Figures 20.19 for preprocedure marking, status, and a representative 1-day result. Creating 4–5 lesions is associated with a 12- to 18-month effect, and creating 6–8 lesions is associated with a 2-year or even permanent effect.

FOREHEAD

Toxin

The bulk of the frontalis is much larger and may require double the dosage of the glabella for complete paralysis. However, overinjection of the lateral frontalis often leads to eyebrow drooping laterally and should be performed cautiously. Dosage may be up to 30 units, but generally is 12–15 units. In my experience, most patients prefer a minimally but not nonmobile frontalis. Anatomically,

the frontalis may have a shallow "v" shape in the superior midline but rarely demonstrates a complete split into two lateral portions as often seen in standard anatomy texts. Respectively, Figures 20.22 and 20.23 show contracted and Figures 20.24 and 20.25 show relaxed close-up preprocedure and at 2 months postinjection of the forehead, corrugators, and lateral orbicularis. Figures 20.26 (contracted and relaxed, pre- and postprocedure, respectively) show the same patient in a full-face view to highlight the overall rejuvenating effect.

Radiofrequency

In my mapping hundreds of nerves, there is a generally apparent pattern of innervation. The temporal branch splits in the temporal fossa into a high branch found just anterior to the hairline; this innervates the medial and superior portion of the muscle and a lower branch found in the supraorbital region halfway between the brow and the hairline. This innervates the frontalis more laterally. Some fibers of

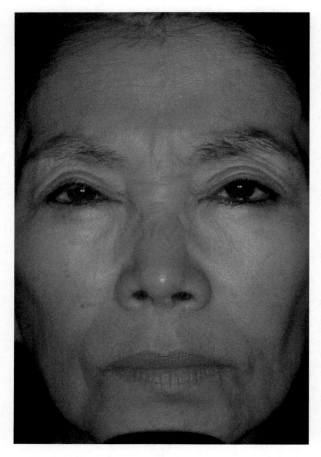

Figure 20.8. Thirteen consecutive months, postoperative view at 3 months of "contracted" corrugators (notice mild recurrence of procerus lines and the "11's" and minimal recurrence of lower forehead).

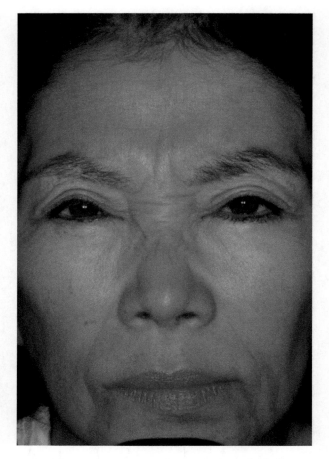

Figure 20.9. Thirteen consecutive months, postoperative view at 4 months of "contracted" corrugators (notice moderate recurrence of procerus lines and the "11's" and mild recurrence of lower forehead).

the supraorbital branch (see earlier discussion) seem to innervate the inferior medial frontalis as well where it courses inferiorly into the region of the glabella.

This means the frontalis can be regionally or selectively treated in many cases. The same schema of map, insert the probe, advance, stimulate, inject, and treat works for the frontalis as in the corrugators. Real-time assessment allows for adjusting the results mid-procedure.

The method of treatment is the same as in the glabella—at least 5 lesions at 1 minute each at 85°C, cooling the skin with a gauze soaked with room temperature saline as needed. In my experience, this is required more often in the forehead than the glabella.

EYEBROW AND CROW'S FEET

Toxin

As shown by Kane,[9] injection in the medial frontalis and superior lateral brow at the orbicularis can elevate the brow

by as much as 6 mm. The principle of a weakened medial frontalis experiencing stronger contractions laterally as a compensation is now well appreciated due to his work. Overinjection of the medial frontalis can weaken it sufficiently to cause strong lateral frontalis contraction, thus overarching the brow in a "Mr. Spock" look. Injecting the superior lateral frontalis can induce stronger contraction in the inferior lateral orbicularis, thus elevating the brow as well.

In addition, a weakened lateral superior orbicularis allows the contracting inferior lateral frontalis to be relatively unopposed for greater lift of the lateral brow. As little as 1.5–3.0 units just under the brow in the orbicularis may achieve excellent brow elevation.

In the crow's feet area, be aware that there are three distinct zones: (1) superior to the lateral canthal line, (2) in the region of the lateral canthal line, and (3) inferior to the lateral canthal line. These three zones should be addressed individually and can be injected alone or in any combination. Generally, the number of units will be less than 10 per

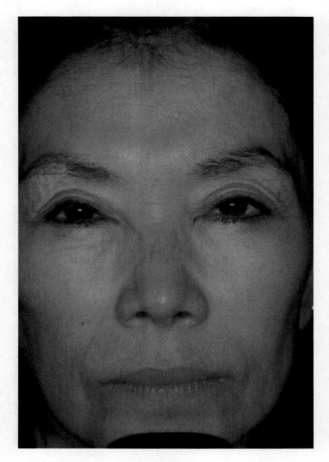

Figure 20.10. Thirteen consecutive months, postoperative view at 4 months, reinjection at 4 months, of "contracted" corrugators (notice minimal presence of procerus lines in addition to the "11's" and lower forehead completely treated).

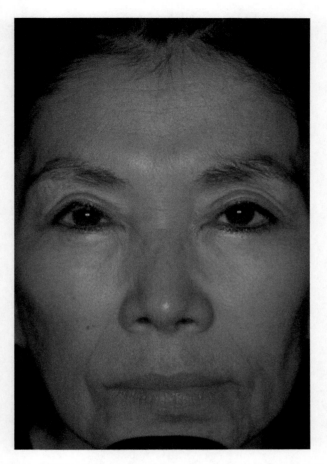

Figure 20.11. Thirteen consecutive months, postoperative view at 6 months, reinjection at 4 months, of "contracted" corrugators (notice minimal presence of procerus lines in addition to the "11's" and lower forehead completely treated).

side. Figures 20.30 and 20.31 show contracted views of the crow's feet prior to and 1 month after injection.

Radiofrequency

This area is particularly challenging for the RF method; however, the results can be spectacular and long-lasting. The principle is to immobilize the muscle at 85°C. Then the physician can shorten the muscle and tighten the skin at 60°C for a dual effect. The key is to remember the axiom, "if you can map it, you can treat it." That is the challenge. It is not always possible to isolate an individual branch to the lateral superior orbicularis. If not, the nerve should not be treated. The innervation may continue along one branch from the crow's feet to the supratarsal orbicularis. This risks an eyelid ptosis, although there has not yet been one reported in the literature.

On successful mapping, the technique is similar to that used for the glabella with the ASIT acronym applying (advance, stimulate, inject, treat). One to two cycles are adequate in the crow's feet.

NASAL MUSCLES (PROCERUS, NASALIS)

Toxin

Direct injection in the procerus muscle generally requires less than 5 units in my hands. This injection not only smooths wrinkles and relaxes the nasal muscles, but helps prevent excessive depression of the media brow that gives the "mad scientist" look.

Radiofrequency

This area is much more straightforward and reliable than that for the crow's feet. The results can be satisfying and long-lasting. The principle is the same: to immobilize the muscle at 85°C. Often, it is possible to isolate the angular branch from a separate branch to the nasalis about 1 cm medial to the vertical line of the pupil and 1 cm inferior to the medial canthus. On successful mapping of one or two nerves, treatment can proceed. The key is to remember

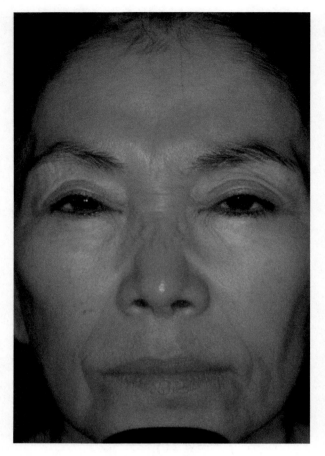

Figure 20.12. Thirteen consecutive months, postoperative view at 7 months, reinjection at 4 months, of "contracted" corrugators (notice mild presence of procerus lines in addition to minimal recurrence of the "11's" and lower forehead completely treated).

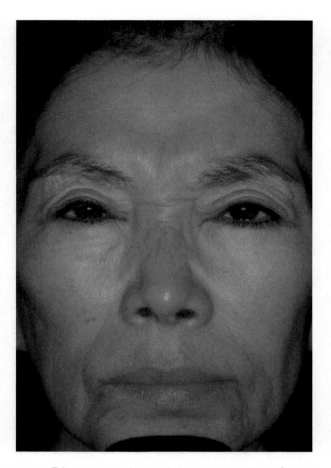

Figure 20.13. Thirteen consecutive months, postoperative view at 8 months, reinjection at 4 months, of "contracted" corrugators (notice moderate presence of procerus lines in addition to mild recurrence of the "11's" and lower forehead completely treated).

the axiom, "if you can map it, you can treat it." Fortunately, in this area, mapping is easier to achieve. If not, the nerve should not be treated. The angular branch is reliably mapped and treated. The only caveat is that the skin near the medial canthus is thin and often requires a moist saline gauze for cutaneous cooling while performing the internal heating. Untoward clinical results from errant nerve lesions are exceedingly rare in this area.

On successful mapping, the technique is similar to that used for the glabella with the ASIT acronym applying (advance, stimulate, inject, treat). One to two 1-minute cycles are generally adequate in the nasal region.

PERIORAL AND CHIN

This is a region where toxin is superior as it can target very small areas with fractional doses, dilution, partial muscle effects, and increased safety. Traditional doses of 2.5 u/0.1 mL are much too high in the perioral region. Dilution of the dosing to 0.5–1.25u/0.1 mL provides great precision

and the ability to "blend" or partially immobilize a muscle over a large area. For RF, remember the muscle distal to the lesion in the nerve is attenuated. In addition, it is more difficult to isolate small, distal branches like those found in the perioral region. However, RF retains the advantage of tightening or foreshortening the muscle and skin during the same treatment session.

Toxin

For the upper lip, 1–2 units diluted in 1 mL of preservative-free saline can break up and smooth the "smoker's" or vertical lip lines with reasonable safety. For the mentalis, more than 1–2 units may run the risk of dropping the horizontal line of the lower lip and compromising oral closure. Small aliquots of 0.5–1 unit per side in the depressor anguli oris are occasionally used, but great care must be taken to avoid a debilitating asymmetry with difficulty in maintaining oral competence, eating, chewing, and speaking, especially the plosive consonant sounds "B" and "P."

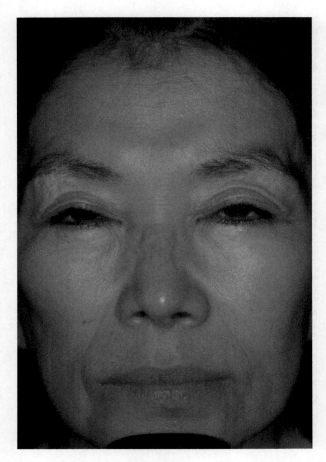

Figure 20.14. Thirteen consecutive months, postoperative view at 9 months, reinjections at 4 and 8 months, of "contracted" corrugators (notice minimal presence of procerus lines in addition to "11's" and lower forehead completely treated).

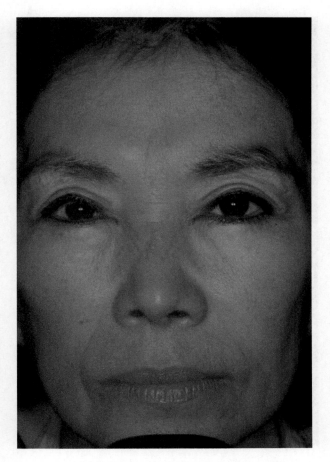

Figure 20.15. Thirteen consecutive months, postoperative view at 10 months, reinjections at 4 and 8 months, of "contracted" corrugators (notice minimal presence of procerus lines in addition to minimal recurrence of "11's" and lower forehead completely treated).

Radiofrequency

The advantage of RF here is the gentle application of heat locally to target the distal end fibers of the buccal branch of the facial nerve in the upper lip. However, there is increased risk of skin injury, and I know of few practitioners who apply this technique. The double benefit is the heat-induced nerve injury and disabling of excessive muscle activity combined with foreshortening of the upper lip by a millimeter or less that compensates for the muscle laxity. The technique is to use the 22-gauge probe from medial to lateral and only medial to the nasolabial fold to avoid disruption of this key aesthetic anatomic boundary.

In my experience, about half of patients have a distinct proximal branch of the marginal mandibular nerve that allows selective targeting of the contractile mentalis. This branch often takes off inferiorly and just laterally to the inferior orbital foramen at the margin of the mandible. Again, the distinct advantage of RF is the lifting and foreshortening of the muscle. This ameliorates the risk of

the complication of a drooping central lower lip from a toxin treatment.

I do not know of any practitioners treating the depressor anguli oris with RF.

NASOLABIAL FOLD

Toxin

This area is well treated by toxin injection, as demonstrated by Kane.[10,11] Its best use is to treat the gummy smile by disabling the excessive contraction of the levator labii superioris and improving the deep medial nasolabial fold near the alar base. After adequate treatment, the superior gingival sulcus is no longer visible, and the smile pattern becomes that of the canine smile. A usual dose is 5–7.5 units, but if there is any doubt about patient sensitivity, doses can be decreased and a second visit scheduled at 2 weeks to evaluate results and the need for additional injection.

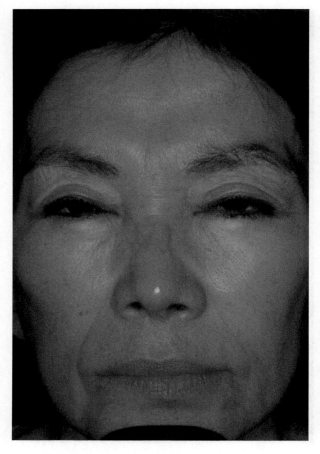

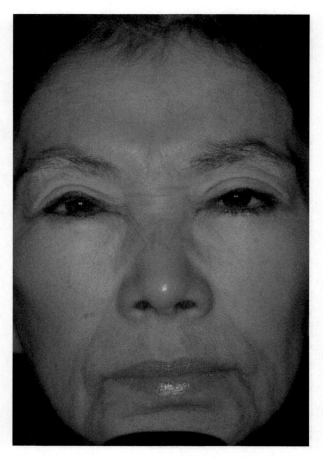

Figure 20.16. Thirteen consecutive months, postoperative view at 11 months, reinjections at 4 and 8 months, of "contracted" corrugators (notice minimal presence of procerus lines in addition to mild recurrence of "11's" and lower forehead completely treated).

Figure 20.17. Thirteen consecutive months, postoperative view at 12 months, reinjections at 4 and 8 months, of "contracted" corrugators (notice mild presence of procerus lines in addition to minimal recurrence of "11's" and lower forehead completely treated).

Radiofrequency

I know of no reports in the literature or personal communications for treatment of the nasolabial fold directly with RF nerve lesioning. However, this is a challenge for future investigation.

NECK

This is an area of very high satisfaction, off-label for the toxins and on-label for RF. A dynamic evaluation technique that is less elaborate than for the upper face can be used. Simply ask the patient to show the bottom teeth to contract the muscles bilaterally as step one and make a face like "smoking a cigar" in one corner of the mouth to contract unilaterally as step two. This triggers the depressor anguli oris (DAO) as well as the platysma. However, the innervation of the DAO is from the marginal mandibular nerve and of the platysma is primarily from the cervical

branch. A great number of patients are not bilateral in my experience. Generally, I find the lateral bands are more contractile and prominent. The medial bands are more often lax in older patients.

Toxin

The most favorable patient is one who has minimal laxity and strong platysmal bands. In addition, postsurgical patients whose skin laxity has been resected are good candidates as well. Patients with lax skin and strong platysmal bands have been treated by many practitioners[12]; however, there is a large risk of increased laxity and an almost certainty of persistent laxity. For the patient with bands without laxity, the success rate is quite high.[13]

Doses of 15–30 units are often recommended, but I find that as little as 15 works quite well in most patients who do not have full lateral and medial bands bilaterally. It is easy to visualize the bands and inject from superior to

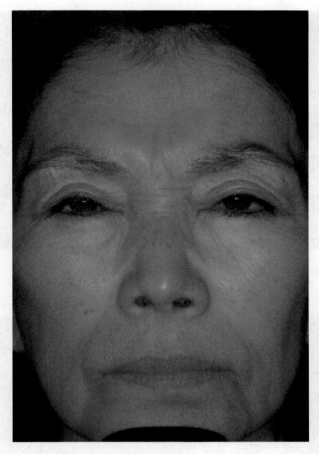

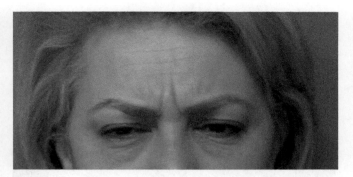

Figure 20.20. Preoperative view of contracted corrugators (note the "11's" and presence of transverse forehead lines).

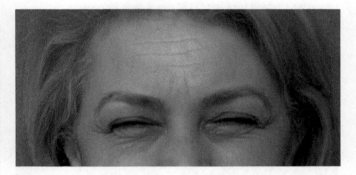

Figure 20.18. Thirteen consecutive months, postoperative view at 13 months, reinjections at 4 and 8 months, of "contracted" corrugators (notice moderate presence of procerus lines in addition to moderate recurrence of "11's" and lower forehead completely treated).

Figure 20.21. Postoperative view at one day of "contracted" corrugators (note the complete treatment of "11's" with residual skin lines due to deep furrows and persistence of untreated transverse forehead lines).

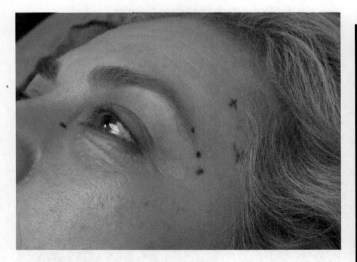

Figure 20.19. Preoperative marking of superior orbital branch of facial nerve with Stimpod nerve stimulator.

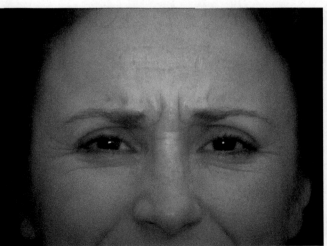

Figure 20.22. Upper face preoperative view contracted.

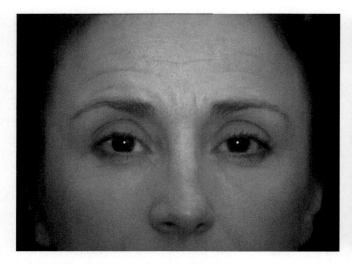

Figure 20.23. Upper face postoperative view at 2 months contracted (note complete correction of procerus and crow's feet lines; mild residual transverse forehead lines and "11's" due to deep furrows).

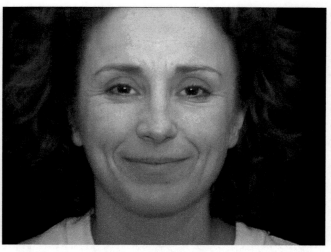

Figure 20.26. Full face preoperative view smiling.

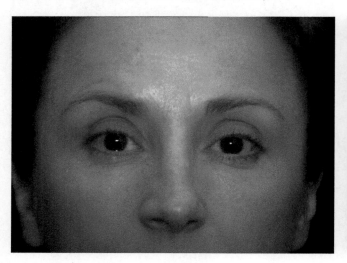

Figure 20.24. Upper face preoperative view relaxed.

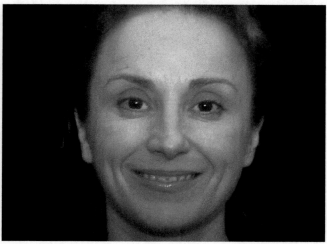

Figure 20.27. Full face postoperative view at 2 months.

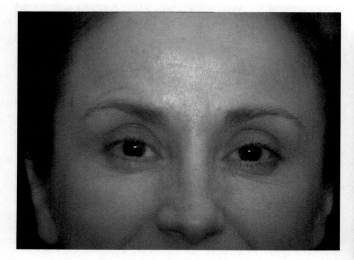

Figure 20.25. Upper face postoperative view at 2 months relaxed (note complete correction of procerus and crow's feet lines; mild residual transverse forehead and corrugator lines).

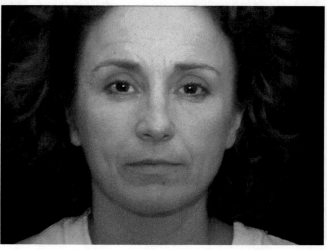

Figure 20.28. Full face preoperative view relaxed.

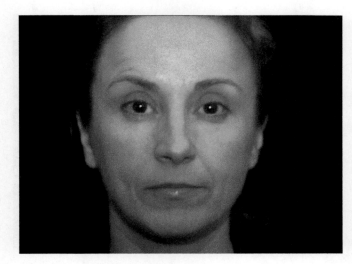

Figure 20.29. Full face postoperative view at 2 months.

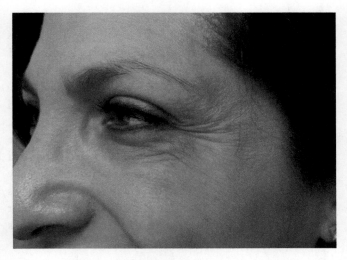

Figure 20.30. Preoperative view, left oblique view, contracted orbicularis oculi at the crow's feet (note full fan configuration).

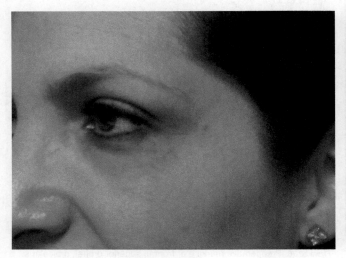

Figure 20.31. Postoperative view at 1 month, left oblique view, "contracted" orbicularis oculi at the crow's feet (note complete correction of full fan).

inferior 3–4 aliquots of 0.05 mL in each band, or a total of approximately 5 units per band. Horizontal lines are improved as well.

Radiofrequency

RF patients with laxity, hyperactive muscles, or both can be treated equally well. This is a distinct advantage of RF over toxin injection: the broader patient selection possible and superior clinical results. The disadvantage is the need for greater clinical skill, more elaborate treatment technique, increased time, and increased risk of burns or marginal mandibular branch injury. Unpublished clinical experience from numerous users reported to me suggests the incidence of burn is estimated at less than 0.1%. The approach is similar to that used for crow's feet but much more reliable and predictable. Generally, in mapping, there are two cervical branches of the facial nerve and they can easily be mapped from the sternocleidomastoid muscle inferior to the angle of the mandible proximally to the midline distally. See Figure 20.32 for details. Again, the effect of RF is immediate. Shown intraoperatively in Figure 20.33, the left-side treatment is evident compared to the yet to be treated right-sided cervical nerve branches. Figure 20.34 show the results after both the left and right side are treated.

The treatment method is consistent with the preceding descriptions: insert the probe, advance, stimulate, inject, treat and repeat 4–5 times over a 2 cm length using moist saline to cool the skin as needed.

The procedure follows those described previously: map; prep; drape; administer minimal local; determine

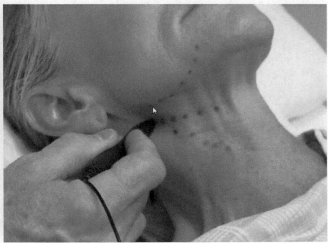

Figure 20.32. Preoperative marking of marginal mandibular nerve and two cervical branches of facial nerve with Stimpod nerve stimulator.

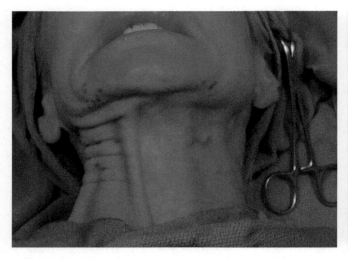

Figure 20.33. Intraoperative view of left cervical branches of facial nerve treated prior to right-sided treatment.

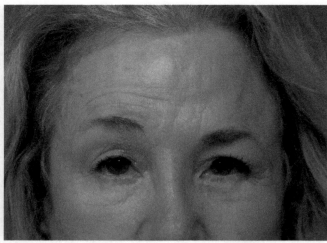

Figure 20.35. Congenital blepharophimosis after four operations and 10 years of botulinum toxin therapy showing persistent asymmetry.

access point; advance; apply internal stimulation; inject 4% lidocaine; treat at 85°C for 1 minute per lesion, usually for 5 lesions over 2 cm; and check the motion/function after each minute for real-time assessment of efficacy (MASIT: map, advance, stimulate, inject, treat).

UNUSUAL CASES

In general, "if you can map it, you can treat it." The principles outlined earlier can apply to unusual cases where blocking the nerve and the distal muscle function is therapeutic. One example is congenital blepharophimosis.

Balancing two sides of the face by creating partial lesions in the nerve serves to harmonize asymmetries. Figure 20.35 shows marked asymmetry in the orbicularis, corrugator, and frontalis. This status was present after a coronal brow lift operation by one surgeon and three brow lift and sling procedures performed by two additional surgeons. Additionally, more than 10 years of toxin injections were performed 3–4 times a year. Finally, the patient had "had enough" and opted for RF treatment. Figure 20.36 show mapping of the various nerve branches. Figure 20.37 shows the immediate post-RF ablation result, which lasted almost 1 year, in keeping with the protocol of creating 2–3 lesions at 85°C for a less than permanent but long-term effect.

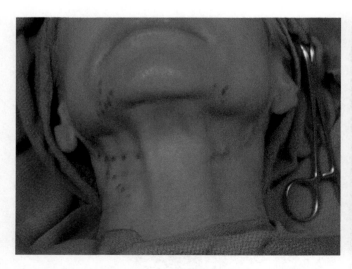

Figure 20.34. Intraoperative view of bilateral treatment of cervical branches of facial nerve.

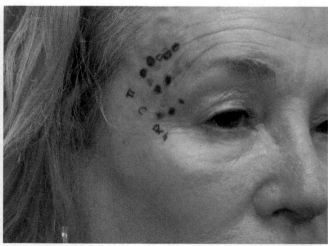

Figure 20.36. Preoperative marking of frontal, superior orbital, orbicularis, and crow's feet branches of facial nerve with Stimpod nerve stimulator.

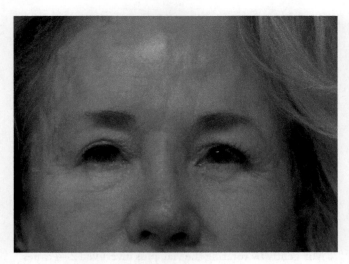

Figure 20.37. Immediate postoperative view after treatment of frontal, superior orbital, and orbicularis branches of facial nerve with Stimpod nerve stimulator.

POSTOPERATIVE CONSIDERATIONS

Fortunately, there are few major postprocedure considerations for either procedure. Each is highly efficacious; however, with the toxin approach, the technical maneuvers are easier to learn. They can be discerned from a healthy knowledge of and respect for the anatomy. While that also is required for the RF approach, the technical maneuvers of mapping and treatment are subtler and require more training. Both techniques are accompanied by low incidences of complications.

TOXINS

There is minimal swelling after toxin injections. Erythema and swelling rarely last more than the rest of the day. Distant effects, while rare, can be manifested by asthenia, generalized muscle weakness, diplopia, dysphagia, dysphonia, dysarthria, urinary incontinence, and breathing difficulties. Fortunately, all these are exceedingly rare occurrences, less than 1%. Eyelid ptosis was 3% in the FDA clinical trial.

Some physicians recommend that patients do not exercise or lie flat on the first day after injection. In my own personal experience, most do not. Many may advise against having a facial massage, laying flat, being inverted, or going into a steam or dry sauna the first few days after injection. Certainly, after a few days, there are essentially no restrictions. Immediate application of cold compresses may minimize edema. Occasionally, a blood vessel may be inadvertently punctured during the injection. Immediate, firm pressure for 5–8 minutes and application of ice will diminish sequelae. Makeup can be applied immediately after injection. Follow-up is generally at 2 weeks. Onset of effect may be as short as 3–5 days. Under no circumstances should a reinjection take place sooner than 2 weeks as a patient may be a late responder and be overdosed if injected earlier.

RADIOFREQUENCY

Immediate swelling with application of RF is directly related to the time of heating—more heat, more swelling. The skin is exceedingly rarely impacted as the volume of the heat zone at the tip of the probe is an estimated 0.1 mL. Treatment occurs deep, and the skin temperature rarely rises above 42–43°C except in the medial canthal area, the crow's feet, and the neck in those patients who have less than 5 mm of pinch thickness. In these locations, the recommended application of saline soaked gauze during the procedure makes problems rare. Burns are estimated at much less than 1%, and this is largely due to continual infrared video monitoring in real time. Dysesthesia or localized anesthesia may occur transiently but usually resolves within a day or two and has not been reported to my knowledge. Demonstrable edema may last 2–3 days in the periorbitum and a day or two less in other locations. No compressive bandages are used, and the analgesic recommended is acetaminophen for 1–3 days.

With an inadequate response, retreatment can take place as soon as the edema is not evident to the careful clinician. This is often after 7 days. It is possible to overinject with lidocaine, thus blocking the motor nerve chemically. This could lead to inadequately heating the nerve and not creating the required lesion.

CAVEATS

For any treatment, an in-depth knowledge of facial anatomy and treatment techniques ensures patient safety and satisfaction.

TOXINS

All Toxins

1. Extra dilution may be ideal for localized effects in the periorbitum or perioral region.

2. Ona- and incobotulinum toxin have essentially the same dosing.

3. Abobotulinum toxin requires approximately 3:1 dosing. To achieve this, mix 3 times as strong and still inject 0.1 mL per location in a serial puncture approach.

4. Off-label, most practitioners store a bottle 7–10 days at 4°C after mixing and will reuse it as a multipatient vial.

5. Potency units are not interchangeable.

6. Potency is determined by each proprietary mouse LD_{50} assay protocol.[14–17]

7. Long-term treatment does not produce additive adverse events.[18]

8. Adverse events are generally technique-dependent and preventable[19] and usually caused by improper placement, dosing, or diffusion into adjacent muscles.

9. Ona- and abobotulinum are complexed with proteins. Incobotulinum toxin is not.

10. Inject the muscle, not the line or wrinkle.

11. Think like pediatrics—dosage/weight—less units for smaller muscles, more units for larger muscles.

12. Remember dilution for blending a dose over a larger area.

Onabotulinum Toxin A (Botox)

1. Store at 36–46°F for 36 months prior to injection.

2. Available in 50 and 100 U per vial.

3. When mixed on label, the syringe has 4 u/0.1 mL.

4. Many or most practitioners mix at 2.5 u/0.1 mL.

5. The standard and the cosmetic formulations are the same. Bottles are 50 and 100 units.

6. Indicated for glabellar lines associated with corrugator and/or procerus muscle activity in adult patients 65 years of age or younger. Also indicated for temporary improvement in the appearance of moderate to severe lateral canthal lines associated with orbicularis oculi activity in adult patients

7. Mix gently by rotating the vial.

8. Onset is 3–7 days.

9. Duration is 3–4 months.

Incobotulinum Toxin A (Xeomin)

1. Store at 68–77°F for 36 months.

2. Available in 50 and 100 U per vial.

3. When mixed on label, the syringe has 4 u/0.1 mL.

4. Many practitioners mix at 2.5 u/0.1 mL.

5. The standard formulation has 200 units per bottle for cervical dystonia and upper limb spasticity. The cosmetic formulation has 100 units per bottle.

6. Indicated for glabellar lines associated with corrugator and/or procerus muscle activity in adults.

7. Mix gently by rotating the vial, plus invert vial 2–4 times to ensure all material is off the rubber stopper.

8. Onset is 3–7 days.

9. Duration is up to 3 months.

Abobotulinum Toxin A (Dysport)

1. Store at 36–46°F for 36 months prior to injection.

2. Available in a 300 unit vial.

3. When mixed on label with 2.5 mL of preservative-free saline, the syringe has 12 u/0.1 mL.

4. Most practitioners do not dilute further.

5. Cosmetic bottle has 300 units per vial.

6. Indicated for glabellar lines associated with procerus and corrugator muscle activity in adult patients 65 years of age or younger.

7. Gently rotate vial until white substance is fully dissolved.

8. Onset is 2–3 days.

9. Duration is up to 4 months.

RADIOFREQUENCY

1. RF generator requires very little maintenance and has high reliability.

2. Store probes in sterile packages, generally with a 2-year expiration.

3. Mapping requires patience and attention to detail but is a quick procedure, and learning curve is easy.

4. Treat the nerve, not the muscle for improvement of lines and wrinkles, balancing muscles.

5. Generally, the proximal nerve innervates the proximal muscles, the distal nerve the distal muscle.

6. RF can be used for nerve, muscle, subcutaneous tissue, and skin in same procedure.

7. Most practitioners prefer to simply heat subcutaneous tissue and skin for tightening and not perform neurolysis at all. This may improve lines and may foreshorten the muscle a small amount.

8. Can be used to create a lesion in any nerve, but regulatory approval otherwise is for soft tissue coagulation and assisting in hemostasis. Off-label use is dominant, and RF is used for muscle, fat, subcutaneous tissue, and skin.

9. Equipment is sturdy and straightforward to use. Understanding anatomy and performing the procedure is not.

10. Onset is immediate for nerves, gradually progressive over 1–6 months for soft tissue.

11. Duration can be permanent if desired.

SELECTED READINGS

1. 2016 Plastic Surgery Statistics Report. https://www.plasticsurgery.org/documents/News/Statistics/2016/plastic-surgery-statistics-full-report-2016.pdf page 5
2. Merriam Webster Dictionary. https://www.merriam-webster.com/dictionary/Botox *"And like thousands of other women who have been Botoxed and were pleased with the results, she's pursuing new and better ways of using a syringe to erase the other signs of aging on her face."—Unmesh Kher, Time, 19 May 2003.*
3. Kim JH, Jeong, JW, Son D, Han K, Lee SY, Choi TH, Chang DW. Percutaneous selective radiofrequency nerve ablation for glabellar frown lines. *Aesth Surg J* 2011;31:747–775.
4. Rivlin D, Personal communication.
5. Rubin LR. The anatomy of a smile: its importance in the treatment of facial paralysis. *Plast Reconstr Surg* 1972;53:384.
6. ElectroThermal 20S Spine Generator, Smith and Nephew, Andover, MA, FDA 510 (k) clearance letter K033981, https://www.fda.gov/cdrh/510k/K033981.pdf; NT-1000NeuroTherm Inc, Middleton, MA, FDA 510 (k) clearance letter K052878, Jan 23 2006, https://www.accessdata.fda.gov/cdrh_docs/pdf5/K052878.pdf; Symphony RF, ThermiGen Inc, Southlake, TX, FDA 510 (k) clearance letter K130689, Nov 15, 2013. https://www.accessdata.fda.gov/cdrh_docs/pdf13/K130689.pdf
7. Fagien S. Botulinum toxin type A for facial aesthetic enhancement: role in facial shaping. *Plast Reconstr Surg* 2003;112(Suppl 5):6S–18S.
8. Eisele KH, Fink K, Vey M, et al. Studies on the dissociation of botulinum neurotoxin type A complexes. *Toxicon* 2011;57:555–565.
9. Emer J, Waldorf H. Neurotoxin update and review, part 1: the science. *Cosmet Dermatol* 2010;23(9):413–418.
10. Kane MAC. Botulinum toxin in plastic surgery indications and operations. In Guyuron B, et al., eds. *Plastic Surgery—Indications and Operations (with DVD)*, Chapter 106, 1379–1380.
11. Kane MAC. The effect of botulinum toxin injections on the nasolabial fold. *Plast Reconstr Surg* 2003;112 (Suppl 5):66–72S.
12. Matarasso A, Matarasso S, Brandt F, et al. Botulinum A exotoxin for the management of platysma bands. *Plas Reconstr Surg* 1999;103:645–652.
13. Kane MAC. Nonsurgical treatment of platysmal bands with injection of botulinum toxin A. *Plast Reconstr Surg* 1999;103:656–663.
14. Thakker MM, Ruvin PA. Pharmacology and clinical applications of botulinum toxins A and B. *Int Ophthalmol Clin* 2004;44:147–163.
15. Ordegren t, Hjaltason H, Kaakkola S et. A double blind, randomised, parallel group study to investigate the dose equivalence of Dysport and Botox in the treatment of cervical dystonia. *J Neurol Neurosurg Psych* 1998; 64:6–12.
16. Annese V, Bassotti G, Coccia G, et al. Comparison of two different formulations of botulinum toxin A for the treatment of oesophageal achalasia. *Aliment Pharmacol Ther* 1999; 13:1347–1350.
17. Albanese A. Discussion of unique properties of botulinum toxins. *Toxicon* 2009;54(5):702–708.
18. Dressler D, Hallett M. Immunological aspects of Botox, Dysport and Myobloc/NeuroBloc. *Eur J Neurol* 2006;13(Suppl 1):11–15.
19. Nettar K, Moss C. Facial filler and neurotoxin complications. *Facial Plast Surg* 2012;28(3):288–293.

21.

LASERS AND ENERGY-BASED DEVICES

Thomas Griffin Jr., Nazanin Saedi, and Christopher B. Zachary

INTRODUCTION

Energy-based devices have offered significant advances in aesthetic surgery in the past several decades since the development of the ruby laser by Thomas Maiman in Howard Hughes's laboratory in 1960, and they are now a mainstay of treatment for a host of medical and surgical conditions. Aesthetic laser therapy is a rapidly expanding field with new technological advances being made on a regular basis.

To provide patients with safe and optimal treatments, the laser surgeon needs to accurately identify the target, select the appropriate device, and then tailor the specific treatment parameters. For lasers and light sources to be effective, their photons must be adsorbed by a certain chromophore, causing focal heating of and damage to that structure. Knowledge of the wavelength, the pulse duration, and the fluence are critical to understanding the likely outcome following this laser–tissue interaction.

This chapter will consider current laser-, light-, and energy-based devices and their applications for aesthetic purposes.

VASCULAR DEVICES AND LASER TISSUE INTERACTIONS

DEVICES

The concept of selective photothermolysis, as first described in 1983 by Anderson and Parish, states that laser pulse duration should approximately match the thermal relaxation time of the targeted tissue.[1] As opposed to the early lasers, which used continuous or quasi-continuous waves, more recent application of selective photothermolysis allowed tailored treatments that targeted specific tissue with limited nonspecific damage to surrounding tissues.

There are four main laser devices and one light source that are currently in use to treat vascular lesions: the pulsed dye laser (PDL), the (frequency doubled Nd:YAG pumped) potassium-titanyl-phosphate (KTP) laser, the alexandrite laser, the neodymium-doped yttrium aluminium garnet (Nd:YAG) laser, and the intense pulse light (IPL)[2-8] (Figures 21.1 and 21.2).

The PDL is considered the optimal treatment for early superficial vascular malformations and can also be used to treat certain types of infantile hemangiomata, though the

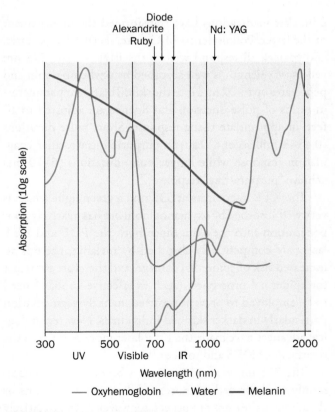

Figure 21.1. Chromophore absorption curve.

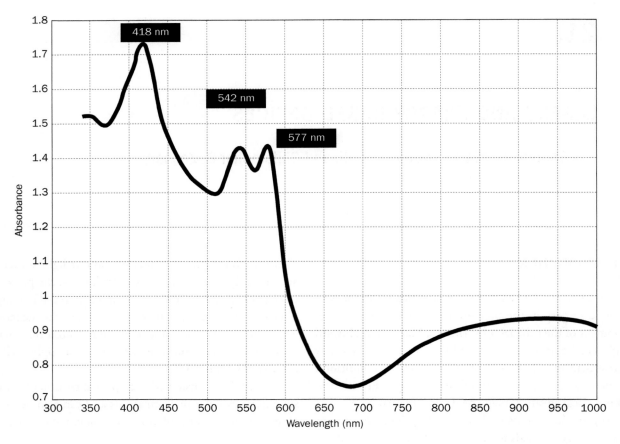

Figure 21.2. Reference hemoglobin spectrum.

β-blocker medications have transformed the management of the latter. Poikiloderma of Civatte, facial telangiectases, and rosacea all respond well to the PDL.[9,10] The 595 nm yellow wavelength is well absorbed by oxyhemoglobin and penetrates up to 1.2 mm into the skin. Treatment parameters in terms of pulse duration and fluence are adjusted to affect an appropriate tissue response. Short pulse durations (0.45–3 millisecond) cause a purpuric intravascular coagulation response while longer pulse durations (6–10 ms) achieve "purpura-free" responses.[7]

The KTP laser emits at 532 nm, a green light which is very well absorbed by oxyhemoglobin but has relatively poor penetration into the skin. Since both the PDL and KTP lasers are competitively absorbed by melanin, there is an increased risk of epidermal damage, and therefore strategies for epidermal protection (such as effective cooling) need to be employed to prevent posttreatment dyspigmentation particularly in darker skinned individuals. New technological advances have made the KTP laser more popular in the treatment of PWS and rosacea.[11]

The 755 nm alexandrite laser is becoming more commonly used for darker, more nodular port wine stains or those that are resistant to other laser wavelengths. Relatively good absorption particularly by deoxygenized hemoglobin and a deeper penetration into the skin are features that assist the alexandrite laser in effective treatment of these venous malformations. Given that the latter wavelength is less well absorbed by melanin, there is somewhat greater safety concerning posttreatment dyspigmentation.

The Nd:YAG 1,064 nm laser, which operates at a wavelength which is beyond the visible color spectrum, has a far greater depth of penetration but significantly less hemoglobin absorption than the PDL, KTP, or alexandrite lasers.[12] Due to its relatively poor epidermal melanin absorption, it is safer to use in darker skinned individuals. However, because of its poor coefficient of absorption by hemoglobin, high fluences and longer pulse widths are required, which creates the potential for volumetric heating, collateral damage, and narrows the patient safety window.[6,13] Cooling is critical for epidermal protection and pain control, as well as to reduce the risk of scarring from nonspecific thermal injury. Every laser surgeon who has had extensive experience with this device has caused some scarring at some stage in his or her career.

The IPL was invented in 1990 (US patent # 5,320,618). Simple in design, this has become the go-to device for many clinicians because its filtered light is capable of treating all the conditions just mentioned including port wine stains and the changes associated with chronic photodamage. Beyond the scope of this chapter is a new invention by Gustavsson: total reflection amplification of spontaneous emission of radiation (TRASER), which is neither a laser nor an IPL but which has a tunable wavelength, a variable pulse width, and very high power with a large spot size, an everyman tool that could replace the PDL, KTP, and long-pulse ruby and alexandrite lasers, all in one box.

CLINICAL APPLICATIONS

TELANGIECTASIAS

Facial telangiectases are most commonly associated with rosacea and chronic photodamage. They are typically located on the nose, cheeks, and chin and measure 0.1–1.0 mm in diameter.

Both the long-pulsed KTP and PDL lasers have been used extensively for the treatment of facial telangiectases. The small (0.7–2 mm) KTP beam diameter can be quite effective in eradicating these vessels with few side effects, little or no bruising, and modest discomfort.[4] In a study by Adrian and Tanghetti, 90% of patients experienced between 75% and 100% clearance of their facial telangiectases after single KTP treatment with no significant side effects or complications.[4] The PDL is also an excellent treatment choice especially for those with extensive facial telangiectases and the underlying blush of rosacea. Using 6–10 msec pulse durations, facial vessels can effectively be treated with nonpurpuric fluences. In those with larger high-flow vessels, multiple passes and/or pulse-stacking techniques may be needed to improve efficacy. It is critical to note that pulse stacking without cooling will cause scarring. Multiple treatment sessions may be required for those with extensive vascularity.[7]

The 1,064 nm Nd:YAG laser can be used to treat the larger-caliber, darker, deeper facial vessels. As described earlier, robust cooling is necessary both for epidermal and superficial dermal protection and to reduce patient discomfort.

Laser pulse durations should be long enough for the heat to cause the surrounding vascular adventitial tissue to shrink. The treatment endpoint for telangiectases is vessel spasm or the change of the vessel color to a more dusky appearance.

POIKILODERMA OF CIVATTE

Poikiloderma of Civatte is characterized by telangiectasia, epidermal atrophy, and actinic dyspigmentation generally involving the lateral aspects of the cheeks, neck, and upper chest. Treatment options include IPL, PDL, and KTP laser in addition to nonablative fractionated devices.

The IPL is often used to treat poikiloderma because its broadband light is effective for both dyspigmentation and telangiectasia. Several studies have reported 50–75% improvement in both the vascular component and the actinic dyspigmentation, with a low side-effect profile.[5] However, care must be taken to avoid a persistent "footprinting" or "honeycomb-like" appearance which occurs when the sapphire crystal is placed without consistent uniformity over the entire treatment zone. This occurs in particular when a one-pass technique is used. The authors generally use a multipass technique, each pass of which is oriented at a different angle to reduce this template appearance. Other adverse effects include scarring with irregular hypopigmentation, postinflammatory hyperpigmentation, posttreatment purpura, mottled appearance, crusting, and erythema. Patients need to be aware that multiple treatment sessions may be necessary to obtain the desired improvement.

LEG VEINS

Venulectasias or "thread veins" are generally red or blue in color, measure 0.2–2 mm in diameter, and develop in dependent areas, predominantly the legs. Leg veins do not respond to lasers as well as vessels on the face because of increased hydrostatic pressure, the anatomy of lower extremity blood vessels, and reduced amount of oxyhemoglobin.[13] Therefore, sclerotherapy remains the first-line therapy, and laser treatment is considered a second-line therapy or for application in those who are needle phobic.[6,13,14]

PIGMENTED LESION DEVICES AND LASER TISSUE INTERACTIONS

Reference has already been made to the role of the KTP and IPL devices for the treatment of chronic photodamage, including lentiginous changes. However, there are additional categories of devices which, by the very nature of their short pulse width, induce a photomechanical disruption of pigmented targets.

Q-SWITCHED LASERS

In the 1980s, quality-switched (Q-switched, QS) lasers revolutionized the way we treat tattoos. Prior treatments with dermabrasion, salabrasion, and continuous wave CO_2 laser all had problematical outcomes including permanent scarring, loss of pigmentation, and, in the case of dermabrasion, unacceptable microdroplets of aerosolized blood which were persistent in the treatment area for hours after the patient had gone home.[15,16]

QS lasers (both nano and pico) store large amounts of energy in the optical cavity until the optical shutter is opened, releasing a high peak power pulse within the nanosecond range (one billionth of a second, 10^{-9} s).[17] The absorbed energy causes rapid expansion/contraction of the target tissue and mechanical fragmentation of pigment particles.[18-20] In the case of a tattoo particle within a macrophage in the dermis, cell membrane rupture allows release of exogenous pigment into the extracellular space which is then eliminated predominantly via the lymphatics.[21] Clinically, the laser tissue reaction is seen as immediate epidermal whitening. These nanosecond QS lasers remain quite effective for many tattoos, though it was understood two decades ago that some of the smaller particle tattoos would need even shorter, picosecond devices to match the thermal relaxation time of these very small structures.[1]

Given that tattoos consist of particles of various sizes, those with larger particles are going to respond best to nanosecond QS lasers. The common misconception that pico devices are optimal for all tattoos is incorrect. However, for those tattoo particles that have a thermal relaxation time of less than 10 ns, the picosecond pulsed lasers should be more effective.[1,22-24] In recent years, several studies have demonstrated that picosecond lasers clear tattoos in fewer treatments when compared to studies using the nanosecond QS lasers.[23-25] It should be known that the current pico devices are actually sub-nano, in the 500–800 psec pulse duration range. Some have called for even shorter pico devices but these have issues with regard to light adsorbing plasma formation.

CLINICAL APPLICATIONS

TATTOOS

A tattoo is the deposition of an exogenous pigmented material into the skin. Once embedded, the exogenous pigment is taken up into lysosomes within dermal fibroblasts, macrophages, and mast cells. As tattoos are becoming increasingly popular, so, too, is removal because of buyer's remorse.

The development of QS nano- and picosecond lasers now allows for the "scar-less" treatment of tattoos. Most patients require a series of treatments spaced approximately 6 weeks apart, with professional tattoos requiring 6–18 or more treatments with the traditional QS nano laser.

Common complications of treatment include hyper- and hypopigmentation and textural changes, which is really a euphemism for scarring. Textural changes may

be present prior to or after the start of laser treatment. Tattoo allergic reactions appear as eczematous, granulomatous, and lichenoid reactions to red (commonly mercury and azo-chemicals), yellow, and occasionally white pigments. Paradoxical darkening can occur when treating flesh-colored tattoos. This occurs immediately after a single laser pulse and is caused by a shift from an oxidized to a reduced state in the tattoo pigment. Thus, "lip liner" might be seen to change from a rouge color to dark brown or black as the ferric oxide tattoo is reduced to ferrous oxide. Similar color changes can be seen with titanium dioxide.

Current evidence suggests that treatment of multi-colored tattoos requires more than one device with multiple wavelength combinations. The hope is that, in the future, the development of true picosecond lasers (10–20 psec) might be colorblind and avoid the need for multiple devices.

LENTIGINES

Lentigines can be effectively treated with an IPL and either the long pulse or QS KTP (532 nm) lasers, and the QS ruby (695 nm) and alexandrite (755 nm) lasers. In Fitzpatrick skin types III and IV, care should be taken to alter parameters to diminish the risk of postinflammatory hyperpigmentation.[26] Patients darker than Fitzpatrick skin type IV can be treated with the QS 1,064 nm Nd:YAG laser. The endpoint is similar to that seen in laser tattoo removal: immediate whitening which results from rapid expansion/contraction of the target chromophore and subsequent gas formation, similar the bends while diving. The lentigines will typically darken over 5–7 days and then fade away. An absolute contraindication to treatment with any QS laser wavelength is a history of gold therapy, as this can result in laser-induced chrysiasis turning the skin a black or gray color.

MELASMA

Melasma is an acquired pigmentary disorder commonly seen in sun-exposed areas of the face and predominantly affecting women of childbearing age. The exact mechanism of melasma has not been fully elucidated, though the activated melanocytes are clearly under hormonal, genetic, and sunlight control.[27] Numerous treatment regimens have been developed over the years, but none has been successful at maintaining lasting results. In addition to mainstays of sun protection, bleaching agents, and topical retinoids, various laser therapies have been utilized. IPL, low-fluence

Q-switched Nd:YAG, and nonablative lasers are the most widely utilized.[8,27–32] Favorable results have been reported with low-fluence Q-switched 1,064 nm and nonablative laser both alone and in combination. These devices are best utilized in combination with topical regimens and strict sun protection in order to maintain results.[33,34] Melasma continues to be a challenging condition to treat since only very minor sun exposure can activate melanocytes.

LASER HAIR REMOVAL

Unwanted hair is a common aesthetic problem. Laser treatment has emerged as a reliable, effective, and permanent method for hair removal and is one of the most popular aesthetic procedures performed. However, lasers are still unable to remove gray or white hair and thus the more traditional methods of electroepilation are still employed for a minority of individuals.

Photoepilation is based on selectively delivering energy to the bulge region of the hair follicle. This energy is converted into heat, which diffuses laterally beyond the actual follicle to the biological "target," namely the stem cells in the bulge region.[12,35,36] Melanin in the hair matrix absorbs wavelengths between 600 and 1,100 nm. The long-pulse ruby (694 nm), long-pulse alexandrite (755 nm), diode (810 nm), long-pulse Nd:YAG (1,064 nm), and IPL (590–1,200 nm) can all destroy hair photothermally.[12]

Device selection is based on skin type. The ideal patient for hair removal is one with lighter skin (phototypes I–III) and dark brown to black hair. Lighter skin phototypes (I–III) respond best to the 755 nm alexandrite or the 810 nm diode laser. When treating darker skin phototypes (IV–VI), it is best to use the 1,064 nm Nd:YAG laser for safety. Most studies have shown comparable efficacy rates when sufficient fluence is used and multiple treatments are performed. Typically, three to eight treatments spaced at 6- to 10-week intervals are recommended. Response rates of 70–90% hair reduction at a 6-month follow-up have been reported.[37]

Patient counseling is important for optimal results and to avoid complications. Patients can shave or use depilatory creams prior to treatment but should avoid plucking, waxing, threading, and electrolysis prior to laser treatment. To avoid burns, scarring, and permanent pigmentary changes, patients with tanned skin should not be treated.

The treatment endpoint is perifollicular erythema. Gray or white epidermal discoloration is an ominous sign as this indicates nonspecific dermal heat injury and is a marker of an inappropriately high fluence. Blister formation and epidermal necrosis may ensue and, in severe cases, may result in dermal necrosis, scarring, and permanent loss of pigmentation.

SKIN RESURFACING

Skin resurfacing lasers target water and can be divided into ablative and nonablative, and further subdivided into fractionated and nonfractionated devices. Ablative lasers predominantly include carbon dioxide (CO2), which operates at a wavelength of 10,600 nm, and the Er:YAG, which operates at 2,940 nm. Traditional nonfractionated ablative treatments remain the gold standard for photorejuvenation, wrinkle reduction, and skin tightening; however, the long downtime, increased susceptibility to infection, long-term skin erythema, potential for scarring, and delayed-onset permanent hypopigmentation have resulted in its use being secondary to the newer fractionated modalities (Figures 21.3 and 21.4).

The development of fractionated lasers has changed the way laser surgeons practice. Based on the concept of fractional photothermolysis (FP), fractionated lasers create microscopic thermal injury or microscopic treatment zones (MTZs).[38] MTZs are calibrated such that the resultant depth, width, and density are defined. Each MTZ is surrounded by normal, unaffected skin, which acts as a reservoir for healing and enables these micro-wounds to resolve quickly, with minimal discomfort. Healing of MTZs results in collagen remodeling and neocollagenesis, a rejuvenating process which lasts for months after treatment.[39,40]

Nonablative fractional resurfacing (NAFR) devices deliver narrow beams of high-energy light from 1,470 to 1,550 nm, targeting tissue water and inducing narrow columns of thermal coagulation without ablating the tissue. The resulting healing process avoids any bleeding or drainage, and consequently the downtime is modest with the exception of redness, swelling, and the development of myriad microscopic epidermal necrotic debris (MENDs).[41]

The original 1,550 nm nonablative fractional laser creates MTZs 100–200 μm in width and 500–1,400 μm in depth. Energy levels can be adjusted from 4 to 70 mJ/MTZ. This deeper penetrating wavelength is ideal for wrinkles, scarring, and other signs of photoaging.[42,43]

Other wavelengths have been added, including the thulium 1,927 nm laser which has greater absorption by water, which limits the depth of penetration to about 200 μm at 20 mJ per pulse. This effectively targets the epidermis and superficial dermis with a thin coagulative zone, similar to a very superficial CO_2 laser but with no

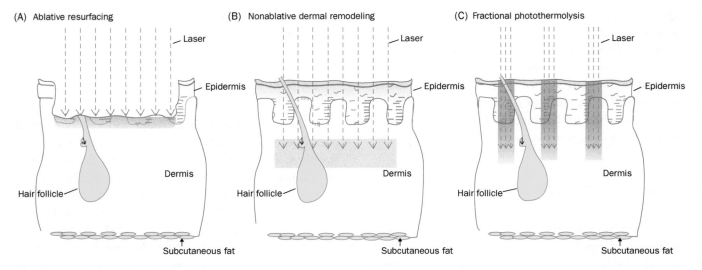

(A) Ablative resurfacing (B) Nonablative dermal remodeling (C) Fractional photothermolysis

Laser — *Epidermis* — *Dermis* — *Hair follicle* — *Subcutaneous fat*

Figure 21.3. Progression of rejuvenation.

bleeding. In addition to applications for dermatoheliosis and dyschromia, this device is quite effective at removing widespread actinic keratoses.[44,45] This provides nice options for more nuanced outcomes, and it can be used in darker skin types such as Asian and Hispanic skin, when accompanied by appropriate bleaching agents.

NAFR has been shown to be an effective treatment for many types of scarring, including inflammatory, traumatic, and surgical, as well as in many other conditions.[42–53]

In addition to fractionated nonablative devices, fractionated *ablative* devices are now available. The three wavelengths most commonly employed—10,600 nm (CO_2), 2,940 nm (Er:YAG), and 2,790 nm (yttrium scandium gallium garnet (YSGG)—are all well absorbed by water such that the treated tissue is rapidly

heated and vaporized. These devices deliver their energy using ingenious delivery mechanisms which can supply up to 2,000 pulses per second in scanners which can be stamped or rolled on the skin. Skin tightening, remodeling of scarring, improvement in texture and tone, and reduction in abnormal skin pigmentation can all be achieved.[53,54]

Most recently, Sciton, Inc. has developed the first commercially available hybrid system they have termed "Halo". This system combines a nonablative 1,470 nm diode wavelength with a 2,940 nm Er:YAG wavelength in a single handpiece that has the ability to deliver both wavelengths in a single pass. The 1,470 nm wavelength is absorbed by water and is capable of penetrating the dermis up to 700 microns. Unique to the Halo is the ability to adjust the penetration depth to as little as 100 microns, thus allowing

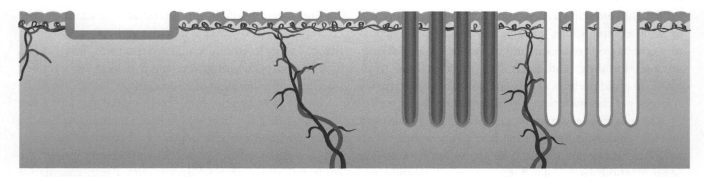

| Ablative Resurfacing (CO2 & 2.94 Erb:YAG) 10-200 mircons | Superficial Fractional Ablative Resurfacing (CO2 & 2.94 Erb:YAG) 10-70 mircons | Non-Ablative Fractional Resurfacing 600-1000 mircons | Ablative Fractional Resurfacing 600-1000 mircons |

Figure 21.4. Resurfacing lasers.

for less aggressive treatment options, but also the ability to more precisely target actinic damage at the 300-400 micron level. This device is significantly less painful than the 1,550 nm nonablative devices and is becoming popular with patients and practitioners alike.

Ablative and nonablative FP offer the opportunity for relatively safe treatment of anatomic regions that were notoriously difficult to rejuvenate with conventional ablative resurfacing. However, significant risks still remain.

Caution should be exercised in treating those with a history of delayed wound healing, history of connective tissue disease, or an immunocompromised status. Isotretinoin use in the prior 6–12 months could theoretically adversely affect wound healing after laser ablation, although this concept is being questioned. Special consideration should be given to any patient with active local or systemic infections and those with keloid scarring. Patients with vitiligo, or a first-degree family history of vitiligo, should avoid these types of procedures as this might activate a latent tendency toward loss of pigmentation.[55]

Resurfacing procedures can be painful without appropriate anesthesia, particularly when using high energies/high density parameters. The application of topical anesthetic ointment and cooling strategies enhance patient tolerance. For ablative procedures, additional anesthesia with nerve blocks, tumescent anesthesia, systemic narcotics, or anxiolytics are often used.

Oral antivirals are generally recommended for herpes simplex virus (HSV) prophylaxis. For ablative procedures, infection remains a significant complication and can lead to permanent scarring; therefore patients should receive antiviral and possibly antibacterial prophylaxis.[56]

Following ablative fractional resurfacing, punctate bleeding and serosanguineous drainage are normal side effects, which dry into a thin keratinous crust within 24–48 hours. Significant edema and erythema of treated skin is observed with both ablative and nonablative fractionated therapies, though the latter is much less evident and of shorter duration. Since the areas of vaporization are minute, and since the skin heals so rapidly, fractionated ablative systems offer an unparalleled safety margin when compared to traditional ablative lasers. Literally, 50% of the skin of the face can be removed with these devices, and yet the skin will heal within 5 days and exhibit no scarring. However, not all areas of skin are created equal. Whereas skin on the cheek, with its thicker dermis and abundant adnexal structures, can tolerate high energies and densities, more modest energy and significantly less fractionated density should be employed on thinner, finer, and less privileged areas.[55] The laser surgeon should possess comprehensive knowledge of local anatomy and skin thickness and also appreciate the composition of the adnexal structures in those locations.

CONCLUSION

Laser devices have come a long way since their inception. There are now numerous devices, wavelengths, and platforms to choose from, each with its own unique abilities. These advances in technology have hinged on several major theoretical breakthroughs which have allowed laser systems to become both more powerful and more specific while at the same time safer. The demand for cosmetic laser procedures increases as our population ages; fortunately, the technology continues to improve. It's critical that these devices are in the hands of those with good judgment and proper training. It is imperative that the laser surgeon understands both the amazing capabilities of these devices, but also the potential side effects and dangers inherently related to them. In this way, physicians and healthcare professionals can continue to provide optimal results in the safest possible way.

REFERENCES

1. Anderson RR, Parrish JA. Selective photothermolysis: precise microsurgery by selective absorption of pulsed radiation. *Science*. 1983;220(4596):524–527.
2. Shimbashi T, Kojima T. Ruby laser treatment of pigmented skin lesions. *Aesthetic Plast Surg*. 1995;19(3): 225–229.
3. Adrian, RM. Treatment of leg telangiectasias using a long-pulse frequency-doubled neodymium:YAG laser at 532 nm. *Dermatol Surg*. 1998;24(1):19–23.
4. Adrian RM, Tanghetti EA. Long pulse 532-nm laser treatment of facial telangiectasia. *Dermatol Surg*. 1998;24(1):71–74.
5. Goldman MP, Weiss RA. Treatment of poikiloderma of Civatte on the neck with an intense pulsed light source. *Plast Reconstr Surg*. 2001;107(6):1376–1381.
6. Lupton JR, Alster TS, Romero P. Clinical comparison of sclerotherapy versus long-pulsed Nd:YAG laser treatment for lower extremity telangiectases. *Dermatol Surg*. 2002;28(8):694–697.
7. Rohrer TE, Chatrath V, Iyengar V. Does pulse stacking improve the results of treatment with variable-pulse pulsed-dye lasers? *Dermatol Surg*. 2004;30(2 Pt 1):163–167; discussion 167.
8. Kim EH, Kim YC, Lee ES, et al. The vascular characteristics of melasma. *J Dermatol Sci*. 2007;46(2):111–116.
9. Glassberg E, Lask GP, Tan EM, et al. The flashlamp-pumped 577-nm pulsed tunable dye laser: clinical efficacy and in vitro studies. *J Dermatol Surg Oncol*. 1988;4(11):1200–1208.
10. Griffin TD Jr., Foshee JP, Finney R, et al. Port wine stain treated with a combination of pulsed dye laser and topical rapamycin ointment. *Lasers Surg Med*. 2016;48(2):193–196.
11. McGill DJ, MacLaren W, Mackay IR. A direct comparison of pulsed dye, alexandrite, KTP and Nd:YAG lasers and IPL in patients with previously treated capillary malformations. *Lasers Surg Med*. 2008;40(6):390–398.
12. Nanni CA, Alster TS. A practical review of laser-assisted hair removal using the Q-switched Nd:YAG, long-pulsed ruby, and

long-pulsed alexandrite lasers. *Dermatol Surg.* 1998;24(12): 1399–01405;discussion 1405.

13. Levy JL, Elbahr C, Jouve E, et al. Comparison and sequential study of long pulsed Nd:YAG 1,064 nm laser and sclerotherapy in leg telangiectasias treatment. *Lasers Surg Med.* 2004;34(3):273–276.

14. Reichert D. Evaluation of the long-pulse dye laser for the treatment of leg telangiectasias. *Dermatol Surg.* 1998;24(7):737–740.

15. Clabaugh WA. Tattoo removal by superficial dermabrasion. Five-year experience. *Plast Reconstr Surg.* 1975;55(4):401–405.

16. Dvir E, Hirshowitz B. Tattoo removal by cryosurgery. *Plast Reconstr Surg.* 1980;66(3):373–379.

17. Kent KM, Graber EM. Laser tattoo removal: a review. *Dermatol Surg.* 2012;8(1):1–13.

18. Anderson RR, Parrish JA. The optics of human skin. *J Invest Dermatol.* 1981;77(1):13–9.

19. Baumler W, Eibler, ET, Hohenleutner U, et al. Q-switch laser and tattoo pigments: first results of the chemical and photophysical analysis of 41 compounds. *Lasers Surg Med.* 2000;26(1):13–21.

20. Izikson L, Farinelli W, Sakamoto F, et al. Safety and effectiveness of black tattoo clearance in a pig model after a single treatment with a novel 758 nm 500 picosecond laser: a pilot study. *Lasers Surg Med.* 2010;42(7):640–646.

21. Saedi N, Green JB, Dover JS, et al. The evolution of quality-switched lasers. *J Drugs Dermatol.* 2012;11(11):1296–1299.

22. Alabdulrazzaq H, Brauer JA, Bae YS, et al. Clearance of yellow tattoo ink with a novel 532-nm picosecond laser. *Lasers Surg Med.* 2015;47(4):285–288.

23. Pinto F, Grosse-Buning S, Karsai S, et al. Nd:YAG (1064-nm) picosecond laser vs. Nd:YAG (1064-nm) nanosecond laser in tattoo removal: A randomized controlled single-blind clinical trial. *Br J Dermatol.* 2016.

24. Torbeck R, Bankowski R, Henize S, et al. Lasers in tattoo and pigmentation control: role of the PicoSure((R)) laser system. *Med Devices (Auckl).* 2016;9:63–67.

25. Saedi N, Metelitsa A, Petrell K, et al. Treatment of tattoos with a picosecond alexandrite laser: a prospective trial. *Arch Dermatol.* 2012;148(12):1360–1363.

26. Wang CC, Chen CK. Effect of spot size and fluence on Q-switched alexandrite laser treatment for pigmentation in Asians: a randomized, double-blinded, split-face comparative trial. *J Dermatolog Treat.* 2012;23(5):333–338.

27. Kang HY, Ortonne JP. What should be considered in treatment of melasma. *Ann Dermatol.* 2010;22(4):373–378.

28. Rokhsar CK, Fitzpatrick RE. The treatment of melasma with fractional photothermolysis: a pilot study. *Dermatol Surg.* 2005;31(12):1645–1650.

29. Tannous ZS, Astner S. Utilizing fractional resurfacing in the treatment of therapy-resistant melasma. *J Cosmet Laser Ther.* 2005;7(1):39–43.

30. Goldberg DJ, Berlin AL, Phelps R. Histologic and ultrastructural analysis of melasma after fractional resurfacing. *Lasers Surg Med.* 2008;40(2):134–138.

31. Ortonne JP, Arellano I, Berneburg M, et al. A global survey of the role of ultraviolet radiation and hormonal influences in the development of melasma. *J Eur Acad Dermatol Venereol.* 2009;23(11):1254–1262.

32. Choi M, Choi JW, Lee SY, et al. Low-dose 1064-nm Q-switched Nd:YAG laser for the treatment of melasma. *J Dermatolog Treat.* 2010;21(4):224–228.

33. Passeron T. Melasma pathogenesis and influencing factors - an overview of the latest research. *J Eur Acad Dermatol Venereol.* 2013;27 Suppl 1:5–6.

34. Dunbar S, Posnick D, Bloom B, et al. Energy-based device treatment of melasma: An update and review of the literature. *J Cosmet Laser Ther.* 2017;19(1):2–12.

35. Grossman MC, Dierickx C, Farinelli W, et al. Damage to hair follicles by normal-mode ruby laser pulses. *J Am Acad Dermatol.* 1996;35(6):889–894.

36. Alster TS, Bryan H, Williams CM. Long-pulsed Nd:YAG laser-assisted hair removal in pigmented skin: a clinical and histological evaluation. *Arch Dermatol.* 2001;137(7):885–889.

37. Lepselter J, Elman M. Biological and clinical aspects in laser hair removal. *J Dermatolog Treat.* 2004;15(2):72–83.

38. Manstein D, Herron GS, Sink RK, et al. Fractional photothermolysis: a new concept for cutaneous remodeling using microscopic patterns of thermal injury. *Lasers Surg Med.* 2004;34(5):426–438.

39. Hantash BM, Bei VP, Kapadia B, et al. In vivo histological evaluation of a novel ablative fractional resurfacing device. *Lasers Surg Med.* 2007;39(2):96–107.

40. Katz TM, Goldberg LH, Marquez D, et al. Nonablative fractional photothermolysis for facial actinic keratoses: 6-month follow-up with histologic evaluation. *J Am Acad Dermatol.* 2011;65(2):349–356.

41. Sukal SA, Geronemus RG. Fractional photothermolysis. *J Drugs Dermatol.* 2008;7(2):118–22.

42. Wanner M, Tanzi EL, Alster TS. Fractional photothermolysis: treatment of facial and nonfacial cutaneous photodamage with a 1,550-nm erbium-doped fiber laser. *Dermatol Surg.* 2007; 33(1):23–28.

43. Saedi N, Jalian HR, Petelin A, et al. Fractionation: past, present, future. *Semin Cutan Med Surg.* 2012;31(2):105–109.

44. Polder KD, Harrison A, Eubanks LE, et al. 1,927-nm fractional thulium fiber laser for the treatment of nonfacial photodamage: a pilot study. *Dermatol Surg.* 2011;37(3):342–348.

45. Weiss ET, Brauer JA, Anolik R, Reddy KK, et al. 1927-nm fractional resurfacing of facial actinic keratoses: a promising new therapeutic option. *J Am Acad Dermatol.* 2013;68(1):98–102.

46. Alajlan AM, Alsuwaidan SN. Acne scars in ethnic skin treated with both non-ablative fractional 1,550 nm and ablative fractional CO2 lasers: comparative retrospective analysis with recommended guidelines. *Lasers Surg Med.* 2011;43(8):787–791.

47. Polder KD. Commentary: A split-face study using the 1,927-nm thulium fiber fractional laser for photoaging and melasma in Asian skin. *Dermatol Surg.* 2013;39(6):889–890.

48. Kim HJ, Kim TG, Kwon YS, et al. Comparison of a 1,550 nm Erbium: glass fractional laser and a chemical reconstruction of skin scars (CROSS) method in the treatment of acne scars: a simultaneous split-face trial. *Lasers Surg Med.* 2009;41(8):545–549.

49. Tanzi EL, Alster TS. Comparison of a 1450-nm diode laser and a 1320-nm Nd:YAG laser in the treatment of atrophic facial scars: a prospective clinical and histologic study. Dermatol Surg. 2004;30 (2 Pt 1):152–157.

50. Erlendsson AM, Anderson RR, Manstein D, et al. Developing technology: ablative fractional lasers enhance topical drug delivery. *Dermatol Surg.* 2014;40 Suppl 12:S142–S146.

51. Yang Q, Huang W, Quian H, et al. Efficacy and safety of 1550-nm fractional laser in the treatment of acne scars in Chinese patients: A split-face comparative study. *J Cosmet Laser Ther.* 2016; 18(6):312–316.

52. Geronemus RG. Fractional photothermolysis: current and future applications. *Lasers Surg Med.* 2006;38(3):169–176.

53. Cho SB, Lee SJ, Cho S, et al. Non-ablative 1550-nm erbium-glass and ablative 10 600-nm carbon dioxide fractional lasers for acne scars: a randomized split-face study with blinded response evaluation. *J Eur Acad Dermatol Venereol.* 2010;24(8):921–925.

54. Alster TS. One-pass CO2 versus multiple-pass Er:YAG laser resurfacing in the treatment of rhytides: a comparison side-by-side study of pulsed CO2 and Er:YAG lasers. *Arch Facial Plast Surg.* 2002;4(4):273–274.

55. Fife DJ, Fitzpatrick RE, Zachary CB. Complications of fractional CO2 laser resurfacing: four cases. *Lasers Surg Med.* 2009;41(3):179–184.

56. Firoz BF, Katz TM, Goldberg L, et al. Herpes zoster in the distribution of the trigeminal nerve after nonablative fractional photothermolysis of the face: report of 3 cases. *Dermatol Surg.* 2011;37(2):249–252.

22.

SKIN OPTIMIZATION STRATEGIES IN PLASTIC SURGERY

Raffy Karamanoukian and Gregory R. D. Evans

Skin aging is a multivariate phenomenon that is influenced by an interdependent and patient-specific footprint of biologic and chronologic aging processes. Biologic aging, or *photo-aging*, is mainly influenced by environmental stress as a result of ultraviolet (UV) light exposure. Chronologic aging, on the other hand, is mainly controlled by the human genome but may be variably influenced by environmental and lifestyle stressors.[1]

The most common patterns of aging include degenerative changes to the skin, muscle, muscle fascia, and adipocyte. The interplay of these four variables is a fundamental focus of a modern plastic surgery practice. In order to remain relevant as leaders in cosmetic rejuvenation, plastic surgeons must be proficient in skin aging pathophysiology and the mechanisms to optimize skin with topical dermatologic monotherapy alone or as a prelude to surgery or laser. The focus of this chapter is twofold: namely, to (1) highlight the importance of skin aging in the global assessment of the cosmetic patient and (2) to elucidate the role of skin optimization in the management of the patient requesting rejuvenative cosmetic surgery.

SKIN OPTIMIZATION IN PLASTIC SURGERY

A dynamic, practical, and open-minded approach to plastic surgery is the core discussion of this textbook. The editor has mindfully incorporated practical plastic surgery principles that can sustain the discipline in the years to come. Plastic surgery has now evolved from a purely surgical discipline to one that embraces pharmaceutical, biologic, nanoparticle, molecular, and technology-driven advancements in medicine. It is this forward-thinking approach that invites a proper discussion of skin care as an elementary and core principle in a thorough plastic surgery consultation and treatment protocol.

The question of whether to incorporate a chapter on skin health correction as the first chapter in a textbook entitled *Operative Plastic Surgery* is insightful. Although plastic surgeons have countless surgical interventions at their disposal, understanding available dermatologic skin therapies may further enhance outcome alone as monotherapy or as an adjunct to cosmetic plastic surgery. The optimization of skin function and health is thus of paramount importance. Ideally, this task is best approached by using a carefully curated protocol of skin health correction prior to plastic surgery and as a maintenance protocol thereafter.

DELAY PHENOMENON IN SKIN OPTIMIZATION

The concept of optimizing skin function and health prior to a surgical procedure is not innovative or new in plastic surgery. The *delay phenomenon* is routinely incorporated prior to surgical flap elevation in order to induce structural and functional changes in flap microvasculature and health. Surgical flap delay remains a reproducible and reliable method to optimize surgical outcome and flap survival. Histologic studies have demonstrated reproducible changes in skin and soft tissue perfusion, improvements in flap surface area survival, and tissue viability as a direct consequence of surgical flap delay.[2]

Modern studies have attempted to reproduce the surgical delay phenomenon using nonsurgical methods, including laser therapy. Odland, RM[3,4] described the use of the Argon tunable dye laser as a nonablative technique to enhance flap survival prior to elevation of a McFarland flap in a rat model. The study demonstrated equivalence between the laser-induced delay technique and surgical delay in optimizing surgical flap survival. Ercocen et al.[5] further elucidated the efficacy of nonsurgical flap delay using the tunable pulsed dye laser on a dorsal rat skin flap model.

Histologically, Ercocen et al. demonstrated changes in microvasculature of the skin including dilation and proliferation of subpapillary and subdermal blood vessels, angiogenesis, and increases in mean flap perfusion after laser therapy. Reichner[6] further supported these findings while studying the utility of Erbium:Yag and CO_2 ablative lasers in optimizing skin flap survival using a nonsurgical delay technique.

Independently, nonsurgical dermatologic skin optimization techniques have consistently demonstrated robust improvements in skin integrity, physiology, and structure using protocol-driven topical regimens.[7] The most notable of these nonsurgical dermatologic skin optimization techniques is seen with the therapeutic use of tretinoin as monotherapy or as a prelude to laser therapy or surgery. As early as 1986, Kligman et al.[8] clearly demonstrated that a topical tretinoin could reproducibly induce changes to both the structure and function of the skin. Based on light and electron microscopy, he demonstrated that tretinoin-treated tissue exhibited numerous salient histologic changes including replacement of atrophic epidermis with hyperplasia, elimination of dysplastic and atypical lesions, dispersion of melanin granules, collagenesis in the papillary dermis, angiogenesis, increased blood flow, increased dermal turnover, and increased fibroblast proliferation and function. These early studies by Kligman have been substantiated and supported by others, attesting to the skin optimization benefits of dermatologic regimens on skin health.

The importance of optimizing skin function prior to a plastic surgery procedure has had variable acceptance in clinical practice. These limitations may be patient-driven, time constraint–driven, or simply overlooked in favor of expediting the scheduling of surgical or laser therapy. Numerous studies have shown increased re-epithelialization rates for skin pretreated with protocol-driven tretinoin regimens and decreased rates of adverse events, including posttreatment dyspigmentation or postinflammatory hyperpigmentation in patients pretreated with tyrosinase-inhibiting topical regimens.[9]

A simple protocol-driven approach to skin optimization may be beneficial to both clinician and patient. In clinical practice, it is important to identify patients with photodamage who would benefit from a corrective skin care regimen. Further stratification of these patients can help identify those patients who require topical skin care *only* as monotherapy and those who may require dermatologic skin optimization as a corrective modality prior to surgery or laser. The latter group may benefit from a "nonsurgical delay" with topical creams in order to improve skin integrity, function, appearance, and health; all of which can further improve patient outcome.[10]

THE AGING SKIN

Identifying patients who would benefit from skin optimization begins with an understanding of the molecular and morphologic changes inherent in aging skin. As the skin ages, it undergoes patterned changes that are influenced by genetics, skin color, and environmental stressors such as ultraviolet (UV) light exposure.

The most common signs of biologic and chronologic aging include the development of wrinkles, changes in skin texture, dyschromias, increased skin laxity, proliferation of surface telangiectasia, and complexion changes. Although it is important to recognize the phenotypical changes of skin aging, it is equally important to understand the molecular pathophysiology that may one day shape future therapies. Modern research has identified patterned cellular and molecular markers that belie these skin changes.

MOLECULAR MECHANISMS OF AGING SKIN

The mechanisms of skin aging are primarily related to (as yet) immutable genetic influences and the chronicity and lifetime exposure to UV light and inflammation. Succinctly stated by Fisher GJ et al.,[11] "UV radiation invokes a complex sequence of specific molecular responses that damage skin connective tissue." These cascading injuries to the skin substrate elicit an increase in reactive oxygen species (ROS) and changes in cell-surface receptors, signal transduction pathways, genome replicative processes, and enzymes that modulate skin integrity, resiliency, and tone.

Studies have demonstrated deleterious UV stimulation of skin matrix-degrading molecules such as metalloproteinase (MMP) 1, MMP-3, MMP-9, and proinflammatory molecules such as interleukin (IL)1β, tumor necrosis factor (TNF)α, IL-6, and IL-8.[11]

The up-regulation of cellular and molecular mechanisms that degrade the integrity of skin structure and function are the deleterious endpoints of the aging process. Simply stated, biologic and chronologic mechanisms of aging cumulatively invoke senescent changes in skin function, degrade the structural matrix of the skin's connective tissue, increase levels of inflammatory mediators, and cause an accumulation of degradative waste byproducts within the skin's substructure. These harmful changes result in a gradual weakening of skin physiology and function.

In the future, advancements in the understanding of the molecular pathways that lead up to skin senescence may ultimately allow us to target specific molecular therapies to combat long-term skin health. Until those molecular targets are identified and targeted with safe and reproducible molecular therapies, the clinician is left with identifying morphologic age-related changes in the skin and utilizing available options for optimizing skin biology in order to achieve an improvement in the skin's appearance.

MORPHOLOGIC CHANGES IN AGING SKIN

The skin undergoes patterned changes as a result of both biologic and chronologic aging. These changes mark milestones in the aging process and can be improved with a protocol-driven therapeutic skin care regimen alone or in combination with a surgical or laser procedure.

Aging skin undergoes characteristic changes as surface fine wrinkles become more deeply embedded within the topography of the skin. Irregular pigmentation, proliferation of skin telangiectasia, atrophic changes to accessory glands, and increased textural roughness predominate on the skin. Functionally, the skin begins to lose its baseline tolerance to environmental stress as the accumulation of degraded matrix molecules affect skin laxity, resiliency, and turgor. The loss of elasticity is likely induced by an up-regulation of proteolytic enzymes within the dermis, dysregulation of the functional basal epidermis and atrophy of accessory eccrine and apocrine glands.[11] The combination of molecular and phenotypic changes in the skin suggests an overpowering dysregulation of skin health and function.

Once recognized, clinicians can exact specific changes in skin physiology, function, and appearance by using an arsenal of topical dermatologic that can up-regulate cellular renewal, stimulate dispersion and exfoliation of melanin, and reverse photodamaged skin.[12] A carefully curated skin protocol begins with an understanding of skin aging and the modalities used to correct each condition individually or together. The goal of these treatments is to improve skin function and morphology as monotherapy or as a prequel to surgery.

RHYTIDS

The development of facial rhytids is influenced by genetics, skin color, cumulative photodamage, conformational skin deformities, collagen and elastin density, and velocity of matrix degradation within the skin. Wrinkles can be characterized by their depth, anatomic location, or function. Terms such as fine wrinkles, deep wrinkles, crow's feet, elevens, laugh lines, and nasolabial folds supplant objective descriptors for facial rhytids. The obfuscatory nomenclature likely stems from the difficulty of objectively characterizing wrinkles by size, depth, or surface area.

Attempts to understand wrinkles from a histopathologic perspective have remained futile. To date, a histologic pathomorphology has yet to be attributed to the wrinkle. Instead, it is thought that wrinkles may represent a conformational change in the skin rather than any pathologic process within it. Kligman et al.[13] analyzed histologic sections of wrinkles and failed to pinpoint reproducible histologic features associated with wrinkles. Based on the study, Kligman concluded that wrinkles represented configurational anomalies on the skin in the absence of any pathologic skin process. Three decades later, Pessa et al.[14] supported Kligman's conclusion that wrinkles represent a configurational skin process rather than a histopathologic one. Pessa hypothesized that wrinkles may be caused by configurational changes on the skin overlying a lymphatic vessel.

SOLAR ELASTOSIS

The effects of biologic aging on the skin elasticity are profound. As a result of cumulative UV damage, the structural matrix of the skin undergoes proliferative changes that are histologically characterized by excessive dermal elastosis caused by the accumulation of elastotic debris trapped within the dermis. This hyperproliferation of dysfunctional elastotic elements is likely related to UV-induced inflammation with the byproduct being an accumulation of glycosaminoglycan and elastotic molecular elements. Histologically, the dermis shows an abundant accumulation of elastotic molecular debris, disorganized tropoelastin, and fibrillin molecules.

Along with a depletion of type I collagen, these pathologic changes in the skin likely contribute to atrophic skin, a loss of skin elasticity, and patterned configurational changes in the skin surface that manifest as wrinkles.

SURFACE TOPOGRAPHIC CHANGES

The topography of the skin can be influenced by hydration, sebum content, compaction of the stratum corneum, pore size, and previous scarring. Textural changes can be caused by atrophy of the skin, wrinkle severity, porosity of accessory glands and pores, photodamage, atrophic skin injury, and previous scarring. These degenerative skin changes are prolific in the setting of chronically photodamaged skin but may be noticeably absent in youthful skin. Topographic surface changes are likely due to cumulative epidermal and dermal changes in the structure and physiology of the skin.

DYSCHROMIA

Pigmentary variegation is a common manifestation of skin aging and represents an intrinsic dysregulation of melanocyte activity that is asymmetric and rarely self-resolving. Age-related precipitors of dyschromia include cumulative UV exposure, irregular patterns of melanocytic hyperplasia and senescence, estrogen and progesterone hormonal load, thyroid dysfunction, inflammation, hemosiderin deposition, and proliferation of surface telangiectasia.

The severity of dyschromia may be further influenced by ethnicity, skin complexion type, genetic variables, photo-sensitizing drugs, lifestyle, and a predisposition to developing pigmentary problems. Hypermelanosis remains the most common cause of premature skin aging and can greatly influence self-esteem. In clinical practice, pigmentary problems are primarily caused by solar-induced melanocytic dysregulation (age spots and complexion variegation), hormonally influenced hyperpigmentation (melasma), and postinflammatory hyperpigmentation.

SOLAR-INDUCED MELANOCYTIC DYSREGULATION

Melanocytic dysregulation is an identifiable result of skin aging, likely influenced by the combination of age-related senescence and UV light-induced dysregulation of melanocyte function. Histologically, there may appear paradoxically adjacent areas of melanocytic depletion coupled with areas of melanocytic hyperplasia, a lack of uniformity in the production of melanin within the skin, and an irregular pattern of melanin deposition found within the epidermis, dermis, and along perivascular dermal channels.

Characteristic findings include solar lentigines, age spots, areas of variegated skin color with pigmentary mottling, hypopigmentation, and notable hypermelanosis. Age-related changes in skin complexion can dramatically diverge from native skin tone depending on a host of variables, most notably lifetime exposure to the sun. These changes are reflected by an patterned loss of skin color uniformity, likely influenced by genetic predisposition and biologic aging.

MELASMA

Melasma is a common postpubertal dyspigmentation characterized by hyperpigmentary macules on the face.[15] The most prevalent anatomic zones of melasma are mandibular (mandible and upper neck), malar (cheek and zygoma), and frontal (forehead and glabella). Development of melasma may often occur in the setting of sun exposure but primarily arises as a result of endogenous or exogenous hormonal influences.

The exact pathogenesis of melasma development remains elusive. Genetically predisposed individuals often experience dyspigmentation in the absence of a precipitating event. A combination of genetics, UV exposure, endocrine abnormalities, photo-sensitizing drug exposure, chemotherapy, and hormonal load are all known to influence the development of melasma.[16]

Women represent 90% of patients with melasma, likely owing to the patterned hormonal influences experienced by women of childbearing age. In the first half of the twentieth century, melasma was known as a "pregnancy mask," as the condition was primarily associated with increases in circulating estrogen and progesterone during pregnancy and lactation. Upon the introduction of oral contraceptives, the demographic of melasma shifted toward nulliparous women of childbearing age. Of note, 10% of melasma cases occur in men with no known endocrine dysfunction.[17]

Unlike age spots, the diagnosis of melasma is based on clinical findings and patient history. Although asymmetric lesions abound, the hyperpigmented macules are uniformly distributed along recognized anatomic patterns on the face along the forehead, cheeks, mandible, and upper lip, independent of sun exposure.

Patients with melasma are often hesitant to associate the patterns of pigmentation with known endogenous and exogenous hormonal influences, opting instead to seek patient-driven single-agent treatment with hydroquinone creams that have limited long-term success. Optimal treatment for melasma includes a cessation of abnormal hormonal influences, sun protection, and multiagent combination therapy with retinoids and melanin-modulating agents as described in this chapter.

POSTINFLAMMATORY HYPERPIGMENTATION

Postinflammatory hyperpigmentation (PIH) is characterized by an abnormal deposition of melanin that occurs during normal wound healing or prolonged inflammation. Unlike normal melanin production and deposition in the epidermis, PIH pigmentary granules are found deep within the dermis, causing long-term dyspigmentation of the skin. It is hypothesized that the abnormal deposition and migration of melanin into the dermis occurs through perivascular channels that are disrupted as a result of inflammation.

Although the primary cause of PIH is inflammation, it appears as though there is a genetic-susceptibility to the development of PIH that may or may not be accentuated by exposure to UV light. Characteristic PIH lesions result from localized inflammation resulting from acne, inflammatory skin conditions such as eczema, thermal burn injuries, iatrogenic laser or chemo-exfoliation, surgery, or skin trauma.

Commonly, PIH produces a process known as *pigmentary framing* in which the skin surrounding an incision becomes hyperpigmented. Histologically, the melanin is usually found in the dermis, alongside perivascular channels, and is deeply embedded within the deeper layers of the skin.

Dysregulation of skin function presents an important and often overlooked dilemma for the plastic surgeon contemplating rejuvenative surgery. On a molecular, cellular, structural, and physiologic level, these described senescent processes of skin aging intimate that the underlying functional health of the skin may benefit from a protocol-driven "delay technique" in order to optimize surgical outcome and induce stimulatory changes to the structure, function, physiology, intrinsic adaptive tolerance, and microvasculature of the supporting skin.

COMMONLY USED PHARMACEUTICAL AGENTS IN SKIN OPTIMIZATION

HYDROQUINONE

Hydroquinone is a water-soluble, aromatic organic phenol[18] that has seen widespread commercial application as a topical skin lightener since the discovery of its dermatologic utility by Oetel in 1936. Its mechanism of action derives from its ability to reversibly disrupt melanogenesis, with a particular affinity to follicular and skin melanocytes.

A common misconception about hydroquinone is that it acts a bleaching agent. In fact, the action of hydroquinone is limited to the suppression of *future* melanin production, but it has no definitive role as a single agent in the treatment of preexisting deposits of melanin. For this reason, hydroquinone is most effective when used simultaneously with other agents to remove old pigmentation and suppress future repigmentation.

Molecular studies on hydroquinone have demonstrated that its primary mechanism of action is primarily twofold, acting as a (1) competitive substrate for tyrosinase and (2) invoking cytotoxic free radical formation within the melanosome itself.[17-19]

Single-agent therapy with hydroquinone is limited. Treatment efficacy is increased when hydroquinone is used with α-hydroxy acids (AHA), retinoids, and natural tyrosinase inhibitors. Hydroquinone is commercially available as a topical cream with concentrations ranging from 2% to 4%. Higher concentrations have yielded a less-than-linear dose-dependent reduction in tyrosinase activity but exhibit higher rates of adverse reactions including skin irritation and, rarely, paradoxic hyperpigmentation as with exogenous ochronosis. By combining hydroquinone with retinoids, non-hydroquinone tyrosinase inhibitors, and exfoliants, the penetrance and reliability of hydroquinone is enhanced while still maintaining a low rate of adverse reactions.

Despite its widespread application as a safe and reversible inhibitor of melanogenesis, a discussion of hydroquinone would not be complete without a discussion of the controversies surrounding hydroquinone. Currently, the European Committee (24th Dir 2000/6/EC) has banned the use of hydroquinone in all cosmetic and over-the-counter (OTC) skin preparations, restricting it to a prescription-only drug, citing the dangers of permanent skin hypopigmentation and exogenous ochronosis. The US Food and Drug Administration (FDA) has issued regulatory changes in its classification of hydroquinone based on the Generally Recognized as Safe and Effective (GRASE) ruling of 1982, which proposed that OTC skin bleaching products containing 1.5–2.0% be generally recognized as safe and effective. In 2006, the FDA proposed to amend the 1982 rule that hydroquinone be GRASE because of evidence indicating that hydroquinone may act as a cancer-causing agent in rodents after oral administration. In the 2006 proposed rule, a recommendation was made that additional studies be conducted by the National Toxicology Program. The 2006 proposal recommended that hydroquinone remain available as an OTC drug.[20,21]

NATURAL SKIN LIGHTENERS

Proposed and enacted restrictions on hydroquinone internationally and in the United States have hastened the search to find alternative ingredients that modulate melanin production and maturation. Ideally, these alternative ingredients should be less melanocytotoxic than hydroquinone, exhibit alternate mechanisms of action to encourage combination treatment regimens, and be readily available or suitable for biosynthesis. Naturally occurring extracts often meet these inclusion criteria and are surprisingly ubiquitous in nature.

Many plant isolates have activity against the tyrosinase enzyme and often have clinically effective antiinflammatory properties.[22] These reversible inhibitors of tyrosinase can be safely employed alongside phenolic hydroquinone to reduce the production and dispersion of melanin within the skin. Herein, we provide a list of non-hydroquinone skin lighteners. The benefits of plant-derived tyrosinase inhibition is the theoretical absence of melanocytotoxicity and the perceived higher safety profile of naturally derived ingredients by the consumer when compared with synthetic pharmaceutical active ingredients.

ARBUTIN

Arbutin is a naturally occurring glucoside derivative of the phenolic tyrosinase inhibitor hydroquinone.[18,22,23] Arbutin competitively inhibits tyrosinase activity and remains cytotoxic to the melanocyte. The action of arbutin derives from its structural similarity to tyrosine, making it a competitive inhibitor of tyrosinase activity. Studies on the efficacy of arbutin, found naturally in bearberry, cranberry, and pear extracts, have demonstrated biosynthetic second- and third-generation homologues of arbutin such as α-arbutin, D-arbutin, deoxy-furan, 2-fluodeoxy-arbutin, and thiodeoxy-arbutin, and which also exert potent tyrosinase inhibition with decreased cytotoxic activity on the melanocyte. The cytotoxic risk profile of arbutin and its homologues are appealing to those patients who desire a non-hydroquinone–based regimen for the treatment of dyschromias.[11]

KOJIC ACID

Kojic acid is a naturally occurring molecule isolated from fungus that has been shown to inhibit tyrosinase enzyme activity. Concentrations of 1–4% have been shown to clinically decrease melanin production, thereby reducing active

hyperpigmentation. Often used a single-agent therapy, kojic acid cream have a low adverse reaction profile and are suitable to use with other skin lighteners to improve skin melanosis.[18,22]

LICORICE

Licorice (*Glycrrhiza glabra*) extract contains several isolates that have effects on melanin production and dispersion. The hydrophobic fraction of licorice is known as glabridin and has been shown to inhibit tyrosinase activity. Glabrene, isoliquiritigenin, licuraside, isoliquiritin, and licochalcone, all isolates of licorice, have also demonstrated activity against the tyrosinase enzyme. Last, liquiritin work on dispersing the melanin and has limited to no activity on the tyrosinase enzyme. Licorice extracts are widely used as nonphenolic alternatives to hydroquinone or as a complement to a hydroquinone based regimen.[18,22]

MULBERRY

Mulberry (*Morus alba*) extract has been shown to inhibit tyrosinase enzyme activity and disrupt melanin maturation. Isolates from mulberry and mulberry twigs include phenolic flavonoids that have been shown to dysregulate melanocyte activity including maclurin, rutin, isoquercitrin, resveratrol, and morin. The action of mulberry also derives from superoxide scavenging activity.[24]

NIACINAMIDE

Niacinamide is the molecular amide of niacin (vitamin B_3) and a precursor of nicotinamide adenine dinucleotide (NADH) and nicotinamide adenine dinucleotide phosphate (NADPH) produced synthetically and found naturally in yeast and the root vegetables. Niacinamide disrupts melanin maturation by inhibiting the transfer of melanosomes to keratinocytes. Secondarily, nicotinamide exhibits broad-based salutary benefits to photodamaged skin, presumably due to the ubiquity of coenzymes NADH and NADPH mechanics in cellular enzyme processes and oxidation-reduction reactions.[25]

Niacinamide has been shown to stabilize transepidermal water loss by fortifying skin barrier function, improve hydration of the horny layer of the skin, stimulate sphingolipid synthesis and keratinocyte differentiation, efface configurational changes and improve skin topography, inhibit photocarcinogenesis, and reduce inflammation.

SALICYLIC ACID

Salicylic acid is a β-hydroxy acid that is synthetically synthesized but is also found naturally in willow bark and sweet birch bark. The action of salicylic acid on hypermelanosis derives from its action of desquamating the skin. Salicylic acid has harsh side effects when used in high concentrations above 10%, but it acts as a mild desquamation agent in low concentrations of 1–2% to eliminate melanin particles from the stratum corneum. It is also used as an effective keratolytic agent which contributes to its use in controlling acneic pustules and limiting postinflammatory hyperpigmentation.

TRETINOIN

Tretinoin belongs to a family of molecules known as retinoids that have been shown to have reproducibly beneficial action profiles on photodamaged skin. On a molecular level, tretinoin binds to a specific nuclear receptor and induces a 70% reduction in AP-1 transcription factor.[12,26] As a result, tretinoin has been shown to improve dermal elasticity and thickness by down-regulating metalloproteinase production and action, inhibiting collagen and dermal matrix degradation, and stimulating type I collagen production. Tretinoin also functions to increase epidermal thickness, induce compaction of the stratum corneum, and promote dispersion of melanin granules. The clinical benefits of tretinoin become self-evident upon usage, with clinical effacement of fine wrinkles, lightening of dyspigmentation, smoothing of textural skin changes, reduction in sebum output and pore size, increased skin elasticity and resiliency, and development of robust neoangiogenesis.

Tretinoin is commercially available as a topical cream in concentrations of 0.025%, 0.05%, and 0.1%. Alternate retinoids such as retinol, retinaldehyde, retinyl palmitate, tazarotene, and adapalene are widely available as OTC or prescription creams with variable efficacy and risk profiles.

The salutary effects of tretinoin are often outweighed, however, by variable compliance rates resulting from patient discomfort known as the *retinoid reaction*. Pruritus, burning, erythema, scaling, and desquamation limit tretinoin use and encourage close patient contact and support to maintain compliance with therapy.

SKIN OPTIMIZATION PROTOCOLS

A protocol-driven corrective skin regimen can help restore the function and health of the skin, thus optimizing outcomes in plastic surgery. The goal of corrective skin restoration is multifold; namely, to (1) reverse senescent changes to skin wrinkling, elasticity, surface topography, and color; (2) restore tolerance to the skin so that it can withstand future laser or surgical treatments; and (3) establish a protocol-driven maintenance regimen to maintain long-term results and retain patients.

Skin optimization may be clinically employed as monotherapy or as a corrective step before a plastic surgery procedure. Evidence-based studies have shown corrective skin care to be complementary to plastic surgery or laser procedures.

Choosing the most appropriate dermatologic regimen for a patient begins with a thorough understanding of the morphologic changes that the skin undergoes as a result of biologic photodamage and chronologic aging. In simple terms, skin aging results in increased skin wrinkling, loss of dermal elasticity, changes in skin topography, and disorganized variegation in skin pigmentation. The most clinically effective dermatologic regimens contain active ingredients that can stimulate cellular renewal in the epidermis and dermis, reduce wrinkling, correct surface topography, and modulate the activity of melanocytes.

Skin aging is an ongoing degenerative process with distinct molecular and cellular patterns of senescence. In choosing an appropriate dermatologic regimen, it is imperative to recommend a protocol-based program that addresses all of the key features of skin aging. Although single-agent regimens may provide some benefit for patients, a combination approach may be better suited for long-term optimization of skin health and function. Single-agent therapy with either hydroquinone or tretinoin incompletely addresses the broad range of molecular and cellular dysregulation that characterize photodamaged skin. Simply correcting wrinkles or pigmentation as an isolated entity mischaracterizes the complexity of photo-aging and limits the potential to optimize the spectrum of dysregulatory mechanisms involved in photo-aging.

The challenge of directing patients to adhere to an established physician-prescribed combination protocol instead of a patient-driven single-agent therapy is ongoing. As with any medical recommendation, patients should understand the basic molecular and cellular processes of aging as well as the targeted goals for treatment. Single-agent skin optimization is poorly thought-out, incomplete, and unreliable in addressing the multifactorial etiology of skin aging.

In the authors' opinion, the most appropriate dermatologic regimen must at least incorporate a retinoid, a phenolic-tyrosinase inhibitor, non-phenolic tyrosinase inhibitors, and an exfoliant.

The Kligman-Willis formula,[18] consisting of hydroquinone 5% cream, tretinoin 0.1% cream, and dexamethasone 0.1% gained early acceptance among clinicians treating hyperpigmentation and melasma. In this formulation, tretinoin allowed enhanced epidermal penetration, encouraged compaction of the stratum corneum, and allowed for increased melanin dispersion from the keratinocyte. Simultaneously, dexamethasone acted as both a modulator of inflammation and a nonselective inhibitor of melanogenesis.

Modifications to the original Kligman-Willis formula exploited the synergy of combination therapy but allowed for modifications in hydroquinone and tretinoin concentrations and for decreased potency of corticosteroids. The limitations of the triple-combination formula became apparent with long-term use, as patients experienced adverse events relating to long-term corticosteroid exposure. Rather than stimulating cellular renewal as a long-term skin optimization regimen, many of these triple-therapies resulted in steroid-induced adverse events such as skin atrophy, proliferation of surface telangiectasia, hypertrichosis, and acne.[27] In addition, higher concentrations of hydroquinone found in specialty-compounded formulas increase the potential for skin irritation and adverse reactions.

The incidence of corticosteroid- and hydroquinone-induced adverse events has curtailed the broad use of triple-therapy in favor of regimens that limit potentially adverse skin reactions. In the author's opinion, the optimal regimen includes a lower dose, hydroquinone 2% cream to disrupt tyrosinase activity while minimizing hydroquinone-induced melanocytotoxicity, coupled with several non-phenolic, non-hydroquinone tyrosinase inhibitors such as kojic acid, mulberry extract, licorice extract, and bearberry extract; a UVA and UVB sunblock; a β-hydroxy acid exfoliant with kojic acid; and tretinoin 0.05% or 0.1% depending on the severity of photodamage. The addition of natural, non-hydroquinone–based skin lighteners is appealing to patients who wish to limit hydroquinone exposure and for clinicians wishing to target abnormal melanocytes using different tyrosinase-inhibiting mechanisms. In the past, rapid retinoid exfoliation became the mainstay of therapy, with patients experiencing prolonged courses of dryness, desquamation, and discomfort. The modern approach optimizes compliance by decreasing dosages and frequency in order to maximize patient adherence to protocol-driven timelines.

It is imperative that patients understand the expected clinical outcome and are aware of the time limitations to achieve clinically significant changes in skin function and health and potential adverse reactions that may limit use.

The most common reasons for noncompliance include skin dryness and desquamation related to the retinoid reaction. Patients are also instructed on the use of sun protection and are given guidelines to avoid direct or indirect sun exposure.

MAINTENANCE REGIMEN

The goal of skin optimization is to redefine the cellular and molecular machinery that drives healthy skin. A protocol-driven dermatologic regimen incorporates stimulatory agents that can reverse photodamaged skin as monotherapy or as a prelude to an impending cosmetic surgery or laser procedure. Patients benefit from a maintenance regimen that allows them to further improve skin health and function, limit future photodamage, and sustain results. A proper skin optimization regimen must therein allow for correction of skin senescence and maintain a platform for continued care. In the authors' opinion, patients are advised to resume maintenance therapy indefinitely, defined by a patient-specific daily program in order to optimize and maintain healthy skin.

CONCLUSION

In order to remain relevant, the modern plastic surgeon must remain proficient in the biologic and chronologic processes of skin aging and their relevance to the global surgical outcome of the patient undergoing a plastic surgery procedure. Nonsurgical methods to optimize the physiology, morphology, and function of the skin may contribute to the overall patient outcome. Prior to discussing options for surgical skin and soft-tissue manipulation, it is the authors' opinion that plastic surgeons should be mindful of skin function and health in optimizing the surgical result. These skin corrective techniques may thus invoke salient improvements that can improve outcome, increase patient satisfaction, and establish a maintenance platform for continued care.

REFERENCES

1. Fisher GJ, Kang S, Varani J, et al. Mechanisms of photoaging and chronological skin aging. *Arch Dermatol* 2002 Nov;138 (11): 1462–1470.
2. Cinpolat A, Bektas G, Coskunfirat N, Rizvanovic Z, Coskunfirat OK. Comparing various surgical delay methods with ischemic preconditioning in the rat TRAM flap model. *J Reconstr Microsurg* 2014 Jun;30(5):335–342.

3. Odland RM, Poole DV, Rice RD Jr, Koobs DH. Use of the tunable dye laser to delay McFarlane skin flaps. *Arch Otolaryngol Head Neck Surg* 1995 Oct;121(10):1158–1161.

4. Odland RM, Rice RD Jr. Comparison of tunable dye and KTP lasers in nonsurgical delay of cutaneous flaps. *Otolaryngol Head Neck Surg* 1995 Jul;113(1):92–98.

5. Erçöçen AR, Kono T, Kikuchi Y, Kitazawa Y, Nozaki M. Efficacy of the flashlamp-pumped pulsed-dye laser in nonsurgical delay of skin flaps. *Dermatol Surg* 2003 Jul;29(7):692–699; discussion 699.

6. Reichner DR, Scholz T, Vanderkam VM, Gutierrez S, Steward E, Evans GR. Laser flap delay: comparison of Erbium:YAG and CO2 lasers. *Am Surg* 2003 Jan;69(1):69–72.

7. Popp C, Kligman AM, Stoudemayer TJ. Pretreatment of photoaged forearm skin with topical tretinoin accelerates healing of full-thickness wounds. *Br J Dermatol* 1995 Jan;132(1):46–53.

8. Kligman AM, Grove GL, Hirose R, Leyden JJ. Topical tretinoin for photoaged skin. *J Am Acad Dermatol* 1986 Oct;15(4 Pt 2):836–859.

9. Chaowattanapanit S, Silpa-Archa N, Kohli I, Lim HW, Hamzavi I. Postinflammatory hyperpigmentation: a comprehensive overview: treatment options and prevention. *J Am Acad Dermatol* 2017 Oct;77(4):607–621. doi: 10.1016/j.jaad.2017.01.036. Review.

10. Gilchrest BA. Treatment of photodamage with topical tretinoin: an overview. *Exp Dermatol* 1995 Jun;4(3):146–154. *J Am Acad Dermatol* 1997 Mar;36(3 Pt 2) S27–S36.

11. Fisher GJ, Kang S, Varani J, et al. Mechanisms of photoaging and chronological skin aging. *Arch Dermatol* 2002 Nov;138(11):1462–1470. Review.

12. Hubbard BA, Unger JG, Rohrich RJ. Reversal of skin aging with topical retinoids. *Plast Reconstr Surg* 2014 Apr;133(4):481e–90e. doi: 10.1097/PRS.

13. Kligman AM, Zheng P, Lavker RM. The anatomy and pathogenesis of wrinkles. *Br J Dermatol* 1985 Jul;113(1):37–42.

14. Pessa JE, Nguyen H, John GB, Scherer PE. The anatomical basis for wrinkles. *Aesthet Surg J* 2014 Feb;34(2):227–234. doi: 10.1177/1090820X13517896.

15. Passeron T, Picardo M. Melasma, a photoagingphoto-aging disorder. *Pigment Cell Melanoma Res* 2017 Dec 29. doi: 10.1111/pcmr.12684. Review.

16. Sarkar R, Arora P, Garg VK, Sonthalia S, Gokhale N. Melasma update. *Indian Dermatol Online J* 2014 Oct;5(4):426–435. doi: 10.4103/2229-5178.142484. Review.

17. Sarkar R, Puri P, Jain RK, Singh A, Desai A. Melasma in men: a clinical, aetiological and histological study. *J Eur Acad Dermatol Venereol* 2010 Jul;24(7):768–772. doi: 10.1111/j.1468-3083.2009.03524.x.

18. Sarkar R, Gokhale N, Godse K, et al. Medical management of melasma: a review with consensus recommendations by Indian Pigmentary Expert Group. *Indian J Dermatol* 2017 Nov-Dec;62(6): 558–577. doi: 10.4103/ijd.IJD_489_17.

19. Haddad AL, Matos LF, Brunstein F, Ferreira LM, Silva A, Costa D Jr. A clinical, prospective, randomized, double-blind trial comparing skin whitening complex with hydroquinone vs. placebo in the treatment of melasma. *Int J Dermatol* 2003 Feb;42(2):153–156.

20. US Food and Drug Administration (FDA). https://www.fda.gov/Drugs/DevelopmentApprovalProcess/DevelopmentResources/Over-the-CounterOTCDrugs/StatusofOTCRulemakings/ucm072117.htm

21. Borovansky J, Riley PA. *Melanins and Melanosomes: Biosynthesis, Biogenesis, Physiological and Pathological Functions*. 2011.

22. Zhu W, Gao J. The use of botanical extracts as topical skin-lightening agents for the improvement of skin pigmentation disorders. *J Investig Dermatol Symp Proc* 2008 Apr;13(1):20–24. doi: 10.1038/jidsymp.2008.8. Review.

23. Miao F, Shi Y, Fan ZF, Jiang S, Xu SZ, Lei TC. Deoxyarbutin possesses a potent skin-lightening capacity with no discernible cytotoxicity against melanosomes.

24. Chang LW, Juang LJ, Wang BS, et al. Antioxidant and antityrosinase activity of mulberry (Morus alba L.) twigs and root bark. *Food Chem Toxicol* 2011 Apr;49(4):785–790. doi: 10.1016/j.fct.2010.11.045.

25. Gehring W. Nicotinic acid/niacinamide and the skin. *J Cosmet Dermatol* 2004 Apr;3(2):88–93.

26. Yamamoto O, Bhawan J, Solares G, Tsay AW, Gilchrest BA. Ultrastructural effects of topical tretinoin on dermo-epidermal junction and papillary dermis in photodamaged skin. A controlled study. *Int J Dermatol* 1998 Apr;37(4):286–292.

27. Majid I. Mometasone-based triple combination therapy in melasma: Is it really safe? *Indian J Dermatol* 2010; 55: 359–362.

PART V.

AESTHETICS

23.

RHYTIDECTOMY

Malcolm D. Paul

INTRODUCTION

The evolution of techniques in facelifting spans nearly 100 years. Early attempts at facial rejuvenation involved limited skin undermining and, frequently, closure under tension resulting in minimal cosmetic improvement and the possibility of tension-related hypertrophic scars (Figure 23.1A, B). The goals have evolved as a clearer understanding of the aging face embraced the concept of both vector-based and volume-based procedures to recapture the heart-shaped face of youth. For the beginner, skin undermining and manipulations of the *superficial musculoaponeurotic system* (SMAS) that do not require undermining are safe and predictable. A journey through the evolution and the variety of SMAS techniques is of value for information, but this does not necessarily suggest that the beginning facelift surgeon embrace and "try" the more advanced techniques.

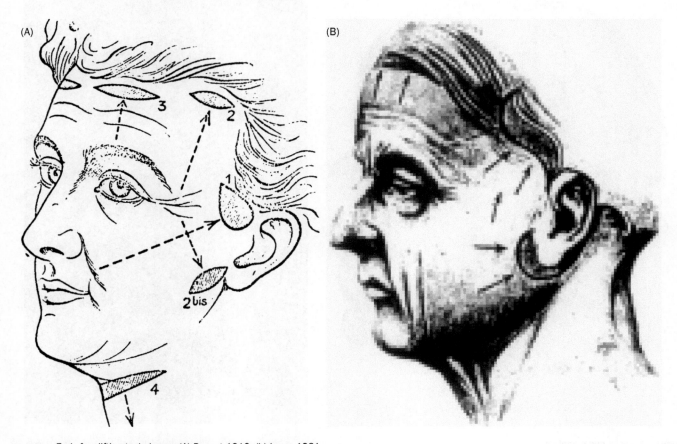

Figure 23.1. Early facelifting techniques: (A) Passot 1919, (b) Lexer 1931.

HISTORY OF SMAS TECHNIQUES

Since its description by Mitz and Peyronie,[1] attention has been directed to various approaches to provide an important foundation for a longer lasting facial rejuvenation than was obtained with skin lifts only. The evolution of techniques regarding the manipulation of the SMAS began with an understanding of the anatomy of the facial nerve and sub-SMAS anatomy (Figures 23.2, 23.3, and 23.4). Techniques involved short anterior dissections[2] and have evolved to SMAS plication and lateral SMAS-ectomy (Figure 23.5),[3] deep plane dissection,[4,5] and high SMAS dissections with flap advancement to fixed structures.[6–8] Each of these approaches relies on an incision in the non-mobile SMAS over the parotid gland or slightly anterior to the parotid gland with anterior and inferior dissection. The goal has been an advancement of the mobile SMAS to the fixed SMAS and, in some techniques, to Lore's fascia (Figures 23.6 and 23.7).[9] Yet one of the most popular approaches to the aging face is the use of pursestring sutures to provide vertical elevation of the ptotic SMAS to correct the jawline and the anterior cheek, the minimal access cranial suspension (MACS) lift (Figure 23.8).[10] Simple plication of the mobile to the non-mobile SMAS[11] and vertical plication of the SMAS[12] are also widely used. Important contributions to the repositioning of ptotic soft tissues incorporating the SMAS include the finger-assisted malar elevation (FAME) procedure[13] and the subperiosteal approach.[14] A thorough understanding of the relevant anatomy as described by Mendelsohn[15] is crucial in safely performing these procedures. The goal of all available options in deep-layer support remains the same: a firm foundation of SMAS, evenly dissected or plicated and advanced to a higher level, mostly superiorly, but also posteriorly as indicated by the clinical findings in each patient.

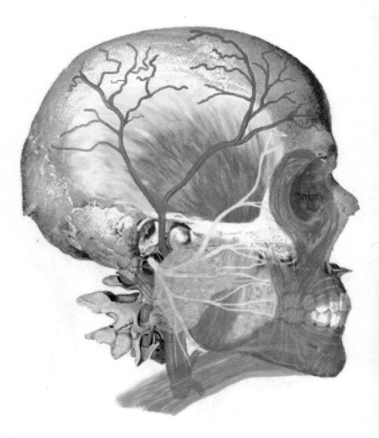

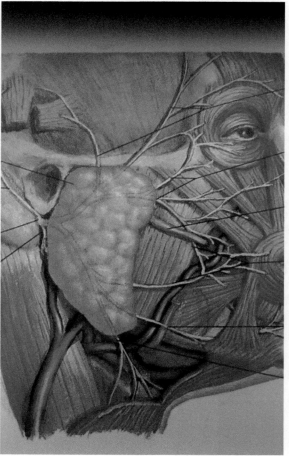

Figure 23.2. Facial nerve anatomy.

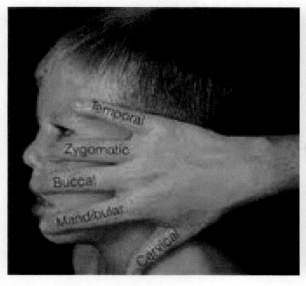
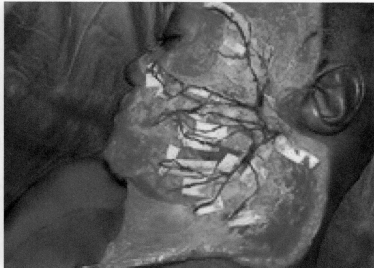

Figure 23.3. Facial nerve anatomy.

ASSESSMENT OF THE DEFECT

As in any planned surgical facial rejuvenation, a thorough history and physical examination is a prerequisite to a favorable patient experience and result. Comorbid

conditions are assessed and appropriate medical clearance is a prerequisite to any elective procedure. Anatomical findings will differ in each age group. However, all patients who are candidates for a facelift procedure have the following clinical findings in varying degrees.

1. Textural changes in the skin (related to genetics, sun damage, and smoking)

2. Cheek laxity and jawline skin laxity

3. Fat atrophy

4. Prominent nasolabial folds

5. Jowl formation

6. Frequently, a downward turned modiolus

7. Irregular contour to the mandibular border

8. Prominent, ptotic, buccal fat pads are seen in many, but not in all patients. Most commonly, prominent buccal fat pads are seen in patients of Latin American, Asian, and Middle-Eastern descent, but Caucasian patients frequently present with similar anatomical findings (i.e., prominent, ptotic buccal fat pads).

9. Laxity of the central neck

10. Visible short or long platysmal bands with a high, middle, or low decussation (fusion of two medial edges of the platysma muscle)

11. Excessive submental fat in one, two, or all three compartments: subcutaneous, interplatysmal, subplatysmal

Figure 23.4. Sub-superficial musculoaponeurotic system (SMAS) anatomy.

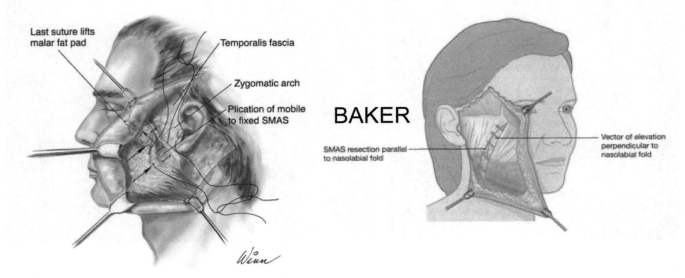

Plication of SMAS

Last suture lifts
malar fat pad

Temporalis fascia

Zygomatic arch

Plication of mobile
to fixed SMAS

BAKER

SMAS resection parallel
to nasolabial fold

Vector of elevation
perpendicular to
nasolabial fold

Figure 23.5. Superficial musculoaponeurotic system (SMAS) plication and lateral SMASectomy.

12. Prominent, ptotic, submaxillary glands

13. Ptotic, hypertrophied, anterior belly of the digastric muscles

Volumetric loss of soft tissue (fat atrophy) in one or more fat compartments is a frequent finding in the aging face. Loss of soft tissue volume will often require augmentation with fat grafting, nonautologous fillers, or facial implants in addition to deep layer (SMAS) advancement and support of the anterior cheek.

Most patients require a direct approach to the age-related changes in their neck depending on the anatomical findings.

INDICATIONS

Facelifting is indicated in patients who show laxity of the facial skin, jowl formation, and laxity along the jawline and the neck with varying degrees of muscle banding and flaccidity in the midline, as well as excessive fat in various compartments of the

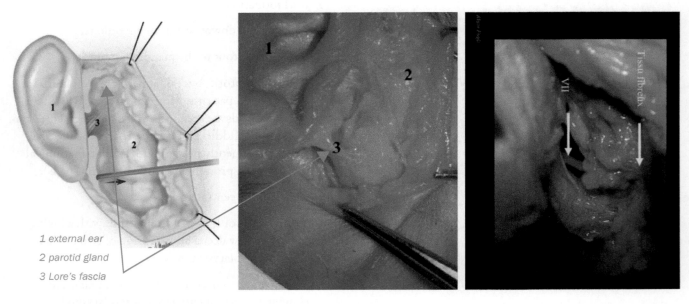

1 external ear
2 parotid gland
3 Lore's fascia

Figure 23.6. Anatomy. The facial nerve emerges at a very deep position anterior to this structure. Lore's fascia is situated approximately 0.7–1 cm beneath the skin surface, whereas the trunk of the facial nerve is situated in 2.5 cm beneath this skin.

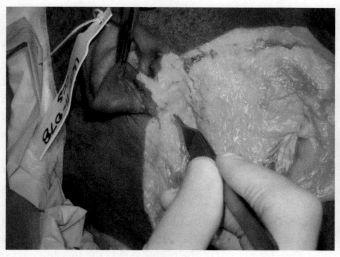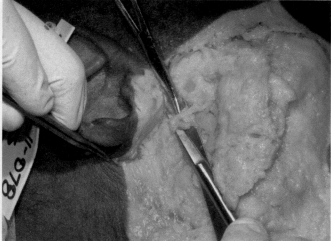

Figure 23.7. Lore's fascia and facial nerve.

central neck. Ptotic soft tissues of the midface are not corrected by skin-only facelifts. Skin-only facelifts rarely achieve long-lasting results and can result in unfavorable scarring when skin tension is used to tighten a face that demonstrates laxity. Young patients rarely achieve long-lasting improvement without some manipulation of the SMAS, and a less invasive SMAS procedure such as a SMAS plication, lateral SMAS-ectomy or a MACS lift will produce a longer-lasting result. Secondary cases and older patients with lax skin and minimal deep tissue laxity as well can obtain improvement with skin lifts if previous sessions included manipulation of the SMAS. Facelifting with manipulation of the SMAS can effectively improve jowling and laxity along the mandibular border as well as reposition the posterior cheek. Modest improvement in the nasolabial fold can be achieved with SMAS manipulation, and alternative treatments may be useful including, but not limited to autologous or nonautologous injections of fillers and subcision release of the crease with simultaneous injection of fillers. Patients who have minimal submental laxity, little subcutaneous fat, and short or absent platysmal bands can often be managed with closed liposuction of the neck without the need for opening the central neck except for a 4 mm stab incision used for access for liposuction. Ptotic and or hypertrophied submaxillary glands can be repositioned with tension applied laterally but often reoccur if not well supported or partially resected.

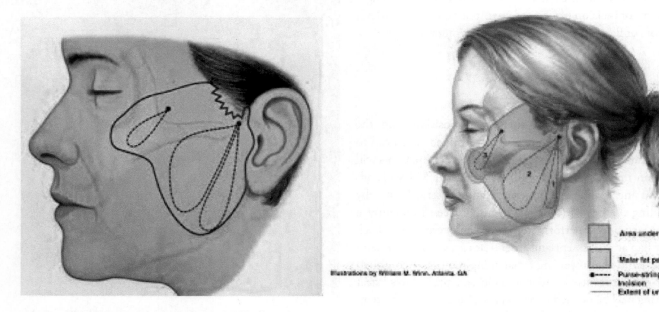

Illustrations by William M. Winn, Atlanta, GA

Area undermined
Malar fat pad
Purse-string suture
Incision
Extent of undermining

Figure 23.8. Minimal access cranial suspension (MACS) lift.

CONTRAINDICATIONS

There are relatively few absolute contraindications to performing a facelift. Those that are more common are:

Noncompensated/untreated cardiopulmonary disease

Uncontrolled hypertension

Systemic diseases; for example, currently being treated for cancer

Bleeding disorders

Conditions that require preoperative medical clearance include a history of cardiovascular disease (stents, bypass, angioplasty, etc.) including hypertension that is controlled. Patients who are smoking have an increased risk of delayed wound healing resulting in unfavorable scarring if they continue to smoke within 3 weeks of having the procedure performed. Patients who continue to smoke are warned of the possibility of problems with wound healing and that the procedures performed will be less aggressive due to the limited undermining that can be performed safely in smokers.

Unstable psychological and psychiatric conditions are a contraindication to having an elective cosmetic surgical procedure. Patients diagnosed with body dysmorphic syndrome (BDS) are unlikely to be satisfied with the results of a cosmetic surgical procedure and can become dangerous to themselves as well as to the surgical team.

All medications currently being taken need to be reviewed. These include aspirin, nonsteroidal antiinflammatory medications (NSAIDs) over-the-counter herbal and anti-aging medications, and large doses of vitamin E.

Patients who have had a prior facelift present challenges in terms of incision placement, manipulation of the SMAS, vectors of flap rotation, and hairline alignment.

PREOPERATIVE PLANNING

Patients are examined in the sitting position, and the planned vectors of correction are determined. The need to add facial fat grafting is individualized as many patients will have an impressive malar fullness when the SMAS is advanced and is anchored superiorly and posteriorly thereby avoiding the need to add fat. In heavy faces, frequently, a SMAS-ectomy is performed to avoid an overly thick cheek after flap advancement and inset. Clearly, we have come to understand that reversing facial aging requires a combination of vector-based and volume-based procedures.[16] Fat grafting may be needed in other areas, for example, the temporal hollows, infrabrow area, lower eyelids, deep anterior

cheek fat compartment, jawline, and perioral areas. These additional procedures are not described in this chapter.

Typically, a 5 cm transverse incision is marked posterior to the submental crease to allow better visualization of the platysma muscles and fat compartments unless only closed liposuction is required, in which case a 5 mm stab incision at or below the crease allows access for suction lipectomy to proceed in the central and lateral neck up to, but not across the jawline. The facelift incision follows the transverse temporal sideburn at the level of the ascending crus helix just within the lower most follicles and is beveled to preserve the follicles or vertically to allow the temporal hair to grow through the scar. The incision courses superiorly and then posteriorly to follow the curvature of the ascending helix. At the superior margin of the tragus, either the incision curves posteriorly to follow the anterior tragal edge, or, mainly in men with a deep pretragal rhytid, will follow the rhytid in front of the tragus. If the incision is made along the tragal edge, a right angle is drawn at the beginning of the tragus, the marking continues along the tragal edge, and then a second right angle is drawn at the lower margin of tragus and then follows the crease in front of the lobule. A 2 mm cuff of skin below the lobule is left on the tragus so that when the flap is inset, the lobule will not appear to be attached to the adjacent skin. The marking continues in the retroauricular sulcus, and, importantly, follows the inverted U-shaped skin onto the concha. In the short scar approach, which is utilized in patients who are younger and have very little work to be done in their neck, the incision ends a short distance behind the lobule following the retroauricular sulcus (Figure 23.9).

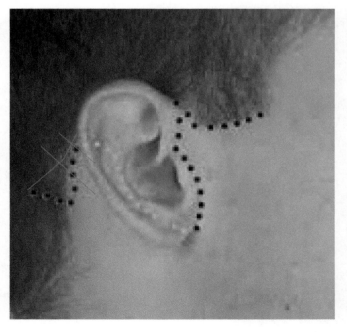

Figure 23.9. Short scar incision.

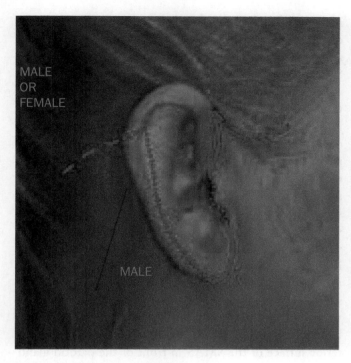

Figure 23.10. Full access facelift incision.

Following this curved line avoids having a vertical scar behind the ear which may become hypertrophic. The incision continues in the sulcus superiorly until the touch point where the helix would touch the scalp. At this point, the incision courses over the hairless skin of the mastoid area and follows the hair transversely in women. In men, the marking follows the lower most hairline because, typically, more skin is advanced in men, which would be raised if the incision was made in the scalp at the same level as is used in females, and, because men do not wear their hair pulled upward, the scar is not visible if the skin is closed carefully without tension. The length of the occipital incision depends upon how low the work has to be performed in the neck (Figure 23.10).

ANESTHESIA, ROOM SETUP, AND INSTRUMENTATION

Many patients can undergo a facelift under oral sedation, oral analgesia, and local anesthesia without the need for intravenous medications or general anesthesia. However, choices are given and include monitored intravenous sedation or general anesthesia with an endotracheal tube in place. Not having an endotracheal tube in place is a welcome benefit of performing these procedures under local anesthesia. Patients with comorbid conditions may require more intense intra- and postop monitoring with

the assistance of a certified registered nurse anesthetist (CRNA) or an anesthesiologist. Patients are given oral or IV antibiotics and steroids preoperatively, which are continued for 5–6 days postoperatively along with oral analgesics and sedatives as needed. Essential monitoring of vital signs is provided throughout the procedure including blood pressure, pulse, and pulse oximetry. A monitor with the capacity for providing a running electrocardiogram (EKG) should be available but is not used routinely. Good overhead and head-mounted lighting is essential. In the alternative, overhead lighting can be supplemented with a lighted fiber-optic retractor.

A standard basic plastic surgery head and neck tray of instruments should be provided. The following instruments should also be available:

4- and 5-prong Freeman Facelift Retractors

Narrow and wide 2-prong skin hooks

Long and short pickups (Adson-Brown)

Short single-tooth Brown pickups

Short and long needle holders, including a Webster flat short needle holder

Short and long straight and curved facelift scissors

Suture scissors

Straight and curved iris scissors

Allis-Adair intestinal clamps (wide Allis Clamps) for grasping the SMAS

4 or 5 mm flat, spatula-type, single-hole suction cannula (with one hole only on the undersurface)

3-0 Vicryl, 3-0 PDS, 5-0 Monocryl, 4-0, 5-0,6-0 Prolene (Ethicon, Summerville, NJ)

Cotton balls dipped in Povidine iodine solution for protecting the ear canals

Skin stapler

½-inch Steri-Strips (3M, Minnesota)

4 × 4 gauze pads

10 mm French silicone suction drains with fluid collection bulbs

Circumferential cotton rolls

4-inch Coban or Ace bandages

Surgipads (ABD pads)

Sterile saline for moistening the gauze pads and Surgipads

1-inch tape

Additional require equipment includes:

Unipolar and bipolar electrocautery unit with short and long flat blades

Grounding pads

Suction machine with disposable tubing and Yankauer suction tips

SURGICAL TECHNIQUE

If performed under oral sedation and analgesia only, the procedure begins with the infiltration of buffered local anesthesia utilizing both 1% and ½% lidocaine with epinephrine, injecting the greater auricular nerve and injecting along the planned incision lines with buffered 1% lidocaine with adrenalin on 27-gauge needles, followed by injections of buffered ½% lidocaine with adrenalin through 22-gauge spinal needles. The concentration of adrenalin is diluted 1:1 with lidocaine without adrenalin in hypertensive patients or those who become hypertensive after the first injections. A submental stab wound incision is made and subcutaneous dissection continues for a few millimeters followed by closed liposuction with a flat, single hole, 4 or 5 mm suction cannula. If the platysma muscle is to be manipulated, the incision is made horizontally for 2.5 cm on either side of the midline (a total length of 5 cm) and subcutaneous dissection continues as far inferiorly as the inferior extent of the bands. The platysma muscles may require additional defatting anteriorly or posteriorly depending on the amount and the location of the fat. The platysma muscles are sutured in the midline with a running or interrupted 3-0 PDS suture followed by interrupted 4-0 nylon sutures staggered at the points of maximal tension. If the platysmal bands are long, they are back-cut for 2–3 cm inferiorly at the desired level of the cervico-mental angle.

Standard tragal edge or pretragal incisions (in patients who have a sharp tragus and well-defined pretragal wrinkle) are joined with a beveled temporal sideburn incision and either a short or a full postauricular incision with or without extension into the occipital hairline as determined by the amount of work to be done on the neck. The cheek dissection proceeds anteriorly subcutaneously to within 2 cm of the nasolabial fold (less anterior dissection

in smokers) and inferiorly to below the angle of the mandible. The length of the inferior dissection depends on the amount of laxity and correction desired in the upper neck. Subcutaneous dissection horizontally along the border of the mandible allows complete release of the mandibular ligament with improvement of the appearance of the jowl. At this point, after obtaining pinpoint hemostasis, a decision is made as to how to manage the SMAS. Young patients and older patients with minimal jowling and anterior cheek laxity can be managed with a plication of the mobile to the nonmobile SMAS using interrupted or running 3-0 Vicryl or 3-0 PDS sutures, a MACS lift (purse string plication of the SMAS), or a lateral SMAS-ectomy, which is marked as an ellipse or as a triangle with the base inferiorly. Patients with midface ptosis and more prominent nasolabial folds and creases are better corrected with sub-SMAS/deep plane techniques. Care must be taken when performing a lateral SMAS-ectomy to not transect branches of the facial nerve which may be close to the posterior surface of the SMAS in front of the parotid gland or adherent to the posterior surface of the SMAS resulting from a prior facelift procedure. A key step to ensure a safe dissection is hydrodissection and a bloodless field. In a patient who is having this procedure under oral sedation and local anesthesia, the flap is injected with, on average, 10 cc of buffered ½% lidocaine with adrenalin. If the patient is under intravenous sedation or under general anesthesia, normal saline can be injected to hydrodissect the flap. Hydrodissection provides an important safeguard as it separates the deep cervical fascia from the SMAS flap, thereby protecting the branches of the facial nerve. Anchoring the SMAS flap to Lore's fascia inferiorly and to the fixed SMAS in the temporal area followed by linear suturing in the preauricular area again to the fixed SMAS over the parotid gland ensures a firm foundation and advancement of the ptotic posterior cheek and jawline soft tissues. Additional sutures are placed along the posterior jawline and subjaw to further tighten the jawline, bringing the SMAS and the platysma fascia to the nonmobile postauricular/mastoid fascia. Open small-cannula liposuction can improve the appearance of the jawline before the skin flap is rotated into position. The entire under-flap surface is irrigated with dilute Povidine iodine solution, and hemostasis is again checked before skin closure. Skin flap inset, excision of excess skin, and closure without tension are performed without tension except for two areas. Tension sutures of 4-0 Prolene or nylon are only placed at the temporal sideburn in front of the ascending helix and the high point in the occipital incision. If a short-scar facelift is planned, the skin flap rotation will be more vertically

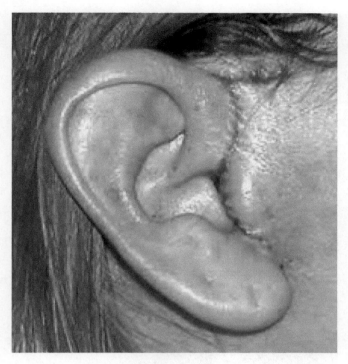

Figure 23.11. Final closure appearance.

oriented and only one tension suture is required at the temporal sideburn directly in front of the ascending helix. The preauricular and submental incisions are closed with running 5-0 Prolene or rapid absorbing sutures (Figure 23.11) The retroauricular incision is closed with 4-0 plain catgut, 4-0 rapid Vicryl, or 5-0 Prolene or nylon. The temporal and occipital incisions are closed with skin staples. Drains are inserted for 48 hours. Saline moist and dry 4 × 4 gauze pads gently embrace the ear followed by a soft cotton roll, Surgipads (one moist and one dry) under the chin, and a circumferential wrap of 4-inch Coban or a 4-inch Ace bandage and tape complete the dressing.

POSTOPERATIVE MANAGEMENT

Most patients are discharged to the care of a responsible adult and do not need to stay in an overnight facility. Older patients, those with comorbid conditions, and those who have undergone several procedures in addition to the facelift may require and/or desire to stay in an overnight facility with monitoring. Intermittent cold compresses are helpful in diminishing swelling and discomfort and may diminish ecchymosis. Patients are seen the following day for a dressing change, at 48 hours for the second dressing change and drain removal, at 1 week, 4–6 weeks, 3 months, 6 months, and at 1 year postoperatively. A supportive dressing is worn for 5–7 days depending on the procedures that were performed on the neck. Patients require oral analgesics for a few days, oral antibiotics for 5–6 days, decreasing doses of Prednisone (Prednisone Dosepak), and a liquid diet then a soft diet for the first few days. Sutures and skin staples are removed at 1 week. The tension sutures are removed at 10–14 days postoperatively.

SEQUELAE AND COMPLICATIONS

Commons sequelae are swelling, bruising, and sensory deficits (due to transecting of the sensory nerves resulting from flap elevation). Unfavorable scarring can occur from excessive tension on the skin, history of smoking, sundamaged skin, and a history of hypertrophic scarring.

Small hematomas can be managed with expression through the suture line or by aspiration and irrigation without the need for a return to the operating room. Large and/or expanding hematomas require urgent exploration to minimize the possibility of impaired circulation in the flaps, which may result in delayed healing and unfavorable scarring. Expanding hematomas in the neck can, when rapidly expanding, apply pressure to the trachea causing lateral movement and airway impairment. If a rapidly expanding hematoma is identified, the sutures should be immediately released and the blood evacuated at the bedside to relieve the pressure on the skin flaps.

Unfavorable scarring, relapse, and/or dissatisfaction due to undercorrection or related to genetic or environmental causes can be corrected, if possible and is warranted, no sooner than 6 months and preferable 12 months postoperatively, when the tissues have softened and the dissection would be somewhat easier to perform.

CONCLUSION

A wide variety of approaches to performing a face and necklift and manipulating the SMAS have as their common goal a harmonious rejuvenation of the aging face, improving the nasolabial folds, smoothing the lax anterior cheek, and addressing the jowls and neck. Each procedure has its proponent(s) and can reliably produce impressive facial rejuvenation. Each patient should be evaluated carefully, and the procedure that is most likely to result in a happy patient and surgeon should be selected. Frequently, this is a less aggressive safe solution which is most likely to obtain a pleasing face and neck rejuvenation.

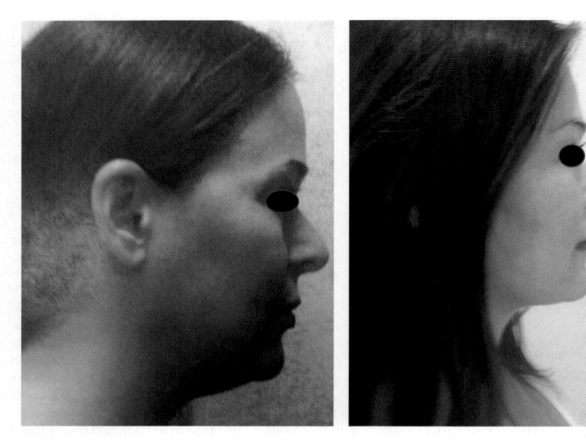

Figure 23.12. Pre and post op temporal browlift, face and necklift.

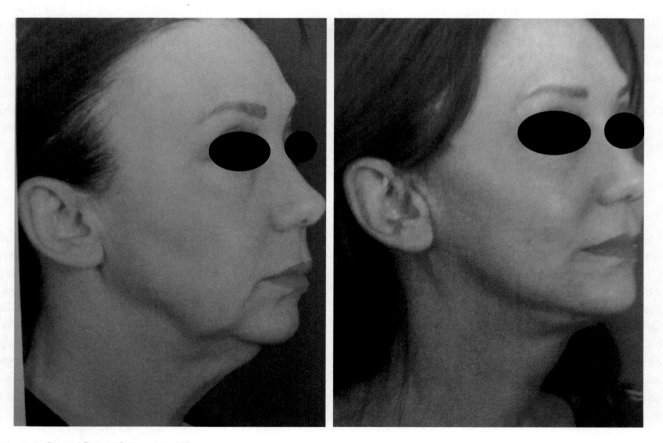

Figure 23.13. Pre and Post op face and necklift.

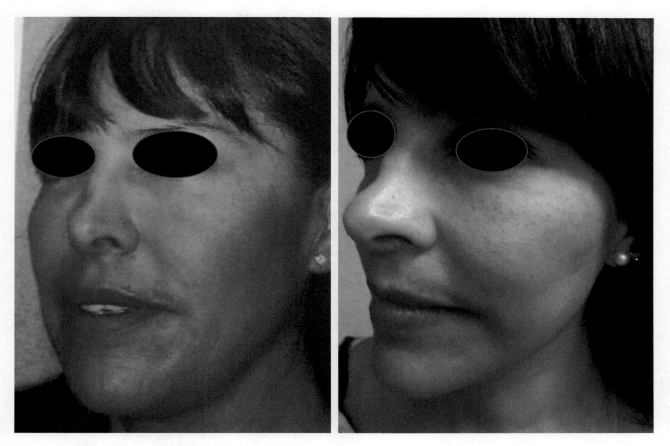

Figure 23.13. Continued.

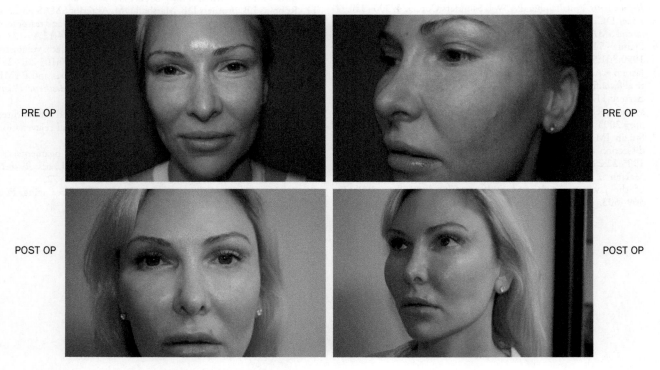

PRE OP

PRE OP

POST OP

POST OP

Figure 23.14. Pre and Post op face and necklift and facial fat grafting.

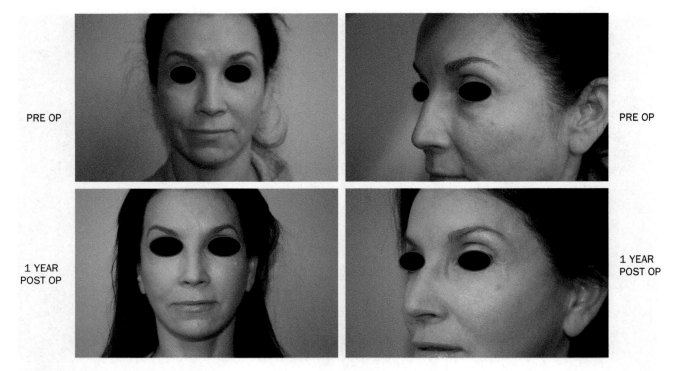

PRE OP

PRE OP

1 YEAR
POST OP

1 YEAR
POST OP

Figure 23.15. Pre and post op face and necklift.

REFERENCES

1. Mitz V, Peyronie M. The superficial aponeurotic system (SMAS) in the parotid and cheek area. *Plast Reconstr Surg* 1976;58:80–88.
2. Skoog TG. The aging face. In: *Plastic Surgery: New Methods and Refinements*. Philadelphia, PA: WB Saunders Co; 1974: 300–330
3. Baker DC. Minimal incision rhytidectomy (short scar face lift) with lateral SMASectomy. *Aesthet Surg J* 2001;21:68–79.
4. Hamra ST. The deep-plane rhytidectomy. *Plast Reconstr Surg* 1990;861:53–61.
5. Jacono AA, Parikh SS. The minimal access deep plane extended vertical facelift. *Aesthet Surg J* 2011;318:874–890.
6. Barton FE Jr., Hunt J. The high-superficial musculoaponeurotic system technique in facial rejuvenation: an update. *Plast Reconstr Surg* 2003;112:1910–1917.
7. Stuzin JM, Baker TJ, Gordon HL, Baker TM. Extended SMAS dissection as an approach to midface rejuvenation. *Clin Plast Surg* 1995;22:295–311.
8. Marten TJ. High SMAS facelift: combined single flap lifting of the jawline, cheek, and midface. *Clin Plast Surg* 2008;35: 569–603.
9. Labbé D, Franco RG, Nicolas J. Platysma suspension and platysmaplasty during neck lift: anatomical study and analysis of 30 cases. *Plast Reconstr Surg* 2006;117:2001–2007.
10. Tonnard P, Verpaele A, Monstrey S, Van Landuyt K, Blondeel P, Hamdi M, Matton G Minimal access cranial suspension lift: a modified S-lift. *Plast Reconstr Surg* 2002;1096:2074–2086.
11. Robbins LB, Brothers DB, Marshall DM. Anterior SMAS plication for the treatment of prominent nasomandibular folds and restoration of normal cheek contour. *Plast Reconstr Surg* 1995;96:1279–1287.
12. Little JW. Three-dimensional rejuvenation of the midface: volumetric resculpture by malar imbrication. *Plas Reconstr Surg* 2000;105:267–285.
13. Aston SJ, Walden JL, Facelift with SMAS techniques and FAME. In: Aston SJ, Steinbrech DS, Walden, JL, eds., *Aesthetic Plastic Surgery*. London: Saunders Elsevier, 2009:73–86.
14. Ramirez OM, Maillard GF, Musolas A. The extended subperiosteal face lift: a definitive soft-tissue remodeling for facial rejuvenation. *Plast Reconstr Surg* 1991;88:227–236.
15. Mendelson BC. Facelift anatomy, SMAS, retaining ligaments, and facial spaces, In: Aston SJ, Steinbrech DS, Walden JL, eds. *Aesthetic Plastic Surgery*. London: Saunders Elsevier, 2009:53–72.
16. Lambros V. Observations on periorbital and midface aging. *Plast Reconstr Surg* 2007;1205:1367–1376.

24

BROWLIFT

Mark E. Krugman

INTRODUCTION

The brow "frames" the face. Probably no facial feature conveys mood and expression as significantly as the brows.

Although there are many factors that influence brow aesthetics,[1] such as other facial features, gender, culture, ethnicity and fashion, there is no "ideal" shape or position that fits everyone. Westmore,[1] an award-winning Hollywood makeup artist, described the arch of the brow peaking on a line tangent with the lateral limbus of the pupil. More recent literature places the brow peak lateral to the lateral limbus.[2]

Paul,[3] in a historical treatise of the evolution of the browlift, attributes the earliest description to Passot in 1919. A series of horizontal ellipses at the forehead were created to elevate the brow.

In the past 20 years, there have been a number of new procedures developed as well as variations on existing procedures and techniques to alter the brow. In this chapter, I will describe two techniques in depth, the coronal and endoscopic lifts. Other methods will be summarized with annotated references for the reader who wishes to explore further Figure 24.1.

NONSURGICAL BROWLIFT

The depressors of the brow are the orbicularis oculi, procerus, and corrugator supercilii. By blocking these muscles with botulism toxin (BoNT-A), the elevator (frontalis) becomes unopposed.[4] Because of the diffusion of the neuromodulator, the depth of injection is not significant.

TRANS-BLEPHAROPLASTY APPROACHES

The depressor muscles of the brow are accessible via a trans-blepharoplasty approach. Ramirez[5] states that this procedure is indicated in patients with male pattern baldness, high foreheads, or hair transplants, and in those who require a blepharoplasty and a browlift. Variations on the trans-blepharoplasty forehead lift are described by Paul,[6] Knice,[7] and Langston.[8] Langston utilizes the absorbable Endotine fixation device (Coajet Systems, Palo Alto, CA) which usually dissolves by 3 months.

BROW-PEXY, TRANSFOREHEAD, LATERAL BROW, AND HAIRLINE (PRE-TRICHIAL) APPROACHES

The brow-pexy or direct browlift is the most powerful of the lifts as it is the closest to the excision of the brow itself. One centimeter of excision equals 1 cm of lift. An elliptical variation of skin is removed from the super brow area (Figure 24.1). It is generally not utilized in cosmetic patients because of the visible scar. It has a place in extremely asymmetrical brow conditions, often associated with unilateral facial paralysis.

The transforehead lift (Figure 24.1) is another method that may have applications in select conditions. The ideal candidate for this procedure would be a bald man with significant brow ptosis and heavy forehead rhytids. After the incision in the deep forehead wrinkle, the procedure proceeds similarly to the lower portion of the coronal lift, which will be described later.

Mahmood and Baker[9] describe a lateral subcutaneous browlift using an updated technique which is focused on patients presenting with lateral brow descent. The technique utilizes shorter temporal incisions and less dissection than a conventional coronal browlift.

The hairline or pre-trichial lift (Figure 24.1) is especially indicated in individuals with brow ptosis and high hairlines. Once the incision is made, the remainder of the

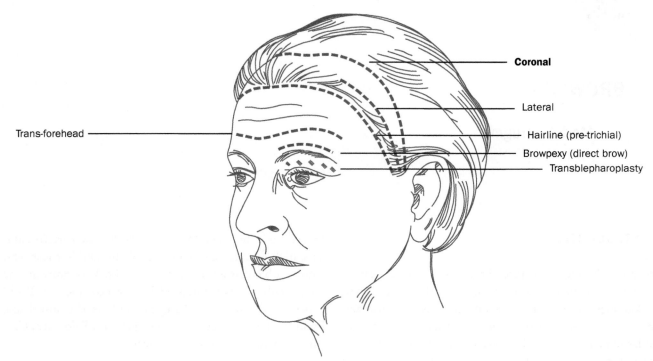

Figure 24.1. Placement of nonendoscopic incisions.

procedure may be carried out similar to a coronal lift. The pre-trichial incision may also be used to lower the hairline by undermining and advancing the scalp and excising superior forehead tissue. This is sometimes referred to as a "reverse" browlift.

Another anterior hairline procedure is described by Pollock and Pollock,[10] The dissection is in the subcutaneous plane. Progressive tension sutures are utilized that provide accurate fixation and eliminate dead space.

BICORONAL BROWLIFT

ASSESSMENT

The bicoronal browlift has been the traditional "work horse" for browlifting. The long incision (Figure 24.1), with its possibilities of hair loss, have led to the creation of the techniques we have previously discussed, as well as the endoscopic browlift, which will be detailed later.

The most important factor in assessing the patient for this procedure is a thorough discussion with the patient about the details of the procedure, including complications, incision placement, and alternative techniques.

EXAMINATION

In considering a bicoronal forehead lift, the patient's hair and hairline are of paramount importance. The patient's preference for hair style must be considered. There must be ample frontal hair (at least 5 cm of hair from the most anterior projecting point). If there is temporal recession, the incision may be modified so that the central bicoronal portion is combined with the lateral or temporal incisions.

The bicoronal incision is at such a distance from the brow that for every 3–4 cm of pull, 1 cm of brow elevation may be expected. Recall that in the brow-pexy or direct browlift the ratio is 1:1.

It is important to assess the amount of brow ptosis as well as blepharochalasis. The classic teaching is that a woman's normal brow position is 1 cm above the supraorbital ridge and for men it is at the supraorbital ridge.

Brow styles are constantly changing and should be part of a thorough patient discussion in front of a mirror or with imaging software before finalizing the approach.

One method of determining the extent of blepharochalasis consists of elevating the brow while simultaneously pinching the eyelid skin. If it is planned to do a simultaneous blepharoplasty, this method is also used to do preoperative markings.

The most accurate way of doing a browlift and blepharoplasty is staging. The browlift must always be done first to prevent an overresection of eyelid skin. The eyelid then can be done after the postoperative brow position has settled, usually in 3 months postoperative. If the staged method is planned, the patient must be agreeable and know the costs in advance. One employed technique is to do the upper eyelid blepharoplasty in 3–6 months following the browlift under local anesthesia with sedation and not charge a surgeon's fee.

Specific contraindications to the coronal browlift are the potential for hairline recession from pattern baldness or a high forehead. The patient must be made aware of and agreeable to hairline elevators, which results in an increased vertical forehead height. Changes in hairstyles must be considered and discussed with the patient. Today, for example, many men and some women have chosen to wear their hair short. If this is a future possibility, other approaches should be considered.

PREOPERATIVE CONSIDERATIONS

The patient is instructed to stop aspirin 3 weeks prior and nonsteroidal antiinflammatories (NSAIDs) 2 weeks prior to surgery. Hair washing with a baby shampoo should be carried out the night before and the morning of surgery. The placement of incisions should be determined prior to the day of surgery.

The patient should be marked in an upright position prior to receiving any sedation. The surgeon should mark the anterior hairline, transverse furrows, glabella frown lines, transverse wrinkles at the nasal root, "bunny" lines, the upper eyelid skin to be resected, and, finally, the proposed incision.

ANESTHESIA

The choice of anesthesia depends on the comfort level of the surgeon in accordance with the patient's concurrence. The options are general anesthesia, either endotracheal or with a laryngeal mask airway (LMA) or monitored anesthesia control (MAC) with intravenous sedation. A preoperative intravenous antibiotic is given. Dexamethasone (Decadron) 10 mg and ondansetron (Zofran) are helpful in reducing postoperative swelling and nausea. Corneal shields and eye lubricant are important.

OPERATIVE TECHNIQUE

A neurological horseshoe support is ideal. Alternatively, a surgical "donut" will suffice. The surgeon is seated at the head of the table with a headlight.

Hair control is a major issue in scalp surgery. Traditionally, a small amount of hair is shaved along the incision line. Many surgeons, including this writer, have moved away from shaving hair and do hair control with multiple small sterile rubber bands and keeping the hair moist during the procedure.

Prior to applying the rubber bands, the hair is washed with a "face safe" prep, such as PHisoHex, and rinsed with sterile water. The incision, anterior scalp, and forehead are infiltrated with 1% lidocaine (Xylocaine) with 1:100,000 epinephrine. Many, including the writer, prefer to inject prior to the prep to allow at least 10 minutes for the epinephrine to have its full vasoconstrictive effect.

INCISION

Respecting the angulation of the hair shafts and follicles, a no. 10 scalpel blade is angulated accordingly. The scalp is well vascularized and will bleed even with epinephrine. It is important to avoid the temptation to cauterize the scalp. Raney clips are very useful, and a bipolar cautery should be used with care on the underlying galeal vessels (Figure 24.2).

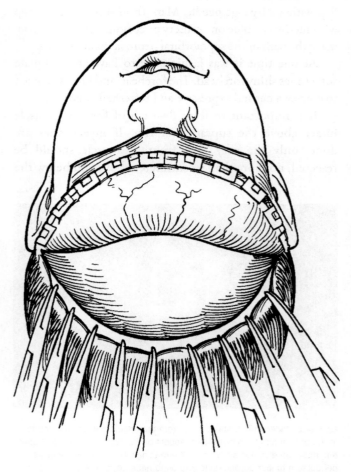

Figure 24.2. Turn down of forehead flap. Raney clips are useful in achieving hemostasis. Note corneal protection.

UNDERMINING

Before undermining, check the corneal protection and place a moist towel over the orbital areas. The dissection should proceed in a subgaleal plane to approximately 4 cm from the supraorbital ridge. At this point, an incision is made through the periosteum from the lateral aspect of one supraorbital ridge to the other.

The subperiosteal dissection proceeds with a wide periosteal elevator such as a 17 mm Langenbeck. Elevation continues to just beyond the ridge and onto the nose beyond the radix (Figure 24.3). In the subperiosteal plane, the supraorbital bundle is more easily visualized and the brow release is more effective.

TRANSLATION OF MARKINGS

In order to perform targeted myotomies or myectomies, it is necessary to translate the external markings internally.

The flap which has been kept folded over the eyes and upper nose is then flipped back into its normal position. The external forehead crease is translated to the underside of the flap with a 21-gauge needle. Mark from superficial to deep with methylene blue or a cautery or coagulation mode. Also, mark the path of the supraorbital neurovascular bundles.

At one time it was fashionable to have an inanimate sometimes shiny forehead. The forehead and brows *do* need to convey a natural expressive and refreshed appearance.

It is important to leave 3–4 cm of forehead muscle intact above the supraorbital rim. If myectomies are done, only the very thin frontalis muscle should be resected, no more than a centimeter above and below the

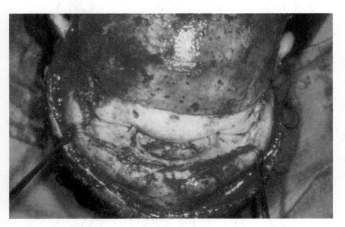

Figure 24.3. Undermining. About 4 cm from the ridge, an incision is made in the periosteum from one lateral aspect of the ridge to the other. Using a periosteum elevator, such as a 17 mm Langenbeck elevator, elevate periosteum to just beyond ridge and on to nose beyond radix.

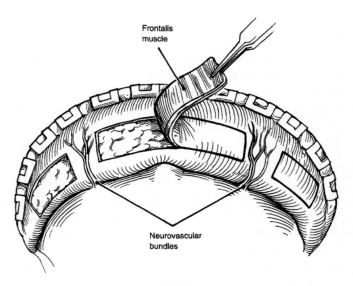

Figure 24.4. After identification of neurovascular bundles, remove thin strip of frontalis muscle. Alternatively, myotomies may be done.

blue marked lines. No more than three or four strips of frontalis should be resected (Figure 24.4). Alternatively, myotomies, a more conservative approach, may be done without removing muscle. Careful incision with cautery is made through galea, and the muscle is teased with a sharp elevator.

The corrugator and procerus muscles may be located in the same fashion and dissected out with a small hemostat. A small amount of the origins of the muscles may be resected or, more conservatively, a myotomy may be done.

SETTING THE TENSION

The scalp should be placed in its anatomical position. Grasp the scalp edges on a line drawn from the lateral limbus of each eye using a D'Assumpcão clamp or other similar device (Figure 24.5). Have an assistant help as the brow position is elevated to 1–1.5 cm above its desired level. Using a no. 11 blade, make three incisions (while maintaining tension on the clamps) lateral to the clamps and in the midline. These three points are then anchored with heavy nylon or Prolene sutures. The excess is then tailored between the tension sutures. Excisions should parallel the direction of the hair shafts and follicles.

CLOSURE

The galea is closed with interrupted Monocryl sutures and the skin edges closed with a running Prolene suture.

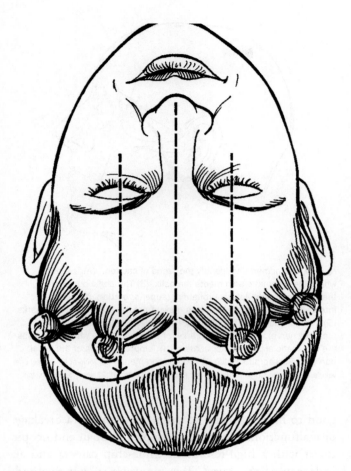

Figure 24.5. Three key sutures: one at midline and two at pupil level.

The hair is again washed with sterile water before the dressing is applied.

A nonadherent dressing, such as Xeroform, is applied, covered by fluffs and Kerlix. A mildly compressive elastic bandage wrap is placed.

POSTOPERATIVE COURSE

The patient is discharged on pain medication and advised to take stool softener, along with the pain medication. A prescription for oral disintegrating ondansetron (ODT) is also given.

The patient is seen either the following day or in 2 days, and the dressing is removed. One of our staff washes out the patient's hair. A hair washing sink in the office is a very useful accessory for facial and scalp surgery.

The patient may then shower, but shouldn't use a hot blow dryer or curlers for at least a month. Chemicals such as hair coloring should be avoided for 6 weeks. The sutures are removed in 1 week.

ENDOSCOPIC BROWLIFTS

The introduction of the surgical endoscope was welcomed by surgeons of every discipline. Plastic surgeons were no exception. The long, traditional bicoronal brow incision resulted in a number of patient complaints,[11] such as numbness behind the incision and hair loss. The endoscopic approach allows the browlift to be performed through smaller incisions, reducing a number of problems that were seen in open procedures.

Two of the pioneers in endoscopic browlift were Ramirez[12] and Isse.[13] The plane was moved from subgaleal to subperiosteal, and the incisions were greatly reduced in size. In addition to being innovators, both of these surgeons were exemplary teachers, not only publishing their techniques, but giving courses and workshops.

ASSESSMENT

Evaluation for the endoscopic browlift is not unlike the earlier described open browlift.

It is important for patients to express their dissatisfaction with their brows and forehead. Which part of the brow are they unhappy with? With the surgeon manually elevating the brows, the patient can reply interactively, and, as in the open browlift, the need for the upper eyelid surgery becomes apparent. The patient should also frown to reveal the activity of the corrugators and procerus, both strong brow depressors, as well as the glabella furrows. Looking up reveals the frontal lines. Balding patients and those with excessively high foreheads will not be candidates for the classic incisions. Some innovative incisions for this category are described by Fisher and Zamboni.[14]

As in the open approach, upper eyelid surgery may be combined with the browlift or staged. The writer prefers to do the upper eyelids as a second procedure in 3–6 months from the time of the browlift. The upper blepharoplasty is done under local anesthesia with sedation. There is no surgeon's fee charged within the 3- to 6-month time frame. The patient is given the costs when quoted for the browlift.

MARKINGS

The temporal crest ligament is an important landmark in this procedure as there are different levels of dissection on each side. Fortunately, the temporal crest is readily palpable and should be marked before the incisions (Figure 24.6).

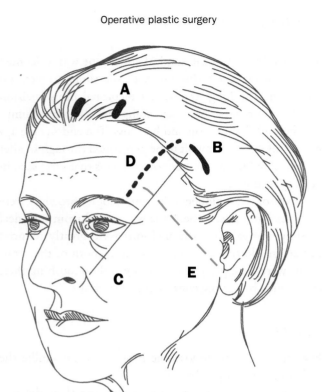

Figure 24.6. Incisions and landmarks for endoscopic brow lift (see text).

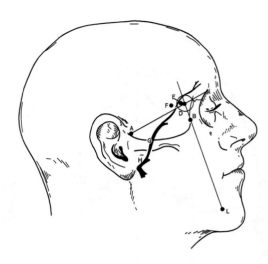

Figure 24.7. Landmarks to identify the "zone of caution." (A) The point where the zygomatic arch meets the helix. (B) The angle between the zygoma and the lateral orbital rim (superior border). (C) Point of intersection between the two lines drawn from the anatomical landmarks. (D) Zone of caution. (E) Sentinel vein. (F) Zygomaticotemporal nerve (sensory nerve). (G) Temporal branch of the facial nerve where it crosses the zygomatic arch (superior border). (H) Temporal branch of the facial nerve. (I) Supraorbital notch. (L) Mental foramen. From Trinei et al. The sentinel vein: surgery in the temporal region. Plast Recon Surg 1998;101:27, used by permission.

There are five incisions made a few millimeters behind the hairline. In the midline is a 1–1 1/2 cm sagittal incision. Five centimeters lateral to the sagittal are right and left parasagittal incisions. These 1.5 cm incisions are roughly on a line tangential to the lateral limbus. They are also a few millimeters behind the hairline. The temporal incisions are coronal, measuring 2–2.5 cm. They are located lateral to the temporal crest and on a line drawn from the ala crease passing through the lateral brow (Figure 24.6).

The muscle activity may be marked as described in the open technique.

The trajectory of the temporal branch of the facial nerve is also marked (Figure 24.6). It is approximately on a line drawn from the lower part of tragus passing about 1.5 cm lateral to the lateral brow and 2 cm above the brow. A detailed description of the nerve and sentinel vein anatomy is described by Trinei (Figure 24.7).[15]

INSTRUMENTATION AND ROOM SETUP

Specialized instrumentation is required for the endoscopic browlift. A 4 or 5 mm rigid 30-degree endoscope is used. The scope is outfitted with a blunt cobra tip. It is

good to have a backup scope in the event of a breakage or malfunction. The scope is coupled with an endoscopic tower with a high-resolution triple-chip camera and an endoscopic light source. Two monitors are not required, but minimize movement of the surgeon and also serve as a backup (Figure 24.8).

Videorecorder and printer are not required, but are helpful in teaching settings and for documentation.

Endoscopic elevators as pictured (Figure 24.9) are necessary. In addition, insulated endoscopic forceps and endoscopic scissors specifically designed for this procedure greatly facilitate the operation.

Our preference for the performance of an endoscopic browlift is general anesthesia. MAC sedation with local is an option depending on preference of the surgeon and anesthesiologist.

The patient who has shampooed the evening prior and the morning of surgery is prepped by washing out the hair with a face-safe prep such as PHisoHex, along with sterile water. The hair is rubber-banded around the incision using sterile bands. Lidocaine (Xylocaine) 0.5% with epinephrine 1:2,000 is injected from 2 cm behind the incisions to the superior orbital and upper lateral orbital rims. Ten to fifteen minutes is allowed to pass between injection and incision time. Injecting prior to prepping and draping is an efficient way of optimizing the anesthesia effect.

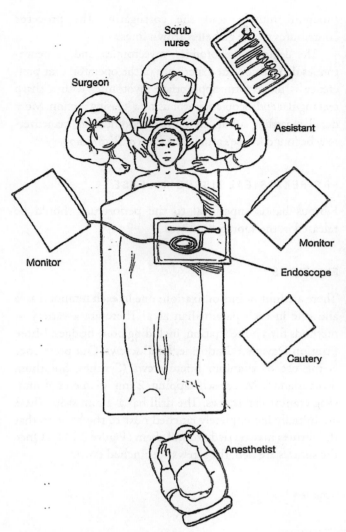

Figure 24.8. Schematic of operating room setup for endoscopic facial procedures. Redrawn from Ramierez OM, Daniel RK. *Endoscopic Aesthetic Surgery. A Video Manual.* New York: Springer-Verlag, 1995:26, fig 3.

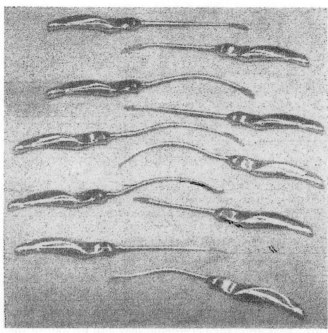

Figure 24.9. Endoscopic instrumentation-specific elevators designed for endoscopic facial procedures.

INCISIONS AND BLIND UNDERMINING

The median and paramedian incisions are made parallel to the hair follicles down to bone. A periosteal elevator is used to undermine 2 cm behind the incisions superiorly to 3 cm above the superior orbital rim inferiorly, to the temporal crest laterally (Figure 24.10).

The temporal incisions are made through the temporoparietal fascia to the deep layer of temporal fascia. We find loupe magnification very helpful in starting this plane. The dissection will stop at least 1 cm above the trajectory of the temporal branch of the facial nerve (Figure 24.10).

The connection of the two planes must always proceed from lateral (temporal) to medial (subperiosteal) to avoid getting under the temporal muscle. The superior portion of the temporal crest ligament may be broken through blindly.

Operative plastic surgery

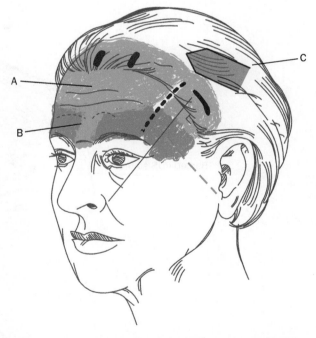

Figure 24.10. Incisions for endoscopic brow lift are shown. (A) "Blind" dissection. (B) endoscopic dissection. Dotted line is temporal crest ligament. Line from inferior tragus to 2 cm above brow represents trajectory of temporal branch of facial nerve. Arrow represents direction of dissection from lateral to medial.

ENDOSCOPIC DISSECTION

The dissection down to the superior orbital rims and medial to the temporal crest ligament continues in a subperiosteal plane with the endoscope. The most central portion of the subperiosteal dissection to the nasal bones may be done blindly as it is central to the neurovascular bundles. The temporal dissection continues down to the sentinel vein. The temporal crest ligament is taken down from lateral to medial with a sharp elevator and/or the endoscopic scissors.

PERIOSTEAL RELEASE

The periosteal release is done in the glabellar and supraorbital areas horizontally. Our preference is to use a sharp rectangular elevator and "tease" the periosteum until it separates. This helps protect the underlying neurovascular bundles. Others use the endoscopic scissors and a laser with a backstop. The periosteum may also be split in the midline. This is especially useful when asymmetries of brow level are present.

MUSCLE MODIFICATIONS

Recall that the principal depressors of the brow are the orbital portion of the orbicularis oculi, the depressor supercilii muscle, and the corrugator. The procerus contributes to the glabellar frown lines.

The degree of myotomies, myectomies, and/or neurotomies depends on the experience of the operator. Our preference is to perform appropriate myotomies with a sharp rectangular endoscopic elevator using a "teasing" action. More detail regarding advanced muscle modification maneuvers may be found in Isse's article in *Clinics of Plastic Surgery*.[13]

PRE-PERIOSTEAL TISSUE RELEASE

Fibrous bands superficial to the periosteum should be released in the supraorbital area.

FIXATIONS

There are four points of fixation; one in each temporal area and one in each paramedian area. There are a variety of methods for a bone fixation, including bone bridges, Mitek Fixation Devices,[16] Endotine,[17] and screws. Our preference is the use of titanium microscrews (Synthes, Solothum Switzerland). We use self-tapping, 2 mm diameter, 4 mm-long craniofacial screws. The drill has a 4 mm stop. These are initially incompletely cinched next to the bone so that the sutures may be tied around them (Figure 24.11). Once the sutures are tied, the screws are cinched down.

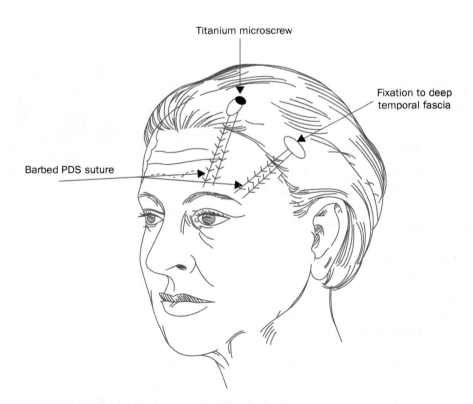

Titanium microscrew

Fixation to deep temporal fascia

Barbed PDS suture

Figure 24.11. Fixation using barbed polydioxanone (PDS) sutures and titanium micro screws.

We prefer barbed sutures of 3-0 polydioxanone (PDO) (Quill Surgical Specialties Corp., Braintree, MA). The barbed suture is threaded through the tissue and exits above the brow. They are mounted on long straight needles. Initially, when we used barbed sutures, we left them long, with the expectation of postoperatively tightening the brows by moving the tissue up on the barbs. We abandoned this maneuver as it was too uncomfortable for the patients. We soon went to cutting off the barbed suture at skin level, then "puckering" up the exit site, which lands the end of the suture under the surface. The major advantage of the barbed suture is that it distributes the points of fixation to multiple areas rather than a single one.

The temporal fixation places the suture to exit above the lateral brow with its superior fixation through the deep temporal fascia.

The incisions are closed with buried Monocryl and skin suture or micro staples.

Care must be taken when applying the light pressure dressing (similar to the open browlift) to avoid disturbing the suture fixation.

The use of micro-screws and PDO barbed sutures has minimized complications and extrusions, as well as providing for a durable fixation.

REFERENCES

1. Gunter JP, Antrobus SD. Aesthetic analysis of the eyebrows. *Plast Reconstr Surg* 1997;99:1808.

2. Bidros RS, Salazar-Reyes H, Friedman JD. Subcutaneous temporal browlift under local anesthesia: a useful technique for periorbital rejuvenation. *Aesthetic Surg J* 2010;30(6):783–788.

3. Paul MD. The evolution of the browlift in aesthetic plastic surgery. *Plast Reconstr Surg* 2001;108:1409.

4. Sneath J, Humphrey S, Carrothers A, Carrothers J. Injecting botulinum toxin at different depths is not effective for the correction of eyebrow asymmetry. *Dermatol Surg* 2015;41:582–587.

5. Ramirez OM. Transblepharoplasty forehead lift and upper face rejuvenation. *Ann Plast Surg* 1996;36:577–584.

6. Paul MD. Subperiosteal transblepharoplasty forehead lift. *Aesthetic Plast Surg* 1996;20:129.

7. Knize DM. Limited-incision forehead lift for eyebrow elevation to enhance upper blepharoplasty. *Plast Reconstr Surg* 1996;97:1334.

8. Langston PR, Williams GB, Rajon R, Metzinger SE. Transblepharoplasty brow suspension with a biodegradable fixation device. *Aesthetic Surg J* 2010;30(6);802–809.

9. Mahmood U, Baker Jr, JL. Lateral subcutaneous browlift updated technique. *Aesthetic Surg J* 2015;35(5):621–624.

10. Pollock H, Pollock TA. Subcutaneous browlift with precise suture fixation and advancement. *Aesthetic Surg J* 2007;27:388–395.

11. Ramirez OM. Anchor subperiosteal forehead lift: from open to endoscopic. *Plast Recontr Surg.* 1995;95:993.

12. Ramirez OM. Anchor subperiosteal forehead lift: from open to endoscopic. Follow-up to Ramierz, O.M. The anchor subperiosteal forehead lift. *Plast Reconstr Surg* 1995;95:993.

13. Isse NG. Endoscopic forehead lift evolution and update. *Clin Plast Surg* Oct 1995;32(4):661.

14. Fisher O, Zamboni WA. Endoscopic browlift in the male patient. *Arch Facial Plast Surg* 2010;12(1):56–59.

15. Trinei FA, Kiewicz J, Nahai F. The sentinel vein: an important reference point for surgery in the temporal region. *Plast Reconstr Surg* 1998;101:27.

16. Fiala TGS, Owsley JQ. Use of the Mitek fixation device in endoscopic browlifting. *Plast Recontr Surg* 1998;101:6.

17. Berkowitz RL, Jacobs DI, Gormon PJ. Brow fixation with the Endotine forehead device in endoscopic browlift. *Plast Reconstr Surg* 2005;116:1761.

25.

BLEPHAROPLASTY

Seanna R. Grob and D. J. John Park

The eyes are vital features that impart the characteristic appearance of a person's face. Dynamic in movement, the eyelids function in ocular protection and lubrication and are capable of expressing a wide range of emotions in nonverbal communication that transcends age, language, and culture. This is made all the more impressive because no two pairs of eyes are the same; in fact, no pair of eyes shares perfect symmetry (a fact that every patient should be reminded of preoperatively). Even among individuals of the same age group, heredity, and sex, there can be tremendous variation in the appearance of the eyes. There are well-known differences in the anatomy between races, sexes, and across age groups that the surgeon should become familiar with in order to customize a surgical plan for the patient.

Despite these nuanced differences, there are sufficient constants in the anatomy of the eyelids such that a systematic understanding is possible. In addition, certain physical features of the eyelids are present in association with other characteristic features of the eyes. For example, individuals with relative proptosis and negative malar vector often have some lower eyelid retraction with scleral show even in the absence of a history of previous surgery or lower eyelid laxity.[1] Older individuals with thin soft tissue and relative enophthalmos often have a deep superior orbital sulcus due to a lack of volume from attenuated pre-aponeurotic fat.

CLINICAL EVALUATION

HISTORY

Patients seeking blepharoplasty can present with any number of chief complaints that can be categorized as functional or aesthetic in nature. The two are, however, intimately intertwined and the surgeon must consider both the function and appearance of the eyelids. Those who present with functional concerns such as constricted visual fields are also concerned about the cosmesis of the blepharoplasty result. Likewise, patients who undergo cosmetic blepharoplasty will not tolerate the functional impairment of dryness, tearing, or blurry vision even with a great cosmetic result. Common functional complaints that may indicate upper blepharoplasty include eye fatigue, difficulty with driving, reading, or watching TV, and even tension-type headaches. These patients tend to be older, although younger patients may also have functional impairment to a degree that would fulfill the health insurance criteria for visually significant dermatochalasis or palpebral ptosis. Common aesthetic complaints include a perception of appearing tired or not having had enough rest, difficulty wearing makeup, dark shadows under the eyes, or asymmetry between the two eyes. Younger Asian patients often present seeking Asian upper blepharoplasty in which an upper eyelid crease and fold is created in a configuration consistent with an Asian upper eyelid crease. It is a commonly held misconception, even among surgeons, that these patients seek a more Caucasian-appearing upper eyelid.

Listening is the first and most important step in the evaluation of a patient who presents seeking blepharoplasty.[2] It is critical to understand what exactly is bothersome to the patient in order to formulate a plan that is in sync with his or her expectations. A patient is likely to be dissatisfied if the surgeon does not take the time to understand what the patient is hoping for. Even a perfectly executed surgical plan misses the mark if the surgeon's perceived target is misaligned with the patient's. Take the time to ask detailed questions. Follow-up with further inquiry. If a patient presents complaining about tired-looking eyes, ask what about their eyes makes them feel as such. Is it the droopy skin that hides the upper lid crease and creates a downward slant to the upper eyelid contour laterally? Is it the shadows under the eyes? For the younger Asian patient, what height and configuration of upper eyelid fold does the patient have in mind: a low-set crease (1–2 mm) or a higher one (3–4 mm)?

Medical and ocular history pertinent to surgical planning should be obtained. Many patients will endorse a history of dry eyes and the use of lubricating drops. How often they use drops and how their eyes feel if they forget to use drops can give the surgeon an idea of the severity of the dryness. Dryness worse upon waking may indicate ocular exposure during sleep, which could worsen after blepharoplasty.[3] Caution should also be taken in patients with a recent history of refractive surgery because corneal sensation is diminished in these patients, and they are at higher risk for dry eyes.[4] A history of preexisting vision problems should be documented as well as drops the patient may be using. Prostaglandin analog drops used for glaucoma (also the active ingredient in bimatoprost ophthalmic solution [Latisse 0.03%, Allergan, Dublin, Ireland]) can aggravate inflammation at the eyelid margin, and their use should be noted.[5] History of prior eyelid or facial surgery should be noted, making note of what was done. A review of the operative note may be necessary in more complex cases. Other pertinent medical conditions include any that would put the patient at undue risk under anesthesia, including but not limited to severe cardiovascular disease, history of stroke, renal or hepatic failure, pulmonary disease with poor reserve, malignant hyperthermia, a history of deep venous thrombosis, or bleeding diathesis. Even patients with relatively poor functional reserve can undergo blepharoplasty under local anesthesia. However, those having surgery under moderate sedation or general anesthesia should have a thorough history, physical, and pertinent laboratory and ancillary studies to assess their fitness for surgery.

The patient's medication list should be reviewed preoperatively. The surgeon should ask about use of any blood thinners or supplements, such as vitamin E, fish oil, garlic, or ginko that can increase bleeding risk. Ibuprofen or aspirin should be stopped for at least 1 week prior to surgery. Retrobulbar hemorrhage is a serious complication associated with blepharoplasty that can cause permanent loss of vision and every precaution should be taken to avoid this complication.

Finally, social history should be reviewed for a history of smoking. Patients who smoke may have issues with postoperative healing, and this should be discussed with the patient prior to surgery.[6]

EXAMINATION

Physical examination for upper blepharoplasty should also include an examination of the whole upper face, and an examination for lower blepharoplasty should also include an examination of the midface.

UPPER EYELIDS

Taking a systematic approach to physical examination will ensure a thorough exam is completed each and every time.

The examination starts with an assessment of skin quality. Eyelid skin is the thinnest on the body thus is much more susceptible to laxity with loss of elasticity compared to thicker skin. Those with thinner eyelid skin also tend to have less robust soft tissue volume and tend to have finer features of their eyes with tapering volume from the brow to the eyelid margin. Those with thicker skin tend to have thicker underlying soft tissue volume with a puffier look to their upper eyelid and eyebrow complex. Thicker eyelid skin tends to be more resistant to wrinkles than thinner skin.

Dermatochalasis conventionally refers to relaxation of the upper eyelid skin, although technically the same term can be used for lower eyelid skin laxity as well. With age, the eyelid skin becomes more inelastic and the eyebrow position tends to droop (although this latter observation has been refuted by some).[7] The result is an apparent excess of the upper eyelid skin with hooding and obscuration of the pre-tarsal platform as the loose skin cascades from the eyelid crease. Almost universally, the hooding is more prominent laterally, imparting a downward slant to the eyes' appearance, reminiscent of a look of fatigue or sadness. In Asians who do not have an upper eyelid crease, the absence of aponeurotic skin attachments allows the loose skin to cascade at the level of the eyelid margin and can cause lash ptosis (analogous to lower eyelid epiblepharon).[8]

The position and shape of the eyebrow should be noted. The position of the eyebrows has a significant effect on the degree of dermatochalasis.[9] Because the position of the eyebrows varies with dynamic expression and because an individual may at baseline subconsciously raise her eyebrows out of habit or to clear her visual axis, the effect on the eyebrows of apparent upper eyelid skin redundancy can be difficult to assess. Secondary dermatochalasis in the presence of moderate to severe eyebrow ptosis may disappear once the eyebrow is manually positioned to an elevated, non-ptotic position. These patients would do better with a brow lift. On the other hand, prominent frontalis compensation with increased tone will mask primary dermatochalasis as the patient maintains an elevated brow position with frontalis contraction. Therefore, it is imperative to examine dermatochalasis with the brows at resting position. This can be done by having the patient close his or her eyes and relax. Light finger pressure on the eyebrows will help them relax. Dermatochalasis is scaled from +1 to +4, with +1 and +2 being very minimal and at a level above the lash line, +3 dermatochalasis rests on the lash line, and, in +4 dermatochalasis, the skin lies below the lash line. Dermatochalasis that extends well beyond the lateral palpebral commissure (Connell's sign) indicates significant lateral brow ptosis. This can be corrected with a temporal brow lift or by extending the blepharoplasty excision pattern further laterally.

Evaluation of dermatochalasis should coincide with evaluation of eyelid ptosis.[2] Eyelid ptosis refers to a drooping of the upper eyelid margin relative to the pupil in straight gaze from involutional, neurogenic, mechanical, or congenital causes. Eyelid ptosis is measured in millimeters as a distance from the central corneal light reflex to the margin of the upper eyelid, also referred to as the margin to reflex distance type 1 (MRD1).[3] MRD2 is a measurement of the distance from the corneal light reflex to the lower eyelid, but it is infrequently used compared to degree of scleral show. With your eyes level with that of the patient, shine a modestly bright light from between your eyes (co-axial) onto the forehead of the patient. Doing so with a dimmer light will prevent reflexive squinting and an artifactual exaggeration of any ptosis. Then, with a millimeter ruler held up next to the patient's eyes, measure the distance from the central corneal light reflex to the upper eyelid margin centrally. Precision of the measurement is 0.5 mm. Levator function is a measure of the excursion of the upper eyelid from downgaze to upgaze with the brow position stabilized. This measurement is important in the assessment for ptosis surgery, a topic that will not be covered in this chapter.

The contour of the eyelid should be assessed as well. The upper eyelid contour should taper up from the medial palpebral commissure and arc gently downward, with the point of maximal height just medial to the pupil. Notches may indicate previous chalazia or infection/inflammation or tumor; peaking, previous levator surgery or tethering; and lateral flare, eyelid retraction related to Graves' disease.

The upper eyelid fold is the fold of skin that cascades from the level of the upper eyelid crease. In other words, an upper eyelid fold cannot exist unless there is an upper eyelid crease and at least some skin that cascades down below the level of the crease. For example, Asians without an upper eyelid crease do not have an upper eyelid fold. In fact, the goal of Asian upper blepharoplasty is to create an upper eyelid fold by the surgical creation of an upper eyelid

crease and to allow for some redundant skin to fold slightly below the newly formed crease.[8] As another example, older Caucasian patients with a progressively deepening superior sulcus from pre-aponeurotic fat atrophy may lose their upper eyelid fold as the skin invaginates into the deep superior sulcus and the redundant skin that had previously folded over the upper eyelid crease gets pulled into the superior orbital sulcus. The position of the upper eyelid fold is measured from the eyelid margin to the level of the fold centrally. The contour should mostly run parallel to the upper eyelid margin, tapering in to a point at the medial palpebral commissure in some instances. With early dermatochalasis, the upper eyelid fold sags laterally, obscuring the pre-tarsal platform on which women apply eyeshadow makeup.

Assessment of the pre-aponeurotic and brow fat follows examination of eyelid ptosis, dermatochalasis, and eyebrow position. Fullness between the eyebrow and the upper eyelid fold may be due to pseudoherniation of the pre-aponeurotic fat pads, of which there are two (central and nasal), prolapse of the lacrimal gland laterally, or prominence of the sub-eyebrow fat pad.[3] Pseudoherniation of the central fat pad with age is uncommon. In fact, involutional atrophy is much more likely in advanced age, exposing a deepened superior orbital hollow. Pinching the eyebrow soft tissue and translating it upward can help distinguish brow fat from orbital fat. Prolapsed lacrimal gland tissue can be visualized upon eversion of the eyelid at the lateral aspect.

In addition to a history of dry eyes, several physical features are associated with an increased risk of exposure and exposure keratitis following upper blepharoplasty: lagophthalmos, poor orbicularis strength, and weak Bell's phenomenon. Lagophthalmos is the inability to completely close the eyes. It is measured in millimeters with the patient closing the eyes gently. Those with even severe lagophthalmos can close completely with forced closure, so it is imperative to make sure lagophthalmos is assessed with gentle eyelid closure. Those with a history of stroke or Bell's palsy have poor orbicularis strength, which increases the risk of exposure postoperatively. With forced closure, the examiner should try to open the eyes. Weakness is graded on the House-Brackmann scale with I being normal function, VI being complete paralysis, and III being moderate weakness. Bell's phenomenon is the upward movement of the eye on eyelid closure. Also known as the *palpebral oculogyric reflex*, this phenomenon protects the ocular surface even in the presence of mild lagophthalmos. An absent or reverse Bell's phenomenon increases the risk of exposure following blepharoplasty. It can be assessed in conjunction with the assessment of lagophthalmos by manually opening the eyelids while the patients tries to close them.

LOWER EYELIDS

Examination of the lower eyelids for blepharoplasty includes assessment of the features associated with age and an assessment of the risk of postoperative eyelid malposition. Lower eyelid retraction and/or ectropion is the most common complication following lower blepharoplasty.[10] In addition to imparting a sickly and unhealthy appearance from exaggerated scleral show and secondary conjunctival injection, there is often ocular irritation and dryness. Prophylactic canthoplasty or canthopexy are often necessary to prevent eyelid malposition in those with lower eyelid laxity or a negative midface vector.

Examination of the lower eyelids in consideration for blepharoplasty starts with assessment of the skin quality. Although the eyelid skin is the thinnest skin on the body, there is significant variation among individuals. Thin skin is more prone to rhytids than thicker skin. Also, the violaceous hue of the underlying orbicularis is also more likely to show through in those with thinner skin. The lower eyelid skin of those of Hispanic, Asian, or South Asian decent will often have darker pigmentation than the surrounding subjacent malar skin. With dermatochalasis of the lower eyelid, the skin gathers and pleats and can impart an even darker hue than if there were fewer wrinkles in the same skin. The surgeon should also note the transition of the thin eyelid skin to the thicker malar skin, which typically follows the arcus marginalis.

Dermatochalasis of the lower eyelid presents as rhytids that run parallel to the orbicularis fibers of the lower eyelid. As with dermatochalasis of the upper eyelids, the apparent redundancy is due to loss of elasticity and lack of skin recoil. In fact, mild dermatochalasis may only be apparent during smiling, at which the malar soft tissue rises and creates bunching of the inelastic skin. Severe dermatochalasis with a history of episodic swelling can manifest as malar festoons. The degree of lower eyelid dermatochalasis is assessed by pinching the eyelid skin.

There are three discrete fat pads of the lower eyelid.[11] The medial and central fat pads are separated by the inferior oblique muscle. The central and lateral fat pads are divided by the arcuate expansion of the capsulopalpebral fascia, a fibrous connective tissue band that spans from the inferior oblique fascia and Lockwood's ligament to the inferolateral orbital wall. The appearance of the fat pads varies, appearing more prominent in upgaze and while upright. In supine position, the pseudo-herniation

is less noticeable. Examine and note the degree of prominence of each of the three fat pads as well as their degree of asymmetry in order to plan how much of the fat to excise. Gentle retropulsion on the eye will bring out more of the pseudo-herniation.

The lower eyelid spans between the anterior and posterior lacrimal crests to the lateral orbital tubercle as a tarsoligamentous sling. With age, laxity at the medial and lateral canthal tendons diminishes the tone of the lower eyelid and can cause rounding of the lateral and medial canthal angle, lower eyelid retraction, and/or ectropion. The degree of laxity can be assessed by the snap back test, in which the eyelid is pulled down and allowed to recoil back into position. Although there is a grading scheme from I to IV, with IV being frank ectropion, a simple normal and mildly or severely prolonged snap back is often sufficient. Even relatively mild laxity at the medial and lateral canthal tendons portends postoperative eyelid malposition. These patients would benefit from adjunctive lateral canthopexy or canthoplasty to prevent secondary eyelid malposition.

Proptosis is an abnormal protrusion or bulging of the eye relative to the orbital walls and is conventionally measured in millimeters from the lateral orbital rim to the point of maximal projection by use of a Hertel exophthalmeter. Even without one, the surgeon should note the degree to which the eye protrudes from the orbit in relation to the inferior orbital rim as this is more clinically relevant. Patients with proptosis tend to have associated lower eyelid retraction even at baseline in the absence of previous surgery. The tarsoligamentous sling dips down in these individuals, much like a belt will tuck under a very protuberant abdomen. Lower eyelid tightening procedures will paradoxically aggravate the retraction. Lower blepharoplasty should be done with extreme caution in these individuals or not at all.[1]

The orbital rim and overlying soft tissue of the midface provides bolster support to the overlying lower eyelid. Much as proptosis portends eyelid retraction, midface retrusion is also associated with a higher risk of postoperative lower eyelid malposition.[1] Also known as a *negative midface vector*, such patients lack the bolstering support that the subjacent orbital rim and soft tissue provides the lower eyelid.

The contour of the malar fat pads and their transition with the eyelid fat pads contributes to an aged appearance.[12] In youth, there is a seamless transition at the lid–cheek junction. Deflation of the malar fat pads will aggravate the appearance of the shadow at the lid–cheek junction. It is not unusual for patients to present for lower blepharoplasty after having lost weight due to loss of facial volume exposing lower eyelid pseudo-herniation. Significant malar deflation should be addressed with adjunctive malar autologous fat grafting or injectable fillers.

PREOPERATIVE PLANNING AND ANESTHESIA

Upper and lower eyelid blepharoplasties are often performed in the outpatient setting under local anesthesia with monitored intravenous sedation.[13] Upper blepharoplasty can safely and comfortably be done under local anesthesia in a procedure room or office setting. General anesthesia is also an option, if necessary, but anesthesia risk must be further assessed. General anesthesia is not a good option if a blepharoplasty is being combined with ptosis repair by levator resection or advancement because it is important to have patient cooperation to check eyelid height intraoperatively. In fact, for upper blepharoplasty, having an awake patient allows the surgeon to assess the appearance of the eyelids with the eyes open.

Numerous techniques for local anesthesia exist, and every surgeon tends to develop his or her own preferences. Local anesthesia often includes a combination of the following: 1–2% lidocaine +/− epinephrine, 0.25–0.75% bupivacaine, and sodium bicarbonate. Saline-diluted or bicarbonate-buffered local anesthetic can help provide a more pain-free injection, as this method normalizes the pH of the anesthetic and lessens the burning sensation. The senior surgeon prefers a 1:1 mixture of 1% lidocaine with 1:100,000 epinephrine and 0.25% bupivacaine. Local anesthesia is given after preoperative marking of the patient. A 30-gauge needle is used and is inserted laterally near the lateral canthus and directed toward the medial canthus while pointing the needle away from the eye. The injection should be subcutaneous, as a suborbicularis injection may result in an unwanted hematoma. Large volumes are not required and may distort the eyelid. If the procedure is being done bilaterally, then equal amounts are injected on both sides to help with the assessment of symmetry. If portions of the fat pads are removed or debulked intraoperatively, additional local anesthesia may need to be injected as excision of the fat pads can be painful.

A drop of proparacaine or tetracaine should be placed in both eyes prior to prepping the patient as Betadine solution can cause significant burning and irritation. The Betadine should be diluted with equal part sterile saline. Sterile balanced salt solution (BSS) is used after the procedure to rinse any remaining Betadine out of the eyes as this can cause a corneal epitheliopathy that can be very uncomfortable for the patient.

SURGICAL TECHNIQUE

UPPER EYELID BLEPHAROPLASTY

Preoperative marking is of critical importance for a good aesthetic result.[14] Marking should be done prior to injection of local anesthesia. The lower incision is marked at 7–10 mm above the lash line. The peak of the crease marking is often higher in females (8–10 mm) and lower in males (7–8 mm) and approximately 4–5 mm in Asians.[3,8] In older patients, with dermatochalasis and its attendant laxity, the final scar can ride higher than intended, so it may be necessary to mark the lower incision 1–2 mm lower than the natural upper eyelid crease. The lower mark along the desired eyelid crease should extend from a point above the punctum medially to the lateral canthus with a varying degree of oblique extension marks medially and laterally depending on the nature and degree of dermatochalasis. The lateral skin excision is especially important for addressing lateral hooding.

Judicious excision of skin from the upper eyelids is key to getting the desired result while avoiding secondary lagophthalmos. The position of the desired upper eyelid fold can be marked when the patient is sitting up. The actual position of the upper incision marking should be slightly lower than this mark. With the skin pinch technique, toothless forceps are used to gently pinch the skin with one end of the forceps at the level of the lower incision marking.[14] Make sure the patient's brow is relaxed during this maneuver. This can be done in several locations along the eyelid and then the dots connected. After the site is marked bilaterally, the markings can be measured for symmetry and the remaining skin can be measured to ensure enough skin is left.

Functionally, the amount of skin that is removed from the upper eyelid is not as important as the amount of skin that is left behind, as overresection of skin can result in exposure keratopathy and vision changes. There should be at least 20–22 mm of skin left between the eyelid margin and inferior aspect of the brow. If the skin pinch technique is utilized, then significant superior rotation of the eyelashes or lagophthalmos should be assessed when the skin is pinched and minimized to prevent exposure issues. A patient can be reassured that additional skin can be removed in a few months if necessary, whereas it is much more difficult to put skin back, with much worse consequences.

After markings are made, local anesthesia is injected and the surgical site is prepped and draped. Blepharoplasty markings can be reinforced using a sterile surgical marking pen or methylene blue.

A no. 15 blade is used to incise the skin along the marked ellipse (Figure 25.1A). Care should be taken to make a shallow incision at the lower edge so as not to inadvertently incise the underlying levator aponeurosis. The surgeon has the option to remove just skin or skin with the underlying orbicularis muscle. The senior author prefers to excise the skin separately from the orbicularis, as often only the lateral portion of the orbicularis is excised (Figure 25.1B). In Asians or in those with particularly thick eyelid tissue, it is preferred to excise the skin and muscle in composite. Excision of the eyelid skin is done under tension, with the eyebrow distracted superiorly. This prevents inadvertent deepening of the excision into the orbicularis or septal plane. For this reason, the senior surgeon prefers excising the skin with cutting monopolar cautery instead of surgical scissors, with which the depth of excision is more difficult to control. Hemostasis with bipolar cautery or monopolar cautery on a low setting will prevent gathering of the tissue with thermal spread.

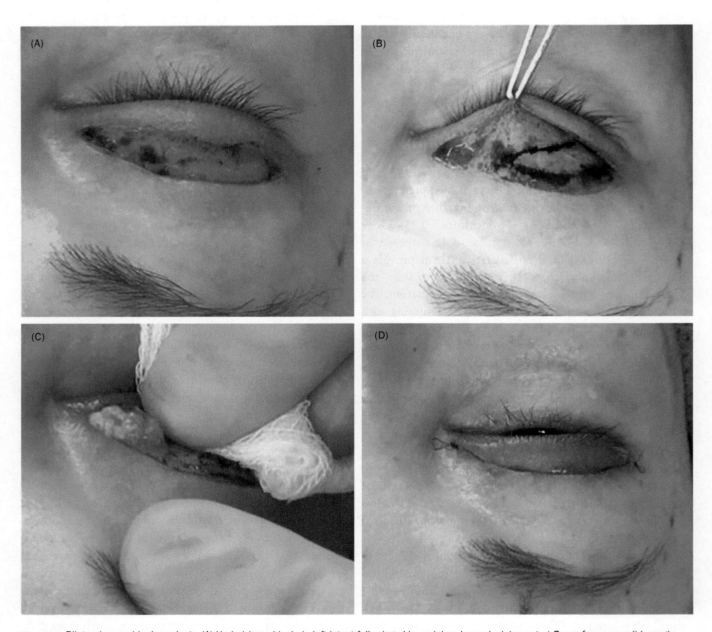

Figure 25.1. Bilateral upper blepharoplasty. (A) Underlying orbicularis left intact following skin excision. Lower incision set at 7 mm from upper lid margin. (B) Pattern for lateral orbicularis muscle excision. For this patient with thinner upper lid tissue, the central orbicularis is preserved. (C) Exposure of the nasal fat pad with retropulsion via small septotomy. (D) Incision is closed with a running subcuticular 6-0 Prolene suture.

There are two fat compartments posterior to the septum in the upper eyelid: the nasal and central pre-aponeurotic fat pads.[3] The lateral is the lacrimal gland, which should not be removed or incised during blepharoplasty. In those with thin eyelid skin and tissue, a prolapsed lacrimal gland can present as a focal prominence laterally and require suspension.[3] This is done by undermining a preseptal dissection to the superolateral orbital rim, incising the septum just off the rim, and securing the lower edge of the prolapsed lacrimal gland to the periosteum with a 5-0 Prolene. Conservative fat resection is critical so as not to create a hollow, deep superior sulcus. Overaggressive fat removal can also cause an unwanted peaking or distortion of the upper eyelid crease. The central fat pad should be excised with extreme caution. Doing so will deepen the superior orbital hollow and can cause unwanted accessory folds to develop. Monopolar cautery can be used to conservatively, and in a controlled fashion, shrink and contour the central fat pad. The nasal fat pad does not respond in this manner and often has to be excised. This is done via a small septal incision nasally, using cutting cautery with the globe in retropulsion. The retropulsion makes the fat pads protrude through the septotomy under pressure (Figure 25.1C). Skin hooks can be placed nasally to place traction on the lid and help with exposure. The nasal fat pad has a whitish color, compared to the more yellow central fat pad. It is not recommended to go digging for orbital fat as there are important orbital structures superonasally, such as the superior oblique muscle and the trochlea through which it passes. Often these fat pads need to be injected with additional local anesthesia as they can be painful to remove or debulk. Hemostasis after fat excision is extremely important. Some surgeons will clamp the fat with a hemostat, cut the excess fat off the hemostat, and then cauterize the remaining stump prior to releasing the hemostat. This is less well tolerated under sedation or local anesthesia. We find that electrocautery is sufficient to excise the fat pads.

Closing of an upper eyelid blepharoplasty is usually achieved with a running suture. 6-0 nylon, Prolene, or fast-absorbing gut can be placed with small bites of skin. The senior author prefers a running subcuticular suture with 6-0 Prolene to avoid milia along the wound (Figure 1D). An inverted interrupted 5-0 Vicryl can be placed to reapproximate the orbicularis at the lateral third junction. If nonabsorbable sutures are used, they should be removed on postoperative day 7.

LOWER EYELID BLEPHAROPLASTY

The goal of lower blepharoplasty is to ablate the prominent lower eyelid bags from orbital fat pseudo-herniation and/or judiciously excise redundant lower eyelid skin. Excision of lower eyelid fat can be achieved through either a transcutaneous or transconjunctival approach. Because much of the lower eyelid pseudo-herniation disappears in the supine position, it is important to assess the amount of fat to be excised preoperatively with the patient in an upright position. With transcutaneous blepharoplasty, a skin muscle flap is elevated in the preseptal plane and allows for wider exposure for adjunctive procedures, such as release of the orbitomalar ligament with fat transposition, and is usually necessary for significant skin laxity or festoons.

The transconjunctival approach to fat excision is associated with a lower risk of secondary eyelid malposition.[15] Although the transconjunctival access provides a tighter exposure, it, too, can be used to reposition fat. When combined with lateral canthoplasty, the exposure becomes much wider. Transconjunctival blepharoplasty is often combined with a skin excision by skin pinch or skin flap elevation,[15] or with ablative laser resurfacing or chemical peel to tighten the lower eyelid skin. Surgeons may prefer one approach over another. A conservative approach with judicious excision or ablation is more important in preventing secondary ectropion than which excisional or ablative approach is taken to address the lower eyelid dermatochalasis. Prophylactic maneuvers such as tightening the lateral canthal tendon and orbicularis suspension are of equal importance in avoiding lower eyelid malposition.

TRANSCONJUNCTIVAL LOWER EYELID BLEPHAROPLASTY

In transconjunctival blepharoplasty, the fat is approached without disruption of the orbicularis and its innervation. It is associated with a lower risk of eyelid malposition than transcutaneous lower blepharoplasty. However, a conservative, careful execution of either technique is more important than the choice of technique in achieving the desired results and avoiding complications.

Transconjunctival blepharoplasty can be used to release the orbitomalar ligament, transpose fat, or remove fat to smooth the contour transition at the lid–cheek junction. The transconjunctival approach is an excellent approach for younger patients with isolated pseudo-herniation with little or no skin laxity. When necessary, this procedure can be combined with a skin excision, laser resurfacing, or chemical peel. Adequate lateral canthal support must be noted or addressed to prevent eyelid malposition.

For the transconjunctival approach, bimanual retraction with an assistant-held Desmarres retractor everting the lower eyelid and a Jaeger lid plate to both protect and retropulse the globe will expose the conjunctival sulcus (Figure 25.2A). Using a cutting monopolar cautery on a needle or Colorado tip, a curvilinear incision is made through the conjunctiva and capsulopalpebral fascia approximately halfway between the inferior tarsal border and the fornix from the

lateral edge of the caruncle toward the lateral canthal angle (Figure 25.2B). A 5-0 Prolene suture can be tagged at the inferior edge of the conjunctiva and retracted superiorly.

The fat pads can be exposed via a preseptal or retroseptal approach. Although the retroseptal dissection is easier,

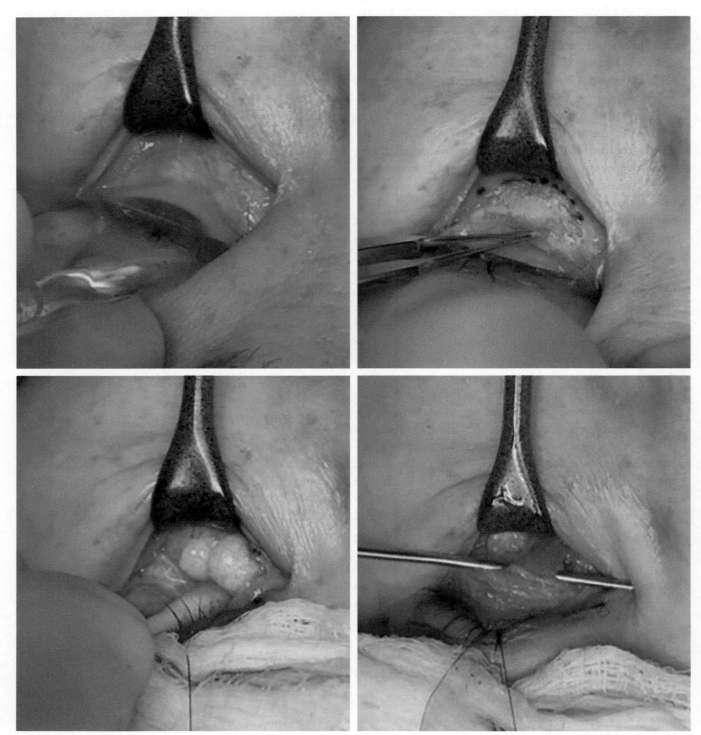

Figure 25.2. Transconjunctival lower blepharoplasty. (A) Exposure of lower lid conjunctival sulcus with bimanual retraction. (B) Curvilinear conjunctival incision and preseptal dissection. (C) Exposure of lower eyelid fat pads with retropulsion via low septotomy. (D) Inferior oblique left undisturbed following conservative fat excision.

the preseptal approach offers superior exposure. For the retroseptal approach, the conjunctival incision is made closer to the conjunctival sulcus, where the capsulopalpebral fascia is not confluent with the septum. The dissection is carried directly through this lower eyelid retractor with the described bimanual retraction, and the septum is left undisturbed. The fat pads are excised with monopolar cautery taking care to ensure meticulous hemostasis before final amputation of the fat because it will retract back into the orbit.

For the preseptal dissection, the conjunctival incision is made slightly higher, where the septum and retractor are confluent (Figure 25.2B). The septum is an avascular diaphanous structure with gossamer-like layers more similar to the parietal temporal fascia than to the temporalis fascia. The dissection is actually carried out within the septal layers so as to leave the orbicularis nerve fibers undisturbed. With cutting cautery, the plane can easily be developed and the lower edge tagged for suture retraction. Two to three cotton swabs replace the Jaeger lid plate in the bimanual retraction for controlled retropulsion and absorption of any bleeding to continue the dissection (Figure 25.2C). The dissection can be carried down to the level of the arcus marginalis and even further for fat transposition.

The inferior oblique sits between the medial and central lower eyelid fat pads. Care must be taken during dissection and excision of fat to avoid injuring this muscle. The oblique muscle is easily visualized with the preseptal dissection but may not be visualized with the retroseptal dissection (Figure 25.2D). The fat pads are excised using monopolar coagulation cautery and can be displayed to ensure approximately equal removal bilaterally (Figure 25.3). Gentle pressure on the globe can assist with fat herniation (Figure 25.2C). The lateral fat pad is more difficult to access through the transconjunctival incision. It usually requires lateral extension of the conjunctival incision. The contour of the lower eyelid should be examined periodically. Gentle

retropulsion mimics the effect of gravity. Set the excised fat pads aside for comparison in order to try to achieve a symmetric result.

Extension of the dissection beyond the arcus marginalis either in a sub-periosteal or pre-periosteal plane, including disinsertion of the orbicularis origin fibers at the inferior nasal orbital rim, softens the contour transition at the lid–cheek junction and allows for transposition of pedicled fat pads into the recesses underlying a clinically noted tear trough deformity. Careful assessment for hemostasis is important prior to closure to prevent retrobulbar hemorrhage. The conjunctiva can be closed with one simple interrupted 6-0 fast-absorbing gut suture or left open to heal by secondary intent.

If a mild amount of skin laxity is noted, the skin can be excised either by skin flap elevation or skin pinch.[15] Alternatively, adjunctive ablative laser or chemical peel can be done to tighten the lower eyelid dermatochalasis. Skin flap elevation is technically more challenging, but it allows for more control to set the incision at the desired distance from the lash line. The skin pinch technique is technically simpler and safer, but the final scar tends to settle slightly lower than the desired subciliary distance.

Skin excision should follow fat excision or transposition. With either approach, the eyelid is tagged at the gray line of the margin centrally with a 5-0 Prolene or equivalent suture and placed on superior traction. Additional local anesthetic injection hydrodissects the subcutaneous plane, and the turgor facilitates a crisp incision.

With a skin flap elevation, a no. 15 or up-turned no. 11 blade is used to make a subciliary incision 1–1.5 mm inferior to the lash line from the level of the punctum to a point 4–8 mm lateral to the lateral palpebral commissure. Sharp dissection starts the flap elevation. The flap can be elevated in this manner, or cutting cautery on low setting can be used to complete the elevation. Extreme care should be taken to prevent button-holing the skin flap. The retraction of the skin with forceps and skin hooks should keep it taut and straight. It is not necessary to carry the elevation all the way to the lid–cheek junction. Typically, not more than 5–6 mm of skin is excised. This is determined by redraping the skin. For good measure, the cheek can be distracted inferiorly to mimic gravity and ensure an even more conservative excision. Excise the skin sharply at the level of the subciliary incision and close with a simple running 6-0 fast-absorbing gut suture.

With skin pinch excision, a T-shaped Converse or Green fixation forceps is used to pinch the subciliary skin after local anesthetic injection without eliciting ectropion. In the absence of the fixation forceps, Brown-Adson forceps

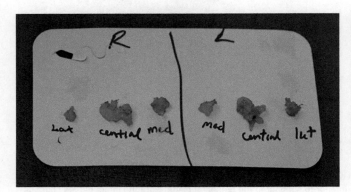

Figure 25.3. Individual fat pads excised from each lower eyelid during bilateral lower blepharoplasty are set aside for comparison.

can be used. Sharp dissection scissors are used to excise the pinched skin at its base. The defect is closed with running 6-0 fast-absorbing gut. With this technique, secondary ectropion is rare. However, the mechanics of pinching the skin makes it somewhat difficult to get very close to the lash line.

Transcutaneous Lower Eyelid Blepharoplasty

In transcutaneous lower eyelid blepharoplasty, a skin muscle flap is elevated in the preseptal plane.[3] It allows for redraping and suspension of the orbicularis, which is very effective at improving the eyelid contour and rhytids.

However, it is associated with a higher rate of secondary malposition, and care should be exercised when excising the skin and muscle.[10] Its superior exposure also makes it more conducive to adjunctive fat transposition or malar fat suspension.[3] For orbital malar festoons, skin excision alone is insufficient, and a skin muscle flap is necessary.

A no. 15 or upturned no. 11 blade is used to make a subciliary incision 1–1.5 mm below the eyelashes under traction (Figure 25.4A). Much lower than this, the scar may be more noticeable postoperatively. This incision is made from the level of the punctum to a point 4–8 mm lateral to the lateral palpebral fissure. When combined

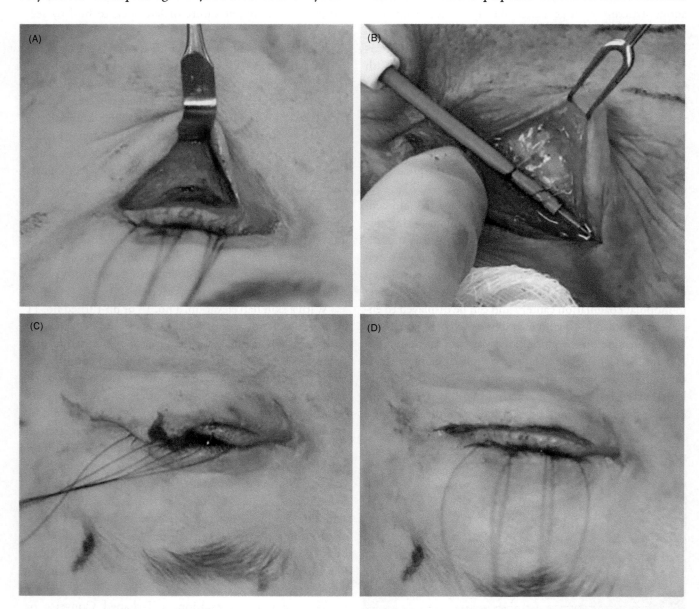

Figure 25.4. Transcutaneous lower blepharoplasty. (A) Preseptal dissection and elevation of lower eyelid skin muscle flap via subciliary incision. Note the pretarsal orbicularis is left intact. (B) Orbicularis motor nerve fibers run from inferior to superior in the preseptal plane. Note the intact nerves coursing toward the pretarsal orbicularis. (C) Superior traction relaxed and skin muscle flap redraped. Dart incision made to precisely determine amount of skin to be excised. (D) Following skin/muscle excision, the edges should be nearly apposed.

with upper blepharoplasty, care should be taken to have the lateral incision extensions at least 8 mm apart. A skin flap is elevated sharply, leaving the pretarsal orbicularis undisturbed (Figure 25.4A). A transverse myotomy is made to begin the skin muscle flap elevation at the tarsal–septal junction (Figure 25.4B). From here, the dissection is in the same plane as the retroseptal transconjunctival dissection. Laterally, just inferior to the lateral pseudo-raphe, the orbicularis is adherent to the lateral orbital rim by way of the superficial portion of lateral canthal tendon. Releasing this greatly widens exposure and allows for more aggressive muscle redraping. However, doing so requires a longer lateral extension of the incision and resuspension of the orbicularis to the underlying periosteum.

With the eyelid margin on upward traction, bimanual retraction with a Desmarres retractor on the skin muscle flap and cotton swabs for upward retraction and controlled retropulsion on the septum facilitates dissection down to the arcus marginalis and beyond if desired. The fat is excised or transposed as described for the transconjunctival blepharoplasty. For fat transposition, the septal incision should be low near the orbital rim, and the eyelid should remain on traction throughout this portion of the procedure. Proper release of the orbitomalar ligament requires disinsertion of the orbicularis at the frontal process of the maxilla. This should be done with cautery and blunt dissection in the pre-periosteal plane or with a Freer elevator in the sub-periosteal plane. Care must be taken while dissecting along the inferior orbital rim to avoid injury of the infraorbital nerve.

With the pre-periosteal extension beyond the rim, the lateral malar fat pad can be suspended with 4-0 PDS suture in a lifted position to the periosteum. The medial malar fat pad is typically diminutive and less amenable to suspension. An intramalar groove separates the two fat pads, runs parallel to the nasolabial fold, and flares into a triangular area of little or no fat near the level of the orbital rim. The superior portions of both malar fat pads are often referred to as the suborbicularis fat pad (SOOF) in the oculoplastic surgery literature. For the senior author, autologous malar fat grafting has largely supplanted fat transposition and malar fat pad suspension as this allows for less extensive dissection, shorter recovery, and the ability to volumize along the entire intramalar groove and diminutive medial malar fat pad.

Next, the skin–muscle flap is redraped and resected (Figure 4C,D). The amount of skin and muscle to be excised is done as described earlier. Excision should bevel such that slightly more orbicularis is excised than the skin to take into account the fact that the pretarsal orbicularis was left intact

at the inset site. An oblique vector superolaterally greatly improves the eyelid contour, but requires a longer lateral extension to reconcile the Burrow's triangle. Preserving the orbicularis adherence near the lateral pseudo-raphe will not allow this oblique vector of pull and precludes the need for orbicularis suspension. To correct the Burrow's triangle after orbicularis suspension, the skin is dissected from the orbicularis muscle laterally and redraped separately. A 4-0 Vicryl suture is used to secure and resuspend the orbicularis muscle to the underlying periosteum lateral to the lateral orbital rim. For more aggressive suspension, the flap can be secured to the superolateral periosteum through suborbicularis tunnel via an upper blepharoplasty defect. The orbicularis suspension is key to supporting the tension of the closure, especially if the native adherence at the lateral rim has been disrupted. The subciliary incision can then be closed with a running 6-0 plain gut suture (or a nonabsorbable suture).

POSTOPERATIVE RECOMMENDATIONS

Dressings are not necessary after a blepharoplasty and they impede eyelid function. Antibiotic ophthalmic ointment is often placed over the incision sites and inside the eye for transconjunctival lower blepharoplasty. Commonly used ointments include erythromycin ophthalmic ointment,[13] Polysporin ophthalmic ointment, tobramycin-dexamethasone ophthalmic ointment (TobraDex), or neomycin-polymyxin b-dexamethasone ophthalmic ointment (Maxitrol). The patient is then sent home with a prescription for the ointment to be placed over the incision site 2–3 times daily for 1 week.

Ice cold compresses applied for the first 4–7 days for 10–20 minutes each hour while awake are very important in reducing postoperative pain and edema. The senior author prefers a moist wash cloth on the eyes with a zipper locked bag of crushed ice or a frozen gel pack. The patient should sleep with his or her head elevated with several pillows.

Some spotting of blood on the wash cloth for the first day or two is typical, and the patient should be informed of such. Patients often will have a variable amount of periorbital ecchymosis and it may be asymmetric. The bruising will travel down the face to the lower lids and cheeks with time. Some patients prefer to wear sunglasses for several days to hide the ecchymosis, but also for sun protection and light sensitivity. Patients are advised that vision may be a bit blurry with ointment. If the eyes swell shut, the patient is advised to call the surgeon immediately as it may portend retrobulbar hemorrhage.

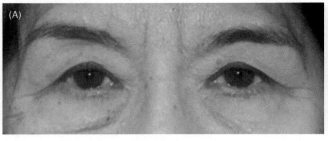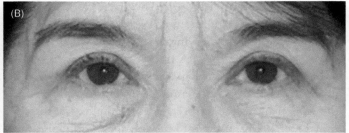

Figure 25.5. Bilateral upper blepharoplasty. (A) Preoperative photo. (B) Postoperative photo.

Patients should avoid any straining, bending over or heavy lifting for at least 1–2 weeks after surgery as these activities could cause rebleeding. Cosmetic products can be resumed at the 2-week mark.

Follow-up is at 1 week for evaluation and/or suture removal. Bruising and swelling typically lasts 10–14 days but may be as prolonged as 3 weeks in some individuals or with extensive dissection.

PRE- AND POSTOPERATIVE RESULTS

A comparison of pre- and postoperative results are seen in Figures 25.5 through 25.8.

COMPLICATIONS

Although not a true complication, undercorrection, overcorrection, and unacceptable asymmetry are far and away the most common reasons that a patient may be unhappy with the result of either upper or lower blepharoplasty.[2,16] It is far more preferable to err on the side undercorrection, as it is easier to revise and excise a bit more fat or skin than to revise an overcorrected result. The margin for error for asymmetry is exceedingly narrow for blepharoplasty, and some minor asymmetry is the rule and not the exception. Patients need to be advised that this is the case and that their expectations should be in keeping with this. The surgeon should expect to revise some of his or her own work on occasion. Fortunately, most revisions can be done in the office setting under local anesthesia.

The most devastating complication associated with blepharoplasty is a retrobulbar hemorrhage causing vision loss. Patients should be educated about this possibility, which, although rare, can be catastrophic. Precautions should be taken to avoid this complication, including a review of medications and cessation of use of blood thinners prior to surgery and for at least 48–72 hours after surgery, meticulous hemostasis,[10] and education about no straining or heavy lifting after surgery. Retrobulbar hematoma presents as a tight, dark contusion which shuts the eye closed and is accompanied by severe pain.[2] Severe asymmetric pain warrants urgent investigation.

Aggressive excision of too much skin either in the upper or the lower eyelid may cause lagophthalmos, eyelid malposition such as retraction or ectropion, and exposure keratopathy. Severe exposure keratopathy after blepharoplasty can also have devastating effects on the vision. Prolonged exposure can cause corneal ulceration, corneal thinning, and permanent scarring. Patients may require more extensive reconstructive eyelid surgery to correct eyelid malposition and exposure, including

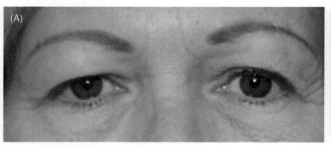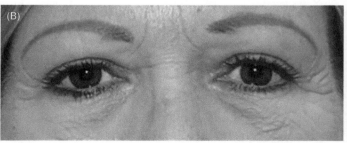

Figure 25.6. Bilateral upper blepharoplasty. (A) Preoperative photo. Note the left-side frontalis compensation. (B) Postoperative photo. Slight apparent undercorrection on the right side due to preserved frontalis compensatory contraction. A few units of botulinum to the left frontalis can correct for this.

AESTHETICS

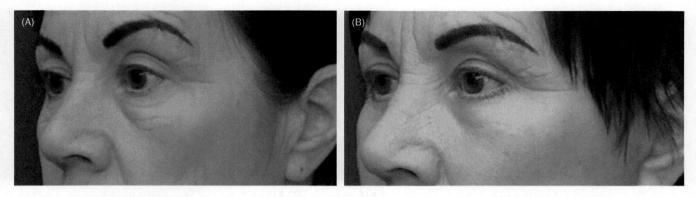

Figure 25.7. Transconjunctival bilateral lower blepharoplasty with skin pinch and lateral canthoplasty. (A) Preoperative photo. (B) Postoperative photo.

middle and posterior lamellar spacer grafts, skin grafts, or tarsorrhaphies. Eyelid malposition is the most common complications following lower eyelid blepharoplasty[10,15] (Figure 25.9). Even if exposure is not an issue, lid retraction, scleral show, or ectropion may be unsightly. Conservative excision of subciliary skin with or without muscle and having a low threshold for prophylactic lateral canthopexy or canthoplasty can help prevent these

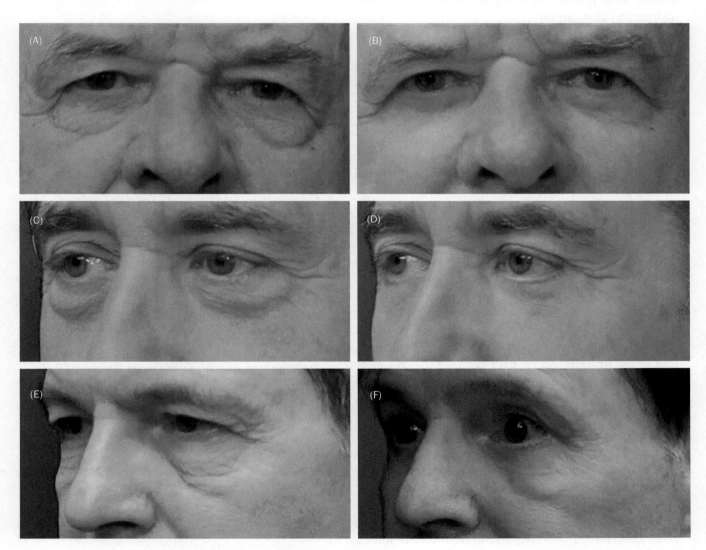

Figure 25.8. Transcutaneous lower eyelid blepharoplasty. Preoperative photos (A,C,E) and postoperative photos (B,D,F) showing significant improvement in lower eyelid dermatochalasis and fat prolapse.

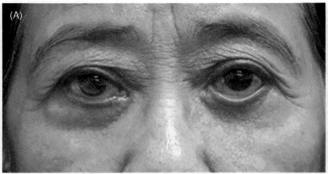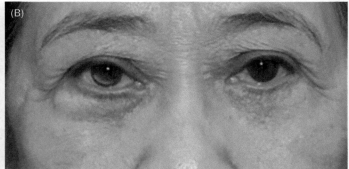

Figure 25.9. Complication following bilateral lower blepharoplasty done elsewhere. (A) Patient with left lower eyelid ectropion from overresection of fat and lower lid retractor dehiscence and right lower eyelid undercorrection laterally. (B) Correction of left lower eyelid ectropion with lateral canthoplasty via tarsal strip and dermis fat graft to left lower eyelid. The patent refused secondary surgery for the right lower eyelid.

complications.[3,10] Caution should be taken in patients with prominent eyes and a negative midface vector as well because these patients are at higher risk for lower eyelid malposition after surgery.

More commonly, patients may experience dry eyes after blepharoplasty. An even more measured approach is necessary for patients with a history of preexisting dry eyes or a recent history of refractive eye surgery. Dry eyes in the early postoperative period is not unusual for the first 1–2 weeks. Patients may improve over time, even over the first few weeks, as the tissue relaxes and orbicularis muscle function improves. Use of artificial tear drops and lubricating eye ointments that can be purchased over the counter can help alleviate the feeling of dryness, "sand in the eye," foreign body sensation, or itchiness and irritation.

Overaggressive excision of fat both in the upper and lower eyelids may lead to a poor aesthetic result. Excision of the central pre-aponeurotic fat pad ablates the apron of volume that contributes to the fullness of the upper lid. Fine contouring with cautery may be judiciously done, but excision often deepens the superior orbital hollow and can lend a skeletal appearance. Over excision of the lower eyelid fat pads can take the convexity of the lower eyelid beyond the desired flat contour to a concavity resulting in a hollowed out appearance. It can result in lower eyelid retraction as well. The lower eyelid fat pads provide bolster support to the lower eyelid, and overexcision may allow the lower eyelid margin to fall even in the presence of adequate tarsoligamentous suspensory support.

Functional orbital structures should be left undisturbed during upper and lower blepharoplasty. The superior oblique or trochlea could be violated during debulking of the nasal fat pad. In the lower eyelid, the inferior oblique separates the nasal and central fat pad and

can be damaged during fat excision, resulting in muscle weakness and diplopia that may be permanent.

REFERENCES

1. Pessa JE, et al. Changes in ocular globe-to-orbital rim position with age: implications for aesthetic blepharoplasty of the lower eyelids. *Aesthetic Plast Surg* 1999;23(5):337–342.
2. Yang P, et al. Upper Eyelid Blepharoplasty: Evaluation, Treatment, and Complication Minimization. *Semin Plast Surg* 2017;31(1):51–57.
3. Codner MA, McCord CD. *Eyelid & Periorbital Surgery.* Second edition.Boca Raton, FL: CRC Press, 2016.
4. Victoria AC, et al. Timing of eyelid surgery in the setting of refractive surgery: preoperative and postoperative considerations. *Curr Opin Ophthalmol* 2011;22(4):226–232.
5. Cunniffe MG, Medel-Jimenez R, Gonzalez-Candial M. Topical antiglaucoma treatment with prostaglandin analogues may precipitate meibomian gland disease. *Ophthal Plast Reconstr Surg* 2011;27(5):e128–e129.
6. Lassig AAD, et al. Tobacco exposure and wound healing in head and neck surgical wounds. *Laryngoscope* 2017.
7. Lambros V. Observations on periorbital and midface aging. *Plast Reconstr Surg* 2007;120(5):1367–1376; discussion 1377.
8. Chen WP. Asian blepharoplasty. Update on anatomy and techniques. *Ophthal Plast Reconstr Surg,* 1987;3(3):135–140.
9. Flowers RS. Periorbital aesthetic surgery for men. Eyelids and related structures. *Clin Plast Surg* 1991;18(4):689–729.
10. Dortzbach RK. Lower eyelid blepharoplasty by the anterior approach. Prevention of complications. *Ophthalmology* 1983;90(3):223–229.
11. Doxanas MT, Anderson RL. *Clinical Orbital Anatomy.* Baltimore, MD: Williams and Wilkins, 1984:xi.
12. Mendelson BC, Muzaffar AR, Adams Jr. WP. Surgical anatomy of the midcheek and malar mounds. *Plast Reconstr Surg* 2002;110(3): 885–896; discussion 897–911.
13. Kossler AL, et al. Current trends in upper and lower eyelid blepharoplasty among American Society of Ophthalmic Plastic and Reconstructive Surgery Members. *Ophthal Plast Reconstr Surg* 2018;34(1):37–42.
14. Tyers AG, Collin JRO. *Colour Atlas of Ophthalmic Plastic Surgery.* Edinburgh/New York: Churchill Livingstone, 1995:x.
15. Baylis HI, Long JA, Groth MJ. Transconjunctival lower eyelid blepharoplasty. Technique and complications. *Ophthalmology* 1989;96(7):1027–1032.
16. Lyon DB, Raphtis CS. Management of complications of blepharoplasty. *Int Ophthalmol Clin* 1997;37(3):205–216.

26.

ADVANCES IN HAIR TRANSPLANTATION

Alfonso Barrera

I incorporated hair transplantation into my practice 25 years, initially for the treatment of male pattern baldness (MPB) but soon thereafter I started finding other applications, particularly in enhancing aesthetics in reconstructive cases of the face and scalp, as in scarring alopecia after facial rejuvenation surgery (the loss of the temporal hairline and sideburn); alopecia due to trauma, burns, and radiation therapy; and even congenital defects (bilateral cleft lip on male patients), thus significantly improving these patients' final aesthetic outcomes.

A complete historic review of hair restoration procedures is beyond the scope of this chapter. Suffice to say that N. Orentreich[1] from New York popularized hair transplantation by introducing the use of punch grafts (hair plugs) in 1959. In addition, he described the "donor dominance" concept more than 40 years ago, which is key to successful hair transplantation. It basically states that each individual hair follicle contains its own unique genetic makeup. When transplanted to another site, these unique genetic properties are preserved regardless of the transplantation site. This enables the hair to grow at the recipient area with the characteristics and longevity of the hair the donor site. Fortunately, most individuals with MPB tend to lose their hair only on the top and crown, sparing the temporal and occipital areas. So, when utilizing these areas as donor sites, we can expect the growth to be as permanent at the recipient site, a most encouraging finding.

We learned a lot from the use of punch grafts; however, the results were often not very natural looking and too clumpy, with 4 mm diameter grafts with great density of hair but empty spaces around and in between them.

The use of single hair grafts is not a new concept; it was described as early as 1943 by Tamura from Japan, who transplanted the pubic area. Then Fujita, also from Japan, reconstructed eyebrows in 1953.

We must always strive to use our technical skills and expertise in an artistic way to provide a final outcome that mimics nature. That is, we must create hairlines consistent with what one would see naturally: a no-line hairline, no clumps, natural feathering of the boundaries, a degree of density that looks aesthetically pleasing, and no visible scarring.

Great advances toward a natural result in hair transplantation techniques occurred in the past three and a half decades. The idea of using a large number of single hair grafts in the front hairline of the scalp was described in 1981 by Nordstrom[2] from Helsinki, Finland, to camouflage the clumpy appearance of punch grafts. It was a tedious, time-consuming effort, and at the time it seemed unrealistic to think about transplanting the whole top of the head in this fashion.

Subsequently, Carlos O. Uebel[3] of Brazil, in 1991, was the first to report in the literature the use follicular unit micrografts and minigrafts to cover the entire area of baldness, doing well over a 1,000 grafts in a single session. Based on his work, I started doing hair transplantation.

For the first time results were able to mimic nature, without the clumpiness and cobblestoning that often accompanied punch grafts (hair plugs), no rows or strips, nor the scars and artificial look of flaps.

In view of the natural results we can obtain using follicular unit micrografts (1- to 2-hair grafts) and follicular unit minigrafts (3- to 4-hair grafts) and the predictability of the results without visible scarring on the recipient scalp and minimal scarring on the donor site, this is my preferred technique of hair transplantation.

I must add that for donor hair harvesting technique, I prefer the strip method, in which a horizontal 1 cm-wide strip is harvested from the occipital area, extending often into the temporal areas (10–25 cm in length or longer, depending on the number of grafts intended). This allows for a tension-free closure, resulting in minimal scarring. I prefer this technique because we can save at least 95% of the hair follicles we harvest. Once the strip is extracted, under magnification we incise parallel to the hair shafts on both edges. We then continue with magnification and background lighting (translumination) to predictably dissect intact follicular unit grafts. In addition, the donor site is camouflaged immediately by combing the hair down (hair is trimmed only on the donor strip itself).

The other technique for donor hair harvesting is follicular unit extraction (FUE), which consists of shaving a wide area of donor hair and using 0.8–1 mm diameter sharp punch knives, either manually or with rotation power or robotics, and extracting the grafts one by one. There are a few selected skilled experts who can do this very well and save most of the hair follicles, but in general it can result in significant wastage of hair follicles (up to 30–40%) because it is very difficult to extract intact follicular unit grafts due to the difficulty of going precisely parallel to the hair shafts along their entire length. Additionally, the donor site can't immediately be camouflaged (as a large area of hair is shaved).

Other surgical techniques described in the past to treat areas of baldness include scalp reduction, scalp flaps, tissue expansion, and the like. These are, for the most part, now out dated; however, in selected cases, tissue expansion or serial excisions can be of benefit.

And it is very important to remember: we are still unable to create new hair follicles, so a prerequisite to be a candidate for this procedure is that the patient must have a sufficient supply of donor hair, with a good supply-to-demand ratio. In general, as we age, the area of demand enlarges and the area of supply shrinks.

HAIR FOLLICLE ANATOMY

When we see vertical histologic sections of skin, as in skin biopsies or when checking margins (for completeness of excision of lesions), we see the epidermis, dermis, dermal appendages,

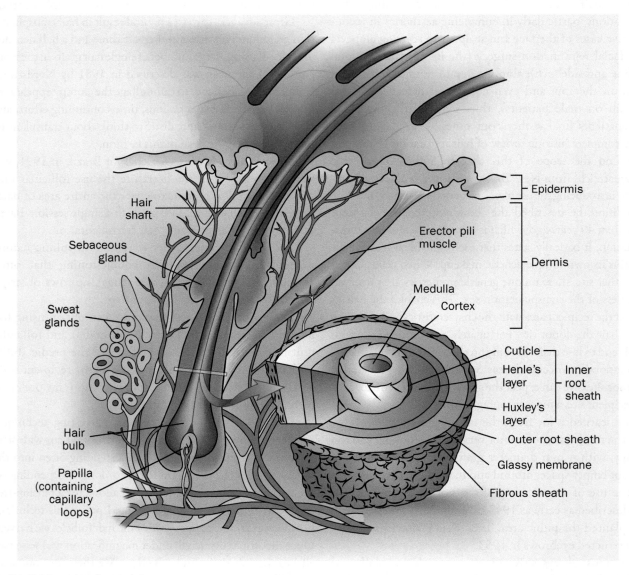

Figure 26.1. Hair transplantation procedure. From Barrera A. *Hair Transplantation: The Art of Micrografting and Minigrafting.* St. Louis, MO: QMP Quality Medical Publishing, 2012; And Second Ed. Alfonso Barrera A, Carlos Oscar Uebel C. *Hair Transplantation: The Art of Follicular Unit Micrografting and Minigrafting,* 2nd ed. St. Louis, MO: QMP Quality Medical Publishing/QMO CRC, 2014.

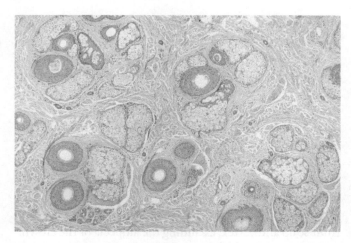

Figure 26.2. Microscopic H & E horizontal section of the scalp to demonstrate how hair grows in follicular units. This section shows several follicular units with varying number of hairs; adjacent to the hair can be seen sebaceous glands, sweat glands, and the piloerectile muscle surrounded by a sheath of collagen.

and subcutaneous fatty tissue (Figure 26.1). These views prevent us from appreciating the fact that hair follicles grow in groups. They grow in follicular units; Headington[4] first described this in his landmark paper in 1984 " Transverse Microscopic Anatomy of the Human Scalp."

There, he states that each "follicular unit" includes 1–4 hairs per unit, each with its own individual sebaceous glands, insertions of erector pili muscles, perifollicular vascular plexus, perifollicular neural net, and perifolliculum circumferential band of fine adventitial collagen that defines the unit (Figure 26.2).

This suggests that a unit is at least to some degree a physiologic entity. Knowing this is very important because, to obtain optimal graft survival and ultimate hair growth, we have learned that it is important to transplant more than just the bare hair shafts. Slightly chubby grafts and follicular unit grafts thrive much better (Figure 26.3).

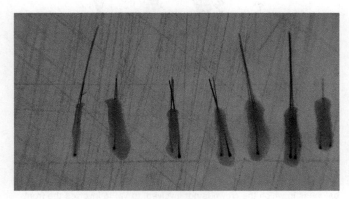

Figure 26.3. Close-up view of dissected follicular unit grafts, from left to right: one-, two-, and three-haired follicular units.

HAIR GROWTH CYCLE

There are four basic phases of hair growth. The living cells at the base of the hair follicle show active mitotic growth. They eventually form a compact column, which extends toward the surface of the skin. A zone of keratinization forms directly above the actively dividing cells. The living cells become dehydrated, eventually die, and are converted into a mass of keratin. The keratin filaments are cemented together by a matrix rich in cystine.

The average rate of growth of scalp hair is about 0.35 mm/day, or about 1 cm/month. The dermal papilla, which is situated just under the actively dividing cells of the follicle, play a very important role in the regulatory control of the hair's growth cycle. The growth cycle phases are as follows:

Anagen: This is the actively growing phase. In this phase, the follicular cells are actively multiplying and keratinizing. In a non-balding scalp, normally about 90% of the hairs are in this phase, which lasts about 3 years.

Catagen: The base of the hair becomes keratinized, forming a club, and separates itself from the dermal papilla. It then moves toward the surface, being connected to the dermal papilla only by a connective tissue strand. This phase lasts 2–3 weeks.

Telogen: Also called *resting phase*. During this phase, the attachment at the base of the follicle becomes weaker until the hair finally sheds. During this period, the follicle is inactive and hair growth ceases. This phase lasts 3–4 months and is very common after hair transplantation. For this reason, we do not see significant growth of the hair grafts until 3–4 months. Additionally, some of the native hair often goes also into catagen and then telogen just from the insult of the surgery. Normally about 10% of hair follicles in a non-balding scalp are in this phase; when the rate of hair loss is greater than the rate of growth, thinning and eventually baldness develops.

The most frequent types of hair loss that I encounter in my practice include:

1. *Male pattern baldness*, being by far the most frequent type, followed by androgenic (pattern) alopecia in females.

2. *Postsurgical alopecia.* This may occur after oncologic resections of the scalp or eyebrows, as well as after facial rejuvenation or craniofacial procedures resulting in loss of sideburns, and frontal, temporal, and/or retroauricular hair loss.

3. *Posttraumatic alopecia.* This includes hair loss due to injuries such as burns and traumatic injuries of the scalp and eyebrows.

4. *Congenital hair loss.* An example is the absence of hair in the prolabium on bilateral cleft lips, and triangular alopecia (triangular area of hair loss in the anterior temporal area).

MPB is basically a gradual conversion of hairs from the terminal (healthy thick) to vellus (clear microscopic) state. It is a hereditary condition that appears to be controlled by a single, dominant, sex-limited autosomal gene.

The expression of this gene is dependent on the level of circulating androgens. The initial signs of thinning clearly correlate with puberty (in males), when the levels of androgens (testosterone) start to rise, gradually converting terminal hair into vellus hair, resulting initially in receding hairlines and, depending on the exact genetic features inherited, may progress to leave only a temporal and occipital fringe.

Testosterone secreted by the testes is the principal androgen circulating in plasma in men, whereas in women the adrenal steroids dehydroepiandrosterone sulfate, androstenediol sulfate, and 4- androstenedione are the most abundant proandrogens.

A proandrogen is a 19-carbon steroid that is converted at the target tissue into active androgen. The enzymatic reduction of testosterone and the listed androgens in the female patient by 5-α-reductase into dehydrotestosterone (DHT) is necessary for the induction of androgenic hair loss both in men and women.

The Norwood classification for MPB is the most commonly seen, going from grade I, the mildest to VII, the most severe (Figures 26.4 and 26.5):

Norwood anterior variant classification involves the front scalp and vertex, excluding the alopecia of the crown.

The keys for a natural result in hair transplantation surgery include:

1. *Small grafts:* 1–2 follicular unit grafts at the front hairline, with 2, 3, or 4 hair follicular unit grafts posterior to that.

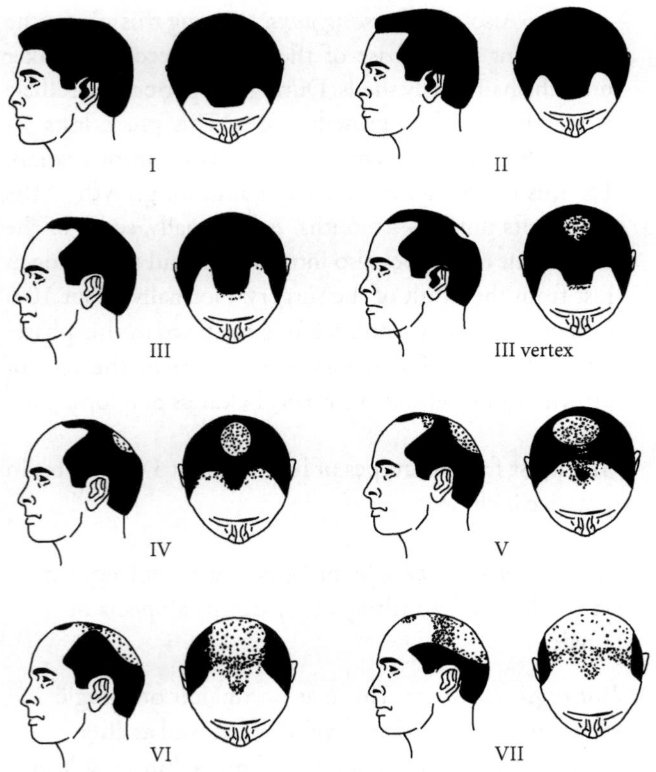

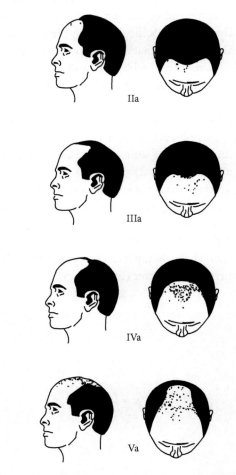

Figure 26.5. Norwood anterior variant. From Ia, which classifies cases of baldness in which the crown is not involved, to Va. Ia involves the front top part of the scalp; numbering increases as the baldness involves the top and extends posteriorly, to Va extending to the crown's anterior boundary.

Figure 26.4. Norwood classification of male pattern baldness (MPB) going from I to VII, with I being the mildest, involving only mild recession of the hairline at the frontotemporal areas, to the VII, the most severe.

2. *Level of the hairline*: There is no magic measurement, the craniofacial proportions vary from person to person, so we must aim for the most aesthetically pleasant level and plan long term (6–9 cm from the eyebrows).

3. *Design*: Slight irregularity is very important to mimic nature.

4. *Density*: We need sufficient density to blend naturally with the neighboring areas, generally a minimum of 70–100 hairs per square centimeter.

5. *Direction of hair growth*: This is very important as well, consistent with residual native hair, particularly at the boundaries of the affected areas (i.e., usually anteriorly at the front hairline at about a 30-degree angle and a slight left or right orientation, sometimes straight upward). On the sideburns and temporal areas, the most optimal direction often is downward, sometimes with a diagonal posterior direction and occasionally an almost straight posterior direction.

6. *Absence of detectable scarring:* Of course, we want no stigma of having had a surgical procedure, with no detectable scarring on the grafted area and only minimal scarring on the donor area. This is accomplished by using ultra-fine blades such as the 15- or 22.5-degree SharPoint blades as we transplant the hair follicular units (Figure 26.9A,B) and doing a slight trichophytic closure of the donor site and closing without tension.

TECHNIQUE

The patient is placed in the supine position, under intravenous sedation with midazolam (Versed) and fentanyl (Sublimaze) and occipital and supraorbital nerve blocks with 0.5% bupivacaine (Marcaine) with epinephrine 1:200,000 (Figure 26.6A–H).

Once the area is locally well anesthetized, we use tumescence infiltration along the donor ellipse. This provides

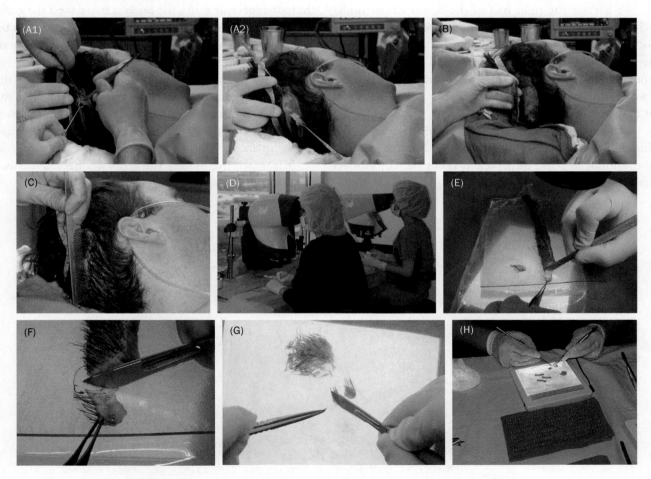

Figure 26.6. (A,B) Harvesting of donor site strip, incising parallel to the hair shafts under 3.5× magnification. (C) Donor site closure, usually without the need to undermine, author uses a continuous running 3-0 Prolene suture. (D) Assistants using the Manthis Microscope (10×) to dissect the grafts. (E–G) Sequence of the dissection, first making slices 1–2 mm thick precisely parallel to the hair shafts; subsequently and with background lighting dissecting the slices into individual follicular unit grafts. (H) The grafts are subsequently lined up in groups of 100 (10 by 10) to keep count of how many grafts are done on each case.

hemostasis, and we believe it assists in the graft dissection. My tumescence solution consists of 120 cc of normal saline with 20 cc of 2% plain Xylocaine, plus 1 cc of epinephrine 1:1,000, plus 40 cc of triamcinolone (Kenalog). The same solution is used to infiltrate both the donor and the recipient areas. By adding Kenalog, we have found significantly less postoperative pain and significantly less postoperative edema.

A horizontal ellipse of scalp is harvested from the occipital area, often extending to the temporal areas, frequently from above the ear on one side to above the ear on the other side.

The ellipse will vary in dimensions depending on the number of grafts planned and the density of the donor site. When planning on 2,000 or more grafts, in my practice, generally, the ellipse will measure 20–25 cm × 1 cm. Always avoid tension at the closure to allow for optimal healing.

Using a no. 10 scalpel blade, incise parallel to the hair shafts.

We harvest the right half of the donor ellipse under 3.5× loupe magnification. Incisions are made precisely parallel to the hair shafts. The plane of dissection is just deep to the hair follicles and superficial enough to avoid injury to significant vessels and sensory nerves, often leaving a little subcutaneous fatty tissues over the galea or fascia.

Usually without the need to undermine, we do a continuous running suture with 3-0 Prolene. Next, the left half of the donor strip will be harvested as our assistants dissect grafts (Figure 26.6D).

Our dissection team starts by processing the donor ellipse into 1.5–2 mm thick slices, parallel to the hair shafts.

Under power of 10× magnification, the initial graft is dissected into thin slivers (1.5–2 mm thick).

With a no. 10 blade and jewelers forceps, the actual grafts are dissected from the slivers. The assistants, under a microscope at 10× magnification (Mantis Microscope), process the donor ellipse into 1.5 mm thick slices and dissect it into follicular unit grafts as the surgeon continues the donor site harvesting and closure. The harvested scalp and all grafts are kept chilled in normal saline until transplanted.

Careful dissection of the thin slices into 1- to 2-hair follicular unit micrografts and 3- to 4-hair follicular unit minigrafts continues and is done with background lighting and using a no. 10 scalpel blade and magnification.

This is the most tedious part of the procedure and one of the most important steps. The grafts obviously need to be handled gently and atraumatically. The darker and thicker the individual hair shafts, the easier it is to dissect the grafts. The ideal grafts have intact hair shafts all the way from the subcutaneous fatty tissue to the scalp surface and contain from one to four hairs each, as they come in nature.

Several hundred grafts will have been dissected at this point. They are lined up in rows on a wet green or blue surgical towel and are now ready for insertion. The process of graft dissection and insertion continues until all the grafts are transplanted.

It is imperative to keep the grafts wet because desiccation damages the hair bulbs.

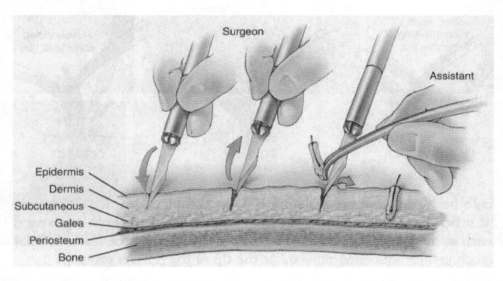

Figure 26.7. Illustration of the stick-and-place technique in which the surgeon makes the recipient site incision and the assistant immediately inserts the graft. From Barrera A. *Hair Transplantation: The Art of Micrografting and Minigrafting.* St. Louis, MO: QMP Quality Medical Publishing, 2012; And Second Ed. Alfonso Barrera A, Carlos Oscar Uebel C. *Hair Transplantation: The Art of Follicular Unit Micrografting and Minigrafting,* 2nd ed. St. Louis, MO: QMP Quality Medical Publishing/QMO CRC, 2014.

GRAFT INSERTION

Infiltration of tumescent solution into the recipient area is important for several reasons, the most important of which is to promote hemostasis and to produce temporary edema of the scalp, which facilitates graft insertion (Figure 26.7).

In a given case, we generally use a total of about 150 mL of tumescence solution throughout the procedure, including in both the donor and recipient sites (Figure 26.8A–D).

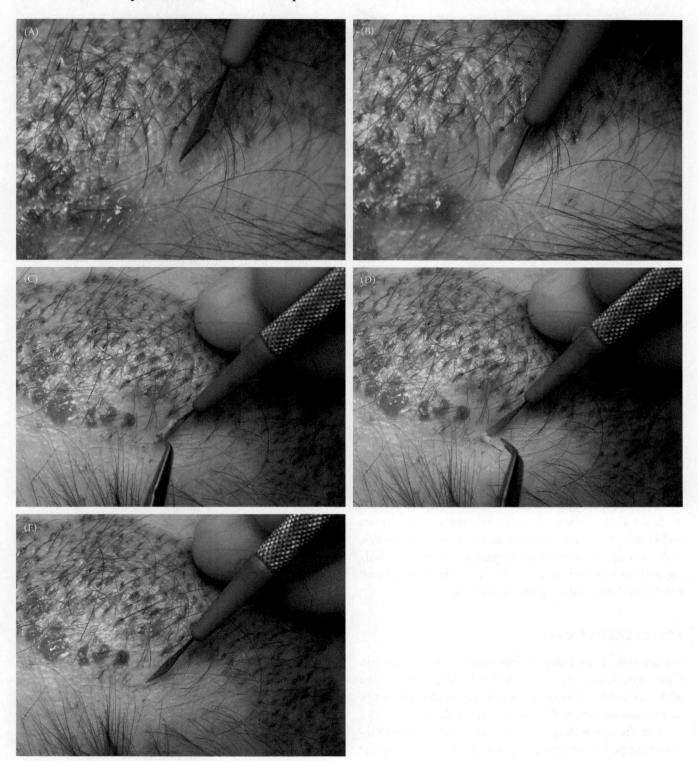

Figure 26.8. (A–D) Demonstration of the stick-and-place technique using 22.5 Sharpoint blade and jeweler's forceps.

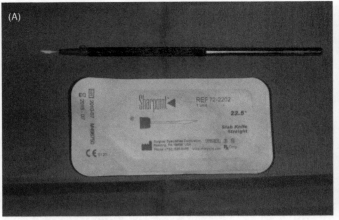
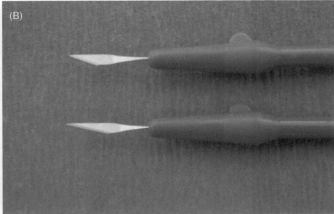

Figure 26.9. Sharpoint blades. (A) A 22.5-degree and (B) a 15-degree Sharpoint blade. The 15-degree blade makes a smaller incision size; the author uses it on the front edge of the hairline.

It is very important to have a good surgical team if these cases are to go smoothly and obtain great results. I have two registered nurses (RNs) and one surgical assistant on my team, with me personally inserting every single graft in all my patients.

One RN under my supervision administers the intravenous sedation (Versed and fentanyl) and circulates, while I harvest the donor strip with the other assistant. I usually see some follow-ups for an hour or so; in the meantime, my other two assistants harvest the grafts. Once they have 500 grafts ready and lined up, we start transplanting them. I am there for every single grafts insertion; I select where the grafts go and incline the blade in the direction I want it to grow. I create the recipient incision, and one of my assistants inserts the graft. This process continues until all the grafts are in. We can't rush it: it usually takes us 4–6 hours, depending on the number of grafts being performed (typically 1,500 to 2,800 per session), depending on the size of the area being grafted and the amount of donor hair available. You can't be in a rush, and we enjoy (my assistants and I) this procedure. The assistants talk while they work, and, if needed, we (including the patient—he or she is only sedated the first hour or two) often will take a short lunch break and then continue grafting until done.

POSTOPERATIVE CARE

For dressing, I use Adaptic impregnated with Polysporin Ointment, Kurlex, and a 3-inch Ace bandage for the first 48 hours. I then allow the patient to gently shampoo daily. The sutures are removed on postoperative day 10.

The aftercare is simple and safe. The main thing is to instruct the patient on being gentle with his or her scalp for the first 2 weeks, after that nothing special is needed, just time. A lot of the transplanted hair will go into telogen (rest phase) and will shed in the first 2–3 weeks; clearly, it is important to make sure the patient understands that. Then, at about 12–14 weeks, it shifts into anagen (growth phase) and the hair begins to grow. By the third to fourth month, it becomes evident that hair begins to grow. Over the next 6–10 months, it gains length and thickness, with the final result usually evident at 1 year postoperatively. Then, if the patient desires greater hair density, additional sessions can be done (Figure 26.10A–J).[5–9]

EXAMPLES

RECONSTRUCTION OF THE LOST SIDEBURN AND TEMPORAL HAIRLINE

Traditionally, facelift incisions can result in a variable degree of cephalic and posterior advancement of the temporal hairline and sideburn, creating an unsightly stigma, a telltale of a poorly performed facelift. These stigmas can predictably and consistently be corrected by the use of modern hair transplantation techniques, specifically follicular unit hair grafting.

It is key to do this in a way that the hair looks natural. To accomplish this, we need very small grafts (single- and double-hair grafts) and have them grow in a consistent and natural direction, downward on sideburns, perhaps in a slightly posterior direction. I initially reported my technique to correct this condition in 1998.[10]

This can effectively remove the stigma (evidence that the patient had a facelift and/or forehead lift procedure), thus complementing immensely the final aesthetic outcome. The objective of this presentation is to briefly describe my personal approach and technique in correcting this condition.

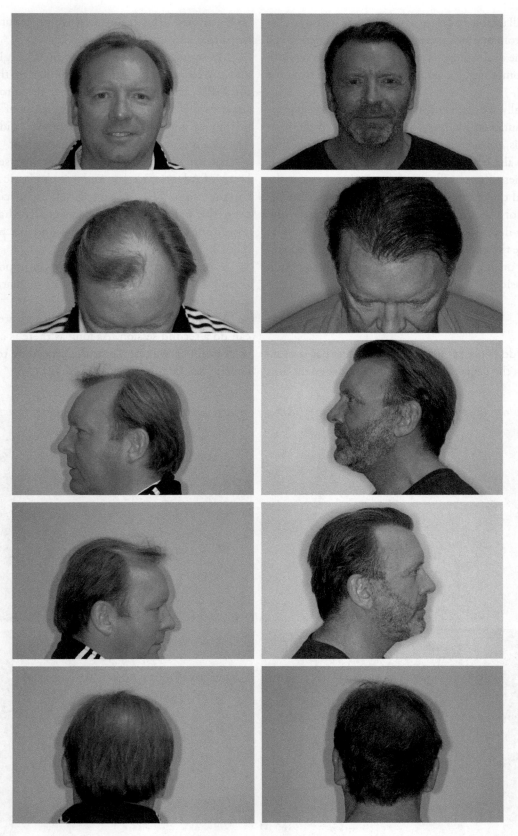

Figure 26.10. 9 year old man with MPB VII, before and then 8 years post operatively after two sessions of Hair transplantation, a total of approximately 5,000 graft, and recent facelift and upper and lower blepharoplasty.

We are still unable to create new hair; we can only redistribute hair from one area to another. So, for a patient to be a candidate, he or she must have enough donor hair to work with. Most commonly, the donor hair is harvested from the occipital area.

Additionally, we often encounter in our practice alopecia of the retro-auricular hairline[11] and elongation of the forehead, which is not uncommon after coronal forehead lifts. Alopecias can also happen after endoscopic forehead lifts.

Most patients have sufficient donor hair to restore the sideburns and the temporal and retroauricular hairline because this is not a large area, but the surgeon must make sure the supply-to-demand ratio is favorable.

Make sure the patient has realistic expectations; explain that it is not uncommon to do a second session to obtain sufficient density.

Technique

We typically do between 300 and 1,500 grafts per session, depending on the degree of alopecia and the size of the area to be covered. This labor-intensive procedure requires an organized and efficient surgical team.

My surgical team consists of three surgical assistants and myself; all steps are quite similar to that described for MPB. The main variant is that this procedure often requires fewer grafts, and the direction of the graft insertion is unique, generally caudally and posteriorly. The idea is to mimic the residual native hair.

For dressings, here, too, I generally use one or two layers of Adaptic, Kerlex, and 3-inch elastic Ace bandage for the scalp. The dressing is left in place for 2 days, then the patient is allowed to gently shampoo daily. The donor site sutures are removed on postoperative day 10.

As in the case of MPB, by the 6 months postoperatively there is a clear and noticeable improvement, and it takes about 1 year for the final result.

At that point, if the patient desires greater density, we can do a second session. As long as there is a good supply of donor hair, we can repeat the procedure to further add density. See (Figures 26.11 and 26.12).

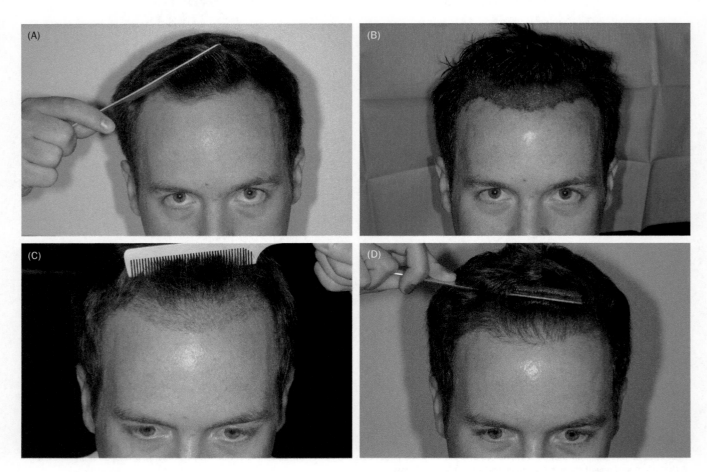

Figure 26.11. (A,B) A 29-year-old patient demonstrates the fast healing and degree of progress early on the postoperative timeline. Shown before, immediately postop, then at 10 days (notice the fast healing), and finally at 6 months postoperatively.

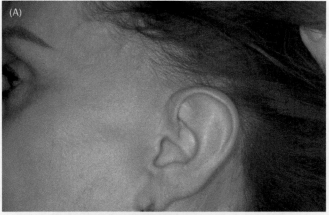

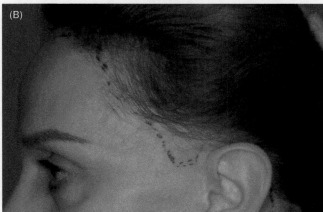

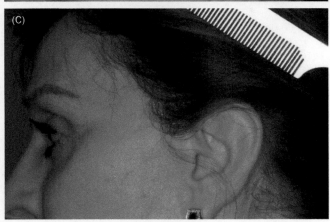

Figure 26.12. (A,B) A 62-year-old woman with scarring alopecia secondary to a facelift procedure. Reconstruction of the sideburn and temporal hairline, before and a year postoperatively.

COMPLICATIONS

Although this is a very safe procedure, minor complications can occur sometimes. The most frequent complication after hair transplantation is *ingrown hairs* and *cysts*. These tend to happen when the grafts are placed too deeply, allowing the recipient scalp to heal on top of the graft and creating

a cyst. When doing 2,000 plus grafts, which is common, you may have just a few that are placed too deeply and that cause this problem. If mild, they are self-resolving, eventually erupting and draining spontaneously, or sometimes requiring a simple squeeze as it matures into a pustule. If deeper, a simple incision and drainage using an 18-gauge needle can be performed.

Widening of the donor site scar is due to tension at the closure and incisions that were not parallel to the hair shafts (resulting in excision of hair roots at the closure). This can usually be avoided by accurate dissection and closure with minimal tension.

Keloids, which are extremely rare, are more likely to occur if harvesting is too caudal (near the lower boundary of the occipital hairline).

CONCLUSION

The use of follicular unit grafts, micrografts, and minigrafts as described is safe and predictable and is very effective in the correction of MPB and female pattern alopecia, including scarring alopecia secondary to facial rejuvenation surgery as well as many other types of scarring alopecias. It results in a great degree of patient satisfaction.

REFERENCES

1. Orentreich N. Autografts in alopecias and other selected dermatological conditions. *Ann NY Acad Sci* 1959;83:463.
2. Nordstrom REA. Micrigrafts for improvement of the frontal hairline after hair transplantation. *Aesthetic Plast Surg* 1981;5:97.
3. Uebel CO. Micrografts and minigrafts: a new approach to baldness surgery. *Ann Plast Surg* 1991;27:476.
4. Headington JT. Transverse microscopic anatomy of the human scalp. *Arch Dermatol* 1984;120:449.
5. Barrera A. Micrograft and minigraft megasession hair transplantation: review of 100 consecutive cases. *Aesthetic Surg J* 1997;17(3):165.
6. Barrera A. Micrograft and minigraft megasession hair transplantation results after a single session. *Plast Reconstr Surg* 1997; 100(6):1524.
7. Barrera A. Refinements in hair transplantation: micro and minigraft megasession. *Perspective Plast Surg.* 1998;11(1):53.
8. Barrera. *Hair Transplantation—The Art of Micrografting and Minigrafting,* 1st edition. Quality Medical Publishing Inc., 2002.
9. Barrera A, Uebel C. *Hair Transplantation—The Art of Follicular Unit Micrografting and Minigrafting.* 2nd edition. St. Louis, MO: Textbook Quality Medical Publishing Inc., 2014. CRC.
10. Barrera A. The use of micrografts and minigrafts for the correction of the post rhytidectomy lost sideburn. *Plast Reconstr Surg* 1998;102(6) 2237–2240.
11. Barrera A. Correcting the retroauricular hairline deformity after face lift. *Aesth Surg J* 2004;24(2) 176–178.

27.

GENIOPLASTY

Leo J. Urbinelli, Ibrahim Khansa, and Mark M. Urata

INTRODUCTION

Genioplasty is a term which refers to the surgical or nonsurgical manipulation of the chin form or the mandibular symphysis. Genioplasty may alter the morphology of the anterior mandible through augmentation, reduction, or asymmetric recontouring. This can be accomplished with autologous techniques (bony reconstruction or autologous fat grafting) or alloplastic techniques (silicone implant or collagen/hyaluronic acid fillers). This chapter focuses on autologous manipulation of the mandibular symphysis through osseous genioplasty.

ASSESSMENT OF THE DEFECT

A thorough history and physical examination of the patient are critical to achieving a satisfactory result that pleases both the patient and the surgeon. It is crucial to ascertain the patient's aesthetic complaints as they relate to their lower face and neck. Take time to specifically evaluate any history of previous orthodontics, orthognathic surgery, facial fillers, and/or facial injuries. Careful examination of the patient's dental occlusion, as well as facial sensation and animation, are always necessary preoperatively. Careful assessment of the facial proportions, including lower facial height, projection, and symmetry, helps the surgeon achieve harmonious results in the osseous genioplasty patient.[1]

Preoperative photography (two- or three-dimensional) and radiographs (posteroanterior and lateral cephalogram with Panorex) are standard in the assessment of the chin deformity. Lateral profile photographs are important in judging the *sagittal position* of the pogonion (anterior-most point on the bony chin) relative to the upper and lower lips and midface. Anterior-posterior photographs are important to assess lower *facial height, width,* and *proportions.*

Preoperative evaluation of the patient's skeletal occlusion is critical to the correct choice of procedure. In a patient with class II skeletal occlusion, a bilateral sagittal split osteotomy, with or without genioplasty, would be indicated.

When considering repositioning the chin point in a sagittal plane, it is useful to utilize the Riedel line, which is a line drawn down through the most prominent points of the upper and lower lips (Figure 27.1).[2] The chin should

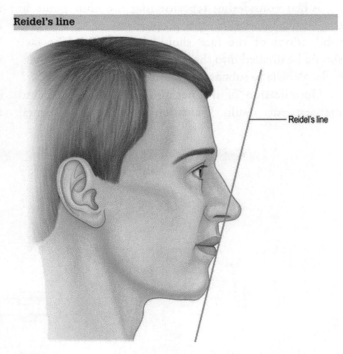

Reidel's line

— Reidel's line

Figure 27.1. Reidel's line connects the most projecting points of the upper and lower lips. The chin should lie on this line. From Guyuron B, Weinfeld AB. Genioplasty, figure 27.13.12. Accessed at https://clinicalgate.com/genioplasty/).

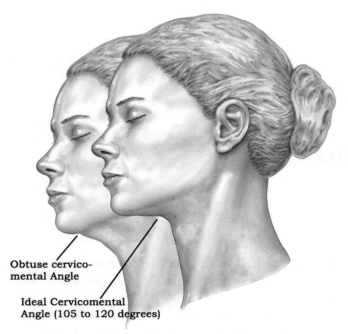

Obtuse cervico-
mental Angle

Ideal Cervicomental
Angle (105 to 120 degrees)

Figure 27.2. Obtuse and ideal cervicomental angles. From Bassichis BA. Neck contouring. *Operat Techn Otolaryngol Head Neck Surg.* 2007;18(3):254–260.

also lie on that line. In general, on lateral profile, the lower lip should lay 2 mm posterior to the upper lip, with the pogonion just slightly posterior to the lower lip in females, and at the same sagittal level as the lower lip in males.

When considering repositioning the chin point in the vertical direction, the proportions of the vertical subdivisions of the face should be assessed. The face should be divided into three equal thirds: trichion to glabella, glabella to subnasale, and subnasale to menton.

Optimization of the neck soft tissues is critical to the aesthetic result. Evaluation of the cervicomental angle (typically 100–115 degrees) is evaluated, and sagittal repositioning of the mandibular symphysis can have dramatic effects in sharpening or blunting this angle (Figure 27.2).

Depth and position of the labial mental fold, best viewed on sagittal photographs, will also impact decision-making when considering sagittal repositioning of the pogonion.[3] Aesthetically, this fold is typically 4–6 mm deep and positioned near the upper third to middle third of the stomion-to-menton distance (Figure 27.3).[4] The depth and height of the labiomental crease should be assessed, and the potential effects of various movements on the crease should be anticipated: moving the chin anteriorly or cephalad deepens the crease, and moving the chin posteriorly or caudad softens the crease.[5]

INDICATIONS

After careful physical examination and assessment of the patient's photos and radiographs, the planned osseous movement of the anterior mandible can be made based on the patient's facial proportions and desired aesthetics. Osseous genioplasty is an excellent operation to (1) correct asymmetries in the symphyseal region of the mandible, (2) vertically augment or reduce the bony mandible, (3) augment a retrogenic mandible in a sagittal plane, or (4) perform a combination of the above movements.

Keep in mind that soft tissue to bony movements tends to harmonize closer to a 1:1 relationship in sagittal advancements and vertical augmentations. In contrast,

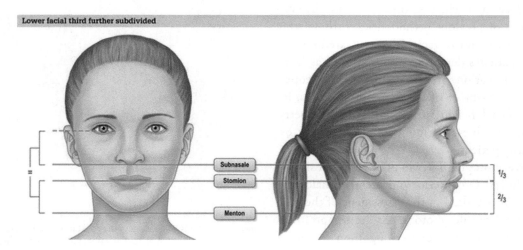

Lower facial third further subdivided

Subnasale

Stomion

Menton

1/3

2/3

Figure 27.3. Aesthetic divisions of the lower third of the face. From Guyuron B, Weinfeld AB. Genioplasty, figures 27.13.10 and 27.13.11. Accessed at https://clinicalgate.com/genioplasty/).

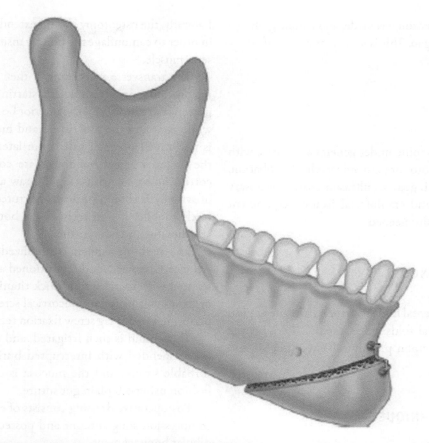

Figure 27.4. A sliding genioplasty where the chin is advanced and vertically shortened. From Baker S, Han K. Genioplasty. In: Taub PJ, Patel PK, Buchman SR, Cohen MN, eds. *Ferraro's Fundamentrals of Maxillofacial Surgery*, 2nd ed. 388, chapter 29, figure 27.29.3.

bony reductions in the vertical and sagittal dimensions do not reduce the soft tissue in such a 1:1 manner and are more challenging to predict.[6]

There are different types of genioplasties, depending on the desired movement[7]:

1. *Sliding genioplasty*: The chin segment is repositioned in any direction while maintaining bony contact with the remaining mandible (Figure 27.4). If two cuts are made, each bony segment can be slid independently. This is known as a *double-step genioplasty* (Figure 27.5).

2. *Jumping genioplasty*: The chin segment is repositioned cranially and anteriorly, so that it is entirely anterior to the remaining mandible.

3. *Reduction genioplasty*: Two parallel cuts are made, and the intervening bone is removed in order to reduce the vertical chin height. To augment the vertical height

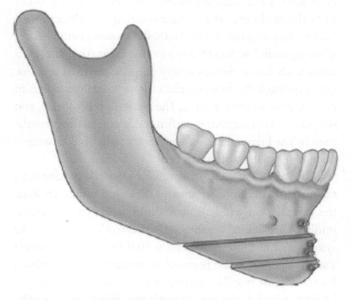

Figure 27.5. Double-step genioplasty. From Baker S, Han K. Genioplasty. In: Taub PJ, Patel PK, Buchman SR, Cohen MN, eds. *Ferraro's Fundamentrals of Maxillofacial Surgery*, 2nd ed. 390, chapter 29, figure 27.29.5.

of the chin, one osteotomy is made, and a bone graft is inserted into the gap. This is known as a *vertical elongating genioplasty*.

ROOM SETUP

The patient is placed supine under general anesthesia with airway maintained via oro- or nasoendotracheal intubation. A handheld reciprocating saw or ultrasonic saw is necessary for the osteotomies, and craniofacial fixation equipment (plates and screws) is also needed.

PATIENT MARKINGS

If changes to the submental fold are planned, the presurgical and planned submental folds are marked. Otherwise, the surgical plan is based upon presurgical photographic and cephalometric data.

OPERATIVE TECHNIQUES

The intraoral mucosa is rinsed with dilute chlorhexidine mouthwash, and the face is prepped with Betadine. A labial buccal sulcus incision is marked. The incision should be at least 4 mm anterior to the attached gingiva in order to facilitate closure. The marked incision is infiltrated with 0.25% bupivacaine with 1:200,000 epinephrine. After allowing sufficient time for vasoconstriction, the incision is made with Bovie electrocautery perpendicular to mucosa. Once through the mucosa, the cautery is straight down to bone, cranial to the mentalis. The mentalis is left intact, and subperiosteal dissection is performed lateral to the mentalis muscle The bilateral mental nerves are visualized, dissected circumferentially, and protected.

The lateral subperiosteal dissection is taken down to the inferior mandibular border. It is important to keep the central chin pad and mentalis attached to the central midline pogonion, creating an inverted-V channel. The symphyseal midline should be scored in order to provide a stable reference. The planned osteotomy is scored with a fissure burr or saw. The course of the mental nerve should be kept in mind: the nerve travels low within the mandibular body before coursing cranially toward the mental foramen. Consequently, the osteotomy should be planned at least 4 mm inferior to the mental foramen. The osteotomy should also be at least 30 mm inferior to the cuspids.

Laterally, the osteotomy should extend to the molar region in order to camouflage the bony transition behind the masseter muscle.

The transverse osteotomy is then carried out using a reciprocating or ultrasonic saw starting laterally and as far posterior as possible on the inferior border of the mandible while guarding the soft tissues and mental nerve. The cut is performed on each side, from lateral to medial. Once the buccal cortical bone cuts are complete, the lingual cortex can be cut with a sagittal saw and the free segment of symphysis should be down-fractured easily and become freely mobile. If not, recheck for bony interferences and attachments and address them.

The free bony segment is mobilized, then, using calipers, advanced, reduced, and repositioned as planned. It is then secured with two 1.0 mm thick titanium angled pre-bent or hand-bent plates and bicortical screws. This can also be performed with a lag screw fixation technique.

The wound is then irrigated, and the mentalis muscle is resuspended with interrupted buried 2-0 braided absorbable suture, and the mucosa is closed in watertight fashion using 4-0 plain gut suture.

Postoperative dressing consists of elastic tape creating a compression sling anterior and posterior to the free mandibular bony segment.

POSTOPERATIVE CONSIDERATIONS

The compression taping remains in place for 3–5 days postoperatively to reduce swelling and ecchymosis. The patient is instructed to avoid pulling down on the lower lip and to maintain a soft diet for 2 weeks. Dilute chlorhexidine mouth rinses are performed twice a day for 2 weeks. Chin anesthesia and paresthesia may last several weeks postoperatively, but are expected to resolve over several months.

CAVEATS

- Examine the occlusion; disguising the malocclusion does not change the skeletal deformity.

- Avoid excessive advancement of the chin; overdoing the sagittal advancement is unattractive.

- Leave a sizable 4–5 mm cuff of mucosa above the buccal sulcus so that reapproximation of these tissues is done easily.

- Avoid overdissection or degloving of mentalis from the central mandible, which can create central soft tissue ptosis and a "witch's chin" deformity.

- Careful osteotomy planning (>4 mm below the mental foramina and 30 mm below the mandibular canine crowns) and soft tissue retraction avoids injury to nerves/teeth.

- Check and recheck that buccal and lingual corticotomies are complete to avoid uncontrolled fractures.

- Permissive hypotension during osteotomies to limit blood loss should be systolic blood pressure (BP) in the 90s and mean arterial BP in the 50s.

- Meticulous closure and resuspension of the mentalis muscle and mucosa are key in avoiding soft tissue ptosis and exposure of hardware.

- Prepare patients for possible postoperative paresthesias; reassure them that nearly all are temporary.

REFERENCES

1. Rosen HM. Aesthetic guidelines in genioplasty: the role of facial disproportion. *Plast Reconstr Surg* 1995;95:463.
2. Guyuron B. *Genioplasty*. Boston: Little, Brown, 1993.
3. Zide BM, Pfeifer TM, Longaker MT. Chin surgery. I. Augmentation—The allures and the alerts. *Plast Reconstr Surg* 1999;104:1843–1853.
4. Michelow BJ, Guyuron B. The chin: skeletal and soft tissue components. *Plast Reconstr Surg* 1995;95:473–478.
5. Guyruron B, Michelow BJ, Willis L. Practical classification of chin deformities. *Aesthetic Plast Surg* 1995;19:257–264.
6. Ferraro JW. Genioplasty. In Evans GRD, ed. *Operative Plastic Surgery*. New York: McGraw Hill, 2000.
7. Baker SB, Genioplasty. In: Weinzweig J, ed. *Plastic Surgery Secrets Plus*, 2nd edition. New York: Elsevier Health Sciences, 2010.

28.

THE AGING NECK

Alan Matarasso and Darren M. Smith

INTRODUCTION

Facelifting is a very common topic in the literature, and the neck is often lifted as a component of facelift surgery. The isolated necklift, however, is less frequently a focus of scholarly attention despite its role as a valuable procedure in the properly selected patient. The neck is generally considered to span from the jawline to the clavicle. Characteristics of a youthful neck have been said to include a well-defined mandibular boarder, a clean sternocleidomastoid border, the absence of jowling, and a cervicomental angle of approximately 105–120 degrees.[1-3]

Signs of aging in the neck often begin to show in the late 30s as the medial platysmal retaining ligaments become attenuated and muscular banding occurs as a result. Other changes of aging include growing prominence of pre- and subplatysmal fat, increasing skin laxity and texture changes, and hypertrophy of the digastric muscles and submandibular glands (which may also become ptotic).

Despite its less prominent role in the literature, the aging neck is a common cause of concern. As we will review here, the aging neck can be dealt with very effectively independently from the face (Figure 28.1). The ability to uncouple neck rejuvenation from facial rejuvenation is fortunate, as the aging of these regions may not coincide or be of equal concern to a given patient.

ASSESSMENT OF THE DEFECT

Several factors contribute to aging the neck's appearance. Each must be considered individually and addressed as appropriate. Skin quality should be assessed independent of skin excess. While excess can be effectively managed with carefully planned vectors of pull and excision, poor skin quality (solar- and tobacco-related changes, certain rhytids) will not be addressed by such maneuvers and necessitate ancillary procedures (peels, laser, etc.).

The presence of subcutaneous and deep fat should be noted and direct excision and/or liposuction should be considered. Deep fat is located in a triangular region defined by the mentum at its apex, the digastric muscles on either side, and the hyoid bone at its base. The deep fat consists of subplatysmal fat and interdigastric fat.

Submandibular gland prominence should be recognized and pointed out to the patient. This prominence may be due to either ptosis or hypertrophy. If not addressed surgically (which we usually do not), ptotic mandibular glands may appear more prominent when the lax surrounding tissues are tightened and the overlying cushion of adipose tissue is thinned. The patient should be advised of this in advance and options discussed.

Finally, the overall appearance of the neck should be considered in relation to surrounding areas (jowls, jawline, midface) to guide any necessary conversations regarding ancillary procedures. Mandible morphology, for example, may favor placement of a chin implant.

PATIENT SELECTION, INDICATIONS, AND CONTRAINDICATIONS

Success in performing a necklift begins with patient selection. To undergo a necklift, patients must accept the necessary incisions, tolerate the recovery period, and understand the relationship between their surgical goals, their anatomy, and the surgeon's ability to reconcile the two. If a patient's goals will not be sufficiently met with an isolated necklift, appropriate ancillary procedures must be discussed. These can range from a facelift to buccal fat pad excision,[4] salivary gland manipulation, or chin implant placement to topical therapies (lasers, peels, etc.). It should be explained

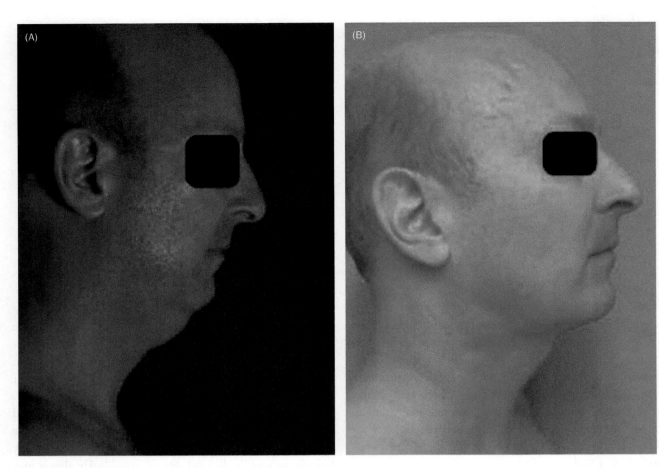

Figure 28.1. Before (A) and after (B) a necklift. Note the clean jawline and the improved cervicomental angle.

to patients that while the nasolabial fold–jowl complex overlaps with the jawline (the most cephalic region treated by a neck lift), an isolated necklift will not completely address this area. Patients that desire neck rejuvenation are favorable necklift candidates if they (1) are not concerned with facial aging, (2) feel their facial aging can be sufficiently treated with nonsurgical modalities, (3) want to avoid a preauricular incision, or (4) are psychologically unable to accept a "facelift."

Contraindications to necklifting are primarily medical in nature and are not different from other major aesthetic surgery procedures.[5,6] Patients with serious comorbidities are not considered for surgery; minor medical problems are optimized and medical clearance is obtained prior to proceeding.

While venous thromboembolism (VTE) is unlikely in the context of a necklift, all generally accepted precautions are taken to avoid this very dangerous entity. These include cessation of all forms of nicotine and female hormone use weeks prior to surgery. Precautions against hematoma formation are taken as well. Factors that might impede normal coagulation (e.g., aspirin and vitamin E) are eliminated,

close attention is paid to hemostasis intraoperatively, and strict control of hypertension is ensured in addition to other measures to reduce hematoma risk.

PREOPERATIVE PLANNING

Once the patient and surgeon have decided to proceed with a necklift, each tissue type (skin, muscle, fat) involved in aging the neck is considered for its role in a given patient's appearance and its amenability to surgical correction. Procedures to rejuvenate the neck represent a cumulative advance up the ladder from liposuction (addresses fat) to submentalplasty (addresses muscle and fat), to full necklift (addresses skin, muscle and fat; the necklift incision is completely postauricular, and addresses the jawline and inferior). An extended necklift (the incision extends slightly cephalically around the lobule and anterior to the ear [Figure 28.2]) allows the jowls to be addressed as well with advancement of the inferior portion of the *superficial musculoaponeurotic system* [SMAS]). A procedure can be downstaged to minimize incision length, discomfort,

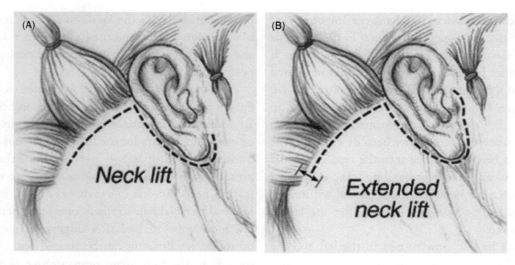

Figure 28.2. The incision for a standard necklift (A) and an extended necklift (B).

recovery, or cost, but the patient must recognize that a "downstaged" procedure will yield a downstaged result. The most extreme form of downstaging, of course, is replacing necklifting altogether with topicals and other nonsurgical options. Tightening energy-based systems, botulinum toxin, and deoxycholic acid may all now offer some degree of neck rejuvenation for the patient who desires improvement while avoiding any form of surgery, but none of these options (together or in combination) will offer results directly comparable to surgical intervention. Ideally, these procedures would be combined to address skin quality (nonsurgical techniques) and skin quantity (surgical interventions).

SURGICAL TECHNIQUE

The operation is performed in an accredited ambulatory operating room with systemic anesthesia administered by

a board certified anesthesiologist. The incisions are marked and wetting solution (1 mL 1:1,000 epinephrine and 100 mL 1% lidocaine in 200 mL of normal saline) is liberally injected. Liposuction is performed as indicated. A 2.4 mm Mercedes cannula is used for neck liposuction, and a 1.8 mm Mercedes cannula is used for jowl liposuction.

Access to the medial borders of the platysma, when required, is achieved via a submental incision caudal or cephalic to the submental skin crease as indicated. The neck is widely undermined with the aid of a lighted retractor in order to identify the medial borders of the platysma and facilitate platysmaplasty, the midline sewing for soft adynamic bands. When redundant medial platysma muscle is present, a strip of excess is excised (Figure 28.3). Conservative subplatysmal fat removal is performed if necessary by either direct excision or melting with ball-tip electrocautery. While deep fat can be safely contoured, if removed, digastric excision and total submandibular gland

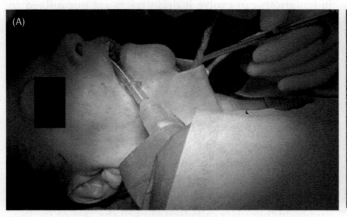
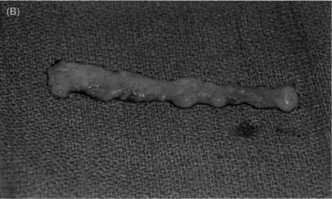

Figure 28.3. Submental access (A) and excision of redundant medial platysma (B).

THE AGING NECK

removal should be considered. A back-cut (myotomy) is made long and low from medial to lateral in the platysma at the level of the cricoid to treat hard dynamic bands. If the muscle can be reapproximated in the midline (based on the extent of separation), it is done with interrupted 3-0 Mersilene sutures (Ethicon, San Lorenzo, Puerto Rico) to achieve a snug, but not tight, approximation. Numerous techniques for platysmal repair have been described.[7,8] The hyoid fascia can be incorporated into the repair with the intention of avoiding recurrent banding.[9] The submental portal is inspected for hemostasis and packed with moist gauze until final inspection and closure after the lateral incisions are closed.

The patient's head is now turned to the left and the right-side necklift incision is performed. The skin flap is widely undermined (usually contiguously with the area undermined via submental access). This dissection proceeds and is completed under direct vision with the scalpel and facelift scissor. The lateral border of the platysma (and lower SMAS in extended neck lifts) identified. If laxity is present, the lateral border of the platysma is undermined and sutured to the sternocleidomastoid (SCM) fascia, avoiding undue tension on the midline platysmal repair. In extended neck lifts, the platysma and lower SMAS are plicated to the SCM fascia at three points to address jowl laxity. Excess skin is redraped, released as necessary from underlying attachments, and excised. The wound is irrigated with the same solution used to infiltrate the skin. Final hemostasis is achieved, a drain (flushed with and soaked in Betadine) is inserted, and the incision is closed. Careful attention is paid to ensure that while redraping and securing the skin the hairline is preserved.

Hair-bearing skin is closed with staples. The region anterior to the drain and between the hair-bearing skin and the postauricular incision is closed with half-buried absorbable mattress sutures. The postauricular crease is closed with 3-0 nylon. A closed-suction drain is placed in the postauricular incision and secured with a suture. The head is turned to the right, and the left side of the necklift is performed. The submental dissection is then inspected for final hemostasis and closed with running deep dermal 4-0 Prolene and simple 5-0 nylon sutures.

DRESSINGS AND POSTOPERATIVE CARE

Antibiotic ointment is applied to all incisions and around the drains. A facelift dressing consisting of three layers of gauze strips covered with a Surginet is placed (Dermapac, Shelton, CT). The dressing and drains are removed on postoperative day 1. The incisions are kept moist with antibiotic ointment during the healing process. The sutures and staples are removed as appropriate during the first 10 postoperative days.

The patient is specifically instructed to avoid neck flexion to minimize the risk of skin flap ischemia. Patients are additionally counseled to refrain from any heavy lifting or strenuous activity for the first 2 weeks and to scale back to normal levels of activity over the third through fourth postoperative weeks. Sun exposure and any topical therapies (facials, peels, etc.) are to be avoided for 2–3 months. Laser removal of facial hair similarly cannot be performed for a few months before and after surgery. Telangiectasias and postoperative bruising can be treated with V-beam laser therapy in the immediate postoperative period. Patients should be inspected frequently for fluid collections, skin ischemia, or other healing issues. Firm subcutaneous areas may be apparent during recovery and can be gently massaged, injected with intralesional steroids, or treated with ultrasound.

Close follow-up is essential in identifying and treating complications. Small, nonexpanding hematomas can be managed outside the operating room. In a sterile environment, the hematoma is suctioned via the necklift incision while the area is irrigated. Gentle pressure is applied. This process is repeated until the suctioned fluid is sufficiently clear.[10] Large or expanding hematomas must be treated emergently in the operating room with wide exposure, ideal lighting, and appropriate instrumentation. When suspicion is sufficiently high, bleeding disorders can be considered and worked up accordingly.

Seromas must be aggressively tapped in a sterile fashion as unresolved seromas can lead to bursa formation and long-term unsightly contour deformities. Small fluid collections can be particularly annoying. They should be serially aspirated until completely resolved. Similarly, indentations can evolve if drain tracts are not milked to empty them of fluid.

Infections are infrequent but must be promptly treated with appropriate antibiotics to minimize the development of potentially severe sequelae, including tissue necrosis. Should skin ischemia occur, the first step in management is to identify and treat reversible causes such as fluid collections, infection, or tension. Dimethyl sulfoxide or nitroglycerine ointment or even hyperbaric oxygen may be utilized in an attempt to mitigate damage to threatened skin.[11] If frank necrosis evolves, standard wound management strategies apply (watchful waiting with local wound care including silver sulfadiazine until the area of involvement is clearly demarcated). Reconstruction as indicated

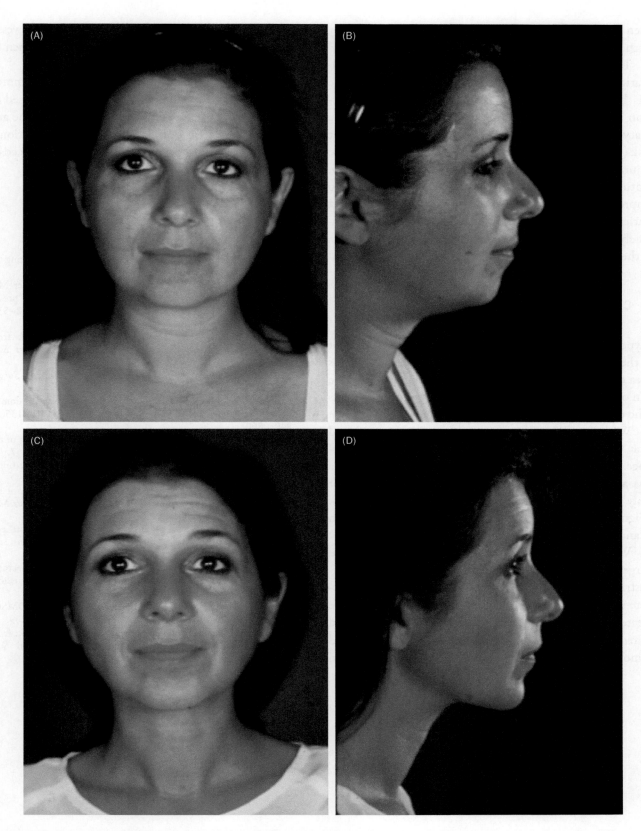

Figure 28.4. Preoperative views (A,B) and postoperative views (C,D) in a patient whose microgenia was addressed with a chin implant and necklift.

then follows. Bovie burns to the skin flaps, should they occur, are treated like tissue ischemia.

There is less risk of facial nerve injury with this operation than in facelifts. The marginal mandibular nerve has been postulated to be compromised from liposuction in the jowl area or subplatysmal dissection. Midline platysmal manipulation can put the cervical branch at risk (especially in secondary interventions). Most of these injuries will resolve spontaneously in 6 months to 1 year. Botulinum toxin can be used on the unaffected side to improve symmetry. Similar management as in facelift patients is advised. Sensory nerve disruption occurs routinely and is self-limiting. Great auricular nerve trauma is the most common nerve injury in necklift procedures.

CAVEATS

Hypertrophic scarring and ischemia are most likely to occur at the apex of the postauricular incision, and tension in this area especially is to be avoided. Midline skin compromise can occur in patients with deep skin creases or in patients who do not hyperextend the neck postoperatively.

With regard to chin implants, patients are advised that the necklift will dramatically improve chin appearance. Chin augmentation is indicated if chin hypoplasia has always been a concern and this appearance did not only evolve secondary to changes of the aging neck (Figure 28.4), though the neck improvement alone can dramatically enhance the appearance of microgenia.

While some authors advocate extensive subplatysmal surgery, in our hands, the submandibular glands and digastric muscles are not routinely resected. In cases of severe submandibular gland hypertrophy, the glands can be treated with botulinum toxin. If the submandibular gland is resected, this is achieved by entering the capsule and removing the inferomedial portion along a caudal and tangential plane, exercising caution to avoid the large vessel in the mid-portion of the gland. The area should then be drained.

Recurrence of platysmal bands is likely more common than thought. This frustrating condition can be caused by "accordioning" of lateral platysma toward the midline and can be managed with botulinum toxin or reoperation.[12] "Bowstringing" of the operated platysma can be reduced by the triangular wedge excision described earlier.

REFERENCES

1. Ellenbogen R, Karlin JV. Visual criteria for success in restoring the youthful neck. *Plast Reconstr Surg* 1980;66:826–837.
2. Greer SE, Matarasso A, Wallach SG, Simon G, Longaker MT. Importance of the nasal-to-cervical relationship to the profile in rhinoplasty surgery. *Plast Reconstr Surg* 2001;108:522–531; discussion 532.
3. Matarasso A. Managing the components of the aging neck: from liposuction to submentalplasty, to neck lift. *Clin Plast Surg* 2014;41:85–98.
4. Matarasso A. Managing the buccal fat pad. *Aesthetic Surg J* 2006;26:330–336.
5. Matarasso A, Smith DM. Combined breast surgery and abdominoplasty: strategies for success. *Plast Reconstr Surg* 2015;135(5): 849e–860e.
6. Matarasso A, Smith DM. Strategies for aesthetic reshaping of the postpartum patient. *Plast Reconstr Surg* 2015;136(2):245–257.
7. de Souza Pinto EB. Importance of cervicomental complex treatment in rhytidoplasty. *Aesthetic Plast Surg* 1981;5:69–75.
8. Ellenbogen R. Pseudo-paralysis of the mandibular branch of the facial nerve after platysmal face-lift operation. *Plast Reconstr Surg* 1979;63:364–368.
9. Yousif J, Matloub H, Sanger J. Hyoid suspension of the platysma: a novel technique for the aging neck. *Plastic Reconstr Surg* 2014;133(4):976
10. Baker DC, Chiu ES. Bedside treatment of early acute rhytidectomy hematomas. *Plast Reconstr Surg* 2005;115:2119–2122; discussion: 2123.
11. Young VL, Boswell CB, Centeno RF, Watson ME. DMSO: applications in plastic surgery. *Aesthet Surg J* 2005;25:201–209.
12. Matarasso A. Managing the components of the aging neck: from liposuction to submentalplasty, to neck lift. *Clin Plast Surg* 2014;41(1):85–98.

PART VI.

RECONSTRUCTIVE FACIAL SURGERY

29.

EYELID RECONSTRUCTION

Seanna R. Grob, Don O. Kikkawa, and D. J. John Park

INTRODUCTION

Eyelid reconstruction is necessary if eyelid defects or eyelid malposition is present. Eyelid defect reconstruction is most commonly necessary after severe trauma to the periocular area or excision of a benign or malignant eyelid lesion. Less commonly, encountered defects may be from congenital eyelid deformities, such as colobomas. With varied sizes of eyelid defects that result from tumor excision, whether by conventional excision or with Moh's micrographic surgery, it is important to be comfortable and flexible with the available options for eyelid reconstruction. Many surgical techniques and procedures have been described for eyelid reconstruction over the years. This also is true for procedures that correct eyelid malposition, such as ptosis, retraction, entropion, and ectropion. Entire textbooks are written on details regarding evaluation and repair of eyelid malposition. The goal of this chapter is not to exhaust all available options but to present some of the more common approaches to eyelid reconstruction and provide the tools for evaluating and planning defect repair.

RECONSTRUCTION OF EYELID DEFECTS

PATIENT EVALUATION

Evaluation of any patient should include a thorough clinical and medical history and complete examination. If the patient presents with trauma, then a thorough trauma survey should take place, and trauma to the globe should be ruled out or addressed before any eyelid reconstruction. Mechanism of injury is also important as a projectile injury might raise concern for an orbital or intraocular foreign body. If the patient presents with an eyelid or periocular tumor, then a thorough history about duration, growth, ulceration, pain, sun exposure, and history of cancer should be elicited. It

also is important to identify certain factors that may impede wound healing, such as history of smoking. Random flaps should be employed more judiciously in patients with known wound healing problems, such as chronic smokers and those with collagen vascular disease. A medication list is important to review as well for use of anticoagulants. Cessation of anticoagulants and antiplatelet agents in preparation for surgery should be coordinated with the patient's primary physician or cardiologist.

An individual's ophthalmic medical history is also important to consider in surgical planning. Monocular patients would be ill-served by a staged procedure in which the seeing eye is obstructed by a flap, as is the case in the Hughes's tarsoconjunctival flap procedure.

A patient's age and social situation may also play a role in the planning process for repair. Older and more infirm patients, who do not have the constitution to undergo a long surgery, may be better served by reconstructive options that require shorter anesthesia time. One-stage procedures, even if it comes at the expense of optimal surgical outcome, may be a better option for these individuals. If patients are homeless, then there may be a greater concern for follow-up or wound infection, which also might alter the surgical plan.

Planning for repair should begin during the initial examination. The surgeon can evaluate the size of an eyelid tumor and attempt to predict the size of the possible defect after excision. The eyelids should be everted to avoid missing a hidden mass underneath the eyelid or extension of a mass. The type of lesion also dictates the extent of the excision and therefore the reconstructive options as well. Benign lesions with a low rate of local recurrence can be excised with little surrounding normal tissue. Lesions that are more locally aggressive, tend to recur frequently, and those that are malignant necessitate wide local excision with a generous margin of normal tissue. Microscopic control of the margins is crucial to ensure complete excision of lesions. This can be achieved by frozen section analysis of the margins. An initial incisional or shave biopsy may suffice for large lesions in which the clinical diagnosis is uncertain, while excisional biopsy may be more appropriate for smaller lesions. Another option to maintain microscopic control of the margins is to coordinate the surgical care with a Mohs micrographic surgeon.

Assessment of the patient's face as a whole is also important. Excess skin or skin laxity may be of benefit in reconstruction. Dermatochalasis, or redundant upper eyelid skin, may be useful if a skin graft is needed in the periocular area. Patients may have scars from previous excisions, which may be a sign of a lack of skin laxity. Patients may also have evidence of diffuse sun damage, and skin grafts may need to be harvested from alternate areas with less sun exposure.

Imaging may be necessary in the setting of trauma or tumor. Malignant lesions associated with stigmata of orbital extension, such as fixation to the underlying periosteum or involvement of the forniceal or bulbar conjunctiva should be evaluated with computed tomography (CT) and/or magnetic resonance imaging (MRI) scans. If there are signs of restriction of extraocular muscle movements or proptosis or patients are complaining of double vision, then imaging is recommended. In the setting of trauma, if there is concern for an open globe, orbital fractures, or orbital or intraocular foreign body, then CT imaging is recommended. MRI should be avoided in the setting of trauma before an orbital or intraocular metallic foreign body is ruled out.

ASSESSMENT OF THE DEFECT

A defect-oriented approach should be performed with eyelid reconstruction. The location and extent of the defect after trauma or following excision of a lesion should be delineated. Reconstruction differs based on location of the defect, whether it is upper or lower eyelid, or if there is medial or lateral canthal involvement. Assessment of the eyelid defect should also include evaluation of the anterior (skin and orbicularis oculi muscle) and posterior (tarsus and conjunctiva) lamella, eyelid margin, lacrimal drainage system, canthal tendons, levator aponeurosis, and eyelid retractor muscles. One must determine which anatomic parts are missing prior to planning a reconstruction. The margins of full-thickness defects may be grasped with small skin hooks or toothed forceps and pulled together to assess the possibility of direct closure or desired tightness of the eyelid margin and the necessary size of any indicated flaps or grafts.

For both the upper and lower eyelids, defects in the medial eyelid may involve the lacrimal drainage apparatus, which may require a more complex reconstruction. Defects in the lateral eyelid may involve a disruption of the lateral

canthal tendon and result in rounding of the lateral commissure unless the eyelid is reattached or re-suspended laterally.

The upper eyelid covers the majority of the eye including the cornea. Deficiencies in the upper eyelid result in loss of its protective nature to the globe, which is essential to preserve vision. Roughness or scarring on the palpebral conjunctiva, exposed sutures, or misdirected eyelashes can cause irreversible damage to the cornea and vision loss. The same can also be true for the lower eyelid.

Casual inspection of the defect will result in an overestimation of the defect due to retraction and shortening of the remaining segments. This necessitates the measuring of the horizontal defect under some tension. For patients who have undergone Mohs surgery, during initial evaluation of the defect, the two ends may be pinched toward each other to assess the laxity of the remaining segments and to assess the actual size of the defect. Intraoperatively, this may be more precisely achieved by grasping the two ends with forceps and bringing the ends toward each other.

Defects involving the eyelid margin require special attention, as the reconstructed eyelid should have a smooth marginal contour and not be irritating to the ocular surface. This is best achieved when the defect can be reapproximated primarily. When the horizontal extent of the defect is less than 25%, it can be reconstructed primarily. In elderly individuals with increased horizontal laxity, 30–40% of defects can often be closed primarily. When this is not feasible, a variety of techniques may be employed to reconstruct the eyelid margin.

While the lines of maximum extensibility are oriented vertically, the eyelids will tolerate only a moderate amount of tension perpendicular to the eyelid margin. This is particularly true of the lower eyelids. Thus, wound or flap tension should be directed parallel to the eyelid margin, when possible, to avoid secondary deformity or lower eyelid ectropion or retraction. Additionally, elective incision lines and closure lines should be placed along natural periocular contour lines to diminish visible scarring whenever possible.

Healing by secondary intention is useful in selected nonmarginal periocular defects.[1] Medial canthal defects evenly distributed above and below the medial canthal tendon are particularly well-suited for spontaneous closure. Very superficial defects along the eyelid margin may also heal by granulation with acceptable results.

INDICATIONS

Traumatic periorbital tissue loss and eyelid defects encountered in the management of periorbital skin cancer

TABLE 29.1 SOFT TISSUE REPLACEMENT TECHNIQUES

Full thickness eyelid flaps
Anterior lamellar flaps or grafts
Posterior lamellar flaps or grafts

are the most common indications for eyelid reconstruction. Congenital anomalies, such as eyelid colobomas; burns; necrotic skin infections; and complications after medical or surgical interventions may require eyelid reconstruction as well. The primary goal of reconstructive surgery is to reestablish functional eyelids that protect the ocular surface and the patient's vision, with a secondary goal of normal to satisfactory aesthetic appearance. Reconstructive techniques depend on the soft tissue that needs to be replaced—full-thickness eyelid defects, anterior lamella (skin and muscle), and posterior lamella (tarsus and conjunctiva) (Table 29.1 and Figure 29.1)

Nonmarginal partial-thickness eyelid defects that are not amenable to direct closure may require development of a local flap for repair. A skin or myocutaneous advancement flap is indicated in pretarsal and preseptal defects, particularly in the eyebrow and medial eyelids. Because of the generous vascular supply of the eyelids, tissue defects ranging up to 10 cm² have been reconstructed with this technique. The rhombic flap and its variants are versatile transposition flaps for the primary repair of medial canthal and lateral periorbital quadrangular or circular defects. A lateral transpositional skin flap is another useful technique in the repair of defects in the area of the lateral canthus involving aspects of both the upper and lower eyelids. If structural support is required, this flap may be used in combination with a periosteal flap or a tarsoconjunctival flap.

The technique chosen to repair full-thickness eyelid defects is based on the size of the defect. Similar techniques can be used for small to medium defects of the upper and lower eyelids, although different techniques are necessary for large and total defects of the upper and lower eyelid. Tables 29.2 and 29.3 provide surgical algorithms based on the size of the eyelid defect.

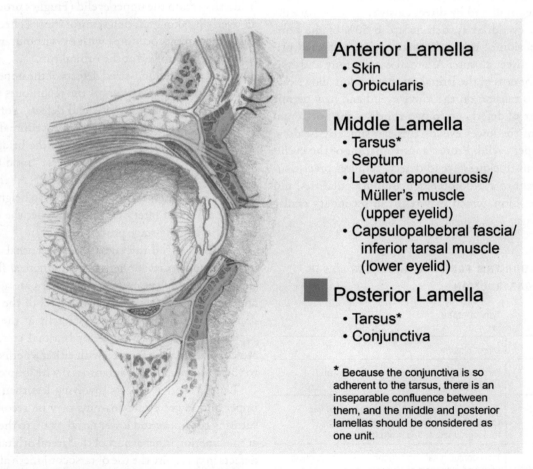

Anterior Lamella
- Skin
- Orbicularis

Middle Lamella
- Tarsus*
- Septum
- Levator aponeurosis/ Müller's muscle (upper eyelid)
- Capsulopalpebral fascia/ inferior tarsal muscle (lower eyelid)

Posterior Lamella
- Tarsus*
- Conjunctiva

* Because the conjunctiva is so adherent to the tarsus, there is an inseparable confluence between them, and the middle and posterior lamellas should be considered as one unit.

Figure 29.1. Sagittal cross-section of the upper and lower eyelids. Deficiency in the middle lamella will cause eyelid retraction, whereas deficiencies in the anterior and posterior lamella will produce ectropion and entropion, respectively.

TABLE 29.2 ALGORITHM FOR FULL-THICKNESS UPPER EYELID RECONSTRUCTION

Size of upper eyelid defect	Type of repair
<25%	Direct closure
25–50%	Direct closure with lateral canthotomy and cantholysis and/or semicircular flap
25–75%	Tarsoconjunctival graft and skin-muscle flap, or semicircular flap with periosteal flap or tarsoconjunctival flap or graft, or tarsal rotation flap with skin-muscle flap
50–100%	Tarsoconjunctival flap (Cutler-Beard or Reverse modified Hughes) and skin graft

Even though vascularized flaps are generally superior to tissue grafts in the eyelids for the same reasons as they are in other parts of the body, grafts also play an important role in eyelid reconstruction (Table 29.4). In cases with full-thickness eyelid repair, at least one of the reconstructed lamella should have a vascular supply.

Closure of lower eyelid margin involving defects that are less than 25–33% of the horizontal length of the eyelid is usually accomplished by direct closure. In older patients with greater eyelid laxity, defects up to 50% of the horizontal dimension of the eyelid may be reconstructed primarily with direct closure. A lateral canthotomy and lysis of the inferior crus of the lateral canthal tendon allows closure with less tension on the lower eyelid and may permit direct closure of defects up to two-thirds of the horizontal dimension of the lower eyelid. This can similarly be done with the upper eyelid. Proper approximation of the eyelid margin in full-thickness eyelid defects requires precise suture placement to avoid notches, margin irregularities, and eyelid malposition, which may result in secondary ocular surface damage.

TABLE 29.3 ALGORITHM FOR FULL-THICKNESS LOWER EYELID RECONSTRUCTION

Size of upper eyelid defect	Type of repair
<25%	Direct closure
25–50%	Direct closure with lateral canthotomy and cantholysis
25–80%	Tarsoconjunctival graft and skin-muscle flap, or semicircular flap +/-periosteal flap or tarsoconjunctival flap or graft
50–100%	Tarsoconjunctival flap (Hughes tarsoconjunctival flap) and skin graft or Mustardé flap

TABLE 29.4 GRAFTS FOR EYELID RECONSTRUCTION

Skin (full-thickness)	Upper eyelid > retroauricular > preauricular > supraclavicular > inner arm[a]
Tarsus	Superior two thirds of the tarsal plate of the upper eyelid, ear cartilage, hard palate mucosa, nasal septal cartilage
Conjunctiva	Bulbar conjunctiva (superior), oral mucous membrane, amniotic membrane

[a] Level of tissue preference from most preferred to least.

Three techniques that are useful in reconstructing defects of 33–66% of the horizontal dimension of the eyelid are the lateral semicircular rotational flap or Tenzel flap, the sliding tarsoconjunctival flap, and the free autogenous tarsoconjunctival graft. Procedures that are widely used in the reconstruction of temporal lower eyelid defects include tarsoconjunctival flaps for the posterior lamella combined with a semicircular rotational flap for anterior lamella replacement.

Reconstructive options for defects of more than 66% of the lower eyelid include a sharing tarsoconjunctival bridge flap from the upper eyelid (Hughes procedure) with an overlying skin graft or a semirotational cheek rotational flap (Mustardé procedure) with or without an underlying periosteal flap hinged at the orbital rim.

Small and medium-sized defects of the upper eyelid may be repaired using variations of the techniques described in the reconstruction of lower eyelid defects. For large upper eyelid defects, a lower lid–sharing procedure developed by Cutler and Beard or modifications of the bridge-flap technique may be performed.[2,3] A "reverse" modified Hughes procedure has recently been advocated.[4,5] Alternatively, if a remnant of superior tarsus that is 3 mm in height remains, it may be advanced inferiorly to reconstruct the upper eyelid margin in a single-stage procedure.[6]

Closure of full-thickness medial canthal defects may be initiated by developing tarsoconjunctival flaps in both the upper and lower eyelids. These flaps are advanced and attached to the periosteum at the level of the desired medial canthal tendon, which is generally at the level of the superior aspect of the posterior lacrimal crest. The tarsal attachments may be secured with either a permanent suture to the periosteum or by a transnasal wire loop or miniplate.

Lateral canthal defects involving less than 30% of the upper and lower eyelid margins may be reconstructed by suturing the upper and lower tarsal plates to the periosteum at the superior, inner aspect of the lateral orbital rim. Larger defects may require the use of tarsoconjunctival flaps. A vertical strip of tarsus can be rotated horizontally and sutured to the periosteum, or a strip of periosteum from the lateral orbital rim can be swung over to attach to the residual tarsal plate. Either flap may then be covered by a transpositional skin flap from the temporal region. If the lateral orbital periosteum is absent, a drill hole may be placed at the desired site of attachment and the tarsal flap anchored to the lateral orbital wall with a nonabsorbable suture.

Canalicular lacerations may occur with tumor resection or trauma. The goal of repair is internal splinting of the torn canaliculus to maintain patency of the remaining lacrimal drainage system. Both bicanalicular and monocanalicular intubation techniques with a Crawford lacrimal intubation set are useful in canalicular reconstruction.[7-9]

CONTRAINDICATIONS

Reconstructive options should take into consideration the age of the patient (e.g., obstruction of the visual axis in children under age 7 years may result in deprivation amblyopia; absence of eyelid laxity in young people hinders reduction of defect size by simple stretching), visual status (e.g., different techniques for only-seeing versus non-seeing eye), preexisting ocular conditions (e.g., corneal surface disease, dry-eye state, glaucoma), and periocular status (e.g., cranial nerve VII dysfunction, previous irradiation or surgery, scars).

PREOPERATIVE PLANNING AND ANESTHESIA

Most eyelid surgery can be performed with local (subcutaneous and subconjunctival) and topical anesthesia with or without intravenous sedation. Topical anesthesia is achieved by instilling proparacaine 1% solution or tetracaine 0.5% solution, a longer acting agent. A small cotton pledget moistened with a 4% solution of topical lidocaine may be applied for improved conjunctival anesthesia or prior to a subconjunctival injection of local anesthesia.

Infiltrative anesthesia is performed with a 30-gauge, 27-gauge, or 25-guage locking needle on a 3–10 cc syringe, taking care to minimize injection pressure. The point of the needle should always be directed away from the patient's eye, in case the needle becomes inadvertently ejected or the patient suddenly moves. Local anesthesia often includes a combination of the following: 1–2% lidocaine +/− epinephrine, 0.25–0.75% bupivacaine, and sodium bicarbonate. Saline-diluted or bicarbonate-buffered local anesthetic can help provide a more pain-free injection, as this method normalizes the pH of the anesthetic and lessens the burning sensation. The senior surgeon prefers a 1:1 mixture of 1% lidocaine with 1:100,000 epinephrine and 0.25% bupivacaine with 1:100,000 epinephrine. Local anesthesia is given after preoperative marking of the patient. Microsurgical instruments should be selected to ensure atraumatic tissue manipulation. Common suture and needle selections are listed in Table 29.5.

The Betadine should be diluted with equal parts sterile saline in the periocular area and on the ocular surface. Sterile balanced salt solution (BSS) is used after the procedure to rinse any remaining Betadine out of the eyes as this can cause a corneal epitheliopathy that can be very uncomfortable for the patient. If a full-thickness skin or cartilage graft is anticipated, the necessary donor site should be inspected, prepared, and draped in the appropriate manner before commencing surgery.

Adequate intraoperative protection of the globe is essential. Artificial tears or BSS should be frequently dropped on the cornea throughout the operation to prevent dryness and corneal abrasions. Protective plastic corneal shields may be lubricated with an ophthalmic ointment and inserted like a contact lens to facilitate globe protection during reconstruction. A malleable retractor can be used to protect the globe when using sharp instruments near the eye as well. Periocular suture knots should be externalized away from the corneal surface, and suture tails are often tied down away for the eye. If this is not possible, softer braided sutures (polyglactin or silk) may result in less ocular surface trauma than more rigid monofilament sutures (nylon or polypropylene).

TABLE 29.5 COMMON SUTURE SELECTIONS IN EYELID SURGERY

Location	Suture choice
Eyelid skin, full-thickness skin grafts	6-0 fast-absorbing plain gut; 6-0 nylon or polypropylene
Subcuticular	6-0 polypropylene
Subcutaneous	4-0 or 5-0 or 6-0 polyglactin
Eyelid margin	6-0 or 7-0 polyglactin or silk
Tarsus	5-0 or 6-0 polyglactin (spatulated needle)
Conjunctiva	6-0 or 7-0 plain gut or chromic gut or polyglactin
Canthal tendons	4-0 or 5-0 Mersilene, polyglactin (half-circle needle), or polypropylene
Lacrimal canaliculi	Crawford silicone tubes; 7-0 or 8-0 polyglactin (pericanalicular tissue)
Levator aponeurosis	5-0 or 6-0 nylon, polypropylene, silk, or Mersilene

SURGICAL TECHNIQUES FOR PARTIAL-THICKNESS DEFECTS

LOCAL SKIN FLAPS FOR PARTIAL-THICKNESS EYELID DEFECTS

Rhomboid Transposition Flaps

Rhomboid flaps are useful in the periocular area, especially in the medial and lateral canthal areas.[10-12] The goal in flap development in these areas is preventing distortion of the eyebrows, eyelid margin, and canthal angles. The key in preventing eyelid malposition after reconstruction with flaps is keeping the vector of tension parallel to the eyelid margin. If the tension is perpendicular or vertical, then ectropion or retraction can result as the wound contracts.

Convert the defect into a rhombic shape with internal angles of 60 or 120 degrees by drawing lines tangential to the defect.[13] (Figure 29.2A), In the periocular area it is important to orient the rhombic flap to place the tension of the donor site closure parallel to the eyelid margin (vertically oriented scar) in order to minimize the chance of eyelid malposition—deformation of the canthi, free eyelid margin, or eyebrow. Mark a line from the center of the 120-degree angles equal in length to the sides of the defect and bisecting the angle. Draw another line, equal in length to any side, at 60 degrees from the end of the extended diagonal in both directions parallel to the rhombic-shaped defect. Of the four potential three-sided flaps, only two flaps exist whose diagonals (lines of closure) are in line with the lines of maximum extensibility for lateral defects or parallel to the eyelid margin for central defects. Proper orientation hides the dipper-shaped scar, places the donor site's tension of closure parallel to the eyelid margin, and minimizes trap-door lymphedema. The flap is elevated and the surrounding area undermined (Figure 29.2B,C). It is then transposed into the defect, and the donor site is closed after wide undermining (Figure 29.2D). The flap is closed in two layers (Figure 29.2E). Closure of the flap in younger patients without skin laxity may produce dog ears, which usually flatten by 6 weeks after surgery or may be excised in standard fashion.

Glabellar or Forehead Transposition Flaps

A glabellar or forehead transposition flap is similar to a typical rhomboid flap and is used commonly for medial canthal partial-thickness defects or medial upper eyelid defects.[13-15] The triangular flap is directed vertically in between the eyebrows with the apex pointing toward the hairline[13] (Figure 29.3A,B). Deep fixation sutures may be necessary to recreate the medical canthal concavity.

Rectangular Advancement Flap

The initial operation begins with conversion of a round to a square defect. A single or a double rectangular flap as wide as the defect is advanced horizontally in the eyelid.[13] The flap's base may be designed slightly wider than its distal portion to maximize the blood supply and to decrease hooding of the skin. The flap usually consists of skin and orbicularis muscle and is created by extensive undermining just anterior to the orbital septum. If the defect is at the medial canthus, deep fixation there helps to recreate the medial canthal concavity, and crossing the apex of the canthal bowl should be avoided as this can prevent webbing and distortion of the concavity. Excision of each Burrow's triangle (lateral to the flap's base) aids in aligning the flap and adjacent wound margins for a smooth closure. The wound is usually closed in two layers.

Blepharoplasty Transposition Flap

A blepharoplasty flap can be created from excess upper eyelid skin with an attachment at the lateral canthal angle.[13] This flap can then be transferred to a defect of the lower eyelid as either a cutaneous or musculocutaneous flap.

FULL-THICKNESS SKIN GRAFT FOR PARTIAL-THICKNESS EYELID DEFECTS

Full-thickness skin grafts can be used for partial-thickness eyelid defects with loss of the anterior lamellae. A well-vascularized wound bed is necessary for graft take. A skin graft for the lower eyelid is ideally taken from excess upper eyelid skin. Alternatively, a graft can be harvested from the retroauricular, preauricular, supraclavicular, and inner arm skin. These areas should be assessed during the clinical exam prior to reconstruction to determine the most ideal location. The defect should be measured. The skin graft should be somewhat larger than the defect to account for primary contracture. The lower eyelid should then be put on traction with a Frost suspension suture prior to measuring the defect, and the graft should be secured with a bolster or pressure patch.

If a full-thickness skin graft is needed for the upper eyelid, the most ideal skin is from the contralateral upper eyelid. The graft should include the entire pretarsal area from the lid margin just superior to the lash line to the eyelid crease. Similar to the lower eyelid, a reverse Frost suture and bolster or pressure patch should be placed over the graft.

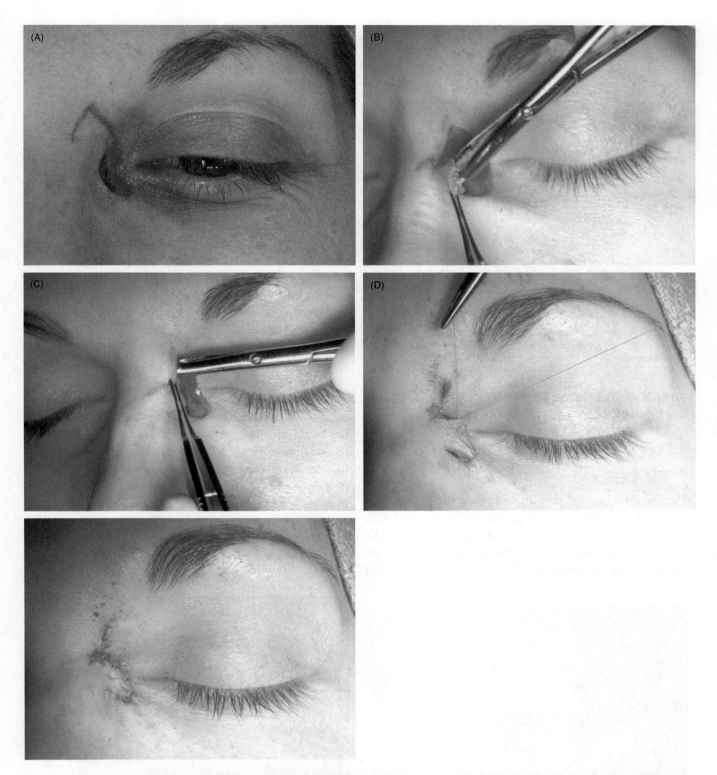

Figure 29.2. (A) Planned rhomboid (Limberg) flap for reconstruction of a left medial canthal defect not involving the canaliculus, medial canthal tendon, or eyelid skin. Bilobed flaps may also be used for larger defects to distribute the tension and transposition across two lobes. If the defect spans both the lateral nasal wall and the medial eyelids, these flaps from the glabella can be combined with horizontal eyelid advancement flaps. (B) The flap is undermined in the subcutaneous plane. (C) A sufficient area around the defect should be undermined to allow for approximation of the edges under minimal tension. (D) Several subcutaneous interrupted 5-0 or 6-0 polyglactin sutures are placed to secure the flap after it has been transposed to fill the defect. (E) The skin edges are then reapproximated, then closed with a fine absorbable or nonabsorbable suture of the surgeon's preference.

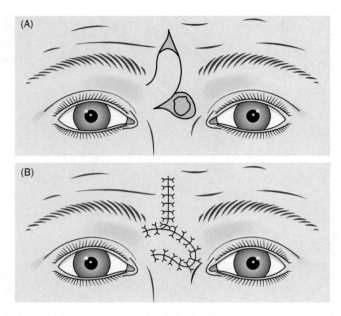

Figure 29.3. (A) Orientation and creating of glabellar flap to fill medial canthal defect. (B) Appearance after transposition of the flap and layered closure.

SURGICAL TECHNIQUES FOR FULL-THICKNESS EYELID DEFECTS

DIRECT CLOSURE

Direct Closure

Defects involving less that 25% of the eyelid margin may be closed primarily.[13,16] With preexisting horizontal laxity, upward of 40% can be closed primarily (Figure 29.4A). Care should be taken to ensure that the edges of the margin are sharp and perpendicular (Figure 29.4A). In cases of

reconstruction following Moh's resection, the edges often need to be recut to produce the sharp, perpendicular edge required at the margin. Reapproximation produces a Burrow's triangle inferiorly, which can be excised inferiorly or with a subciliary incision.

The margin must be reapproximated such that the lash line, gray line, and the mucocutaneous junction line up. One method of accomplishing this involves placement of 2–3 interrupted or vertical mattress 6-0 silk or polyglactin sutures at the margin—at the gray line and the anterior and posterior lash line (Figure 29.5). The suture ends are kept long and subsequently secured under interrupted cutaneous sutures anteriorly and inferiorly so as not to irritate the eye. The mattress sutures can help produce the subtle eversion of the edge necessary to avoid secondary notching. Polyglactin sutures are absorbable, which is an advantage in the young population who may not be able to cooperate for suture removal. Chromic sutures have also been used with the sutures tails cut short (Figure 29.6). With traction applied via the marginal sutures, two partial-thickness interrupted 5-0 or 6-0 polyglactin sutures on spatulated needles reapproximate the tarsal edges (Figure 29.7A,B). This is crucial as tarsal sutures provide the most tensile support to the closure. The overlying skin is then closed with interrupted or running 6-0 fast-absorbing plain gut sutures incorporating the suture tails from the eyelid margin (Figures 29.8 and 29.9) If the lesion is just along the lid margin, then an incision can be made along the upper eyelid crease in the upper eyelid and subciliary in the lower eyelid to redrape the skin and address the dog ear deformities for the best cosmetic result.

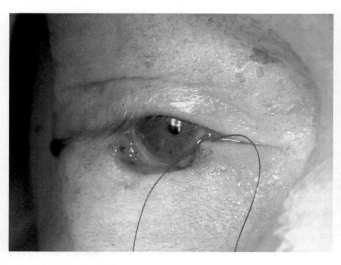

Figure 29.4. (A) Full-thickness pentagonal defect involving just over 25% of horizontal dimension of the lower eyelid. In this case, a lateral canthotomy/cantholysis was performed to recruit additional horizontal length.

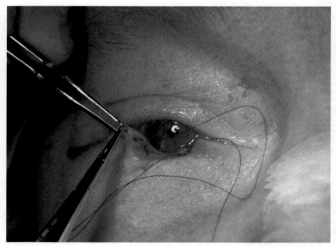

Figure 29.5. A single interrupted 6-0 silk suture is placed at the gray line and left long for use as traction. The margin edges should line up in three dimensions once the suture is secured. An additional suture is placed at the posterior lash line after the tarsal sutures are placed.

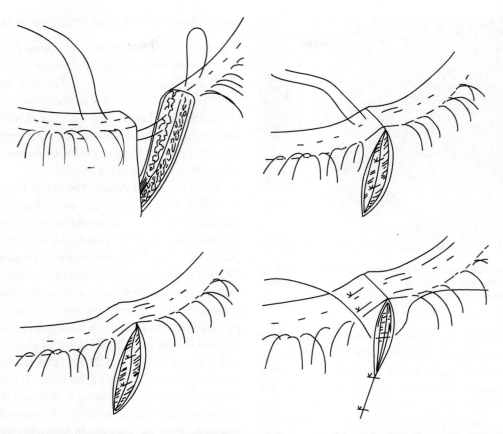

Figure 29.6. Method for direct eyelid margin closure. Two interrupted 6-0 chromic gut sutures (or 6-0 or 7-0 polyglactin or silk) can be placed as a vertical mattress stitch at the gray line and posterior lash line to evert the edges of the lid margin. With secondary wound contraction, the eversion settles down to create a smooth contour. Chromic gut sutures can be cut short, as shown in the figure, but traditionally the suture tails are left long and incorporated into the skin sutures to be directed away from the ocular surface.

Lateral Canthotomy and Cantholysis

With defects involving up to 50% of the central lower eyelid margin that cannot be closed primarily, a variety of approaches may be undertaken to provide additional horizontal length to allow closure of the defect.[17,18] Initially, a lateral canthotomy and cantholysis can be done to provide additional horizontal length to allow for primary closure of the defect (Figure 29.9). A slightly superiorly inclined

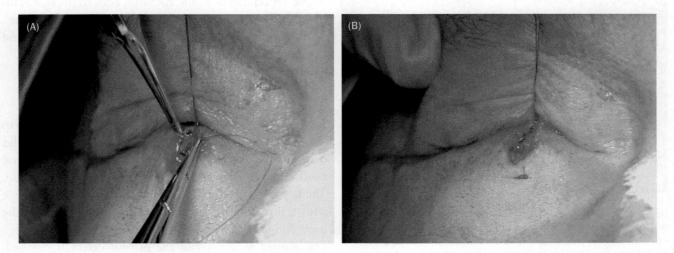

Figure 29.7. (A,B) The tarsus is reapproximated with 1–2 partial thickness interrupted 6-0 polyglactin sutures on a spatulated needle. For analogous defects involving the upper eyelid, three such sutures should be placed to account for the taller tarsus.

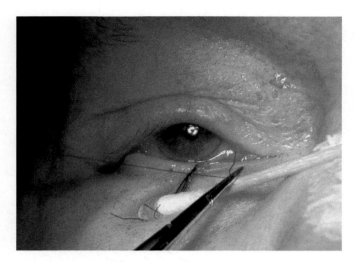

Figure 29.8. The ends of the two 6-0 silk sutures at the margin are trimmed after being folded away from the globe and tied into the knot of a third 6-0 silk suture placed at the anterior lash line.

incision is made from the lateral commissure laterally about 5–8 mm in length through the orbicularis. The canthotomy is performed by dividing the lateral canthal tendon in line with the horizontal axis of the palpebral fissure to isolate the lower lateral canthal tendon from the upper. The cantholysis is accomplished by inserting one blade of a tenotomy or Stevens' scissors under the conjunctiva and the other between the orbicularis and the lateral canthal tendon and then severing the connection. This can also be accomplished with monopolar cautery. This can be done for both the upper and lower eyelid.

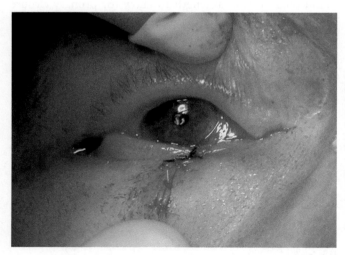

Figure 29.9. The remaining skin defect can be closed with a fine absorbable or nonabsorbable suture. If a dog-ear is present, a Burrow's triangle can be excised. In corresponding defects of the upper eyelid, the dog-ear can be managed by making horizontal relaxing incisions at the upper eyelid crease, medially and laterally, forming a 'T' with the vertical closure.

Lateral Semicircular Rotational Flap or Tenzel Flap

Defects of up to 50% of the horizontal extent of the eyelid that cannot be bridged by canthotomy and cantholysis alone may be closed with a Tenzel lateral semicircular flap[19] (Figure 29.10). This is really the workhorse for reconstruction of lateral eyelid defects of both the upper and lower eyelid. It can be combined with periosteal flaps and tarsoconjunctival flaps or grafts for reconstruction of both the anterior and posterior lamellae.

For lower eyelid defects, the flap is designed to arc superiorly in a semicircular line from the lateral commissure.[17,19] The diameter of the arc should be roughly twice the extent of the defect. The flap is undermined in the suborbicularis plane to allow rotation medially (Figures 29.10A and 29.11). The flap must be done in conjunction with lateral canthotomy/cantholysis for complete release of the eyelid (Figure 29.11). Once the flap is rotated medially in order to provide horizontal length to the lower eyelid, the curvilinear incision should straighten out with a Burrow's triangle at its end (Figures 29.10B and 29.12). This can then be excised in the usual fashion. The marginal defect is closed as described earlier (Figure 29.12). Several deep interrupted absorbable sutures are placed to secure the rotated flap in its new position. The final scar lies in line with the rhytids of the orbicularis muscle, with good aesthetic outcomes (Figure 29.13). The lateral canthus of the upper eyelid is secured to the flap to reconstruct the lateral canthal angle. There must be sufficient tension in the final reconstructed eyelid to maintain apposition to the globe and prevent laxity. In instances in which the Tenzel flap appears markedly thinner than the native eyelid or if additional structural support is needed, a periosteal flap from the maxillary process of the zygoma may be elevated and secured to the posterior aspect of the Tenzel flap or to the cut tarsal edge to provide additional bulk (see lateral canthal anchoring, described later). The conjunctival defect is allowed to re-epithelialize and heal by secondary intention.

McGregor Z-Plasty Flap

A McGregor Z-plasty flap is similar to a semicircular flap and is used for reconstruction of full-thickness lower eyelid defects.[13,20] The flap is also done in conjunction with lateral canthotomy/cantholysis for complete release of the eyelid. The flap is designed starting from the lateral canthal angle with a line directed superiorly and ending lateral to the brow with a Z-plasty fashioned laterally. The flap is elevated and rotated medially and the margin defect is repaired. The triangles from the Z-plasty are transposed as the flap is

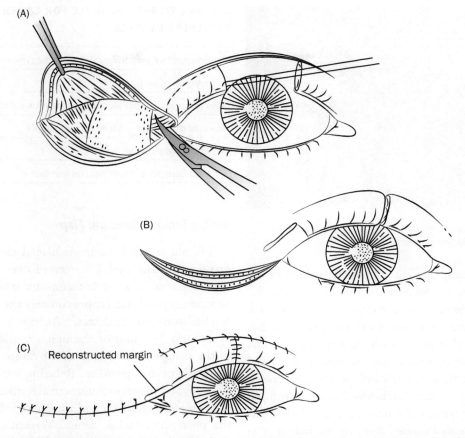

Figure 29.10. For upper eyelid defects, the Tenzel flap is designed with the arc curving inferiorly. For corresponding defects of the lower eyelid, the arc should curve superiorly. (A) The flap is undermined in the suborbicularis plane. A complete upper lateral cantholysis is required for maximal mobilization into the defect. (B) The flap is rotated into the defect medially. (C) The eyelid margin is closed primarily, as described previously, and the donor site closed with simple running or interrupted sutures. The flap should be secured to the periosteum at the lateral orbital rim and the commissure redefined with a single 6-0 plain gut suture. Because the Tenzel flap tends to be thinner than the eyelid margin, it can be combined with a periosteal flap to add bulk in the posterior lamella.

rotated medially. The lateral canthus of the upper eyelid is secured to the flap to reconstruct the lateral canthal angle in a similar fashion to that with the semicircular flap. The flap is closed with superficial and deep sutures.

Semirotational Cheek Advancement Flap: Mustardé

The Mustardé semirotational cheek flap can be helpful for reconstructing large, nasal, lower eyelid defects.[21–23] A semicircular flap is developed beginning at the lateral

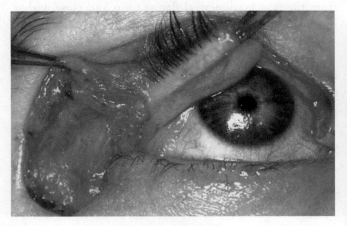

Figure 29.11. Right upper lid defect between 25% and 50% of the lid margin. A Tenzel semicircular flap elevated and lateral canthal tendon transected. Note medial distraction of the eyelid with disinsertion of the canthal tendon.

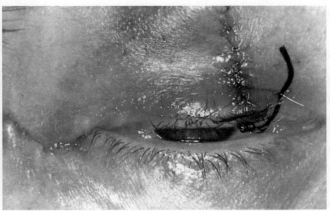

Figure 29.12. Appearance immediately following reconstruction of the lid margin and closure of the lateral canthal defect.

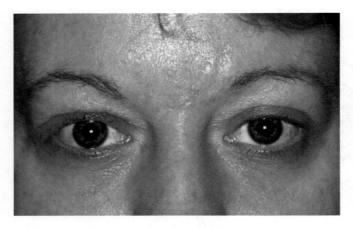

Figure 29.13. Appearance several months later, following right upper lid reconstruction with Tenzel semicircular flap.

TABLE 29.6 TISSUE AVAILABLE FOR LOWER EYELID POSTERIOR LAMELLA

Tarsoconjunctival graft from upper eyelid (has mucous membrane lining)
Autologous ear cartilage
Autologous hard palate mucosa (has mucous membrane lining)
Acellular crosslinked collagen dermal matrix
Nasal chondromucosal
Intraoral lower lip or cheek mucous membrane

canthus, curving gently upward at least to the level of the brow, and extending to the area anterior to the auricular tragus.[21] The cutaneous flap is completely undermined, taking care to maintain hemostasis and avoid the branches of the facial nerve that lie beneath the superficial fascia. If posterior lamellae reconstruction is necessary, a nasal chondromucosal graft, auricular cartilage graft, free tarsal graft, or sharing tarsoconjunctival bridge flap can be sutured to the remaining conjunctival mucosa, using 6-0 plain gut suture, with the mucosal surface abutting the bulbar conjunctiva and inferior cornea. The rotational cheek flap is mobilized to fill the anterior lamellar defect. The dermis of the flap is anchored to the external aspect of the lateral orbital rim periosteum with two or three 4-0 non-absorbable sutures. The lateral canthus is reformed by suturing the dermis of the cheek flap and the lateral aspect of the chondral graft/tarsus to the periorbita just inside the lateral orbital rim. The tarsus or the posterior lamellar graft is sutured to the posterior aspect of the rotational flap at the new lower eyelid margin, using a running 6-0 or 5-0 plain gut suture. The wound is closed in two layers. It is often necessary to excise redundant skin at the lateral edge of the flap.

POSTERIOR LAMELLAE RECONSTRUCTION

Posterior lamellar reconstruction requirements are different in the upper compared to the lower eyelid. In the upper eyelid, the posterior lamellae is touching and rubbing directly against the cornea, so a much softer, smooth epithelial surface is required to avoid corneal damage.[6,13,24] This is not the case for the lower eyelid that is often away from the cornea and does not require a mucous membrane surface in reconstruction. The tissue available for reconstruction of the posterior lamella for the upper (Table 29.6) and lower (Table 29.7) eyelids is listed below.

Sliding Tarsoconjunctival Flap

A 4-0 silk traction suture is placed through the eyelid margin, and the eyelid is everted over a Desmarres retractor. Tarsal relaxing incisions are made to fashion an adequately sized flap (approximately the width of the defect) adjacent to the defect.[25] At least 2 mm of the lower eyelid and 3–4 mm of the upper eyelid tarsus adjacent to the margin is left intact at the donor site to maintain eyelid shape and position. Relaxing incisions should extend beyond the tarsoconjunctival border. Elevate the flap with careful dissection and transpose it horizontally into the posterior lamellar defect. Vertical overcorrection is desirable since the flap frequently settles postoperatively, creating an eyelid margin depression. Suture the free edges of the tarsal flap to the tarsus at the edges of the defect as described for direct closure. For lesions near the lateral canthus, it may be necessary to suture the flap to the periosteum of the lateral orbital rim or remnants of the lateral canthal tendon. The flap should have good apposition to the globe. The anterior lamella is reconstructed with a full-thickness skin graft or an advancing myocutaneous flap. Recess the skin graft or myocutaneous flap 1 mm from the tarsoconjunctival flap margin and close with a running 6-0 plain gut or fast gut stitch.

TABLE 29.7 TISSUE AVAILABLE FOR UPPER EYELID POSTERIOR LAMELLA

Conjunctival or tarsoconjunctival flap/graft from lower eyelid (has mucous membrane lining)
Free tarsoconjunctival graft from contralateral upper eyelid
Buccal mucous membrane graft
Sliding upper lid tarsoconjunctival flap
Hard palate mucosa
Nasal chondromucosal

Free Autogenous Tarsoconjunctival Graft

To harvest a free autogenous tarsoconjunctival graft, the upper eyelid or contralateral upper eyelid can be used as a donor site.[26,27] The upper eyelid is everted over a Desmarres retractor with a 4-0 silk traction suture. A full-thickness tarsal incision, equal to the length of the recipient defect, is made parallel to the eyelid margin, leaving 3–4 mm of intact tarsus along the entire eyelid margin. Vertical tarsal cuts to the upper border of the tarsus complete the tarsal incisions. The levator aponeurosis is dissected off the anterior surface of the tarsal plate, and the graft is excised at its conjunctival attachment superiorly. The donor site is not closed. The donor tarsoconjunctival graft is positioned in the recipient defect and sutured to the conjunctiva of the fornix with 6-0 mild chromic or plain gut sutures and to the host tarsus with 6-0 polyglactin partial-thickness sutures. For upper eyelid defects, the levator aponeurosis is attached to the donor tarsus. The anterior lamella is reconstructed with a vertically advancing or transpositional myocutaneous flap. A bipedicle skin–muscle flap from the superior defect margin is useful for large defects of the upper eyelid. Recess the myocutaneous flap 1 mm from the tarsoconjunctival graft margin and close with a running stitch. The donor skin–muscle defect can be closed with a full-thickness skin graft if necessary.

A Hewes-Beard Flap

A Hewes-Beard flap is a tarsoconjunctival transposition flap from the upper lid that can be used to bridge lateral lower eyelid full-thickness defects greater than 10 mm horiztontally[28] (Figure 29.14). It is an axial flap based laterally on the superior palpebral arcade and transposed to

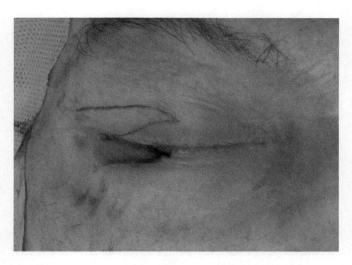

Figure 29.15. The anterior lamella is reconstructed with a Tripier flap, which is a myocutaneous transposition flap from the upper eyelid.

the lateral lower eyelid for reconstruction of the posterior lamella. The skin flap, such as a Tripier flap, is marked (Figure 29.15). The Hewes-Beard flap is marked over an everted upper eyelid (Figure 29.16). The horizontal extent should just bridge the defect, as measured with lateral traction on the residual eyelid. The superior limit of the flap should be approximately 2 mm superior to the upper border of the tarsus centrally in order to ensure inclusion of the superior vascular arcade. As in the Hughes's flap, 3–4 mm of tarsus should be left in the upper lid adjacent to the margin to prevent notching or instability of the upper eyelid. The flap is elevated and dissected laterally, taking care not to disrupt the vascular arcade (Figure 29.17). It can then be transposed inferiorly and the

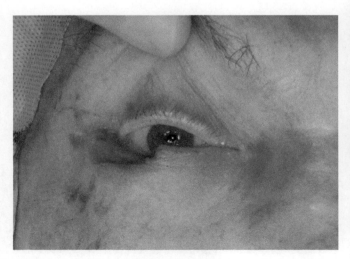

Figure 29.14. Full-thickness defect of the right lateral lower eyelid including the canthus with no residuum of eyelid laterally.

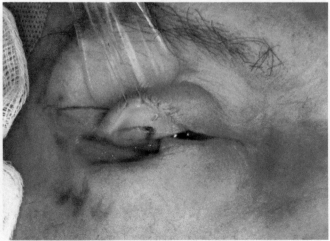

Figure 29.16. The posterior lamella is reconstructed with the Hewes flap, a tarsoconjunctival transposition flap with a laterally based pedicle. At least 4 mm of vertical tarsal height should remain in the upper eyelid centrally.

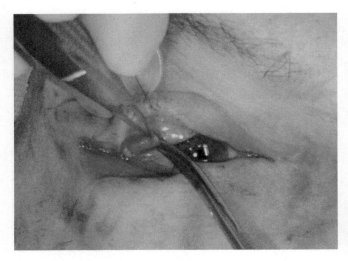

Figure 29.17. The flap is elevated with sharp dissection, taking care to preserve its laterally hinged base.

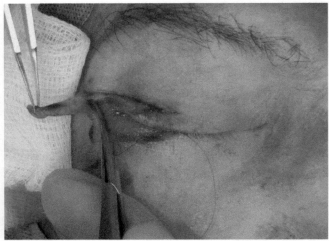

Figure 29.19. The Tripier flap is then elevated in the suborbicularis plane.

edges of the recipient and donor tarsus secured to the recipient bed (Figure 29.18). Although the Hewes-Beard flap has a more robust vascular supply than the periosteal flap, it does not have enough inherent perfusion to support a full-thickness skin graft. Therefore, the anterior lamella is usually reconstructed with a modified Tripier flap from the upper eyelid (Figures 29.19–29.21) or semicircular flap.

Lid-Sharing Tarsoconjunctival Bridge Flap: Hughes Procedure

Large defects, greater than 50%, of the lower eyelid margin require a different approach to reconstruction of the

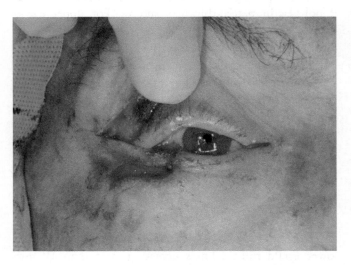

Figure 29.20. The Tripier flap is trimmed and transposed to fill the cutaneous defect. The skin can be closed with fine absorbable or nonabsorbable sutures. A single interrupted 6-0 plain gut suture is used to define the new lateral commissure.

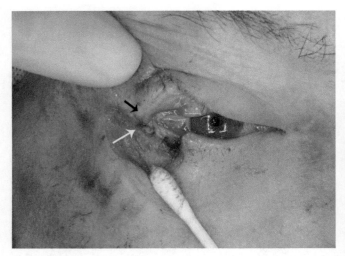

Figure 29.18. The flap is secured to the recipient defect with 5-0 or 6-0 Vicryl sutures. To reconstitute support laterally, the Hewes flap is secured to the remnant of the lateral canthal tendon (*white arrow*). A thin bridge of conjunctiva from the lateral upper eyelid should be de-epithelialized (*black arrow*).

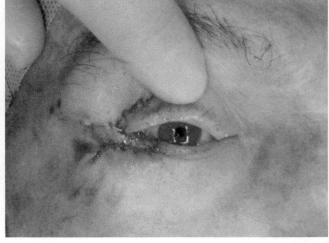

Figure 29.21. Appearance immediately following reconstruction with Hewes tarsoconjunctival flap.

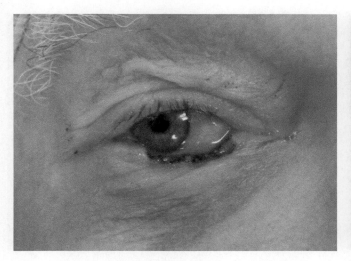

Figure 29.22. Hughes Stage I. Full-thickness defect of the lower eyelid involving well over 50% of its horizontal limit. The canthal tendons and canaliculus are intact.

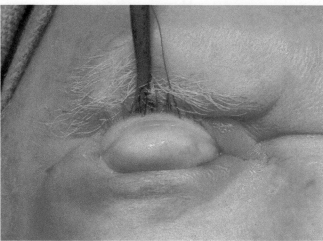

Figure 29.23. A 4-0 silk suture is placed at the upper eyelid margin for traction. The conjunctival surface of the tarsus is exposed by everting the upper eyelid over a Desmarres retractor.

anterior and posterior lamellae of the eyelid (Figure 29.22). This is accomplished by the use of two separate flaps: a tarsoconjunctival flap to reform the posterior lamella and a full-thickness skin graft or a local flap for the anterior lamella. One of these flaps must bring its own vascular supply in order to support the other flap.

The Hughes's flap is a tarsoconjuctival flap advanced from the upper eyelid.[29] Wendell Hughes initially described the procedure in 1937.[29] The transverse tarsal segment of the flap is connected at its base to the forniceal conjunctiva, whence it gets its blood supply. Once advanced inferiorly, it provides conjunctiva and tarsus necessary to fill the lower eyelid defect. The resulting bridge of conjunctiva occludes the visual axis. At 6–12 weeks, this conjunctival bridge can be severed in a second-stage operation. A full-thickness skin graft may then be used to reconstruct the anterior lamella. Medial and lateral periosteal flaps may be needed to tether the tarsoconjunctival flap in complete defects of the lower eyelids.

The horizontal dimension of the Hughes's flap may be determined by measuring the residual defect once the two marginal edges are drawn together. A 4-0 silk traction suture is placed at the gray line of the upper lid and the eyelid is everted over a Desmarres retractor (Figure 29.23). The exposed tarsal conjunctiva is dried and a transverse mark is made parallel to the margin, 4 mm superior to it. At least 3–4 mm of tarsus must be left undisturbed so as to avoid upper eyelid notching and other contour abnormalities. The transverse incision is made just through the tarsus, slightly shorter than the measured horizontal defect, and over the central aspect of the tarsus where it is tallest (Figure 29.24). Vertical incisions are made at the flanking ends of the

transverse incision, and the tarsal flap is elevated sharply. Dissection is then carried superiorly to separate the conjunctiva from the Müller's muscle (Figure 29.25), which is quite adherent to the conjunctiva. Gentle hydrodissection with sterile saline on a 30-gauge needle between the conjunctiva and Mullers muscle makes dissection in the plane significantly easier. As the dissection is carried superiorly, relaxing vertical incisions in the conjunctiva should be made to the fornix (Figure 29.26). These incisions should splay outward slightly, such that the base is wider than the end of the flap.

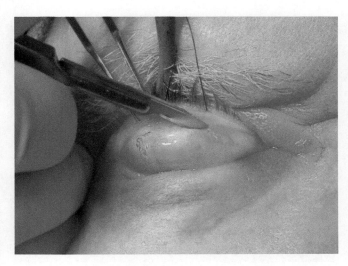

Figure 29.24. The tarsal portion of the flap is incised with a no. 15 blade. The horizontal dimension is determined by the horizontal dimension of the defect. At least 4 mm of vertical tarsal height should be preserved in the upper eyelid to prevent secondary buckling of the upper eyelid margin. As a result of the curved contour of the upper tarsus, the tarsal portion of the flap is tallest at its center.

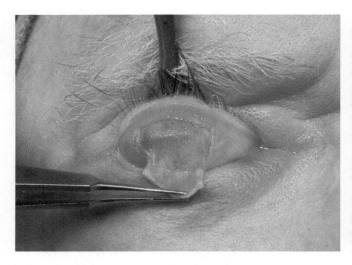

Figure 29.25. The tarsal flap is sharply elevated from its underlying attachments, consisting of the orbicularis oculi muscle and the confluence of the septum and levator aponeurosis.

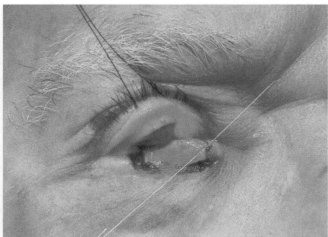

Figure 29.27. Two partial-thickness interrupted 5-0 or 6-0 polyglactin sutures on a spatulated needle are used to approximate the tarsal portion of the flap to the tarsal edge of the recipient defect. The superior limit of the tarsal portion of the flap should be in line with the eyelid margin of the defect.

The tarsal component of the Hughes's flap can then be secured to fill the lower eyelid defect. The vertical edges of the Hughes's flap are sutured to the edges of the marginal defect with partial-thickness 5-0 or 6-0 polyglactin sutures through both the donor and recipient tarsus (Figure 29.27). The inferior edge of the tarsoconjunctival flap is secured to the edge of the residual conjunctiva of the lower eyelid with running 6-0 plain gut or polyglactin suture, thereby completing reconstruction of the posterior lamella (Figure 29.28). There should be minimal tension after securing the tarsoconjunctival flap (Figure 29.29). The anterior lamellar defect can be reconstructed with a full-thickness skin graft (Figure 30A–D), and a bolster is positioned to hold the graft in position (Figure 29.31). Alternatively, a small vertical myocutaneous advancement flap, if the vertical extent of the skin defect is minimal, is an option. The latter option under normal circumstances is less than ideal as it exerts a downward force on the lower eyelid and will produce retraction. In this situation, however, the Hughes's flap provides counterbalancing traction superiorly. For this reason, the second stage should be delayed to prevent secondary eyelid retraction.

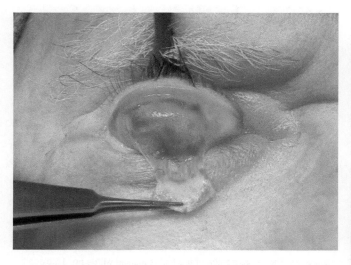

Figure 29.26. Flanking vertical relaxing incisions are made in the conjunctiva as the flap is sharply developed between the plane of the conjunctiva and Müller's muscle. Because a natural areolar plane does not separate the two structures, saline or a local anesthetic can be injected to hydrodissect between the planes and facilitate dissection.

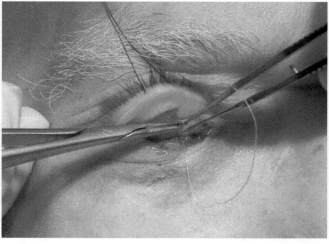

Figure 29.28. An additional 5-0 or 6-0 polyglactin suture is used in a running fashion to approximate the inferior edge of the tarsoconjunctival flap to the edge of the conjunctiva and lower eyelid retractors of the defect.

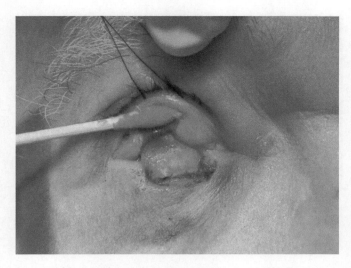

Figure 29.29. After inset of the Hughes flap into the defect, there should be minimal tension.

The conjunctival pedicle is normally divided postoperatively at 6–12 weeks, but can be done as early as 2 weeks (Figure 29.32). This is done by sliding a Crawford tube grooved director or the handle end of a Desmarres retractor under the flap to protect the globe. A no. 15 Bard Parker blade or scissor is used to incise the flap slightly higher than the lower lid margin and beveled anteriorly, such that the conjunctiva can be draped anteriorly and the new mucocutaneous junction can be recreated away from the globe (Figure 29.33). Alternatively, a blunt scissor can be used to open the flap. The residual pedicle on the upper lid can be amputated at its base so as not to irritate the ocular surface (Figure 29.34). Eyelid margin contouring may be necessary at a later visit. Artificial lashes, eyeliners, or a tattoo are recommended instead of eyelash transplantation.

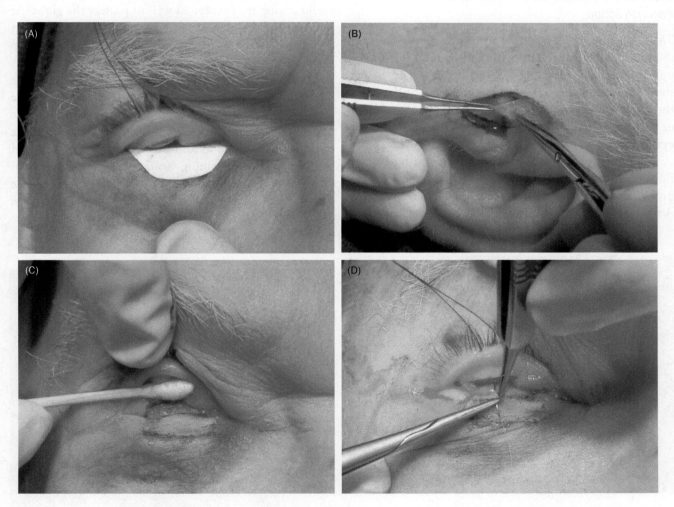

Figure 29.30. (A) A template can be used to determine the size and shape of the full-thickness skin graft. (B) The skin graft can be harvested from the eyelid, preauricular skin (as in this case), or from the postauricular or supraclavicular areas. (C) The skin graft is sutured into position with a commination of interrupted and running plain gut sutures. (D) The superior edge of the skin graft is secured to the conjunctival flap with 6-0 fast-absorbing gut in an interrupted fashion with partial-thickness bites.

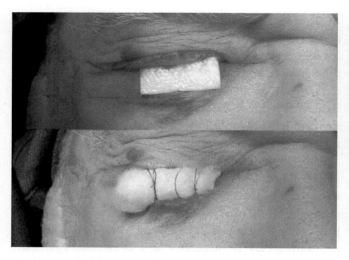

Figure 29.31. A bolster dressing with first Telfa and then cotton balls is tied over the skin graft with several 5-0 silk sutures.

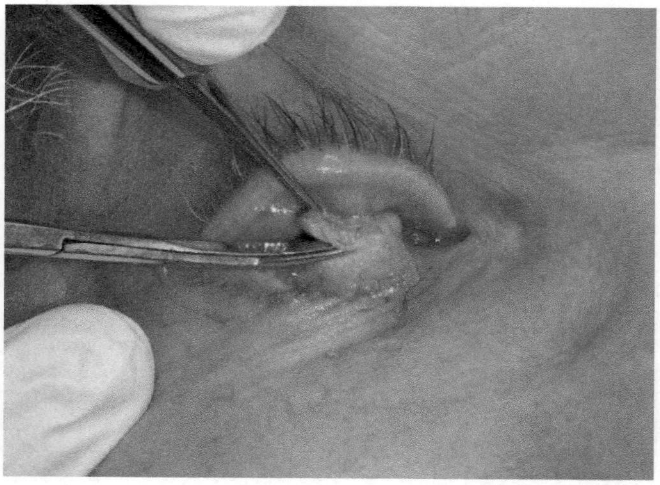

Cutler-Beard Bridge Flap for Upper Eyelid Reconstruction

The Cutler-Beard Flap is used to reconstruct wider full-thickness defects of the upper eyelid or total loss of the upper eyelid[2] (Figure 29.35). The upper eyelid defect should be trimmed in a rectangular fashion. The flap from the lower eyelid should be approximately the same width or just slightly narrower than the defect of the upper eyelid.

A corneal protector is placed and then a horizontal full-thickness incision is made in the lower eyelid approximately 5 mm below the margin (Figure 29.36A). A malleable or similar instrument can be placed under the

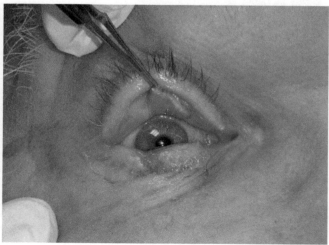

Figure 29.33. The Hughes flap is released just slightly above the planned eyelid margin. With further healing, the flap contracts will be in line with the native eyelid margin.

eyelid during the incision as well to protect the globe. At the edges of the incision, full-thickness vertical incisions are carried to the inferior fornix (Figure 29.37). The flap is then put on stretch with skin hooks, and the conjunctiva layer of the flap is then dissected off the posterior edge of the flap. This conjunctival flap is then pulled under the lower eyelid margin and is sutured to the conjunctiva of the upper eyelid defect (Figure 29.36B). A graft of ear cartilage or other tissue is used to reconstruct the missing tarsus and is sutured to the remaining tarsus or remnants of the medial or lateral canthal tendons (Figure 29.36C). Then, the myocutaneous flap is pulled under the lower eyelid bridge

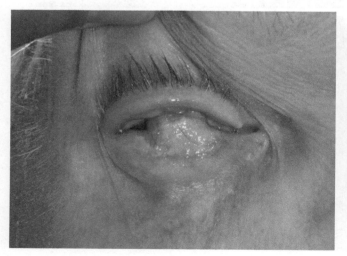

Figure 29.32. Hughes Stage II. Appearance 6 weeks after first-stage reconstruction with a Hughes flap. Notice how the margin of keratinized epithelium has migrated proximally on the flap.

Figure 29.34. The remaining proximal portion of the flap is severed from the upper eyelid, and hemostasis is achieved with cautery.

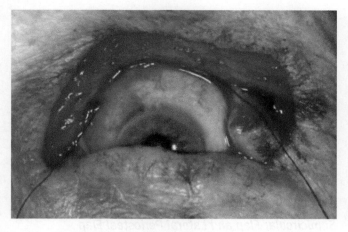

Figure 29.35. Near total full-thickness defect of the left upper eyelid. Some residual eyelid is present laterally.

and is sutured to the skin edges of the upper eyelid defect (Figure 29.36D).

Separation of the flap is then carried out about 4–6 weeks later (Figure 29.36E). The incision to separate the flap is marked about 2 mm below the desired location of the new upper eyelid margin. The posterior conjunctiva is rotated anteriorly and sutured over the margin. If needed in the upper eyelid, an eyelid crease can be made with full-thickness silk or Vicryl sutures in a horizontal mattress technique. Then the donor side of the eyelid is revised and the lower eyelid margin bridge is sutured back to the lower eyelid skin (Figure 29.36F). Patients have a functioning eyelid with a good aesthetic result after opening of the flap (Figure 29.38).

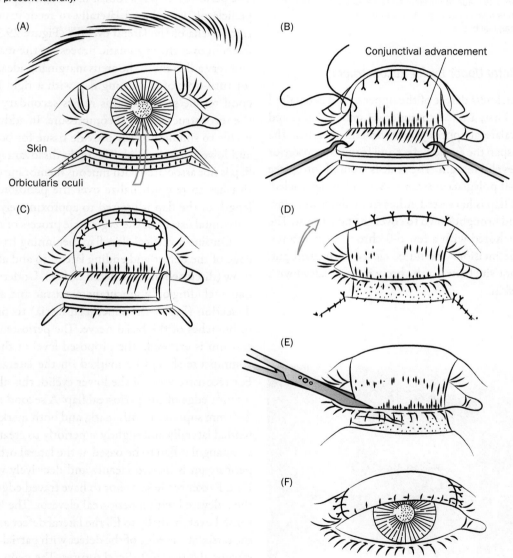

Figure 29.36. Large full-thickness defects of the upper eyelid can be closed with a Cutler-Beard flap, a cross-eyelid flap advanced under a bridge of intact lower eyelid margin. (A) A full-thickness transverse blepharotomy is made 5–6 mm below the eyelid margin, leaving the lower palpebral arcade intact. Relaxing incisions are made extending inferiorly. (B,C) The flap is split in the subconjunctival plane to prepare a bed for a free graft with contralateral tarsus, cartilage, or alloplastic dermal matrix. (D) The anterior layer of the flap is draped over the free graft and secured to approximate the defect. (E,F) At 4–6 weeks, the flap is divided, the eyelid margin contoured, and the donor site in the lower eyelid reconstructed.

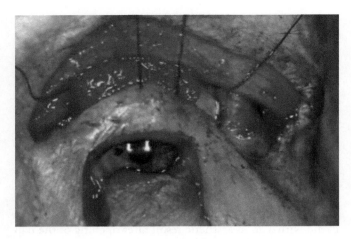

Figure 29.37. Cutler-Beard Stage I. A full-thickness transverse blepharotomy with relaxing incisions is made to develop the Cutler-Beard flap. The transverse incision is made below the vascular arcade to preserve perfusion to the marginal bridge.

Single-Stage Total Upper Eyelid Reconstruction

A total, full-thickness defect of the upper eyelid is repaired in three steps. First, a tarso-conjunctival graft is harvested from the contralateral upper eyelid as described earlier. The graft is used to span the eyelid defect and forms the posterior lamella at the eyelid margin. The graft is sutured into place using 5-0 or 6-0 polyglactin sutures. Second, a bipedicled, myocutaneous flap is harvested either from above or below the eyebrow and brought down to cover the tarsal graft. The flap may be anchored with a few 6-0 chromic gut sutures, but most of the incisions should be closed with plain gut. Third, the donor site beneath the brow is free-grafted with full-thickness skin.

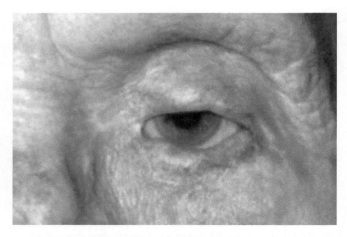

Figure 29.38. Cutler-Beard Stage II. Appearance 2 months following second-stage division of the Cutler-Beard flap.

LATERAL CANTHAL ANCHORING

A simple lateral eyelid defect can be closed with a Tenzel flap rotated along the eyelid margin as described earlier. The orbicularis can be attached to the lateral orbital rim and can help create and reconstruct the lateral canthal angle without a graft or flap. If additional bulk is needed or more extensive defects are present with disruption of the lateral canthal tendon, then a lateral periosteal flap can be used to reconstruct the lateral canthal tendon for both the upper and lower eyelid.

Semicircular Flap and Lateral Periosteal Flap

The periosteal flap is a robust flap that can provide a strong pedicle of tissue based laterally to reconstruct the posterior lamella of the lateral eyelid[30] (Figure 29.39). The periosteum over the zygomatic process of the maxilla is dense and very adherent to the arcus marginalis, ideal as a fulcrum for turn-over of the strong flap with a rigid base that has good tensile strength. This resists secondary rounding of the reconstructed lateral commissure. In addition, the flap is able to simultaneously provide tissue for both the upper and lower lateral eyelid. The main disadvantage is that the flap is not associated with mucous membrane (the conjunctiva has to re-epithelialize over the periosteum), and the length of the flap is limited to approximately 10 mm (the horizontal extent of the zygomatic process of the maxilla).

Outline a vertical skin flap, beginning from the lateral edge of the defect and ending lateral to and above the eyebrow (discussed in more detail earlier). Undermine the skin flap, including only subcutaneous tissue and avoiding deep dissection (below the superficial fascia) to prevent injury to branches of the facial nerve. The periosteum of the lateral rim is exposed. The proposed level of the new lateral commissure should be marked on the lateral orbital rim. For reconstruction of the lower eyelid, this also marks the inferior edge of the periosteal flap. A second mark is made 4–5 mm superior to this mark, and both marks are then extended laterally and slightly superiorly to create the lines of a rectangular flap to be based at the lateral orbital rim. The periosteum is incised cleanly and decisively with a no. 15 Bard Parker blade so as not to have frayed edges. The flap is then elevated with a periosteal elevator. The hinged flap is turned over medially to fill the lateral defect and secured to the tarsus at the edge of the defect with partial-thickness interrupted 5-0 or 6-0 Vicryl sutures. The main disadvantage is that the flap is not associated with mucous membrane (the conjunctiva has to re-epithelialize over the periosteum) and the length of the flap is limited to approximately

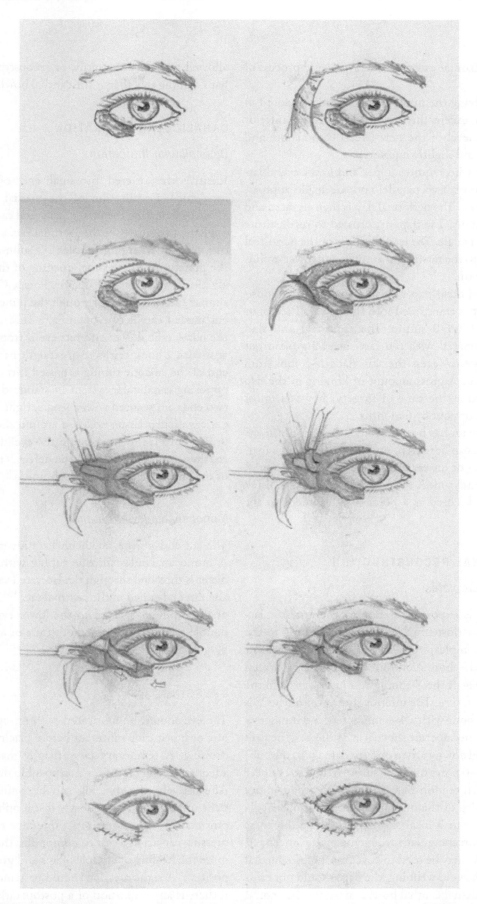

Figure 29.39. For defects of the lateral lower eyelid, a periosteal flap can be used to reconstruct the middle and posterior lamella. (B) The periosteal flap is a rectangular flap up to 10 mm in length and is folded over its base at the arcus marginalis. The distal margin is at the junction of zygoma and temporalis. (C,D) A Tripier suborbicularis transposition flap from the upper eyelid is elevated to reconstruct the anterior lamella. (E–G) The periosteal flap is designed in a superior oblique direction, just above the desired position of the lateral commissure. This flap provides excellent tensile support for the reconstructed lateral commissure. (H) The distal edge of the periosteum is secured to the tarsal edge of the defect with two interrupted partial-thickness 6-0 Vicryl sutures. The edge of the lateral canthal tendon from the upper eyelid is secured to the flap to define the lateral commissure. Additionally, the base of the flap can be secured for additional support. (I) The Tripier flap is trimmed to size, inset into the defect, and approximated with interrupted and running 6-0 absorbable or nonabsorbable sutures.

10 mm (the horizontal extent of the zygomatic process of the maxilla).

Defects involving the upper lateral eyelid are closed in a similar fashion, except the periosteal flap is just inferior to the proposed level of the new lateral commissure and extends laterally and slightly inferiorly.

For a patient who requires upper and lower eyelid lateral canthal support, two parallel cuts are made approximately 1.5 cm apart. The periosteal flap is then elevated and bisected horizontally. The flaps are crossed to reconstitute the lateral canthal angle. The leading edges of the periosteal flaps are sutured to the tarsus of the upper and lower eyelids with 6-0 polyglactin.

Once the periosteal flap(s) is in the appropriate position, the skin flap is transposed into the defect. The donor area is closed with 6-0 suture. The periosteal and skin flaps are approximated with 6-0 fast-absorbing plain gut suture, taking care to recess the skin flaps 1–2 mm from the eyelid margins. A gross amount of kinking in the flap may be addressed at the time of surgery; however, most irregularities smooth out by 6 months.

If the periosteum has been resected, then a drill in the lateral orbital rim can be used to suture the remaining tarsus (if enough laxity) or an ear cartilage or a free fascia graft to the lateral orbital rim. A suture anchor, such as a Mitek anchor, can also be used as a point of attachment to the orbital rim.

MEDIAL CANTHAL RECONSTRUCTION

Cantilevered Microplates

The nasal bone is exposed anterior to the anterior lacrimal crest. The periosteum is reflected posteriorly to the nasoethmoidal complex. A Y-shaped microplate is bent to conform to the bony contour of the medial orbital wall.[31] The long leg of the Y should rest just inferior to the frontoethmoidal suture. The inferior short arm of the Y is fixed to the nasal bone with a 4–5 mm screw. A 4 mm screw is used to fasten the superior short arm of the Y. (The drill should be directed downward to prevent damage to the cribriform plate.) A 4-0 polypropylene suture is used to connect the medial canthal tendon remnants directly to an empty hole in the long leg of the miniplate. The anterior lamella is reconstructed with a local skin flap or a full-thickness skin graft. Often, rectangular myocutaneous advancement flaps (Figure 23.1) may be used to cover most of the medial canthal defect. To avoid webbing, the flaps should not cross the apex of the medial canthal bowl concavity. The central concavity may be covered with a full-thickness skin graft,

allowed to heal secondarily, or reconstructed by multiple flaps coming together at the canthal bowl apex.

CANALICULAR INTUBATION

Bicanalicular Intubation

Identify the severed proximal end of canaliculus (or canaliculi). Localization of the medial opening may be aided by irrigating the intact ipsilateral canaliculus with air, applying pressure over the lacrimal sac, and noting the location of the emerging bubbles in a submerged field. Dilate the punctum and proximal opening of the transected canaliculus with a punctal dilator. Pass a Crawford tube, or similar silicone tubing, through the punctum and into the cut medial canalicular opening.[32] Thread the stent down the nasolacrimal duct and retrieve it from the inferior meatus with a hook retriever or straight hemostat. The other end of the silicone tubing is passed through the ipsilateral opposing canalicular system in standard fashion, and the two ends are secured with a single, tight, square knot. The pericanalicular tissue is closed around the tubing with 6-0 or 7-0 polyglactin sutures and the eyelid margin and skin repaired as necessary. The eyelid defect is repaired using one of the previously illustrated techniques.

Monocanalicular Intubation

The cut ends of the canaliculus are identified and dilated. A monocanalicular silicone tubing without a wire introducer is threaded through the lacerated sections of the canaliculus and coiled in the lacrimal sac.[33,34] The proximal end of the tubing is secured to the lower eyelid with a single double-armed 7-0 polyglactin suture or a monocanalicular plug system.

DRESSINGS

The eye should be lubricated with an ophthalmic antibiotic or lubricating ointment before placing a light-pressure dressing. A temporary tarsorrhaphy may be necessary if adequate eyelid closure is not possible under the dressing. Alternatively, the dressing can be omitted and the patient or family may frequently instill ophthalmic drops or ointment. In addition to its protective role, a well-placed dressing can act as a cast to immobilize the eyelids and promote the healing of complex flaps and grafts in the desired position. A tight dressing should be removed immediately if there is any indication of a postoperative orbital hemorrhage (e.g., severe retrobulbar pain, periorbital ecchymosis and tenseness, vomiting). Liberal use of ophthalmic ointment, a nonadherent dressing, or ophthalmic ointment–impregnated fine gauze covered by one or two soft absorbent eye pads taped to the cheek and forehead usually provides a proper eyelid dressing.

Steri-Strips may provide additional postoperative support in areas of increased wound tension (e.g., lateral canthal suspension). Compactly rolled cotton (dental rolls) may be useful if focal compression is required (e.g., medial canthal concavity, full-thickness skin graft bolsters).

POSTOPERATIVE CARE AND RECOMMENDATIONS

Dressings are not always necessary after eyelid reconstruction. Pressure dressings or bolsters are often placed over periocular skin grafts to help with healing. Antibiotic ophthalmic ointment is often placed over the incision sites and inside the eye if any ocular surface or conjunctival surgery was done. Commonly used ointments include erythromycin ophthalmic ointment, Polysporin ophthalmic ointment, tobramycin-dexamethasone ophthalmic ointment (Tobradex), or neomycin-polymyxin b-dexamethasone ophthalmic ointment (Maxitrol). The patient is then sent home with a prescription for the ointment to be placed over the incision site 2–3 times daily for 1 week.

Ice cold compresses for the first 4–7 days for 10 minutes each hour while awake is very important in reducing postoperative pain and edema. The senior author prefers a moist wash cloth on the eyes with a zipper locked plastic bag of crushed ice or a frozen gel pack. The patient should sleep with his or her head elevated with several pillows.

Some spotting of blood on the wash cloth for the first day or two is typical, and the patient should be informed of such. Patients often will have a variable amount of periorbital ecchymosis. The bruising will travel down the face to the lower lids and cheeks with time. Some patients prefer to wear sunglasses for several days to hide the ecchymosis, but also for sun protection and light sensitivity. Patients are advised that vision may be a bit blurry with ointment. If the eyes swell shut, the patient is advised to call the surgeon immediately as it may portend retrobulbar hemorrhage.

Patients should avoid any straining, bending over, or heavy lifting for at least 1–2 weeks after surgery as these activities could cause rebleeding. Bruising and swelling typically lasts 10–14 days but may be as prolonged as 3 weeks in some individuals or with extensive dissection.

Follow-up is at 1 week for evaluation and/or suture removal. Nonabsorbable periorbital skin stitches are usually removed 4–7 days postoperatively. Eyelid margin sutures are removed after 10–14 days.

REPAIR OF ECTROPION, ENTROPION, EYELID RETRACTION, AND ACQUIRED BLEPHAROPTOSIS

PATIENT EVALUATION

The type and anatomic cause of eyelid malposition must be determined before choosing the appropriate corrective surgical procedure. Patients may present with *ectropion*, turning out of the eyelid; *entropion*, turning in of the eyelid; *retraction*, abnormal elevation of the upper eyelid and abnormal lowering of the lower eyelids; or *ptosis*, drooping of the upper eyelids. A detailed periocular and ocular examination is necessary to determine the cause of each of these types of eyelid malposition.

Ectropion of the lower eyelids can be involutional, cicatricial, mechanical, or paralytic. Surgical treatments vary depending on the cause of ectropion. Involutional lower eyelid ectropion may result from canthal tendon laxity, laxity of the pretarsal or preseptal orbicularis muscle, and/or disinsertion of the lower eyelid retractors. A simple pinch test, in which the eyelid is pulled from the globe, is an effective method of determining the degree of eyelid laxity. More than 6 mm of laxity is abnormal. Another method is the snapback test, in which the lower eyelid is pulled away from the globe and allowed to retract. A slow return to normal position is indicative of poor eyelid tone. Deficiency of eyelid skin may result in cicatricial ectropion, which is commonly seen after excess skin is excised in lower eyelid blepharoplasties. If the eyelid margin cannot be pulled superiorly at least 2 mm above the inferior limbus, vertical insufficiency of the eyelid exists, and the patient may require a skin graft to replace insufficient tissue.

Lower eyelid retraction may occur with or without lower eyelid ectropion. Eyelid retraction may be caused by canthal tendon laxity, posterior lamellar (conjunctiva and eyelid retractors) insufficiency, proptosis, thyroid ophthalmopathy, shallow orbits, or large globes, as seen in high myopia. Clinical signs of retraction are lowering of the eyelid resulting in an increase in the inferior scleral show.

Involutional entropion is a result of horizontal eyelid laxity, overriding of the preseptal orbicularis oculi muscle, or disinsertion of the lower eyelid retractors.[35,36] With dehiscence of the lower eyelid retractors, excursion of the lower eyelid may be diminished in down-gaze. Occasionally, the edge of the attenuated lower eyelid retractors is seen as a white band paralleling the eyelid margin in the inferior fornix. An overriding orbicularis muscle is often evident on forced closure of the eyelids, which results in worsening of the entropion. Cicatricial entropion is caused by a vertical shortening of the posterior tarsoconjunctival lamella of the eyelid. Therefore, the inferior fornix should be carefully evaluated for cicatricial changes as treatment for this could range from replacement of the foreshortened fornix or systemic treatment of an inflammatory condition such as ocular cicatricial pemphigoid.

Ptosis, or drooping of the upper eyelid, may be a result of disinsertion or injury to the levator aponeurosis or from a neurological process such as Horner's syndrome or a third cranial nerve palsy.[37,38] It is extremely important to determine the cause of ptosis on clinical exam to rule out a potentially life-threatening cause such as a posterior communicating artery aneurysm causing a third-nerve palsy or a carotid dissection causing a Horner's syndrome. Levator dehiscence may be caused from involutional changes, trauma, prior ocular surgery, or prolonged contact lens wear. Patients with aponeurotic ptosis typically demonstrate normal levator function (>10 mm), an elevated eyelid crease, and thinning of the eyelid appearance. The degree of ptosis may be quantitated by measuring the margin reflex distance (MRD) or the position of the upper eyelid margin relative to the corneal light reflex. A normal MRD is 3.5–4.5 mm, and an MRD lower than this, especially when affecting peripheral vision, is a good indicator of visually significant ptosis. Small amounts of ptosis can also be evaluated using a phenylephrine test. Photos of the eyelid position with the brows stabilized should be taken and then a drop of phenylephrine is placed in both or the affected eye. If improvement in ptosis is noted with the phenylephrine drop, then the ptosis can be repaired using a posterior ptosis approach. The presence or absence of Bell's phenomenon is important to note preoperatively as well as determining if the patient has issues with dry eye syndrome because a poor Bell's reflex and dry eye syndrome preoperatively may increase the risks of corneal exposure and dry eye postoperatively.

INDICATIONS

Most cases of involutional ectropion have a component of lateral canthal tendon laxity which can often be corrected by horizontally tightening the eyelid with a lateral tarsal strip (LTS) procedure.[39] The LTS may also be an approach in the management of some forms of paralytic ectropion, along with a tarsoconjunctival onlay flap or a lateral tarsorrhaphy.

Anterior lamellar insufficiency may be corrected by full-thickness skin grafts or rotational myocutaneous flaps. A LTS by itself or as an adjunct to skin grafting may be effective for patients with lower eyelid or lateral canthal malposition, no eyelid laxity, or shortage of the anterior lamella.

Posterior lamellar inadequacy causing entropion or retraction is managed with lysis of any cicatrix or symblepharon, recession of the lower eyelid retractors, and placement of an appropriate spacer graft. Hard palate mucosa,[40,41] autogenous cartilage,[42] irradiated donor cartilage, porcine acellular dermal matrix (Enduragen), and porous polyethylene curved spacers are all useful as interpositional supports.

Reinsertion of the lower eyelid retractors and resuspension of the lateral canthus may be performed through an infraciliary or a transconjunctival approach in the correction of involutional entropion. In cases of mild to moderate eyelid margin entropion and trichiasis, a transverse tarsotomy procedure is extremely useful for patients with or without trachoma. For moderate cases of cicatricial entropion, an interpositional hard-palate mucosal graft can be used to lengthen the middle and posterior lamellae.

Levator aponeurosis advancement through an external approach is the most commonly employed technique in the repair of aponeurotic defects with good levator muscle function. An upper eyelid crease incision allows excellent intraoperative exposure and facilitates postoperative revisions. A mullerectomy may be indicated with smaller amounts of ptosis and with a good response to topical phenylephrine.

CONTRAINDICATIONS

Surgical management of involutional ectropion should be considered only if medical treatment has failed. Aggressive ocular lubrication will often result in improvement of eyelid margin position if ectropion is of recent onset. Lubrication and punctal occlusion may also reduce the symptoms of exposure seen in lower eyelid retraction. Postoperative eyelid retraction may be improved with eyelid massage performed within a few weeks of surgery. Ectropion may be mechanical or cicatricial from the growth of a periocular skin cancer. The area should be carefully evaluated for any concerning lesions that may be causing the eyelid malposition. Sometimes they can be subtle, and a slit lamp microscope or loupes may assist in the examination. Loss of eyelashes in areas along the eyelid margin may be a concerning sign for a possible malignancy as well.

If a LTS will result in lateral displacement of the punctum toward the nasal limbus, medial canthal tendon laxity exists and should be addressed before horizontally tightening the eyelid.

Cicatricial entropion may be caused by inflammatory conditions that should be addressed prior to repair. Cicatricial changes can be a result of ocular cicatricial pemphigoid, chronic glaucoma drops, chemical exposure, and the like. It is important to determine the cause of the scarring before surgical intervention.

Patients with good levator function whose ptosis resolves after the instillation of a 10% solution of phenylephrine may not require levator aponeurosis advancement. Müller's muscle-conjunctival resection is adequate in these cases of mild ptosis, often seen in Horner's syndrome patients. Advancement of the levator aponeurosis is inadequate in cases of myogenic congenital ptosis and other manifestations of severe ptosis with minimal or no levator function. Frontalis suspension techniques should be used in these patients.[43]

Avoid creating any lagophthalmos in patients at risk for corneal decompensation. The mnemonic BADD (poor Bell's phenomenon, anesthetic cornea, dry eye, denervated seventh nerve) is useful to identify patients at risk for postoperative corneal problems. Lagophthalmos should also be avoided in patients with rheumatoid arthritis or contact lens intolerance or who are of advanced age.

Another concern in ptosis surgery is appropriate preoperative evaluation of eyelid position. Herring's law of motor correspondence is important to remember in patients with unilateral ptosis. Repair of unilateral ptosis may exacerbate undetected contralateral ptosis.

ROOM SETUP

The instruments and anesthesia techniques used in eyelid malposition surgery are the same as those previously described for general eyelid reconstruction.

The importance of corneal protection during eyelid reconstruction cannot be overemphasized. The use of a corneal protector during any eyelid or periocular surgery is strongly encouraged.

PATIENT MARKINGS

The upper eyelid crease should be measured and marked with a fine-tipped skin marker in cases of ptosis repair and full-thickness skin graft harvest. If a blepharoplasty is done simultaneously, then the eyelids will need to be marked accordingly as well.

The eyelid crease should be 4–5 mm above the superior punctum, 8 mm (in men) to 10 mm (in women) above the central eyelid margin, and 6–7 mm superior to the lateral canthal angle. If a unilateral procedure is being performed, the eyelid crease should match the contralateral upper eyelid. Excess skin superior to the crease marking may be pinched up and marked if a graft is to be harvested or a concomitant blepharoplasty is to be performed. It is helpful to use the aesthetic subunits of the eyelid as boundaries for flaps and incision lines. Please see the blepharoplasty chapter for details regarding this procedure.

TECHNIQUES

Surgical Technique: Lateral Tarsal Strip

A lateral canthotomy is performed with a no. 15 scalpel blade or straight, sharp iris scissor. The skin incision is 3–5 mm long. A lateral cantholysis is carried out using a straight iris scissor to incise the inferior crus of the lateral canthal tendon. The tendon can be "strummed" and attachments snipped until the lower eyelid is free to be distracted inferiorly. The amount of lid shortening should be measured and marked. The eyelid is split along the gray line into anterior and posterior lamellae; the split is 3–10 mm long, depending on the amount of lid shortening necessary. The lower eyelid retractors and conjunctiva are cut at the plane of the inferior tarsal border to free the lateral tarsus. The mucocutaneous junction is trimmed along the eyelid margin, and the conjunctival epithelium is debrided from the bulbar surface of the tarsus with a no. 15 scalpel blade. The lateral canthal tendon remnant is excised and the lateral tarsus shortened, depending on the degree of horizontal laxity. The new tarsal margin is reanastomosed to the periosteum on the inner aspect of the lateral orbital wall with a 4-0 polyglactin, Mersilene, or Prolene suture on a semicircular needle. The amount of lid shortening may be varied by the placement of the suture in the LTS or by the amount of shortening performed on the LTS. An initial slight overcorrection in vertical lid position is desirable. (The lateral canthal angle is generally about 2 mm superior to the medial canthal angle.) Excess anterior skin and muscle are excised, and the lateral canthotomy is closed in a single layer.

Eyelid Reconstruction with a Hard-Palate Mucosal Graft

A lateral canthotomy and inferior cantholysis are performed. Sharp dissection is used to release the scarred and contracted conjunctiva and lower eyelid retractors from the inferior tarsus. Once the incision reaches the medial area inferior to the puncta, it is directed inferiorly for about 3 mm. Dissection in the plane between the posterior lamella and the orbital septum and posterior orbicularis fascia is used to free the lower eyelid retractors from any overlying cicatrix. A hard-palate mucosal graft is harvested in standard fashion. With the mucosal side of the graft oriented toward the globe, a running 6-0 mild plain gut suture is used to fixate the graft first to the recipient inferior tarsal edge (in order to bury the knot under the graft) and then to the recessed conjunctiva. The lateral canthus is resuspended. Other available options for spacer grafts for treatment of eyelid retraction or deficiency of the posterior lamella can be inserted in a similar fashion in the same location.

Cicatricial Ectropion Repair of the Lower Eyelid with Skin Graft

Mark the subciliary incision approximately 2–3 mm below the eyelashes and lid margin extending for 2–3 mm beyond the contracted area. Undermine the retracted skin until the ectropion of the lower eyelid is fully corrected and the lid margin can be elevated freely. It is important to release any scar tissue or bands. The dissection can continue all the way down to conjunctiva if necessary to release scar tissue or adhesions. If there is significant eyelid laxity, then eyelid shortening may be necessary. Measure the size of the defect. Mark the area of the full-thickness graft, which is ideally tissue of the upper eyelid that can be marked as a blepharoplasty incision and then trimmed as necessary. Otherwise, post-auricular tissue is often the next best option. The graft is thinned as necessary, depending on the location it was harvested from, and then it is sutured into position with a combination of interrupted and running sutures. A Frost suture tarsorrhaphy is then placed for upward traction on the lower eyelid, and a pressure patch +/− bolster is secured over the skin graft.

Transcutaneous Entropion Repair of the Lower Eyelid: Retractor Reinsertion and Lateral Canthoplasty

A lateral canthotomy and inferior cantholysis is performed. An infraciliary incision is made in typical fashion and a skin–muscle flap is elevated. The orbital septum is opened, exposing the lower eyelid retractors. The retractors are sutured to the inferior edge of the lower eyelid tarsus with two or three 6-0 silk or polyglactin sutures with the knots oriented anteriorly. Pretarsal orbicularis is resected.

Horizontal shortening with an LTS is performed to correct for coexisting eyelid laxity.

Transconjunctival Entropion Repair of the Lower Eyelid: Retractor Reinsertion and Lateral Canthoplasty

A lateral canthotomy and inferior cantholysis is performed. The conjunctiva and retractor band are incised with a straight iris scissor along the inferior tarsal border following the contour of the tarsus. Often a disinserted white retractor band can be seen in the fornix. The retractors are dissected off of the conjunctiva, taking care not to buttonhole the conjunctiva. A small amount of orbicularis is excised just inferior to the tarsal border to address the overriding orbicularis. The retractors are then reinserted on the inferior border of the tarsus using buried 6-0 polyglactin interrupted sutures. The conjunctiva is then closed with a running 6-0 fast gut or plain gut suture. Horizontal shortening with an LTS is performed to correct for coexisting eyelid laxity.[44]

Transverse Tarsotomy and Lid Margin Rotation for Cicatricial Entropion

Two 4-0 silk sutures are passed through the lower eyelid margin to provide traction, allowing distraction of the eyelid away from the globe. A horizontal incision is made from the conjunctival surface 2 mm from the lid margin full-thickness through the tarsus but not through the orbicularis. The incision should be several millimeters long but should not be carried medially beyond the punctum. If necessary, sharp dissection in the postorbicularis fascial plane may be performed to release any scarring between the anterior and middle lamellae. Each arm (spaced 3–4 mm apart) of a double-armed 6-0 chromic gut suture is passed through the superior edge of the lower fragment of the tarsal plate and through the orbicularis and skin to exit anterior to the lash line. For greater rotational effect, the sutures should exit closer to the lash line. Up to three or four double-armed sutures spaced 4–5 mm apart may be used, depending on the length of the affected eyelid margin. Modest overrotation is the desired end point.[45]

Levator Aponeurosis Advancement

An incision is made in the eyelid crease through the skin and the orbicularis muscle. The orbital septum, which inserts onto the aponeurosis 3–5 mm above the superior tarsal border, is identified and opened with a scissor. Preaponeurotic orbital fat is retracted superiorly with a Desmarres retractor, and the levator aponeurosis is located.[46] Sharp dissection of the anterior tarsal surface is performed to bare the tarsal plate before placement of the tarsal sutures.[47] Sutures of 7-0 polypropylene or silk or polyglactin are passed in interrupted fashion partial-thickness through the tarsus about 3 mm from the upper tarsal border and then through the lower edge of the aponeurosis. Two sutures placed centrally and slightly nasal to the pupillary line often give adequate eyelid margin contour.[48] No ptosis formula for quantitating the amount of levator advancement required is exact, and the surgeon will be best served by adapting published recommendations to his or her own method. The eyelid position should be checked intraoperatively, if possible with the help of the patient, to evaluate for symmetry and good eyelid margin contour. The patient may be raised to an upright position during the operation to assess eyelid height and contour as well. The appropriate adjustments should be made until the surgeon is satisfied with the symmetry and appearance. The skin incision is closed in standard fashion. Two or three deep interrupted sutures passing through the skin, pretarsal orbicularis, and the edge of the levator aponeurosis may be placed to help reform the eyelid crease in certain cases.

Posterior Ptosis Repair with Conjunctival Mullerectomy

Anesthetize the upper eyelid using pretarsal and subconjunctival local anesthesia or a frontal nerve block. Place a traction suture, such as a 4-0 silk suture, through the skin, orbicularis, and tarsal plate 2 mm adjacent to the lid margin. Evert the upper eyelid using a Desmarres retractor. Measure the planned amount for conjunctival resection. The initial report described by Putterman[49] recommended that if the response to phenylephrine was elevation to a normal level, then 8.25 mm of Muller's muscle and conjunctiva would be resected. A 6.25–9.75 mm graded resection would be completed if the ptotic eyelid elevated to slightly higher or lower than the normal or ideal eyelid position,[49, 50] whereas Dresner[51] recommends 4 mm of resection for every 1 mm of ptosis. Therefore, 8 mm of resection would be used for the treatment of 2 mm of ptosis. The caliper is set depending on the amount of resection required. There are several options for marking. One option is to place the caliper at half the amount planned for resection (for an 8 mm resection, place the caliper at 4 mm). Measure for the superior border of the tarsus and either make a mark or place a marking suture at the halfway mark, approximately 7 mm nasally and temporally. Two toothed forceps can be used to firmly grasp the conjunctiva and Muller's muscle medially

and laterally, or, alternatively, if a suture was used (often passed several times along the mark through conjunctiva and Muller's muscle) this can be lifted and the Putterman clamp is placed and locked. The clamp should be relatively centered along the tarsus. Take care to ensure no skin is trapped in the clamp. The clamp is held vertically and a 6-0 double-armed plain gut suture is run in a horizontal mattress technique back and forth approximately 1–1.5 mm below the clamp from temporal to nasal. A no. 15 blade is used to excise the tissue by cutting between the suture and the clamp (touching the clamp while excising to avoid cutting your suture). The nasal end of the suture is then run back temporally approximating the two edges of conjunctiva and then the knot is buried temporally or can be externalized to the skin of the upper eyelid and tied.

DRESSINGS

The principles of wound care and ocular protection previously described for general eyelid reconstruction also apply to eyelid malposition surgery. One or two double-armed 4-0 silk sutures passed through the lower eyelid margin (Frost sutures) and fixed to the forehead with Steri-Strips (e.g., spacer grafts for lower eyelid retraction) for 4–7 days may help prevent contracture of the lower eyelid after reconstruction. An extended-wear bandage soft contact lens might be considered in patients at risk for mechanical damage to the cornea (e.g., hard-palate mucosal graft or posterior ptosis surgery). If a hard-palate mucosa graft has been harvested, a palate obturator worn for up to 1 week postoperatively greatly diminishes donor site morbidity.

POSTOPERATIVE CARE

Patients should be seen about 5–7 days after surgery or sooner if there are any issues or concerns. The postoperative instructions listed earlier for eyelid reconstruction apply to cases of eyelid malposition repair as well.

REFERENCES

1. Harrington JN Reconstruction of the medial canthus by spontaneous granulation (laissez-faire): a review. *Ann Ophthalmol* 1982;14(10):956–60, 963–6, 969–70.
2. Cutler NL, Beard C. A method for partial and total upper lid reconstruction. *Am J Ophthalmol* 1955;39(1):1–7.
3. Dutton JJ, Fowler AM. Double-bridged flap procedure for nonmarginal, full-thickness, upper eyelid reconstruction. *Ophthal Plast Reconstr Surg* 2007;23(6):459–462.
4. Sa, HS, Woo KI, Kim YD. Reverse modified Hughes procedure for uppereyelid reconstruction. *Ophthal Plast Reconstr Surg* 2010;26(3):155–160.

5. Mauriello JA Jr, Antonacci R. Single tarsoconjunctival flap (lower eyelid) for upper eyelid reconstruction ("reverse" modified Hughes procedure). *Ophthalmic Surg* 1994;25(6):374–378.

6. Jordan DR, Anderson RL, Nowinski TS. Tarsoconjunctival flap for upper eyelid reconstruction. *Arch Ophthalmol* 1989;107(4):599–603.

7. Dortzbach RK Angrist RA. Silicone intubation for lacerated lacrimal canaliculi. *Ophthalmic Surg* 1985;16(10):639–642.

8. Hawes MJ, Segrest DR. Effectiveness of bicanalicular silicone intubation in the repair of canalicular lacerations. *Ophthal Plast Reconstr Surg* 1985;1(3):185–190.

9. Reifler DM. Management of canalicular laceration. *Surv Ophthalmol* 1991;36(2):113–132.

10. Borges AF. The rhombic flap. *Plast Reconstr Surg* 1981;67(4):458–466.

11. Bullock JD, Koss N, Flagg SV. Rhomboid flap in ophthalmic plastic surgery. *Arch Ophthalmol* 1973;90(3):203–205.

12. Bullock JD, Hamdi B. Double rhomboid flap in ophthalmic plastic surgery. *Ophthalmic Surg* 1980;11(7):431–434.

13. Codner MA, McCord CD. *Eyelid & Periorbital Surgery*, 2nd edition. Boca Raton, FL: CRC Press, 2016.

14. Kim JH, Kim JM, Park JW, et al. Reconstruction of the medial canthus using an ipsilateral paramedian forehead flap. *Arch Plast Surg* 2013;40(6):742–747.

15. Patrinely JR, Marines HM, Anderson RL. Skin flaps in periorbital reconstruction. *Surv Ophthalmol* 1987;31(4):249–261.

16. Divine RD, Anderson RL. Techniques in eyelid wound closure. *Ophthalmic Surg* 1982;13(4):283–287.

17. Jordan DR, Anderson RL, Holds JB. Modifications to the semicircular flap technique in eyelid reconstruction. *Can J Ophthalmol* 1992;27(3):130–136.

18. Lewis CD, Perry JD. Transconjunctival lateral cantholysis for closure of full-thickness eyelid defects. *Ophthal Plast Reconstr Surg* 2009;25(6):469–471.

19. Tenzel RR, Stewart WB. Eyelid reconstruction by the semicircle flap technique. *Ophthalmology* 1978;85(11):1164–1169.

20. McGregor IA. The z-plasty. *Br J Plast Surg* 1966;19(1):82–87.

21. Callahan MA, Callahan A. Mustarde flap lower lid reconstruction after malignancy. *Ophthalmology* 1980;87(4):279–286.

22. Baker SR. *Local Flaps in Facial Reconstruction*, 3rd edition. Philadelphia, PA: Elsevier/Saunders, 2014:xii.

23. Cies WA, Bartlett RE. Modification of the Mustarde and Hughes methods of reconstructing the lower lid. *Ann Ophthalmol* 1975;7(11): 1497–1502

24. Leone CR, Jr. Tarsal-conjunctival advancement flaps for upper eyelid reconstruction. *Arch Ophthalmol* 1983;101(6):945–948.

25. Kersten RC, et al. Tarsal rotational flap for upper eyelid reconstruction. *Arch Ophthalmol* 1986;104(6):918–922.

26. Hawes MJ. Free autogenous grafts in eyelid tarsoconjunctival reconstruction. *Ophthalmic Surg* 1987;18(1):37–41.

27. Stephenson CM, Brown BZ. The use of tarsus as a free autogenous graft in eyelid surgery. *Ophthal Plast Reconstr Surg* 1985;1(1):43–50.

28. Hewes EH, Sullivan JH, Beard C. Lower eyelid reconstruction by tarsal transposition. *Am J Ophthalmol* 1976;81(4):512–514.

29. Hughes WL. Total lower lid reconstruction: technical details. *Trans Am Ophthalmol Soc* 1976;74:321–329.

30. Leone CR, Jr. Lateral canthal reconstruction. *Ophthalmology* 1987;94(3):238–241.

31. Howard GR, Nerad JA, Kersten RC. Medial canthoplasty with microplate fixation. *Arch Ophthalmol* 1992;110(12):1793–1797.

32. Crawford JS. Intubation of obstructions in the lacrimal system. *Can J Ophthalmol* 1977;12(4):289–292.

33. Long JA. A method of monocanalicular silicone intubation. *Ophthalmic Surg* 1988;19(3):204–205.

34. Patrinely JR, Anderson RL. Monocanalicular silicone intubation. *Arch Ophthalmol* 1988;106(5):579–580.

35. Dryden RM, Leibsohn J, Wobig J. Senile entropion. Pathogenesis and treatment. *Arch Ophthalmol* 1978;96(10):1883–1885.

36. Jones LT. The anatomy of the lower eyelid and its relation to the cause and cure of entropion. *Am J Ophthalmol* 1960;49:29–36.

37. Kersten RC, de Conciliis C, Kulwin DR. Acquired ptosis in the young and middle-aged adult population. *Ophthalmology* 1995;102(6):924–928.

38. Paris GL, Quickert MH. Disinsertion of the aponeurosis of the levator palpebrae superioris muscle after cataract extraction. *Am J Ophthalmol* 1976;81(3):337–340.

39. Anderson RL, Gordy DD. The tarsal strip procedure. *Arch Ophthalmol* 1979;97(11):2192–2196.

40. Cohen MS, Shorr N. Eyelid reconstruction with hard palate mucosa grafts. *Ophthal Plast Reconstr Surg* 1992;8(3):183–195.

41. Kersten RC, et al. Management of lower-lid retraction with hard-palate mucosa grafting. *Arch Ophthalmol* 1990;108(9):1339–1343.

42. Baylis HI, et al. Autogenous auricular cartilage grafting for lower eyelid retraction. *Ophthal Plast Reconstr Surg* 1985;1(1):23–27.

43. Carter SR, Meecham WR, Seiff SR. Silicone frontalis slings for the correction of blepharoptosis: indications and efficacy. *Ophthalmology* 1996;103(4):623–630.

44. Dresner SC, Karesh JW. Transconjunctival entropion repair. *Arch Ophthalmol* 1993;111(8):1144–1148.

45. Kersten RC, Kleiner FP, Kulwin DR. Tarsotomy for the treatment of cicatricial entropion with trichiasis. *Arch Ophthalmol* 1992;110(5):714–717.

46. Anderson RL, Beard C. The levator aponeurosis. Attachments and their clinical significance. *Arch Ophthalmol*, 1977;95(8):1437–1441.

47. Anderson RL, Dixon RS. Aponeurotic ptosis surgery. *Arch Ophthalmol* 1979;97(6):1123–1128.

48. Jones LT, Quickert MH, Wobig JL. The cure of ptosis by aponeurotic repair. *Arch Ophthalmol* 1975;93(8):629–634.

49. Putterman AM, Urist MJ. Muller's muscle-conjunctival resection ptosis procedure. *Ophthalmic Surg* 1978;9(3):27–32.

50. Putterman AM, Fett DR. Muller's muscle in the treatment of upper eyelid ptosis: a ten-year study. *Ophthalmic Surg* 1986;17(6):354–360.

51. Dresner SC. Further modifications of the Muller's muscle-conjunctival resection procedure for blepharoptosis. *Ophthal Plast Reconstr Surg* 1991;7(2):114–122.

30.

FOREHEAD FLAP FOR NASAL RECONSTRUCTION

Evan Matros and Julian J. Pribaz

CONCEPTUAL CONSIDERATIONS

The forehead flap is an important part of any reconstructive surgeon's armamentarium. Successful execution involves thoughtful consideration and inclusion of a number of basic plastic surgery principles.[1] Because the procedure involves multiple stages, a longitudinal vision and plan needs to be carefully established. The surgeon must also work in conjunction with the patient to explain the process and ensure reconstructive expectations and goals are aligned. Although the forehead flap may be the gold standard for complex nasal defects, some patients may seek a more expeditious reconstruction with lesser aesthetic goals. A skin graft to simply close the defect may be satisfactory; therefore, careful and effective communication is essential to a successful outcome.

Prior to initiating any reconstruction, a thorough history and physical exam should be performed. Because a significant number of nasal reconstructions occur in the setting of skin cancer associated with senescence, medical comorbidities are often a consideration along with the safety of general anesthesia. Active smoking needs to be discussed and should be considered a strong relative contraindication. Previous scars on the face should be closely examined, especially on either the forehead or nose, as some patients will have had previous surgery. The height of the forehead is a consideration as well since a low hairline can place hair in areas where it is not normally present. Confirmation of negative tumor margins is necessary prior to proceeding with surgery. For patients with aggressive tumors or those likely to receive adjuvant irradiation, delayed reconstruction is encouraged with temporary closure using skin grafts.

SKIN QUALITY

The skin quality of the nose changes dramatically over a relatively small area. As one proceeds in a caudal direction from the radix to the nasal tip, the skin transitions from being thin, compliant, and pliable, to thick, pitted, and sebaceous. The zone of thick skin is generally confined to the anatomic nasal tip and ala, whereas the thin skin is present on the sidewalls and dorsum. The difference in tissue quality is best exemplified by the fact that small defects of the upper nose can be closed primarily whereas defects as small as a few millimeters on the tip or ala will cause significant distortion if closed similarly. The columella, alar margins, and soft triangles are also made up of thin and pliable skin.

THE SUBUNIT CONCEPT

The combination of skin quality along with the underlying subsurface architecture of the nose, including the bone and the cartilage, creates subtle but important convexities and concavities when the nose is viewed externally.[2] The transition between these adjacent areas creates light reflections and shadows that define the commonly referred to subunits of the nose: tip, dorsum, columella, sidewalls, alae, and soft triangles (Figure 30.1).[3] The shadow between adjacent subunits represents an opportunity for the reconstructive surgeon to place incisions at these border regions thereby minimizing their appearance. Each patient has a uniquely shaped nose with different proportions and shape to the anatomical subunits. Delineating them in the operating room may not accurately mimic the way light is transmitted when patients are viewed upright; therefore, it may be beneficial to outline subunits in the preoperative area.

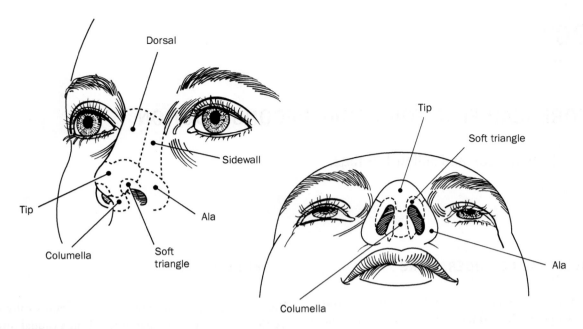

Figure 30.1. Topographic nasal subunits.

A secondary aspect relevant to the subunit concept that needs consideration is trapdoor healing. Myofibroblasts recruited to an area of flap healing tend to create a bulge or pincushion appearance above the nasal surface. As such, the properties of wound healing can be harnessed to improve the reconstructive outcome in areas which are naturally convex, such ala and tip subunits. Whereas poor contour should always be avoided because of its obvious nature, scarring when thoughtfully considered is not problematic and can be used to enhance the aesthetic result.

Because the distinct form of each subunit defines normal nasal appearance, the reconstructive outcome is often improved when an entire, rather than partial, subunit is replaced. Partial subunit replacement will often place a scar along an area of maximal convexity in the middle of a subunit, rather than the more ideal position within the concavity between adjacent subunits. For this reason, if a defect involves more than 50% of a subunit, the remainder is often removed; therefore, the flap is designed to replace the entire subunit exactly. This approach minimizes the patch-like appearance more commonly associated with partial subunit reconstruction (Figures 30.2 and 30.3).

COVER, LINING, AND SUPPORT

Thinking about the nose in three separate layers anatomically positioned from superficial to deep facilitates the reconstructive process: skin cover, cartilaginous or bony support, and nasal mucosal lining. Each layer has specific considerations. Similar to the unique qualities of skin in different regions just described, the subsurface support of bone and cartilage throughout the nose contributes to the distinct appearance of each subunit.[4] Therefore, thoughtful

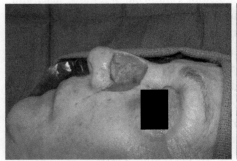 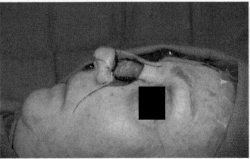 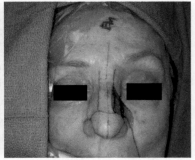

Figure 30.2. Application of the subunit concept in nasal reconstruction. Soft tissue defect of the nose (left). Delineation of subunits highlights missing portions of nasal dorsum and cheek in addition to entire sidewall (center, right).

RECONSTRUCTIVE FACIAL SURGERY

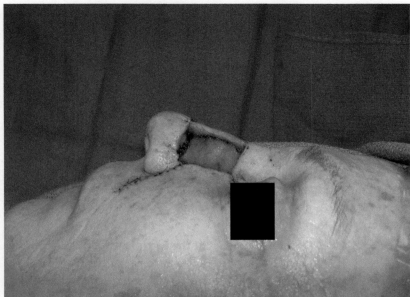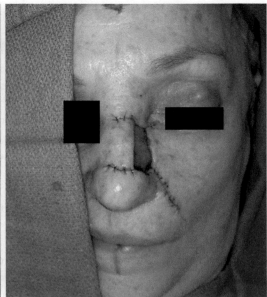

Figure 30.3. Local advancement flaps of cheek and nasal dorsum can be performed to confine the defect to the left nasal side wall only.

reconstruction should attempt to replace like with like to maintain normal appearance. The nasal dorsum and sidewall subunits, because of their linear shape, are often replaced with rigid grafts harvested from rib or the nasal septum. In contrast, the nasal tip, because of its curved shape, requires an underlying framework that is more malleable. For this reason, cartilage is almost always used. Reconstruction of the nasal alar is unique in that the fibrofatty tissue normally present allows for a curved appearance but with enough intrinsic rigidity to avoid airway collapse during inhalation. Once the ala is manipulated surgically in any way, it almost always loses this quality, leading to external valve collapse. As such, ala reconstruction requires nonanatomic cartilage graft placement using the conchal bowl. Regardless of the anatomic area, cartilaginous or bony support should be anticipated with placement during the primary reconstruction. Once the cover and lining have healed to one another with scar formation, they are rarely compliant enough to allow room for delayed cartilage placement or to transmit the shape of the underlying cartilage construct through a stiffened skin envelope.

Composite defects that include nasal lining are the most complex since replacement of all three lamina is required.[5] In general there is a limited amount of spare nasal lining that can be used to replace missing areas. Lining can be obtained from high in the nasal vault in the form of a bipedicle bucket handle flap for reconstruction of small ala or alar margin lining defects. Larger amounts of mucosa can be obtained from the septum. Septal flaps can hinge anteriorly off a branch of the labial artery that supplies the

columella or alternatively can be obtained from the contralateral side in the form of a turnover flap. These flaps can be useful for midvault, not tip, reconstruction; however, they are technically challenging, with a potential for distortion of remaining normal anatomy, so should be only performed in those with sufficient experience.

The simplest option for nasal lining is a skin graft placed on the undersurface of a forehead flap. The skin graft can be placed at the time a forehead flap is turned, or, alternatively, it can be prelaminated while on the forehead in a separate procedure. Skin grafts have two principal drawbacks. First, secondary contracture tends to distort the overlying skin envelope. Second, it is difficult to place intervening cartilage without devascularizing the graft.

Perhaps the simplest and most reliable option for small and moderate size lining defects is use of an additional flap. Considerations are turnover of remaining external skin, nasolabial, facial artery musculomucosal (FAMM), or a folded forehead flap. Whereas the fathers of modern nasal reconstruction originally espoused septal flaps, the folded forehead flap has become the workhorse for repair of lining defects.[6] Additional tissue can be harvested at the distal extent of forehead flap within the hair-bearing scalp and folded for use as lining. No thinning of the forehead flap is performed at the initial stage, with reconstruction generally completed in three operations. Whether a folded forehead or septal flap, vascularized lining is superior for long-term outcomes when compared to grafts especially in younger patients.

Heminasal and subtotal lining defects generally require a free radial or ulnar forearm flap repaired to the facial artery.

TWO VERSUS THREE STAGES

Reconstruction using a forehead flap can be performed in either two or three stages depending upon the complexity of the defect.[7-9] Each stage is performed approximately 3 weeks apart. For straightforward defects of the nasal side wall or mid-vault that require only resurfacing, thinning of the forehead flap can be accomplished at the time it is rotated, eliminating the need for an intermediate stage. However, if cartilage placement is required or the forehead flap involves folding on itself for lining, an intermediate stage for contouring or separation of the cover and lining portions is necessary. In three-stage reconstructions there is little benefit to thinning the flap at the first operation. Because the flap has already been delayed, it can be thinned aggressively at the intermediate operation as it is re-elevated. The frontalis muscle and excess subcutaneous fat transferred at the first operation are removed, sculpting is performed, and cartilage grafts are placed. The flap attached by its original pedicle is returned to cover the newly contoured subsurface architecture. Three weeks later, the flap pedicle is divided. The authors prefer the three-stage operation in the majority of cases for its vascular reliability and superior ability to contour at the intermediate operation.

DELAY PROCEDURE

A surgical delay is talked about more often than it is performed. Unless the patient has recently quit smoking or there are transverse scars on the forehead, most flaps can be transferred to the nasal defect in one operation. In actuality, the three-stage forehead flap serves as a delay ensuring vascular reliability. In the rare instance that a delay is indicated, the flap should be "sufficiently challenged" such that its blood supply is improved for when it is rotated.

COMBINED DEFECTS

Not uncommonly, nasal defects may include adjacent structures, such as the upper lip or medial cheek. In such instances, the forehead flap should only be used for the nasal portion of the reconstruction. Cheek or nasolabial flaps should be used ensuring a subunit approach to each distinct structure on the face. It is also best to perform reconstruction of adjacent areas in a separate operation prior

to the forehead flap.[10] The platform on which the nose is situated needs to be entirely stable. Too many moving parts at one time leads to unpredictable outcomes.

INDICATIONS

A detailed algorithm for nasal reconstruction is beyond the scope of this chapter; however, options include full-thickness skin grafts, and miter, glabellar, V-Y, nasolabial, bilobe, and forehead flaps.[11]

The following concepts can be broadly considered:

1. Unique properties of the proximal and middle third of the nose, which affect reconstructive decision-making, include its thin nonsebaceous skin, intrinsic laxity, and underlying rigid support braced by the nasal bone. For these reasons, unlike the distal third, proximal and middle defects may be amenable to primary closure or a full-thickness skin graft. As defect size increases, local flaps to employ are the V-Y, miter, or glabellar flaps.

2. Distal third defects positioned laterally at the ala or along the alar groove are commonly amenable to closure with nasolabial or V-Y flaps. In contrast, distal-third defects positioned centrally can be closed with a bilobe flap.

3. As distal defects exceed approximately 1.5 cm in diameter, there is insufficient tissue remaining on the nasal surface to redistribute without causing significant distortion. Moreover, when more than one nasal subunit is involved, consideration needs to be given to regional tissues outside the nose, such as the forehead flap.

CONTRAINDICATIONS

Contraindications to performing forehead flap nasal reconstruction are few. Probably the most important is active smoking. For the most part, the procedure is elective, so clinical conditions should be optimized to ensure favorable outcomes. Other relative contraindications include previous surgery or radiation to the area, collagen vascular diseases, ongoing need for anticoagulation which cannot be stopped safely for surgery, or medical comorbidities which preclude general anesthesia.

PATIENT AND ROOM SETUP

Patients are generally placed under general anesthesia to perform the procedure. An oral ray tube is preferred to minimize obstruction of the operative field. It is important that the endotracheal tube is taped to the lower lip without any traction or displacement of the upper lip or nasolabial creases. The entire face as well as ears are prepped into the operative field. The eyes need to be protected with either a temporary tarsorrhaphy stitch, plastic eye shields, or Steri-Strips. Local anesthetic with epinephrine can be used to minimize bleeding, although this can prevent feedback about flap vascularity.

STAGE 1: SURGICAL TECHNIQUE

The procedure begins be defining the defect. For wounds that have been temporarily skin grafted or allowed to contract substantially prior to reconstruction, the defect needs to be recreated to its original size. Skin at the defect margin can be re-elevated to allow structures to return their anatomic position. All debris is removed sharply until bleeding vascularized tissue is present.

Once this preparatory step is complete, the surgeon needs to determine which subunits have been affected by the extirpative procedure. All of the nasal subunits are drawn with temporary marker or blue dye to determine which structures need to be replaced. As described, if 50% or more of a subunit is missing, the remainder is sharply removed. Even for partial subunit replacement, a small amount of remaining tissue can be removed to place scars

at the border region between adjacent subunits. Thus, the final defect is not determined until after the subunit unit concept has been incorporated into the reconstructive decision making process (Figure 30.4).

Next, a template should be made of the defect for transfer to the forehead. For lateral defects, the template should be taken from contralateral uninvolved structures such as the hemi-tip, ala, soft triangle, and nasal sidewall. Construction of a template based on the defect itself will underestimate the extent of soft tissue needed because it does not account for absent soft tissue thickness or convexity of the subunit. Midline defects are more challenging because no normal structure exists on which to create a template. Sometimes bone wax or other material can be used to temporarily build up the surface of a midline defect such as the nasal tip before the template is taken. Templates can be created in a variety of ways. The simplest way is to free-hand contour the foil of a suture packet with scissors. Dr. Menick has outlined a more precise way. The margin of the defect or normal subunits are carefully outlined with marker followed by placement of Steri-Strips beyond the drawn border. Collodion is placed on top of the Steri-Strips, allowing it to harden. Once dry, the Steri-Strip cast is removed with temporary markings tattooed to the undersurface. The Steri-Strip cast is then placed on foil and scissors are used to cut along the subunit margin of the Steri-Strips and foil simultaneously. The Steri-Strip cast is discarded, with the foil being used for the reconstruction (Figure 30.5). The newly created foil template can be checked against the normal remaining subunit (lateral) or defect (central) allowing for minor secondary trimming. Still another method of template creation, preferred by Dr. Pribaz, is

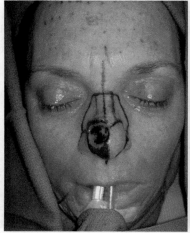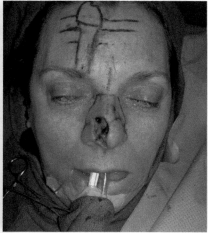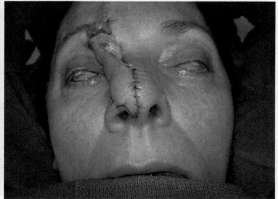

Figure 30.4. Nasal defect involving approximately 60% of right hemi-tip (*left*). Subunit excision of remaining hemi-tip (*center*). Forehead flap reconstruction of right hemi-tip (*right*). Note preservation of soft triangle to avoid notching.

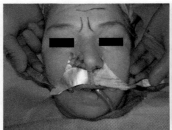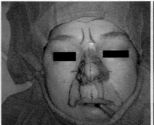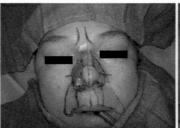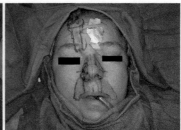

Figure 30.5. Steri-Strip and collodion cast created from normal left upper lip is converted to foil to determine position of right alar base inset (*left*). Foil template created from left normal ala and sidewall (*center left*). Foil template is compared to actual defect of right hemi-nose (*center right*). Foil template is transferred to ipsilateral forehead, including an extension for nasal lining (*right*).

through the use of thick DuoDERM. The adhesive surface is placed directly on the nose, with precise trimming to the size of the defect to be reconstructed. The benefit of DuoDERM compared to foil is that its thickness and pliability are more similar to normal nasal tissues. Regardless of the technique used, because the template has been precisely and carefully prepared, no further adjustments are made to the flap at the time of transfer. If the forehead flap is to be folded for nasal lining, a second template can be made free-hand for this as well (Figure 30.6). Alternatively, a local flap can be used for lining replacement, prior to the forehead flap transfer.

Identification of the supratrochlear artery, which serves as the flap pedicle, is performed next using a Doppler probe. It generally lies vertically above the level of the medial canthal tendon. The pedicle for the flap can start immediately above the eyebrow; however, it's very common to have to cut through the medial aspect of the brow to lengthen the pedicle for the flap to reach the nasal defect. A pedicle approximately 13–15 mm wide is drawn. A wider pedicle is unlikely to improve vascularity as the forehead flap is highly reliable. Moreover, a wider pedicle will effectively shorten the arc of rotation. The pedicle should be oriented vertically, not obliquely, to maximize axial vascularity of the skin island on the forehead even if this incorporates hair with the reconstruction. Remaining

hair follicles are easily ablated during flap thinning at the second stage. For cases requiring an extension of the forehead flap for nasal lining, this portion of the reconstruction is always harvested from within the hair-bearing scalp. Hair is normal on the nasal lining in the form of vibrissae so this should be well tolerated. The authors prefer using the paramedian forehead tissue ipsilateral to the defect with medial flap rotation to shorten the pedicle length required (Figures 30.4 and 30.6). Once the foil template is outlined on the forehead, reference marking stitches of 6-0 nylon can be placed at key points of the flap to assist in anatomic placement during the insetting. These sutures correspond to important features such as the junction between subunits.

Flap elevation is performed after the perimeter of the flap and its pedicle are incised. Because the authors prefer an intermediate stage for thinning in the majority of cases, the flap is elevated deep to the frontalis muscle along its entire course. For cases that do not require an intermediate stage, the portion of the flap used in the actual defect reconstruction is elevated in the subcutaneous fat superficial to the frontalis. Thereafter, the remainder of the flap is elevated deep to the frontalis to maximize vascularity. Whether the reconstruction is performed in two or three stages, the most caudal 1 cm of flap elevation is performed in the subperiosteal plane to avoid damage to the vascular

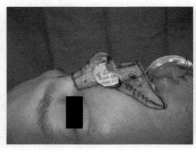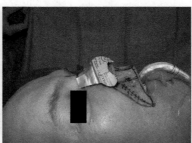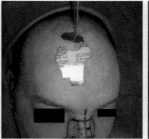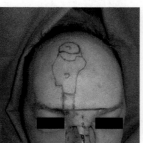

Figure 30.6. Foil template of alar lining defect (*left*). Foil template of cover including ala and sidewall (*center left*). Placement of cover and lining templates on ipsilateral forehead (*center right*). Drawn forehead flap with pedicle. Note subunit excision of previous skin graft on right nasal sidewall (*right*).

RECONSTRUCTIVE FACIAL SURGERY

pedicle. The surgeon can lengthen the pedicle further below the brow as needed until the flap reaches the defect with no tension.

Once rotated, the flap is inset at the nasal defect. The previously placed 6-0 nylon marking sutures are aligned at key anatomic points. No changes to flap are made to fit the defect since it should already be the correct size based on the accuracy of the templates. During insetting, there should be no tension anywhere along the suture line. Capillary refill should be ensured around every stitch. If there is blanching at a stitch that does not reperfuse, then the stitch needs to be replaced. The smallest caliber stitch that gets the job done is usually best. For cases in which an intermediate stage is planned, the flap can be quite bulky. If necessary, portions of the flap do not necessarily need to be inset as it will heal secondarily to the defect surface. A Xeroform dressing can be loosely secured to the raw surface of the flap with chromic sutures. Alternatively, a skin graft can be used, but will subsequently be discarded (not preferred).

The forehead is reapproximated in anatomic fashion. Horizontal hash marks can be drawn with ink across the forehead prior to the flap elevation to ensure anatomic realignment at the time of closure. Extensive undermining above the galea and periosteum can be performed if primary closure is achievable. Often there is a standing cone deformity at the hair-bearing scalp that needs to be excised to improve contour. Bare areas of the forehead with exposed periosteum should be dressed with Xeroform and allowed to epithelialize secondarily. The subsequent widened scar at the forehead can be revised in the future during any planned nasal revision. Skin grafts are not placed at the forehead.

POSTOPERATIVE CARE

Patients usually spend 1 night in the hospital following the procedure. During the early postoperative period, there can be mild serosanguineous drainage from the flap that can benefit from experienced nursing care. Patients are allowed to shower 24 hours after surgery to allow for gentle mechanical debridement of dried blood. Sutures are removed at 5–7 days. Antibiotics are usually limited to 24 hours postoperatively unless cartilage grafts are used, in which case the duration is 5 days. For patients who wear glasses, they can be suspended from the forehead with a piece of tape placed around the bridge for 1 week.

COMPLICATION

Complications are uncommon. In the immediate postoperative period, capillary refill should be monitored. Mild venous congestion is common. This can be tolerated as it will improve within the first few days. If it appears to be getting progressively worse in the recovery area, then consideration needs to be given to replacing the flap in anatomic position on the forehead. This is a safe and easy maneuver if there is any uncertainty about viability. The flap can be returned to the nasal defect in 3–5 days following the vascular delay. Whereas some mild degree of venous congestion is expected, ischemic complications are rare except in smokers. If the flap is inset tension-free and sutures are carefully manipulated to avoid local ischemia, partial flap loss is uncommon. Vascular reliability is ensured further if no thinning of the flap is performed at the initial operation. Infection is also unusual, although may be more common when grafts are placed.

STAGE 2: AN INTERMEDIATE OPERATION

Three weeks after the initial operation, contouring of the flap and nasal substance is performed in an outpatient procedure. The vascular reliability at this point enables a superior ability to thin the flap and is the principal reason the authors prefer an intermediate operation in the majority of the cases. Conceptually, it is easiest to think of the flap as a thin skin cover which will allow the underlying subsurface

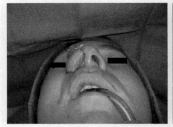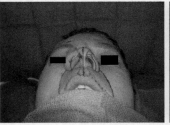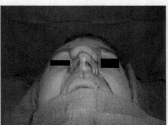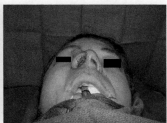

Figure 30.7. Bulky full-thickness folded forehead flap at time of initial flap transfer (*left*). Subunits are drawn demonstrating separation of cover and lining portions of forehead flap (*center left*). Forehead flap is elevated at 2–3 mm in thickness and remains attached to its pedicle. Lining portion has neovascularization from remaining nasal tissues. Nonanatomic cartilage graft is placed (*center right*). Thinned forehead flap is returned to nasal defect (*right*).

FOREHEAD FLAP FOR NASAL RECONSTRUCTION

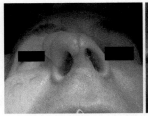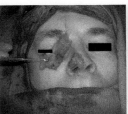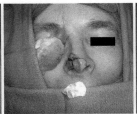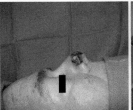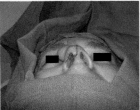

Figure 30.8. Right hemi-tip and partial ala reconstruction 3 weeks following initial forehead flap transfer. No thinning of flap was performed (*left*). Forehead flap is re-elevated at 2–3 mm in thickness while remaining attached to its pedicle (*center left*). Nasal subunits are redrawn to allow for contouring (*center*). Nonanatomic cartilage graft (*center right*). Thinned forehead flap is returned to nasal defect (*right*).

architecture to penetrate through. Therefore, during the second operation, the flap should be uniformly elevated at 2 mm in thickness in the superficial subcutaneous plane with a scalpel. At this point any reconstruction used for the nasal lining, such as skin grafts or the folded portion of the forehead flap, are effectively separated from their original blood supply, being vascularized only by the nasal substance itself (Figure 30.7). Once it is re-elevated, the remainder of the forehead flap subcutaneous fat and frontalis muscle is adherent to the surface of the original nasal defect. The forehead flap, attached only by its vascular pedicle, is wrapped in gauze while the rest of the operation proceeds.

Contouring of the original nasal defect is performed next. The nasal subunits are redrawn. Foil templates created at the initial operation can be resterilized to identify correct anatomic position of the nasal subunits. Sculpting of remaining tissue on the nasal surface is then performed according to which units are being reconstructed. Whereas areas such as the tip require a certain amount of fat present, thinner areas such as the sidewall need to be thinned down to the nasal lining or bone. Cartilage and bone grafts are harvested and placed at this time as well (Figure 30.8). Conchal ear cartilage can be placed at the ala to prevent external valve collapse. Septal cartilage is more rigid, so can be used for tip support or to brace the nasal sidewall.

Intermittently during the sculpting process, the forehead flap can be returned to the nasal defect to check the appearance. The reconstruction should be inspected from all viewpoints including the worm's view. Once the surgeon is satisfied, the flap is secured to the margin of the nasal defect with fine nonabsorbable sutures similar to the initial operation.

STAGE 3: PEDICLE DIVISION

Three weeks after contouring and placement of nasal support, the pedicle is ready for division. Neovascularization has occurred, with the flap no longer dependent on its axial blood supply from the supratrochlear artery. The flap is transected sharply in its midportion. The flap at the nose will be observed to refill retrograde from the nasal substance. The base of the flap is then inset into the medial brow by converting it to an inverted-V or pennant shape. It is contoured to match the surrounding tissues and inset with nonabsorbable sutures. At the nose, additional contouring can be performed as necessary although it is generally not needed. As long as the approximately 50% of the flap surface area remains adherent to the nose, the flap can be partially re-elevated for thinning. The flap margin is then

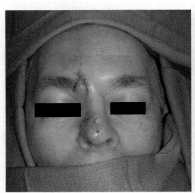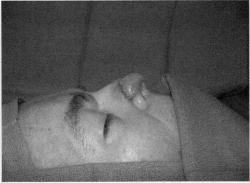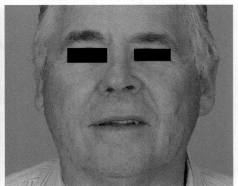

Figure 30.9. Appearance immediately following division and inset (*left and center*). Long-term outcome of same patient (*left*).

RECONSTRUCTIVE FACIAL SURGERY

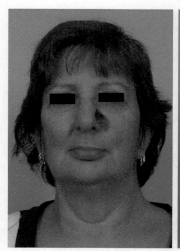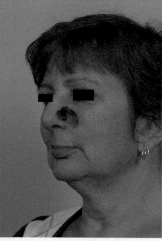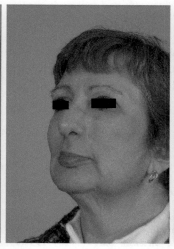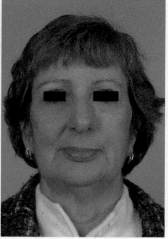

Figure 30.10. Preoperative images of left medial cheek and nasal side wall full-thickness defect (*left and center left*). Long-term outcome following cheek advancement flap followed by three-stage forehead flap with full-thickness skin graft for nasal lining (*center right and right*).

carefully tailored to meet the nasal margin without tension for insetting using nonabsorbable sutures (Figure 30.9).

REVISIONS

A minimum of 4–6 months should be allowed to pass before revisions are considered. The soft tissue swelling will take time to resolve before the final appearance becomes apparent (Figures 30.10 and 30.11). Minor secondary procedures include (1) placement of direct scars along the junction of nasal subunits such as the ala and sidewall, (2) additional flap thinning, (3) alar base elevation or narrowing in the form of a V-Y flap, (4) thinning of nasal lining flaps along the alar margin to improve airflow, and (5) placement of additional cartilage grafts to brace against scarring, which occurs over time.

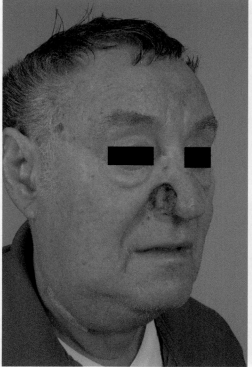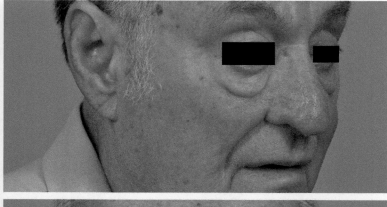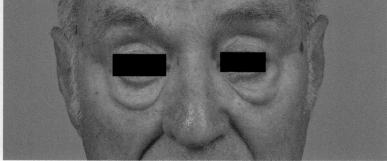

Figure 30.11. Preoperative images of right alar and partial sidewall defect (*left*). Long-term outcome following three-stage forehead flap with nonanatomic conchal cartilage graft (*top and bottom right*).

FOREHEAD FLAP FOR NASAL RECONSTRUCTION

CAVEATS

Beyond sound surgical technique and judgment, perhaps the strongest recommendation is to seriously consider performing forehead flap nasal reconstruction in three, not two, stages.

REFERENCES

1. Millard DR. *Principlization of Plastic Surgery*. Boston: Little Brown and Company, 1986.
2. Gonzalez-Ulloa M, Castillo A, Stevens E, Alvarez Fuertes G, Leonelli F, Ubaldo F. Preliminary study of the total restoration of the facial skin. *Plast Reconstr Surg* (1946) 1954;13:151–161.
3. Burget GC, Menick FJ. The subunit principle in nasal reconstruction. Plastic and reconstructive surgery 1985;76:239–247.
4. Burget GC, Menick FJ. Nasal support and lining: the marriage of beauty and blood supply. *Plast Reconstr Surg* 1989;84:189–202.
5. Burget GC, Menick FJ. Nasal reconstruction: seeking a fourth dimension. *Plast Reconstr Surg* 1986;78:145–157.
6. Menick FJ. A new modified method for nasal lining: the Menick technique for folded lining. *J Surg Oncol* 2006;94:509–514.
7. Burget GC, Menick FJ. *Aesthetic Reconstruction of the Nose*. St. Louis: CV Mosby, 1994.
8. Carpue J. *An Account of Two Successful Operations for Restoring a Lost Nose*. London: Longman H, Rees, Orme and Brown, 1816.
9. Kazanjian VH. The repair of nasal defects with the median forehead flap; primary closure of forehead wound. *Surg Gynecol Obstetr* 1946;83:37–49.
10. Menick FJ. Defects of the nose, lip, and cheek: rebuilding the composite defect. *Plast Reconstr Surg* 2007;120:887–898.
11. Guo L, Pribaz JR, Pribaz JJ. Nasal reconstruction with local flaps: a simple algorithm for management of small defects. *Plast Reconstr Surg* 2008;122:130e–139e.

31.

NASOLABIAL FLAP

Michael Budd, Melissa Kanack, and Michael Lee

Nasal restoration may be one of the earliest forms of reconstructive surgery, and the nasolabial flap has been part of the nasal reconstruction lexicon for centuries. Many variations of this flap have been described in the effort to expand the uses of this versatile tissue. The fundamental reasoning for selecting any reconstructive technique is to recreate the shape, color, and texture of the damaged structure while maintaining any physiologic function. The nasolabial flap supplies well-vascularized tissue of sufficient color, texture, and volume for reconstructing most commonly the nasal ala area.[1] However, it has also been described as a possible choice for various other areas of the nose, lips, oral cavity, and tongue.[2] We will review the nasolabial flap's indications, anatomy, design, operative technique, and any special considerations.

ASSESSMENT OF THE DEFECT

The nose is a complex aesthetic and functional structure with concave and convex contours that are composed of thin to thick skin with varying concentrations of adnexal structures as well as complex air flow patterns that are difficult to maintain after reconstruction. In particular, defects of the nasal ala pose a unique reconstructive quandary in that care must be taken to maintain support of the external nasal valve while preventing alar rim notching and preservation of the alar-facial groove.[3]

Defect analysis is vital in determining the appropriateness of using the nasolabial tissue for reconstructing an area. When evaluating wounds, the surgeon must consider several key factors including which aesthetic zones are involved (alar, tip, dorsum, etc.), the percentage of aesthetic zones removed (more or less then 50%), which layers are damaged (skin, lining, support structure), thickness of tissue required to fill the defect, and the ability of the nasolabial flap to easily reach

the most distal portion of the wounds without undue tension.[4] In planning the reconstruction, all layers must be replaced with equivalent tissue, and special attention to structural support must be given to improve aesthetics and function.

INDICATIONS

The nasolabial flap is primarily used for nasal reconstruction and most frequently for alar reconstruction due to the tissue's location, texture, color, and bulk. Its natural tendency to contract creates a more rounded and mounded appearance, which can help recreate the alar shape and develop a new alar groove which is very difficult to reconstruct.[5] However, this can be overpronounced, creating a "pincushion" affect requiring secondary revision surgery (Figure 31.1). The nasolabial flap may provide tissue for skin coverage, lining, or both in limited application by folding the flap. This requires extensive thinning of the flap, particularly in the distal portion which will be used in the alar region. Care must be taken with younger patients where the donor site for the nasolabial flap may be more obvious even when precisely located (Figure 31.2) due to the shallow nasolabial fold as compared to older patients.

Small, skin-only defects of the ala may be more optimally reconstructed with skin grafts or local flaps, such as a rhomboid or bilobed.[6] However, deeper defects of the ala that require more bulk and support are uniquely qualified for a nasolabial flap reconstruction. In addition, defects that are greater than 50% of the alar aesthetic unit will have a better result with complete removal of the alar subunit and placement of a nasolabial flap.[4] Careful flap design to strategically place scars along the borders of the aesthetic zones optimizes the cosmetic outcome.[7]

Even though some of the inherent qualities of the nasolabial flap favor it as a primary choice for large

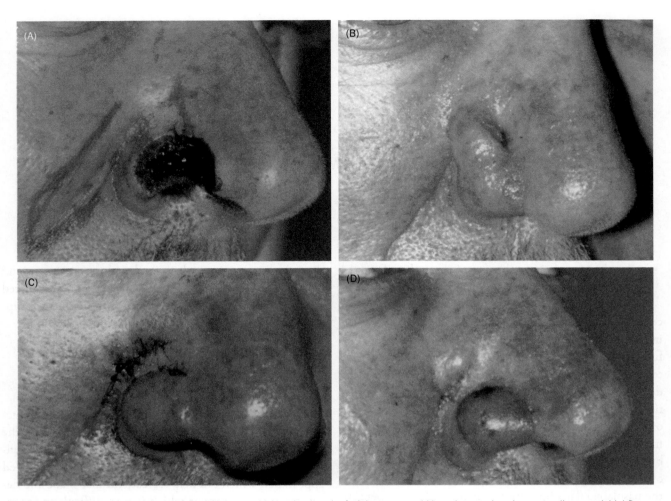

Figure 31.1. Alar defect. (A) Note that remaining alar base, which maintains alar-facial groove, could have been reduced more to allow nasolabial flap to recreate more of the alar aesthetic unit. (B) Flap in place, rolled on itself to recreate alar rim. (C) Secondary division of flap and initial insetting, with preservation of skin bridge to define superior extent of ala. (D) Two weeks after insetting, flap demonstrates pincushion appearance. Flap will be thinned to flatten superior aspect and create more anatomic contour because the ala is not completely convex.

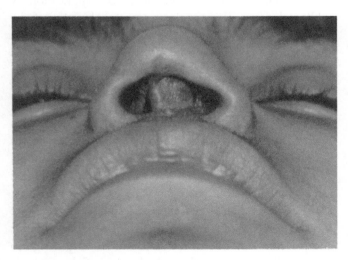

Figure 31.2. Columellar defect in a 9-year-old girl that resulted from repeated trauma. Washio flap was used to reconstruct the defect. Potential donor site scar from nasolabial flap was considered unacceptable.

and deep alar defects, there are other areas in certain circumstances that may also benefit from this technique. The superiorly based nasolabial flap may have application in four other areas of the nose: the nasal tip, columella, septum, and the sidewall. The nasolabial flap may be used as a single-staged transpositional flap for the sidewall (Figures 31.3 and 31.5), while the nasal tip (Figure 31.4), columella, and septal reconstructions usually require a second procedure in order to divide the vascular pedicle and complete the inset of the flap.[8,9] Reconstruction of the columella may require bilateral nasolabial flaps, which will create some nasal obstruction until they are divided 2–3 weeks later.[10] Septal reconstruction can be performed to a limited degree by means of tunneled bilateral nasolabial flaps. Their use results in keratinized epithelium being introduced into the nasal cavity, but, over time, the problem resolves as the flaps mucosalize. The nasolabial flap can also be used for dedicated nasal lining by turning

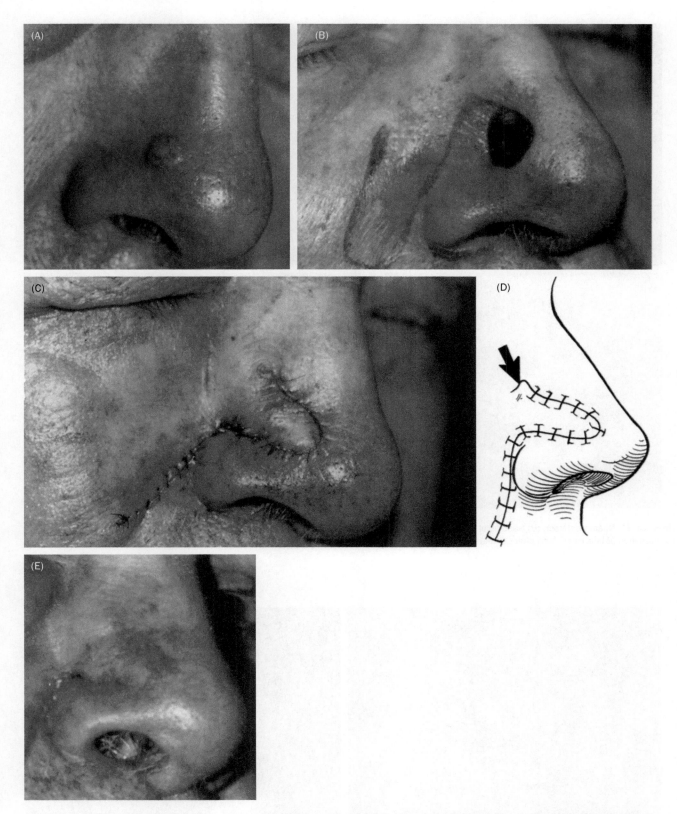

Figure 31.3. (A) Basal cell carcinoma of side of nose. (B) A sidewall defect with intervening skin, which will require excision for one-stage procedure. Ala is preserved. Incisions are placed to avoid compromising nasofacial groove. (C,D) Nasolabial flap in place, with standing cone at point of rotation. (E) Donor site is well-healed, with slightly raised appearance of flap.

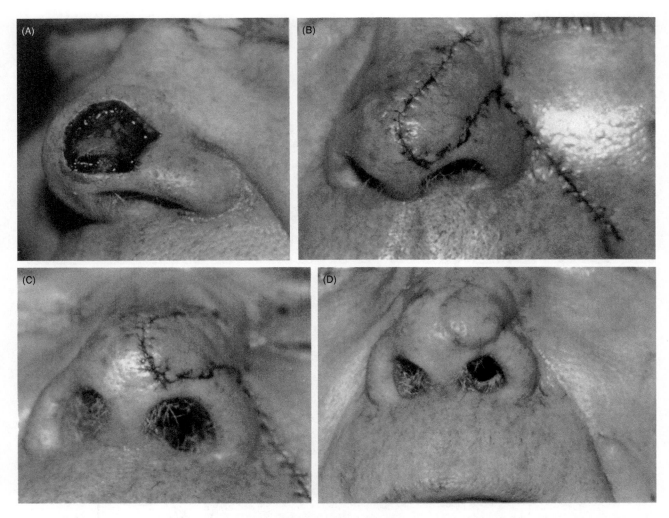

Figure 31.4. (A) Nasal tip defect. (B) Nasolabial flap requires excision of intervening skin for one-stage procedure. (C) Note that contour is acceptable. (D) Presence of late pincushion effect and standing cone at inferior aspect of donor site.

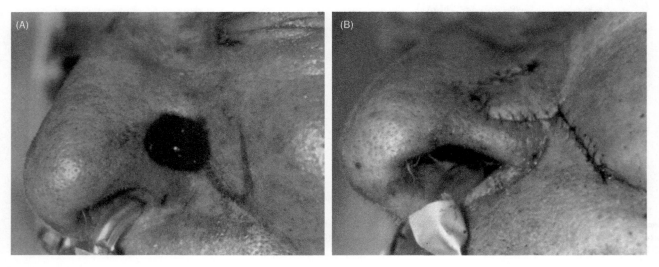

Figure 31.5. (A,B) Nasal alar and sidewall defect repaired with rhomboid flap from nasolabial fold.

the flap over and positioning the skin on the intranasal aspect of the nose. In cases of total reconstruction, this option may be combined with a forehead flap. However, thick dermis and subcutaneous fat create a bulky lining, which often results in airway obstruction requiring multiple debulking or thinning procedures.

The inferiorly based nasolabial flap has been described for lip, oral cavity, and tongue reconstructions. The flap can be rotated as a single-staged procedure for the ipsilateral lateral lip and oral commissure areas. However, for tongue and oral cavity reconstructions, the flap has to be tunneled through the cheek to reach these defects.[11] There are also well-described primary techniques for the lip, oral cavity, and tongue such as skin or vermillion grafts, lip sharing, mucosal flaps, or cheek advancement techniques. However, there are many reasons that these "first choice" techniques may not be available, ranging from patient preferences to previous surgery or radiation therapy.[12] Therefore, the nasolabial flap can be used as a secondary choice but each case requires individual analysis and treatment.

ANATOMY

The nasolabial fold is created by the superficial musculo-aponeurotic system (SMAS) and mimetic musculature as they fuse with the orbicularis oris muscle. Lateral to the fold, there are no cutaneous muscle attachments (i.e., no support), while medial to the fold, mimetic muscles insert on skin and support against gravity and the aging process. Redundant skin is created by gravity pulling the skin and adipose tissues inferiorly against the pull of the mimetic musculature.[13] The nasolabial flap is created from this skin and subcutaneous tissue superior and lateral to the fold. Typically, 2–3 cm of skin can be harvested from the fold and still allow for primary closure. The exact location of the nasolabial fold in children may be difficult to identify, even in animated patients.

Muscular perforators arising from the angular branch of the anterior facial artery, as well as anastomotic branches from the internal maxillary artery, the transverse facial artery, and the labial artery, provide primary vascular supply to the nasolabial flap by way of the subdermal plexus. Care must be taken to preserve these underlying vascular connections at the base of the flap because it is usually raised superficially to the mimetic muscles. The nasolabial flap is thus an axial pattern flap, but it can be converted to a more random pattern flap if the deep connections are not maintained.[14] In any case, for large flaps, or long flaps with a narrow skin base, care must be taken to preserve these perforating branches. If the flap will extend past the midline

or is folded on itself, the perforators should be maintained or delay considered. The cheek skin is drained by the angular vein (among others) and care must be exercised to avoid putting the flap under tension, especially over a convexity, where venous drainage may be compromised and result in flap congestion and the potential for flap loss.

CONTRAINDICATIONS

As previously discussed, aesthetically, there are better choices than the nasolabial flap for nasal, lip, oral cavity, and tongue reconstructions with the notable exception of deep or full-thickness alar defects. Remember, caution should be used in younger patients due to the visibility of the donor site scar. On the other hand, effacement of the nasolabial fold may occur in the elderly, creating significant cheek asymmetry. Care must also be taken when considering tunneling the pedicle, which could disrupt key aesthetic structures like the alar-facial sulcus and the philtral columns of the lip.[2]

However, there are certain nonaesthetic considerations that may eliminate the nasolabial tissue for transfer. Primarily, while the nasolabial area is a desirable donor site due to tissue redundancy, there may not be enough tissue for larger defects, and this area should be avoided. In addition, there is some controversy with regards to the exact nature of the flap's blood supply. Some argue that it is a random flap based on the subcutaneous and subnormal plexus of the cheek, while others describe perforators from the facial and angular arteries. Either way, damage to the medial cheek tissue (superiorly based) or oral commissure tissue (inferiorly based) from surgery or radiation therapy would compromise the use of this flap. The anatomic location of the defect is also an important consideration because undue tension on the flap will cause necrosis of the tissue. The glabellar and medial canthal regions are well out of the arc of rotation of this flap. Care must be taken when dividing the pedicle as well as overly aggressive debulking at this time will cause necrosis of the flap. Finally, patients who have a history of smoking or have diabetes are particularly prone to flap failure. For these patients, the skin bridge and underlying perforators should both be preserved while aggressive thinning of the flap should be reserved for a second procedure. Active smokers should stop prior to undergoing this technique.

ROOM SETUP

The vast majority of nasolabial flap nasal reconstructions may be performed under local anesthesia with sedation.

However, patients with significant medical problems may be better served in a formal operating room setting with the assistance of an anesthetist. More extensive procedures, including multiple flap procedures, may be more easily accomplished under general anesthesia.

The patient is usually placed in the supine position with the head toward the back table to allow access to both sides of the face. The patient is prepped with 50% dilute Betadine. A complete face prep is performed to allow wide draping and prevent oxygen trapping under the drapes. The eyes are irrigated to remove any of the prep solution. A split drape is placed over the rest of the patient.

PATIENT MARKINGS

Regardless of whether the flap will be superiorly or inferiorly based, the critical component of the patient marking is placement of the medial incision in the nasolabial or nasofacial crease. In older patients, the location of the site may be determined with the patient supine and under general anesthesia, but younger patients require facial animation to determine scar placement. Normally, the crease can be located by having the patient grimace. The lateral incision may be 2–3 cm from the medial incision, depending on the amount of tissue required, and should usually be shorter than the medial incision to allow for as broad a pedicle skin base as possible. This may not always be possible, or necessary, if the deep perforators are maintained and a secondary procedure is planned to detach and inset the flap. A foil template of the defect can be used to facilitate marking in order to determine the size of flap required. The flap is usually designed just above the level of the oral commissure. This allows for enough length to easily reach the anterior ala. If the tip requires coverage, this flap may need to be designed more inferiorly to provide enough length. Care must be taken not to unduly efface the nasolabial or nasofacial crease. The superolateral portion of the upper lip should be avoided (Figure 31.6). Finally, at the time of flap marking, the decision needs to be made whether the reconstruction will be performed in one or more stages. Most often, secondary pedicle division is undertaken to avoid deformities created by pedicle tunneling.

TECHNIQUE

Once the appropriate flap has been chosen and the appropriate incisions outlined, the periphery of the flap is infiltrated with 1% lidocaine solution with epinephrine

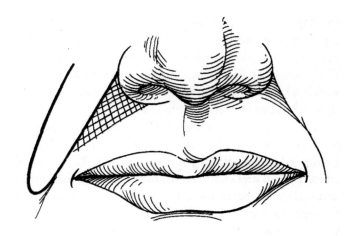

Figure 31.6. When designing the flap, the superolateral portion of upper lip should be avoided.

1:100,000. Care is taken not to infiltrate the actual flap or the base of the flap, which may compromise the vascularity of the tissue to be transferred. The skin is incised down to the muscles proximally and more superficial distally. The proximal lateral incision is kept shorter than the medial incision to maintain a wider base, thus preserving important segments of the subdermal blood supply (Figure 31.7). This typically occurs when the incisions are carried more superiorly in the nasofacial region. This is not necessary if the flap is going to be elevated on a subcutaneous pedicle alone.

The flap is elevated from distal to proximal. The level of dissection is relatively superficial distally, maintaining 2–3 mm of subcutaneous adipose tissue, and at the level of

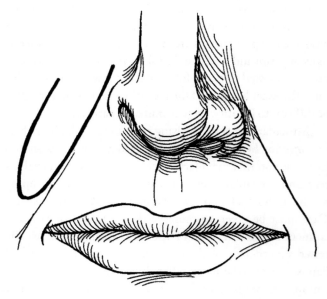

Figure 31.7. Lateral incision is kept more inferior than medial incision to maintain wider base and preserve subdermal plexus. Medial incision is made in nasolabial sulcus.

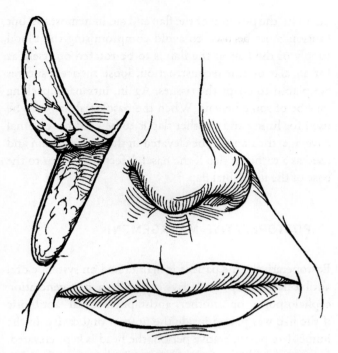

Figure 31.8. Distally, flap can be elevated in a more superficial plane and deeper as base and perforators are approached. Dissection should be superficial to mimetic muscles.

the muscles proximally (Figure 31.8). More tissue can be elevated distally, but this area will need to be judiciously thinned in most cases before in-setting of the flap takes place. The flap should be thinned symmetrically, not just on the periphery. When the flaps are thinned on the periphery only in order to preserve the vascular supply of the flap, the disparity in thickness between the flap and subcutaneous tissue at the recipient site will predispose the flap to a more biscuit-like appearance in the long term; the combination of flap contraction and underlying fat compression can give the flap a pincushion appearance. Either the flap should be thinned evenly or a revision performed at a later date to address the persistence of the centrally located subcutaneous fat.[15]

As the flap is elevated toward the base, more tissue is maintained on the flap to preserve any potential perforating blood vessels. This area will not be used in the actual reconstruction, but serves to maintain the viability of the flap. In all cases, the flap elevation takes place superficial to the orbicularis oris muscle and mimetic muscles, as well as the facial artery and angular vessels. When the superiorly based flap is elevated in the nasofacial region superiorly, thinning of the flap may need to be more aggressive to conform to the thinner soft tissue of the lateral wall of the nose.

Alar structural support is most commonly provided by conchal bowl cartilage grafts because of their similar shape to the ala but septal cartilage may be used as well. These

may be placed at the time of flap rotation or delayed to a subsequent procedure.[16] If cartilage grafts are placed during the initial surgery, vascularized lining is required to sandwich the cartilage graft and completely cover it with well-perfused tissue. In full-thickness defects, mucosal flaps must be used and not skin grafts to provide total coverage over the cartilage graft. However, if the cartilage is placed later, a skin graft may be used for lining at the initial surgery. In either situation, the thinned distal flap is rolled over the edge and sutured to the inner mucosa or skin graft, thus hiding the scar in the nasal vestibule.

The decision to perform the reconstruction in one, two, or three stages is very important at this time. During a three-stage procedure the flap is initially rotated, then thinned, and finally the pedicle is divided in three separate steps. This allows for delay of the flap with subsequent aggressive whole-flap thinning. If a two-stage procedure is planned, less aggressive thinning of the flap will be achieved during the second stage because a portion of the flap cannot be re-elevated, preserving the vascular supply after the pedicle is divided. Future thinning may be required once the flap has further settled. If a one-stage procedure has been chosen, intervening skin should be removed to allow for insetting of the flap (Figure 31.9).

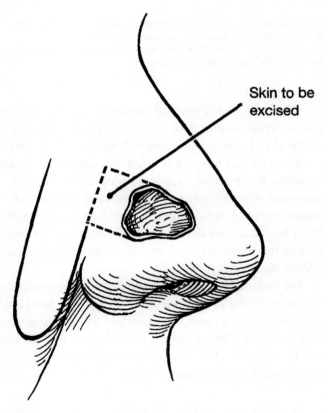

Skin to be excised

Figure 31.9. One-stage procedure will require excision of intervening skin.

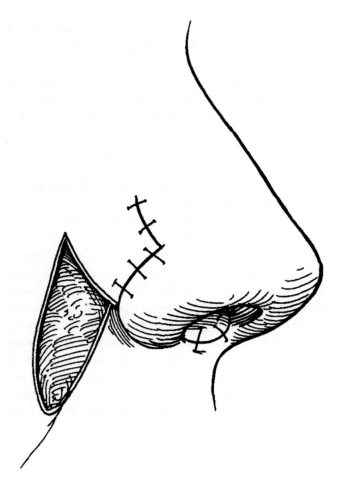

Figure 31.10. Incision is made in alar groove, through which the superiorly or inferiorly based nasolabial flap is passed into nose for septal or columellar reconstruction. Skin island flap can also be considered, which would alleviate need for secondary division.

maintain the position of the flap and aid in hemostasis, but caution must be used to avoid compromising the blood supply of the flap. If the flap is to be rotated on itself, as for an alar or rim reconstruction, loose mattress sutures are placed to coapt the tissues. Again, intranasal packing may be of some benefit. When the nasolabial flap is to be used for lining and another flap is to be used for external coverage, the flap may be elevated in the usual fashion and used as a turnover flap if the nasal defect is adjacent to the base of the nasolabial flap.[17]

POSTOPERATIVE MANAGEMENT

Postoperatively, the patient is maintained on systemic oral antibiotics for up to 7 days, typically a first-generation cephalosporin or another antistaphylococcal antibiotic if the flap was placed inside the nose or oral cavity. In the immediate postoperative period, the head is kept elevated. Intranasal packing, if placed, is routinely removed within 24 hours. Skin sutures are removed within 7–10 days. Two-stage procedures usually undergo division and final inset 2–3 weeks after the initial procedure. Revisions are delayed for 2–3 months to allow for settling of the soft tissue. Strategies for flap revision often focus on recreating the nasolabial fold or alar facial groove, which are important aesthetic landmarks, as well as additional debulking of the flap if needed. As discussed previously, cartilage grafts may also be placed at this time if indicated.

CAVEATS

The nasolabial flap is a workhorse flap for lower nasal reconstruction. In the younger patient, consideration must be given to the donor site scar. Care must be taken to avoid excessive tension and thinning at the base of the flap to preserve the blood supply. Likewise, while the tip of the flap may be thinned judiciously at the initial insetting, a secondary revision several months after flap division is perhaps a more prudent course, particularly in a patient with risk factors such as tobacco use or diabetes. Finally, caution must be exercised to prevent undue tension on the flap, especially if the flap is used across the midline, because the convexity of the dorsum and tip could compromise the distal blood supply.

When the flap is elevated, regardless of whether the reconstruction is one, two, or three stages, the donor site is closed in layers with interrupted sutures of 5-0 Vicryl or Monocryl and 5-0 or 6-0 nylon. No drains are usually required. For external nasal reconstructions, the flap is contoured appropriately and sutured in place with interrupted sutures or a running stitch with 5-0 or 6-0 nylon. Many buried sutures should be avoided to prevent disruption of the blood supply. External or internal splints are seldom used.

For intranasal (septal) or columellar reconstructions that are planned to be done in two stages, an alar-facial incision is made to pass the nasolabial flap into the nose (Figure 31.10). This prevents distortion of the ala and will be repaired when the flap is divided in the second-stage procedure. Intranasal packing may be used to help

REFERENCES

1. Day TA, Stucker FJ. Regional and distant flaps in nasal reconstruction. *Facial Plast Surg* 1994;10:349–357.
2. Baker SR, Johnson TM, Nelson BR. The importance of maintaining the alar-facial sulcus in nasal reconstruction. *Arch Otolaryngol Head Neck Surg* 1995;121:617–622.
3. Hoasjoe DK, Stucker FJ, Aarstad RF. Aesthetic and anatomic considerations for nasal reconstruction. *Facial Plast Surg* 1994; 10:317–321.
4. Burget GC, Menick FJ. *Aesthetic Reconstruction of the Nose.* St. Louis: CV Mosby, 1992:544–591.
5. Barton FE. Acquired deformities of the nose. In: McCarthy JG, ed. *Plastic Surgery.* Philadelphia: WB Saunders, 1990:1987–2035.
6. Lawrence WT. The nasolabial rhomboid flap. *Ann Plast Surg* 1992;29:269–273.
7. Spear SL, Kroll SS, Romm S. A new twist to the nasolabial flap for reconstruction of lateral alar defects. *Plast Reconstr Surg* 1987;79:915–920.
8. Cameron RR. Nasal reconstruction with nasolabial cheek flaps. In: Grabb WC, Myers MB, eds. *Skin Flaps.* Boston: Little, Brown, 1975:323–335.
9. Klingensmith MR, Millman B, Foster WP. Analysis of methods for nasal tip reconstruction. *Head Neck* 1994;16:347–357.
10. Ozkus I, Cek DI, Ozkus K. The use of bifid nasolabial flaps in the reconstruction of the nose and columella. *Ann Plast Surg* 1992;29:461–463.
11. Uglesic V, Virag M. Musculomucosal nasolabial island flaps for floor of mouth reconstruction. *Br J Plast Surg* 1995;48:8–10.
12. Yanai A, Nagata S, Tanaka H. Reconstruction of the columella with bilateral nasolabial flaps. *Plast Reconstr Surg* 1986; 77:129–132.
13. Larson DL. An historical glimpse of the evolution of rhytidectomy. *Clin Plast Surg* 1995;22:207–212.
14. Hynes B, Boyd JB. The nasolabial flap: axial or random. *Arch Otolaryngol Head Neck Surg* 1988;114:1389–1391.
15. Steenfos H, Tarnow P, Blomqvist G. Experience with the modified defatted nasolabial transposition flap in nasal reconstruction. *Scand J Plast Reconstr Surg* 1995;29:51–52.
16. Barton FE. Reconstruction of the nose. In: Georgiade GS, Georgiade NG, Riefkohl R, Barwick WJ, eds. *Textbook of Plastic, Maxillofacial and Reconstructive Surgery.* Baltimore: Williams & Wilkins, 1992:539–550.
17. Ariyan S, Chicarilli Z. Cancer of the upper aerodigestive system. In: McCarthy JG, ed. *Plastic Surgery.* Philadelphia: WB Saunders, 1990:3439–3440.

32.

NASAL FRACTURES

REDUCTION

Christine J. Lee and Raj M. Vyas

The nose has several vital functions, including respiration and olfaction. The nose, as the leading point of the face, is without protective covering and is the least resistant of the facial bones to the application of a directional mechanical force. The cartilaginous and bony pyramidal structures of the nose absorb externally applied energy, thereby reducing the transmission of external forces to the cranial vault. Nasal fractures are therefore the most common facial fractures caused by trauma and the third most common fracture of the human body. Furthermore, the nose tends to be a very personal and characteristic facial feature, helping to distinguish each individual's unique identity. The management of isolated nasal fractures, therefore, requires a systematic approach to diagnosis, treatment, and follow-up care to ensure optimal functional and aesthetic results while minimizing complications.[1]

ASSESSMENT OF THE DEFECT

ANATOMY

The adult nose is composed of a bony and cartilaginous pyramid with a midline septum bordered by two nasal passages. The paired nasal bones join the frontal bone superiorly, the ascending process of the maxilla laterally, and the nasal septum medially. The nasal septum is composed of both a cartilaginous and bony segment. The bony septum includes the perpendicular plate of the ethmoid and the vomer. The bone is thick at the base and becomes progressively thinner at the distal margins. The rest of the nasal septum is predominantly composed of a quadrangular septal cartilage that has three distinct angles in relationship to the nasal

spine: anterior septal, midseptal, and caudal septal. The cartilaginous pyramid of the nose is also composed of the upper and lower lateral cartilages. The paired upper lateral cartilage segments are attached to the nasal bones proximally and to the quadrangular cartilaginous septum medially. The lower lateral alar cartilage segments are C-shaped and free-floating, and they are encased in the mobile nasal tip by enveloping soft tissue. The area where the lateral crura of the lower lateral cartilages arch over the distal ends of the upper lateral cartilages and the medial crura begin to descend into the columella of the nose functions to support the nasal tip (Figure 32.1).

The nerve supply to the skin covering the nose is through the infraorbital and supratrochlear branches of the trigeminal (fifth) cranial nerve. Facial muscles in the glabella and along the sides of the nose are innervated by the facial nerve (seventh cranial). The nerve supply to the nasal mucosa is from branches of the trigeminal nerve. The lateral nasal wall mucosa is innervated by the anterior ethmoidal branch of the ophthalmic nerve division anteriorly; the internal nasal branch of the infraorbital nerve caudally; the anterior superior alveolar branch of the maxillary nerve, which supplies the anterior end of the inferior concha; and the posterior nasal branch of the maxillary nerve, which passes through the sphenopalatine foramen and supplies the lateral nose posteriorly (Figure 32.2). The nasopalatine nerve originates in the pterygopalatine ganglion and exits through the sphenopalatine foramen to supply the posterior margin of the nasal septum. The remainder of the septum is primarily innervated from the anterior ethmoid nerve and the internal nasal branches of the infraorbital nerve (Figure 32.3). The olfactory region consists of the superior nasal concha and the upper third of the nasal septum (Figure 32.3). It is innervated by the

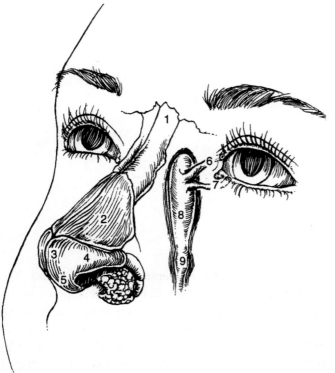

1. Nasal bone
2. Upper lateral cartilage
3. Nasal dome
4. Lateral crura of lower lateral cartilage
5. Medial crura of lower lateral cartilage
6. Superior canaliculi
7. Inferior canaliculi
8. Lacrimal sac
9. Lacrimal duct

Figure 32.1. Normal architecture of nasal pyramid. Lacrimal system is deeply situated medially, within the lacrimal groove of the medial orbital wall.

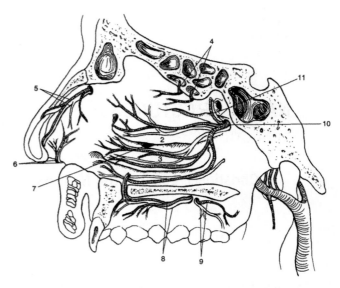

1. Superior concha
2. Middle concha
3. Inferior concha
4. Posterior ethmoid arteries
5. Anterior ethmoid nerve and artery
6. Internal nasal branch of infraorbital nerve
7. Middle meatus—nasal opening of lacrimal duct
8. Greater palatine nerve and artery
9. Lesser palatine nerve and artery
10. Sphenopalatine artery and branches of sphenopalatine ganglion
11. Posterior septal artery and nerve

Figure 32.2. Vascular and neural supply of lateral nose.

olfactory nerve, which enters the cranial cavity through the cribriform plate of the ethmoid bone and terminates in the olfactory bulb.

The blood supply of the nose consists of the anterior and posterior ethmoidal branches of the ophthalmic artery, derived from the internal carotid. The remainder of the blood supply arises from the external carotid artery with the predominant blood supply to the nose arising from the sphenopalatine artery. It enters through the sphenopalatine foramen, sends lateral nasal branches anteriorly and caudally along the conchal surfaces, and forms the posterior septal artery. The greater palatine branch of the maxillary artery sends a terminal branch through the incisive canal to reach the caudal portion of the nasal septum. The facial artery also contributes by three external skin branches: the septal branch of the superior labial artery; branches from the lateral nasal artery, which pierce the ala to supply the lateral vestibular region; and anastomoses from the ascending palatine branch (Figures 32.2 and 32.3).

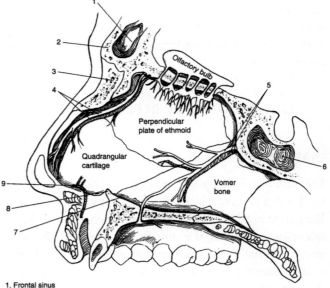

1. Frontal sinus
2. Nasal process of frontal bone
3. Nasal bone
4. Anterior ethmoid nerve and artery
5. Nasopalatine nerve and artery
6. Sphenoid sinus
7. Maxillary crest
8. Nasal spine
9. Septal branch of superior labial artery

Figure 32.3. Neurovascular network of nasal septum.

CLASSIFICATION AND PATHOPHYSIOLOGY

Nasal fractures can be broadly classified as either simple or complex. Simple nasal fractures are those confined to only the nasal structures; complex fractures include adjacent facial bone fractures. Most simple nasal fractures can be treated with closed reduction techniques with little difficulty; complex injuries may require surgical correction and produce a higher rate of morbidity.[1–3]

The scope of this discussion focuses on simple fractures, which can be further categorized as angulated, depressed, or comminuted. Angulated nasal fractures result from an oblique lateral force and are the most common. A minimal force often does not result in significant disruption between the osseous and cartilaginous components of the nose. Distortion involves either a medial collapse of the lateral side of the nasal pyramid (Figure 32.4) or displacement of the entire nasal pyramid away from the direction of the blow. The septum is usually not involved. A greater frontal force, however, can cause the cartilaginous septum to buckle, with potential displacement from the vomerine groove (Figure 32.5). The patient in this case typically displays a C- or S-shaped deformity of the nasal dorsum.[2]

Depressed nasal fractures are caused by direct frontal trauma, resulting in significant septal injury (Figure 32.6).

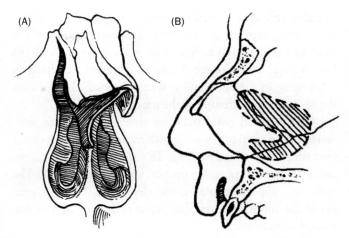

Figure 32.5. (A) Lateral angulated force with combined frontal force, creating significant buckling of nasal septum with displacement from vomerine groove. (B) sagittal view. Note overriding fractures of cartilaginous septum, perpendicular plate of ethmoid bone, and vomerine groove.

The fracture can involve the nasal tip, nasal dorsum, septum, and anterior nasal spine and can potentially involve the frontal processes of the maxilla, lacrimal, and ethmoid bones. Stranc subcategorized these fractures into three planes that directly correlate with the impact of injury. Plane 1 injuries involve the cartilaginous components of the nose distal to the anterior nasal spine and the distal end of the bony septum; Plane 2 injuries involve not only the cartilaginous but also the bony structural components of the nose; and Plane 3 injuries involve not only the nose

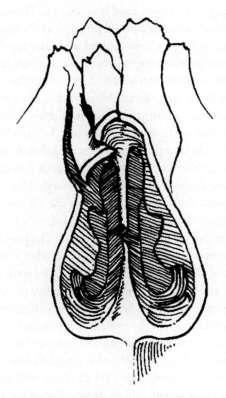

Figure 32.4. Laterally deviated nasal fracture without significant disruption of cartilaginous components.

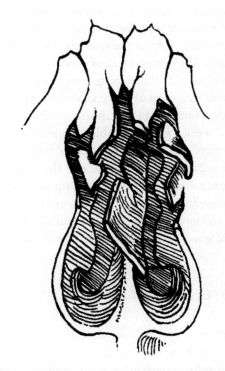

Figure 32.6. Severe frontal force, creating comminuted nasal fracture.

but also orbital or cranial structures. A significant fracture of the nasal septum and the cephalad bony portion of the nose causes the nasal bones to be pushed inward and the lateral nasal bones to be displaced outward, resulting in telescoping of the surrounding fracture ends and significant depression and flattening of the nasal bridge.

Comminuted nasal fractures result in complete shattering of the nasal bones and result most often from a direct frontal impact (Figure 32.6). This condition also occurs more frequently in older people with brittle bones. The nose may appear angulated and depressed, which is generally the result of septal distortion or fragmented or impacted nasal bones.[4]

INDICATIONS AND CONTRAINDICATIONS

The institution of compulsory seat belt laws in Canada and the United States in recent years appears to have reduced the number of isolated facial injuries from motor vehicle accidents. In addition, the rapid retrieval and survival of patients with life-threatening trauma resulting from severe and complex craniomaxillofacial fractures appears to be increasing.[5]

The presence of concomitant injuries in any patient presenting with facial trauma must be carefully assessed. The standard priorities in the initial evaluation of trauma victims include maintaining a patent airway, controlling hemorrhage, initiating fluid volume resuscitation, and managing neurosurgical, thoracic, and abdominal injuries, all of which take precedence over the management of facial fractures. The management of nasal fractures in selected patients without life-threatening emergencies may be coordinated with the repair of trauma to other organ systems. If early repair is not possible, definitive repair can be deferred for up to 2 weeks, allowing stabilization of the patient and the reduction of facial edema and ecchymosis. Waiting longer than 2 weeks, however, allows the fracture sites to heal, creating a more difficult and arduous reduction and repair. Early exploration and repair is essential in children, who have an increased osteogenic potential, which results in more rapid bone healing and adherence of fracture sites.[3–5]

PREOPERATIVE EVALUATION

A careful history and physical examination are always important in the initial evaluation of any patient presenting with a potential nasal fracture. The history should document the nature of the injury and the direction of the traumatic force. Patients must also be thoroughly questioned regarding previous nasal trauma, nasal deformity, or nasal obstruction. The examiner should not assume that all existing nasal deformity is the result of the most recent nasal trauma.

The physical examination includes both an external and internal nasal evaluation. The nose should be inspected visually for any deviation and then palpated for displacement, step-offs, crepitance, and tenderness. Examination of the internal nose should be performed with a nasal speculum with the addition of lighting and suction. Assessment of the mucosa should determine the presence of mucosal lacerations, septal hematoma, bone displacement, and exposed cartilage. If there is a small
segment of exposed septal cartilage and the mucosa is intact on the contralateral side, further management is not required. However, if both sides of the septum are without mucosal coverage, a perforation may develop secondary to cartilage necrosis, and septal coverage with a mucosal flap must be performed. A septal hematoma can be recognized by its bluish, boggy appearance and is the only condition that warrants urgent intervention. Immediate evacuation of the hematoma and nasal packing must be done to avoid mucosal or septal necrosis, which can occur in as little as 24 hours. A small vertical incision is made through the septal mucosa, and the blood is evacuated. The mucosa can then be returned to its normal position and maintained by intranasal packing. Unrecognized and untreated, a septal hematoma can lead to septal necrosis and result in a saddle-nose deformity with retraction of the columella.

When there is significant nasal trauma, the patient must be examined for additional adjacent injuries. Injuries to the posterior wall of the frontal sinus and the cribriform plate of the ethmoid may produce cerebrospinal rhinorrhea. This can be determined by using a glucose stick test to measure the glucose content of the nasal drainage. Furthermore, a cerebrospinal leak should be suspected in patients with a "ring sign," detected by allowing a drop of nasal fluid drainage to fall on a piece of filter paper. The positive sign is a characteristic central area of blood encircled with concentric rings of clearer fluid. Patients should be started on prophylactic antibiotics to avoid the possibility of intracranial infection until the dural tear seals. Associated orbital and maxillary fractures may be present; signs include periorbital tenderness and swelling, a palpable step-off in the orbital rim, infraorbital nerve anesthesia, enophthalmos, and evidence of orbital entrapment. Telecanthus, with the appearance of an epicanthal fold, suggests disruption of one or both medial canthal tendons. The lacrimal apparatus may also be injured by severe nasal trauma. If injury is suspected, the integrity and patency of the lacrimal system must be verified using a lacrimal probe or a fluorescein test to identify stained tears in the nose.[1–3]

Radiographs of isolated nasal fractures are of little clinical value, since most displaced nasal fractures can be diagnosed by a thorough history and physical.[6] A prospective study by Clayton and Lesser reported that radiographs of the nasal bones had no influence on the eventual treatment received by patients and therefore were not indicated in the routine management of nasal fractures. Complex facial injuries involving the nasoorbital maxillary structures, however, can be accurately identified by a single 30-degree occipitomental radiograph, which is often augmented with subsequent computed tomographic (CT) imaging to provide greater fracture detail prior to surgical correction.[7]

OPERATIVE TECHNIQUE

MANAGEMENT PRINCIPLES FOR CLOSED REDUCTION

Closed reduction of nasal fractures by manipulation, followed by external splinting, is the most common treatment for nasal fractures. The technique is simple, of short duration, and has a low rate of morbidity. Due to the heterogeneity of nasal fractures, careful patient selection for closed reduction is necessary to attain satisfactory results.[8] Closed reduction should be performed on deformities limited to simple displaced fractures with no septal injury and can be performed in the emergency room if clinical examination clearly defines the deformity, the injury is acute, and the patient is stable. Swelling rarely prevents accurate reduction if the patient is seen within 3 hours of the injury. When there is excessive nasal swelling, reduction should be performed 4–5 days after injury, when the majority of swelling has subsided, but before fracture healing, which occurs after 14 days in adults and after 7–8 days in children.[9] The results of closed nasal fracture reduction 1 week after injury are equal to those performed acutely in the emergency room in an ideal patient who has sustained a compressed ipsilateral nasal bone fracture. Closed reduction is less satisfactory, however, if the nasal bone fractures are significantly comminuted or involve the maxillary-orbital complexes.[3,10,11]

PROCEDURE FOR CLOSED REDUCTION

The correct use of sedation and local anesthesia to reduce nasal fractures is important for patient relaxation and cooperation. A recent study[12] documented no difference in the cosmetic and functional outcome of nasal fractures reduced under local anesthesia compared to those reduced under general anesthesia. More importantly, there was no difference in the reoperation rates for nasal obstruction or external deformities. Local anesthesia in the emergency room or in the clinic should therefore be considered as the first-line treatment for displaced nasal fractures.[12]

Topical anesthesia may be administered by spraying a 4% solution of oxymetazoline hydrochloride (Neo-Synephrine) on the nasal mucosa followed by a 4% solution of lidocaine. Additional levels of topical anesthesia and vasoconstriction can be obtained by applying cotton pledgets soaked in a 4% solution of cocaine. The nose should be infiltrated, following the application of topical anesthesia, with local anesthetic using a 0.5% solution of bupivacaine (Marcaine) with 1:100,000 epinephrine. Local anesthesia is injected along the nasal dorsum and anterior maxilla and at the base of the septum to block the infratrochlear, infraorbital, and nasopalatine nerves (Figure 32.7). Performing a nasal block with local anesthesia allows improved visualization and control of bleeding and enhances postoperative pain control.[12]

Manipulation should be performed in a well-lighted room to minimize distorting shadows on the nose. A simple depressed unilateral nasal bone fracture can be reduced with a Boies elevator, Asch forceps, or the handle of a knife. The instrument is inserted beneath the nasal dorsum, and, with

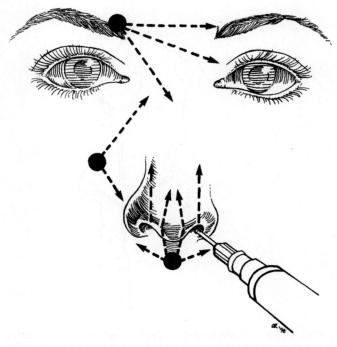

Figure 32.7. Anesthetic infiltration sites used for nasal block.

a slowly elevating force, the nasal bone is out-fractured and elevated (Figure 32.8A). Careful determination should be made to ensure that the cephalad portion of the instrument is placed just beneath the depressed nasal bone segment and not inserted into the cribriform plate. The external distance from the angle of the glabella to the tip of the nose should be used to approximate the depth of insertion and the instrument subsequently placed just short of this distance. External pressure exerted by the contralateral hand molds the fragments to their appropriate positions, and the degree of elevation is controlled simultaneously with the inserted instrument. If this procedure is unsuccessful, a Walsham forceps may be used by grasping the depressed bone, with one blade internally and the other externally, to disimpact the in-fractured bone (Figure 32.8B). The bone can then be elevated and shifted with more control, overcoming distortional forces to restore a normal anatomic position.

Frequently, the contralateral nasal bone may be shifted medially, in which case appropriate digital compression inward can achieve optimal pyramid position.[3,10,11]

The septum should be evaluated after reduction of the nasal bones and should be restored to the anatomic midline after elevation of the nasal dorsum. Deformity can recur despite adequate reduction of the nasal bones if the septum is not reduced correctly. The septum may be buckled, fractured, or displaced from the vomerine groove. The septum can be repositioned with the blades of the Asch forceps by grasping both sides of the septum and elevating it anteriorly and cephalad until it is replaced back into the midline (Figure 32.8C). This procedure will maintain the height of the nasal bridge in depressed fractures and provide an architectural scaffold to support the molding of comminuted nasal bone fractures. The septum must be reinspected after the procedure to ensure that no mucosal

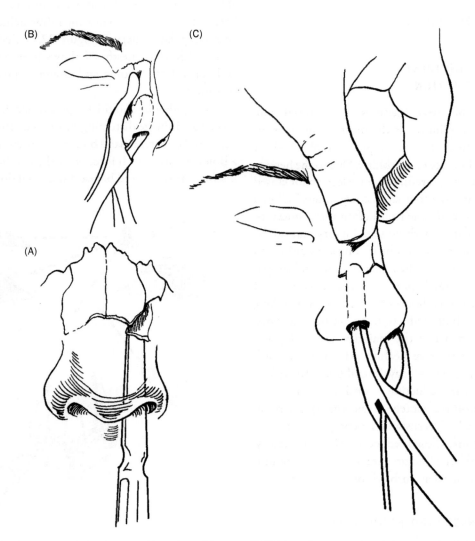

Figure 32.8. (A) Bovie elevator used to elevate depressed lateral nasal fracture. (B) Walsham forceps used to disimpact and reduce lateral nasal fracture. (C) Asch forceps used to anteriorly elevate depressed nasal septum.

lacerations or hematomas have developed. If the septum is severely disrupted and does not remain in the anatomic midline after reduction, internal splints using polyethylene plates (Doyle II nasal septal splints) or antibiotic ointment–coated nasal tampons can be inserted into each nostril and secured to the columella using a 4-0 nylon mattress suture. The suture should be placed caudal to the intermembranous septum and not through it. Care should be taken to tie the suture loosely to avoid pressure necrosis of the septum. It may be necessary to surgically wire the septum to the nasal spine if the reduction cannot be maintained.[10,13]

Fracture stabilization with internal and external splints is critical to maintain and protect an anatomic nasal reduction and plays a large role in obtaining a successful final result. The external splint is necessary to maintain lateral pressure and can be made of plaster of Paris, aluminum, heat-malleable plastic sheets, or other materials, as chosen by the individual surgeon. Before application of external splints, Steri-Strip tape should be placed transversely across the entire dorsum of the nose and across the nasal tip to hold the nose in an anatomically correct position. The skin must be clean and coated with an appropriate adhesive solution (e.g., benzoin). If plaster is used, it is placed in warm water and quickly molded to conform to the shape of the nose, extending from the intercanthal area to the cephalad portions of the lower lateral cartilages. External splinting should be applied for 7 days to provide optimal results in maintaining the shape of the external nose.

Internal nose packing with antibiotic-impregnated gauze has long been considered an essential component of fracture management because it holds the reduction, provides added stability, and prevents synechia formation. However, these functions come at the price of significant patient discomfort as well as potential for packing-related morbidities such as headache, dry mouth, septal perforation, and difficulty in removal. Recent studies have shown that minimal packing duration as little as 1 day had comparable outcomes to longer packing durations while reducing patient discomfort. The patient should be treated with oral antibiotics while the internal nasal packing is in place. Patients must be advised that staphylococcal toxic shock syndrome is a potential infection risk, and if significant fever occurs 1 or 2 days after the injury, the packing must be removed.[14]

The nasal bones may be unstable laterally in some comminuted nasal fractures after reduction. The surgeon should consider using external retention plates in such patients, placed along the sides of the nose and secured for 2 weeks with through-and-through sutures or wires. The plates are composed of thin malleable lead sheets. Silastic sheets cut slightly larger should be placed under the lead plates as a protective cushion. This technique may also be beneficial in patients with a cerebrospinal leak; in such patients, the use of nasal packing is contraindicated because of the increased risk of infection.[13]

When reduction of the septum is unattainable after Asch forceps manipulation, the surgeon should perform an acute submucosal resection, which involves resecting telescoped or buckled portions of septum overriding the fracture sites. However, awareness of the potential complications associated with an acute septal or mucosal resection is essential. Traumatized septal mucosa may not tolerate the wide undermining required for a submucosal resection. This may result in mucosal necrosis with subsequent septal perforation. Furthermore, cartilage that is removed during the acute stage may eventually be needed at a later date for reconstruction during a secondary rhinoplasty. If cartilage is removed inferiorly without knowing the condition of the dorsal septal cartilage, a saddle-nose deformity can result. An extensive acute submucosal resection is therefore rarely indicated. Acute correction of the deformity, however, provides the optimal time to produce a straight septum before scarring occurs and permanently deviates the septum.

The nose, in time, may gradually return to a distorted position, despite the appearance of an adequate reduction. The cause of this late distortion is often attributed to inadequate correction of a bony septal deviation.[7,8] Investigators believe residual displacement of the bony septum may cause unrelenting stress on the reduced cartilaginous septum, contributing to subsequent redisplacement. Additionally, Fry proposed that fractures in the cartilaginous septum, which occur during septal buckling at the time of initial injury, weaken the internal stress on the side of the injury, resulting in the septum deviating away from the side of the tears.[15] The patient should be advised that, regardless of the reasons for a suboptimal result, a secondary corrective rhinoplasty may be required. This should be performed no earlier than 3 months after the injury, when residual edema and ecchymosis have resolved and the acute inflammatory phase has ended. The nasal deformity can then be precisely defined. Furthermore, submucosal resection can be performed at this time without concern for potentially losing dorsal septal support, and the osteotomy sites can be placed away from old fracture lines, avoiding refracture and possible comminution.[1]

INDICATIONS FOR OPEN REDUCTION

The majority of nasal fractures can be successfully reduced by closed reduction techniques, with stabilization using internal and external splinting. There are some situations, however, that may require an open reduction. Nasal bone fractures that are severely comminuted with telecanthus, fractures that extend into the frontal process of the maxilla or frontal bones, presence of dorsal depression or septal bone and cartilage injury, and any fracture that fails to remain stable after a manual closed reduction usually require an open reduction.[8] Attempting a closed reduction on a fracture with a significant lateral nasal deviation may require excision of a C-shaped piece of septal cartilage and bone (see Figure 32.5B). This technique is used to prevent the interlocked, fractured septal edges from distorting the mobile lateral nasal bone fragments toward their initial displaced position. These situations may benefit from several open reduction techniques designed to correct the specific pathologic condition.

In addition to adequate reduction of the deformity, focus should be directed at stabilization of the structural framework. Davis et al. employ the use of "open structure stabilization," which describes the application of open structural rhinoplasty techniques to acute fracture management. The use of autologous structural grafts and suture fixation techniques can restore and even improve the damaged skeletal tissue.[16]

PROCEDURE FOR OPEN REDUCTION

A membranous marginal incision is performed to approach the septum between the caudal portion of the septum and the columella (Figure 32.9A). The incision can be extended laterally just inside the nostril rims or inferiorly to the junction of the septum with the maxillary crest. This allows access to the floor of the nose and the lateral crura of the lower lateral cartilages. Mucoperichondrial flaps and, if needed, mucoperiosteal flaps are elevated on both sides of the septum once the cartilage is identified (Figure 32.9B). The mucosal flaps should be elevated beyond the fracture site. Complete visualization of the septum can be achieved with the aid of a nasal speculum. Once the fracture site is visualized and the extent of deviation determined, the septum can be reduced or partially resected under direct vision. An irreducible septal fracture can be straightened by dislocating the septum from the vomerine grove and performing a low horizontal resection along the vomerine groove or a vertical incision along the cephalic margin of the cartilaginous septum to restore anatomic alignment. Rongeurs can be used to remove portions of displaced cartilage or bone along the length of the septum (Figure 32.9C). Care must be taken, however, to avoid removing the entire fractured segment or potentially injuring the cribriform plate. A curved septum can be straightened by scoring the cartilage with a beaver knife on the concave

side (Figure 32.9D). These relaxing incisions overcome the internal stress of the deformed cartilage, causing it to bend away from the incisions. Stability of the straightened cartilage can be reinforced to prevent recurrence of the curvature, which can occur with healing, by using chromic sutures placed in a figure-of-eight fashion through the straightened cartilage. The mucosal septal incision is closed with chromic sutures and nasal packing, or internal splints are used to hold the mucosal flaps against the repositioned septum and to obliterate the dead space. A chromic suture introduced with a straight (Keith) needle can also be sewn continuously in a cephalad to caudal direction across the entire septum to hold the mucosal flaps in place.[3,11,17]

The elevation of mucoperichondral flaps along the nasal floor is a useful approach for septal fractures involving the maxillary crest. The displaced septum usually requires excision of approximately 3–4 mm of the inferior cartilage to achieve reduction. This allows the septum to swing back to its original position along the vomerine groove. If the maxillary crest is displaced and cannot be reduced or is significantly unstable, excision of the displaced fragment should be performed. A 4-0 chromic suture is placed between the periosteum of the anterior nasal spine and the caudal portion of the inferior septum to stabilize the reduction. Internal nasal packing can also add support after reduction.

Fractures primarily involving the nasal pyramid that require open reduction can be approached by either a coronal or a direct glabellar incision. The coronal approach is often preferred in patients with combined craniofacial injuries or nasal fractures extending to the frontal-ethmoid region, since it provides a larger operative field for fracture visualization. A direct open approach using an "open sky" incision or a simple horizontal incision in the glabellar region is useful for patients with isolated or comminuted nasal fractures.[18] The original wound can often be used to gain access to the nasal pyramid in patients with preexisting frontonasal lacerations by reopening or extending the old scar. The medial canthal portion of the open sky exposure must be a zigzag to prevent subsequent webbing as the scar matures. This technique is useful in assessing the medial canthal tendon when correcting telecanthus or the nasolacrimal duct as it passes into its bony canal. Acute dacryocystorhinostomy should be considered if significant injury to the lacrimal apparatus is present. Once exposure is obtained, the depressed nasal bone fragments are stripped of their periosteal attachments to improve visualization of all fracture sites. All fracture fragments should be preserved and a precise anatomic reduction and stabilization performed by wiring the small fracture fragments together

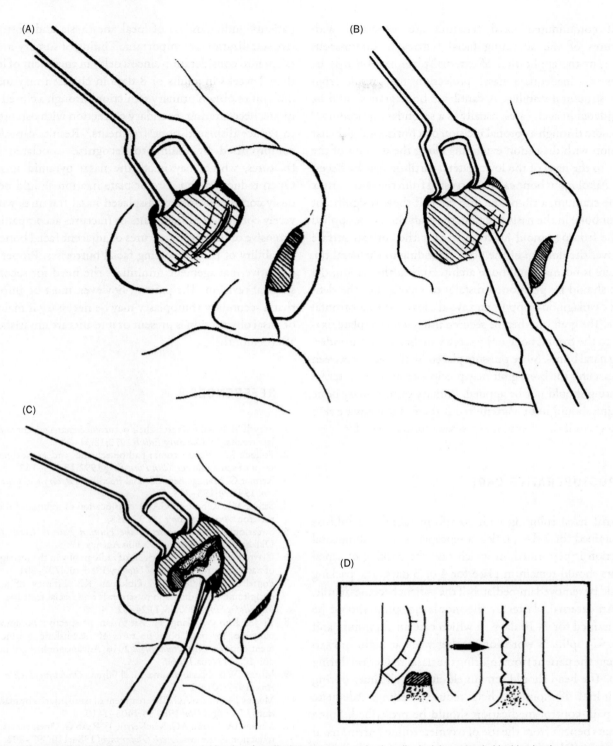

Figure 32.9. (A) mucosal incision placed between caudal border of cartilaginous septum and columella. Incision extended inside alar rim or across nasal floor to allow complete exposure of juncture between cartilaginous septum and maxillary crest. (B) Elevation of septal mucoperichondrial flaps, allowing adequate exposure of fracture sites. (C) Rongeurs used to resect irreducible displaced portions of septal cartilage (submucosal resection). (D) Scoring concave side of curved septum (septoplasty) and tangentially osteotomizing vomerine groove to align septum.

to create larger bony segments, which facilitates the overall reduction. Small bone fragments can be stabilized by placing multiple wires in different directions through one drill hole to help prevent excessive weakening of fragile bone segments by use of multiple drill holes. The fragments can then be linked together to provide rigid fixation.[13,17] Alternatively, large fragments can be repositioned and held with miniplate or screw fixation.[18]

If comminuted nasal fractures are associated with fractures of the adjoining facial buttresses, interosseous wiring or the application of external plate fixation may be necessary. Inadequate nasal projection may result from poor structural stability. A cantilever bone graft should be considered in such cases, usually as a secondary procedure.[19] Exposure through a coronal incision or a horizontal glabellar incision with dissection extending along the dorsum of the nose, to the level of the lower lateral cartilage may be necessary. Autologous bone can be harvested from the outer cortex of the cranium, a rib or the iliac crest. If there is significant loss of bone in the nasion region, the graft should be applied to the frontoethmoid junction so that the cortical surface lies over the dorsum of the nose, extending to the nasal tip. If there is normal nasal bone architecture at the nasion, the graft should be positioned distally to reconstruct the deficient cartilaginous support and avoid a loss of the nasofrontal angle. The graft can then be secured using screw or plate fixation to the frontal bone or by screws anchored to the underlying nasal bones. Since pressure placed on the tissue between the cast and the bone graft may precipitate necrosis, external splinting should not be applied. Primary or secondary bone grafting should not be attempted if there is inadequate skin coverage or if the wound is excessively contaminated.[20]

POSTOPERATIVE CARE

Internal nasal splinting with Xeroform packing should be maintained for 2 days, unless a septoplasty or a submucosal resection is performed, in which case the packing or septal splints should remain in place for 4 or 5 days. The packing should be removed immediately if the patient becomes febrile.

An external plaster or thermoplastic splint should be maintained for 7–10 days, in which case an aluminum and moleskin splint is worn for another week at night only to prevent the patient from injuring the nasal reduction during sleep. The head should remain elevated at all times during the initial 48 hours to help reduce swelling. Adequate oral pain control medication should be prescribed. Some patients benefit from the use of oxymetazoline (Afrin) nasal spray every 8 hours for 3 days after removal of internal nasal packing to decrease mucosal swelling and drainage.

CAVEATS

Good results can usually be obtained from a closed reduction of most nasal fractures in appropriately selected patients. Judicious use of local anesthesia and postoperative stabilization are important. Timing of surgery must be taken into consideration since a delay in treatment of longer than 2 weeks in adults or 8 days in children may make it difficult to obtain primary reduction through a closed technique, necessitating secondary correction with osteotomies to reduce displaced bone fragments.[9] Results can also be compromised by failing to recognize associated facial fractures, which may make the nasal pyramid unstable. Open reduction and wire or plate fixation should be seriously considered in very displaced nasal fractures with severely comminuted fragments or fractures accompanied by extensive or displaced fractures of adjacent facial bones and instability of the supporting facial buttresses. Proper early operative management minimizes the need for secondary surgical revision. The patient, however, must be informed that a secondary rhinoplasty may be necessary if malunion or nasal obstruction is present or if results are unsatisfactory after 3 months.

REFERENCES

1. Mayell M. Nasal fractures: their occurrence, management and some late results. *J R Coll Surg Edinb* 1973;18:31–36.
2. Pollock RA. Nasal trauma: pathomechanics and surgical management of acute injuries. *Clin Plast Surg* 1992;19:133–147.
3. Renner G. Management of nasal fractures. *Otolaryngol Clin North Am* 1991;24:195–213.
4. Stranc MF, Robertson GA. A classification of injuries of the nasal skeleton. *Ann Plast Surg* 1979;2:468.
5. Swearington JJ. *Tolerances of the Human Face to Crash Impact.* Oklahoma City: Federal Aviation Agency, 1965.
6. Clayton MI, Lesser TJ. The role of radiography in the management of nasal fractures. *J Laryngol Otology* 1986;100:797–801.
7. Pogrel MA, Podlesh SW, Goldman KE. Efficacy of a single occipitomental radiograph to screen for midfacial fractures. *J Oral Maxillofac Surg* 2000;58(1):24–32.
8. Yi JS, Kim MJ, Jang YJ. An Asian perspective on improving outcomes for nasal bone fractures by establishing specific treatment options. *Clin Otolaryngol* 2016. Advance online publication. doi: 10.1111/coa.12660.
9. Moran WB. Nasal trauma in children. *Otolaryngol Clin North Amer* 1977;101:95.
10. Murray JA, Maran AG. The treatment of nasal injuries by manipulation. *J Laryngol Otol* 1980;94:1405–1410.
11. Murray JA, Maran AG, MacKenzie IJ, Raab G. Open versus closed reduction of the nose. *Arch Otolaryngol* 1984;110:797–802.
12. Owen GO, Parker AJ, Watson DJ. Fractured nose reduction under local anesthesia: is it acceptable to the patient? *Rhinology* 1992;30:89–96.
13. Illum P, Kristensen S, Jorgensen K, Pedersen CB. Role of fixation in the treatment of nasal fractures. *Clin Otolaryngol* 1983;8: 191–195.
14. Choi DS, Lee JW, Yang JD, Chung HY, Cho BC, Choi KY. Minimal packing duration for close reduction for nasal bone fracture treatment. *J Plast Surg Hand Surg* 2015;49(5):275–279.
15. Fry H. Nasal skeletal trauma and the interlocked stresses of the nasal septal cartilage. *Br J Plast Surg* 1967;20:146–158.

16. Davis RE, Chu E. Complex nasal fractures in the adult—a changing management philosophy. *Facial Plast Surg* 2015;31(3):201–215.
17. Kurihara K, Kim K. Open reduction and interfragment wire fixation of comminuted nasal fractures. *Ann Plast Surg* 1990;24:179–185.
18. Converse JM, Hogan M. Open-sky approach for reduction of naso-orbital fractures. *Plast Reconstr Surg* 1970;46:396.
19. Frodel JL. Management of the nasal dorsum in central facial injuries: indications for calvarial bone grafting. *Arch Otolaryngol Head Neck Surg* 1995;121:307–312.
20. Gruss JS. Complex nasoethmoid-orbital and midfacial fractures: role of craniofacial techniques and immediate bone grafting. *Ann Plast Surg* 1986;17:377.

33.

REPAIR OF LIP DEFECTS WITH THE ABBE AND ESTLANDER FLAPS

Howard N. Langstein and Stephen S. Kroll

ASSESSMENT OF THE DEFECT

Lip defects can usefully be classified as either small, medium, or large, based on reconstructive needs. Small defects are those that can be closed primarily without significant anatomical distortion. This group would usually include defects of up to one-fourth of an upper lip or one-third of a lower lip, depending on the size of the patient's mouth and the extensibility of the tissues. Medium-sized defects are those that can be repaired with a single flap from the remaining lip. These would normally include defects of one-half to three-fourths of an upper or lower lip. Large defects are too big to repair with a single local flap and require either a staged reconstruction or a flap of distant tissue. The Abbe and Estlander flaps are lip switch procedures that are appropriate for medium-sized defects of the upper or lower lip.

THE ABBE FLAP

INDICATIONS

The Abbe flap is a highly useful flap that can be used to repair almost any moderate-sized defect of the upper or lower lip. It is most useful, however, in three specific situations: (1) a moderate sized central defect of the upper lip, especially the philtrum (Figure 33.2); (2) a moderate-sized defect of the lower lip that is off-center but spares the commissure (Figure 33.1); and (3) to restore symmetry to a relatively small lower lip as part of a staged reconstruction of a large lower lip defect (Figure 33.3).

CONTRAINDICATIONS

The Abbe flap cannot be used when there is insufficient remaining lip to allow reasonably normal function of the donor lip after harvesting of the flap. It is therefore not appropriate for very large lip defects. The Abbe flap is usually not the best choice for midline lower lip defects because, in that situation, the Karapandzic technique usually gives superior results in one stage. Previous irradiation of the donor lip can also be a contraindication.

ROOM SETUP

Operating room setup is not especially critical in this operation. Ideally, however, an oral endotracheal tube should be avoided (in favor of a nasotracheal or tracheostomy tube) since the oral tube distorts the lip, makes it difficult to judge lip symmetry and can be in the way of the surgery.

MARKINGS AND DESIGN

The Abbe flap is a staged cross-lip flap based on the coronal branch of the labial artery, which is located a few millimeters from the lip border, just deep to the mucosal surface (Figure 33.4). It is usually based medially so that, after rotation, the flap will rest comfortably in the defect without torsion on the pedicle (Figure 33.5). The surgeon should attempt to position the flap so that the thickness of the vermilion of the donor site matches, if possible, that of the lip segment that is being replaced. The flap is usually designed to be one-half the width of the defect, so that the tissue deficiency will be shared equally between the upper and lower lips. When a discrete aesthetic unit in the upper

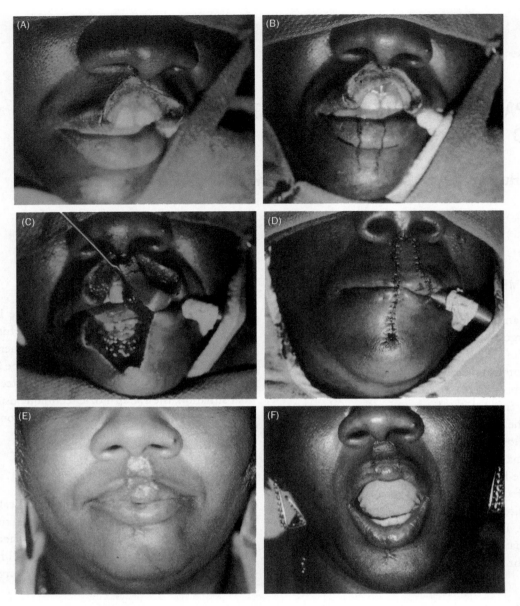

Figure 33.1. (A) Midline defect of upper lip. (B) Abbe flap is designed on lower lip. (C) Flap is transferred to upper lip. (D) Immediately after flap transfer. (E,F) Five months later: although scars are hypertrophic, lip contour is good. (F) Oral aperture and lip function are excellent.

lip (such as the philtrum) is being replaced, however, the flap width should be designed so that the normal size of the aesthetic unit is restored. The extended Abbe flap can carry additional tissue from the white portion of the upper or lower lip or even chin tissue.

TECHNIQUE

The vermillion should be marked with methylene blue before incision. The skin incision is made with a scalpel while an assistant pinches the lip on either side of the incision to minimize bleeding. One should incise the lip opposite the pedicle first to ascertain where the coronal

branch of the labial artery is located and ligate both sides. Then the incision is made on the pedicle side. Because the labial artery is deep to mucosa and near the orbicularis oris muscle, the incision can be carried through part of the vermilion surface without jeopardizing the arterial blood supply, making the flap pedicle appear very narrow on the frontal view and making it easier to inset the flap after rotation (Figure 33.6). This technique also improves the early cosmetic appearance of the repair and makes repair of the vermilion borders more accurate. Hemostasis is obtained with electrocautery, using a needle tip or bipolar current to minimize charring. The mucosal part of the pedicle should be left fairly wide so

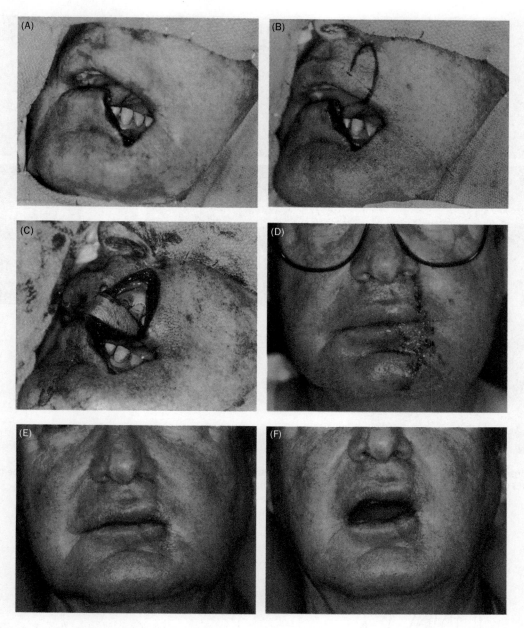

Figure 33.2. (A) Off-center defect of lower lip. (B) Abbe flap design. (C) Flap being transferred to lower lip. (D) Early result, before pedicle division. (E,F) After pedicle division.

that adequate venous return is maintained because, although a discrete artery is included in the pedicle, there is no corresponding vein.

After the flap is mobilized and rotated, a considerable effort should be made to approximate the vermilion borders accurately. Although inaccurate approximation can be corrected later, it is far easier to repair the vermilion edges correctly before scar tissue has had a chance to develop. Accurate repair of the vermilion is naturally easier if the surgeon has extended the incision on the pedicle side of the flap onto the vermilion surface, as described earlier.

Once the flap has been rotated, both the donor and recipient sites are closed in layers. Horizontal mattress sutures of 4-0 or 5-0 absorbable suture in the mucosa are useful to minimize the risk of developing leaks. More attention should be focused on the repair of the lower lip, where gravity encourages accumulation of saliva and a fistula is more likely. The lip muscle is closed in a separate layer, usually using 3-0 or 4-0 Vicryl (or equivalent), to restore continuity to the orbicularis oris muscle. The skin closure is completed with of 5-0 monofilament, using either absorbable or permanent suture, depending on the surgeon's preferences. The pedicle is left intact, connecting the upper

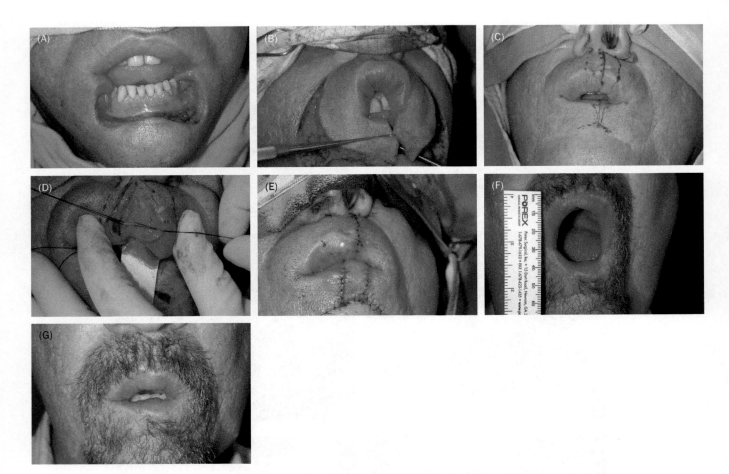

Figure 33.3. (A) Large defect of lower lip. (B) After repair of large defect with Karapandzic flaps creating microstomia. (C) Design of Abbe flap. (D) Division of coronal artery. (E) Inset of Abbe flap. (F) Result in repose. (G) Result with maximal opening demonstrating adequate stomal opening.

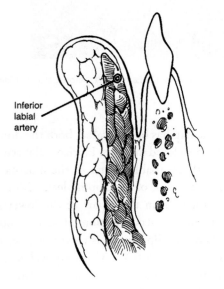

Figure 33.4. Anatomic drawing of cross-section of lower lip, showing coronal branch of labial artery.

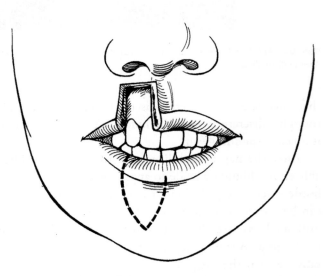

Figure 33.5. Design of Abbe flap.

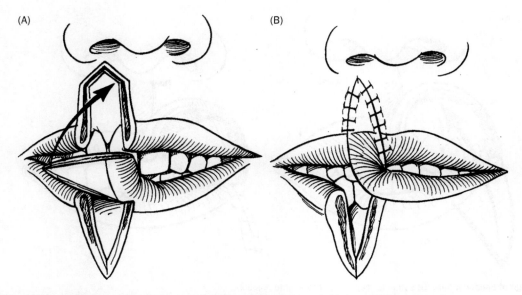

Figure 33.6. (A,B) Extending incision onto vermilion, but preserving wide pedicle on mucosal side to maintain venous return.

and lower lips together temporarily (Figure 33.1C). The vermilion should be approximated with 5-0 Vicryl, which is softer and more comfortable in this sensitive location than a stiff monofilament suture would be.

POSTOPERATIVE CARE

No dressings or splints are required. Local application of antibiotic-containing ointments may be useful for a few days. A clear liquid diet is advisable for the first day, after which a full liquid diet is permitted. The use of a toothbrush is avoided until flap division; a Water-Pik appliance is helpful for dental hygiene, which otherwise would be difficult because of the limited oral aperture.

PEDICLE DIVISION

After a period of 3 weeks, the Abbe flap pedicle can be divided. The flap donor site can be aggressively revised at this stage to line up the vermilion borders as well as possible, but revision of the flap itself is usually best deferred until the blood supply is more securely established.

THE ESTLANDER FLAP

INDICATIONS

The Estlander flap is simply a lateral one-stage lip switch. It is most useful in medium-sized lateral defects of the upper or lower lip that include the commissure. It is most often used, however, for upper lip defects. It is especially useful in upper lip defects that include part of the adjacent cheek because the flap can be extended to transfer additional skin. It is similar to the Abbe flap, but because it does not have to preserve an intact commissure, it can be a one-stage procedure. In some cases, however, a commissuroplasty may subsequently be required to widen the oral aperture and improve symmetry between the left and right sides of the mouth.

CONTRAINDICATIONS

Like the Abbe flap, the Estlander flap is contraindicated if there is insufficient residual lip to allow harvesting the flap without creating unacceptable deformity in the donor lip, but this is seldom the case since the defect is lateral. It is therefore usually not appropriate for large lip defects, which are better suited by Karapandzic flaps.

MARKINGS AND DESIGN

The flap is usually designed to be one-half the width of the actual defect so that the tissue deficiency will be shared equally between the upper and lower lip (Figure 33.7). If necessary, extensions of the flap can be designed to repair adjacent defects of the cheek (Figure 33.8). The pedicle itself is just like that of an Abbe flap, except that the incision does not ordinarily

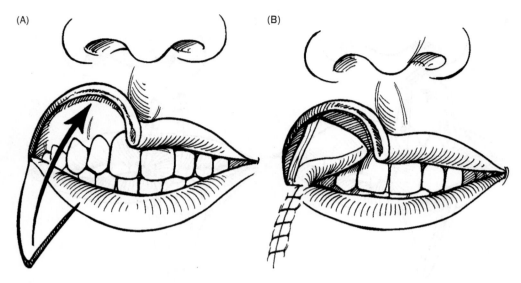

Figure 33.7. (A) Design of Estlander flap. (B) Estlander flap being rotated into position.

extend onto the vermilion since the pedicle becomes the new commissure.

TECHNIQUE

The flap is elevated just as in an Abbe flap and rotated into the defect (Figure 33.7B). Closure of the donor defect is performed in layers, just as in the Abbe flap, but temporary bridging of the oral aperture by the pedicle is not necessary to create a permanent and definitive closure. Careful repair of the muscle laterally will create some lateral tension, which will serve to pull on the new commissure. The surgeon should take care to accurately line up the vermilion borders and to suture the orbicularis oris muscle layer securely (with 4-0 Vicryl or equivalent) to avoid muscle separation and notching.

POSTOPERATIVE CARE

Postoperative care is simpler than that of the Abbe flap because the oral aperture is not temporarily interfered with. A clear liquid diet is advisable for the first day, after which a normal diet is permitted. Local application of an antibiotic-containing ointment during the first week will help to keep the suture line clean. The patient should exercise care when performing oral hygiene during the first 2 weeks to avoid excess tension on the flap.

Subsequent revision of the oral commissure may be necessary in some cases, if the width of the vermilion is excessive or the oral aperture is insufficiently wide, but this is rare. No splints or physical therapy are required.

CAVEATS

Although only a narrow pedicle is necessary to maintain arterial blood supply to the flap, the mucosal base of both the Abbe and Estlander flaps should be maintained to ensure adequate venous return. In both procedures, an attempt should be made to line up the vermilion borders as accurately as possible in the first stage, when there is a minimum of scarring and edema, since it will be more difficult to do later.

For the Abbe flap, a second stage is always necessary for division of the flap pedicle. Although some reports suggest that this can be performed as early as 11 days after flap transfer, there is usually no pressing reason to divide the pedicle so quickly, and it is safer to wait 3 weeks. After division of the pedicle, only a minimum amount of reopening of the incision between the flap and adjacent lip can be performed without jeopardizing flap survival, so a perfect completion of the flap inset is usually not possible at that time. For this reason, it may be necessary to revise the vermilion border (at the pedicle site) at a third stage several weeks later if an optimal aesthetic result is desired. If the vermillion border was aligned adequately at the first stage, then the flap division is simply within the red lip and any abnormalities related to residual pedicle scar can be easily addressed later in the office.

As in all flaps, reduced flap perfusion and a higher incidence of complications should be expected in patients who smoke. Smoking should be absolutely prohibited after both techniques for the first postoperative week and, in the case of the Abbe flap, is best avoided until at least a week after the pedicle has been divided. If the patient smokes, the pedicle of the flap may be made wider than usual in an attempt to compensate for the reduced blood flow.

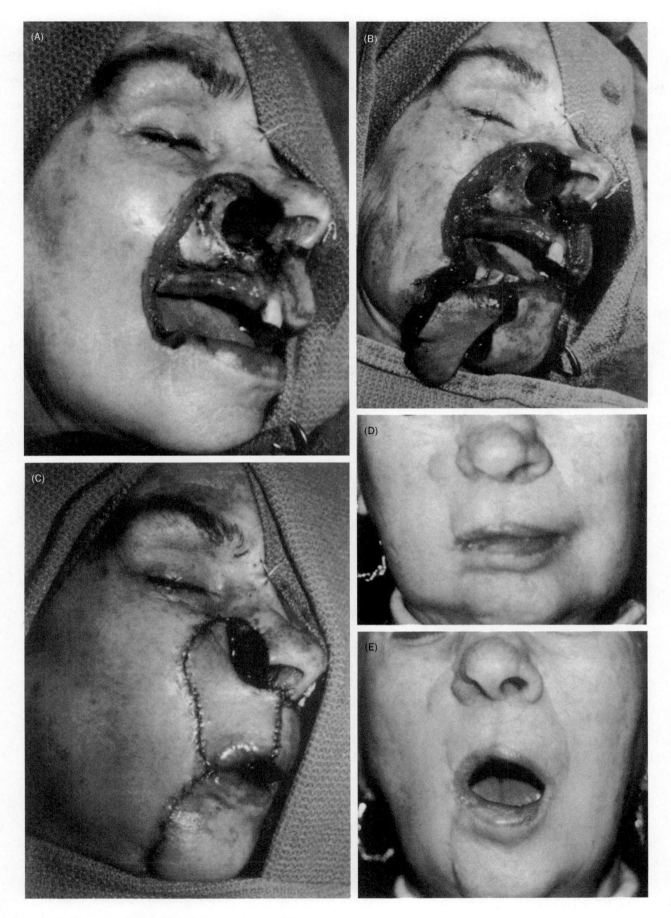

Figure 33.8. (A) Moderately large defect of upper lateral lip, cheek, and part of nose. (B) Modified Estlander flap designed to repair lip and cheek and form base for subsequent nasal repair. (C) Flap after transfer and inset. (D,E) Result 6 months later. From *Adv Plast Surg* 1993;9:127.

SELECTED READINGS

Abbe RA. A new plastic operation for the relief of deformity due to double harelip. *Med Rec* 1898;53:477.

Estlander JA. Eine Methode aus der einen Lippe Substanzverluste der anderen zu ersetzen. *Arch Klin Chir* 1872;14:622.

Kroll SS. Staged sequential flap reconstruction for large lower lip defects. *Plast Reconstr Surg* 1991;88:620–625.

Kroll SS. Lip reconstruction. In: Kroll SS, ed. *Reconstructive Plastic Surgery for Cancer.* St. Louis: CV Mosby, 1996:201–209.

Langstein HN, Robb GL. Lip and perioral reconstruction. *Clin Plast Surg* 2005;32(3):431–435.

34.

TRAUMATIC TOTAL OR PARTIAL EAR LOSS

Jenna Martin Bourgeois and Keith A. Hurvitz

INTRODUCTION

Acquired ear defects are becoming increasingly more common following trauma, which can include motor vehicle accidents, assaults, and workplace injuries. Reconstruction of the external ear following traumatic amputation remains an extremely challenging procedure for plastic surgeons. Numerous reconstructive techniques have been utilized throughout history, with the mainstays of treatment being composite grafting, peri-auricular tissue flaps, pocket principles, cartilage banking, and microsurgical techniques. This chapter discusses current concepts for managing traumatic total or partial ear loss and complements the previous published work by Eugenio Aguilar III.[1]

The external ear is a complex structure with multiple aesthetic subunits and planes (helix, scapha-antihelix complex, posterior conchal wall, and conchal floor).[2] The anterior ear skin is fixed to the perichondrium, whereas the posterior ear has a thin layer of subcutaneous tissue between the skin and perichondrium. The blood supply can be variable but is generally dominated by branches of the superficial temporal and auricular vessels.[3] Due to the ear's unique anatomic structure and thin skin adherent to the perichondrium, an aesthetic reconstruction following complete or partial ear loss is difficult and relies on a surgeon's knowledge of the full spectrum of techniques for ear reconstruction.

CLINICAL ASSESSMENT OF THE DEFECT AND CLASSIFICATION OF INJURY

Prior to proceeding with ear reconstruction, the plastic surgeon must evaluate the overall condition of the patient, including any associated head trauma or life-threatening injuries. At times, patients may have sustained trauma that precludes immediate intervention for a traumatic ear injury because life-saving interventions must be performed first. Additional factors that play a role in determining proper treatment of traumatic ear injuries include timing of the injury (acute, subacute, or delayed presentation) and mechanism of injury, such as human/animal bite, assault, burn, traffic accident, or crush injury.

When evaluating the traumatized ear, the surgeon must assess the size of the amputated portion, condition of tissues amputated, and condition of the stump and surrounding tissues.[4] Defects can be divided anatomically into injury or loss of the upper third, middle third, lower third/lobule, or total loss of the auricle. Further classification of the degree of auricular injury has been described by Weerda.[5] First-degree injuries include abrasions or superficial trauma without significant cartilage involvement that will likely heal with conservative management and wound care. Second-degree auricular injuries have a skin tear with a nutrient skin pedicle that continues to provide sufficient blood supply to the remainder of the ear. Third-degree injuries include partial or total avulsion, and fourth-degree injuries include amputation of the auricle with complete loss of the auricle. Second-, third-, and fourth-degree injuries are most commonly addressed by the plastic surgeon with evaluation in the emergency department followed by operative management.[3]

ACUTE MANAGEMENT

As discussed earlier, the overall condition of the patient is the most important factor prior to proceeding with ear reconstruction. After determining the mechanism of injury, it is important to irrigate the wound copiously, debride devitalized tissues, and evaluate the ear for tissue bridges, skin and cartilage viability, and underlying infection risk factors. For example, bite injuries are often severe crush injuries with a very high risk for infection. Patients often require additional aggressive wound irrigation and appropriate antibiotic therapy targeted against oral flora. When concerned for infection or immediate closure is not feasible, one should cleanse the wound and keep tissues moist with frequent dressing changes. In patients who do not possess an allergy to sulfa drugs, mafenide acetate (Sulfamylon cream) can be useful for wounds with exposed cartilage due to its increased cartilage penetration.[6]

Additionally, it is important to monitor for auricular hematoma due to blunt auricular trauma. If untreated, this will result in cauliflower ear, with potential infection or cartilage necrosis. Treatment is dependent on the severity of injury and includes needle aspiration, open drainage, and/ or drain placement. Bolster dressings are then applied to prevent recurrence of hematoma.[6]

It is important to determine optimal time for treatment, including replantation with composite grafting of the traumatized segment or use of microsurgical techniques. Many of the grafts and local advancement flaps described in this chapter can be performed in a delayed fashion if the initial reconstruction is unsuccessful or is not possible due to patient instability. Additionally, patients may present to the plastic surgeon in a delayed fashion after initial treatment by debridement, approximation, or transplantation at an outside facility. However, with each additional insult or failure of reconstruction, achieving an aesthetic or normal appearing result becomes more difficult.

PARTIAL AMPUTATION

TUBES

Interest in ear reconstruction began in the mid-1800s and was further progressed with the use of local flaps, most commonly mastoid, postauricular, or cervical tube flaps. The use of cervical tubes involves the creation of skin and subcutaneous tissue tubes that are kept attached at the proximal and distal end, with closure of the center of the tube. Each stage includes a delay of approximately 3 weeks while the tube matures, followed by division of the distal end with continued advancement or "walking" of the tube to the level of the auricle for reconstruction of the defect. As microsurgical and local flap options have improved, the technique of tube flap reconstruction has fallen out of favor.[1]

COMPOSITE GRAFTS

For small to moderate defects of the helix and upper to middle third of the ear, composite grafts from the contralateral ear are an excellent match of contour and tissue. This reconstructive method is especially advantageous if the patient has a large or protruding contralateral ear. A wedge-shaped graft of 1–2.5 cm in width is resected from the contralateral ear and is transplanted to a clean cut defect on the affected ear. The perichondrium should be closed with small absorbable sutures, and the skin should be closed with small nonabsorbable sutures. Skin sutures should not be placed too closely or tied too tightly to prevent skin necrosis.

The success of this technique depends on a small-size composite graft and a well-vascularized tissue bed. Composite grafts can also be combined with local advancement flaps to increase vascularization. Composite grafts are a simple reconstructive technique despite the propensity toward a decrease in graft size after transplantation.[7]

LOCAL ADVANCEMENT FLAPS

For partial traumatic defects of the ear, local advancement flaps with the use of healthy surrounding ear structures and peri-auricular skin are the mainstays of reconstruction. These techniques are extremely useful in the upper and middle third of the helix.

The tunnel technique of Converse involves making an incision through the edge of the auricular defect and then through the skin of the mastoid area.[8] A subcutaneous

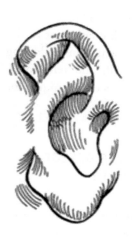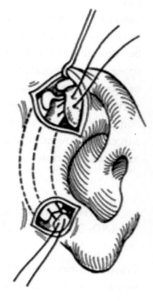

Figure 34.1. Tunnel technique of Converse.

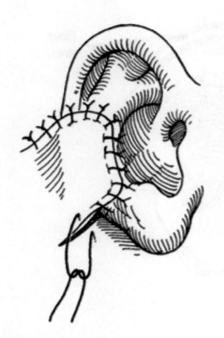

Figure 34.2. Dieffenbach flap.

tunnel in the mastoid area is then created, and the superior and inferior edges of the mastoid skin incision are approximated to the superior and inferior edges of the ear defect. A cartilage graft from the traumatized segment or contralateral ear is then placed in the subcutaneous pocket. The reconstructed auricle will then be elevated off the mastoid skin at a later stage (Figure 34.1).

An additional technique for reconstruction of the middle third of the ear with local tissue is the multistage technique of Dieffenbach.[9] It utilizes a posteriorly based mastoid flap which is elevated to cover the auricular defect. The flap is subsequently divided and folded on itself at a secondary stage, with skin grafting of the donor site (Figure 34.2).

A frequently utilized reconstructive tool for upper and middle third helical defects is the chondrocutaneous advancement flap, also known as the *Antia-Buch flap.*[10] This technique utilizes an advancement flap of the adjacent intact helical margin based on a wide post-auricular skin paddle. The incision in the anterior helical sulcus extends through the anterior skin and cartilage but does not violate the posterior skin. The incisions can extend into the lobule if necessary, with a back cut for additional advancement (Figure 34.3). The cartilage should be reapproximated with interrupted absorbable sutures followed by skin closure. This flap will result in a smaller sized ear, but the result will have a good contour. A staged reduction of the contralateral ear can also be performed in the future for better symmetry.

For large composite upper helical defects, pre-auricular banner flaps based off the preauricular skin can be utilized. Davis described his technique for superior helical reconstruction whereby he elevated an anteriorly based pedicled flap of skin and cartilage from the root of helix and conchal bowl.[7,11] The composite flap is then transposed to its new location at the top of the ear. Skin grafting of raw surfaces completes the process (Figure 34.4).

Lower third and lobule defects are most commonly reconstructed with adjacent tissue. First descriptions in the early 1900s included local rotational flaps from the neck and posterior auricular area.[12] One of the more popular and time-tested techniques was first described by Gavello in 1907.[13,14] This reconstruction utilizes an anteriorly based horizontal bilobed flap of skin and subcutaneous tissue obtained from the infra-auricular and post-auricular region. After raising the tissues, the posterior flap is folded onto the anterior flap to create the posterior surface of the

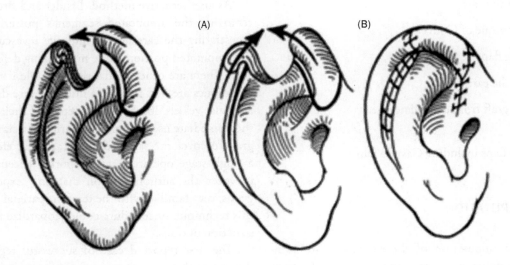

(A)   (B)

Figure 34.3. Antia-Buch technique.

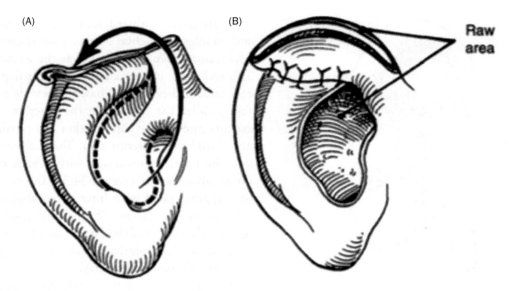

(A)   (B)   Raw
                                                    area

Figure 34.4. Conchal composite graft.

new lobule and is then sutured in place. This technique has been modified to include the addition of cartilage grafts to provide shape and volume to the newly created earlobe.[15]

TECHNIQUE CHOICE BY LOCATION OF INJURY

Upper ear:

Composite graft from contralateral ear

Antia-Buch advancement flap

Composite flap (Davis)

Tunnel technique of Converse

Middle third of the ear:

Tunnel technique of Converse

Dieffenbach flap

Lower third of the ear:

Composite graft from contralateral ear
Lobule:

Local tissue flaps including Gavello flap

TOTAL AMPUTATION

Total traumatic amputation of the ear is a more complex and challenging problem, with numerous options

proposed. Prior to microsurgical techniques, there were reported successes of reattachment of a complete ear amputation merely as a composite graft. The first well-documented report of survival of a free graft occurred in 1898, by W. J. Brown, with continued reports throughout the literature.[16] However, many cases have been fraught with complications of partial or complete necrosis. Another method of reconstruction, the *pocket principle*, utilizes the retroauricular pocket and amputated cartilage segment. The amputated auricular segment is cleaned, denuded of skin with dermabrasion, and then buried in an elevated retroauricular pocket with later elevation at a subsequent stage. Complications of this technique include significant resorption of the buried cartilage, poor definition and stability of the auricular cartilage, and destruction of the retro-auricular skin for any future procedures if reconstruction fails.[17]

As an alternative method, Baudet and Brent described removing the amputated segment's posterior skin and fenestrating the cartilage to improve revascularization of the amputated portion while minimizing deformity of the ear.[18] There are other modalities available if microsurgical techniques are not an option due to severe damage to the auricular vessels. Ibraham et al. reported their success with the immediate use of a temporoparietal fascia flap and skin graft to cover the salvaged amputated ear element.[19] It is a single-stage operation with reported acceptable results; however, the authors caution that only experienced surgeons, very familiar with the temporoparietal flap, attempt this technique since failure could jeopardize future reconstruction options.

The first reported case of successful replantation of the ear with microvascular anastomosis was performed in 1980 and utilized the superficial temporal artery with vein grafting to a superior post-auricular artery and vein grafting to two small veins near the inferior pole of the ear.[16] Excellent targets for microvascular replantation often include the superficial temporal artery and the posterior auricular arteries. In 2004, a review of the literature was performed and found only 37 cases of microsurgical repair, with 14 of these cases having no venous anastomosis performed. Due to frequent, significant damage to the small auricular vessels in traumatic amputations, there is often an inability to perform a venous anastomosis, with resultant venous congestion. Thus, microsurgical ear replantations may require anticoagulation, leech therapy, or hyperbaric oxygen therapy.[20,21] Ultimately, the cosmetic result obtained with microvascular replantation is far superior when compared to the pocket method or composite grafting techniques.

Using the valuable skills gained from craniofacial surgery and microtia reconstruction, multistage delayed autologous rib cartilage reconstruction can be performed in combination with local tissue flaps, temporoparietal flaps, and skin grafting with great success. This method of reconstruction would likely be undertaken in the delayed or subacute setting after early attempts at reconstruction were not possible or have failed.[2]

POSTOPERATIVE CARE

Postoperative care of the reconstructed ear requires frequent monitoring (especially in microsurgical replantation) with dressings that apply no pressure on the reconstructed ear. In ear replantation cases with or without microsurgery, 80% of surgeons reported leeching, with improvement of venous congestion. Although there is no standardized regimen, many surgeons will frequently use systemic heparin, aspirin, and/or dextran, which is more controversial.[22]

Hyperbaric oxygen therapy may also lead to augmented survival of compromised tissue and may be beneficial if available following replantation of a complete or partial ear amputation.[22]

THE FUTURE OF EAR RECONSTRUCTION

Total ear reconstruction remains a challenge. Alloplastic materials such as silicone, hydroxyapatite, and porous polyethylene have been utilized for reconstruction in lieu of autologous tissues, but this can lead to disastrous results with infection or immunogenicity. In delayed reconstruction, autologous rib cartilage reconstruction for the auricular framework has been the standard of care, but there is significant donor site morbidity from rib harvest. In search of a nonimmunogenic and inert scaffold for auricular framework, numerous studies in tissue engineering have been using chondrocytes and stem cells with a three-dimensional scaffold.[23] Continued research is ongoing to develop a framework with long-term sustainability to assist in complex delayed ear reconstruction.

REFERENCES

1. Aguilar E A. Traumatic total of partial ear loss. *Operat Plast Surg*: 308–313.
2. Brent B. technical advances in ear reconstruction with autogenous rib cartilage grafts: personal experience with 1200 cases. *Plast Reconstr Surg* 1999;1–4(2):335–338.
3. Siegert R, Magritz R. Reconstruction of the auricle. *Head Neck Surg* 2007;6:1865–1871.
4. Brent B. Reconstruction of the auricle. In: McCarthy G, ed. *Plastic Surgery*. Vol 3, part 2. Philadelphia: WB Saunders, 1990:2094–2152.
5. Weerda H, Siegert R. Classification and treatment of acquired deformities. *Face* 1998;6:79–82
6. Marcus JR. *Essentials of Craniomaxillofacial Trauma*. St. Louis: Quality Medical Publishing, 2012.
7. Davis J. Reconstruction of the upper third of the ear with a chondrocutaneous composite flap based on the crus helix. In: Tanzer RC, Edgerton MT, eds. *Symposium on Reconstruction of the Auricle*, Vol. 10. St. Louis: CV Mosby Company, 1974:246–247.
8. Converse JM. Reconstruction of the auricle. *Plast Reconstr Surg* 1958;2:150–153.
9. McCarthy JG. *Plastic Surgery*, Vol. 3. Philadelphia: WB Saunders, 1990:2094–2152.
10. Antia NH, Buch VI. Chondrocutaneous advancement flap for the marginal defect of the ear. *Plast Reconstr Surg* 1967;39:472–477.
11. Ha RY, Hackney F. Plastic surgery of the ear. *Selected Readings* 2005;5(10)
12. Carver GM. Reconstruction of the ear lobule. *Plast Reconstr Surg* 1946;12(3):203–207.
13. Gavello P. *Les Autoplasyies*. Paris: G Stenheil, 1907. Quoted by Nelation C, Ombredanne L.
14. Chattopadhyay D, Gupta S, Murmu M, Guha G, Gupta S. Revisiting Gavello's procedure for single stage reconstruction of the earlobe: the vascular basis, technique and clinical uses. *Can J Plast Surg* 2012;20(2):22–24.
15. Cabral AR, Alonso N, Brinca A, Vieira R, Figueiredo A. Earlobe reconstruction by the Gavello technique and bilobed flap. *An Bras Dermatol* 2013;33(2):272–275.
16. Pennington DG, Lai MF, Pelly AD. Successful replantation of a completely avulsed ear by microvascular anastomosis. *Plast Reconstr Surg* 1980;65(6):820–823.
17. Pearl RA, Sabbagh W. Reconstruction following traumatic partial amputation of the ear. *Plast Reconstr Surg* 2011;127(2):621–629.
18. Baudet J. A propos d'un procede original de reimplantationd'un pavilion de l'oreille totalement separe. *Ann Chir Plast* 1972;17:67.
19. Ibrahim, SMS, Zidan A, Madani S. Totally avulsed ear: new technique of immediate ear reconstruction. *J Plast Reconstr Aesthet Surg* 2008;61:S29–S36.

20. Steffen A, Katzback R, Klaiber S. A comparison of ear reattachment methods: A review of 25 years since Pennington. *Plast Reconstr Surg* 2005;118(6):1359–1364.

21. O'Toole G, Bhatti K, Massod S. Replantation of an avulsed ear, using a single arterial anastomosis. *J Plast Reconstr Aesthet Surg* 2008;61:326–329.

22. Komorowska-Timek E, Hardesty RA. Successful reattachment of a nearly amputated ear without microsurgery. *Plast Reconstr Surg* 2008;121(4):165e–169e.

23. Nayyer L, Patel KH, Esmaeili A, et al. Tissue engineering: revolution and challenge in auricular cartilage reconstruction. *Plast Reconstr Surg* 2012;129(5):1123–1137.

35.

SCALP RECONSTRUCTION

Joseph J. Disa and Edward Ray

ASSESSMENT OF THE DEFECT

The scalp serves both protective and aesthetic functions. Injury or loss of the scalp may lead to desiccation and osteonecrosis of the underlying calvarium as well as potentially life-threatening osteomyelitis and meningitis. Causes of scalp defects include trauma (e.g., avulsion, animal bites), thermal burns, radiation, infection, and malignancy, as well as congenital deformity. The method of scalp reconstruction chosen depends on multiple factors, including the depth of the defect and mechanism of injury.

Scalp reconstruction starts with a systematic approach, beginning with definition of the defect and identification of the reconstructive priorities (Figure 35.1). Factors that will influence the final result need to be considered carefully, including the presence of devitalized tissue requiring debridement; the magnitude of the defect; the presence of contaminated or infected material; the presence or need for hardware, allografts, or prosthetic materials in reconstruction; the effects of radiation (past or future) on the tissue; and the presence of dead space, as well as patient comorbidities and environmental factors (e.g., heart disease, diabetes, smoking). Necrotic or infected tissue will need debridement, and contaminated hardware should be removed. Implanted hardware and exposed bone should be covered with vascularized tissue. Dead space should be obliterated. Failure to address these issues will lead to a unacceptable rate of local sepsis and wound breakdown.

Radiotherapy causes chronic and cumulative changes to skin, resulting in a fragile epidermis, increase in collagen production, and damage to elastic fibers, as well as loss of follicular structures, hyperkeratosis, and increased risk of secondary malignancies. Infection, including cellulitis, is more common in irradiated skin due to locally impaired immune function and diminished lymphatic flow. Irradiated skin does not tolerate tension due to poor elasticity, which limits the utility of expansion or skin flap rotation. Full-thickness burns are sometimes reconstructable with skin grafts alone, once a suitable wound bed is present. Skin that has been grafted or that has healed secondarily will be inelastic, precluding its use in future skin flaps. Scalp defects resulting from traumatic avulsion may afford an opportunity to replant missing tissue by microvascular repair. The time span following trauma, as well as the quality of the injured tissue and blood vessels, has a bearing on the chances of a successful replantation.

Whenever possible, patients should be evaluated by the plastic surgeon before surgical debridement or tumor resection, to assess the anticipated tissue needs (e.g., bone, soft tissue, dura) as well as the availability of local, regional, and distant donor sites, accounting for the presence

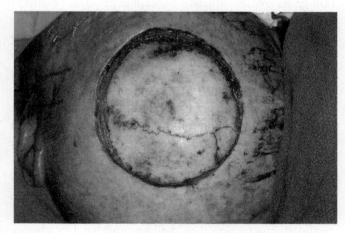

Figure 35.1. Malignant fibrohistiocytoma of scalp. Resection left a large defect that was reconstructed with latissimus dorsi muscle flap.

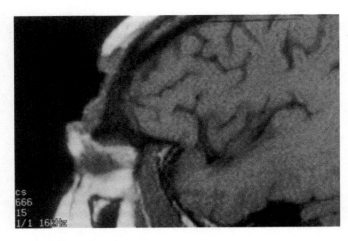

Figure 35.2. Advanced squamous cell carcinoma of left forehead that has invaded cranium. Reconstruction proceeded with rectus abdominis free tissue transfer after surgical resection.

of irradiated tissue or prior surgical scars (Figure 35.2). A more complex reconstructive option (i.e., free tissue transfer) is warranted when these circumstances preclude durable reconstruction with simpler techniques.

INDICATIONS

The primary goals of scalp reconstruction are to reestablish the appearance and function of the scalp. This entails the restoration of durable soft tissue coverage to protect vital structures (i.e., the brain and calvarium), restore contour, and optimize aesthetic appearance, in order of importance. Following evaluation of the wound characteristics and consideration of the injury mechanism, a stepwise approach to identify the simplest and most appropriate technique to achieve these goals is warranted. When local flaps or skin grafts are not sufficient or feasible, regional or distant flaps will be needed. Practical considerations, such as the patient's aesthetic concerns (e.g., the ability to use a wig to cover the reconstructed scalp) should be weighed along with the other advantages and disadvantages of a particular technique.

The indications, risks, benefits, and alternatives for each appropriate option should be discussed with the patient in order to obtain informed consent before undertaking any procedure.

Once a technique is chosen, thorough planning is essential. Patient positioning, donor and recipient site issues, the postoperative care plan, and potential obstacles to successful reconstruction should all be considered in advance of surgical management. Several different algorithms have been developed to assist in planning scalp reconstruction based on defect size and location as well as the availability of local tissues.

When soft tissue is the only tissue requiring replacement, the defect is small, and local skin is of good quality, *primary closure* or *local and regional soft tissue flaps* should be considered first due to the low morbidity and technical ease of these approaches. Local flaps do, however, require careful geometric planning. Due to limited soft tissue elasticity and the convexity of the cranium, simple closure of scalp wounds is often not feasible.

Larger soft tissue defects may benefit from staged procedures such as *tissue expansion, dermal substitution grafts* (e.g., acellular dermal matrices), and *skin grafting*, particularly in patients who are not candidates for free tissue transfer. The curvature of the cranium limits the reach of local flaps, which may prompt consideration of tissue expansion to increase flap dimensions and vascularity. Extensive defects or composite defects (e.g., in patients with advanced malignancy) pose a significant challenge and often require *free tissue transfer. Free flaps*, while requiring more meticulous planning and adequate recipient vessels, provide multiple options for reliable and abundant tissue transfer, usually in a single stage, and are thus often the best choice for large and/or more complex defects of the scalp.

CONTRAINDICATIONS

As with any operative procedure, the health and comorbidities of the patient may alter the decision to pursue a more invasive or prolonged surgical approach. Tissue and wound characteristics, as well as mechanism of injury, may preclude some reconstructive options. For example, prior irradiation and surgical scars limit the utility of local flaps or recipient vessel availability when free tissue transfer is being considered. A necrotic wound bed or active infection should always be addressed before undertaking reconstruction. Positive tumor margins and/or the need for postoperative irradiation of the tumor bed can create a dilemma for the reconstructive surgeon. In palliative situations, immediate reconstruction is sometimes considered, keeping in mind the underlying risks of local cancer recurrence and altered wound healing.

TIMING OF RECONSTRUCTION

Immediate scalp reconstruction following tumor extirpation or trauma has several advantages over delayed repair.

First, the effects of scarring and wound contracture are preempted. The defect is likely well-defined and thus the tissue requirements are readily apparent. Cost and quality of life factors are optimized, minimizing the need for repeated hospitalizations and additional surgical procedures. The psychological benefits of a more prompt restoration of function and bodily integrity should also not be underestimated.

Some situations either preclude or mandate immediate coverage. An open craniotomy requires prompt coverage to achieve dural continuity and brain coverage. As previously mentioned, active infection should be addressed prior to attempting soft tissue repair. When debridement cannot be completed without confidence that the wound bed will support tissue coverage, repair should be delayed until necrotic material, especially in a contaminated wound, can be completely removed.

PATIENT POSITION AND ROOM SETUP

The positioning of the patient depends on the need for transfer of tissue from distant sites, as well as any simultaneous reconstructive procedures. Simple anterior and lateral defects may be addressed with the patient in a supine or slightly rotated position, with the head supported by a soft foam ring or an adjustable neurosurgical "horseshoe" headrest. The latter can be used with the patient supine or prone and provides wide access to surrounding tissues. The table can be positioned in a reverse Trendelenburg position to give the surgeon optimal exposure when standing at the head. If the need for microvascular anastomosis is anticipated, recipient vessels are carefully identified and preserved, especially branches of the external carotid artery and internal jugular vein.

OPERATIVE TECHNIQUE

ANATOMY

The scalp comprises five layers. Skin, with its hair follicles, is the outermost. Beneath the skin is a layer of connective tissue containing blood vessels. Deeper still is the galea aponeurosis, a tough musculofascial layer that bridges the frontalis muscles anteriorly to the occipitalis muscles posteriorly. The galea is contiguous with the superficial temporal fascia laterally and with the superficial musculoaponeurotic system (SMAS) of the face. Avulsions

of adjacent tissues occur at predictable locations such as the supraorbital, temporal, auricular, and occipital areas, where muscles insert on bony prominences. This explains why eyebrows, forehead skin, and the external ears are often traumatically avulsed in continuity with the scalp. Loose areolar tissue, the fourth and weakest layer, is susceptible to shearing forces. The pericranium is the deepest layer of the scalp, adhering to the skull, and can support a skin graft when better options for reconstruction are not available.

The blood supply of the scalp is provided by the supraorbital and supratrochlear arteries (from the ophthalmic artery) as well as the superficial temporal, posterior auricular, and occipital arteries (from the external carotid artery). A thorough understanding of this vascular anatomy is essential for planning local flaps. The superficial temporal artery is the most accessible and reliable of the scalp vessels for microvascular anastomosis, though it is by comparison more fragile than the branches of the external carotid artery found in the neck. The entire scalp can be revascularized by a single superficial temporal artery because of the extensive collateral circulation within scalp tissue.

ADJUNCTS TO RECONSTRUCTION

The use of negative pressure wound therapy (NPWT) became popular with the introduction of commercially available vacuum-assisted wound closure devices in the 1990s. NPWT is purported to improve local circulation, expedite revascularization of wound beds (i.e., promote granulation), stimulate wound contraction, and isolate clean wounds from external contamination. This modality provides one option for temporizing wounds that cannot be immediately repaired or in preparation for a skin graft. NPWT is also frequently employed as a protective bolster over skin-grafted wounds and can be left in place for 5–7 days. NPWT is contraindicated for wounds that are grossly infected, necrotic, or that contain unresected neoplasm.

Acellular dermal matrices (e.g., AlloDerm and Flex-HD) as well as engineered dermal substitutes (such as Integra) have been used as a first stage in reconstruction, prior to skin grafting, in order to achieve a thicker neodermis and potentially more durable wound covering. Integra is a bilayer biologic substrate shown to produce a scalp wound surface that will support a skin graft following vascular ingrowth and incorporation over the pericranium or other sufficiently vascularized tissues.

PRIMARY CLOSURE

For very small defects (<3 cm wide), primary closure is sometimes feasible. Wide undermining and scoring of the galea (cuts placed parallel to the defect, 15–20 mm apart) facilitate this approach, sparing the patient a more extensive reconstructive procedure and minimizing the risk of alopecia. Generally, scalp tissue is more lax further from the vertex. A two-layer closure allows most of the tension to be placed in the galeal plane so that the skin can be approximated under less tension.

SKIN GRAFTS

Placing grafts over bone can be problematic due to poor vascularity of the wound bed. Staged cranial wound preparation techniques have been developed to promote the vascularity of the recipient site before skin graft placement. These involve either drilling 2 mm holes in the outer table or using a mechanical burr to remove the entire outer table, enabling granulation to develop from the exposed diploë. This technique can only be applied where the cranium is sufficiently thick, and care must be exercised to avoid iatrogenic dural tears, cerebrospinal fluid leak, brain injury, or excessive bleeding. Because skin grafts lack dermal elements, alopecia should be expected. In addition, graft stability following radiation and chemotherapy may be tenuous. Dermal substitutes may be of benefit when skin grafting is required, as described previously.

LOCAL AND REGIONAL FLAPS

Larger scalp defects that are not amenable to primary closure or grafting, or that require more durable coverage, will sometimes be reconstructable with local or regional flaps. Because the scalp has poor pliability, local and regional flap choices are limited to defects less than 100 cm² and must be carefully planned. Scoring of the galea in a linear fashion, perpendicular to the direction of desired stretch, will improve the reach of scalp flaps.

The *temporoparietal flap* is based on the frontal and parietal branches of the superficial temporal artery. This flap may be used to repair anterior or posterior scalp defects and can provide vascularized coverage for bone grafts. The temporoparietal muscle and fascia are thin and arise anterior to the ear. The superficial fascia supplied by the superficial temporal vessels is an extension of the galeal aponeurosis. Dissection is begun by locating the superficial temporal artery with a Doppler probe. The axis of rotation is taken at the preauricular fold anterior to the helix crus. Dissection

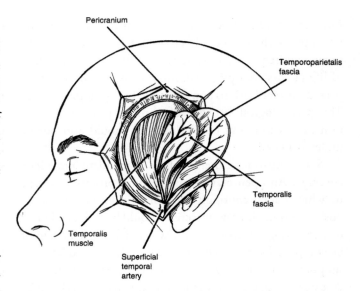

Figure 35.3. Elevation of temporoparietal flap. Dissection of fascia near posterior base of pedicle should hug cartilaginous margin of crus helix to avoid injury to primary vessels.

proceeds through the dermis in a plane that leaves the temporal vessels exposed on the surface of the temporoparietal fascia. Posterior dissection is continued until a 5 cm base is obtained. The galea and temporoparietal fascia are divided distally along the lateral margins, and elevation of the fascia in a plane superficial to the pericranium and anterior to the fascia of the temporalis muscle is achieved. Dissection of the fascia near the posterior base of the pedicle should hug the cartilaginous margin of the crus helix to avoid injury to the primary vessels (Figure 35.3). The flap is rotated and inset through the subcutaneous plane.

The *Juri* or *temporoparieto-occipital* flap, is used for treatment of frontal or frontoparietal alopecia and defects. The flap is supplied by the parietal branch of the superficial temporal artery. The base of the flap, typically 4 cm wide, is determined by the location of the superficial temporal artery, located by palpation or with the assistance of the Doppler probe, 2–3 cm above the zygomatic arch. The flap is raised in the subgaleal plane, then rotated into the defect and sutured in place with absorbable subcutaneous suture and nonabsorbable skin sutures or staples (Figure 35.4).

Multiple large flaps (three or four) may be designed as originally described by Orticochea. *Orticochea flaps*, based on constant vascular pedicles, are expanded by parallel and perpendicular galeotomies and may be used to cover large areas (up to 30% of the scalp) with hair-bearing skin. The anterior pedicle is made up of the collateral branches of the ophthalmic vessels. The lateral pedicle contains the superficial temporal vessels, and the posterior vessels are composed of two groups corresponding to the lateral and medial branches

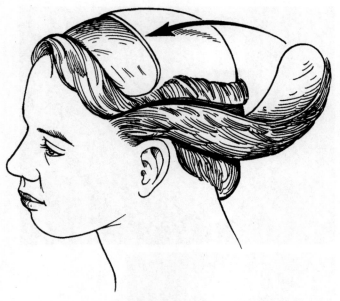

Figure 35.4. Elevation and delay of temporoparieto-occipital flap (by Juri).

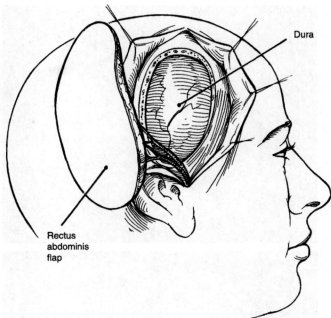

Figure 35.5. Insetting of rectus abdominis muscle. Superficial temporal vessels are used for anastomosis.

of the occipital arteries. To cover large defects of the scalp, forehead, and nape of the neck, flaps can be elevated in a three- or four-flap technique. Each flap must have its own vascular pedicle to ensure adequate circulation. Disadvantages of this technique include scalp scarring, interruption of scalp circulation, disturbance in hair follicle orientation, possible alopecia, and the potential need for additional skin grafts.

MICROSURGICAL FLAPS

Free tissue transfer is often the most reliable choice for large (>100 cm^2) and/or composite scalp defects. The options for free flap reconstruction include free muscle flaps covered with skin graft versus free fasciocutaneous or myocutaneous flaps. The *rectus abdominis muscle flap* can be used for smaller reconstructions, while the *anterior lateral thigh (ALT) fasciocutaneous flap* or *latissimus dorsi muscle flap* can cover larger defects. Furthermore, the latissimus dorsi may be combined with other tissues supported by the thoracodorsal system. Alternative, but less commonly used free flaps for scalp reconstruction include the *omental, scapular,* and *radial forearm.* Although still controversial due to the inherent long-term risks and cost involved, face and scalp transplantation has been proved feasible in a limited number of highly selected patients.

RECTUS ABDOMINIS FLAP

The rectus abdominis flap can provide a large amount tissue with a long vascular pedicle. The flap is suitable for

filling deeper defects and for covering moderate defects (<60 cm^2). The advantages of this selection are that the patient need not be moved for muscle harvest and that two surgical teams may work simultaneously. Inset of the rectus abdominis muscle is illustrated in Figure 35.5 using superficial temporal recipient vessels.

LATISSIMUS DORSI FLAP

The latissimus dorsi muscle or myocutaneous flap can provide a large amount of tissue sufficient to cover the entire scalp. It also may be transferred together with the serratus anterior or scapular flap, using a common vascular pedicle comprising the subscapular-thoracodorsal or circumflex scapular system. Frequently, a muscle flap with skin graft is used for scalp coverage, though some surgeons include a paddle of skin to monitor flap viability during the early postoperative period. Figure 35.6 shows a large scalp defect reconstructed with a latissimus dorsi muscle flap and skin graft.

OMENTAL FLAP

Omentum covered with a split-thickness skin graft was one of the first free flaps described for scalp reconstruction. The main indication for using the omental flap is the need for skin resurfacing in large defects of the skull where other tissues are unavailable or inadequate. One

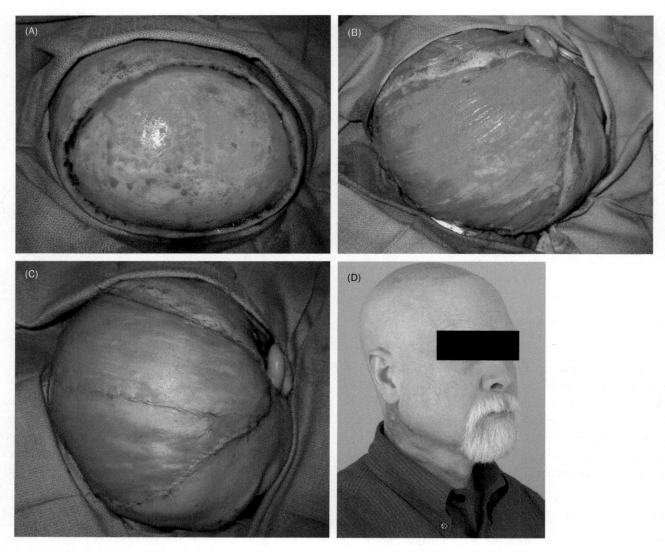

Figure 35.6. Latissimus dorsi muscle free flap used for reconstruction of a large scalp defect. (A) Scalp defect following resection of a poorly differentiated sebaceous carcinoma in a 49-year-old man. (B) Following inset of the free latissimus dorsi muscle flap. (C) Final result after split-thickness skin graft applied to the latissimus flap. (D) Patient at 1-year follow-up.

advantage of this flap is its abundant blood supply, which makes it ideal to improve circulation and limit infection in the recipient area. With less invasive flap options now available, the omental flap has somewhat fallen out of favor because a laparotomy is required, and the flap can be difficult to secure.

Technique of Dissection

An upper midline incision is made and is deepened to the abdominal fascia. After entry into the peritoneal cavity, the omentum is delivered outside the abdomen and the gastroepiploic vessels are identified (Figure 35.7). The vessels directed to the greater curvature of the stomach are ligated and divided, and the omentum is separated from the transverse colon in an avascular plane. The left gastroepiploic artery is divided from the splenic artery and the omental flap is retracted to expose the right gastroepiploic pedicle (Figure 35.8). If the defect to be covered is long, the flap can be extended by interrupting the gastroepiploic artery just beyond the right omental artery. The middle omental artery can also be interrupted, which enables obtaining a long flap without damaging the blood supply. The microvascular anastomosis proceeds as previously described. Following flap transfer, the abdominal fascia is closed with no. 1 running or interrupted suture and the skin is closed with nonabsorbable suture or staples.

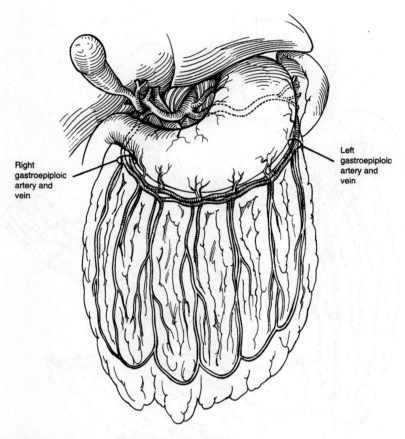

Figure 35.7. Omentum is delivered outside abdomen. Note gastroepiploic vessels.

Right gastroepiploic artery and vein

Left gastroepiploic artery and vein

FASCIOCUTANEOUS FLAPS

Thin fasciocutaneous flaps, most notably the scapular, lateral arm, and radial forearm flaps, have been employed successfully for scalp coverage. The scapular flap is highly versatile, providing various combinations of skin, fascia, muscle, and bone. The radial forearm flap can be harvested either as a fasciocutaneous flap or, when a small amount of bone is also needed, as an osteocutaneous flap (Figure 35.9).

ANTERIOR LATERAL THIGH FLAP

The anterolateral thigh (ALT) fasciocutaneous perforator flap has found increased popularity for scalp reconstruction due to its potential to transfer a large amount of skin with less donor site visibility and morbidity than that of alternative flaps. The thickness of the thigh's subcutaneous fat layer, especially in patients with a higher body mass index (BMI), sometimes limits the utility of the ALT. The flap may be modified to include fascia lata (for dural repair) by incorporating the transverse branch of the lateral femoral circumflex artery which provides the blood supply to this

tissue. Figure 35.10 shows an example of a large scalp defect reconstructed with a free ALT flap.

RECIPIENT VESSEL CHOICE

The greatest difficulty in free tissue transfer to the scalp is the availability of suitable vessels for microvascular anastomosis. An important consideration guiding vessel choice is the site of the reconstruction. Postoperative positioning of the patient and potential compression of the flap pedicle should also be considered when deciding which recipient vessels to use.

The superficial temporal vessels are often a suitable choice for the microvascular reconstruction of the scalp. It is helpful to locate and mark this pedicle using a pencil Doppler. An incision is placed in the skin crease anterior to the ear from the upper level of the external auditory meatus and extending into the temporal area. The temporoparietal and deep parietal fascia are incised and the vascular pedicle isolated. Alternatively, the occipital artery can be used for reconstruction.

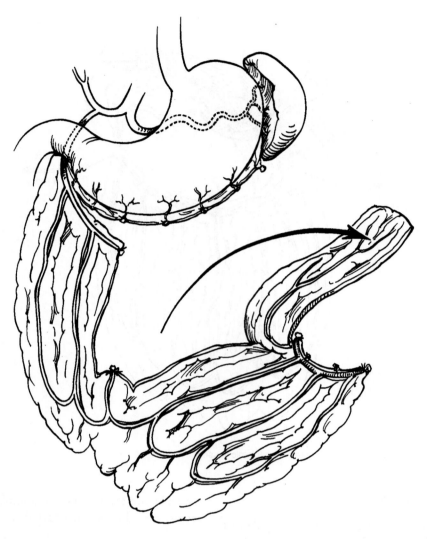

Figure 35.8. Division of left gastroepiploic vessels from splenic artery. If defect to be covered is long, flap is extended by interrupting gastroepiploic artery just after right omental artery.

If the external carotid artery and the internal jugular vein are used, the neck is extended and the head rotated to the contralateral side. An incision is made following the anterior margin of the sternocleidomastoid muscle from the mastoid process to the mid-portion of the muscle. The platysma and the cervical fascia are incised and upper and lower skin flaps are developed. The anterior margin of the sternocleidomastoid is identified, dissected, and retracted, exposing the facial vein. The facial vein is also retracted or ligated and divided to expose the carotid sheath. After opening the sheath, the internal jugular vein is identified, isolated, and retracted using vessel loops. The carotid bulb is easily noted, and the external carotid artery is recognized by the presence of collateral branches. The dissection of the external carotid artery should be performed proximally to identify the hypoglossal nerve. Branches of the external carotid artery are isolated and retracted using vessel loops.

If pedicle length is a concern, a vein graft can be harvested and anastomosed to the external carotid artery and internal jugular vein. This arteriovenous (AV) loop is allowed to perfuse while the free flap dissection is completed. The AV loop is divided and the free flap vessels anastomosed into the respective arterial and venous segments of the graft. An alternative technique is to place vein graft extensions on the free flap vessels prior to anastomosis to the neck vessels.

CRANIOPLASTY

When dura mater requires repair (beyond primary closure) to prevent cerebrospinal fluid leak and to protect the brain, autologous tissues are readily obtained for use as grafts, including pericranium, temporalis fascia, and fascia

POSTOPERATIVE MANAGEMENT

In addition to routine postoperative care, special precautions must be taken to monitor flaps. The patient's head must be maintained in a neutral position to avoid mechanical compression of the vascular pedicle. When neck vessels are used in free flaps, tracheostomy tube ties or oxygen masks with elastic bands that encircle the neck should be avoided. The flaps should be fully exposed, without dressings, to allow for regular inspection. Free muscle flaps with skin grafts should not have compressive dressings. Flap perfusion must be monitored hourly for the first 2 days, assessing color, capillary refill, and tissue turgor. Flaps that appear pale and have prolonged capillary refill may have compromised arterial inflow. Blue discoloration, more rapid capillary refill, and rapid, dark bleeding upon pinprick suggest a problem with venous outflow. Additional information on the condition of the flap may be obtained by assessing the pedicle or perforators within the flap using a percutaneous Doppler device. Various other monitoring devices, such as transcutaneous oxygen saturation monitors and implantable Dopplers, may also be helpful. With most cutaneous reconstructions, however, a significant portion of the flap is exposed for clinical assessment and sophisticated adjuncts are not usually needed for monitoring.

If abnormal arterial or venous blood flow is suspected following free tissue transfer, the flap requires immediate surgical exploration. In the event of pedicle thrombosis, it may be possible to salvage the flap if the blood supply is

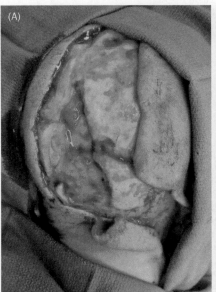

Figure 35.9. Inset of radial forearm flap in scalp defect from sarcoma resection in a 73-year-old man.

lata. A variety of materials have been employed to replace missing bone: split calvarium, split-rib, and iliac crest, as well as nonautogenous material (e.g., methylmethacrylate, titanium, and demineralized bone).

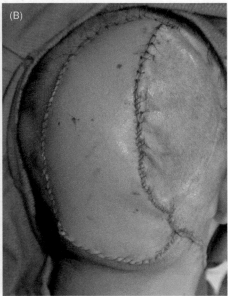
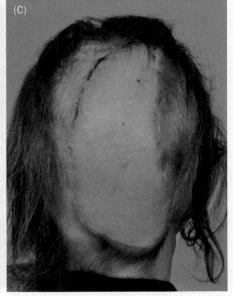

Figure 35.10. A 48-year-old woman with history of radiation for malignancy exhibiting a large full-thickness scalp defect. (A) Following debridement of a failed scalp rotation flap. (B) Defect reconstructed with a fasciocutaneous anterior lateral thigh (ALT) flap. (C) One month postop.

restored and any anatomic or technical causes of pedicle compromise are promptly corrected. Because undue pedicle compression can lead to vascular thrombosis, patient positioning in the postoperative period must be monitored diligently. Drains are usually left in place until the output is less than 30 mL over 24 hours. Patients should be counseled about protection from damaging ultraviolet (UV) light using sunscreen and hats.

CAVEATS

Scalp reconstruction requires careful decision-making due to the variety of techniques available and the potentially devastating consequences of a failed reconstruction. Knowledge of the vascular anatomy is critical for local flap elevation and microvascular transfer. Limitations on scalp rotation should be considered for defects that have been exposed to radiation and prior surgical trauma. The prevention of postoperative pressure on the flap and vascular pedicle is vital to avoid flap compromise. Finally, in cases of alopecia, autologous hair transplantation may be an option for some patients and is covered elsewhere in this text.

SELECTED READINGS

Angelos PC, Downs BW. Options for the management of forehead and scalp defects. *Facial Plast Surg Clin North Am* 2009;17(3):379–393.

Antonyshyn O, Zuker R. Tissue expansion in head and neck reconstruction. *Plast Reconstr Surg* 1988;82:58–68.

Arashiro K, Ohtsuka H, Ohtani K, et al. Entire scalp replantation. *J Reconstr Microsurg* 1995;11:245.

Arnold PG, Lovich SF, Pairolero PC. Muscle flaps in irradiated wounds: an account of 100 consecutive cases. *Plast Reconstr Surg* 1994;93:324–327.

Baker S, Johnson TM, Nelson BR. Technical aspects of prolonged scalp expansion. *Arch Otolaryn Head Neck Surg* 1994;120:431.

Beasley NJP, Gilbert RW, Gullane PJ, et al. Scalp and forehead reconstruction using free revascularized tissue transfer. *Arch Facial Plast Surg* 2004;6:16–20.

Bernstein EF, Sullivan FJ, Mitchell JB, et al. Biology of chronic radiation effect on tissues and wound healing. *Clin Plast Surg* 1993;20:435–453.

Bo B, Qun Y, Zheming P, et al. Reconstruction of scalp defects after malignant tumor resection with anterolateral thigh flaps. *J Craniofac Surg* 2011;22:2208–2211.

Borah GL, Hidalgo DA, Wey PD. Reconstruction of extensive scalp defects with rectus free flaps. *Ann Plast Surg* 1995;34:281–287.

Brown GED. Indirect deltopectoral flap. *Br J Plast Surg* 1976;29:122.

Browning FSC, Eastwood DS, Price DJE, et al. Scalp and cranial substitution with autotransplanted greater omentum using microvascular anastomosis. *Br J Surg* 1979;66:152.

Chao AH, Yu P, Skoracki RJ, et al. Microsurgical reconstruction of composite scalp and calvarial defects in patients with cancer: A 10-year experience. *Head Neck* 2012;34:1759–1764.

Cohen SR, Bartett SP, Whitaker LA. Reconstruction of late craniofacial deformities after irradiation of the head and face during childhood. *Plast Reconstr Surg* 1990;86:229–237.

Desai SC, Sand JP, Sharon JD, et al. Scalp reconstruction: an algorithmic approach and systematic review. *JAMA Facial Plast Surg* 2015;17(1):56–66.

Fischer JP, Sieber B, Nelson JA, et al. A 15-year experience of complex scalp reconstruction using free tissue transfer—analysis of risk factors for complications. *J Reconstr Microsurg* 2013;29:89–98.

Furnas H, Lineaweaver WC, Alpert BS, et al. Scalp reconstruction by microvascular free tissue transfer. *Ann Plast Surg* 1990;24:431–444.

Gordon L, Buncke HJ, Alpert BS. Free latissimus dorsi muscle flap with split-thickness skin graft cover: a report of 16 cases. *Plast Reconstr Surg* 1982;70:173.

Gundeslioglu AO, Selimoglu MN, Doldurucu T, et al. Reconstruction of large anterior scalp defects using advancement flaps. *J Craniofac Surg* 2012;23:1766–1769.

Harii K. Clinical application of free omental flap transfer. *Clin Plast Surg* 1978;5:273.

Hoffmann JF. Management of scalp defects. *Otolaryngol Clin North Am* 2001;34(3):571–582.

Imanishi NN, Minabe T. The arterial anatomy of the temporal region and the vascular basis of various temporal flaps. *Br J Plast Surg* 1995;48:439.

Kaixiang C, Su Z, Kecheng J, et al. Microsurgical replantation of the avulsed scalp: report of 20 cases. *Plast Reconstr Surg* 1996;97:1099.

Khan A, Chipp E, Hardwicke J, et al. The use of dermal regeneration template (Integra) for reconstruction of a large full-thickness scalp and calvarial defect with exposed dura. *J Plast Reconstr Aesthet Surg* 2010;63:2168–2171.

Kinsella CR, Grunwaldt LJ, Cooper GM, et al. Scalp reconstruction: regeneration with acellular dermal matrix. *J Craniofac Surg* 2010;21:605–607.

Koenen W, Goerdt S, Faulhaber J. Removal of the outer table of the skull for reconstruction of full-thickness scalp defects with a dermal regeneration template. *Dermatol Surg* 2008;34:357–363.

Kwee MM, Rozen WM, Ting JWC, et al. Total scalp reconstruction with bilateral anterolateral thigh flaps. *Microsurgery* 2012;32:393–396.

Lai CS, Lin SD, Chou CK, et al. Subgalea-periosteal turnover flap for reconstruction of scalp defects. *Ann Plast Surg* 1993;30:267.

Larson DL. Long-term effects of radiation therapy in the head and neck. *Clin Plast Surg* 1993;20:485–490.

Lesavoy MA, Dubrow TJ, Schwartz RJ, et al. Management of large scalp defect with local pedicle flaps. *Plast Reconstr Surg* 1993;91:783.

Lu MM. Successful replacement of avulsed scalp. *Plast Reconst Surg* 1969;43:231.

Maillard GF, Landolt A. Penetrating Marjolin's ulcer of scalp. *Br J Plast Surg* 1984;37:463.

Manders EK, Graham WP, Schenden MJ, et al. Skin expansion to eliminate large scalp defects. *Ann Plast Surg* 1984;12:305.

Mehrara BJ, Disa JJ, Pusic A. Scalp reconstruction. *J Surg Oncol* 2006;94:504–508.

Momoh AO, Lypka MA, Echo A, et al. Reconstruction of full-thickness calvarial defect: a role for artificial dermis. *Ann Plast Surg* 2009;62(6):656–659.

Miller MJ, Janjan NA. Treatment of injuries from radiation therapy. In: Kroll SS, ed. *Reconstructive Plastic Surgery for Cancer*. St. Louis: CV Mosby, 1996;17–36.

Mustoe TA, Porras-Reyes BH. Modulation of wound healing response in chronic irradiated tissues. In: Granick MS, Solomon MP, Larson DL, eds. *Clinics of Plastic Surgery: Management of Chronic Radiation Wounds*. Philadelphia, PA: WB Saunders, 1993;465–472.

Nahai F, Hurteau J, Vasconez LO. Replantation of an entire scalp and ear by microvascular anastomoses of only one artery and one vein. *Br J Plast Surg* 1978;31:339.

Oishi SN, Luce EA. The difficult scalp and skull wound. *Clin Plast Surg* 1995;22:51.

Orticochea M. New three-flap scalp reconstruction technique. *Br J Plast Surg* 1971;24:184.

Ranev D, Chindarsky B. Operative treatment of deep burns of the scalp. *Br J Plast Surg* 1969;24:309–312.

Sakai S, Soeda S, lshii Y. Avulsion of the scalp: which one is the best artery for anastomosis? *Ann Plast Surg* 1990;24:350.

Sanger JR, Matloub HS, Gosain AK, et al. Scalp reconstruction with prefabricated abdominal flap carried by radial artery. *Plast Reconstr Surg* 1992;89:315.

Shanoff E, Tsur H. Fenestration and delayed skin grafting for the cover of the exposed inner table of the skull. *Br J Plast Surg* 1981;34:331.

Shenoy AM, Nanjundappa A, Nayak UK, et al. Scalp flap. *J Laryngol Otol* 1993;107:324.

Snyderman CH, Janecka IP, Sekhar LN, et al. Anterior cranial base reconstruction: role of galeal and pericranial flaps. *Laryngoscope* 1990;100:607.

Sosin M, DelaCruz C, Bojovic B, et al. Microsurgical reconstruction of complex scalp defects: An appraisal of flap selection and the timing of complications. *J Craniofac Surg* 2015;26:1186–1191.

Terranova W. The use of periosteal flaps in scalp and forehead reconstruction. *Ann Plast Surg* 1990;25:451.

Thomas A, Obed V, Murarka A, et al. Total face and scalp replantation. *Plast Reconstr Surg* 1998;102:2085–2087.

Wei FC, Dayan JH. Scalp, Skull, Orbit, and Maxilla Reconstruction and Hair Transplantation. *Plast Reconstr Surg* 2013;131: 411e–424e.

Wieslander JB. Repeated tissue expansion in reconstruction of a huge combined scalp-forehead avulsion injury. *Ann Plast Surg* 1988;20:381.

Zhou S, Chang T, Guan WX, et al. Microsurgical replantation of the avulsed scalp: report of six cases. *J Reconstr Mlcrosurg* 1993;9:121.

PART VII.

HEAD AND NECK SURGERY

36

MODIFIED AND RADICAL NECK SURGERY

Edward A. Luce

INDICATIONS

Radical neck dissection, the en bloc resection, dependent on definition, of the major lymph node–bearing areas of the neck, has been the cornerstone of extirpative head and neck cancer. Whether performed in isolation or in conjunction with resection of a primary within the upper aerodigestive tract, the performance of a neck dissection should be an elegant demonstration of the combination of an intimate knowledge of neck anatomy and technical proficiency. The classical radical neck dissection was described by Crile in 1906, but was eclipsed to some degree by the advent of therapeutic radiation or radiotherapy. Dissatisfied with radiotherapy as the primary treatment modality for head and neck cancer, Grant Ward in Baltimore and Hayes Martin in New York in separate publications returned to an operative focus in descriptions of the radical neck dissection. The radical neck dissection as described by Ward and Martin consisted of the dissection and removal of all of the lymphatic drainage of the neck, the jugulodigastric and anterior cervical chain, and the submandibular and the posterior cervical triangles with retention of the principal nerves—vagus, hypoglossal, lingual, and phrenic—as well as the underlying muscular floor.

Modification of the standard or full neck dissection awaited the description by Boca of preservation of the sternocleidomastoid for cosmetic outcomes, the spinal accessory nerve to avoid the often disabling effect of a denervated trapezius, and the internal jugular vein to minimize the occurrence of cerebral edema. A selective neck dissection limits the scope of the dissection based on the assumption of the lymphatic drainage of the primary, such as a supraomohyoid for a carcinoma of the lower lip or anterior dissection for a thyroid cancer.

CONTRAINDICATIONS

Contraindications to the performance of a radical neck dissection usually hinge on the criterion of resectability. Involvement of the essential structures of the base of skull, carotid artery, and vertebral spine have conventionally been considered a contraindication to the en bloc resection of neck dissection because of unresected and residual tumor. As with all cancer contraindications or criteria of unresectability, each of these, most particularly including the carotid artery, has been bent in the past.

The purpose of this chapter is to illustrate the technique of a standard "classical" radical neck dissection with an emphasis on unit, or compartmental, approaches to the dissection, including an outline of the important anatomic structures of each compartment.

ROOM SETUP AND PATIENT MARKINGS

Performance of the neck dissection, either with or without a composite component, requires the surgeon to be on the ipsilateral side and the assistant on the opposite side, with an additional assistant to the surgeon's side. An endotracheal tube for standard neck dissection can be placed only above and to the opposite side of the surgical field, with anesthesia personnel at the head of the table. Tracheostomy requires some modification of that placement but also can be accomplished by moving the anesthesia personnel to the opposite side and inferiorly.

Proper exposure requires draping the majority of the face, the entire neck, and the upper chest within the operative field to prepare for any contingency that may arise during the procedure. Additional areas for reconstruction, such as a pectoralis, fibula, rectus, or radial forearm flap, obviously require additional draping and exposure (Figure 36.1).

The selection of a proper incision blends the criteria of adequate exposure and the provision of sufficient blood supply. Incisions most commonly used are the vertical, single, or double Y and the transverse parallel incisions of McFee. We prefer a "lightning bolt" modification of the single Y incision, zigzagging the vertical component to avoid neck skin contracture. The topographic landmarks described are palpated, and a point is selected two fingers breadth below the midportion of the body of the mandible, connecting the mastoid posteriorly with the midline of the submental region by a gently curving line that traverses this point below the mandible and outlines the transverse or hyoid crease incision. The vertical incision is outlined by palpation of the carotid pulse superiorly and the midclavicle line inferiorly. The incision begins posterior to the carotid pulse to allow skin coverage of this structure by the anterior flap, which is better vascularized than the posterior skin, if a posterior compartment dissection is included in the operation (Figures 36.2 and 36.3).

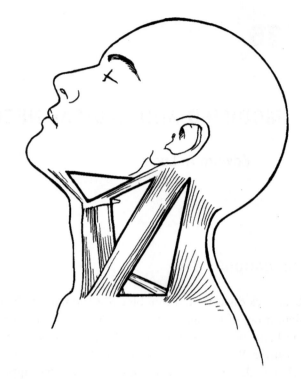

Figure 36.1. Triangles of neck.

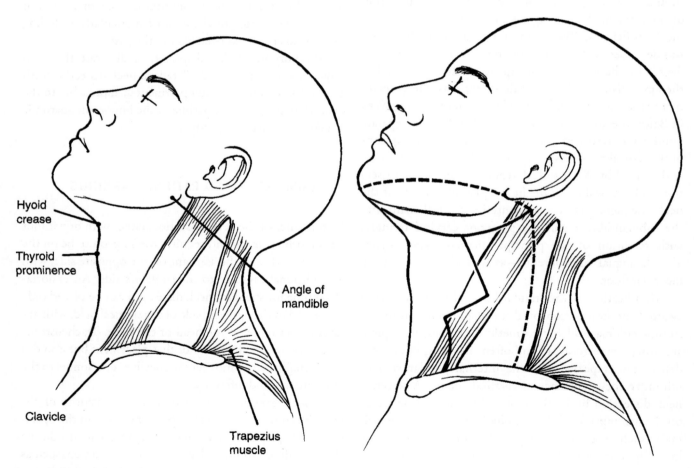

Figure 36.2. Anatomic landmarks.

Figure 36.3. Incision and area of dissection.

HEAD AND NECK SURGERY

If a skin resection of a previous biopsy site must be included, modifications are fairly easily done with this combination of incisions. If the neck has been previously irradiated, we prefer parallel transverse incisions, using the hyoid crease incision superiorly and a parallel incision one and half to two fingers breadth above the clavicle inferiorly. This bipedicle flap approach is known as the *McFee incision*. Anterior cervical primaries and cancer of the larynx or thyroid are approached with a cervical apron flap, often with posterior inferior extensions to permit radical exposure of the neck contents.

SURGICAL TECHNIQUE

The anatomic compartments included in the neck dissection are those of the posterior cervical triangle, subdivided into a superior and inferior subcompartment by the course of the spinal accessory nerve; the anterior cervical triangle, subdivided by the inferior belly of the omohyoid; and the submandibular and submental triangles. The pertinent anatomic landmarks define the limits of the dissection and aid in selection of incisions. The limits of the dissections are palpated and include the angle of the mandible as the superior limit (the landmark for location of the marginal mandibular branch of the seventh cranial nerve), the thyroid cartilage as the anterior limit, the clavicle as the inferior limit, and the anterior border of the trapezius as the posterior limit. The sternocleidomastoid muscle divides the anterior from the posterior compartment or triangle. Flaps are raised beneath the platysma muscle superiorly to above the body of the mandible and taken anteriorly to the thyroid prominence, inferiorly to the clavicle, and posteriorly to the trapezius.

Structures seen at this juncture are the facial artery and vein, anterior and just below the angle of the mandible; the marginal mandibular nerve at the angle; and the external jugular vein and greater auricular nerve, crossing the body of the sternocleidomastoid from inferior to superior. Initial dissection begins in the posterior compartment (Figure 36.4). The superior limit of the triangle is defined by identifying the intersection of the anterior border of the trapezius with the posterior border of the sternocleidomastoid (Figure 36.5A). The spinal accessory nerve

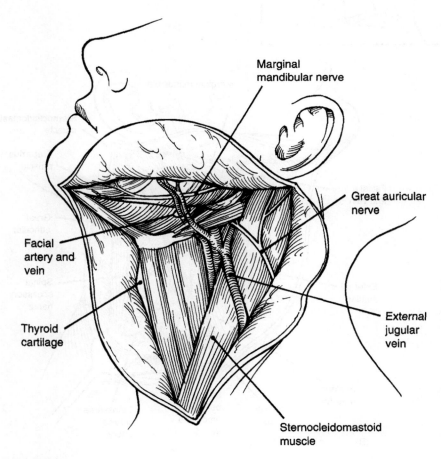

Figure 36.4. Reflected flaps/exposure.

enters the triangle at the midportion of the posterior aspect of the sternocleidomastoid and crosses the compartment, coursing inferiorly and posteriorly to the trapezius muscle. The inferior belly of the omohyoid marks the transition of the dissection from the posterior compartment to the supraclavicular fossa compartment and is also a landmark for identification of the transverse cervical artery, the blood supply to the lower trapezius. The brachial plexus and posterior and middle scalene muscles inferiorly will be barely discernible at the completion of the posterior compartment dissection.

The posterior triangle is initially dissected superior to inferior to expose the entire anterior border of the trapezius muscle, and then the triangle is dissected from posterior to anterior. Identification of the spinal accessory nerve, if it is to be preserved, is accomplished with a nerve stimulator, and the nerve is dissected superiorly until it courses beneath the sternocleidomastoid muscle. The posterior and inferior dissection of the posterior compartment is made more tedious by the necessity to preserve the nerve and also by the anatomic necessity that multiple small blood vessels run at right angles to the plane of dissection (Figure 36.5B).

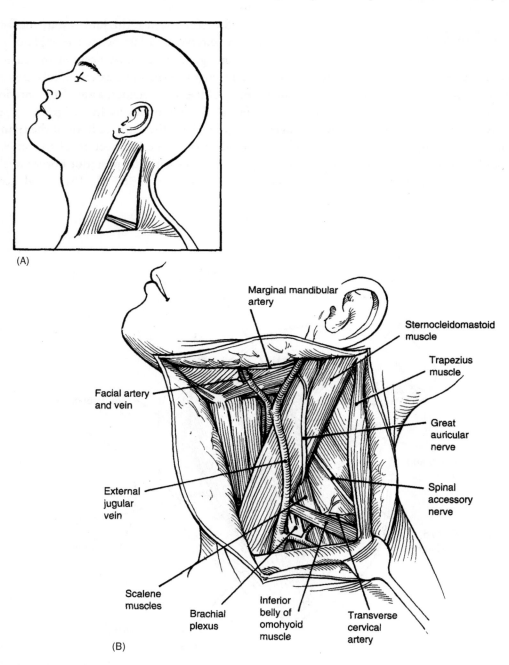

(A)

(B)

Figure 36.5. Posterior triangle. (A) Boundaries. (B) Flaps reflected.

HEAD AND NECK SURGERY

Once the inferior belly of the omohyoid is clearly exposed in the supraclavicular fossa and the distal attachment sacrificed, the supraclavicular fossa compartment can be dissected from posterior to anterior quite easily, ending at the posterior aspect of the clavicular insertion of the sternocleidomastoid muscle. The course of the transverse cervical artery is highly variable, and although it parallels the clavicle at times, it can be seen as far as 6 cm superior to the clavicle. The artery can be an important source of blood supply to the trapezius muscle, but, perhaps more importantly, it can be the source of troublesome bleeding deep within supraclavicular fat if it is inadvertently injured. As dissection proceeds, the brachial plexus, the levator scapulae, and the middle and anterior scalene muscles will be exposed on the floor of the dissection. Finally, at the medial anterior edge of the compartment is the phrenic nerve, crossing the anterior scalene muscle. If the thin fascia that overlies the nerve is carefully preserved, the nerve will not be lifted from the underlying floor or scalene muscle and is more easily dissected free of damage (Figure 36.6).

Dissection of the anterior triangle is facilitated considerably, because the previous dissection has been from posterior to anterior of the posterior and supraclavicular compartments. The sternocleidomastoid muscle is still intact at this juncture, and, if it is to be preserved, the dissected contents are brought beneath the sternocleidomastoid muscle. If the muscle is to be sacrificed, division of the two portions—clavicular and sternal heads—is accomplished by

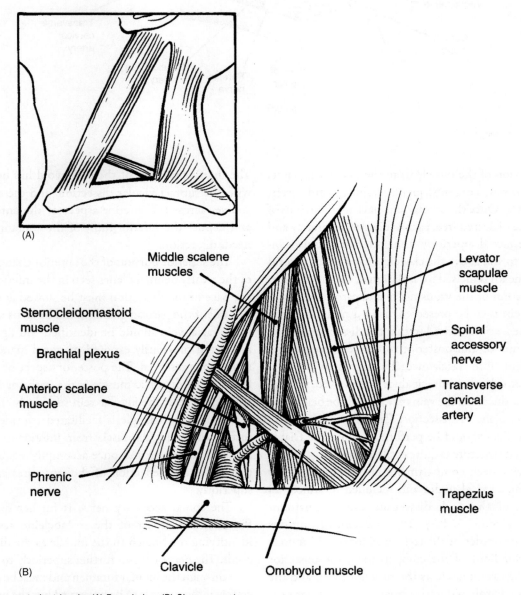

(A)

(B)

Middle scalene muscles

Sternocleidomastoid muscle

Brachial plexus

Anterior scalene muscle

Phrenic nerve

Clavicle

Omohyoid muscle

Levator scapulae muscle

Spinal accessory nerve

Transverse cervical artery

Trapezius muscle

Figure 36.6. Inferior posterior triangle. (A) Boundaries. (B) Close-up anatomy.

MODIFIED AND RADICAL NECK SURGERY

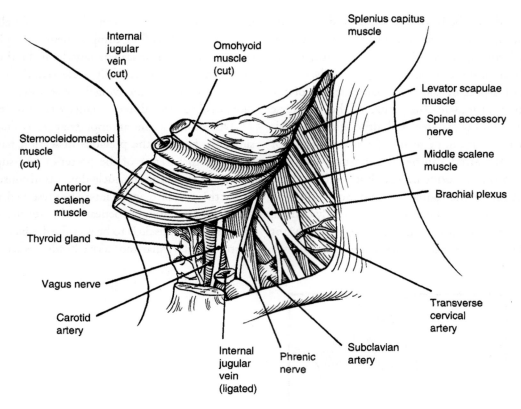

Internal jugular vein (cut)

Omohyoid muscle (cut)

Splenius capitus muscle

Sternocleidomastoid muscle (cut)

Levator scapulae muscle

Spinal accessory nerve

Middle scalene muscle

Anterior scalene muscle

Brachial plexus

Thyroid gland

Vagus nerve

Carotid artery

Internal jugular vein (ligated)

Phrenic nerve

Subclavian artery

Transverse cervical artery

Figure 36.7. Posterior triangle.

careful dissection of the muscle from the underlying fascia and the important contents, jugular vein, carotid artery, and vagus nerve. Once the sternal and clavicular portions of the muscle are dissected free, each is divided separately and the muscle retracted superiorly. The underlying fascia is incised parallel to and above the clavicle, exposing the carotid sheath. The sheath is incised for isolation of the jugular vein and identification of the vagus nerve and carotid artery. If the jugular vein is to be preserved, as in a modified neck dissection, the fascia is incised so that the dissection will be taken both anterior and posterior to the vein, requiring a separate incision of the fascia medially (Figure 36.7).

On the left side, the thoracic duct is preserved, but the entrance of the duct into the vein may actually be below and inferior to the plane of dissection. Therefore, no discrete search for the duct should be performed, since the friable and thin-walled structure is quite easily injured.

The anterior neck compartment, encompassing levels 2 and 3 of the cervical nodes and included in almost all modifications of the neck dissection, can be anatomically defined (Figure 36.8A). The anatomic definitions are the anterior border of the sternocleidomastoid muscle as the posterior limit of the compartment, the posterior belly of the digastric muscle as the superior limit, and the strap muscles (thyrohyoid and sternal thyroid) anteriorly.

The inferior portion of the omohyoid has been sacrificed with the supraclavicular dissection, and the superior belly courses across the inferior aspect of the anterior triangle and defines the inferior limit of the supraomohyoid that needs dissection.

The superior portion of the anterior triangle lacks some of the clearly defined planes seen in the inferior aspect, and the pace of the dissection must be slowed at this juncture. The tail of the parotid gland should be transected, the posterior facial vein should be identified and ligated, and the associated previously exposed marginal mandibular nerve should be preserved. The posterior aspect of the posterior belly of the digastric muscle is the path for identification and exposure of the jugular vein superiorly. The dissection of the anterior triangle is facilitated considerably by dissection of the jugular fascia from inferior to superior as a separate maneuver, and once accomplished, by division of that fascia and reflection of the structures anteriorly and superiorly.

The spinal accessory nerve is further dissected from the posterior aspect of the sternocleidomastoid muscle, identifying the branch to the muscle as the dissection proceeds. The nerve courses further superiorly to exit with the vein through the jugular foramen and must be dissected discretely if the nerve is to be preserved but the vein sacrificed.

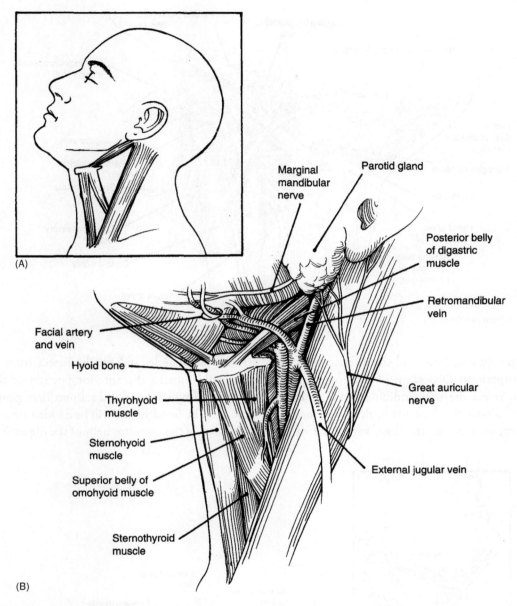

Marginal
mandibular
nerve

Parotid gland

Posterior belly
of digastric
muscle

Retromandibular
vein

Facial artery
and vein

Hyoid bone

Thyrohyoid
muscle

Sternohyoid
muscle

Superior belly of
omohyoid muscle

Sternothyroid
muscle

Great auricular
nerve

External jugular vein

(A)

(B)

Figure 36.8. Anterior triangle. (A) Boundaries. (B) Close-up anatomy.

If a standard neck dissection is to be performed with sacrifice of both muscle and vein, after transection of the tail of the parotid, the mastoid origin of the sternocleidomastoid muscle is divided and the dissection along the posterior aspect of the posterior belly of the digastric muscle is done to the point of the jugular vein, as described above. The jugular vein is ligated at that juncture, and the spinal accessory nerve is pushed posteriorly out of the further anterior dissection.

At this time, completion of the anterior superior portion of the dissection of the anterior compartment is done by identification and ligation of the superior thyroid artery and vein. Ordinarily, except in instances of laryngeal and hypopharyngeal carcinoma, the superior thyroid artery and the accompanying superior laryngeal nerve deep to the artery are left undisturbed. The hypoglossal nerve is traced anteriorly through its course across and lateral to the bifurcation of the carotid and to the entrance into the submandibular triangle. The posterior belly of the digastric is further defined to its tendinous insertion into the hyoid. At this stage, the dissection of the anterior compartment is completed, and the specimen is still attached to the submandibular and submental triangles (Figures 36.8B and 36.9).

The submandibular triangle, or compartment (Figure 36.10), is defined by the posterior belly of the digastric and stylohyoid muscles posteriorly and inferiorly, the anterior

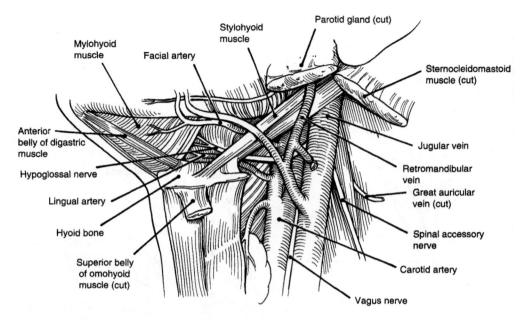

Figure 36.9. Anterior triangle relationships.

belly of the digastric anteriorly, and the inferior aspect of the mandible superiorly. Dissection of the compartment will expose and resect the submandibular gland, transect Wharton's duct, dissect the contents of the posterior submandibular compartment off the floor composed of the styloglossus muscle, and finally dissect from beneath the mylohyoid muscle, the anterior portion of the compartment. The lingual nerve and submaxillary ganglion will be exposed. The facial vessels will be divided for a second time at the level of the posterior belly of the digastric muscle after

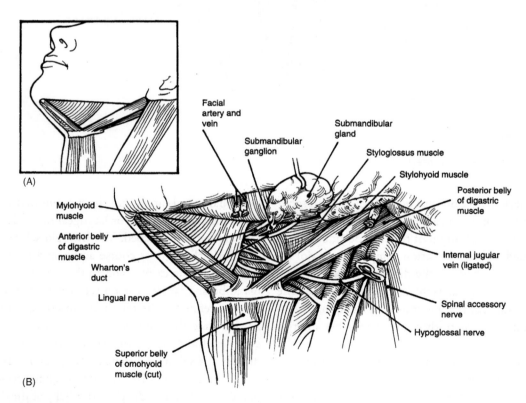

Figure 36.10. Submandibular triangle. (A) Boundaries. (B) Close-up anatomy.

HEAD AND NECK SURGERY

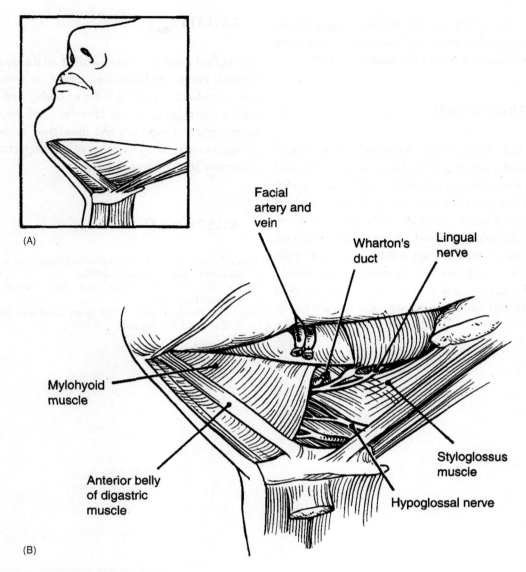

(A)

Facial artery and vein

Wharton's duct

Lingual nerve

Mylohyoid muscle

Styloglossus muscle

Anterior belly of digastric muscle

Hypoglossal nerve

(B)

Figure 36.11. Submental triangle. (A) Boundaries. (B) Anatomy.

entrance into the compartment inferiorly from their origin at the carotid artery and jugular vein.

The important structure of the submandibular compartment, the lingual nerve, can be easily injured unless care is taken to identify the nerve during the dissection. Inferior traction on the submaxillary gland will distinguish the parasympathetic innervation of the gland from the submaxillary ganglion and the association of the latter structure with the lingual nerve more superiorly. With continued traction on the gland, the parasympathetic branches can be ligated and divided, allowing the nerve to retract superiorly out of harm's way.

The submental triangle is the smallest compartment in the neck, defined by the anterior belly of the digastric laterally, the mandible superiorly, and the hyoid inferiorly (Figure 36.11A). Discrete dissection of this compartment

is usually done in cases of carcinoma of the lower lip or in cancer of the anterior floor of the mouth (Figure 36.11B).

WOUND CLOSURE AND DRESSINGS

Wound closure is accomplished over suction catheters. Two suction catheters are placed transversely in the neck, one superiorly and one inferiorly, and brought out through separate stab incisions over the mastoid and clavicle posteriorly, respectively. Wound closure is facilitated by the use of scratch marks so that flaps can be placed back into their original beds. Layers of the incisions are closed discretely with a layer of absorbable sutures for platysma closure and skin sutures or stapling. Wounds are dressed openly to allow inspection of flaps and drainage. Patients who have had a neck dissection performed that was not in conjunction with intraoral or mandibular resection can be fed the following day. Suction catheters are left in place until drainage is minimal, usually 2–3 days.

POSTOPERATIVE CARE

The recovery and rehabilitation of head and neck patients is facilitated considerably by the early introduction of physical therapy. Even in the absence of sacrifice of the sternocleidomastoid muscle or spinal accessory nerve, the patient's level of functioning can be enhanced by a short course of physical therapy. If the spinal accessory nerve has been sacrificed, physical and occupational therapy will be prolonged by the necessity to teach the patient to use other muscles for abduction of the arm. In this way, problems with shoulder joint adhesions and secondary musculoskeletal pain can be minimized.

CAVEATS

The radical neck dissection, similar to dissection of other regional lymph node–bearing tissues, is a technical procedure and accomplished most smoothly and proficiently with a thorough anatomic knowledge of the sequence of compartmental exposure and dissection, accompanied by an innate sense of the location of the important anatomic structures of each compartment.

SELECTED READINGS

Bocca E, Pignatoro O. A conservative technique in radical neck dissection. *Ann Otolaryngol* 1967;76:975.

Martin H. *Surgery of Head and Neck Tumors*. New York: Hoeber-Harper, 1957.

Ward GE, Hendrick JW. *Tumors of the Head and Neck*. Baltimore: Williams and Wilkins, Baltimore, 1950.

37.

PAROTIDECTOMY

Tjoson Tjoa and William B. Armstrong

INTRODUCTION

The major salivary glands exist as paired structures in the upper neck and primarily serve to secrete saliva, which plays a major role in lubrication, digestion, swallowing, bacterial defense, and taste modulation. The parotid gland is the largest of the major salivary glands, positioned in the upper neck and pre-auricular area, wrapping around the mandibular ramus. While the parotid gland is the most common site of salivary neoplasms, surgery of the parotid gland is performed for a variety of neoplastic, infectious, and inflammatory conditions.

When performing surgery on the parotid gland, it is essential to have a comprehensive understanding of facial nerve anatomy. During development, as the epithelial buds of the parotid gland grow and branch, they extend between the divisions of the facial nerve.[1] Thus, the extratemporal branches of the facial nerve become surrounded by the parenchyma of the gland, with approximately 80% of the gland lying superficial to the nerve. Parotidectomy involves meticulous dissection to identify and preserve the branches of the facial nerve while extirpating the necessary tissue to meet the goals of the operation.

ANATOMY

The parotid glands are located in the upper neck. Each gland overlies the masseter muscle, wraps posteriorly around the ramus of the mandible, and is closely related to the zygoma superiorly, the ear canal cartilage posteriorly, the parapharyngeal space medially, and the sternocleidomastoid muscle and posterior belly of the digastric muscle inferiorly (Figure 37.1).

The facial nerve originates at the pontomedullary junction and contains motor fibers that control the muscles of facial expression and the posterior belly of the digastric, stylohyoid, and stapedius muscles, as well as conducting sensory and parasympathetic fibers that contribute to taste, salivation, and lacrimation. The main trunk of the facial nerve courses through the temporal bone and exits the skull at the stylomastoid foramen, directly into the substance of the parotid gland. From there, however, its extratemporal anatomy and branching pattern has significant variability. In fact, no two facial nerves exhibit the exact same branching pattern and course—it is this variability that makes the parotidectomy such a unique and sometimes challenging surgery. Additionally, while the facial nerve is a surgical landmark that separates the superficial from the deep lobe of the parotid gland, there does not exist a defined fascial plane between the two lobes. This phenomenon has clinical and surgical relevance and is the reason why neoplastic processes can extend both superficial and deep to the facial nerve rather than honoring strict definitions of superficial and deep parotid lobes.

PREOPERATIVE WORKUP

Parotid masses typically present with a painless lump in the area of the gland. Because the differential diagnosis of parotid lesions is so broad, including autoimmune, obstructive, infectious, inflammatory, and neoplastic etiologies, it is important to take a comprehensive history with attention to each of these possibilities. A physical exam with attention to the characteristics of the lesion, facial nerve function, and associated skin lesions or neck masses is also of the utmost importance.[2]

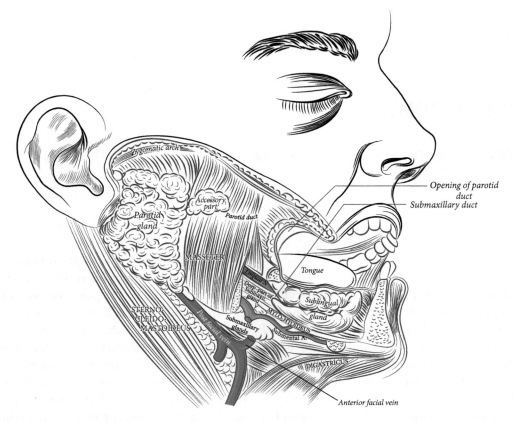

Figure 37.1. Location of the parotid gland relative to the structures of the upper neck and face. From *Gray's Anatomy* The Classic Collectors Edition. Henry Gray Copyright 1977. Bounty Books, New York.

In addition to a complete history and physical exam, various imaging modalities may be helpful.

Axial imaging using either magnetic resonance imaging (MRI) or computed tomography (CT) scans are commonly used. MRI images can provide high-resolution soft tissue detail demonstrating deep lobe extent, neural involvement, and cortical bone invasion.[3,4] CT scans can help to identify sialoliths, or stones within the salivary duct that appear hyperdense. CT scan can also delineate the fibrofatty tissue plane that distinguishes the medial aspect of the deep lobe of the parotid from the soft tissues of the parapharyngeal space.[5] Ultrasound is a noninvasive, cost-effective imaging modality that can provide information about lesions of the superficial parotid lobe, and it is often used to guide fine-needle aspiration (FNA) biopsies.[6]

The utility of FNA cytology in the workup of parotid neoplasms is debated; at this time, few parotid tumors are treated with nonsurgical management, so opponents of FNA biopsies argue that it rarely alters the treatment plan. Additionally, it is subject to sampling error and requires the presence of an expert cytologist. However, in the presence of qualified cytologists, an adequate sample can aid in diagnosis by distinguishing benign from malignant lesions. Many malignant parotid tumors will present initially as an asymptomatic mass, and identification of these tumors preoperatively aids tremendously in surgical planning and patient counseling.[7]

Although 80% of parotid masses are benign, the patient must be counseled preoperatively in the event of malignant histologic analysis results.[8] A superficial parotidectomy provides a complete biopsy specimen and is adequate treatment for most patients. The histopathologic specimen can be examined at the time of operation by frozen section analysis to rule out or confirm malignancy. Thus, the possibility, albeit remote, of the need for total parotidectomy, facial nerve resection, and ipsilateral neck dissection are discussed before surgery. Also, possible complications such as sialocele, gustatory sweating (Frey's syndrome), upper neck and earlobe numbness, and hematoma, are presented as part of the preoperative informed consent.

ROOM SETUP AND PREPARATION

The patient should be positioned supine with a shoulder roll and the head extended and turned to the opposite side of the parotidectomy. Slight elevation of the head can help to decrease venous pressure during surgery. The table is positioned to allow for complete access to the entire head, and general anesthesia is administered via orotracheal intubation. Long-acting muscle relaxants are avoided so that the facial nerve may be tested intraoperatively. It is necessary to inquire throughout the course of the operation whether paralytic agents have been given because anesthesia staffing frequently changes, and the surgeon's assumption that normal facial nerve conductivity was preserved throughout the procedure can lead to disastrous consequences. Facial nerve monitoring can be performed with the assistance of an intraoperative nerve monitor, with either 2-channel or 4-channel leads, commonly placed in the mentalis, orbicularis oris, orbicularis oculi, and frontalis. Regardless of whether a formal nerve monitor is used, it is important to expose the entire hemiface so that direct visualization of the musculature can be performed throughout the surgery to observe for stimulation of the nerve branches. This can either be prepped into the field or covered with a clear drape.

The exposed surgical field includes the hemiface, ear, and neck, which should be prepped to below the clavicle. Again, because of the small possibility of malignancy with any parotid lesion, the neck should be exposed should a neck dissection be necessary after frozen section analysis. The most commonly used incision for a parotidectomy is a modified Blair incision, which begins in a natural preauricular crease and extends from the tragus to the lobule, at which point it curves posteriorly and inferiorly to follow the anterior border of the sternocleidomastoid muscle to a point 2 cm below the mandible, typically in a natural cervical skin crease (Figure 37.2). This incision allows for

full visualization of the entire parotid gland and can easily be extended onto the neck, if cervical lymphadenectomy becomes necessary. Although it is possible to perform a parotidectomy through a facelift incision, that approach potentially compromises additional surgery if it is required. Plain 1:100,000 dilution of epinephrine can be injected into the subcutaneous tissues along the planned incision to decrease skin bleeding. Lidocaine injection into the parotid bed is avoided because it may result in transient facial nerve paralysis, rendering nerve monitoring useless.

OPERATIVE TECHNIQUE

SUPERFICIAL PAROTIDECTOMY

The modified Blair incision is made using a no. 15 blade, as outlined earlier. Any bleeding points are cauterized using a bipolar or Bovie electrocautery. It is important to carry the preauricular incision 1–2 mm inferior to the crease made by the lobule of the ear in order to prevent a satyr (pixie ear) deformity. Skin flaps are then raised by establishing a plane just superficial to the parotid fascia, which is just deep to the superficial musculoaponeurotic system (SMAS). Alternatively, a thick subcutaneous flap can be raised, with "fat up, fat down," superficial to the SMAS plane. In such cases, the SMAS can be raised separately off the parotid fascia and used in an advancement flap fashion at the end of the case to help reconstruct the defect and potentially decrease the occurrence of Frey's syndrome by providing a barrier between the parotid and sweat gland fibers in the subcutaneous flap.

The flaps are raised anteriorly and posteriorly to visualize the entire border of the parotid gland and lateral surface of the sternocleidomastoid muscle. At this point, skin flaps are held in position with skin hooks and are kept moist with saline throughout the procedure. The greater auricular nerve is usually encountered during the initial incision in the posterior aspect of the wound overlying the sternocleidomastoid muscle, approximately 1 cm posterior to the external jugular vein. Branches of the greater auricular nerve to the parotid gland are ligated, and, unless involved with tumor, the remainder of the nerve is left intact to avoid anesthesia of the ear. The great auricular nerve can also serve as donor graft material in the case that a portion of a branch of the facial nerve is involved in tumor and requires resection. The posterior border of the gland is dissected off the sternocleidomastoid muscle and the cartilage of the external ear canal (Figure 37.3). This can typically be done with the aid of Bovie or bipolar electrocautery. The

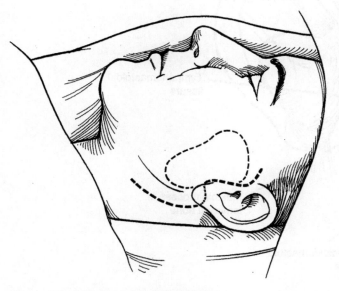

Figure 37.2. Modified Blair incision with parotid gland outlined.

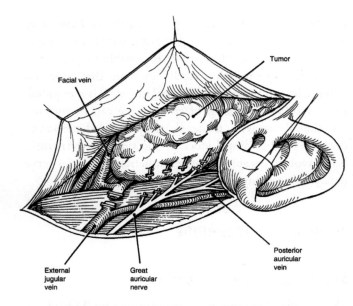

Figure 37.3. Posterior edge of parotid prior to mobilization off the sternocleidomastoid muscle. The external jugular vein and branches of the greater auricular nerve have been ligated.

posterior belly of the digastric muscle is identified below the parotid gland and followed posteriorly toward the mastoid tip to free the parotid gland and delineate the inferior extent of dissection.

Once the lobule and ear canal cartilage is freed from the gland, a skin hook is used to retract the lobule superiorly. A small bridge of tissue typically remains between the sternocleidomastoid muscle and the ear canal cartilage. This can carefully be bluntly dissected out and any small veins ligated using a microbipolar electrocautery. All soft-tissue dissection is performed before nerve identification and dissection.

Identification of the facial nerve begins with a thorough understanding of its anatomy. The main trunk exits the stylomastoid foramen posterolateral to the styloid process and enters the posterior border of the gland, where it appears as a white structure approximately 2 mm in diameter. Multiple landmarks are useful to assist in the identification of the nerve at this point, each of which is described later (Figure 37.4).

1. The tragal cartilage of the external ear canal forms a "pointer" as it extends deeply, at the bony–cartilaginous junction, which is palpable after the gland is dissected off the cartilage. The nerve typically lies in an area between 1 and 1.5 cm deep and slightly anterior and inferior to this tragal pointer.

2. The attachment of the posterior belly of the digastric muscle is along the digastric groove of the medial

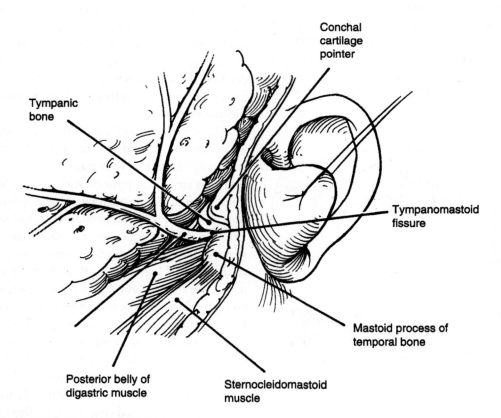

Figure 37.4. Landmarks for identification of the facial nerve.

HEAD AND NECK SURGERY

surface of the mastoid bone. The digastric muscle can typically be found with blunt dissection in a superomedial direction after separating the posterior parotid from the sternocleidomastoid muscle. The nerve lies approximately 1 cm deep to the attachment of the upper border of the digastric muscle.

3. The tympanomastoid suture line is a constant bony landmark that can be palpated between the tympanic and mastoid bones. The main trunk of the nerve is typically found between 6 and 8 mm distal to the endpoint of this suture line. A branch of the posterior auricular artery is frequently seen in close proximity to the nerve in this area. While helping to localize the nerve, it can also become a source of nuisance bleeding. A nerve stimulator may aid in pinpointing the nerve if it is not readily visible.

4. The styloid process is deep to the nerve, so it should be used cautiously as a palpable landmark since the nerve passes superficial to the styloid process as it exits the stylomastoid foramen.

5. If access to the proximal main trunk of the facial nerve is blocked by tumor or inflammation, retrograde dissection can be performed by identifying one or more distal branches of the nerve and following them proximally. The marginal mandibular branch can typically be found overlying the angle of the mandible, and it courses distally along the inferior border of the mandible within the fascia overlying the submandibular gland. The zygomatic branch can be identified by careful dissection anterior to the parotid gland over the zygomatic arch. Excellent hemostasis with bipolar cautery and good exposure is required to locate the branches. Loupe magnification aids in this process.

6. When necessary, the facial nerve can be identified more proximally in the mastoid bone via a mastoidectomy and followed peripherally. This approach is usually reserved for large or recurrent lesions with clinical evidence of proximal nerve involvement and requires expertise in performing otologic surgery.

The surgeon should be well versed in the various anatomic landmarks and nerve identification techniques to facilitate gland removal with minimal risk of nerve injury based on the characteristics of the lesion to be removed. No matter what method of nerve identification is used, the greater the exposure, the more likely a safe and successful dissection will occur. Whatever technique is chosen, the parotid fascia should not be incised until the nerve is visualized to avoid injuring a superficial nerve, especially when a tumor distorts the gland architecture, displacing the nerve laterally.

Once the main trunk of the nerve is identified, a nonlocking, smooth-tipped, angled nerve dissector instrument can be used to follow it distally. Loupe magnification of 2.5× or greater is extremely helpful for this and subsequent stages of dissection. Within the proximal parotid parenchyma, the main trunk usually bifurcates at a point called the pes anserinus into superior (temporofacial) and inferior (cervicofacial) divisions. The temporofacial branch further divides into the temporal, zygomatic, and buccal branches. The temporal branch supplies the frontalis muscle and generally follows a line drawn from 0.5 cm anterior to the tragus to 1.5 cm lateral to the eyebrow (Pitanguy's line). The zygomatic and buccal branches supply facial muscles of the midface, including the periorbital and upper lip. These three branches may have small peripheral anastomoses and can provide cross-innervation in the event of injury. The inferior division splits into the marginal mandibular branch, which innervates the lower lip depressors, and the cervical branch, which descends to innervate the platysma. The marginal mandibular branch is almost invariably seen as it crosses superficial to the posterior facial vein, but it may have several fine strands and lies just below the border of the mandible. This nerve branch is the most intolerant of manipulation, has no cross-innervation, and is especially susceptible to transient paresis postoperatively. While this is the typical branching pattern of the nerve, there is considerable variability in the number of peripheral branches, and often there are anastomosing branches within the parotid gland, so it benefits the surgeon to be continuously vigilant for nerve branches during the remainder of the dissection (Figure 37.5).

The initial technique used to dissect along the nerve is to spread parallel to the course of the nerve just at the edge of the gland with the tips of the dissector pointed down. Once the nerve is clearly delineated, it can be followed with a fine-tipped dissector gently on the nerve, traveling from proximal to distal along each branch. The parotid tissue lateral to and superficial to the plane of the nerve can be divided with a knife, a bipolar electrocautery device, or an ultrasonic scalpel. Following the nerve branches in such a manner slowly unveils the branches and allows for them to be followed distally as the parotid tissue is separated superficial to them. While some authors rely on visual observation of twitches in the face, other authors choose to use a nerve stimulator to test for nerve activity before dividing the parotid tissue each time. Regardless, some form of monitoring of the facial musculature should be performed during the

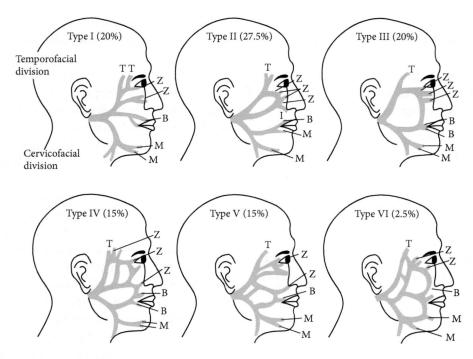

Figure 37.5. Common branching patterns of the extratemporal facial nerve.

dissection in order to help identify and preserve the nerve branches.

The typical approach is to start following the branches at the pes anserinus, beginning at either the lowermost branch of the lower division or the uppermost branch of the upper division, depending on where the lesion to be removed is located. As the parotid parenchyma is freed from each branch, the next branch inferiorly or superiorly is followed and the parotid tissue is released. This is performed, branch by branch, until all nerve branches in the area of the lesion are dissected free and the portion of the parotid with the enclosed mass is mobilized for removal. Once the entire course of the nerve is freed, the superficial portion of the gland is completely resected. The specimen is then sent to pathology for permanent examination in most cases or submitted for frozen section analysis in cases where a malignant diagnosis is suspected and requires confirmation.

TOTAL PAROTIDECTOMY

Removal of the entire parotid gland may be indicated for gross tumor invasion of the deep lobe or high-grade malignant tumor anywhere within the parotid gland. A superficial parotidectomy is first performed as described earlier. The overlying facial nerve is then teased away from the deep lobe. Nerve hooks can be used to gently retract the branches of the nerve, and sharp scissors are used to release the fascial connections between the nerve and the gland

deep to it. The portion of the gland overlying the masseter muscle is the elevated off the surface of the muscle back beyond the angle of the jaw. This deep lobe tissue is then dissected from its fibrous attachments to the mandible and the stylomandibular ligament. Inferiorly, the gland is elevated off the stylohyoid muscle. The posterior facial vein is divided, and the external carotid artery is identified as it passes beneath the angle of the mandible before branching into the maxillary and superficial temporal arteries; these vessels may need to be ligated when involved with tumor. After the deep lobe is freed, it is gently displaced from beneath the facial nerve.

RECONSTRUCTION AND POSTOPERATIVE CARE

Once the resection is complete and any necessary repair or grafting of the facial nerve has been performed, attention is turned to closure. Defects caused by resection of large portions of the parotid gland sometimes necessitate reconstruction. The primary goals of reconstruction are (1) to restore normal facial contours, (2) to cover any raw exposed gland surface so as to prevent aberrant reinnervation of the skin by parasympathetic nerve endings, and (3) to provide external skin coverage in cases where the disease process necessitates resection of skin.[9,10] Many techniques have been described for reconstruction. In small resections, the parotid capsule can often be closed primarily. Local flaps using the superficial musculoaponeurotic system (SMAS) flap, temporoparietal fascia flap, or the sternocleidomastoid muscle flap can be used. Cervicofacial advancement flaps generally provide enough tissue to close large cutaneous defects.[11] In larger resections, the defect can be filled with autologous abdominal fat or acellular dermis. For larger resections with skin defects, regional pedicled flaps such as the supraclavicular or submental flap, as well as soft tissue free flaps such as the anterolateral thigh or radial forearm, can be used.

Prior to closure, the wound is inspected for bleeding and hemostasis is achieved using bipolar cautery. A small-diameter, closed-suction drain is placed in the wound and brought through the skin through a separate stab incision behind the ear. Subcutaneous absorbable tacking sutures may be used to align the incision. The skin is then closed, using any method that properly approximates the skin edges. Antibiotic ointment is applied and the patient is awakened from anesthesia.

Facial nerve function is observed during extubation and retested in the early postoperative period. In the case of incomplete eye closure, an aggressive regimen of eye lubrication is recommended to prevent corneal abrasions. If expected to be permanent, a gold weight placement and canthopexy can be performed to assist in eye closure. The wound is inspected for hematoma, which, if it occurs, should be drained early to prevent skin flap loss. The patient is kept overnight in the hospital and discharged the following day. Suction drains are usually kept in place for 2–3 days postoperatively to prevent seroma or sialocele and to facilitate healing of the skin flap down onto the parotid bed. Sutures are removed within 7 days, and further follow-up is dictated by histologic diagnosis and treatment protocols.

CAVEATS

Parotidectomy remains the gold standard for definitive diagnosis and treatment of parotid tumors, as well as the preferred treatment for various inflammatory conditions of the parotid gland. The key to successful parotidectomy is expert knowledge of facial nerve anatomy in order to safely identify the nerve, followed by careful and meticulous dissection to avoid weakness to the face. Key landmarks that aid in the identification of the main trunk of the nerve include the posterior belly of the digastric muscle, the tragal pointer, and the tympanomastoid suture line, which should be identified early in the dissection. Wide exposure is necessary to promote safe identification of the nerve and is one of the keys to optimizing surgical outcome.

REFERENCES

1. Walvekar RR, Loehn BC, Wilson MN. Anatomy and physiology of the salivary glands. In: Johnson JT, Rosen CA, eds. *Bailey's Head and Neck Surgery—Otolaryngology*. 5th ed. Baltimore: Lippincott Williams and Wilkins, 2014:91–700.
2. Bartels S, Talbot JM, DiTomasso J, Everts EC, Andersen PE, Wax MK, Cohen JI. The relative value of fine-needle aspiration and imaging in the preoperative evaluation of parotid masses. *Head Neck* 2000;22:781–786.
3. Lee YY, Wong KT, King AD, Ahuja AT. Imaging of salivary gland tumours. *Eur J Radiol* 2008 Jun;66(3):419–436.
4. Kuan EC, Mallen-St Clair J, St John MA. Evaluation of parotid lesions. *Otolaryngol Clin North Am* 2016;49:313–325.
5. Som PM, Brandwein-Gensler MS. Anatomy and pathology of the salivary gland. In Som PM, Curtin HD, eds. *Head and Neck Imaging*. 5th ed. St. Louis, MO: Elsevier, 2011:2525–2535.
6. Haidar YM, Moshtaghi O, Mahmoodi A, Helmy M, Goddard JA, Armstrong WB. The utility of in-office ultrasound in the diagnosis of parotid lesions. *Otolaryngol Head Neck Surg* 2017 Jan;156(3):511–517. Epub ahead of print.
7. Cohen EG, Patel SG, Lin O, Boyle JO, Kraus DH, Singh B, Wong RJ, Shah JP, Shaha AR. Fine-needle aspiration biopsy of salivary gland lesions in a selected patient population. *Arch Otolaryngol Head Neck Surg* 2004 Jun;130(6):773–778.
8. Spiro RH. Salivary neoplasms: overview of a 35-year experience with 2,807 patients. *Head Neck Surg* 1986 Jan-Feb;8(3):177–184.
9. Witt RL, Pribitkin EA. How can Frey's syndrome be prevented or treated following parotid surgery? *Laryngoscope* 2013 Jul;123(7):1573–1574.
10. Emerick KS, Herr MW, Lin DT, Santos F, Deschler DG. Supraclavicular artery island flap for reconstruction of complex parotidectomy, lateral skull base, and total auriculectomy defects. *JAMA Otolaryngol Head Neck Surg* 2014 Sep;140(9):861–866.
11. Irvine LE, Larian B, Azizzadeh B. Locoregional parotid reconstruction. *Otolaryngol Clin North Am* 2016 Apr;49(2):435–446.

38.

THE RADIAL FOREARM FLAP

Brogan G. A. Evans and Gregory R. D. Evans

ASSESSMENT OF THE DEFECT

Squamous cell carcinoma and other malignancies frequently arise in the oral cavity. Contact of the oral mucosa with alcohol and tobacco are known contributing

factors in the development of head and neck cancer. The abuse of these promoters often lead reconstructive surgeons to encounter defects of the oral cavity found at the base of tongue, floor of the mouth, and retromolar trigone (Figure 38.1). Upon initial inspection, an

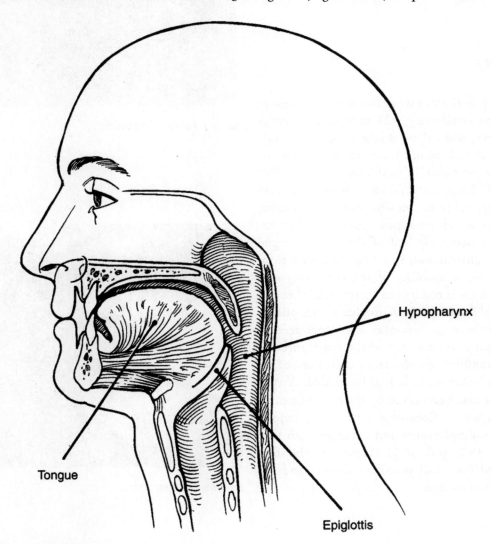

Hypopharynx

Tongue

Epiglottis

Figure 38.1. Anatomy of head and neck area.

assessment is always important in determining the appropriate flap for closure of these defects. In some cases, the defects are composite and extensive, including the mandible, skin of the cheek or neck, and even the orbit. However, in the majority of cases, these defects are confined to the intraoral mucous membranes and require both a replacement lining and variable quantities of underlying soft tissue for repair. In addition to an initial assessment, it is critical to evaluate additional factors from a reconstruction concern, such as previous surgery, radiotherapy, and chemotherapy. In patients with previous radiation injury, treatment necessitates the use of well-vascularized tissue. Additionally, when radiation injuries are seen in combination with previous surgery, the fibrosis and diminished oxygen tension in the tissue often leads to poor wound healing. The use of a free tissue transfer with the radial forearm flap can obviate this poor wound healing and replace previously irradiated tissue with well-perfused normal fascia and skin.

INDICATIONS

The goals of intraoral reconstruction are (1) to ensure good speech and swallowing, (2) to ensure coverage of vital structures, and (3) to obtain good cosmesis.[1-15] With these goals in mind, it is evident that one of the primary determinants in oral function is in fact tongue function. Thus, the total amount of tongue remaining after surgical resection determines the amount of function that is achieved postoperatively. For example, in cases where only half of the native tongue remains after reconstruction, it is vital to have a thin, pliable flap to ensure mobility of the remaining segment. Ultimately, these results can be achieved through the use of a radial forearm flap to provide a thin, pliable fasciocutaneous tissue for intraoral soft tissue defects. It is these optimal characteristics of the radial forearm flap—tongue mobility and the large diameters of its recipient vessels—that make it highly reliable. A typical example of a case best served by the radial forearm flap is a patient with a floor-of-mouth cancer requiring marginal mandibulectomy and coverage with soft tissue (Figures 38.2 and 38.3). However, the flap can also be used for small maxillary defects and for esophagocutaneous fistulas.

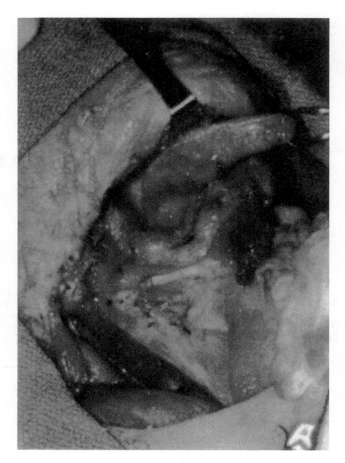

Figure 38.2. Floor-of-mouth defect.

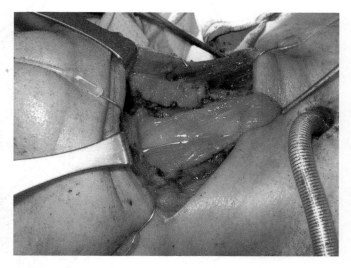

Figure 38.3. Laryngeal defect.

HEAD AND NECK SURGERY

CONTRAINDICATIONS

For total or subtotal defects of the tongue, the radial forearm flap does not provide the bulk necessary for reconstruction. Atrophy will occur during the postoperative period, and the remaining portion of the flap may be too small to allow for functional speech or swallowing.

A poor result on Allen's test necessitates further evaluation of the upper extremity vasculature, and if it is suspected that the radial artery is the dominant vascular supply to the hand or if the palmar arch is not patent, an alternative flap should be considered.

PATIENT MARKINGS AND ROOM SETUP

The operation is begun with the patient in the supine position on the operating table. The table should be placed straight, usually 180 degrees from anesthesia, allowing access to both sides of the neck by the extirpative surgeons. The nondominant hand is chosen unless there is a contraindication precluding its use, such as previous surgery, the patient's occupation, or the lack of a patent palmar arch. As an alternative, the table may be turned to allow ease of access to the operated side, but, during the microvascular anastomosis, the surgeon and the assistant must have access to the operative microscope by standing on both sides of the table. The surgical defect is marked in the head and neck, and the cephalic vein

and radial artery are marked on the nondominant forearm. The anesthesia and phlebotomy staff must know which arm will be used during surgery to avoid intravenous access and phlebotomy sticks in that arm (Figure 38.4). Variations in anatomy may occur in the division of the vascular distribution of the ulnar and radial sides of the hand.

Preoperatively, surgeons must perform an Allen's test, as it is essential that any obstruction within the radial, ulnar, or digital arteries be known before the flap is elevated. The absence of collateral circulation precludes the use of this flap or, at least, demands vascular reconstruction. A tourniquet is placed on the upper arm and wrapped in sterile drapes. Alternatively, a sterile tourniquet can be placed and included in the field. The arm is placed on one or two arm boards and is prepared within the field along with the head and neck area. Simultaneous harvest and tumor extirpation may be performed, especially if the tumor is contralateral to the flap harvest. However, this is often difficult, and frequently the harvest of the radial forearm flap must await completion of the extirpation.

OPERATIVE TECHNIQUE

ANATOMY

The anatomic basis of the radial forearm free flap is the vascularity supplied by the radial artery.
This artery runs longitudinally along the volar aspect of the forearm and gives off perforating branches to the skin,

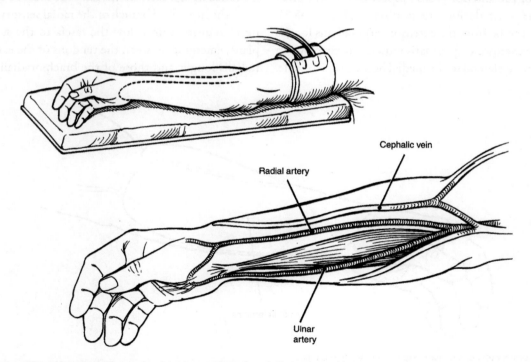

Figure 38.4. Patient positioned on table with tourniquet in place and arm board. Note vein markings.

subcutaneous tissue, muscle, and bone. The flap's cutaneous septal perforators lie between the flexor carpi radialis and the brachioradialis muscles. The entire flap may be raised on this septal stalk with maintenance of vascularity. Reconstruction of the radial artery with vein grafts is usually not required, but if insufficient flow to the radial side of the hand through the palmar arch is noted, a radial artery replacement can be achieved by using one of the many veins in the forearm (Figure 38.4).

The flap's venous drainage is through three separate venous systems, including the cephalic vein, the basilic vein, and the venae comitantes that run adjacent to the artery. The venae comitantes are the veins most frequently used for flap transfer, but they are occasionally too small. Consequently, it is advisable to elevate a cephalic or basilic vein with the flap in case an alternative venous drainage pathway is required (Figure 38.4).

Sensory innervation of the flap is provided by the medial and lateral antebrachial cutaneous nerves of the forearm, as well as by sensory branches of the radial nerve. If a sensate flap is desired, one of these branches can be harvested with the flap and sutured to the lingual or another cutaneous nerve in the neck (Figure 38.4).

TECHNIQUE

Defect type and tissue requirements dictate the design of the flap. The territory of the flap may be extended from the lower third of the anterior (volar) aspect of the arm proximally to the wrist flexion crease distally (Figure 38.5). Distal width can be from the extensor carpi radialis longus muscle to the extensor carpi ulnaris muscle. Proximal width may vary from the lateral to the medial humeral epicondyle.

If pedicle length is desired, flap design is placed distally on the extremity. If pedicle length is not an issue, dissection places the distal edge of the flap 2–5 cm proximal to the wrist crease. By doing this, it offers a thicker flap skin for reconstruction and less exposure of the flexor tendons after flap elevation. A tourniquet is placed on the upper arm, and, once the limb is exsanguinated with an Esmarch bandage, the tourniquet pressure is maintained at 250 mm Hg (tourniquet time should average 1 hour or less). While there are currently several techniques reported regarding flap elevation, we prefer to identify structures at the distal border first. Once the flexor tendons, radial artery and vena comitantes, cephalic vein, brachioradialis, and median nerve are all noted, the elevation can begin on either the radial or ulnar side of the forearm, with our preference being initial ulnar elevation (Figure 38.6). The antebrachial fascia is incised, and dissection proceeds just below this fascia, along the flexor tendons. Care must be taken to preserve the paratenon for adequate skin graft "take." Suturing the antebrachial fascia to the skin can prevent shearing; however, this is uncommon. Dissection is continued radially under the antebrachial fascia until the radial vessels are identified. Special attention should be given to avoid damage to the fasciocutaneous branches as they emerge from the intermuscular septum (Figure 38.6). The radial vessels are divided distally, and the dissection continues toward the extensor carpi radialis longus muscle. The antebrachial fascia is incised over the brachioradialis muscle if the flap design extends this far. Care must be taken to preserve the superficial branch of the radial sensory nerve. This nerve transits from below the fascia to the subcutaneous plane, emerging between the tendons of the extensor carpi radialis longus and those of the brachioradialis tendon at

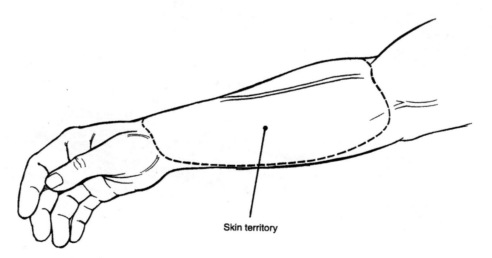

Figure 38.5. Skin territory that can be harvested with radial forearm flap.

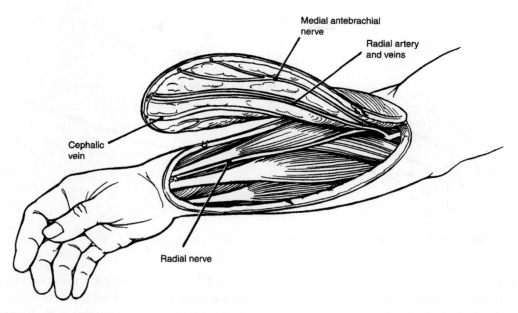

Figure 38.6. Elevation of flap with superficial veins and cutaneous nerves. Vessels are ligated near antecubital fossa to obtain pedicle length and large-diameter vessels.

about the juncture of the distal and middle third of the forearm. The nerve may exit anywhere from as far distally as a few centimeters proximal to the radial styloid to the midportion of the forearm (Figure 38.7).

The sensory radial nerve lies superficial to the radial artery and arborizes after reaching its superficial location (Figure 38.7). If used, the superficial veins (cephalic or basilic) are also divided distally (Figure 38.6). The flap is then elevated from a distal to proximal direction on its radial artery pedicle with venae comitantes and the superficial vein intact. The deep investing fascial components

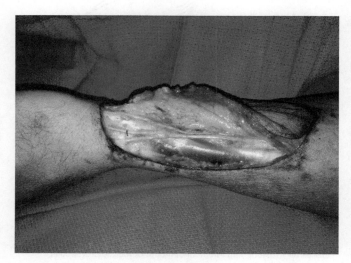

Figure 38.7. Radial sensory nerves that arborize usually into three branches. Care must be taken to avoid injury.

at the wrist below the radial artery and vena comitantes are left intact for wrist stability. An incision may be extended up the forearm to the bifurcation of the ulnar artery if a long vascular pedicle is required. The increased vessel diameter (2–4 mm) around the antecubital fossa facilitates microvascular anastomoses (Figure 38.6). After dissection, tourniquet compression is released and the vascularity of the hand is again assessed. If arterial reconstruction is required, numerous upper extremity superficial veins can be used.

Alternatively, the flap may be elevated ulnarly and radially to the fascial septum over the radial artery, allowing for continued blood flow through the artery until the defect is prepared for flap transfer. The radial artery is then divided distally, the flap is elevated with the radial pedicle, and the radial artery is reconstructed appropriately. Closure of the forearm proceeds simultaneously with flap insetting, and adequate hemostasis is essential if the skin graft is to be successful. Reactive hyperemia may occur for 5–10 minutes once the tourniquet is released. Dermal absorbable sutures are used to close as much of the wound as possible. Full- or split-thickness unmeshed skin grafts are placed over the remaining open wound (Figure 38.8). Paratenon must be intact, and every effort to advance muscle over the tendons should be made before skin grafting. The superficial sensory nerves should be covered in the closure with native arm skin as opposed to direct placement of a skin graft on the nerve if possible. Dressings and a volar splint are applied with the

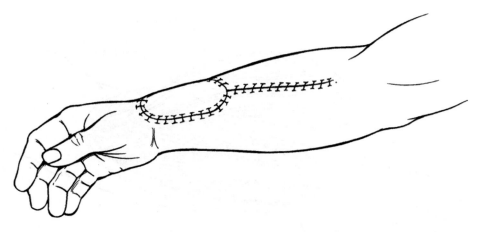

Figure 38.8. Closure of forearm with skin graft placed distally and primary approximation used proximally.

hand in either a neutral position or position of function. This provides adequate stabilization to prevent shearing until neovascularization of the skin graft can occur (Figure 38.9). Dressings are usually maintained for 5 days, at which time splints are reapplied for an additional week to protect the skin graft from shearing in the early postoperative period. Once the splint is removed, active and passive motion is begun. Skin grafts are kept moist with cream postoperatively.

Three-dimensional defects are easily filled, and the flap can be rotated on itself for insetting. While insetting requires adequate exposure and traditionally necessitates lip-splitting incisions along with mandibulotomies, over the past 5 years we have attempted surgical resection without lip-splitting incisions and have received much more aesthetic results. Ultimately, although insetting maybe more challenging, the overall result is marked improvement in patient aesthetic outcomes. Mattress or closely placed interrupted sutures (Vicryl) are required to secure a "water-tight" closure (Figures 38.10 and 38.11). Insetting is usually completed before performing the anastomosis to allow for accurate placement of sutures without bleeding or flap edema. Microvascular anastomoses are performed to large, high-flow vessels, as we typically attempt to utilize branches from the external carotid or internal jugular vein in an end-to-end fashion. When this is not possible, end-to-side anastomoses with the external carotid or internal jugular vein can be performed utilizing a 2.5–2.7 mm aortic punch for the arterial arteriotomy. Furthermore, an end-to-end anastomosis can be performed between the cephalic vein and the external jugular vein. Care must be taken, however, with tracheotomy ties as they can frequently compress this venous anastomosis. In irradiated tissue, blood flow must be assessed before the anastomosis, and arterial and venous dissection must proceed with both care and limited manipulation.

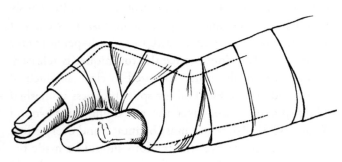

Figure 38.9. Dressing and splint applied to forearm with hand in position of function. Note that splint includes distal interphalangeal (DIP) joint immobilization to prevent tendon movement and enhance skin graft adherence.

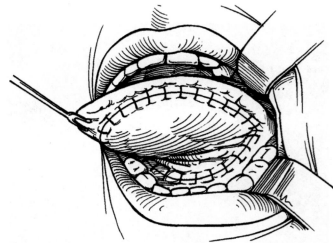

Figure 38.10. Insetting flap into floor-of-mouth defect. Microvascular anastomosis to external carotid artery and internal jugular vein is performed after insetting flap.

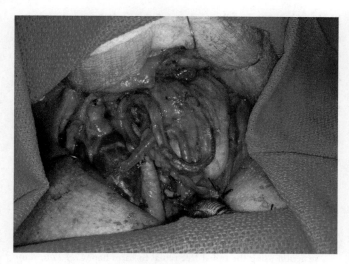

Figure 38.11. Insetting flap laryngeal defect.

OSSEOUS COMPONENT

An anterolateral segment of the radial bone (up to 10 cm) that lies between the insertions of the pronator teres and the brachioradialis muscle can be included in the radial forearm free flap. This flap allows nourishment to the radius by two fascioperiosteal branches through the intermuscular septum and musculoperiosteal branches through the flexor pollicis longus and pronator quadratus from the radial artery. The flap is raised in a similar fashion while leaving the intermuscular septum intact. Medially, the muscle bellies of the flexor pollicis longus and pronator quadratus are divided and elevated to reach the periosteum. This allows access to incise the periosteum longitudinally beyond the attachment of the septum to the radius. Bony cuts are made in a beveled fashion, and special attention must be made to preserve radial bone stability. This is done by limiting the bony excision to one-third the diameter of the radius. The osteocutaneous flap is then elevated, with attention paid to preserving the intermuscular septum with the flap and intact radius.

We have found this bone to be thin and poor for mandibular reconstruction. Successful placement of dental implants into this bone is unreliable, and we recommend other options if large mandibular bony reconstruction is required. We have found, however, that the radius is excellent for midface, palatal, and nasal reconstruction. In order to prevent radial bone fracture, we have begun routinely plating the radial bone following osteotomy.

SENSORY INNERVATION

The lateral and medial antebrachial cutaneous nerves provide sensation to the forearm and the potential for a sensate flap. The lateral antebrachial cutaneous nerve is a continuation of the musculocutaneous nerve that passes deep to the cephalic vein at the elbow and then descends along the radial border of the forearm to the wrist. Its innervation is to the skin over the lateral half of the anterior surface of the forearm.

The medial antebrachial cutaneous nerve pierces the deep fascia with the basilic vein at about the middle of the forearm where it divides into an anterior and posterior branch. The anterior branch supplies the skin over the medial half of the anterior surface of the arm, while the posterior branch lies anterior to the medial epicondyle of the humerus and supplies the skin over the medial third of the posterior surface of the forearm. In dissecting the radial forearm flap, frequent division of the lateral or medial antebrachial cutaneous branches is required. Patients should understand the potential for sensory loss when this flap is used. Nerve ends should be buried into muscle to prevent the potential for painful neuromas.

POSTOPERATIVE CARE

After surgery, patients are observed closely in the surgical intensive care unit. Frequently, the patients have undergone tracheostomy, making observation and monitoring of the flap easier. The flap is monitored with a handheld Doppler device, and a place on the skin paddle must be found to measure the Doppler signal. The radial artery and vein are quite large, and both signals should be audible. The signal is marked by a Prolene stitch, allowing ease and consistency of obtaining the Doppler signal. Absence of the arterial or venous signal or the appearance of an ecchymotic flap demand reexploration. If the flap is "buried" with no observable skin paddle, an implantable Doppler device (20 MHz) is placed around the vein. Wires are brought through the neck incision or through a separate incision and are maintained for 3 weeks after surgery, at which time they are removed. Alternatively, if the pedicle is directly below the neck skin, a Prolene stitch can be placed in the skin that allows monitoring of the vessels. One must ensure, however, that one is listening to the correct vessels.

Feeding is begun through a feeding tube placed at the time of surgery. Oral feedings are usually deferred for 7–10 days, depending on the location, as well as previous surgical and adjuvant therapy history of the patient. A modified barium swallow is performed before initiation of feeding.

The upper extremity is maintained in a splint for 5 days (Figure 38.9), allowing for good fixation of the skin graft. The splint is placed back on for another week to give additional protection to the graft. Once the splint is removed, local skin graft care resumes and range of motion is increased. If an osseous component is harvested, beveling the osteotomy sites and limiting bony resection to one-third of the radius diameter reduces the risk of fracture. Immobilization for 6–8 weeks has been routine. However, recently, we have begun routinely plating the radial bone following osteotomies. This allows early motion and prevents possible fracture of the remaining radius. If reconstruction of the radial artery is necessary or if the radial sensory nerve is exposed, rotational flaps may be required to cover these exposed structures. We have avoided meshing split-thickness skin grafts used for coverage.

CAVEATS AND COMMENTS

Remember during dissection that the radial sensory nerve is quite superficial. Care in elevation of the flap is mandated. If the nerve is injured, microvascular repair should proceed.

Because it is our choice to use the superficial venous system, the flap dissection is more dorsal than anticipated. The superficial veins are quite consistent and provide large calibers with sufficient length for the anastomosis.

Paratenon must be intact over the tendons to allow an adequate bed for the adherence of the skin graft. Hemostasis must be meticulous to prevent elevation of the graft. Frequently, this portion of the operation is relegated to less-experienced surgeons on the operating team, when, in fact, careful closure of the donor defect can prevent postoperative tendon exposure and complications.

Frequently, patients experience paresthesias or anesthesias over the radial dorsum of the hand. This is most likely secondary to dissection of the radial sensory nerve or the lateral antebrachial cutaneous nerve. Sensation frequently returns over time; however, some patients may experience a permanent loss.

In our opinion, the radial forearm free flap offers a consistent form of oral lining replacement provided that bulk or bone is not required. With the flap's versatility and ease of execution, it has become a workhorse for intraoral reconstruction for cancer-related defects.

REFERENCES

1. Anthony JP, Singer MI, Mathes SJ. Pharyngoesophageal reconstruction using the tubed free radial forearm flap. *Clin Plast Surg* 1994;21:137–147.
2. Buncke HJ. *Microsurgery: Transplantation-Replantation. An Atlas Text.* Philadelphia: Lea & Febiger, 1991.
3. Cormack GC, Lamberty BGH. A classification of fasciocutaneous flaps according to their patterns of vascularization. *Br J Plast Surg* 1984;37:80–87.
4. Evans GRD, Schusterman MA, Kroll SS, et al. The radial forearm free flap for head and neck reconstruction: a review. *Am J Surg* 1994;168:446–450.
5. Hentz VR, Pearl RM, Grossman JAI, et al. The radial forearm flap: a versatile source of composite tissue. *Ann Plast Surg* 1987;19:485–498.
6. Juretic M, Car M, Zambelli M. The radial forearm free flap: our experience in solving donor site problems. *J Craniomaxillofac Surg* 1992;20:184–186.
7. Lind MG, Amander C, Gylbert L, et al. Reconstruction in the head and neck regions with free radial forearm flaps and split-rib bone grafts. *Am J Surg* 1987;154:459–462.
8. Mackinnon SE, Dellon AL. *Surgery of the Peripheral Nerve.* New York: Thieme, 1988.
9. Schusterman MA, Kroll SS, Weber RS, et al. Intraoral soft tissue reconstruction after cancer ablation: a comparison of the pectoralis major flap and the free radial forearm flap. *Am J Surg* 1991;162:397–399.
10. Song R, Gao T, Song Y, et al. The radial forearm flap. *Clin Plast Surg* 1982;9:21.
11. Strauch B, Yu HL. *Atlas of Microvascular Surgery: Anatomy and Operative Approaches.* New York: Thieme, 1993.
12. Swanson E, Boyd JB, Mulholland RS. The radial forearm flap: a biomechanical study of the osteotomized radius. *Plast Reconstr Surg* 1990;85:267–272.
13. Swartz WM, Banis JC. *Head and Neck Microsurgery.* Baltimore: Williams & Wilkins, 1992.
14. Yang G, Chen B, Gad Y. Forearm free skin flap transplantation. *Chung-Hua I Hsueh Tsa Chih [Chinese Medical Journal]* 1981; 61:139.
15. Evans GRD. The radial forearm flap. In Evan GRD, ed. *Operative Plastic Surgery.* New York: McGraw Hill, 2000: 354–361.

39.

THE RECTUS ABDOMINIS FLAP

Melissa Mueller and Gregory R. D. Evans

OVERVIEW

Tobacco, alcohol, and human papillomavirus make squamous cell carcinoma most common in the oral cavity. The first step in reconstructing defects within the oral cavity is to understand the nature of the cancer and, subsequently, the margins for resection. Squamous cell carcinoma may involve the base of the tongue, the floor of the mouth, and the retromolar trigone. As the tumor grows, it may invade the mandible, cheek, or neck, resulting in the need not only for skin but for other composite tissues as well. In determining the nature of the defect, one must consider the requirements for mucosa and skin. If mucosa is the only lining to be replaced, the skin paddle of the rectus flap can be placed intraoral. If external skin is required, options include placing the skin paddle externally and skin grafting the internal component or, alternatively, allowing the internal muscle to remuscosalize. If the subcutaneous tissue provides too much bulk, the skin and soft tissue can be removed, and the rectus muscle, along with its accompanying fascia, can be placed intraoral.

Adjuvant therapy may require alternative planning for the rectus abdominis flap. Radiotherapy demands careful observation regarding patency of the recipient vessels. Previous radiation injury necessitates the use of well-vascularized tissue. Free tissue transfer with the rectus abdominis flap can obviate poor wound healing and replace previously irradiated tissue with well-perfused fascia and skin. Previous surgery and radiotherapy may preclude the local closure of neck flaps because of the potential loss of skin after surgical elevation. A larger skin paddle designed on the rectus abdominis may be required to replace the neck skin. Alternatively, this defect may be skin-grafted because the rectus muscle provides a well-vascularized bed for adherence.

INDICATIONS

The rectus abdominis myocutaneous (RAM) flap is ideal for defects needing large, soft tissue bulk without bony

reconstruction. In particular it is selected for defects of the tongue, orbits, maxilla, cheek, posterior mandible, and cranial base. Although ALT may be the current preferred method, RAM remains the authors' flap of choice for total glossectomy reconstruction. In extensive craniofacial reconstruction, it may be combined with an additional free or regional flap. Despite overlapping indications with the anterolateral thigh (ALT) flap, the rectus abdominis flap remains an essential reconstructive option for head and neck reconstruction.

For glossectomy defects of greater than 70%, the radial forearm flap provides insufficient soft tissue volume making the rectus or ALT flap preferable selections. For such defects, a surface cover and bulk are needed to facilitate a functional swallow. Creating additional volume in the adynamic, neotongue allows for contact with the palate during deglutition and assists with propulsion of food into pharynx. Wider, thicker flaps improve speech and swallow outcomes while minimizing aspiration risk. To accomplish this, the flap is designed larger than the defect and the desired final size to account for atrophy. The flap may be made sensate with anastomosis of intercostal nerve to lingual nerve but its benefit is not well established. Laryngeal suspension sutures securing hyoid and mandible prevent neotongue prolapse and improves functional outcomes.

The rectus abdominis flap also provides ideal coverage for large skull base defects. For large defects, the rectus abdominis flap will provide the necessary soft tissue volume to obliterate dead space. Re-establishing a central nervous system (CNS) barrier over dural closure is essential to prevent CSF leak and infection. A skin paddle is unnecessary unless a concurrent palatal defect is present. For smaller skull base defects, radial forearm flap (RFF), ALT, and local flaps may provide enough soft tissue bulk.

The rectus abdominis flap should also be considered to reconstruct large or combined orbital exenteration defects. If soft tissue provided by a radial forearm fasciocutaneous flap is inadequate to address size of orbital defect, the RAM flap is indicated.

Reconstructive goals are to obliterate sinuses, cover exposed dura, restore mid-face volume, and accommodate ocular prosthesis, if possible. For extended defects involving maxilla and/or palate, goals of reconstruction also include to provide nasal lining, to close the nasal cavity, to prevent sinonasocutnaeous fistula, and to provide palatal coverage (Figure 39.1).

Another common indication for the rectus abdominis flap is a posterior mandibular defect. The RAM flap provides sufficient soft tissue bulk to achieve acceptable cosmetic appearance of the lower face and provides a skin paddle to reconstruct large oral mucosa defects. In such defects, reconstruction of the large oral lining defect contributes more to the restoration of function than does the replacement of the bone. Disruption of the pterygoid muscles from their mandibular insertions leads to mandibular deviation (crossbite), which is frequently not resolved even

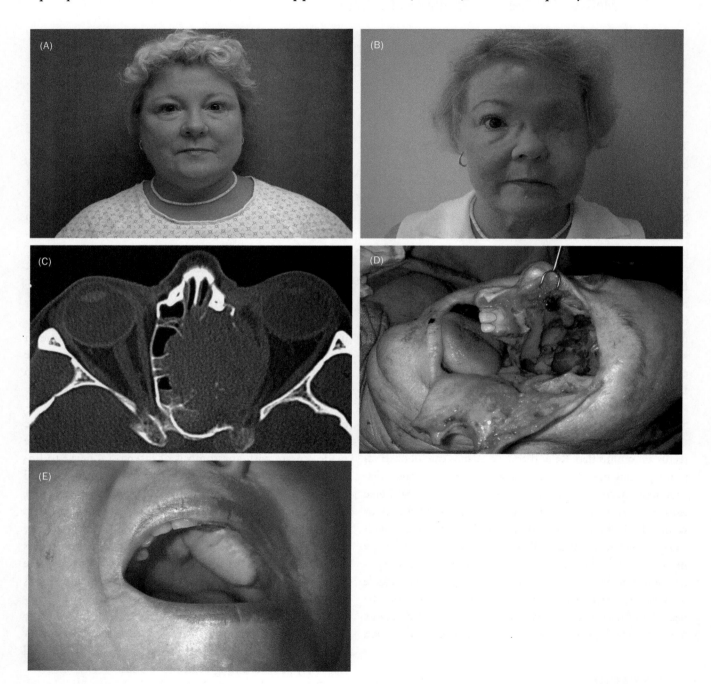

Figure 39.1. Pre- and postop photos (A,B) of patient with tumor invading maxilla, nasal cavity, hard palate, and orbit. (C) A rectus abdominis myocutaneous flap was used to fill the large mid-face defect. (D) Skin paddle was used for intraoral defect. (E) rectus abdominis myocutaneous (RAM) was used to restore midface volume, provide nasal lining, close the nasal cavity, prevent sinonasocutnaeous fistula, and provide palatal coverage.

HEAD AND NECK SURGERY

with bony replacement. Malocclusion is also inherent in reconstruction, even in bony reconstruction, because of disruption of the condyle, temporomandibular joint (TMJ), and masseter muscle insertion. Despite this malocclusion, RAM reconstruction leads to little alteration in functional outcomes of speech and swallow. RAM reconstruction is indicated in cases of insufficient condyle and subcondylar ramus, when titanium hardware or vascularized bone reconstruction cannot be utilized. RAM provides reasonable functional and cosmetic outcomes and should be strongly considered for posterior mandible reconstruction in patients who are not candidates for vascularized bone reconstruction. If a limited posterior mandibular defect is combined with a palatomaxillary defect, a single RAM may be used to reconstruct both.

The RAM flap is ideal for extensive, combined defects as well as multilaminar defects, in which a multi-island vertical rectus abdominis myocutaneous (MI-VRAM) or an additional free flap may be required. The RAM flap is well suited to reconstruct posterior palatomaxillary defects with the goal of preventing oronasal fistula. Floor of mouth defects with a significant amount of submandibular dead space may be more appropriate for RAM compared to ALT, particularly in patients with thin body habitus. RAM flap is also indicated for buccal mucosa defects and large through-and-though defects of the cheek. The later can be reconstructed with two skin paddles to mimic buccal mucosa and external cheek skin. The MI-VRAM flap is created by excising all intervening skin and subcutaneous fat down to the anterior rectus fascia between intended skin paddles. Multiple skin paddles can be used in the midface to recreate palate, nasal lining, periorbital, cheek mucosa, and external cheek skin and in the lower face to recreate tongue, buccal mucosa, floor of mouth, lateral pharyngeal wall, and external skin. For extended and combined defects, such as a maxillary and mandibular defect or a mandible and glossectomy defect, fibula reconstruction can be utilized for mandibular reconstruction and RAM can be used for soft tissue bulk, buccal reconstruction, and neotongue formation. As exhibited by the varied indications, RAM flaps are ideal for large soft tissue defects that do not require bony fixation.

CONTRAINDICATIONS

America's worsening obesity epidemic may limit future flap utility in head and neck reconstruction. In instances of excessive flap bulk, the skin paddle can be removed and the muscle and fascia used in the closure of the defect. The intraoral muscle or fascia can be skin-grafted or allowed to remuscosalize. Alternatively, delayed flap thinning or liposuction may be performed. However, defects requiring skin paddles in obese and morbidly obese patients may require reconstruction with alternate flaps. Gender-specific adipose distributions make the RAM flap more useful among males with a mid-range body mass index. On the other extreme of body habitus, extremely thin body habitus with less than a centimeter of abdominal subcutaneous thickness may not benefit from flap harvest if the flap has insufficient soft tissue bulk.

Previous abdominal surgery may preclude the use of the flap secondary to scarring and vascular compromise. If upper abdominal surgery has been performed, the inferior epigastric pedicle may be viable and flap transfer can proceed. If lower abdominal surgery has been performed, the inferior epigastric vascular system may be injured. In both of these instances, exploration of the vessels should proceed before flap elevation to assess whether the flap transfer is possible. Bilateral absence of a suitable perforator precludes flap use. A midline incision may not preclude flap harvest, granted no vascular disruption. On preoperative examination, patients should have been examined for prior umbilical hernia repairs and vascular surgery involving femoral vessels for atherosclerotic disease. History should inquire regarding prior trauma and surgeries. Those patients with a history of coagulopathy and medical status unable to withstand long operations will not be candidates for any free flap reconstruction. Patients should also be screened for connective disorders, vasculitis, peripheral vascular disease, venous insufficiency, and any disorder than impacts coagulation and wound healing.

ADVANTAGES

The rectus abdominis flap is one of the most versatile flaps in the armamentarium of the microvascular surgeon given its logistical advantages, its inherent characteristics, and its wide range of applications.

The rectus abdominis flap allows for logistical convenience because repositioning is unnecessary, and a two-team approach can be utilized. Simultaneous flap harvest and tumor extirpation reduces operative time and anesthetic risks. The harvest is straightforward and within the technical purview of most plastic surgeons given its widespread use in breast reconstruction. This combination allows for relatively quick harvest.

The rectus abdominis flap provides a reliable and consistent flap option for head and neck reconstruction. The pedicle is long and of large caliber, and variations in vascular anatomy are rare (Figure 39.2). If necessary, the pedicle length can allow reconstruction contralateral to the anastomosis. The wide distribution of musculocutaneous perforators allows for a variety of skin paddle designs. This ability to vary the three-dimensional architecture allows better conformation to the defect and obliteration of dead space. The robust musculocutaneous perforators allow for a large skin paddle. In fact, the RAM flap has the largest number of cutaneous perforators of all soft tissue flaps. Available muscle for harvest is up to 8 × 30 cm, and it can be harvested segmentally or in full depending on the reconstructive needs. The well-vascularized, robust muscle promotes wound healing, particularly important in the setting of previous radiation; brings vital tissue into areas frequently prone to poor wound healing; and facilitates delivery of chemotherapeutic agents within the tumor field. The muscle and soft tissue bulk tolerates irradiation and

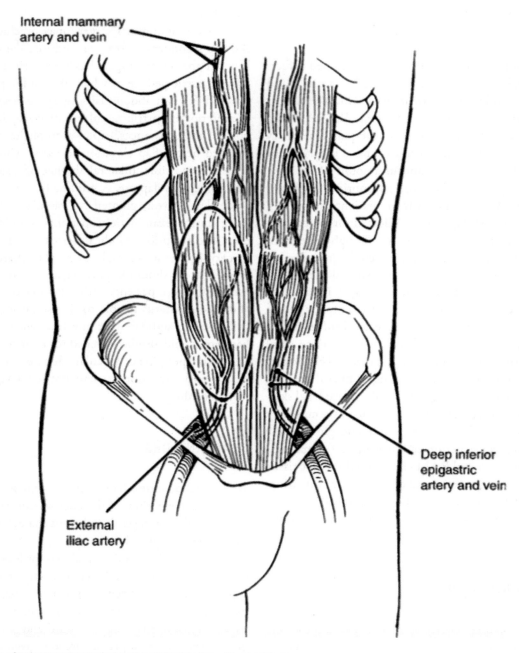

Figure 39.2. Outline of myocutaneous vertical rectus abdominis flap with vasculature.

HEAD AND NECK SURGERY

protects the underlying anastomosis and neck vasculature. The rectus abdominis flap provides the largest volume of soft tissue based on a single pedicle, making it ideal for elimination of significant dead space. The donor site is easily hidden by clothing and is less conspicuous than forearm and leg donor sites.

The flap's versatility in inset allows for a wide range of non-bony reconstructive applications. It can reconstruct single anatomic defects, combined defects, and multilaminar defects. It can be folded onto itself, allowing for reconstruction of complex, three-dimensional defects. It can provide the continuous closure of the anterior pharynx, along with repair of an intraoral defect or the formation of a neotongue (Figure 39.3). Because of its robust perforator supply, it can be designed with multiple skin islands to reconstruct multilaminar defects, for example providing surface cover for mucosa, cheek skin, orbit lining, nasal lining, and neotongue surface. This is a clear advantage over the ALT flap, in which only two-thirds have adequate perforators to perform a double skin island flap.

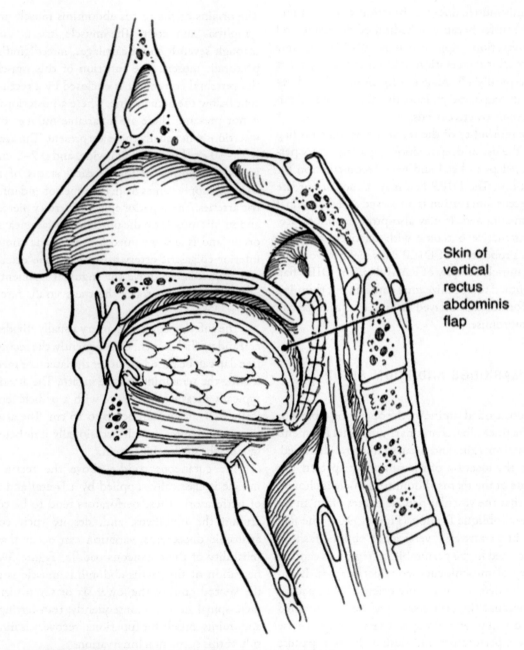

Skin of vertical rectus abdominis flap

Figure 39.3. Vertical rectus abdominis flap placed intraorally. Note how skin becomes neotongue.

DISADVANTAGES

The predominant disadvantage of the rectus abdominis flap is donor site morbidity, namely abdominal bulge, abdominal weakness, abdominal hernias, functional deficits, and pain. These potential outcomes can be mitigated by minimizing harvest of anterior rectus sheath, limited to only immediate vicinity of perforators, and by avoiding all anterior rectus sheath harvest below the level of the arcuate line. Harvest can be performed using medial row perforators to potentially minimize disruption of intercostal innervation and subsequent functional deficits. The rectus abdominis muscle does not function well as a functional muscle transfer because of its limited excursion and segmental innervation. Approximately 20–30% volume atrophy occurs after denervation. Although the flap's soft tissue bulk is typically advantageous for head and neck reconstruction, among obese patients the size of the flap can often surpass reconstructive needs.

Donor site morbidity of the rectus myocutaneous flap has prompted the use of deep inferior epigastric artery perforator (DIEP) flaps in head and neck reconstruction for similar indications. The DIEP flap may reduce donor site morbidity if rectus innervation is preserved and abdominal wall fascia is maintained. It may also provide a more predictable reconstructive outcome with relatively constant size over time. Proponents of DIEP flaps seek to avoid the unpredictable muscle atrophy of RAM flap. The DIEP flap may also be thinned to optimize final contour, but thinning should be performed in a delayed fashion to minimize risk of vascular compromise.

PATIENT MARKINGS AND ROOM SETUP

The patient is positioned supine on the operating table. For orientation, the linea alba, semilunaris, inguinal ligament, symphysis, costal margin, and arcuate line are identified. Depending on the location of the tumor extirpation, the appropriate side of the rectus abdominis muscle is chosen, remembering that the vascular pedicle comes off in an inferior and lateral oblique fashion (Figure 39.2). The flap may be raised in a transverse, vertical, or oblique fashion but must be situated in the periumbilical region to capture highest density of musculocutaneous perforators. If appropriate for the defect, a vertically oriented skin paddle is preferable because the entire skin paddle is contained within perfusion zone one. Preoperative imaging may be utilized to mark perforators and design the skin paddle

before surgery. The extirpative team and the reconstructive team may work together to allow for more efficient use of operative time. Once the flap is elevated, perfusion through the inferior epigastric vessels allows for equilibration of the vascular system after the superior vasculature is ligated.

FLAP HARVEST

ANATOMY

The origins of the rectus abdominis muscle are the pubic symphysis and crest. The muscle inserts into the fifth through seventh costal cartilages, interdigitating with the pectoralis muscle. The function of this muscle is to flex the vertebral column. It is enclosed by a rectus sheath, except below the arcuate line, where a posterior fascial cover is not present. There are a variable number of tendinous insertions, but usually three are present. The average muscle is 25–30 cm long, 4–8 cm wide, and 0.7–2 cm thick, but varies depending on the physical status of the patient. Arterial supply comes from the superior and inferior epigastric arteries. The superior epigastric artery pierces the rectus abdominis muscle on the posterior surface near the muscle's origin and is accompanied by two venae comitantes. The inferior epigastric artery arises from the external iliac artery immediately above the inguinal ligament. It ascends obliquely and penetrates the transversalis fascia from the arcuate line.

The inferior epigastric artery usually divides into a lateral and medial branch. Consequently, the rectus abdominis free flap can be raised on either the lateral or medial branch, leaving the remaining muscle in situ. The arterial diameter typically measures 3–5 mm, with a pedicle length of typically 6–8 cm but can be up to 15 cm. The artery has two venae comitantes, which occasionally join before their origin off the external iliac vein.

The cutaneous paddle above the rectus abdominis muscle is classically supplied by a lateral and medial row of perforators. These perforators tend to be concentrated around the umbilicus, and, despite their constancy in anatomic dissections, variation can occur that alters the reliability of the cutaneous paddle (Figure 39.4). The innervation of the rectus abdominis muscle is supplied by the ventral rami of the lower six or seven segmental thoracic spinal nerves. Consequently, transferring the rectus abdominis muscle for functional recovery is limited as a result of this segmental innervation.

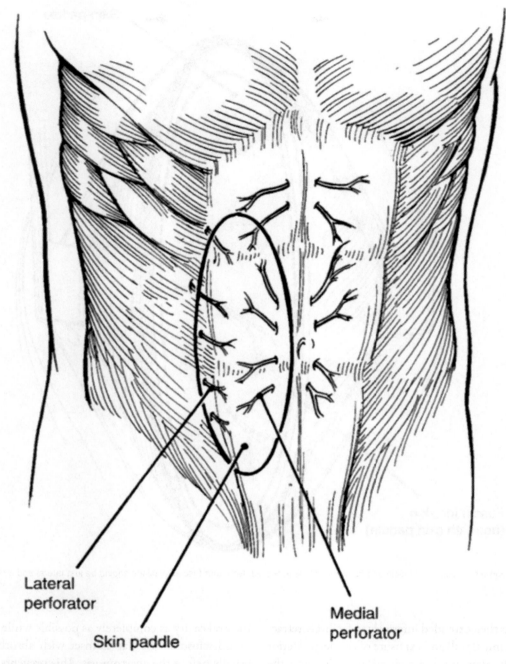

Lateral perforator

Skin paddle

Medial perforator

Figure 39.4. Skin paddle with medial and lateral perforators.

TECHNIQUE

The dissection is begun with the outline of the skin paddle on the abdomen. If the patient is a smoker or if there is concern about the skin perfusion from the vascular perforators, the flap can be designed so that more perforators are included around the umbilicus. If the skin paddle is vertical, adequate perforators usually accompany the flap elevation and skin viability is maintained. The flap design should include excess volume, accounting for expected muscle atrophy during the first 6 months postoperatively. The subcutaneous excision can be beveled outward to ensure maintenance of the maximal number of perforators to the skin paddle. The skin is incised and the anterior rectus fascia is exposed. The fascia is incised just lateral to the perforators, then reflected laterally to expose the rectus muscle (Figure 39.5). The fascial incision extends to below the lowest perforator, then turns and heads superiorly, circumscribing the fascia that includes the perforating vessels that will be removed with the flap. The

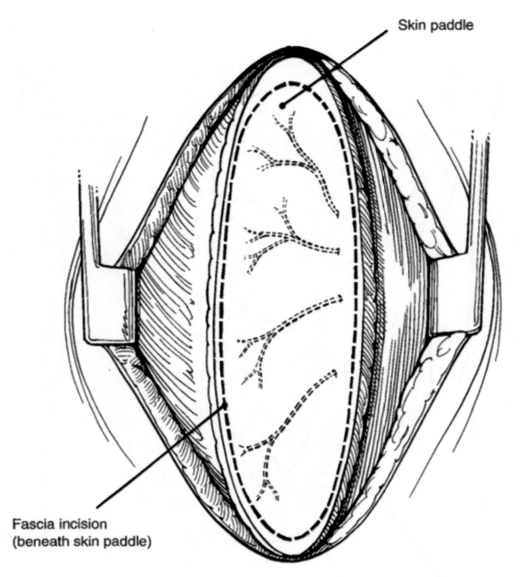

Skin paddle

Fascia incision
(beneath skin paddle)

Figure 39.5. Skin incision with exposure of fascia and fascial incisions indicated. Note that fascial incisions should be just lateral and medial to perforators.

fascial incision is then extended inferiorly to facilitate retraction of the abdominal wall and exposure of the deep inferior epigastric vessels, allowing direct visual dissection and the creation of a long vascular pedicle (Figure 39.6).

Once the pedicle has been isolated, the muscle is divided above and below the flap. Fibers of the rectus muscle lateral to the perforating vessels, like the fascia, can be preserved in situ. Alternatively, if most of the perforators are lateral, the muscle can be preserved medially. The surgeon should include in the flap only as much muscle as necessary to maintain the blood supply because excess muscle bulk tends to interfere with flap insertion. The flap can also be dissected on the perforators above, without muscle.

For glossectomy reconstruction, the rectus abdominis flap can be folded to maximize the amount of volume and fill the oral cavity as completely as possible while still allowing mouth closure. The flap is inset with absorbable sutures, usually before the anastomosis. This prevents the bleeding and edema that follow revascularization from securing the flap to the intraoral tissue and also establishes appropriate pedicle length for anastomosis. If multiple skin islands are utilized, the skin island closest to the pedicle should be used for intraoral closure, placing the distal, less dependable island externally to facilitate monitoring and for ease in management in the event of vascular compromise. If radiation therapy is required postoperatively, the rectus abdominis flap may swell further, leading to problems with speech and swallow. The edema usually resolves at the conclusion of the radiation therapy, and flap atrophy proceeds along with normal healing.

HEAD AND NECK SURGERY

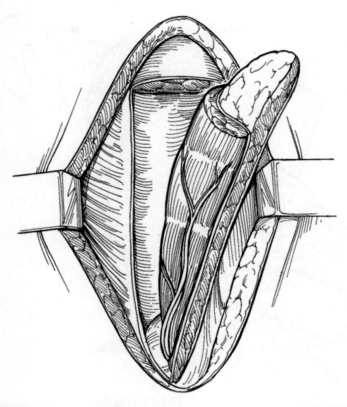

Figure 39.6. Lateral fascial incision with exposure of rectus muscle and inferior epigastric vessels. Flap is elevated in cranial-to-caudal direction after a similar dissection of a medial portion of rectus muscle.

Although many recipient vessels are potentially available in the head and neck, the authors prefer end-to-side anastomoses to the internal jugular vein and the external carotid artery (Figure 39.7). The high flow rates offered by these vessels tend to wash away platelet plugs, decreasing the incidence of thrombosis. However, if appropriately sized branches are present that lend themselves to a technically easier anastomosis, an end-to-end anastomosis can be performed.

If the oral defect is limited to one-half to two-thirds of the tongue, an alternative reconstruction can often be accomplished by using a rectus abdominis muscle and fascia without a skin paddle. Split thickness skin grafts may be used directly on the muscle, or the anterior fascial coverage of the muscle can be used, which will remucosalize. Although this reconstruction will use denervated muscle that is susceptible to atrophy, the smaller defect often lends itself to such a reconstruction with adequate maintenance of bulk for more lasting results.

Donor site closure begins with anterior rectus sheath fascia. Fascia is approximated with interrupted, figure-of-eight 0-Ethibond stitches. This is followed with a running Quil suture or 1-Prolene. Harvest of the flap is adjusted to preserve fascia to minimize need for mesh in abdominal fascial closure. However, when mesh is required, biologic

is preferred. A drain is left above the fascia, and abdominal subcutaneous tissue is closed in a typical multilayer fashion. Scarpa's fascia is closed with 2-0 PDS, dermal sutures placed with 3-0 Monocryl, and the epidermis is approximated with a running 4-0 Monocryl.

POSTOPERATIVE CARE

The patients and flaps are monitored in the surgical intensive care unit for 1–2 days and subsequently in a step-down unit for another 2–3 days. It is important to mark the location of the Doppler signal on the skin paddle with a Prolene stitch to facilitate consistent monitoring. Loss of the arterial or venous signal or the appearance of an ecchymotic flap demands re-exploration. If the flap is buried with no visible skin paddle, an implantable Doppler device (20 MHz) is placed around the vein. Wires are brought through the neck incision or through a separate incision and maintained for 3 weeks postoperatively.

Feeding is begun through a feeding tube placed at the time of surgery. Oral feedings are usually deferred for 7–10 days, depending on the location and previous surgical and adjuvant therapy history of the patient.

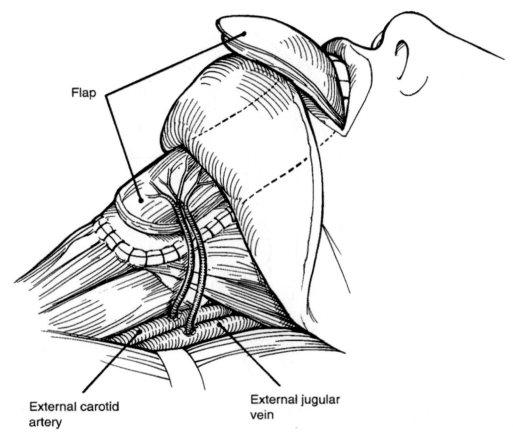

Flap

External carotid
artery

External jugular
vein

Figure 39.7. Insetting of flap into head and neck. Anastomosis to internal jugular vein and external carotid artery.

Over the next 6 months, flap bulk will remarkably diminish. Patients should be counseled preoperatively regarding flap atrophy, and revision surgery, if necessary, should be avoided until the edema resolves. Radiation therapy can accentuate the flap and facial edema, which usually resolves after the conclusion of the adjuvant therapy.

CONCLUSION

Although a wide variety of options are available for reconstruction of the oral cavity, the rectus abdominis free flap is an ideal choice for defects needing large, soft tissue bulk without bony reconstruction, particularly for defects of the tongue, orbits, maxilla, cheek, posterior mandible, and cranial base. Its ability to be folded upon itself and harvested with multiple skin paddles makes it versatile for complex three-dimensional and multilaminar defects. Its pedicle size and length and consistent vascular anatomy make the flap a reliable choice for head and neck reconstruction.

SELECTED READINGS

Cappiello J, Piazza C, Taglietti V, Nicolai P. Deep inferior epigastric artery perforated rectus abdominis free flap for head and neck reconstruction. *Eur Arch Otorhinolaryngol* 2012 Apr;269(4):1219–1224.

Chana JS, Odili J. Perforator flaps in head and neck reconstruction. *Semin Plast Surg.* 2010 Aug;24(3):237–254.

Hanasono MM. Reconstructive surgery for head and neck cancer patients. *Adv Med* 2014:795483. Epub 2014 Nov 9.

Hurvitz KA, Kobayashi M, Evans GR. Current options in head and neck reconstruction. *Plast Reconstr Surg* 2006 Oct;118(5):122e–133e.

Kim EK, Evangelista M, Evans GR. Use of free tissue transfers in head and neck reconstruction. *J Craniofac Surg* 2008 Nov;19(6):1577–1582.

Neligan PC, Lipa JE. Perforator flaps in head and neck reconstruction. *Semin Plast Surg* 2006 May; 20(2):56–63.

Patel NP, Matros E, Cordeiro PG. The use of the multi-island vertical rectus abdominis myocutaneous flap in head and neck reconstruction. *Ann Plast Surg* 2012 Oct;69(4):403–407.

Syme DB, Shayan R, Grinsell D. Muscle-only intra-oral mucosal defect reconstruction. *J Plast Reconstr Aesthet Surg* 2012 Dec;65(12):1654–1659.

Wei FC, Mardini S. *Flaps and Reconstructive Surgery.* New York: Saunders, 2009.

Zhang B, Li DZ, Xu ZG, Tang PZ. Deep inferior epigastric artery perforator free flaps in head and neck reconstruction. *Oral Oncol* 2009 Feb;45(2):116–120.

40.

MICRONEUROVASCULAR RECONSTRUCTION FOR FACIAL REANIMATION

Michael Klebuc

Free functional muscle flaps provide an effective means of reanimating the paralyzed mid-face and perioral region. The technique is well suited for individuals whose native muscles of facial expression have failed to develop in utero, undergone irreversible atrophy, sustained significant trauma or have been sacrificed during oncologic resection. Functional muscle flaps have played a prevalent role in the treatment of developmental facial paralysis. Free gracilis muscle flaps innervated by the masseteric nerve have become the preferred reconstruction for children with Moebius syndrome at many centers.[1] The technique is also well suited to individuals with long-standing facial paralysis because the potential to restore innervation and achieve forceful contraction in mimetic muscles with denervation periods of greater than 18 months is limited.

A series of different donor muscles have been utilized for smile restoration and eye closure including the serratus anterior, latissimus dorsi, pectoralis minor, rectus femoris, and platysma. The free gracilis muscle flap enjoys wide popularity for facial reanimation, and its use for smile restoration will be a principle focus of this chapter. The gracilis muscle's long fibers, reliable neurovascular anatomy, well-concealed skin incision, and limited functional loss make it well suited for this purpose.

Over the past decade, there has been considerable interest in reducing muscle flap bulk in an effort to achieve more natural, aesthetically pleasing reconstructions, and the technical aspects of small segment flap design will be considered later in the chapter.

Motor innervation is an additional topic that warrants significant consideration. The facial nerve and masseteric nerve are frequently used to power free muscle flaps; however, the spinal accessory and hypoglossal nerves can be employed in select cases.[2] The contralateral facial nerve is frequently utilized in conjunction with a cross-face nerve graft as a source of motor innervation. The principle benefit of the facial nerve donor site is the ability to deliver spontaneous, emotionally mediated facial motion. Unfortunately, the facial motion produced by a cross-face nerve graft and free muscle flap can be weaker than the unaffected side. This is not unexpected as the motor axons must cross two sites of microsurgical nerve repair and traverse a graft that is often more than 20 cm in length. Recently, there has been interest in suturing the downstream end of the cross-face nerve graft to infraorbital nerve branches. The ingrowth of sensory nerve fibers into the graft is thought to prevent senescence of the Schwann cells, which in turn may enhance motor axon growth through the graft.[3] Early animal data support this concept; however, the exact benefit in the clinical arena is yet to be determined.

Attempts have also been made to utilize the contralateral facial nerve as part of a single-stage reconstruction.[4] The motor nerves to the latissimus dorsi and rectus femoris flaps are capable of spanning the face; however, long muscle denervation times while awaiting nerve growth often yields weak contraction. This can be compensated by utilizing larger flaps; however, excess bulk and a diminished aesthetic result can occur.

The ipsilateral facial nerve can also be employed to neurotize free muscle flaps as part of a single-stage reconstruction. In select oncologic cases, functional mapping of the facial nerve can be performed prior to tumor resection. The proximal facial nerve branches producing contraction of the zygomaticus major are marked for later co-optation.

The masseter nerve is frequently used to innervate free muscle flaps in cases of developmental facial paralysis and can reliably achieve smile restoration in a single stage. The nerve has a dense population of myelinated motor fibers (main trunk 2,700/descending branch 1,550) that can produce powerful facial motion.[5,6] Flap volumes can be significantly reduced when the masseter is selected as the source of innervation. Small muscle flaps often produce good commissure excursion with minimal cheek fullness.

Unfortunately, in a significant number of individuals, the masseter nerve has no connections with the emotional centers in the brain. Clenching of the teeth will initially be required to generate a smile; however, with diligent practice over a 2–3 year period, one can expect that approximately 80% of patients will smile without biting and around 50% will develop a reflexive almost spontaneous-appearing smile.[7] These changes are likely a result of cerebral neuroplasticity; however, recent electromyographic (EMG) studies suggest that up to 40% of the population show electrical activity in the masseter muscle with normal smiling, suggesting communication between the fifth and seventh cranial nerves.[8,9] Although the motion produced by the masseter nerve is powerful, it can have an "on-off" quality and can fail to provide the functional muscle flap with sufficient resting tone.

CONTRAINDICATIONS

Free functional muscle flaps are generally contraindicated in patients with hypercoagulable disorders. Additionally, the hypoglossal nerve should usually be avoided as a nerve donor in individuals with Moebius syndrome as its transection can produce severe problems with swallowing. The age of the patient must be given consideration when selecting facial reanimation procedures. Cross-face nerve grafts and free muscle flaps have successfully been performed on very young children; however, the blood vessels are miniaturized and the children often lack the maturity to comply with the requested restrictions in their postoperative activities. Performing the cross-face nerve graft at 5 years of age and the free muscle flap the following year overcomes these issues and completes the reconstruction by the time that the child starts to be aware of physical differences. Issues can also arise on the opposite end of the age spectrum. The potential for nerve growth and regeneration drops off significantly after 50 years of age. Although there are no hard and fast rules regarding advanced age and the use of cross-face nerve grafts, the technique may be less successful after 50 years of age especially in individuals with multiple medical comorbidities. The masseter nerve may prove a better nerve donor site in this subset of patients. Additionally, microvascular procedures have similar flap survival rate regardless of age; however, increased rates of major cardiovascular and pulmonary events are witnessed in older patients.

Finally, the masseter nerve should be avoided as a nerve donor site in unmotivated individuals as diligent, lengthy postoperative physical therapy is paramount to achieving a good result.

ROOM SETUP

The room setup should include two different tables and sets of instruments. One setup will be used to work in the head and neck region (clean contaminated) where there is communication with the mouth and nose. The second setup (clean) will be reserved for harvesting nerve grafts and muscle flaps from the lower extremities. This configuration will also permit two surgical teams to work simultaneously.

The operating table is usually not turned; however, an extension is applied to the anesthetic circuit to facilitate the creation of ample working space. General nasotracheal intubation is preferred, and the endotracheal tube is sutured to the columella and padded. Care is taken to avoid pressure on the nasal alae that may produce ulceration during these lengthy procedures. The avoidance of long-acting muscle-relaxing agents during induction is also of paramount importance. If the subcutaneous tissue is to be infiltrated with a hemostatic solution, it is important to verify that it does not contain a local anesthetic. The use of a narrow head rest attachment to the operating table will facilitate access to the head and neck. Additionally, a gel-filled shoulder roll can help draw the neck into gentle extension.

The mouth is cleansed with chlorhexidine gluconate 0.12% oral rinse, and, after the skin preparation is completed, the eyes are treated with white petrolatum ophthalmic ointment and covered with transparent film dressings. Sterile sequential compression devices and forced air warming blankets are liberally utilized.

TWO-STAGE RECONSTRUCTION

FIRST STAGE

Patient Markings

The principal goal of the first stage is to identify the zygomatic/buccal branches on the unaffected hemiface that produce isolated contraction of the zygomaticus major muscle. Once isolated, a branch can be selectively divided and a microsurgical repair performed to a cross-face nerve graft.

The desired branch can usually be identified at the midway point between the helical root and oral commissure (Figure 40.1). This landmark is often referred to as Zuker's point and is marked preoperatively.[10]

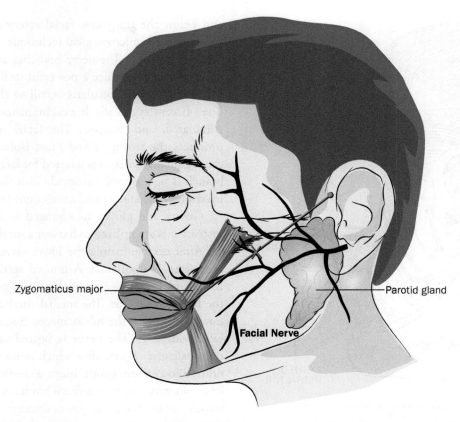

Zygomaticus major — — Parotid gland

Facial Nerve

Figure 40.1. Location of facial nerve branch to zygomaticus major found half way between the root of the helix and the commissure (Zuker's Point).

Operative Technique: Cross-Face Nerve Graft

The first stage of the reconstruction includes exploration of the uninjured facial nerve and placement of a cross-face nerve graft. If a single cross-face nerve graft is to be performed for smile restoration, then a limited preauricular access incision is planned with a proximal extension into the sideburn. If additional cross-face grafts will be placed for treating the lower third of the face, then a submandibular extension is included to provide better access to the lower buccal and marginal mandibular branches of the facial nerve (Figure 40.2).

The subcutaneous tissues are infiltrated with a solution containing 1:100,000 epinephrine. After allowing ample time for the hemostatic effect, the pre-auricular incision with the sideburn extension is created and facelift scissors are utilized to elevate a broad base skin flap in the zygomatic and buccal region extending the dissection approximately 2 cm past the medial boarder of the masseter muscle. At this juncture, a superficial musculoaponeurotic system (SMAS) flap is elevated, leaving the parotid fascia intact. The cephalic border of the SMAS flap is released near the lower edge of the zygomatic arch and reflected inferiorly enhancing the exposure (Figure 40.3). The zygomatic branches of the

facial nerve can now be identified emanating from the anterior border of the parotid gland and are often enveloped by a fascial arcade and enshrouded by adipose tissue. The zygomatic branches of the facial nerve lying directly above

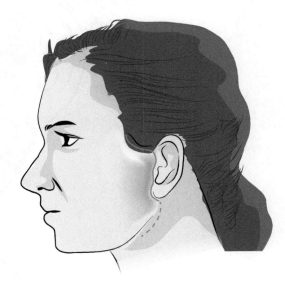

Figure 40.2. Preauricular incision for exploration of temporofacial branches of the facial nerve. A submandibular extension is added if cervicofacial branches are to be identified.

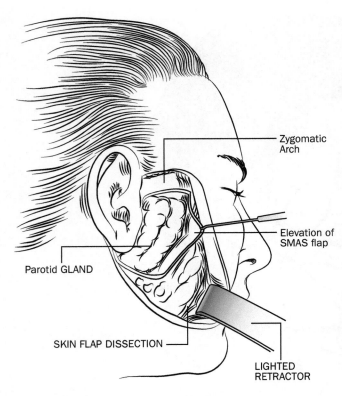

Figure 40.3. Skin and SMAS flap elevation for facial nerve exposure.

and below the transverse facial artery are identified and dissected with microsurgical technique, utilizing the operating microscope. The nerve branches are then stimulated and frequently produce a powerful smile with little or no activation of the orbicularis occuli or the orbicularis oris. The adjacent zygomatic/buccal branches are now explored, stimulated, and mapped. The facial nerve branch that produces the strongest and most isolated contraction of the zygomaticus major is selected for later transection. This branch is now traced retrograde into the parotid gland to maximize its diameter and axon count (Figure 40.4).

Gowns and gloves are changed and a separate set of instruments are utilized to harvest a sural nerve graft.

After exsanguinating the lower extremity, a pneumatic tourniquet is insufflated. A limited vertical access incision is now created 1.5–2 cm behind the posterior border of the lateral malleolus. The medial sural cutaneous nerve is now identified in the subcutaneous tissue deep to the lesser saphenous vein. The nerve is ligated and divided in the retromalleolar region, after which point a nerve stripper is utilized to perform gentle, blunt dissection. Resistance may be encountered near the inferior border of the gastrocnemius muscles where the nerve passes through a fibrous arcade to

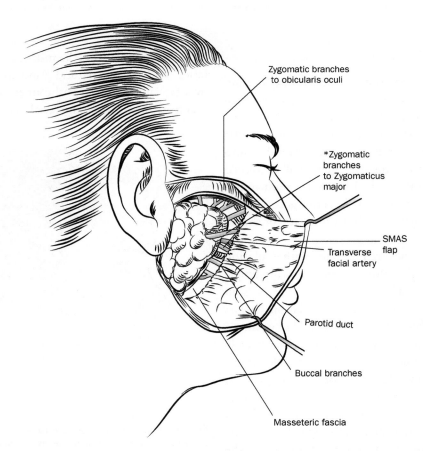

Figure 40.4. Zygomatic facial nerve branches producing activation of the zygomaticus major and levator labii superioris muscles coursing above and below the transverse facial artery.

follow a subfascial course. Overly vigorous dissection with the nerve stripper may result in transection of the nerve or injury to its internal architecture. It is advisable to create an additional access incision to release the fascia or a tethering nerve branch (sural communicating branch) so as to achieve an atraumatic dissection. Once the nerve has been mobilized to the inferior border of the popliteal fossa it can be divided with the swivel knife at the end of the nerve stripper, yielding a nerve graft ranging from 25 to 30 cm in length.

The nerve graft is now delivered to the head and neck region and drawn through a deep subcutaneous tunnel spanning the face with the aid of tendon-passing clamps. The nerve is reversed to limit axon escape through side branches during the regenerative process. An additional access incision may be created through the mucosa of the upper lip to facilitate passage of the nerve graft and to provide access to sensory nerve branches (infraorbital nerve) if an end-to-side neurotrophic anastomosis is desired. The distal end of the nerve is marked with a heavy Proline suture and banked in the contralateral preauricular region. At this juncture, the previously isolated facial nerve branch is selectively transected and a tension free, end-to-end, epineurial nerve repair is performed to the cross-face nerve graft with interrupted 10-0 nylon sutures and utilizing the operating microscope (Figure 40.5).

The SMAS flap is now resecured in its native position, and a closed suction drain is inserted into the subcutaneous space prior to skin closure.

The patients are maintained on clear liquids for 48–72 hours followed by a soft diet for 4 weeks. Oral rinse is recommended over brushing of the teeth, and strenuous activity is avoided for 6–8 weeks.

SECOND STAGE: FREE MICRONEUROVASCULAR MUSCLE FLAP

Patient Markings

Preoperative markings play an important role in the second stage of the reconstruction. In the upright sitting position, the nasolabial fold and dominant smile vector are marked on the unaffected side. Mirror image markings are now created on the paralyzed hemi-face. The most commonly encountered smile vector follows a line joining the commissure to the root of the helix; however, a more oblique risorius dominant smile can be encountered and thoughtful study of each smile is required prior to surgery (Figure 40.6). Additionally, the site of the Tinel's sign is marked to facilitate identification of the distal cross face nerve graft.

Operative Technique: Free Microneurovascular Muscle Flap

Ten to twelve months after a successful first-stage operation a positive Tinel's sign should be present in the zygomatic region on the paralyzed side indicating that it is appropriate to proceed with a free muscle flap.

If the superficial temporal vessels are selected as recipients, then a limited preauricular incision with an extension into the sideburn is created. However, the facial artery and vein are more frequently utilized as recipient vessels, and their exposure is enhanced by extending the incision into the submandibular region. At this juncture, the cross-face nerve graft is identified with aid from its distal marking suture, and the terminal portion is excised and sent for frozen section pathological evaluation to verify the

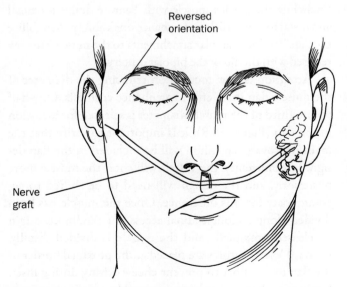

Figure 40.5. Cross face nerve graft with distal marking suture for later identification.

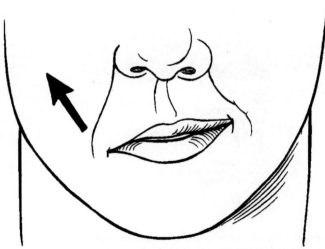

Figure 40.6. Smile vector and nasolabial fold marked preoperatively. Vector usually extends from the commissure to supra-helical, temporal region.

presence of myelinated nerve fibers. Once the course of the nerve graft has been ascertained, a thick skin flap with generous subcutaneous tissue is elevated in the temporal, zygomatic, and buccal regions terminating the dissection at the lateral border of the orbicularis oris. A robust flap is important to facilitate gliding of the muscle flap and prevent unsightly dermal adhesions.

This broad exposure provides unfettered access to the facial artery and vein that are mobilized to a point near the modiolus. A thorough dissection is essential as the increased vessel length offers greater flexibility with flap positioning. In an effort to reduce later fullness in the cheek, a segment of the buccal fat pad can be resected. A series of 2-0 PDS anchoring sutures are now placed into the lateral border of the orbicularis oris muscle. The sutures should enter the orbicularis oris on its superficial surface and exit on its deep surface. This placement will facilitate later anchoring of the muscle flap as the knots will be tied in a more superficial, unobstructed plane (Figure 40.7). Gentle traction on these sutures should produce a pleasing facsimile of a smile and

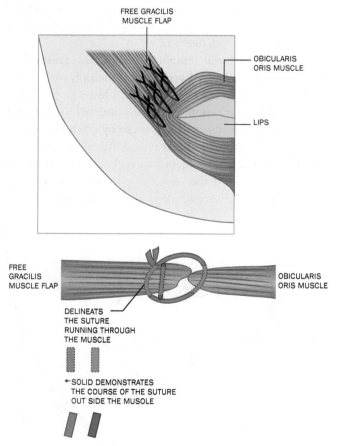

FREE GRACILIS
MUSCLE FLAP

OBICULARIS
ORIS MUSCLE

LIPS

FREE
GRACILIS
MUSCLE FLAP

OBICULARIS
ORIS MUSCLE

DELINEATS
THE SUTURE
RUNNING THROUGH
THE MUSCLE

*SOLID DEMONSTRATES
THE COURSE OF THE SUTURE
OUT SIDE THE MUSOLE

Figure 40.7. Medial anchoring sutures are placed superficial-to-deep in an effort to facilitate later suture tying. Heavy, horizontal mattress, polyglactin sutures are placed in the muscle flap to prevent suture cheeswring during inset.

adjustments are frequently required. Proper placement of the medial anchoring sutures is essential to obtaining an aesthetic result and is best achieved at this time as later revisions can prove challenging. The distance from the medial suture anchors to lateral fixation site in the temporal region is measured and 2 cm is added to determine the length of the free muscle flap.

Attention is now focused on harvesting the free gracilis muscle flap. Gowns and gloves are changed and a different set of instruments are employed. The lower extremity contralateral to the paralyzed hemi-face is abducted into a frog leg position. A stack of sterile towels is utilized to buttress the lateral knee to prevent a traction injury to the sciatic nerve. The proximal, tendinous portion of the adductor longus muscle is palpated and a parallel, vertical access incision is planned 2 cm posterior to this landmark. The skin is incised, and the dissection is propagated through the subcutaneous tissue down to the adductor fascia. A perforator is often encountered 8–10 cm inferior to the pubic tubercle. This frequently corresponds to the level of the main vascular pedicle and can be incorporated along with adjacent subcutaneous tissue to provide soft tissue volume if required. The adductor fascia is now widely incised and the dominant nutrient pedicle is identified coursing between the adductor longus and brevis muscles. A single artery and two vena comitantes are usually identified entering the gracilis muscle on its deep surface near its anterior border. The anterior branch of the obturator nerve is identified coursing on top of the vascular pedicle. After verifying its function with a nerve stimulator, the nerve is mobilized proximally and divided. The vascular pedicle is now skeletonized and great care is taken to ligate and divide the branches radiating to the adductor longus that can produce troublesome bleeding. Encircling the gracilis muscle with Penrose drains proximal and distal to the pedicle can enhance one's ability to mobilize the flap. The loose areolar attachments to the muscle are now released with the aid of the bipolar cautery.

Attention is now focused on reducing the diameter of the muscle flap in an effort to enhance cosmesis. One-half to one-third of the muscle diameter is selected for inclusion in the flap (Figure 40.8). It is important to verify that the main neurovascular hilum will be included in the flap design. Intermittently, the vessels will enter the muscle more posteriorly, and the design will need to be shifted to accommodate for this difference. Once the muscle has been divided along its longitudinal access, the tendinous origin is released proximally and the muscle is divided distally. Heavy 0 Vicryl sutures are placed at the proximal border of the flap in an effort to prevent cheese-wiring during inset. Little or no benefit has been achieved by placing sutures in the muscle to mark resting tension.

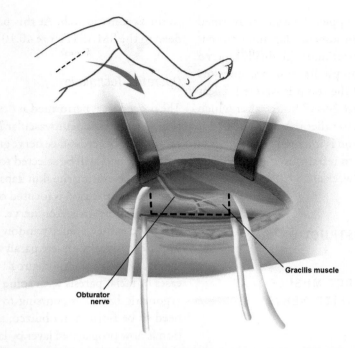

Figure 40.8. Gracilis muscle exposed via a medial thigh incision 2 cm below the adductor longus tendon. Obturator nerve crosses the vascular pedicle prior to muscle entry. One half to one quarter of the muscle's diameter is incorporated into the flap design.

If a segment of the gracilis tendon is desired for additional static support, it is now harvested via a small access incision in the distal, medial thigh.

The vascular pedicle is ligated and divided, and the artery is irrigated with heparinized saline until a clear venous effluent is present. The muscle flap is delivered to the surgical site in the head and neck, where it is secured to the medial anchoring sutures. In cases where significant upper dental show is desired a slip of gracilis fascia can be sutured to the medial orbicularis oris via a small vertical incision in the vermillion. Gentle lateral traction is now placed on the muscle flap. The production of slight motion at the commissure signals that proper tension has been achieved and the lateral flap edge is secured to the temporal fascia with 2-0 PDS sutures. The microvascular anastomosis is now completed. Once the muscle flap is revascularized, the obturator nerve can be stimulated to verify that the proper smile vector has been obtained.

A microsurgical nerve repair is now undertaken joining the obturator nerve to the cross-face nerve graft. This is performed with 10-0 nylon in an interrupted, epineurial fashion. It is important for the nerve repair to reside below the muscle flap as this positioning will facilitate later revision surgery if required (Figure 40.9). The incisions are now repaired over a small closed suction drain. A transcutaneous Doppler signal can be reliably identified in most cases. Alternately, an implantable venous Doppler can be utilized. Antibacterial ointment is applied to the incisions, and additional dressings that could produce unwanted compression are avoided.

POSTOPERATIVE CARE

The patients are maintained on one and a half times their hourly intravenous maintenance fluids for the first

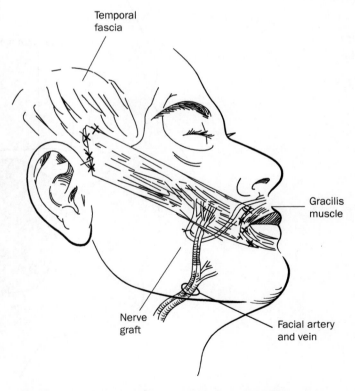

Figure 40.9. Free gracilis muscle flap inset. Vascular anastomosis to the facial artery and vein. Cross face nerve graft coursing below the muscle to facilitate later debulking if required. Proximal suture anchoring to the temporal fascia. Medial suture anchoring to the orbicularis oris.

postoperative day, and hourly Doppler checks are performed in an enhanced monitoring environment (flap unit or intensive care unit). Fluids and monitoring are gradually tapered over the 4–5 day period of hospitalization. Vasopressors and diuretics are avoided, and the room is warmed. Clear liquids are provided for the first 24–48 hours, after which the patient is transitioned to a soft diet that is followed for 4 weeks. Progressive mobilization is initiated after 72 hours of bed rest. Patients are asked to refrain from heavy lifting and sporting activities for 6–8 weeks.

SINGLE-STAGE RECONSTRUCTION

OPERATIVE TECHNIQUE: FREE MUSCLE FLAP NEUROTIZED BY THE MASSETER NERVE

Operative Markings

The identification of the motor nerve branch to the masseter has been facilitated by the description of topographic landmarks. The main trunk of the nerve can reliably be isolated at a point 3 cm anterior to the tragus and 1 cm inferior to the zygomatic arch. At this point, the nerve lies 1.5 cm deep to the SMAS (Figure 40.10).[5,11,12]

Operative Technique

The procedure is performed as describe in the preceding section ("Free Microneurovascular Muscle Flap") with several exceptions. No cross-face nerve graft will be present, and the masseter nerve will be selected to innervate the free muscle flap. After elevating the skin flaps and mobilizing the recipient vessels, attention is focused on isolating the descending branch of the masseter nerve. Utilizing the landmarks described earlier, a small window of SMAS will be resected. In patients with complete paralysis, the dissection proceeds rapidly down to the aponeurosis of the masseter muscle. In cases of facial paresis with some preserved eye closure, the zygomatic branches coursing to the orbicularis oculi will need to be isolated, mobilized, and preserved. The dissection is now propagated layer by layer with a fine right-angle clamp and bipolar cautery into the deeper portion of the masseter muscle. Judicious use of electrical stimulation will help guide the exploration. The masseter muscle has three lobes, and the nerve will be found resting on the superficial

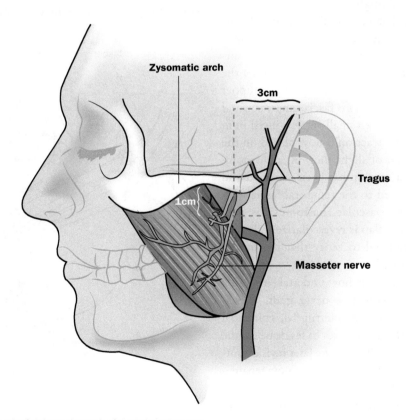

Figure 40.10. Cutaneous landmarks for the main trunk of the masseter nerve.

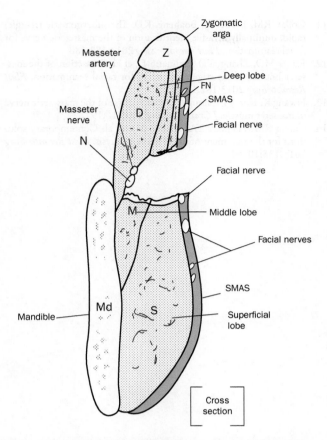

Figure 40.11. Cross sectional anatomy demonstrating the 3 lobes of the masseter muscle. The main trunk of the masseter nerve lies on the superficial surface of the deep lobe.

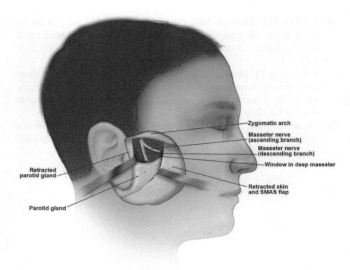

Figure 40.12. Surgical exposure of the masseter nerve. The descending nerve branch is mobilized and selectively transected. An end-to-end microsurgical nerve repair is then created between the masseter nerve branch and the motor nerve of the free gracilis muscle flap (obturator nerve).

surface of the deep lobe (Figure 40.11).[13,14] The descending branch of the masseter nerve charts a deep, oblique course running toward the anteromedial border of the muscle. This branch is skeletonized and selectively transected. Fully mobilizing the branch will allow it to be transposed into a more superficial plane, thus facilitating the later nerve repair (Figure 40.12). The proximal branches of the masseter nerve are preserved to prevent muscle atrophy that could produce a cosmetic deformity. The muscle flap inset is then performed; however, it is often beneficial to repair the obturator nerve to the masseter nerve prior to the microvascular anastomosis or lateral flap anchoring to facilitate exposure. In addition, the masseter nerve often produces inadequate muscle flap resting tone, and the provision of extra static support with fascial grafts can prove beneficial.

Rehabilitation

In general, some motion will start to be visualized around the sixth postoperative month. At that time, facial exercises will be initiated. Patients are asked to spend a minimum of 30 minutes per day in front of the mirror working to achieve maximal excursion and symmetry. The postoperative rehabilitation is critical when the masseter nerve is utilized.

REFERENCES

1. Zuker RM, Goldberg CS, Manktelow RT. Facial animation in children with Möbius syndrome after segmental gracilis muscle transplant. *Plast Reconstr Surg* 2000;106:1.
2. Klebuc M, Shenaq S. Donor nerve selection in facial reanimation surgery. *Seminars Plast Surg* 2004;18:53.
3. Placheta E, Wood MD, Lafontaine C, et al. Enhancement of facial nerve motoneuron regeneration through cross-face nerve grafts by adding end-to-side sensory axons. *Plast Reconstr Surg* 2015;135:46.
4. Takushima A, Harii K, Asato H, et al. Fifteen-year survey of one-stage latissimus dorsi muscle transfer for treatment of longstanding facial paralysis. *J Plast Reconstr Aesthet Surg* 2013;66:29.
5. Borschel GH, Kawamura DH, Kasukurthi R, et al. The motor nerve to the masseter muscle: An anatomic and histomorphometric study to facilitate its use in facial reanimation. *J Plastic Reconstr Aesthet Surg* 2012;65:363.
6. Coombs CJ, Ek EW, Cleland H, et al. Masseteric-facial nerve coaptation-an alternative technique for facial nerve reinnervation. *J Plast Reconstr Aesthet Surg* 2009;62:1580.
7. Manktelow RT, Tomat LR, Zuker RM, et al. Smile reconstruction in adults with free muscle transfer innervated by the masseter motor nerve: effectiveness and cerebral adaptation. *Plast Reconstr Surg* 2006;118:885.

8. Lifchez SD, Matloub HS, Gosain AK. Cortical adaptation to restoration of smiling after free muscle transfer innervated by the nerve to the masseter. *Plast Reconstr Surg* 2005;115: 1472.

9. Schaverien M, Moran G, Stewart K, et al. Activation of the masseter muscle during normal smile production and the implications for dynamic reanimation surgery for facial paralysis. *J Plast Reconstr Aesthet Surg* 2011;64:1585.

10. Dorafshar AH, Borsuk DE, Bojovic B. Surface anatomy of the middle division of the facial nerve: Zuker's point. *Plast Reconstr Surg* 2013;131:253.

11. Collar, RM, Byrne, PJ, Boahene, KD. The subzygomatic triangle: rapid, minimally invasive identification of the masseteric nerve for facial reanimation. *Plast Reconstr Surg* 2013;183;188.

12. Fisher MD, Zhang, YD, Erdmann D, et al. Dissection of the masseter branch of the trigeminal nerve for facial reanimation. *Plast Reconstr Surg* 2013;131:1065.

13. Hwang K, Kim YJ, Chung IH, et al. Course of the masseteric nerve in masseter muscle. *J Craniofac Surg* 2005;16:197.

14. Garcia RM, Hadlock TA, Klebuc MJ, et al. Contemporary solutions for the treatment of facial nerve paralysis. *Plast Reconstr Surg* 2015;135:1025e.

41.

ALT FLAPS

Jonathan A. Zelken and Ming-Huei Cheng

INTRODUCTION

The anterolateral thigh (ALT) flap was introduced in Asia more than 30 years ago and has gained widespread popularity throughout the global shift toward microvascular reconstruction. Song first described the ALT flap in 1984.[1] Ever since, it has evolved as one of the most versatile and most reliable of the thigh-based free flaps. The ALT donor site is easily concealed when it is primarily closed and needs not violate a functional motor unit, resulting in minimal potential cosmetic deformity and disability. It has become the workhorse flap for head and neck reconstruction, with increasing utility in limb, trunk, and perineal reconstruction. The ALT flap is indicated for reconstruction of a diverse range of defects of various surface areas and depths; it can be used "ultra-thin" for resurfacing, rolled up for reconstruction of tubular structures or taken with muscle to obliterate dead space or to provide bulk. The flap has been used in trauma salvage as a flow-through flap, as a tissue carrier to "piggy back" additional flaps. The flap can be raised pedicled (proximally or distally) or free, supra- or subfascial, thinned, or harvested with muscle or additional tissue components. Despite the "pendulum effect" to which many new techniques are prey, the ALT flap has withstood the test of time.

INDICATIONS AND CLASSIFICATION

The ALT flap has become popular for providing ample soft tissue and can be modified to include various quantities of skin, fat, fascia, and muscle. It is inherently pliable, and this quality can be further modulated with thinning procedures and suprafascial harvest. Although the ALT flap was originally developed as a free flap, it may also be raised as a proximally pedicled flap for perineal or abdominal reconstruction or as a distally-based pedicled flap with reverse flow for knee traumatic defects or to optimize amputation stumps.

Flaps are defined by their vascular supply as either myocutaneous or septocutaneous. The distinction is significant since the "true" perforator flap relies on intricate dissection of the myocutaneous perforator passing through the vastus lateralis muscle.[2] A septocutaneous flap may portend an easier harvest with shorter, more direct vessels penetrating the septum between rectus femoris and vastus lateralis. Alternatively, the ALT flap may be defined by its tissue components: skin, fat, fascia, muscle, or nerve. The ALT flap may be raised as a compound myocutaneous flap with simple en-bloc elevation of the overlying skin, or the skin paddle may be dissected separately of the underlying muscle based on the perforators. The versatility of the ALT flap is reflected by the extensive spectrum of defects to which it is routinely applied. An algorithm outlining the different ALT flap types suitable for various defects is outlined in Figure 41.1).

Thin flaps with a large surface area are ideal for resurfacing or for draping over three-dimensional or mobile structures. Such "ultra-thin" ALT flaps are also suitable for defects where a bulky contour deformity would be undesirable cosmetically (i.e., face) or functionally (i.e., dorsum of foot, ankle, hand). The ALT flap is pliable enough to be folded, tubed, or packed into cavities, and its convenience of harvest and predictable anatomy make it an excellent first-line emergency flap. Myocutaneous ALT flaps may be raised with skin and muscle intact or with the tissue components separated on individual perforators for more flexible insetting of the flap. Nearby tissues such as iliac crest bone, tendon, fascia, or nerve may be included in an extended composite ALT flap based on the shared lateral circumflex femoral artery system.[3] The ALT perforator flap may be divided to provide multiple tissue paddles,[4] two

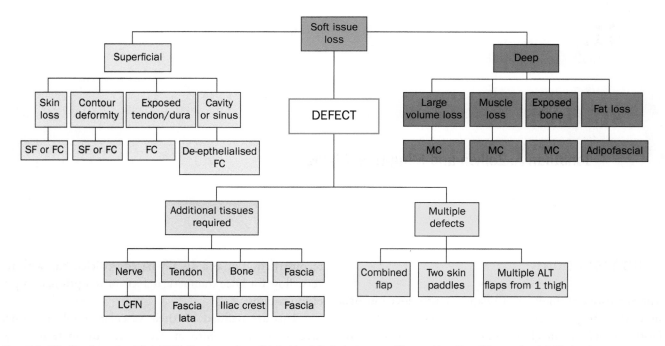

Figure 41.1. Algorithm for anterolateral thigh flap harvest as dictated by defect size, composition, and location. SF, suprafascial; FC, fasciocutaneous; LCFN, lateral cutaneous femoral nerve; MC, musculocutaneous; ALT, anterolateral thigh. From Ali RS, Bluebond-Langner R, Rodriguez ED, Cheng MH. The versatility of the anterolateral thigh flap. *Plast Reconstr Surg* 2009;124:e395-407.

smaller sized ALT flaps raised from one thigh,[5] or multiple flaps raised based on the lateral femoral circumflex artery (LCFA) to fill multiple defects by way of a single vascular anastomosis.[6]

HEAD AND NECK RECONSTRUCTION

ALT flaps are routinely used in head and neck reconstruction. They are favored for three-dimensional defects, particularly those that exceed 5 cm in any dimension. At the senior authors' institution, the ALT flap has become commonplace since defects resulting from oral cancer (often secondary to betel nut chewing) tend to be large. The thin and sizable, sometimes hairless ALT fasciocutaneous flap is ideal for resurfacing intra-oral defects and can be folded to line complex three-dimensional defects. When the flap is divided into multiple paddles, each supplied by individual perforator(s), complex defects such as through-and-through defects can be simplified and reconstructed safely.[4] Alternatively, de-epithelialization of the skin paddle can achieve a similar effect by enabling the flap to be buried to efface contour deformities and obliterate dead space.[7]

Composite mandibular defects are increasingly reconstructed with osteocutaneous flaps such as the fibula flap to replace missing tissues, optimize function, and combat effects of radiotherapy. The fibula osteocutaneous flap may be combined with an ALT flap for vast composite

tissue defects, for instance, after segmental mandibulectomy with through-and-through soft tissue defects (Cheng Class III).[8]

The ALT flap is suitable for external resurfacing, and the fibula is used for mandibular and oral lining reconstruction. In these cases, we recommend harvest of both flaps from the same extremity with simultaneous recipient site preparation. If there are insufficient candidate recipient vessels following cancer recurrence, revision, or radiotherapy, the ALT flap can be used to "piggy back" a second flap or serve as a flow-through flap.

Maxillary defects are often complex and three-dimensional and demand multiple tissue components for reconstruction. The myocutaneous ALT flap is ideal for complex maxillary defects. Vastus lateralis muscle or de-epithelialized skin or fascia may be used to obliterate the sinus and fill dead space. Skin paddle may be used to resurface the nasal lining and cutaneous defects, and separate anatomic compartments. After partial glossectomy, a pliable fasciocutaneous ALT flap may be used to replace the lost tongue. Fasciocutaneous ALT flaps can preserve residual tongue motion and enhance speech and swallowing. Total or near-total glossectomy defects may require additional muscle bulk, and this can be provided by vastus lateralis included with the myocutaneous ALT flap. Co-aption of the lateral femoral cutaneous nerve to the lingual nerve to provide sensation has been performed, however, long-term advantage of this additional step is yet to be determined.[9]

Many surgeons favor fasciocutaneous flaps over the free jejunal flap for pharyngoesophageal reconstruction. Fasciocutaneous flaps from the forearm, arm, and thigh have been described. The authors favor the ALT and anteromedial thigh (AMT) flaps for ease of harvest and well-tolerated donor site morbidity. A wide ALT flap may be harvested to fabricate a long, wide-bore tube that generates more intelligible, less "wet" sounding speech than the jejunum. Harvesting additional fascia facilitates three-layered closure of the neo-tube resulting in a safer, watertight closure that reduces postoperative complications such as stricture, leakage, and fistula formation. Other pearls include orienting the incision lines away from the anastomosis, lining the irradiated neck vessels with a dermal tail, and including a skin paddle for monitoring (Figure 41.2).[7]

The fasciocutaneous ALT flap is particularly useful during calvarial reconstruction. Fasciocutaneous flaps are thought to undergo less soft tissue contraction than muscle-bearing flaps. The harvest of additional fascia can be used to reconstruct and fortify the dura mater, and a pliable thinned-skin paddle will conform to complex topographic features of the skull.[3] Frontonasal fistulas may be obliterated with specially designed ALT myocutaneous flaps.[10] Defects incorporating the facial nerve can be treated with a composite ALT flap that employs fascia to create a static sling and branches of the lateral femoral cutaneous nerve (LFCN) for interpositional facial nerve grafts. Alternatively, sensory branches via the LFCN can be co-apted to branches of the trigeminal nerve to restore sensation to these flaps. Finally, fasciocutaneous ALT flaps can be used to restore facial asymmetries seen in hemifacial microsomia, after tumor resection and radiation. Flaps with large surface area can be raised thin enough to be buried under facial flaps and include fascia that provides a gliding surface over the deeper muscles of facial expression.

LOWER ABDOMEN, AND PELVIS RECONSTRUCTION

Pedicled ALT flaps may be used to reconstruct defects of the lower abdomen, perineum, trochanter, and gluteal and ischial tuberosity in a single stage (Figure 41.3).[11] The composition of the flap is tailored to the defect. At the authors' institution, wounds of the lower abdomen are generally approached differently from those of the groin and perineum.

For abdominal defects, the thickness of the defect is considered first. For full-thickness abdominal defects, the quality of the surrounding tissue and wound environment is evaluated. A hostile wound bed warrants bulky, vascular coverage using a muscle-bearing flap. Conversely, a partial-thickness traumatic defect surrounded by healthy skin may be managed with a fasciocutaneous flap, sometimes using the fascia to repair the abdominal wall defect in a tension-free fashion. If the lower abdominal defect is partial-thickness and there is no exposed bowel, the quality and hostility of the wound bed should be examined, as well as the presence of prosthetic material. When the surrounding soft tissue

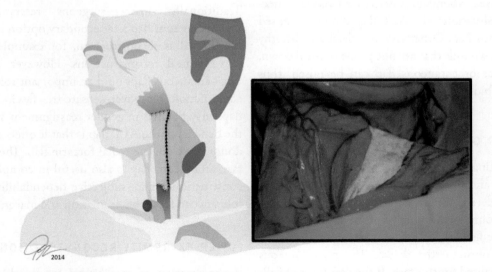

Figure 41.2. Left: Hypopharyngeal reconstruction after left-sided neck dissection. In this example, the flap was designed to shield the diseased neck from toxic leakage and radiation, protecting vulnerable tissues like the carotid artery. The suture line was oriented away from the contralateral neck. The skin paddle was at the most distal end of the flap, theoretically enhancing sensitivity to perfusion changes. *Right*: Intraoperative photograph of the same.

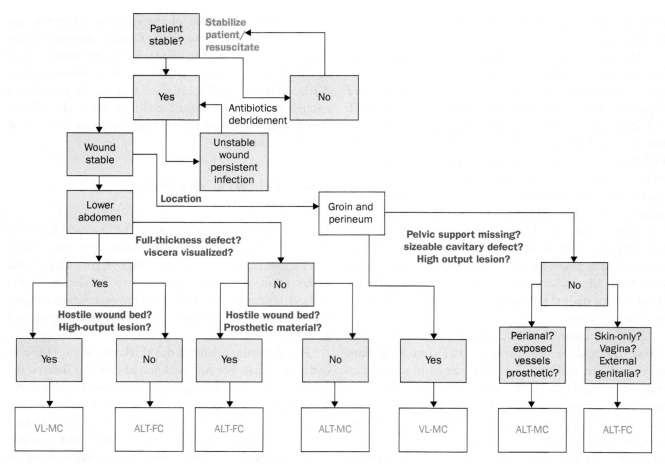

Figure 41.3. Algorithm for reconstruction of lower abdominal, groin, and perineal are using the pedicled anterolateral thigh (ALT) flap. VL-MC, vastus lateralis myocutaneous flap; ALT-FC, anterolateral thigh fasciocutaneous flap; ALT-MC, anterolateral thigh myocutaneous flap. From Zelken JA, Al-Deek NF, Hsu CC, Chang NJ, Lin CH, Lin CH. Algorithmic approach to lower abdominal, perineal, and groin reconstruction using anterolateral thigh flaps. *Microsurgery* 2014.

is poorly perfused or has been irradiated, or if prosthetic material is exposed, abundant vascularized tissue is necessary. In these situations, the ALT flap should be raised as a myocutaneous flap. Otherwise, for clean and healthy partial-thickness wounds that are not prone to breakdown, a fasciocutaneous or cutaneous flap can be raised, thus minimizing morbidity and unwieldy or superfluous bulk.

PERINEAL AND GROIN DEFECTS

When approaching defects of the perineum and groin, the competence and integrity of pelvic support structures should be considered. When there is a loss of pelvic support, a hostile wound bed, or high-output lesions (i.e., urinary leak, enteric fistula), bulky tissue should be recruited to reinforce or obturate the defect. The myocutaneous ALT flap is well suited for this task. If the defect is not full-thickness, a less bulky alternative may be used, such as a fasciocutaneous or cutaneous ALT flap.[11]

PHALLUS AND PERINEUM

Traditionally, many surgeons reserved the ALT fasciocutaneous flap as a secondary option in patients with failed phallus reconstruction, for example, or for complex perineal reconstructions. However, pedicled ALT fasciocutaneous flaps hold an important role in phallus reconstruction. Moreover, sensate-free fasciocutaneous ALT flaps may be used in gender reassignment surgery. One of the benefits of the ALT flap is that it offers a more discreet donor scar than the radial forearm flap. The pedicled ALT fasciocutaneous flap is also useful in complex perineal reconstruction for its subjective dependability and relative tolerance to fecal contamination and maceration.[12,13]

LOWER EXTREMITY RECONSTRUCTION

Reconstruction of the injured leg should preserve limb length, function, and appearance. Extremity wounds have variable soft tissue requirements for which local tissue may not suffice. The thigh is a veritable warehouse of donor tissue based primarily on branches of the circumflex femoral arteries.[6] The ALT flap is based on the LFCA, which boasts a long vascular pedicle that should not compromise distal perfusion when ligated. In contrast, a flow-through flap designed on a short vascular pedicle can restore arterial flow in a single-vessel limb or in those with peripheral vascular disease.[14] Distally based reverse-flow ALT flaps have been successfully used to repair soft tissue defects of the ipsilateral knee with and without venous supercharge.[15–17]

The anatomy of thigh flaps allows the surgeon to harvest tissue from the distally injured leg if it is indicated. The skin paddle of ALT flaps routinely exceed 20 cm in length and 10 cm in width. Flap composition should reflect the location and nature of the defect as well as anticipated functional demands. For example, wounds involving the malleoli require thin coverage to facilitate footwear fitting. Deeper wounds, or those in the setting of osteomyelitis, require bulk for obliteration of dead space. The ALT flap offers sufficient area of skin and the ability to tailor additional muscle.

Another advantage of the ALT flap for lower limb reconstruction is that epidural anesthesia can be used in patients unfit for general anesthesia. Fasciocutaneous flaps do not sacrifice an entire motor unit and are encouraged for all cases that do not necessitate the added bulk of a myocutaneous flap. Reported indications for a myocutaneous ALT flap include, but are certainly not limited to, reconstruction of avulsed plantar heel tissue, amputation stump revision, and length preservation and immediate reconstruction of the Achilles tendon with vascularized fascia lata.

UPPER EXTREMITY RECONSTRUCTION

The goals and principles of lower extremity reconstruction apply to upper extremity reconstruction. When possible, fasciocutaneous flaps are favored to minimize donor site morbidity and superfluous bulk that can impair recipient site function. Special considerations in upper extremity reconstruction include coverage of exposed tendons and the preservation of grip and dexterity. Vascularized fascia lata can be used to ensheath exposed tendons and can even be used to restore joint motion in cases of severe bursitis.[18] Functional restoration of elbow flexion and extension following degloving injury and concomitant biceps and triceps tendon injuries has been achieved using a free ALT flap and fascial extension.[19] Although free flaps are traditionally used, the pedicled ALT flap may play an important role in reconstruction of the degloved hand and other mutilating hand injuries[20] (Figure 41.4). In a recent series, the pedicled ALT and groin flaps were used to resurface the dorsal and palmar surfaces and then divided in a second stage. The proposed benefit of pedicled groin and thigh flaps for reconstruction of hand injuries is preservation of existing vasculature for use in toe-to-hand and other subsequent reconstructions.

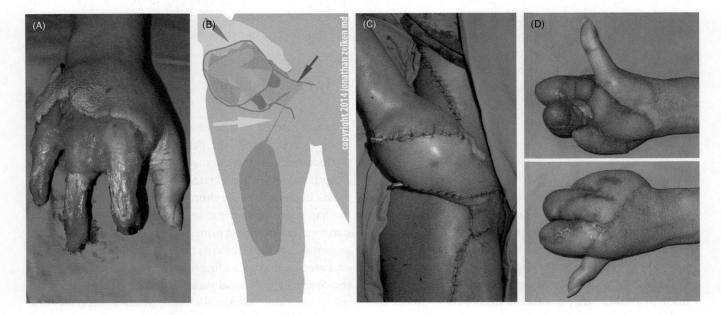

Figure 41.4. The pedicled anterolateral thigh-and-groin flap sandwich flap for resurfacing the degloved and mutilated hand. (A) Crush and degloving injury following debridement. (B) The pliable groin flap (*blue arrow*) provided palmar coverage. The anterolateral thigh (ALT) (*red arrow*) pedicle was dissected as proximally as possible, delivered through the wound extension (*yellow arrow*), and gently draped over the dorsum, providing total wound coverage. (C) The tissues were closed in a tension-free manner. (D) Postoperative view after 2 syndactyly releases and debulking. From Zelken JA, Chang NJ, Wei FC, Lin CH. The combined ALT-groin flap for the mutilated and degloved hand. *Injury* 2015;46:1591–1596.

BURN INJURY

The burned extremity may require extensive resurfacing for reconstruction of vital structures and restoration of function. Release of disabling contractures results in sizable tissue defects and may require microvascular tissue transfer. The ALT fasciocutaneous flap offers a large skin paddle; bilateral ALT flaps have been used to salvage the severely burned leg.[21] When the thigh is involved in the burn injury or there is local soft tissue trauma, the thigh may not be a dependable donor source for tissue transfer. However, there are case reports of the previously burned anterolateral thigh skin being used for microvascular transfer.[22] When more tissue is needed than the thigh(s) can safely provide, tissue expansion should be considered. In these cases, tissue expanders are inserted subcutaneously, lateral to the perforators, and expanded over the course of several months. The expanded skin allows for harvest of even larger ALT flaps and facilitates closure of the donor site.[23, 24]

BREAST RECONSTRUCTION

Although not commonly considered part of the autologous breast reconstruction armamentarium, the ALT flap may be considered for some women[25,26] (e.g., women with low body mass index and insufficient abdominal tissue who prefer not to sacrifice gluteal contour and wish to avoid implants). In most women, adipofascial ALT flaps are not as voluminous as abdominal flaps, but in larger patients, larger flaps can be raised. Ultimately, ALT flaps may not be ideal for breast reconstruction and indications are limited. However, the ALT is a defensible option for women seeking autologous reconstruction who are not candidates for abdominal-based reconstruction or in whom previous abdominal flaps have failed.

CONTRAINDICATIONS

Not all patients are candidates for free tissue transfer. Patients must be medically stable and able to tolerate an extensive operation and significant blood loss might be not encountered. There is no accepted age cutoff, but calcified vessels and advanced peripheral vascular disease may predispose to technical difficulty and flap demise. Patients with hyper and hypocoagulable tendencies should be treated prior to reconstruction. Patients must be compliant, and willing and prepared to adhere to strict rehabilitation protocols and guidelines. Although there are exceptions, an ALT flap cannot be raised if the site has been previously harvested. Since they share the same source vessel, an ALT cannot be raised if an AMT or tensor fascia lata (TFL) flap has been raised on the ipsilateral thigh if the prior harvest extended to the femoral vessels. Although preoperative angiography is not routinely performed, it is an important resource that provides reassurance and may save time. Previous operations or injuries of the groin and thigh warrant angiographic studies to ensure appropriate perfusion along the planned vascular axis.

ROOM SETUP

The operating suite should be set up with the recipient site in mind, preferably in a way that allows a two-team approach: one team is designated to flap harvest while the second prepares the recipient site. For flap harvest, the patient must be supine with the donor extremity prepped from umbilicus to toe. The genitals and anus are excluded from the operative site. A sandbag or padding may be placed under the ipsilateral buttocks and trunk to facilitate internal rotation of the thigh and vessel exposure in the groin. The operating room should be equipped with a Doppler probe, self-retaining retractors, monopolar and bipolar electrocautery, fine dissecting instruments, surgical loupes (2.5× magnification or greater), 9-0 or finer nylon suture, and a surgical microscope. Skin grafting instruments should be accessible. Optional instruments may include intraoperative perfusion imaging devices, vessel coupling devices, wound closure devices and transcutaneous oximeters for spot-checking in real time and postoperatively.[27]

PATIENT MARKINGS

Flaps are marked to account for and overcorrect the defect being reconstructed. The patient is marked in the supine position with the hip internally rotated and knee extended. Length and width are dictated by defect parameters, and, in most circumstances the short axis of the defect determines the flap width. In many cases, donor sites that are 8 cm or narrower can be closed primarily. Flaps are designed as long as possible to facilitate coverage, up to 26 cm. Thigh flaps are based on the descending branch of the LFCA. Although the course of that vessel varies, it can be reliably predicted using anatomic landmarks: the anterior superior iliac spine (ASIS) and the patella. A line drawn from the ASIS to the superolateral patellar edge represents the course of the LFCA. A point halfway between the ASIS and patella

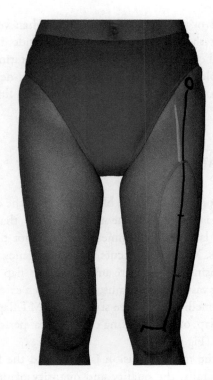

Figure 41.5. Traditional anterolateral thigh (ALT) flap markings. A 10 × 20 centimeter flap is marked (*blue ellipse*), centered around perforators (*red dots*) that are confirmed with ultrasound. The anterior superior iliac spine (ASIS)–patellar axis (*black line*) predicts the position of the septum and deep branches of the source vessel. The lateral cutaneous femoral nerve (*yellow line*) is often used to sensitize the flap.

estimates the origin of a central perforator. Two additional points 5 cm proximal and distal to the midway mark can predict the position of additional perforators; reassuring Doppler signals will confirm the actual perforator position (Figure 41.5). Designs that are based on a geometrical template of the defect that includes the pedicle direction may be preferred. In emergency cases where an ALT flap had not been anticipated, an ALT flap can be marked empirically and the medial edge elevated to allow visual confirmation of suitable perforators.

OPERATIVE TECHNIQUES

FLAP HARVEST

The medial border is incised down to or through fascia, depending on the preferred plane of dissection. Suprafascial flaps are raised superficial to the fascia and may be technically more demanding.[28] The flap is elevated laterally until the perforators supplying the skin paddle are identified. Intramuscular dissection of the selected perforator(s) proceeds in a retrograde fashion to connect with a source

vessel that exists in a relatively avascular plane, deep to the vastus lateralis muscle. If the source vessel is the transverse branch of the LCFA, this may require an extended intramuscular dissection. The ALT flap is classically thought of as a septocutaneous flap, though this may not always be the case. Septocutaneous perforators are more likely to be located proximally and follow a direct route to the source vessel; this permits rapid and straightforward dissection of the ALT flap. Myocutaneous perforators may take a more circuitous route, requiring 5–6 cm of meticulous dissection from the surrounding muscle. Precise hemostasis is encouraged since a bloodstained field impairs visualization of perforator anatomy.

The senior author has observed partial rectus femoris necrosis following ligation of the ALT source vessel proximal to its branch to rectus femoris. Despite this, the authors do not advocate routine pedicle ligation distal to this branch. The motor nerve and branches to the vastus lateralis arise from the femoral nerve and parallel the vascular pedicle. It is important to identify and preserve the femoral nerve and its branches during intramuscular perforator dissection. This is particularly true for muscle-sparing or true perforator ALT flaps. If the motor nerve runs between multiple perforators, the motor nerve can be preserved and the components of ALT flap are divided based on separate perforators and taken as a chimeric-style flap.[3,4] Alternatively, the motor nerve may be divided if it facilitates flap elevation and then repaired with a fine nylon suture. A third alternative is to preserve the motor nerve and harvest the flap using a single perforator.

FLAP INSET

Flap inset is dependent on the location and nature of the defect. Pearls of wisdom and other technical maneuvers vary by reconstructive site, but several principles should be respected for all flaps: (1) ALT flaps can tolerate more ischemic time when less muscle is included. (2) Flaps should be insetted without tension. (3) Flap inset should be planned after careful observation of the position, direction, and length of both recipient pedicle vein and artery. Particularly when partial inset of the flap is done prior to the anastomosis of the pedicles. (4) Deep and transcutaneous drains are generally placed at the authors' institutions. Transcutaneous drains are generally impervious fingers (crafted from Penrose drains or surgical gloves) that allow fluid egress at the donor-recipient interface. (5) Deep drains should emerge from preexisting wounds. It remains controversial whether one or two venous anastomoses should be attempted. (6) Generally, one venous anastomosis is sufficient, but when two can be performed with relative ease without imposing additional donor morbidity, then two should be performed. One study suggests that flaps with a single anastomosis are more likely to require take-back than flaps with two.[29]

DONOR SITE MANAGEMENT

Primary closure of the donor site generally results in minimal pain or paresthesia, acceptable scar cosmesis, good thigh contour, and rapid return to ambulation. Patients may report transient numbness in the distribution of the LFCN but seldom report any discernible weakness in the authors' experience. That said, objective assessment has demonstrated a 10–30% reduction in strength of knee extension, and tethering of the underlying muscle has been described with the use of skin grafts.[30–32] Reported techniques for donor site closure include skin grafting, preexpansion of the flap, local advancement flaps, and locoregional transposition flap. Possible donor site complications include wound infection, dehiscence, bulging and herniation of the thigh, seroma, sensory disturbances, compartment syndrome, and unacceptable cosmetic appearance. Seromas can be prevented with external compression and closed suction drainage and are uncommon. Donor site scar cosmesis is optimized when tissues are closed primarily, and this is often the case for flaps that are less than 8 cm wide. Larger flaps may be closed primarily for part or all of the length. The remaining defect should be skin grafted with a split-thickness graft. In younger or female patients, skin grafting should be avoided when possible, as healed grafts are objectively less attractive than a linear scar.

POSTOPERATIVE CONSIDERATIONS

As with any free flap, postoperative monitoring is critical for early detection of compromised flaps and initiation of appropriate management, and potentially salvage of the flap. A skilled nursing team is the cornerstone of a successful reconstruction program, but skilled nurses may not always be available. This is particularly true for the private sector. In these cases, the operating surgeon should extensively train his postoperative nursing staff prior to embarking on free flap reconstruction. Doppler signals are relatively easy to monitor, but flap turgor, color, and capillary refill must be documented. Color cards and smartphones can facilitate communication when changes are identified,[33] and commercially available transcutaneous monitoring can be studied remotely for an extra layer of protection.[27] The

authors advocate operative exploration whenever there is doubt, but there may be times when bedside diagnostics facilitate the decision to return to the operating theater. For example, portable near-infrared imaging devices may predict intraoperative findings when clinical findings are indistinct.[34]

CAVEATS

In the majority of cases, the blood supply to the cutaneous ALT flap is via myocutaneous perforators that traverse the vastus lateralis. Sometimes there will not be suitable perforators. When this occurs, the contingency plan may include raising a composite myocutaneous flap using the underlying vastus lateralis muscle as a carrier, extending the dissection medially as a "free-style" free AMT flap, laterally as a TFL flap, or reattempting contralateral perforator dissection[35,36] (Figure 41.6).

After the medial incision is made and the flap is reflected laterally, the quality and quantity of perforating vessels is assessed. If no perforating vessels are identified in the lateral intermuscular septum or distal vastus lateralis, perforating branches of the oblique and transverse branches are explored; the TFL flap is an attractive alternative. When fascia is desired, the TFL may be the only choice. If no perforators are found after extensive exploration, or they appear unreliable, dissection proceeds medially along the superficial plane of the rectus femoris. Efforts are made to identify perforating vessels of the AMT flap. When a promising vessel is discovered, the AMT flap can be designed about that perforator and raised. If a large flap (>25 cm of length) is needed, neither the TFL nor AMT will suffice. In these cases, it may be best to convert to the contralateral vastus lateralis myocutaneous composite flap, taking special care not to undermine the skin paddle. Another option is to harvest a distant flap like the latissimus dorsi when the contralateral thigh is not an option.

If perforating vessels are present but injured, the etiology of injury must be considered. Vessel injury attributed to the inciting trauma makes the ipsilateral ALT unreliable. In such cases, the contralateral thigh is chosen unless it too exists within the zone of injury. When both thighs are compromised, distant alternatives are the best option. Iatrogenic vessel injury warrants careful evaluation of remaining blood supply and circumstances leading to injury. One or two perforators are generally sufficient to supply a modest-sized ALT flap and dissection may proceed. However, if there is any concern of compromised or

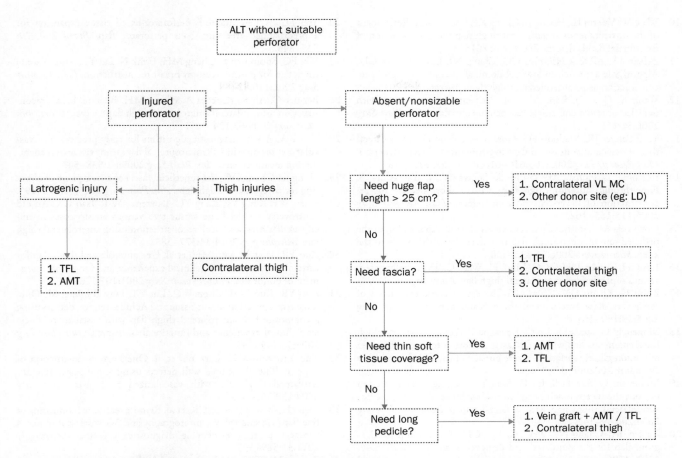

Figure 41.6. Algorithm for contingency flap harvest when anterolateral thigh(ALT) perforators are unreliable, damaged, or nonexistent. TFL, tensor fascia lata flap; AMT, anteromedial thigh flap; VL-MC, vastus lateralis myocutaneous flap; LD, latissimus dorsi flap. From Lu JC, Zelken J, Hsu CC, et al. Algorithmic approach to anterolateral thigh flaps lacking suitable perforators in lower extremity reconstruction. *Plast Reconstr Surg* 2015;135:1476–1485.

insufficient inflow after iatrogenic injury, a TFL or an AMT flap should be attempted.

CONCLUSIONS

The anterolateral thigh flap is versatile, taken either as a cutaneous or myocutaneous flap, and can be transferred microsurgically or transposed as a pedicled flap. It may include other tissue components such as tensor fascia lata, partial iliac bone, or lateral femoral cutaneous nerve. The recipient sites include scalp, head and neck, trunk, perineal, and upper and lower extremities, and the donor site morbidity is minimal.

REFERENCES

1. Song YG, Chen GZ, Song YL. The free thigh flap: a new free flap concept based on the septocutaneous artery. *Br J Plast Surg* 1984;37:149–159.

2. Wei FC, Jain V, Suominen S, Chen HC. Confusion among perforator flaps: what is a true perforator flap? *Plast Reconstr Surg* 2001;107:874–876.

3. Ali RS, Bluebond-Langner R, Rodriguez ED, Cheng MH. The versatility of the anterolateral thigh flap. *Plast Reconstr Surg* 2009;124:e395–e407.

4. Huang JJ, Wallace C, Lin JY, et al. Two small flaps from one anterolateral thigh donor site for bilateral buccal mucosa reconstruction after release of submucous fibrosis and/or contracture. *J Plast Reconstr Aesthet Surg* 2010;63:440–445.

5. Chou EK, Ulusal B, Ulusal A, Wei FC, Lin CH, Tsao CK. Using the descending branch of the lateral femoral circumflex vessel as a source of two independent flaps. *Plast Reconstr Surg* 2006;117:2059–2063.

6. Lin CH, Wei FC, Lin YT, Yeh JT, Rodriguez Ede J, Chen CT. Lateral circumflex femoral artery system: warehouse for functional composite free-tissue reconstruction of the lower leg. *J Trauma* 2006;60:1032–1036.

7. Zelken JA, Kang CJ, Huang SF, Liao CT, Tsao CK. Refinements in flap design and inset for pharyngoesophageal reconstruction with free thigh flaps. *Microsurgery* 2015.

8. Cheng MH, Huang JJ. Chapter 12: Oral Cavity, tongue and mandibular reconstructions. In PC Neligan, ed. *Plastic Surgery*, Vol. 3, 3rd ed. Oxford: Elsevier, 2013.

9. Engel H, Huang JJ, Lin CY, et al. A strategic approach for tongue reconstruction to achieve predictable and improved functional and aesthetic outcomes. *Plast Reconstr Surg* 2010;126:1967–1977.

10. Wu CW, Valerio IL, Huang JJ, Chang KP, Cheng MH. Refinement of the myocutaneous anterolateral thigh flap for reconstruction of frontonasal fistula defects. *Head Neck* 2015.

11. Zelken JA, AlDeek NF, Hsu CC, Chang NJ, Lin CH, Lin CH. Algorithmic approach to lower abdominal, perineal, and groin reconstruction using anterolateral thigh flaps. *Microsurgery* 2014.

12. Wang X, Qiao Q, Burd A, et al. Perineum reconstruction with pedicled anterolateral thigh fasciocutaneous flap. *Ann Plast Surg* 2006;56:151–155.

13. Yu P, Sanger JR, Matloub HS, Gosain A, Larson D. Anterolateral thigh fasciocutaneous island flaps in perineoscrotal reconstruction. *Plast Reconstr Surg* 2002;109:610–616; discussion 617–618.

14. Koshima I, Fujitsu M, Ushio S, Sugiyama N, Yamashita S. Flow-through anterior thigh flaps with a short pedicle for reconstruction of lower leg and foot defects. *Plast Reconstr Surg* 2005;115:155–162.

15. Gravvanis AI, Tsoutsos DA, Karakitsos D, et al. Application of the pedicled anterolateral thigh flap to defects from the pelvis to the knee. *Microsurgery* 2006;26:432–438.

16. Lin CH, Zelken J, Hsu CC, Lin CH, Wei FC. The distally based, venous supercharged anterolateral thigh flap. *Microsurgery* 2015.

17. Zhou G, Zhang QX, Chen GY. The earlier clinic experience of the reverse-flow anterolateral thigh island flap. *Br J Plast Surg* 2005;58:160–164.

18. Muneuchi G, Suzuki S, Ito O, Kawazoe T. Free anterolateral thigh fasciocutaneous flap with a fat/fascia extension for reconstruction of tendon gliding surface in severe bursitis of the dorsal hand. *Ann Plast Surg* 2002;49:312–316.

19. Muneuchi G, Suzuki S, Ito O, Saso Y. One-stage reconstruction of both the biceps brachii and triceps brachii tendons using a free anterolateral thigh flap with a fascial flap. *J Reconstr Microsurg* 2004;20:139–142.

20. Zelken JA, Chang NJ, Wei FC, Lin CH. The combined ALT-groin flap for the mutilated and degloved hand. *Injury* 2015;46:1591–1596.

21. Huang CY, Lin SH, Chuang SS. Salvage of the severely burned leg with anterolateral thigh flaps. *Burns* 2005;31:524–529.

22. Das-Gupta R, Bang C. Anterolateral thigh perforator flap from previously burned skin for secondary reconstruction of neck with post burn sequelae, new limits explored. *J Plast Reconstr Aesthet Surg* 2006;59:628–630.

23. Hallock GG. The preexpanded anterolateral thigh free flap. *Ann Plast Surg* 2004;53:170–173.

24. Tsai FC. A new method: perforator-based tissue expansion for a preexpanded free cutaneous perforator flap. *Burns* 2003;29:845–848.

25. Wei FC, Suominen S, Cheng MH, Celik N, Lai YL. Anterolateral thigh flap for postmastectomy breast reconstruction. *Plast Reconstr Surg* 2002;110:82–88.

26. Bernier C, Ali R, Rebecca A, Cheng MH. Bilateral breast reconstruction using bilateral anterolateral thigh flaps: a case report. *Ann Plast Surg* 2009;62:124–127.

27. Keller A. A new diagnostic algorithm for early prediction of vascular compromise in 208 microsurgical flaps using tissue oxygen saturation measurements. *Ann Plast Surg* 2009;62:538–543.

28. Hong JP, Chung IW. The superficial fascia as a new plane of elevation for anterolateral thigh flaps. *Ann Plast Surg* 2013;70:192–195.

29. Chen WF, Kung YP, Kang YC, Lawrence WT, Tsao CK. An old controversy revisited-one versus two venous anastomoses in microvascular head and neck reconstruction using anterolateral thigh flap. *Microsurgery* 2014;34:377–383.

30. Kuo YR, Jeng SF, Kuo MH, et al. Free anterolateral thigh flap for extremity reconstruction: clinical experience and functional assessment of donor site. *Plast Reconstr Surg* 2001;107:1766–1771.

31. Kuo YR, Kuo MH, Chou WC, Liu YT, Lutz BS, Jeng SF. One-stage reconstruction of soft tissue and Achilles tendon defects using a composite free anterolateral thigh flap with vascularized fascia lata: clinical experience and functional assessment. *Ann Plast Surg* 2003;50:149–155.

32. Kuo YR, Kuo MH, Lutz BS, et al. One-stage reconstruction of large midline abdominal wall defects using a composite free anterolateral thigh flap with vascularized fascia lata. *Ann Surg* 2004;239:352–358.

33. Engel H, Huang JJ, Tsao CK, et al. Remote real-time monitoring of free flaps via smartphone photography and 3G wireless Internet: a prospective study evidencing diagnostic accuracy. *Microsurgery* 2011;31:589–595.

34. Zelken JA, Tufaro AP. Current trends and emerging future of indocyanine green usage in surgery and oncology: an update. *Ann Surg Oncol* 2015.

35. Lu JC, Zelken J, Hsu CC, et al. In-flap anastomosis as back-up option for anterolateral thigh flaps lacking suitable perforators. *Plast Reconstr Surg* 2015.

36. Lu JC, Zelken J, Hsu CC, et al. Algorithmic approach to anterolateral thigh flaps lacking suitable perforators in lower extremity reconstruction. *Plast Reconstr Surg* 2015;135:1476–1485.

42

LATISSIMUS DORSI FREE FLAPS

David H. Song, Deana S. Shenaq, and Jesse Smith

INTRODUCTION

The latissimus dorsi free flap remains one of the most widely popular choices for complex head and neck reconstruction since its original description as a pedicled option in 1978 by Quillen[1] and later as a free flap by Watson in 1979.[2] This is due in part to its versatility, especially in the setting of the complex anatomy of the head and neck region.[2,3] Early reconstructive techniques involved the use of local tissue in a staged fashion for reconstruction. Unfortunately, these initial efforts resulted in aesthetically poor outcomes, complications, and the need for several revision surgeries. The trend has moved toward immediate, single-stage reconstruction using free tissue transfer.

The benefits of free tissue transfer in the setting of head and neck reconstruction include (1) transfer of tissue with a robust blood supply and reliable vascular pedicle, allowing for easier microvascular anastomosis; (2) more sufficient bulk as compared to local–regional flaps; (3) ability to create various flap designs; and (4) potential for composite flaps that offer greater potential to restore integrity and function, with a degree of complexity that parallels that of the multitude of defects seen in the head and neck region.

ASSESSMENT OF THE DEFECT

Head and neck defects amenable to reconstruction with the latissimus dorsi free flap may result from trauma, burns, infection, congenital abnormalities, and oncologic resection. In trauma situations, one must consider that the actual zone of injury may be larger than appreciated at the time of initial assessment as marginal tissue is allowed to demarcate. Oncologic reconstruction can be complicated by the nature of the medical therapy, and thus more aggressive treatments have resulted in defects of increasing complexity and size.

Even more so, extensive radiation injury increases the difficulty of recipient vessel harvest in addition to increasing the risk of wound healing complications, infection, and reconstructive failure.[4] Examples of common defects amenable to reconstruction using the latissimus dorsi free flap include skin defects of the neck, pharyngoesophagus, oral cavity (including through-and-through defects), parotid region defects, and scalp.

INDICATIONS

Commonly cited advantages to the latissimus dorsi free flap include ease of flap elevation, minimal donor site morbidity, ability for primary donor site closure, potential for immediate reconstruction of large defects without the need for tissue expansion given the availability of a large skin island (25 × 40 cm) devoid of hair, a long vascular pedicle (5–15 cm) that remains protected in the setting of extensive neck dissection, and the large-caliber pedicle (artery 2–4 mm and vein 2.5–4.5 mm), which allows for easier microsurgical anastomosis. Furthermore, the latissimus dorsi muscle is one of the thinnest muscles in the human body. With denervation atrophy over time, it eventually acquires the characteristics of a fasciocutaneous flap.

One indication of this broad and flat muscle is in scalp reconstruction. It can be used to cover large scalp defects as a muscle-only flap, and, when used with an overlying skin graft, it has the potential to provide good contour over time (Figure 42.1).[5]

It has also been described as a myofascial flap for coverage of the skull base, and, with inclusion of the thoracolumbar fascia, it can be used to repair dural defects. Harii published its use in facial reanimation, as he connected the thoracodorsal nerve to the facial nerve for this purpose.[6] The latissimus dorsi flap is also particularly suitable for

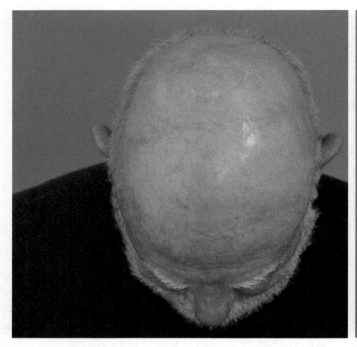 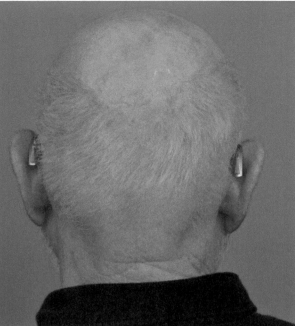

Figure 42.1. Postoperative photographs of a scalp reconstruction utilizing a latissimus dorsi muscle flap and nonmeshed, split-thickness skin graft at 10-month follow-up. Note the good contour that can be achieved. Photo courtesy of Michael A. Howard, MD.

coverage of large through-and-through defects of the oral cavity. In these instances, two skin paddles may be utilized, one supplied by the transverse branch and the other by the vertical branch of the thoracodorsal artery.[7]

For skin-only defects, the thoracodorsal artery perforator (TAP) flap is a useful modification. This flap was introduced by Angrigiani et al. in 1995,[8] and is a fasciocutaneous flap based on musculocutaneous perforators from the thoracodorsal system. It provides a relatively thin and pliable skin paddle. A single perforator may supply a skin paddle with dimensions up to 15 × 8 cm. If the patient is thin, the flap ranges from 1 to 2 cm in thickness but is variable based on the amount of subcutaneous fat present. Advantages over the traditional latissimus flap include decreased risk of seroma formation, donor-site contour deformity, and shoulder immobility postoperatively.

Another well-described modification is the muscle-sparing (MS) latissimus dorsi flap,[9] which involves harvesting a partial strip of the latissimus dorsi muscle that contains a descending branch of the thoracodorsal vessels with the flap. The transverse branch of the thoracodorsal artery and the main thoracodorsal nerve are left in situ. Including a partial strip of muscle affords the added benefit of decreased incidence of partial flap loss in addition to the benefits of decreased donor site morbidity.[10] Full strength on manual evaluation at 2 months follow-up has been reported.

The inclusion of scapular bone or rib with the latissimus dorsi muscle elevation allows for an osteomyocutaneous transfer and has been used for reconstruction of the mandible or other parts of the facial skeleton and calvarium.[11] Advantages of the latissimus-serratus-rib osteomyocutaneous free flap include its long vascular pedicle that contains large-caliber vessels that are rarely involved by occlusive disease. Furthermore, the flap pairs a long segment of vascularized bone with the option to tailor the latissimus myocutaneous component to match an overall low-volume or high-volume soft tissue defect. The main disadvantage is that the bone has a relatively thin cortical component, which is an important caveat to consider for patients who will eventually require osteointegrated dental implants.

CONTRAINDICATIONS

Preoperatively, it is necessary to review coexisting medical problems and undercover comorbidities that are potentially reversible or at least modifiable in order to best optimize the patient for surgery. Examples of important modifiable comorbidities include obesity, poor blood glucose control, malnutrition, and tobacco use. Patients with significant comorbid health issues may not be candidates for free flap reconstruction. Previous surgery, trauma, and/or local tissue damage secondary to radiotherapy may present limitations in the availability of quality donor tissue and the use of recipient vessels for free flap reconstruction. Body habitus is also a significant consideration, as patients who are obese with short necks and/or radiation fibrosis may increase the difficulty of flap harvest, inset, and final orientation.

Interestingly, the functional deficit from loss of the latissimus dorsi muscle can be upwards of 7% in most individuals. Typically, if the other muscles of the shoulder girdle are intact, then the loss of muscular function is rarely noticeable for activities of daily living. However, in paraplegics or crutch-dependent individuals, lack of latissimus dorsi function may severely weaken functional mobility and transfers. Those with neuromuscular disorders such as poliomyelitis may experience pelvic instability.[12] Therefore, in these instances, it may be prudent to pursue the muscle-sparing or TAP modifications versus another donor site altogether.

Also important in head and neck reconstruction in general is the consideration of the availability of recipient vessels. Reviewing preceding operative reports is essential. Previous surgeries such as thyroidectomy, parotidectomy, cosmetic procedures of the face and neck, submandibular gland surgery, tracheostomy, carotid endarterectomy, cervical spine fusions via an anterior approach, and neck dissections will impact the amount of scar tissue present and the availability of recipient vessels. A history of previous microvascular reconstructions will be important to note. Recognizing the inherent factors individual to each patient is critical so that the reconstruction may be tailored.

It is often assumed that superior outcomes are achieved when choosing the more sophisticated and complex option for reconstruction; however, early recognition of the contraindications to free tissue transfer during planning stages is arguably the most significant part of improving the likelihood of a successful outcome. Thoughtful and thorough consideration of all the options available is demanded of the surgeon at the time of initial assessment to identify the type of reconstruction best suited for the patient and his or her overall state of health and fitness.

ROOM SETUP

Traditionally, the latissimus dorsi flap is harvested in either the lateral decubitus or prone position. Positioning the patient in lateral decubitus allows the surgical team to raise the entire muscle, including an osseous component if necessary. The main disadvantage of this approach is the inability for two surgical teams to work synchronously in certain situations. Typically, if the recipient site is the calvarium, this can be prepared at the same time as flap harvest with greater ease than if the flap is being transferred to the neck. If the two teams are unable to work synchronously, then both ischemia time as well as the total time under general anesthesia will be lengthened. This is an important consideration during flap planning, especially for patients with extensive comorbidities.

If harvesting in lateral decubitus position, the patient is placed on his or her side using a deflatable beanbag with the operative side facing up. We prefer to rotate the table 180 degrees to allow ample room for assistants and another surgical team if feasible. Good communication with anesthesia providers is essential to ensure that the endotracheal tube is secured and there is ample extension on the circuit so that it is not tethered, particularly with neck movement (Figure 42.2).

When possible, the laterality of the donor site is ipsilateral to the recipient site to minimize repositioning. Care should be taken to avoid positioning the beanbag

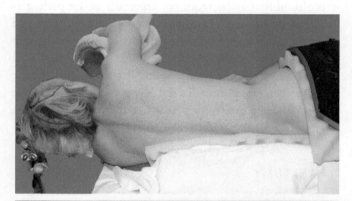

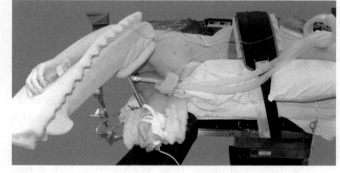

Figure 42.2. The patient is positioned in lateral decubitus with the ipsilateral arm abducted and padded on an airplane device. Shown is the contralateral arm extended and padded on an arm board with a slight bend in the elbow to prevent unnecessary hyperextension. In preparation for scalp reconstruction, the head is placed in a horseshoe device to allow for circumferential access, and the cervical spine is in a neutral position. As the bed was rotated 180 degrees to increase the amount of space available for the operative teams, an endotracheal tube circuit extension was added and secured with tape to the operative table. A seatbelt was placed over the hips. Photo courtesy of Michael A. Howard.

higher than the spinous processes posteriorly, which will serve as a landmark for flap elevation. Several unfortunate complications have been described resulting from lateral decubitus positioning, including brachial plexus, radial nerve, and other motor and sensory injuries. Therefore, an axillary roll should be placed at least three fingers breadth below the contralateral axilla in attempt to safeguard against these complications. When prepping the patient, prep the back slightly past midline. It is not necessary to include the entire arm, but we prefer to keep it in the surgical field by utilizing a sterile stockinet and placing it on an airplane device. This allows the arm to be ranged during the course of the dissection to facilitate easier pedicle harvest. Particularly useful in scalp reconstruction is positioning the head on a separate horseshoe headrest, which can provide additional cranial support while allowing more exposure. Typically, these headrests are padded to reduce the incidence of pressure necrosis and are adjustable for various head sizes. It is imperative to assure that the cervical spine is in a neutral position.

Depending on the location of the defect, intraoperative repositioning may be required, especially if the patient is positioned prone. If repositioning is necessary, then the donor site can either be closed immediately after the flap has been raised (during ischemia time) or postponed until after microvascular anastomosis and flap inset. If the donor site is to be closed immediately, it is our common practice to place the flap in a sterile plastic bag and on ice, utilizing a slurry machine to preserve the flap during ischemia time.[13]

ANATOMY

The latissimus dorsi is a large, fan-shaped muscle that arises from the spinal processes of T7–T12, the thoracolumbar fascia, the iliac crest and the lower 3–4 ribs. It inserts into the floor of the intertubercular sulcus of the humerus between the pectoralis major and teres major, allowing for adduction, medial rotation, and extension of the arm at the glenohumeral joint. The most superior aspect of the muscle and its tendon of insertion make up the posterior axillary fold, along with the teres major.

The latissimus dorsi is a Mathes and Nahai type V muscle, with its dominant arterial supply via the thoracodorsal artery (arising from the subscapular artery, supplying the proximal and lateral two-thirds of the muscle) and the perforating branches of the intercostal arteries (supplying the distal and medial portions). The lower portion of the muscle is supplied by lumbar perforators. There is typically a single venae comitantes accompanying the thoracodorsal and subscapular arteries. It is innervated via the thoracodorsal nerve, a branch of the posterior cord of the brachial plexus. The thoracodorsal nerve closely accompanies the thoracodorsal artery.

The thoracodorsal vessels course along the deep surface of the latissimus dorsi muscle along the lateral thoracic wall, consistently giving off a branch to the serratus anterior, which can serve as the vascular pedicle if the thoracodorsal vessels are inadvertently ligated. Intramuscularly, the pedicle reliably divides into two branches: the transverse branch and the vertical (or lateral) branch.[14,15] Both branches travel from the deep surface of the muscle to become intramuscular. This constant vascular anatomy is the rationale for the ability to divide the flap into two separate skin paddles.

The TAP flap is supplied by one or more perforators off the distal main thoracodorsal artery and/or its lateral branch. The first perforator is typically located 6–8 cm below the posterior axillary fold. This perforator may either branch off the distal thoracodorsal artery or arise from its lateral branch. Dissecting inferiorly, as many as three additional perforators arise at 1.5–4 cm intervals along the course of this lateral branch. Each perforator is accompanied by two venae comitantes as it travels obliquely through the muscle, coursing 3–5 cm before penetrating through the dorsal thoracic fascia to supply the overlying skin and subcutaneous tissue. The diameter of each perforating artery is approximately 0.3–0.6 mm.

Aside from the aforementioned serratus branch, extramuscularly, the thoracodorsal pedicle routinely gives off another branch to the inferior scapular angle (angular branch), which can support a bone flap based on the scapular tip. Additionally, when there is a need for an osseous component to the reconstruction, the latissimus and serratus may be easily transferred on a single vascular pedicle that includes a segment of rib. Several cadaveric studies have demonstrated the reliability of the blood supply to the rib provided by the thoracodorsal artery. The pedicle is ligated proximal to the serratus branch. Distally, the serratus branch gives rise to common slip arteries, each of which supplies adjacent slips of serratus muscle. Muscle slips 5 through 9 are consistently supplied by a single dominant branch of the thoracodorsal system. These common slip arteries measure approximately 9.5 cm in length, allowing multiple slips of muscle to be harvested and orientated independently. Communication between these vessels and the rib periosteum are most abundant near the anterior axillary line. The length of rib available for harvest varies, with lengths of 9–10 cm reported in the literature.

PATIENT MARKINGS

Important landmarks to identify and mark include (1) the anterior border of the latissimus dorsi muscle, (2) the scapular tip, (3) midline spinous processes (Figure 42.3).

It may be easiest to identify these landmarks preoperatively by asking patients to stand with their hands pressed against their hips to emphasize the anterior border of the latissimus dorsi. This border may be especially difficult to identify in obese patients. If the border is not easily identifiable, then a line may be drawn between the dorsal axillary fold and the midline of the iliac crest. Mark the superior edges of the latissimus dorsi muscle as well, if apparent. The maximum dimensions of the latissimus dorsi muscle that may be harvested are typically 20 × 40 cm.

The skin island can be designed anywhere overlying the muscle but, when possible, it should be planned along the upper two-thirds of the latissimus dorsi muscle. This is the region with the highest density of myocutaneous perforators according to anatomical studies. To facilitate primary closure of the donor site, the skin paddle should not exceed 10 cm in width.

For the muscle-sparing version, the skin island can be oriented horizontally, vertically, or obliquely. We prefer a vertical pattern for the TAP flap modification (see Figure 42.3). Before outlining the skin island, use a Doppler probe to identify perforators in a vertical direction; this step is typically unnecessary in the conventional harvest of the entire muscle given its consistent vascular anatomy. When searching for these perforators, start lateral to the anterior border of the latissimus dorsi. Ideally, identify and mark three perforators but no less than two. Measure the defect size and grossly determine the size of the skin island required. To add volume, it is essential to capture as much subcutaneous fat as possible by beveling outward, gathering an "apron" of tissue.

If planning to harvest rib, there are a few significant differences to consider in regards to markings. The surgical prep should proceed more anteriorly to the hemithorax, taking into account that communication between these distal vessels to the thoracodorsal system and the rib periosteum are most abundant near the anterior axillary line. With the patient in the lateral decubitus position, mark ribs 5 though 9 along the anterior axillary line prior to incision. This will facilitate matching the overlying skin and soft

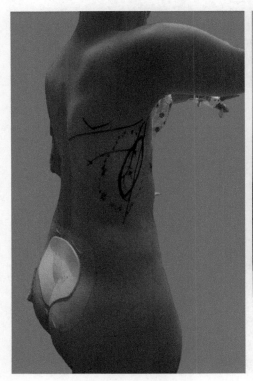
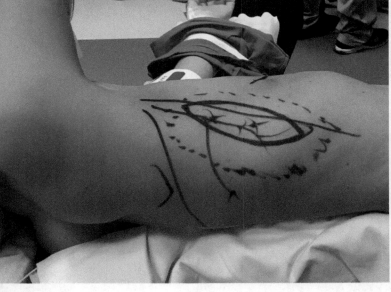

Figure 42.3. Landmarks for latissimus dorsi flap harvest include the scapular tip, the midline spinous processes, and the anterior border of the latissimus muscle. For the thoracodorsal artery perforator modification, the authors prefer a vertically oriented skin paddle (also pictured) with identification of at least two skin perforators via hand-held Doppler. Dotted lines indicate the planned undermining to capture additional subcutaneous fat in order to add volume and bulk to the reconstruction.

tissue to its corresponding rib, which can become skewed as tissues begin to shift during harvest.

OPERATIVE TECHNIQUE

If incorporating a skin paddle, the incision should begin through the skin and upper levels of the dermis and proceed through the subcutaneous tissue to the deep fascia overlying the latissimus dorsi muscle. Beveling outward from the skin edge will help to capture additional subcutaneous fat and avoid disruption of the musculocutaneous perforators. After the skin island is incised in its entirety and the deep muscular fascia is clearly visualized, flaps are raised overlying the remainder of the latissimus dorsi muscle. Proceed initially in the inferolateral and then the superomedial direction to encompass the desired amount of muscle. Dissection should continue to the most anterior aspect of the latissimus dorsi muscle in order to dissect the muscle off the serratus anterior. Distally, the latissimus dorsi muscle fibers fuse with the anterior slips of the serratus anterior muscle. Therefore, it is easier to establish a plane of dissection between these two muscles more proximally. When an adequate amount of tissue is dissected, then the latissimus dorsi muscle may be transected distally and medially.

The superior fibers of the latissimus dorsi may be identified by elevating the inferolateral border of the trapezius off the latissimus dorsi muscle. The superior aspect of latissimus dorsi is transected moving from medial to lateral, over the inferior aspect of the scapula and dissected off the adjacent teres major muscle. With the majority of the

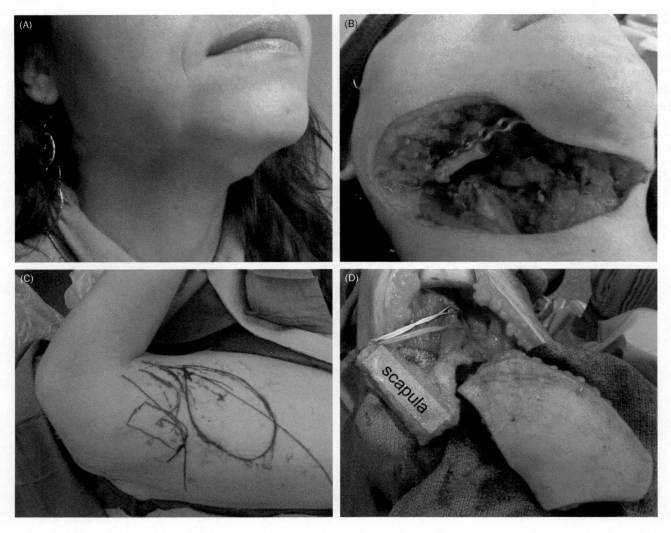

Figure 42.4. (A) A 33-year-old woman presented with a recurrent fibromyxosarcoma that was invading the mandible. A scar at the right neck was present from a prior resection. (B) The resection specimen included skin with the preexisting scar, muscle, and a segment of anterior mandible. The remaining defect is shown. (C,D) The patient was a professional dancer and preferred to avoid a fibular donor site. A latissimus osteomyocutaneous flap was planned, including a segment of scapula to reconstruct the mandibular defect. Photo courtesy of Lawrence J. Gottlieb, MD, FACS

latissimus dorsi muscle freed, the muscle is then folded upward and outward to allow dissection of its vascular pedicle with maximum exposure of the thoracodorsal system. After careful dissection of the vascular pedicle, the flap should be checked for color and bleeding at its edges prior to ligation of the pedicle to ensure its viability.

Specific to the TAP modification, the lateral edge of the skin island should be marked 1–2 cm lateral to the anterior border of the latissimus dorsi muscle to include the perforators of the descending branch of the thoracodorsal artery. Incision should proceed as described earlier until the level of the deep fascia overlying the latissimus dorsi muscle. At this level, the muscle should then be split vertically along its natural muscle fiber orientation. Dissection should begin 1 cm medial to the descending branch of the thoracodorsal artery and stop proximal to the bifurcation of the main pedicle into the descending

and transverse branches, approximately 5 cm from the posterior axillary fold. The transverse branch does not need to be included. The more inferior that the skin island is positioned on the back, the longer the pedicle length. In the muscle-sparing modification, the latissimus dorsi muscle is split longitudinally along the muscle fibers medial to the descending branch of the thoracodorsal artery. The width of this strip of muscle does not need to exceed 3 cm. Including a strip of muscle may decrease the incidence of partial flap loss.

To harvest a latissimus dorsi osteomyocutaneous chimeric flap, including rib and/or scapula, we prefer to begin the dissection by making an incision at the anterior border of the latissimus dorsi muscle.[16] The thoracodorsal vessels and its perforators to the overlying skin should be identified and preserved. Following the pedicle proximally and distally, intercostal perforators and the serratus and angular

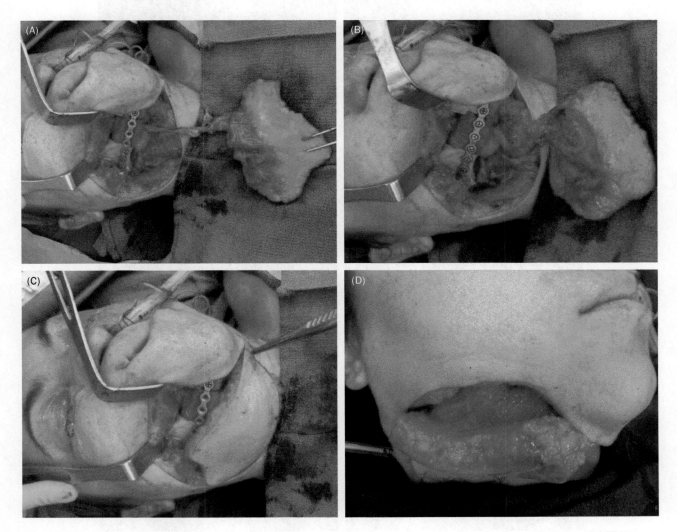

Figure 42.5. (A) The latissimus osteomyocutaneous flap with thoracodorsal pedicle has been ligated in preparation for free tissue transfer. (B) The scapular bone is inset first, prior to microvascular anastomosis. (C) The remainder of the flap is then inset, and (D) muscle is used to cover the reconstruction plate. Photo courtesy of Lawrence J. Gottlieb, MD, FACS.

branches are found. If ribs are to be harvested, typically ribs 8, 9, and/or 10 are included and dissected off the intercostal muscles. Care should be taken to preserve the intercostal nerves. When scapula is to be harvested, the angular branch of the thoracodorsal artery should be followed distally as it travels to the lateral border and tip of the scapula. The scapula is dissected free of the surrounding musculature and cut to the size of the defect. If reconstruction of a dural defect is necessary, the serratus anterior fascia supplied by the serratus branch can be included as a vascularized dural replacement. The thoracodorsal vessels should be dissected

proximally to its origin from the subscapular artery to maximize pedicle length. Once the pedicle is fully dissected and tagged with a vessel loop, the skin paddle containing the thoracodorsal perforators and the latissimus dorsi muscle can be designed based on a template of the defect size (Figures 42.4, 42.5, and 42.6).

Multiple possibilities for recipient vessels exist in the head and neck region. The superior thyroid vessels are generally a good option for lower face defects, even with concomitant neck dissections. The artery is well protected within the carotid sheath and is generally undisturbed by

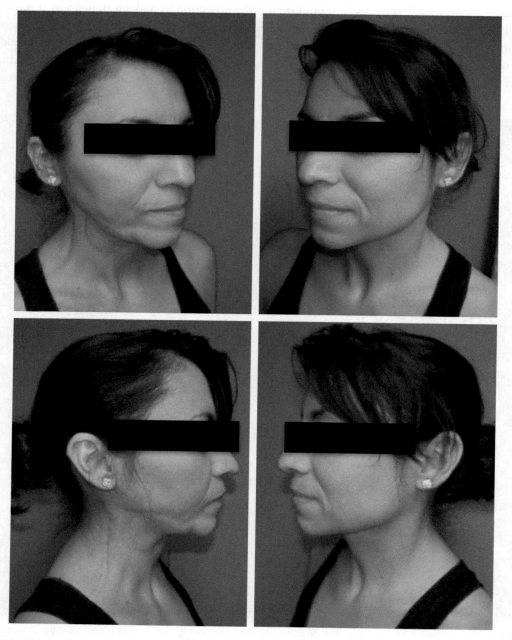

Figure 42.6. The patient subsequently underwent radiation therapy and is pictured at 3-year follow-up with a stable reconstruction. Photo courtesy of Lawrence J. Gottlieb, MD, FACS.

HEAD AND NECK SURGERY

resection and/or dissection. It must be mobilized sufficiently to provide adequate length.

The facial vessels are another good option and are easily localized by palpation against the body of the mandible. The artery can be exposed using a small incision, typically 3 cm in length centered directly over the vessel just below the body of the mandible. Take care to avoid and protect the marginal mandibular branch as it crosses over the artery. In certain cases, such as mandibulectomy, these vessels may have been ligated during the resection but often a stump of sufficient length to facilitate microvascular anastomosis may have been preserved.

If there is a history of head and neck radiotherapy, finding recipient vessels outside of the radiation zone may be necessary. The superficial temporary artery is easily localized by palpation anterior to the ear above the zygomatic arch. Given its location and reliable anatomy, it is a good choice for either upper or lower head and neck defects. However, the caliber of its terminal branch is smaller than other branches of the external carotid artery.

The transverse cervical vessels tend to be less affected by radiotherapy and are of larger caliber than the superficial temporal vessels, usually greater than 2 mm in diameter. These vessels are generally less affected by atherosclerosis as well. The transverse cervical artery originates from the subclavian artery and is located at the base of the neck just lateral to the lower third of the sternocleidomastoid muscle. When operating on the left side of the neck, there is potential for injury to the thoracic duct, and the surgeon should be mindful of this risk. One should also be prepared to explore the contralateral neck for recipient vessels and harvest a vein graft if needed.

POSTOPERATIVE CARE

The donor site is generally closed primarily in a layered fashion over a drain to reduce the risk of postoperative seroma formation, which is a common complication of full muscle harvest.

In certain instances, particularly when extended latissimus flaps have been harvested, the donor site may not close primarily or primarily closure may result in too much tension across suture lines, causing increased risk of dehiscence. Rather than using a skin graft closure, a local perforator flap can be designed to enhance the aesthetics of the donor site. Typically donor site scars can be concealed within clothing and shoulder function remains full (Figure 42.7).

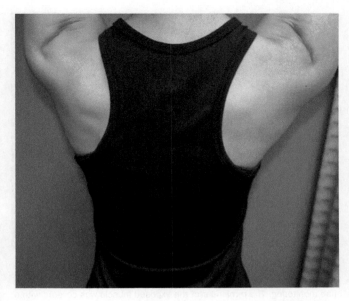

Figure 42.7. Donor site scars are well-concealed within clothing, and patients typically do not experience shoulder dysfunction. Photo courtesy of Lawrence J. Gottlieb, MD, FACS.

Postoperative care for the recipient site is variable depending on the defect and its etiology. The skin island is monitored closely in the early postoperative period. A hand-held Doppler probe is used as a supplement to clinical exam findings, allowing the user to monitor the patency of the arterial and venous anastomoses. Continuous, transcutaneous tissue oximetry (e.g., ViOptix) may also be considered in the perioperative period. If detected early, prompt re-exploration for any signs of vascular insufficiency may allow for a higher rate of flap salvage.

Prophylactic systemic antibiotics, prophylactic heparin subcutaneous injections, and conventional analgesics are used according to standard of care. Evaluation and treatment by a physical therapist can begin the first postoperative day, with a focus on early mobilization and reconditioning. Patients should be encouraged to range their shoulder to avoid stiffness.

CAVEATS

Using a latissimus dorsi muscle flap with an overlying skin graft eliminates the contour deformity and bulkiness that ensues with a skin paddle and a thick layer of subcutaneous tissue, particularly in scalp reconstruction; however, postoperative monitoring and durability of the skin may be impaired. Some surgeons choose to initially incorporate a small island of skin to facilitate flap monitoring Figure 42.8).

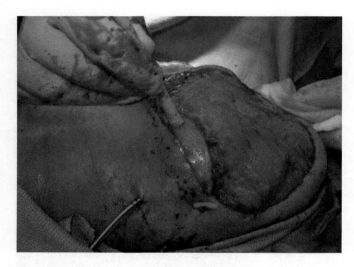

Figure 42.8. A latissimus dorsi myocutaneous flap has been used to reconstruct a scalp defect, and a small skin paddle was taken to facilitate flap monitoring. The remainder of the exposed muscle was covered with a skin graft. Photo courtesy of Lawrence J. Gottlieb, MD, FACS.

REFERENCES

1. Quillen CG, Shearin JC, Georgiade NG. Use of the latissimus dorsi myocutaneous island flap for reconstruction in the head and neck area: case report. *Plast Reconstr Surg* 1978 Jul;62(1):113–117.
2. Watson JS, Craig RD, Orton CI. The free latissimus dorsi myocutaneous flap. *Plast Reconstr Surg* 1979 Sep;64(3):299–305.
3. Shestak KC, Schusterman MA, Jones NF, Johnson JT. Immediate microvascular reconstruction of combined palatal and midfacial defects using soft tissue only. *Microsurgery* 1988;9(2):128–131.
4. Robson MC, Zachary LS, Schmidt DR, Faibisoff B, Hekmatpanah J. Reconstruction of large cranial defects in the presence of heavy radiation damage and infection utilizing tissue transferred by microvascular anastomoses. *Plast Reconstr Surg* 1989 Mar;83(3):438–442.
5. Gordon L, Buncke HJ, Alpert BS. Free latissimus dorsi muscle flap with split-thickness skin graft cover: a report of 16 cases. *Plast Reconstr Surg* 1982 Aug;70(2):173–178.
6. Harii K. Refined microneurovascular free muscle transplantation for reanimation of paralyzed face. *Microsurgery* 1988;9(3):169–176.
7. Baker SR. Closure of large orbital-maxillary defects with free latissimus dorsi myocutaneous flaps. *Head Neck Surg* 1984 Mar;6(4): 828–835.
8. Angrigiani C, Grilli D, Siebert J. Latissimus dorsi musculocutaneous flap without muscle. *Plast Reconstr Surg* 1995 Dec;96(7):1608–1614.
9. Schwabegger AH, Harpf C, Rainer C. Muscle-sparing latissimus dorsi myocutaneous flap with maintenance of muscle innervation, function, and aesthetic appearance of the donor site. *Plast Reconstr Surg* 2003 Apr 1;111(4):1407–1411.
10. Kim H, Wiraatmadja ES, Lim S-Y, et al. Comparison of morbidity of donor site following pedicled muscle-sparing latissimus dorsi flap versus extended latissimus dorsi flap breast reconstruction. *British Journal of Plastic Surgery* Elsevier Ltd; 2013 May 1;66(5): 640–646.
11. Seitz I, Adler N, Odessey E, Reid R, Gottlieb L. Latissimus dorsi/rib intercostal perforator myo-osseocutaneous free flap reconstruction in composite defects of the scalp: case series and review of literature. *J Reconstr Microsurg* 2009 Aug 13;25(09):559–567.
12. Germann G, Ohlbauer M. Latissimus Dorsi Flap. In: Wei F-C, Mardini S, eds. *Flaps and Reconstructive Surgery.* New York: Elsevier Health Sciences, 2009.
13. Francel TJ, Vander Kolk CA, Yaremchuk MJ. Locally applied hypothermia and microvascular muscle flap transfers. *Ann Plast Surg* 1992 Mar;28(3):246–251.
14. Tobin GR, Schusterman M, Peterson GH, Nichols G, Bland KI. The intramuscular neurovascular anatomy of the latissimus dorsi muscle: the basis for splitting the flap. *Plast Reconstr Surg* 1981 May;67(5):637–641.
15. Bartlett SP, May JW, Yaremchuk MJ. The latissimus dorsi muscle: a fresh cadaver study of the primary neurovascular pedicle. *Plast Reconstr Surg* 1981 May;67(5):631–636.
16. Lee JC, Kleiber GM, Pelletier AT, Reid RR, Gottlieb LJ. Autologous immediate cranioplasty with vascularized bone in high-risk composite cranial defects. *Plast Reconstr Surg* 2013 Oct;132(4):967–975.

43.

ULNAR FOREARM FLAP

Arthur Salibian

INTRODUCTION

The ulnar forearm flap was first reported by Lovie et al.[1] in 1984, 3 years after the description of the radial forearm flap by Yang et al.[2] Since then, significant clinical experience has been gained in the use of the ulnar forearm flap for comparison with its more popular counterpart, the radial forearm flap. The advantages attributed to the ulnar forearm flap include relatively hairless skin on the ulnar aspect of the forearm, thicker flap, better skin graft take over the donor site, less visible scarring on the inside of the forearm, and less donor site morbidity.[3] Disadvantages of the ulnar forearm flap relate to its shorter vascular pedicle and the proximity of the ulnar nerve to the ulnar artery, requiring careful dissection to avoid functional deficits in the hand.

The ulnar forearm flap has been mostly used as a microvascular free flap for reconstruction of head and neck defects[4] and less often for coverage of extremity defects, penile reconstruction, or as a pedicled flap[5] for hand and forearm reconstruction. I have found the ulnar forearm flap particularly helpful in microvascular reconstruction of large head and neck defects and intraoral defects that require bulk for functional reconstruction.[6,7]

ANATOMY

The forearm flap based on the ulnar artery is harvested distal to the origin of the common interosseous artery that is located 1 cm away from the bifurcation of the brachial artery into the ulnar and radial arteries. Proximally, the ulnar artery runs deep to and between the flexor digitorum superficialis and the flexor carpi ulnaris, sending off septocutaneous or musculocutaneous perforators to the skin via the medial intermuscular septum. These perforators are longer and sparser than the distal perforators, averaging two to three in number. Proximally, the median nerve is readily visible

crossing the ulnar artery, whereas the ulnar nerve cannot be visualized because of its location deep to the flexor carpi ulnaris. The ulnar nerve joins the ulnar artery distally and runs in close proximity to the artery into the wrist. The ulnar nerve gives off the dorsal sensory branch to the hand 8–9 cm from the pisiform bone. The course of the neurovascular bundle distally is more superficial, having shorter arterial perforators that directly supply the skin and the periosteum of the ulna.

The venous drainage of the ulnar forearm flap consists of a deep system comprising the venae comitantes accompanying the ulnar artery and a superficial system that includes the basilic vein, the median antebrachial vein, or other unnamed superficial veins exiting the flap proximally. The course of the basilic vein along the ulnar aspect of the forearm and its multiple tributaries draining the volar forearm are consistent. The size of the basilic vein in the antecubital area is 6 mm compared to the larger of the two venae comitantes that measures 2.5 mm.

A rare 1–6% anomaly of the ulnar artery is its superficial course proximally over the flexor carpi ulnaris and the superficial flexors of the digits. The superficial location of the artery facilitates the proximal dissection and allows the use of a longer arterial pedicle. Another more common neuronal variation (22.9%) in the proximal forearm is the Martin-Gruber anastomosis between the median and ulnar nerves.[4] The importance of these neuronal crossovers lies in their preservation to avoid motor/sensory deficits in the hand.

PREOPERATIVE EXAM AND PLANNING OF ANTEGRADE VERSUS RETROGRADE FLOW FLAP

Preoperatively, Allen's test and Doppler examination determine the patency of the ulnar and radial arteries. The superficial veins are examined in the proximal forearm, in particular the basilic vein, if they are to be used. Ultrasound exam may help in identifying patent superficial veins that are not readily visible.

The ulnar forearm flap may be used as an antegrade flow flap based on the proximal ulnar artery or as a retrograde flow flap using the distal end of the ulnar artery, depending on the size of the flap and location of the defect with respect to the recipient vessels. For transfers of small to medium-sized flaps in proximity to the recipient vessels, the proximal ulnar artery is used for the anastomosis. Larger flaps located 7–8 cm away from the recipient artery are based on the distal ulnar artery to utilize the larger surface area of the proximal forearm for coverage.

For reverse-flow flaps, the basilic vein has to be used to drain the flap because a long vein is needed to reach the recipient vein that is usually located adjacent to the recipient artery. In scalp reconstruction, a longer basilic venous pedicle may be used for a venous anastomosis to the contralateral neck.

TECHNIQUE OF FLAP ELEVATION

The following describes the harvesting of a large, distally based ulnar forearm flap covering the volar surface of the forearm. For larger flaps, the ulnar border of the flap may be safely extended three-quarters of the way over the dorsum of the forearm. The ulnar forearm flap is outlined over the ulnar artery that runs along a line drawn from the pisiform bone to a point 4 cm lateral to the medial epicondyle. In thin individuals, the groove between the flexor digitorum superficialis and the flexor carpi ulnaris may be palpated

to mark the course of the artery. The proximal border of the flap is placed 2 cm below the antecubital crease and the distal margin 2 cm proximal to the distal wrist crease. For a reverse-flow flap requiring a longer vascular pedicle, a narrow 3 cm segment of the distal forearm may be preserved in continuity with the proximal flap to include the distal cutaneous perforators.

The ulnar forearm flap is harvested under tourniquet control. Prior to inflating the tourniquet, the flap is marked, including the location of the basilic vein and superficial veins in the proximal forearm. A transverse incision is made over the proximal forearm to explore the superficial venous system and verify the patency of the basilic vein and other superficial veins draining the flap. If there are no patent superficial veins, harvesting of the flap is aborted and the opposite forearm is explored for the presence of patent veins. In the initial superficial dissection, the medial cutaneous nerve is preserved if the flap is to be used as a sensory flap.

The radial aspect of the flap is first raised suprafascially to reach the ulnar border of the flexor digitorum superficialis and identify the perforating vessels coursing through the medial intermuscular septum between the flexor digitorum superficialis and the flexor carpi ulnaris. Here the fascia is incised and the flexor digitorum superficialis retracted laterally to expose the origin of the perforators from the ulnar artery (Figure 43.1). The median nerve crossing the ulnar artery at this point is retracted laterally to expose the takeoff of the common interosseous artery. Three to four perforators originate 3–4 cm distal to the common interosseous artery and

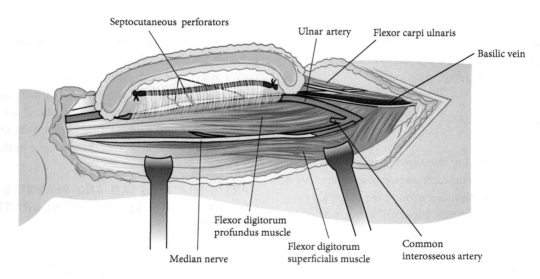

Figure 43.1. Radial aspect of raised ulnar forearm flap showing takeoff of the common interosseous artery from the radial artery and the proximal septocutaneous perforators.

course over the flexor carpi ulnaris. Proximally, the ulnar nerve cannot be visualized as it lies deep to the flexor carpi ulnaris and medial to the ulnar artery. As the dissection proceeds distally, the ulnar nerve joins the ulnar artery and accompanies it into the wrist

Next, the ulnar aspect of the flap is raised suprafascially to include the basilic vein and its tributaries draining the flap. Distally, care is taken not to injure the dorsal sensory branch of he ulnar nerve. The dissection of the ulnar artery starts distally by incising the deep fascia over the flexor carpi ulnaris and retracting the muscle medially to visualize the ulnar nerve and separate it from the ulnar artery and venae comitantes. Arterial branches to the muscle and nerve are coagulated with the bipolar current and divided. The dissection then moves proximally to identify the origin of the dorsal branch of the ulnar nerve followed by the proximal perforators running over the flexor carpi ulnaris (Figure 43.2). These perforators, which are longer than the distal ones, are carefully dissected away from the flexor carpi ulnaris. For intramuscular perforators, a cuff of muscle is included to preserve the continuity of the vessel to the skin. The flexor carpi ulnaris is then retracted medially to identify the takeoff of the common interosseous artery.

Prior to ligating the ulnar artery, the tourniquet is released and the circulation to the hand is inspected by manually occluding the distal radial artery and confirming the pulses in the digits with the Doppler instrument. The ulnar artery is then ligated distal to the common interosseous artery. If a long basilic vein is to be used, a longitudinal incision is made along the medial aspect of the arm to

harvest the vein. Other superficial veins in the antecubital area draining the flap and joining the basilic vein are also preserved.

The forearm defect is covered with a split-thickness skin graft from the thigh or a full-thickness skin graft obtained in an elliptical fashion from the groin or lower abdomen. A pressure dressing is applied over the skin graft, and the wrist and elbow are immobilized in a volar fiberglass splint. Another alternative to avoid immobilization of the forearm is to apply a vacuum-assisted compression dressing.

The design and elevation of a small ulnar forearm flap based on one or two perforators is basically the same as just described except that, prior to circumscribing the flap, the location of the proximal ulnar artery perforators is determined to ensure that they supply the flap. After siting the flap, a 6 cm incision is made along the radial border of the outlined flap to partially raise the flap and visualize the location of the proximal perforators. The design of the flap is then adjusted, moving it distally or proximally, to include the perforators supplying the flap. For small flaps, the venae comitantes are used for the venous anastomosis. The larger basilic vein may be used if superficial veins are noted to exit the flap and join the basilic vein.

Different structures, such as muscle, tendon, and bone, may be incorporated in the ulnar forearm flap for function, bulk, or structural support. If the flexor carpi ulnaris or the palmaris longus are to be included in the flap, the proximal perforators supplying the muscles are preserved. A 12 cm anterior segment of the ulna may be incorporated in the flap by preserving the distal subcutaneous perforators that

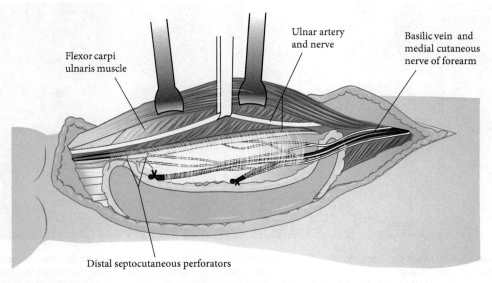

Flexor carpi ulnaris muscle

Ulnar artery and nerve

Basilic vein and medial cutaneous nerve of forearm

Distal septocutaneous perforators

Figure 43.2. Ulnar side of the flap showing the ulnar nerve completely separated from the distal septocutaneous perforators.

supply the periosteum. When obtaining a bone graft, the ulna is plated to prevent fractures.

The ulnar forearm flap may be used as a fat flap for facial contouring in hemifacial microsomia. The flap utilizes the thicker layer of fat in the proximal forearm for the facial augmentation. To harvest the fat flap, a longitudinal incision is made along the course of the ulnar artery and the skin is lifted off the subcutaneous fat to contour the fat.

INTRAORAL AND FACIAL RECONSTRUCTION

The ulnar forearm flap is most commonly used in head and neck reconstruction because of the availability of recipient vessels in the proximity of the oral or facial defect. When used as a relatively small antegrade flow flap, the short vascular pedicle of the ulnar forearm flap will reach the neck or temporal vessels for coverage of an intraoral or cheek defect (Figure 43.3). For larger intraoral defects, such as total or subtotal tongue defects or oropharyngeal-palatal defects, a reverse flow flap with a longer leash is preferable to utilize the larger and thicker proximal portion of the forearm flap for coverage. The proximal flap can be safely folded on itself to provide the necessary bulk in the oral cavity to eliminate dead space and improve function. Here, flap volume must be larger than the defect because of anticipated flap atrophy, particularly in patients who are to undergo postoperative radiotherapy. In reverse-flow flaps, in which the proximal border of the flap is situated in the oropharynx, a long basilic extended vein graft is needed to reach the neck. For large through-and-through cheek defects requiring folding of the flap for external and internal lining, a reverse-flow flap

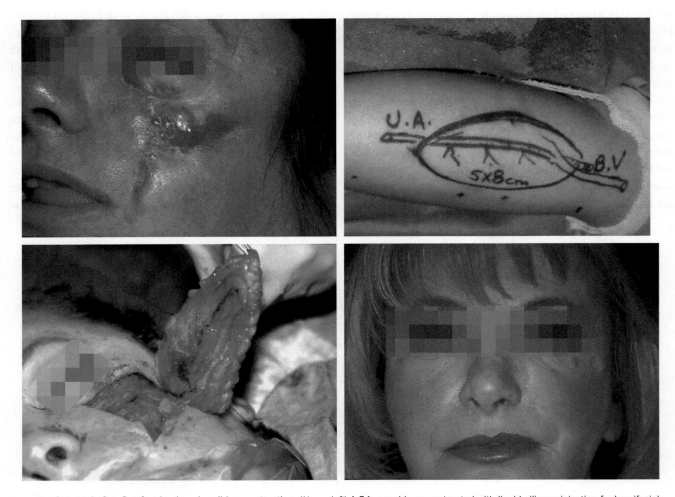

Figure 43.3. Antegrade flow flap for cheek and eyelid reconstruction. (*Upper left*) A 54-year-old woman treated with liquid silicone injection for hemifacial microsomia; the silicone extruded through the cheek and eyelid many years later. (*Upper right*) Markings of a relatively small antegrade flow flap based on the proximal perforators. (*Lower left*) Cheek defect being covered with the thick proximal forearm flap. (*Lower right*) Result at 4 years.

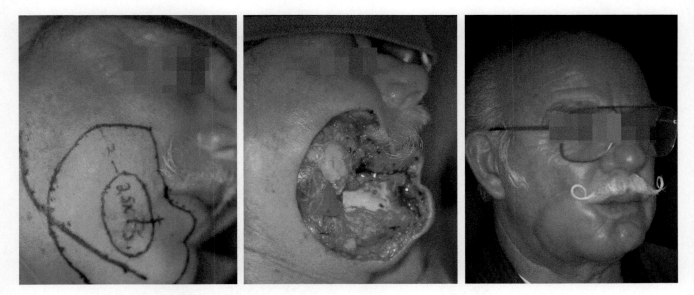

Figure 43.4. Large folded flap for through-and- through cheek defect. (*Left*) Outline of a 5 × 2.5 cm sarcoma of the cheek requiring wide excision. (*Center*) Through-and-through soft tissue defect. (*Right*) Folded large reverse-flow flap anastomosed to the external carotid artery and internal jugular vein.

is desirable to optimize the use of the thicker portion of the flap (Figure 43.4).

SCALP RECONSTRUCTION

Reconstruction of a large scalp defect may be problematic if the defect is located in the vertex and suitable recipient superficial temporal veins are not available. The superficial temporal artery, although small in caliber, is a reliable recipient artery. In contrast, the superficial temporal vein may be small and not suitable for an end-to-end anastomosis to a larger caliber vein.

For major defects involving the vertex of the scalp, a 7 cm arterial pedicle is needed to reach the defect. If used as a reverse-flow flap based on the distal ulnar artery, the wider proximal portion of the flap covers the defect, and a long basilic vein pedicle exiting the proximal end of the flap may be used to drain into the opposite neck (Figure 43.5). The distal narrower part of the flap is de-epithelialized for 7 cm and tunneled retrogradely from the scalp defect into the preauricular area. The 15 cm long basilic vein on the contralateral side is then tunneled subcutaneously in front of the ear into the opposite neck for an end-to-end anastomosis to the external

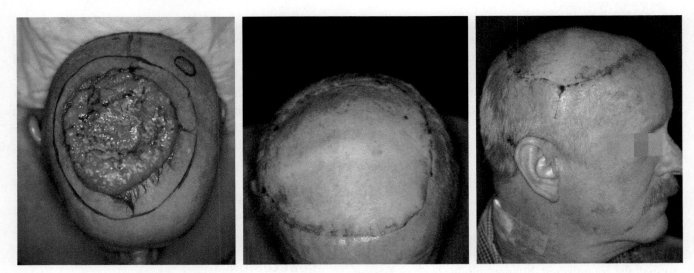

Figure 43.5. Scalp vertex reconstruction. (*Left*) Extensive squamous cell carcinoma involving the calvarium. (*Center*) Reconstruction with a reverse-flow flap using the right temporal donor artery and the left external jugular vein. (*Right*) The distal flap has been de-epithelialized and buried beneath the right temporal skin.

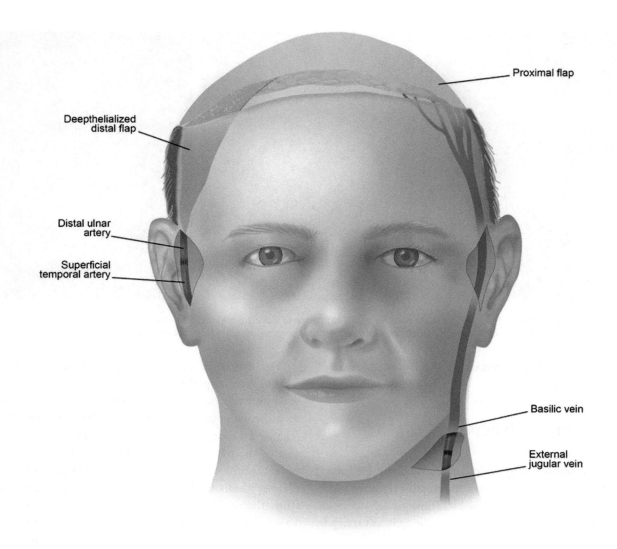

Proximal flap

Depthelialized
distal flap

Distal ulnar
artery

Superficial
temporal artery

Basilic vein

External
jugular vein

Figure 43.6. Large retrograde-flow flap covering the scalp with the basilic vein tunneled subcutaneously to the opposite neck for an end-to-end anastomosis to the external jugular vein.

jugular vein (Figure 43.6). A counterincision in the contralateral preauricular area facilitates the delivery of the vein into the neck. The venous anastomosis in the neck is performed first, followed by the arterial anastomosis in the preauricular area to minimize the clamping time of the superficial temporal artery.

TOTAL LOWER LIP RECONSTRUCTION

The size and thickness of a reverse-flow proximal ulnar forearm flap is well suited for total lower lip reconstruction. Usually a 14 cm long flap having a width of 8 cm is needed to span the commissural distance and line both surfaces of the lip by folding the flap on itself. The long axis of the flap is oriented horizontally across the proximal forearm, using the radial half of the flap for external coverage and the ulnar

half for inner lining. The ulnar end of the flap may be rolled in a "jelly roll" fashion to add bulk to the upper border of the folded flap. An acellular dermal matrix sling is then passed through the rolled flap, tunneling the ends subcutaneously through the cheeks for anchoring to the lateral infraorbital rims. The basilic vein, exiting the flap on the opposite side, is also tunneled subcutaneously into the neck for suturing end-to-end to the external jugular vein (Figure 43.7). Although this type of lower lip reconstruction provides only a static oral cavity dam, excellent oral competency and range of motion can be achieved (Figure 43.8).

CONCLUSION

The ulnar artery supplies 77% of the forearm skin with consistent proximal septocutaneous perforators.[8] This vascular

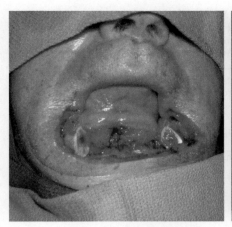 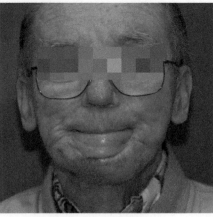 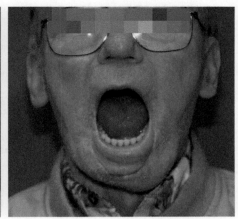

Figure 43.7. Total lower lip reconstruction in a composite defect. (*Left*) Surgical defect following resection of an invasive squamous cell carcinoma of the lip. The bone was reconstructed with an iliac crest graft, and an 8 × 14 cm ulnar forearm flap was used to reconstruct the lip. (*Center*) Complete lip apposition for oral seal. (*Right*) Full jaw opening and retention of dentures.

pattern can be used to advantage in head and neck reconstruction for coverage of large defects or contouring for bulk and functional intraoral reconstruction. For large defects, a reverse-flow flap is used with the venous outflow on the opposite end of the artery requiring the use of a long basilic vein. The basilic vein may be routed in two ways for the venous anastomosis: (1) rotate the vein from the proximal forearm end of the flap back into the distal end for a venous anastomoses adjacent to the recipient artery, or (2) route the basilic vein to the opposite neck for an end-to-end anastomosis to the external jugular vein or an end-to-side anastomosis to the internal jugular vein.

Of the more than 200 microvascular head and neck ulnar forearm flap transfers, I have always used the external carotid artery for an end–to–side arterial anastomosis, rather than an end-to-end anastomosis to the branches of the external carotid artery to avoid recipient artery spasm and possible arterial occlusion. I also prefer the superficial venous system for flap drainage because of the larger caliber vein.

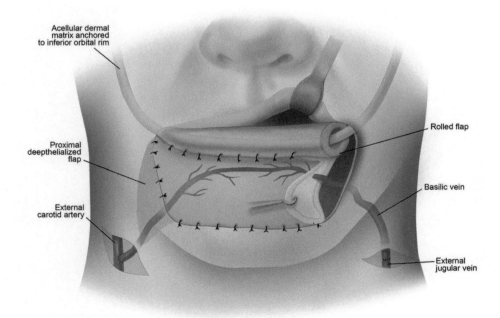

Figure 43.8. Retrograde-flow flap measuring 8 × 14 cm for total lower lip reconstruction with the basilic vein anastomosed to the contralateral external jugular vein. The radial aspect of the flap may be rolled for additional bulk along the upper border of the reconstructed lip.

REFERENCES

1. Lovie MJ, Duncan GM, Glasson DW. The ulnar artery forearm free flap. *Br J Plast Surg*. 1984;37:486–492.
2. Yang G, Chen P, Gao Y, et al. Forearm free skin flap transplantation. *Natl Med J China* 1981;61:139–141.
3. Hekner DD, Abbink JH, van Es RJ, Rosenberg A, et al. Donor-site morbidity of the radial forearm free flap versus the ulnar forearm free flap. *Plast Reconstr Surg* 2013;132:387–393.
4. Hakim SG, Trenkle T, Sieg P, Jacobsen HC. Ulnar artery-based free forearm flap: review of specific anatomic features in 322 cases and related literature. *Head Neck* 2014;36:1224–1229.
5. Glasson DW, Lovie MJ. The ulnar island flap in hand and forearm reconstruction. *Br J Plast Surg* 1988;41:349–353.
6. Salibian AH, Allison GR, Armstrong WB, et al. Functional hemitongue reconstruction with the microvascular ulnar forearm flap. *Plast Reconstr Surg* 1999;104:654–660.
7. Salibian AH, Allison GR, Krugman ME, et al. Reconstruction of the base of the tongue with the microvascular ulnar forearm flap: a functional assessment. *Plast Reconstr Surg* 1995;96:1081–1089.
8. Hekner DD, Roeling TA, Van Cann EM. Perforator anatomy of the radial forearm free flap versus the ulnar forearm free flap for head and neck reconstruction. *Int J Oral Maxillofac Surg* 2016;45:955–959.

44.

THE FREE FIBULA FLAP

Matthew T. Houdek and Steven L. Moran

INTRODUCTION

The free vascularized fibula flap, originally described by Taylor in 1975, has become the most common microvascular flap option for long bone and mandibular reconstruction following trauma and tumor extirpation.[1,2] The free fibula flap can provide up to 26 cm of straight, cortical bone and has acceptable donor site morbidity.[3,4] Published series have noted high rates of reconstructive success, with primary bony union rates of up to 80% and overall union of 97% following supplemental nonvascularized bone grafting*.[4–8]

The peroneal artery provides the vascular supply to the fibula flap, as well as to the surrounding skin and soft tissue; as such, the bone flap can be harvested with skin, muscle, and tendons supplied by the peroneal artery, allowing the surgeon to create a variety of composite flaps. Wei described in detail the peroneal artery perforators to the skin surrounding the fibula allowing for the elevation of the osteoseptocutaneous fibula flap; these skin perforators have been further studied by Yu and colleagues.[3,9] The flap can be harvested with a skin island as large as 200 cm². A reliable skin island has allowed the osteoseptocutaneous flap to become the standard for mandibular reconstruction where intraoral and extraoral coverage are often needed. The skin paddle also provides a reliable means of monitoring postoperative flap perfusion. In cases where sensation needs to be restored, the skin island of the fibula can be elevated with the lateral sural nerve to provide a neurotized septocutaneous flap. In addition, the flap can be transferred with portions of the flexor hallucis longus, soleus, and peroneus muscles to provide extra bulk for extensive soft tissue defects.

If the vascularity to the periosteum is preserved, the fibula can be osteotomized, which allows the creation of

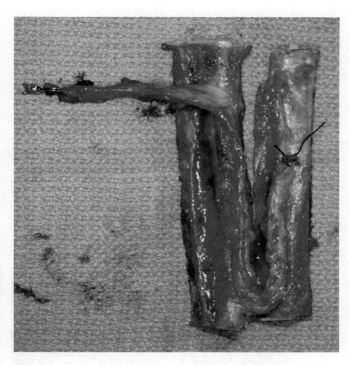

Figure 44.1. An example of a double-barrel fibula graft. Note the peroneal pedicle is attached to both segments of the bone.

several smaller vascularized bony segments attached by a common peroneal pedicle. These vascularized segments can be folded to create a double- or triple-barrel fibular strut graft, which is valuable for reconstruction of the femur, spine, and humerus (Figure 44.1). Using this technique the fibula can also be reshaped to create a neomandible.[10–12] Finally, the vascularized fibula is capable of hypertrophy over time, thus its diameter can increase, allowing it to bear increasing load in the lower extremities.[2,10] In this chapter, we provide our indications for the use of the free fibula and free fibula

* No conflicts of interest are declared by any author on this study. No disclosures of funding were received for this work from NIH, Wellcome Trust, or HHMI.

osteoseptocutaneous flap with techniques for safe and reliable dissection.

SURGICAL INDICATIONS

For reconstruction of the upper and lower extremities, utilization of the free fibula graft is usually reserved for defects longer than 5 cm in length. For bone defects less than 5 cm, nonvascularized cancellous or cortical cancellous grafts can be used for bone reconstruction. For specific areas like the humerus or femur, substantial shortening of the bone can be tolerated with minimal functional deficit, thus obviating the need for bone graft in some cases; however, decisions to shorten bones should be made in consultation with an orthopedic surgeon. Other indications for vascularized bone grafts include those circumstances where the potential for bony healing is compromised within the wound environment, such as in cases of soft tissue infection, osteomyelitis, radiation, and avascular necrosis. In these circumstances, a free fibula flap or other form of vascularized bone graft may be required to achieve bony union despite a bone defect of less than 5 cm. Other choices for vascularized bone graft include the medial femoral condyle flap, the lateral femoral condyle flap, the iliac crest bone flap, scapular flap, and vascularized rib grafts.[13] A description of each of these flaps is beyond the scope of this chapter, but each flap has its own

benefits and specific donor site morbidity. All vascularized bone options should be considered when evaluating any bony defect to provide the patient with the best reconstructive outcome. Our current recommendations for the use of the vascularized fibular graft in the adult are (1) bone defects greater than 5 cm in length; (2) defects less than 5 cm in size, but in areas of compromised bone healing; and (3) composite defects requiring both skin and bone. Indications for the use of the vascularized fibula graft within specific anatomic regions are described in the following sections.

UPPER AND LOWER EXTREMITIES

The diaphysis of the radius and ulna are similar to the size and shape of the fibula, allowing for straight segmental reconstruction within the forearm. For forearm reconstruction, the use of a free vascularized fibula has been associated with 85–89% graft union.[5,8,14,15] Likewise, diaphyseal bone defects of the humerus can be reconstructed with a fibula graft; however, the diameter of the fibula is smaller than the humerus, which can prove challenging for bone fixation, and its use can be associated with a high rate of graft fracture (Figure 44.2).[16,17] To limit the chance of fracture in cases of humeral reconstruction, we advocate for the use of a rigid compression plates.

In the lower extremity, the fibula can be used to reconstruct the tibia and femur in the setting of segmental bone

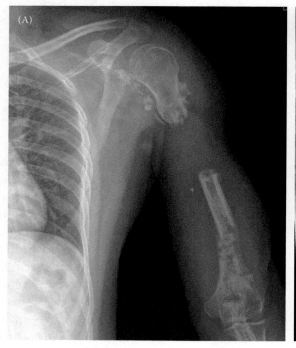
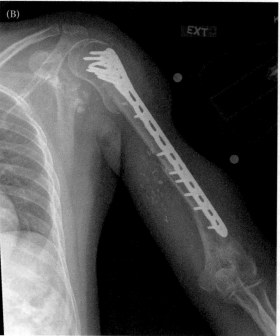

Figure 44.2. Reconstruction of the humerus using a vascularized fibula and a spanning plate. (A) The original segmental defect can be seen in this anteroposterior (AP) radiograph. (B) A vascularized fibula was used in conjunction with a spanning locking plate for reconstruction. AP radiograph shows result at 4 months. Note that fibula was intussuscepted into the native bone ends, and unicortical screws were used for fixation of graft.

loss, pathologic fracture, failed allograft, and radiation-induced nonunions. Intercalary reconstruction of the femur and tibia with the fibula alone can result in repeated fibular stress fractures due to the fibula's poor size match for the diameter of the native bone. Due to this biomechanical mismatch, our preference is to perform these reconstructions with (1) the use of a double barrel fibular construct, (2) utilize a spanning locking plate or intramedullary nail to augment any remaining native bone, or (3) in oncologic cases supplement the fibula with a bulk structural allograft (historically described as the Capanna technique).[18]

In the setting of traumatic bony defects of the lower extremity, the timing to reconstruction has been debated. Recent reports suggests that radical debridement and reconstruction with immediate vascularized bone grafts leads to high salvage rates and low levels of postoperative infection.[19,20] We advocate for free tissue transfer at the time of definitive fixation if the wound bed is clean and the patient is medically appropriate for free tissue transfer. Unlike the upper extremity, where amputation is associated with poor clinical outcomes, in the lower extremity, the treating surgeon must determine if it is technically possible to save the lower extremity and if salvaging the limb is in the best interest of the patient. If limb salvage resulted in a painful or chronically unstable leg, this may hinder functional recovery, and the patient may be better served with an amputation.

For oncologic reconstruction, the use of Capanna technique combines the biological benefits of the vascularized free fibula and the structural support of cortical allograft. Currently, this is our preferred technique to reconstruct pediatric oncologic defects of the lower extremity.[21] Recent publications have note a 94% limb salvage rate utilizing the Capanna technique for reconstruction of intercalary defects of the tibia and femur following tumor extirpation in the pediatric age group[22] (Figure 44.3).

AVASCULAR NECROSIS OF THE FEMORAL HEAD

The vascularized fibula flap has been used to treat osteonecrosis of the femoral head for several decades. In these cases the fibula is placed into the center of the femoral head in an intramedullary fashion; these cases are most often performed without the use of a skin paddle.[23] Experimental models have shown that vascularized bone flaps are capable of repairing necrotic bone through a process of neovascularization and bone growth from the vascularized flap into necrotic areas.[24] Clinical studies by Urbaniack and others have shown clinical and radiographic improvement in the femoral head following flap transfer for avascular necrosis (AVN).[23] Long bone nonunions, secondary to

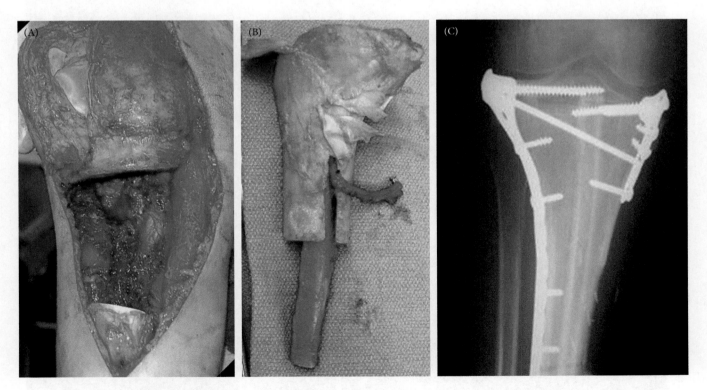

Figure 44.3. An example of the Capanna technique in a 15-year-old boy with Ewing's sarcoma of the tibia. (A) Intercalary defect of tibia. (B) The Capanna construct, which consists of a vascularized fibula doweled inside a massive cadaveric allograft. (C) Anteroposterior (AP) radiograph of tibia showing healing at the proximal metaphyseal junction at 3 months.

THE FREE FIBULA FLAP

osteoradionecrosis, have also been shown to heal following treatment with vascularized fibular grafts.[6]

AXIAL SKELETON AND PELVIS

Autologous bony reconstruction of the axial skeleton and pelvis may be required following resection of multiple vertebrae or large portions of the pelvis and sacrum. The free fibula can be used to enhance or restore the structural integrity of the spine, sacrum, and pelvis.[25,26] For spinal reconstruction, the fibula can be placed either in an anterior or posterior position to enhance stability and accelerated bone graft incorporation.[25,26] For sacropelvic reconstruction, following partial or total sacrectomy a single- or double-fibula transfer is often used to provide structural support to the pelvis[26] (Figure 44.4).

MANDIBULAR RECONSTRUCTION

The free fibula is the first choice for mandibular reconstruction following tumor extirpation. The fibula can be used in all patients, including those who require replacement of

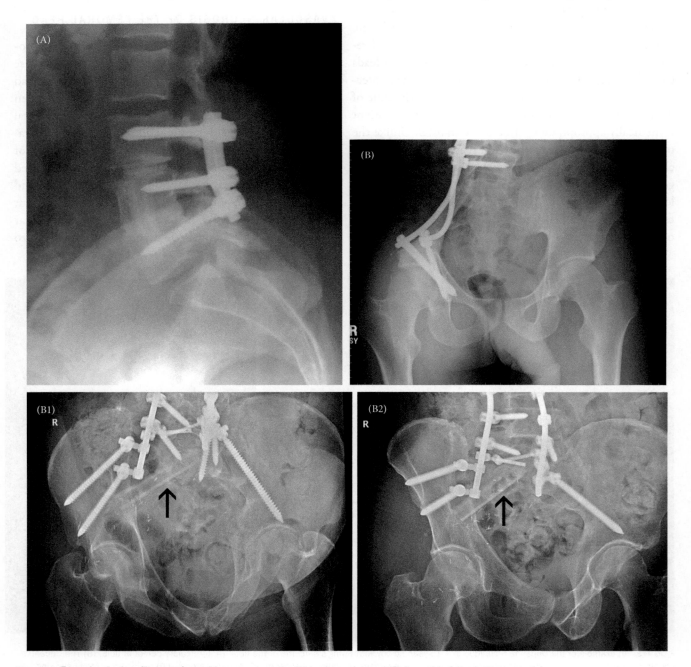

Figure 44.4. Example of a free fibula graft used to reconstruct the (A) lumbar spine and (B) the pelvis following tumor excision.

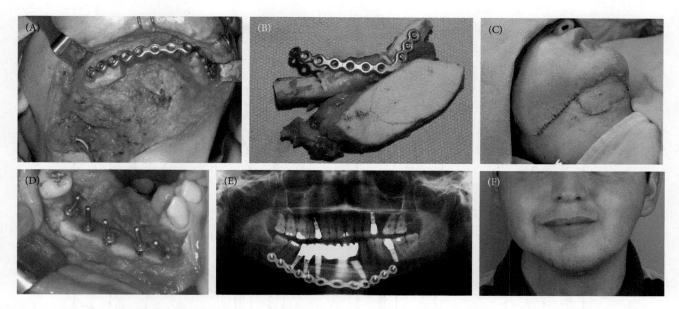

Figure 44.5. (A) Mandible reconstruction with a free fibula in a 26-year-old solider following loss of his parasymphyseal region in an explosion. (B) Three osteotomies are used to construct a new mandible, which is fit to the precontoured reconstruction plate shown in (A). (C) A skin paddle is used to close the external soft tissue defect. (D) In a second stage, osteointegrated implants are placed allowing for correction of occlusion (E) and improved cosmetic appearance (F).

the overlying skin, intraoral mucosa, or both (Figure 44.5). Excellent results can be obtained in patients with benign pathologic conditions or low-grade malignancies affecting the mandible where only the bone needs to be excised. These patients may also be candidates for primary placement of osteo-integrated dental implants during the initial surgery.

Advanced carcinomas of the mandible are frequently associated with involvement of adjacent internal and external soft tissue structures. Treatment of these cancers can result in large soft tissue defects. In such cases, the skin provided by fibula osteocutaneous flap alone may be inadequate for total reconstruction. To overcome these situations, another free flap may be required in combination with the fibula osteoseptocutaneous flap. The free fibula is used for bony reconstruction and coverage of one surface (intraoral or extraoral), and an anterolateral thigh flap or radial forearm flap is used to provide bulk and cover the other surface. The second flap may be anastomosed to the distal runoff of the peroneal vessels or to a separate recipient artery and vein.

Reconstruction of the mandibles complex anatomy has been simplified with the use of three-dimensional printed models and templates. Prior to this technique, surgeons relied on the intraoperative evaluation and free-hand cutting to create a new mandible, which could lead to imperfect results. Now computer-aided design (CAD) software can be used to create precision cutting guides which can be used in the operating room to improve postoperative occlusion and aesthetic outcome.[27]

CONTRAINDICATIONS

Contraindications to using the vascularized fibula flap include technical inability to harvest the flap due to previous fibular fracture or fibula surgery. Any history of injury to the peroneal artery may prevent successful harvest of the flap. Also, one must rule out the presence of vascular occlusive disease and vascular anomalies such as the peroneal magnus artery, which would prevent peroneal arterial sacrifice. While controversial, we perform a computed tomography (CT) angiogram on all patients prior to fibula harvest to rule out peroneal artery occlusion, confirm the presence of a peroneal magnus artery, and verify adequate inflow to the foot through the posterior tibial and anterior tibial artery, thus allowing sacrifice of the peroneal artery without concern for foot ischemia (Figure 44.6).

SURGICAL PLANNING

Careful preoperative planning is essential for a successful procedure. Planning can be significantly aided with a thorough clinical exam of the extremity, plain radiographs, CT angiogram, and cross-sectional imaging (CT, CT angiogram, or magnetic resonance imaging [MRI]). Recently, modeling with three-dimensional printed templates has

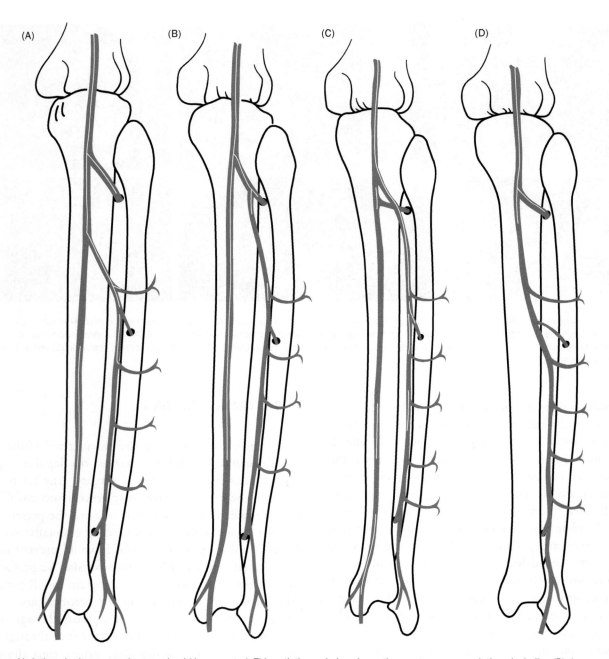

Figure 44.6. Variations in the peroneal artery should be expected. This artistic rendering shows the most common variations including (B) the peroneal artery originating from the anterior tibial artery, (C) the peroneal artery arising from the popliteal artery, and (D) the peroneus magnus artery, in which case the peroneal artery replaces the posterior tibial artery.

significantly aided preoperative planning by allowing the surgeon to visualize the potential defect and adequately plan and template for the procedure.[28]

Depending on the indication for the free fibula flap, consultation with a multidisciplinary surgical team is recommended. In the setting of an oncologic resection, our preference is for immediate reconstruction following tumor extirpation if the wound is clean and the tumor surgeon is satisfied with the surgical margins. For traumatic

defects, we recommend serial debridements followed by subsequent flap coverage at the time of definitive bone fixation. If the wound bed is considered to be "dirty" in either the oncologic or traumatic setting, a negative-pressure wound dressing is used for temporary wound coverage in conjunction with an external fixator. Serial debridements are then performed until the wound is clean, at which point we proceed with reconstruction and definitive bony fixation.

FLAP ANATOMY

The blood supply to the fibula is based on an endosteal and periosteal vascular network. The endosteal blood supply arises from a branch of the peroneal artery. The peroneal artery originates from the posterior tibial artery distal to the popliteal fossa. It branches from the posterior tibial artery approximately 3 cm distal to the popliteal muscle and the take off the anterior tibial artery (Figure 44.7). At a level approximately 7 cm below the head of the fibula, the peroneal vessel passes between the soleus and the tibialis posterior muscle. The peroneal artery then runs dorsal and posterior to the tibialis posterior muscle and anterior and ventral to the flexor hallucis longus muscle as it abuts the fibula (Figure 44.8). The nutrient artery to the fibula is typically found 6–14 cm distal to the peroneal take off. This nutrient artery typically enters in the middle third of the bone's diaphysis and divides into ascending and descending branches. In addition to supplying the fibula, the

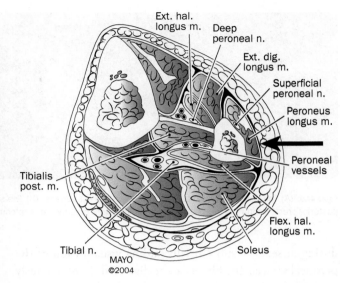

Figure 44.8. Cross-sectional anatomy of vascularized fibular bone graft. Harvest of the fibula is usually performed through a lateral approach in the interval created between the peroneus longus and soleus muscles. The peroneus muscles are elevated to the anterior crural septum, which is divided to elevate the anterior compartment muscles.

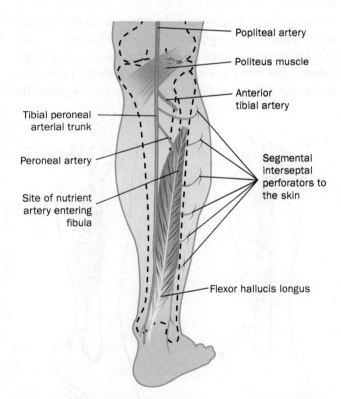

Figure 44.7. Artist's rendering of the vascular anatomy of the posterior leg. In most cases, the peroneal artery arises from the posterior tibial artery 3 cm below the popliteal muscle and the take-off of the anterior tibial artery. The artery courses between the posterior tibialis muscle and the flexor hallucis longus (FHL) as it gives off a nutrient artery to the fibula. (1) popliteal artery (2) tibial peroneal arterial trunk (3) peroneal artery (4) anterior tibial artery (5) site of nutrient artery entering fibula (6) Segmental interseptal perforators to the skin (7) Flexor hallucis longus (8) politeus muscle.

peroneal artery sends multiple perforating vessels to the skin of the lateral lower leg and muscles of the deep compartment of the leg.

The peroneal artery's diameter at its origin from the posterior tibial artery can range from 1.5 to 4 mm. The artery is usually accompanied by two venae comitantes, which are typically larger in diameter than the artery. If the flap is going to be harvested as an osteoseptocutaneous flap, the dominant cutaneous perforators to the skin overlying must be included in the flap. These perforators are typically located in the lower two-thirds of the leg over the posterior border of the fibular shaft.[9] These perforators run within the posterior crural septum.

FLAP HARVEST

PATIENT POSITIONING

The patient is typically positioned supine; however, in cases of posterior reconstruction (such as in cases of sacral, spinal, or pelvic reconstruction), the fibula harvest can be performed with the patient in the prone position. The flap can be harvested under tourniquet control. When the patient is positioned supine, we prefer to place the knee in mild flexion. Flexing the knee allows the soleus and posterior compartment musculature to fall away from the fibula

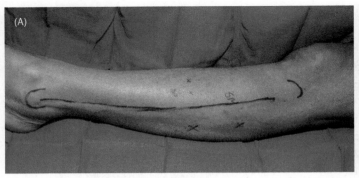
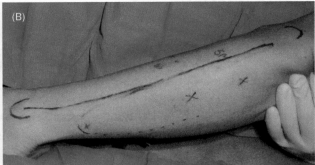

Figure 44.9. (A) The contour of the fibula is marked on the leg surface. (B) The skin island is centered over the posterior long axis of bone, where the posterior crural septum is located. Cross mark indicates presence of septocutaneous perforator, identified with hand-held Doppler.

during dissection, substantially adding visualization of the peroneal vessels. The fibula can be dissected simultaneously while the extirpative team is working on the involved extremity or in the mouth. The ipsilateral or contralateral fibula can be harvested; however, in cases of lower extremity trauma or tumors involving the tibia, we rarely harvest the ipsilateral fibula as this may contribute to further ipsilateral leg instability.

Flap Design

The flap is outlined with the patient in supine position. Although it might not necessarily be used for soft tissue coverage, a small skin island is always included with the fibula flap as a means of monitoring the flap's viability in the postoperative period. Skin markings begin by outlining the contour of the fibula over the skin surfaces (Figure 44.9). The long axis of the skin island is centered over the posterior border of the fibula at the junction between the middle and distal third of the fibula; this junction is where most of the septocutaneous perforators are localized.[9] A hand-held Doppler can be used to identify the septocutaneous perforators in this area. One or two sizable septocutaneous perforators are generally sufficient to provide blood supply to a skin island 22–25 cm in length and 10–14 cm in width (Figure 44.10). If the skin island exceeds 3–4 cm in width, direct closure of the donor site defect in the leg may not be possible; in such cases, we recommend a split-thickness skin graft for coverage of donor site to avoid excessive tension during closure. Excessive tension during closure can result in the development of a compartment syndrome and thus should be avoided. At least 6–8 cm of the distal fibula should be left intact to prevent ankle instability. Proximally, an osteotomy just below the neck of the fibula facilitates dissection of the peroneal vascular pedicle and maximizes fibular length.

FLAP DISSECTION

There are two described methods for fibula harvest: a posterior approach was originally described by Taylor but we prefer a lateral approach, which has gained popularity with most surgeons.[1,29] To begin the lateral approach for an osteocutaneous fibular flap, the outlined skin island is incised over the anterior border down to the deep fascia. Once the fascia is visualized, dissection is carried superior and inferior in this suprafascial plane to allow one to identify the interval between the soleus and the peroneus longus muscle. This is the interval through which the perforators to the skin will pass within the posterior crural septum. The

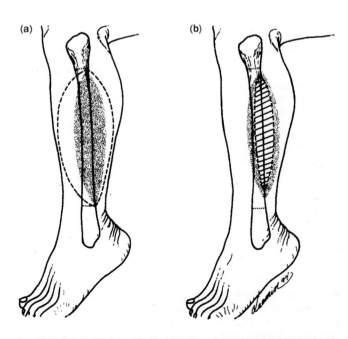

Figure 44.10. (Large skin island (dotted line, A) or small skin island (striped area, B) can be included with fibula bone, centered on posterior crural septum. However, in both instances, anterior incision of fascia (shaded area) should always be localized posterior to anterior crural septum to prevent injury to deep peroneal nerve; posterior incision should preserve the sural nerve.

location of the septum can be identified through the fascia by the presence of a fat stripe on the posterior aspect of the peroneus longus tendon adjacent to the posterior crural septum. It must be emphasized that the perforators to the skin island run within this septum and must be preserved if a skin island is to remain viable (Figure 44.11).

Once the septum is identified, the fascia of the skin island overlying the peroneus muscles can be incised. This allows one to raise the skin island to the anterior border of the crural septum. At this point, one will see the perforators entering the skin flap. The posterior incision of the skin flap may now be made down to the deep fascia. The deep fascia

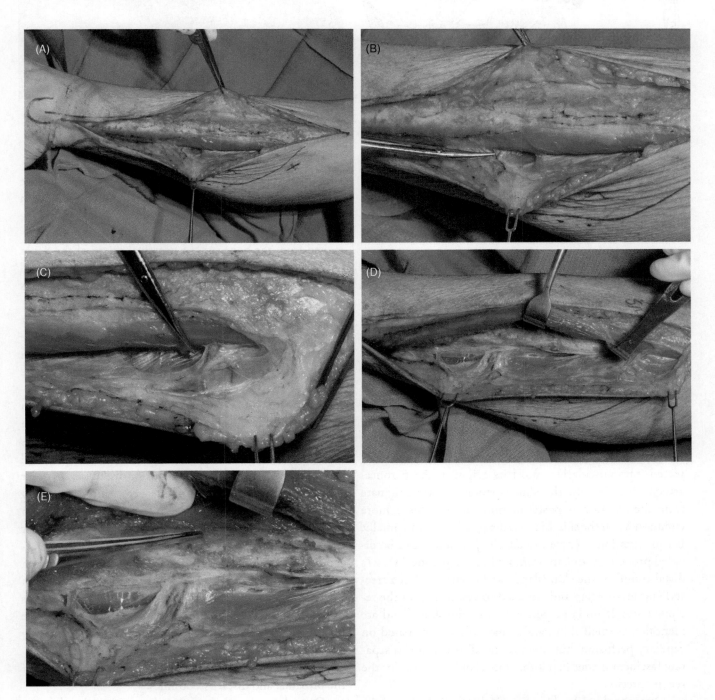

Figure 44.11. (A,B) Dissection begins by elevating the anterior aspect of the incision until one identifies the interval between the peroneus muscles and the soleus. The fascia covering the peroneus muscle is elevated to reveal the perforators passing posterior to the fibula in the posterior crural septum (C). Once the perforators are clearly identified, the posterior margin of the skin island can be dissected. The fascia is elevated, moving toward the interval between the peroneus and soleus. Once one is sure the perforators are protected, one may elevate the lateral and anterior compartment muscles off the fibula (D,E).

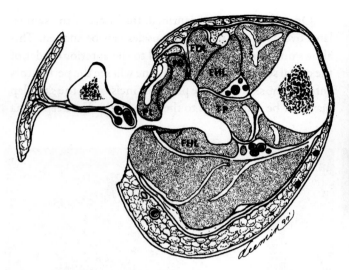

Figure 44.12. The skin island is preserved within the posterior crural septum. Image shows artist's rendering of a transverse section through proximal third in left leg. Anatomic relations of fibula and muscles divided during dissection of flap. PL, peroneus longus muscle; PB, peroneus brevis muscle; EDL, extensor digitorum longus; EHL, extensor hallucis longus; TP, posterior tibialis; FHL, flexor hallucis longus.

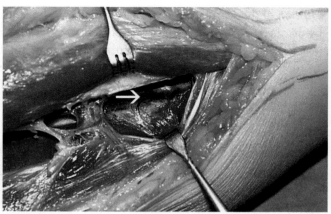

Figure 44.13. The peroneal vessels (arrow) can be visualized at flexor hallucis longus (FHL) origin.

of the skin flap is elevated off the gastrocnemius and soleus muscle. The sural nerve and lesser saphenous vein should be preserved during this portion of the dissection to minimize donor site morbidity. The skin island will now be attached to the leg only by the thin transparent posterior crural septum (Figures 44.11 and 44.12).

Although rare, anatomic variations in the blood supply to the skin island may be encountered; these include the absence of septocutaneous perforators with the presence of myocutaneous perforators only and the absence of both septocutaneous and myocutaneous perforators.[9] In the first instance, the myocutaneous vessel can be dissected intramuscularly toward its origin in the peroneal artery. Occasionally, the skin perforators may originate from the anterior or posterior tibial artery; this is more common when the skin island is designed more proximally. If this situation is encountered, the perforator can be divided proximally and anastomosed to the peroneal vessel's distal runoff or the skin island can be harvested as a free-style perforator flap and attached to vessels within the recipient site. If no large perforators to the skin island are identified, a small skin paddle may still survive based on capillary perfusion, but one may need to consider a separate fasciocutaneous flap if the skin island is critical for the reconstruction.

Once the skin island has been isolated, dissection of the fibula precedes by bluntly developing a plane between the soleus and peroneus muscles. The thick fibrous attachments of the proximal soleus are then separated from the fibula.

Large perforating branches from the peroneal vessels to the soleus must be ligated. Once the soleus muscle has been separated from the fibula, the thin membrane over the flexor hallucis longus muscle is divided and the muscle is detached from the bone. At the proximal origin of the flexor hallucis longus muscle one can now visualize the peroneal vessels as they pass anterior to the flexor hallucis longus muscle (Figure 44.13).

At this point, we now dissect the lateral compartment off the fibula. The peroneus longus and brevis muscles are lifted from the bone to expose the anterior crural septum between the lateral and anterior compartment muscles. The anterior crural septum is divided and the extensor muscles (digitorum and hallucis longus) are detached from the bone. Extraperiosteal dissection is performed leaving a 1–2 mm cuff of muscle on the bone until the interosseous membrane is identified. Superiorly, the common peroneal nerve is identified and protected during dissection. In order to protect the deep branch of the peroneal nerve during the cephalad portion of the fibula dissection, we perform subperiosteal dissection over the proximal anterior border the fibula as we pass below the proximal portion of the extensor hallucis longus muscle and the extensor digitorum muscles (Figure 44.14). One can identify the branches from the peroneal nerve running on the deep posterior surfaces of these muscles. The interosseous membrane can now be identified and if adequately visualized it may be sharply divided. In some cases, division of the interosseous membrane can be performed more easily following creation of the proximal and distal osteotomies.

Once the peroneal vessels have been exposed and the interosseous membrane has been identified, one may create the proximal and distal osteotomies. The osteotomy sites are marked and the periosteum is stripped off a few millimeters

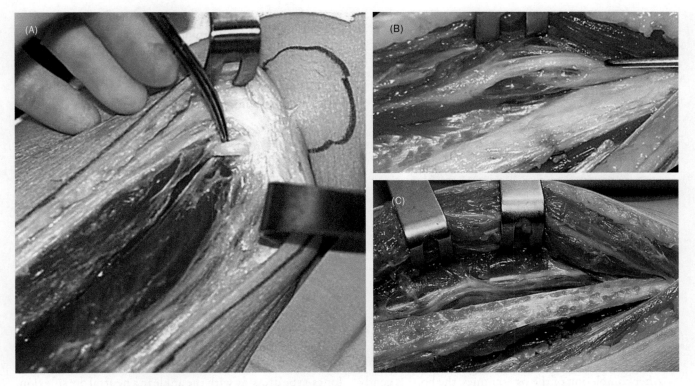

Figure 44.14. (A) The common peroneal nerve is identified at the superior margin of the incision prior to dissection of the lateral compartment muscles. (B) The deep peroneal nerve runs close to the anterior fibular surface. In an effort to protect the nerve, subperiosteal dissection can be used at this level until the deep peroneal nerve and anterior tibial vessels are clearly visualized (C).

from the bony circumference. Care is taken to leave a large periosteal cuff for later transfer to the recipient site. We prefer to perform the distal osteotomy first. Large Chandler retractors are placed below the bone to protect the underlying peroneal artery. A Gigli saw or oscillating saw is used to create the osteotomy. The proximal osteotomy is made in a similar fashion (Figure 44.15). The proximal osteotomy is made just distal to the neck of the fibula; this proximal osteotomy can help with the exposure and dissection of

the peroneal vascular pedicle. Careful attention is paid to protecting the peroneal vessels during the osteotomy as small veins can tear and bleed during this portion if one fails to adequately mobilize the vessels prior to the osteotomy. At least 6 cm (typically 7–8 cm) of the distal fibula should be left intact to prevent valgus ankle instability. In children, a distal tibiofibular arthrodesis (syndesmosis) should be performed in order to prevent late ankle instability during growth (Figure 44.16).

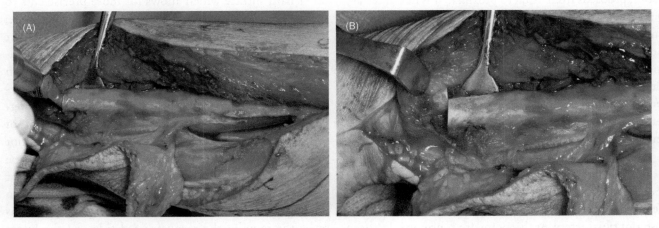

Figure 44.15. (A) Chandler retractor is used to protect the underlying structures as the distal osteotomy is created made. (B) Bone end following distal osteotomy.

THE FREE FIBULA FLAP

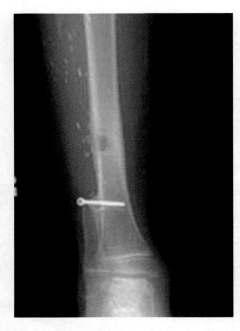

Figure 44.16. An example of a syndesmosis screw used to fuse remaining stump of fibula to the tibia.

After completion of the osteotomies, the bone is gently retracted outward from the leg distally and proximally using bone clamps (Figure 44.17). This maneuver facilitates exposure of any remaining anterior compartment muscles attached to the bone. The interosseous septum is now more easily identified and divided. Once the interosseous membrane is divided, the outward traction applied to the bone is maximized to enhance the pedicle dissection. During this dissection, the distal ends of the peroneal artery and vein are identified, ligated, and divided (Figure 44.18). The posterior tibialis muscle is sectioned close to the bone. The peroneal vessels lie in close contact with the deep surface of the muscle, surrounded by a thick membrane, which should be opened carefully to expose the vessels. Vessel dissection proceeds from distal to proximal. It is not necessary to include part of the posterior tibialis or extensor hallucis longus muscles in the dissection of the peroneal vessels, but the septocutaneous perforators must be carefully preserved since they pass from the peroneal vessels to the septum within these muscles, close to the bone. If considered prudent, a minimal cuff of muscle could be included with the peroneal vessels to prevent sectioning the septocutaneous perforator vessels to the skin.

The vessel dissection is carried to the level of the origin of the flexor hallucis longus tendon, which is divided from the fibula. The vessels are followed to the tibial peroneal trunk. Here, we verify the location of the posterior tibial nerve and posterior tibial artery. At this point, if a tourniquet has been used for dissection, the tourniquet is released and perfusion to the fibula and foot are confirmed. The flap is allowed to reperfuse for at least 20 minutes prior to separation of the flap. During this time, hemostasis is obtained. The peroneal artery and venae comitantes are then clamped and ligated as proximally as possible. The graft is then transferred to the recipient site for implantation.

DONOR SITE CLOSURE

The donor site is carefully examined for any signs of bleeding prior to closure. The flexor hallucis longus muscle is sutured back to the posterior tibialis muscle and interosseous membrane with absorbable sutures. If the flexor hallucis longus muscle is devitalized, we prefer to excise the muscle entirely rather than risk the development of late muscle necrosis, possible infection, or a great toe flexion contracture. A suction drain is placed between the anterior and posterior compartment muscles. The skin incision is either primarily closed or skin-grafted, depending on the size of the skin paddle that was removed. The patient is then placed in a bulky Robert Jones-type dressing with the ankle in a neutral dorsiflexion position. This is then removed 72 hours postoperatively and converted to a walking-boot. If no other orthopedic contraindications exist, the patient is allowed to weight-bear as tolerated.

OSTEOTOMIES AND FIXATION

In cases of mandibular reconstruction and where a double-strut fibula is required, fibular osteotomies will be required following flap dissection. Osteotomies can be made with the fibula left in situ in the leg or on the back table in the operating room. We prefer to move the flap to the back table so we may work on a bone board or other hard surface which allows for more precise cuts to the fibula. Regardless of where the osteotomies are made, preparation for bone cuts is made by deciding what part of the bone will be used according to the proper orientation of the donor vessels and the skin island. The length of each bone segment and the osteotomy sites are determined using the acrylic templates or the specimen as a reference. Usually, one osteotomy is made for recreation of the mandible angle and one or two more for the anterior body; these three cuts are adequate to simulate the shape of the lower jaw in reconstruction of hemimandibular defects. To achieve facial symmetry, the distance between the angle of the mandible and the midsagittal plane has to be the same in the reconstructed side and the intact hemimandible.

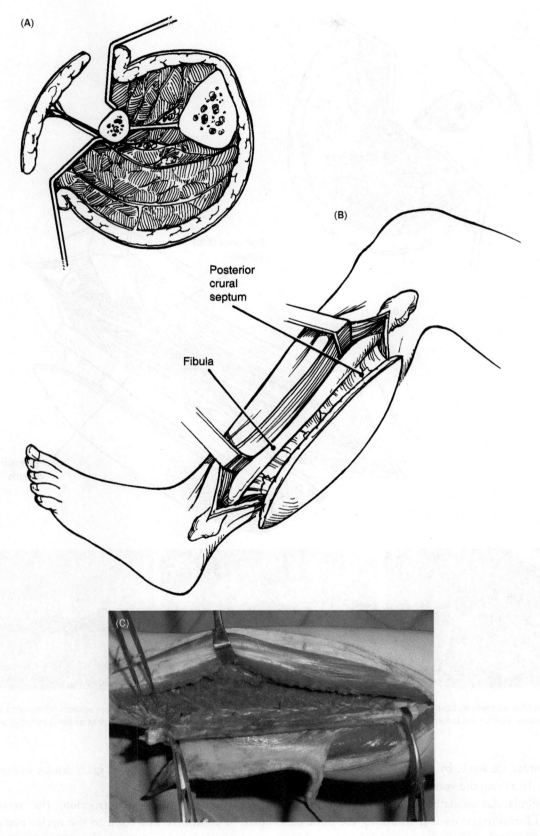

Figure 44.17. (A,B) After completing osteotomies, bone is gently retracted outward to expedite dissection of muscles in anterior and deep posterior compartment of leg. (C) Bone retractors allow for gentle retraction on fibula which can aid in exposing the interosseous membrane and peroneal vessels.

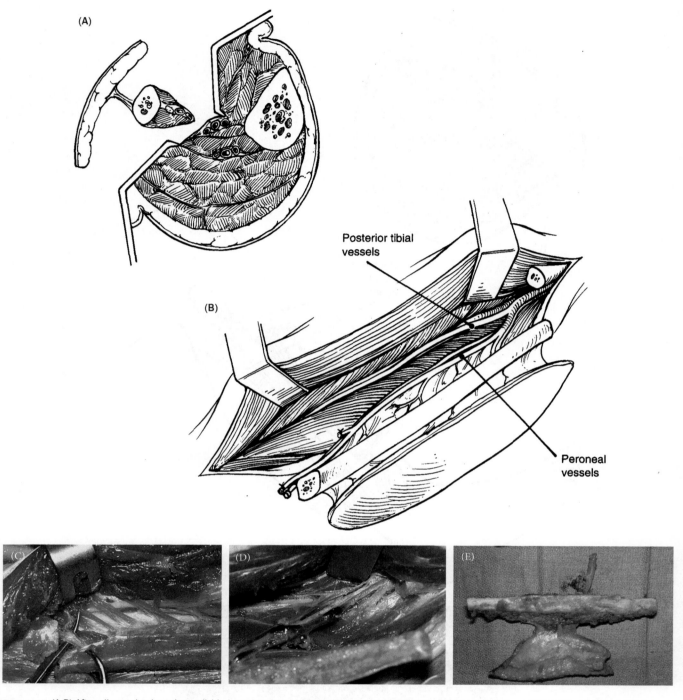

(A)

(B)

Posterior tibial vessels

Peroneal vessels

(C) (D) (E)

Figure 44.18. (A,B) After all muscles have been divided, peroneal vessels are dissected to their origin. (C) The peroneal vessels are isolated and divided distally. The vessels are then dissected proximally to their origin (D). The flap is then divided and carried to the back table for creation of any shaping or osteotomies (E).

Osteotomies are made by carefully stripping the periosteum and dissecting the vessels away from the area to be cut on the fibula. An oscillating saw is used to create the osteotomy. Liberal irrigation is used during the bone cuts to prevent excessive heat from injuring the remaining bone ends. No gap should be left between the bone segments, and a smooth contact surface between the ends of the native mandible and fibular graft can be obtained with a high-speed burr.

For mandibular reconstruction, the reconstruction plate is contoured and fixed to the native mandible prior to removal and is used to template the curvature and shape of the fibular graft. The spatial orientation of the bone graft has to be assessed also in relation to the maxillary arch and the occlusion plane; otherwise, dental prosthetic rehabilitation, whether immediate or secondary, will be difficult. The lateral surface of the fibula should be placed facing the reconstruction plate using one or two screws in each bony segment. It is always desirable to reproduce the inferior mandibular border contour. However, because of the shorter height of the fibula compared with the native mandible, there is no major difference when the bone graft is fixed up to 1.0 cm higher than the normal inferior border. This technical modification is particularly useful to place osteointegrated dental implants simultaneously or at second-stage surgery (Figure 44.5).

If the skin island is used for intraoral reconstruction, it is completely inset at this time; otherwise, the oral mucosa is closed and the skin island is fixed partially outside. When both an intraoral and external soft tissue defect need reconstruction, the skin island is fixed in the oral cavity, a strip of skin in the middle is de-epithelialized, and the rest of the skin is fixed partially in the exterior surface. Meticulous caution should be taken before performing the vascular anastomoses to be sure that the septocutaneous perforators are not kinked or twisted and that the peroneal vessels are in good position for the vascular anastomoses.

For fibula graft stabilization in long bone reconstruction, the fibula can be intussuscepted within the native bone ends. This technique works best in the humerus and femur (Figure 44.2). Alternatively, the fibula may be used as an onlay graft. We prefer to minimize bicortical screw placement within the fibula to avoid iatrogenic pedicle injury; 3.5 mm screws work best for stabilization of the graft and can be placed in a lag type fashion if the fibula is being used as an onlay graft. Intercalary reconstructions are stabilized with a spanning locked plate in which 2–4 screws can be placed into the fibula.

POSTOPERATIVE MANAGEMENT

The reconstructed extremity is immobilized with the skin island exposed so that hourly Doppler exams can be performed. If no skin island is included with the flap, or if there is only an intraoral skin island, the flap should be monitored with an implantable Doppler device. Any changes in the perfusion should prompt exploration of the anastomosis in the operating room. We monitor the flap hourly for the first 48 hours following surgery, and then evaluate the flap every 2 hours for the next 24 hours.[30] We do not routinely anticoagulate patients following free tissue transfer, but we do use deep venous thrombosis prophylaxis with either aspirin or subcutaneous heparin until the patient is ambulating regularly.

COMPLICATIONS

The most devastating complication following surgery is flap loss due to anastomotic failure. Thrombosis of the pedicle has been reported to occur in as many as 10% of cases.[31] We recommend close monitoring of the pedicle with either an easily visualized skin island or an implantable Doppler device. Early identification of thrombosis or flap trouble increases the likelihood of flap salvage. If flap loss is encountered, we would recommend another attempt at vascularized bone with the contralateral fibula or other types of bone flaps.

Nonunion can occur despite patent anastomosis and can be due to the local wound environment, inadequate debridement, and poor fixation.[31] Smoking and chemotherapy have both been linked to nonunion and delayed union.[21,32] In such cases, we would recommend attempts at nonvascularized grafting (autologous cancellous graft) of the nonunion site as this has been associated with conversion to union in greater than 95% of cases.[31,32] It is important to remember that union times are affected by the location of the recipient site. Union times vary from 6 to 8 weeks in the jaw, 2 to 3 months in the upper limb, 3 to 4 months in the femur and tibia, and 4 to 9 months in the spine.[2,33] The diagnosis of nonunion should be made with the aid of serial radiographs and CT imaging.

Stress fractures of the fibula can occur in as many as in 15–20% patients when the fibula is used for lower extremity reconstruction.[19,31] Treatment may involve simple casting or, in more severe cases, application of an external fixator until healing. Stress fractures do help to promote hypertrophy but can be disabling to the patient. In order to prevent fracture, we advocate for the use of rigid, spanning locked plates for fixation of the graft when possible.

Donor site complications are not uncommon. These can include Flexor hallucis longus muscle (FHL) contracture, peroneal nerve palsy, compartment syndrome, valgus ankle malalignment, and tibial stress fractures.[19,31] A recent systematic review of donor site complications noted wound dehiscence occurring in 7% of patients, delayed wound healing in 17% of patients, partial skin graft loss in 8% of patients, and total skin graft loss occurring in 4.7% of patients. Late donor site morbidities included chronic pain in 6.5% of patients, ankle instability in 5.8% of patients, limited range of motion in the ankle reported in 11.5% of patients, claw toe in 6% of patients, and a sensory deficit in almost 7% of patients. The final mean American Orthopaedic Foot and Ankle Society score was found to be 85.5% following flap harvest.[34]

TIPS FOR SUCCESSFUL DISSECTION

1. Although controversial, a CT angiogram is obtained in all patients in preparation for free fibular transfer. The CT angiogram does not add any additional significant morbidity while providing information on inflow and outflow vessels in both legs. This identifies the rare peroneal artery–dominant arterial supply to the leg (peroneal arteria magna), and, in such cases, the contralateral leg or another source of a bone graft should be considered for flap harvest.

2. All flaps are planned to include a skin paddle in the flap design. The skin paddle can always be discarded if not needed and returned to the donor site as a full-thickness skin graft.

3. Six to eight centimeters of the distal fibula must remain intact to stabilize the ankle. In children with an open physis, we always place a tibia–fibular syndesmotic screw following fibula harvest to allow for stable ankle development.

4. Iatrogenic deep peroneal nerve injury can be prevented by clear identification of the peroneal nerve prior to lateral compartment dissection and a subperiosteal dissection over the proximal fibula until the peroneal nerve is identified. The dissection can then be continued superficial to the periosteum once the nerve is protected.

5. A cuff of periosteum can be kept at the distal and proximal portion of the fibula. If the vascular supply to the periosteum is maintained, it can be wrapped around the bone of the donor site to speed bony union.

6. The nutrient vessel to the fibula should be preserved during flap harvest and subsequent osteotomies.

7. The surgeon should always verify the location of the tibial nerve and posterior tibial artery prior to ligation of the peroneal vessels.

8. If the flexor hallucis longus muscles has been injured or devascularized following fibula harvest, the muscle belly should be debrided in its entirety. This helps to prevent postoperative hallux contracture secondary to FHL fibrosis.

9. For osteocutaneous flaps, a meshed skin graft is always used to cover the donor site. Attempts at primary closure have been associated with compartment syndrome in the donor leg.

REFERENCES

1. Taylor GI, Miller GD, Ham FJ. The free vascularized bone graft. A clinical extension of microvascular techniques. *Plast Reconstr Surg* 1975;55:533–544.
2. Taylor GI, Corlett RJ, Ashton MW. The evolution of free vascularized bone transfer: a 40-year experience. *Plast Reconstr Surg* 2016;137:1292–1305.
3. Wei FC, Chen HC, Chuang CC, Noordhoff MS. Fibular osteoseptocutaneous flap: anatomic study and clinical application. *Plast Reconstr Surg* 1986;78:191–200.
4. Lin CH, Wei FC, Chen HC, Chuang DC. Outcome comparison in traumatic lower-extremity reconstruction by using various composite vascularized bone transplantation. *Plast Reconstr Surg* 1999;104:984–992.
5. Han CS, Wood MB, Bishop AT, Cooney WP, 3rd. Vascularized bone transfer. *J Bone Joint Surg Am* 1992;74:1441–1449.
6. Wood MB. Femoral reconstruction by vascularized bone transfer. *Microsurgery* 1990;11:74–79.
7. Heitmann C, Erdmann D, Levin LS. Treatment of segmental defects of the humerus with an osteoseptocutaneous fibular transplant. *J Bone Joint Surg Am* 2002;84-A:2216–2223.
8. Jupiter JB, Gerhard HJ, Guerrero J, Nunley JA, Levin LS. Treatment of segmental defects of the radius with use of the vascularized osteoseptocutaneous fibular autogenous graft. *J Bone Joint Surg Am* 1997;79:542–550.
9. Yu P, Chang EI, Hanasono MM. Design of a reliable skin paddle for the fibula osteocutaneous flap: perforator anatomy revisited. *Plast Reconstr Surg* 2011;128:440–446.
10. Wei FC, El-Gammal TA, Lin CH, Ueng WN. Free fibular osteoseptocutaneous graft for reconstruction of segmental femoral shaft defects. *J Trauma* 1997;43:784–792.
11. Chen MC, Chang MC, Chen CM, Chen TH. Double-strut free vascularized fibular grafting for reconstruction of the lower extremities. *Injury* 2003;34:763–769.
12. Jones NF, Swartz WM, Mears DC, Jupiter JB, Grossman A. The "double barrel" free vascularized fibular bone graft. *Plast Reconstr Surg* 1988;81:378–385.
13. Houdek MT, Wagner ER, Wyles CC, Nanos GP, 3rd, Moran SL. New options for vascularized bone reconstruction in the upper extremity. *Semin Plast Surg* 2015;29:20–29.
14. Soucacos PN, Korompilias AV, Vekris MD, Zoubos A, Beris AE. The free vascularized fibular graft for bridging large skeletal defects of the upper extremity. *Microsurgery* 2011;31:190–197.
15. Kremer T, Bickert B, Germann G, Heitmann C, Sauerbier M. Outcome assessment after reconstruction of complex defects of the forearm and hand with osteocutaneous free flaps. *Plast Reconstr Surg* 2006;118:443–454; discussion 455–446.
16. Rose PS, Shin AY, Bishop AT, Moran SL, Sim FH. Vascularized free fibula transfer for oncologic reconstruction of the humerus. *Clin Orthop Relat Res* 2005;438:80–84.
17. Rashid M, Hafeez S, Zia ul Islam M, Rizvi ST, ur Rehman S, Tamimy MS, et al. Limb salvage in malignant tumours of the upper limb using vascularised fibula. *J Plast Reconstr Aesthet Surg* 2008;61:648–661.
18. Capanna R, Campanacci DA, Belot N, Beltrami G, Manfrini M, Innocenti M, et al. A new reconstructive technique for intercalary defects of long bones: the association of massive allograft with vascularized fibular autograft. Long-term results and comparison

with alternative techniques. *The Orthopedic clinics of North America* 2007;38:51–60, vi.

19. Yazar S, Lin CH, Wei FC. One-stage reconstruction of composite bone and soft-tissue defects in traumatic lower extremities. *Plast Reconstr Surg* 2004;114:1457–1466.

20. Peat BG, Liggins DF. Microvascular soft tissue reconstruction for acute tibial fractures--late complications and the role of bone grafting. *Ann Plast Surg* 1990;24:517–520.

21. Moran SL, Shin AY, Bishop AT. The use of massive bone allograft with intramedulary free fibular flap for limb salvage in a pediatric and adolescent population. *Plast Reconstr Surg* 2006;118:413–419.

22. Houdek MT, Wagner ER, Stans AA, Shin AY, Bishop AT, Sim FH, et al. What is the outcome of allograft and intramedullary free fibula (Capanna technique) in pediatric and adolescent patients with bone tumors? *Clin Orthop Relat Res* 2016;474:660–668.

23. Urbaniak JR, Coogan PG, Gunneson EB, Nunley JA. Treatment of osteonecrosis of the femoral head with free vascularized fibular grafting. A long-term follow-up study of one hundred and three hips. *J Bone Joint Surg Am* 1995;77:681–694.

24. Willems WF, Alberton GM, Bishop AT, Kremer T. Vascularized bone grafting in a canine carpal avascular necrosis model. *Clin Orthop Relat Res* 2011;469:2831–2837.

25. Ackerman DB, Rose PS, Moran SL, Dekutoski MB, Bishop AT, Shin AY. The results of vascularized-free fibular grafts in complex spinal reconstruction. *J Spinal Dis Techn* 2011;24:170–176.

26. Moran SL, Bakri K, mardini S, Shin AY, Bishop AT. The use of vascularized fibular grafts for the reconstruction of spinal and sacral defects. *Microsurgery* 2009;29:393–400.

27. Monaco C, Stranix JT, Avraham T, Brecht L, Saadeh PB, Hirsch D, et al. Evolution of surgical techniques for mandibular reconstruction using free fibula flaps: The next generation. *Head Neck* 2016;38 Suppl 1:E2066–E2073.

28. Hanasono MM, Skoracki RJ. Computer-assisted design and rapid prototype modeling in microvascular mandible reconstruction. *Laryngoscope* 2013;123:597–604.

29. Gilbert A. Free vascularized bone grafts. *Int Surg* 1981;66:27–31.

30. Salgado CJ, Moran SL, Mardini S. Flap monitoring and patient management. *Plast Reconstr Surg* 2009;124:e295–e302.

31. Minami A, Kasashima T, Iwasaki N, Kato H, Kaneda K. Vascularised fibular grafts. An experience of 102 patients. *J Bone Joint Surg (Brit vol)* 2000;82:1022–1025.

32. Houdek MT, Bayne CO, Bishop AT, Shin AY. The outcome and complications of vascularised fibular grafts. *Bone Joint J* 2017;99-B:134–138.

33. Moran SL, Bakri K, Mardini S, Shin AY, Bishop AT. The use of vascularized fibular grafts for the reconstruction of spinal and sacral defects. *Microsurgery* 2009;29:393–400.

34. Ling XF, Peng X. What is the price to pay for a free fibula flap? A systematic review of donor-site morbidity following free fibula flap surgery. *Plast Reconstr Surg* 2012;129:657–674.

45.

THE EVOLUTION OF THE ILIAC CREST FLAP

Peirong Yu and Mark V. Schaverien

INTRODUCTION

The deep circumflex iliac artery (DCIA) osteomusculo-cutaneous flap with iliac crest bone was the gold standard for many years for mandibular reconstruction, providing a large vascularized bone stock of similar shape to the hemi-mandible.[1-9] Despite the increasing popularity of the fibula osteocutaneous flap, which allows for more re-fined reconstruction and permits multiple osteotomies, the iliac crest free flap remains an important option in the armamentarium for mandibular reconstruction and has also been used for maxillary reconstruction.[10,11] It is particularly useful for through-and-through defects involving intraoral mucosa, bone, and external skin to avoid the requirement for a second skin flap. The fixed anatomical configuration and the lack of segmental blood supply limits the precision to reconstruct some defects, particularly those of the anterior mandible, and total mandibulectomy defects may require bilateral iliac crest flaps. The donor site scar is well hidden, and the bone is thick and will readily accept osseointegrated dental implants.

The flap was originally described as an osteomusculo-cutaneous flap, limitations of which include excessive bulk of the muscle carrier, unreliability of the skin paddle when separated from the muscle, and gait disturbance and abdominal wall weakness resulting from the de-tachment of abdominal and thigh muscles from the iliac crest.[1-7] The relative immobility of the skin paddle in re-lation to the bone component can make intraoral inset of the skin paddle challenging, and the internal oblique muscle may need to be used to provide intraoral lining. The conventional flap often produces a block-like ap-pearance, without the refined contour of the fibula flap. Subsequently, there have been modifications to the orig-inal flap design to address these disadvantages. Safak et al.

introduced a modified harvest technique for the iliac crest flap without the "obligatory" muscle to reduce the bulk of the soft tissue,[12] and Kimata et al. later popularized this as the DCIA perforator flap.[13] Bergeron et al. later reappraised the perforator anatomy of the DCIA in an effort to increase the reliability of the skin flap.[14] Shenaq et al. described the harvest of the inner cortex only of the iliac crest, preserving the outer cortex and therefore maintaining the thigh muscle attachments and reducing donor site morbidity.[15]

ANATOMY

VASCULAR ANATOMY

Taylor et al. and Sanders and Mayou were the first to dem-onstrate that the DCIA is the dominant blood supply to the anterior ileum via endosteal and periosteal mechanisms, as well as giving rise to perforators that course through the abdominal wall musculature to nourish the skin over-lying the anterior ileum.[1-3] Later studies revealed that the ascending branch of the DCIA supplies the internal oblique muscle.[16] The main trunk of the DCIA arises from the posterolateral aspect of the external iliac artery, just deep and superior to the inguinal ligament where the deep inferior epigastric artery branches medially (Figure 45.1): however, rarely it may arise from the femoral artery slightly below the inguinal ligament. It then ascends on the medial aspect of the iliac bone toward the anterior superior iliac spine (ASIS), giving off one or two ascending muscular branches to the abdominal wall within 1 cm of the ASIS, sandwiched between the transversus abdominis and the internal oblique muscles. After piercing the transversalis fascia, the ascending branch terminates on the undersurface of the internal oblique muscle. Various

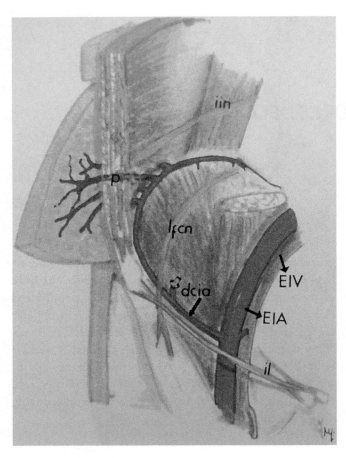

Figure 45.1. Anatomy of the deep circumflex iliac artery (DCIA). The DCIA is a branch of the external iliac artery (EIA) that travels approximately 2 cm above the inguinal ligament and is crossed by the lateral femoral cutaneous nerve anterior to the anterior superior iliac spine (ASIS).

perforator in 30%.[12] Bergeron et al. found perforators to be present in 92% of specimens with a mean of 1.6 (range 0–5) perforators, located in a 6 × 4 cm rectangular area superior to the iliac crest, 5 cm posterior to the ASIS.[14] The main trunk terminates with anastomoses with the lumbar and iliolumbar arteries. There are some anatomic variations of the DCIA and its ascending branch: the DCIA may be duplicated; and the ascending branch may originate from the main trunk of the external iliac artery, may be multiple in number, and may serve as the dominant vessel to the iliac bone with only a minor contribution from the DCIA. Venae comitantes accompany the DCIA and its perforators, joining to form a single vein 2–3 cm lateral to the external iliac artery at the level of the inguinal ligament. It crosses either in front of or behind the external iliac artery to reach the iliac vein. The accompanying vein usually has a diameter of 2–3 mm. The DCIA is typically 1.0–1.5 mm in caliber, with a pedicle length of 6–8 cm. In cases where the DCIA is absent or unsuitable, the superficial circumflex iliac artery (SCIA) can be harvested to rescue the skin paddle.

NEURAL ANATOMY

Important sensory nerves in the groin region should be preserved during flap elevation. Sensory innervation of the flap is not possible. The lateral femoral cutaneous nerve and the ilioinguinal nerve travel in the territory of the flap and should be carefully identified and preserved. In the groin, between the external iliac vessels and the ASIS, the lateral femoral cutaneous nerve lies lateral to the ilioinguinal nerve. The lateral femoral cutaneous nerve (L2, L3) travels through the inguinal ligament approximately 1 cm lateral to the ASIS. This nerve further descends along the line connecting the ASIS and the superolateral corner of the patella to supply sensation to the anterior lateral aspect of the thigh. Entrapment of this nerve may cause severe pain of the thigh and groin. Division of the nerve will result in permanent numbness in the thigh.

The ilioinguinal nerve originates from the L1 ventral ramus. It pierces the transversus abdominis and the internal oblique, and then traverses the inguinal canal below the spermatic cord. The nerve emerges with the spermatic cord from the superficial inguinal ring to supply the proximal medial skin of the thigh and the skin over the root of the penis and upper part of the scrotum in males or the skin covering the mons pubis and the adjoining labium majus in females. Entrapment of the nerve during surgery may cause recurrent pain in this distribution.

amounts of the internal oblique muscle can be included in the flap based on the ascending branch. The DCIA continues along the medial surface of the iliac crest as the transverse branch, traveling between the insertion of the transversus abdominis and the internal oblique muscles. Multiple small branches are given off to the periosteum of the medial cortex of the iliac crest near the ASIS, allowing reliable harvest of the split iliac crest. It then sends off small branches to the iliacus muscle, which also eventually reach the underlying periosteum and anastomose with other periosteal vessels to supply the bone, with harvest of up to 14 cm of bone length possible, although with limited capability to perform osteotomies. The DCIA eventually pierces the transversus abdominis muscle and then gives rise to one or two musculocutaneous perforators that supply a cutaneous territory of 12 × 6 cm over the iliac crest. Taylor et al. found a mean of six cutaneous perforators supplying this cutaneous vascular territory,[1,2] and Safak et al. reported multiple musculocutaneous perforators in 70% of dissections and a single dominant

OPERATIVE APPROACH

CHOOSING THE SIDE FOR FLAP HARVEST

For posterior mandibulectomy defects including the condyle, ramus, and posterior body, the ipsilateral iliac crest flap should be chosen. The outer surface of the iliac crest should face extraorally with the reconstructive plate fixed to this external surface. The inner surface of the bone flap and pedicle should face intraorally. The ASIS becomes the angle of the mandible, and the anterior inferior iliac spine becomes the condyle of the mandible facing the temporomandibular joint. The iliac crest bone itself should be used to reconstruct the body of the mandible. The vascular pedicle will be situated behind the new angle of the mandible.

CONVENTIONAL ILIAC CREST FLAP

The skin paddle is marked two-thirds above and one-third below the line of the anterior iliac crest (Figure 45.2). The medial skin incision is made 1 cm above the inguinal ligament and extends laterally along the superior border of the outlined flap. The spermatic cord or round ligament is retracted upward and medially to expose the inguinal floor. The external iliac vessels and the origin of the deep circumflex iliac vessels are then exposed (Figure 45.3). By following the vessels laterally, the internal oblique and the transversus abdominis muscles are divided from the inguinal ligament. Near the ASIS, the ascending branch and the lateral femoral cutaneous nerve should be identified. The ascending branch is divided if the internal oblique muscle is not needed (Figure 45.4). The three layers of the abdominal wall muscles are divided exposing the vascular pedicle between the overhanging transversus muscle and the iliacus muscle. The iliacus muscle is then divided below the vessels. The DCIA along the inner cortex is palpable or a Doppler device can be used to identify it.

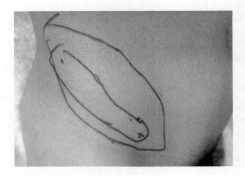

Figure 45.2. A skin paddle is outlined over the iliac crest lateral to the anterior superior iliac spine.

Next, the lower lateral incision is made to separate the thigh muscle attachments to the iliac crest. Care should be taken to preserve some of the muscle/tendon attachments to the iliac crest to minimize functional disturbance. The inguinal ligament is detached from the ASIS. The lateral femoral cutaneous nerve and the ilioinguinal nerve should be identified and preserved. Using an oscillating saw, the outer cortex of the iliac crest is cut, followed by the inner cortex through the already divided iliacus muscle. The cut should be about 2 cm below the palpable vascular pedicle.

MODIFIED FLAP HARVEST TECHNIQUES

Inner Cortex Iliac Crest Flap

Harvest of full-thickness iliac crest bone creates a disruption of the abdominal wall muscle and thigh muscle attachment, and this disruption may result in abdominal hernia formation and gait disturbance. To minimize the risk of these donor site complications, the inner cortex only can be harvested with a rim of the iliac crest bone, without detaching the thigh muscles. After making the lower lateral skin incision, the periosteum of the outer rim of the iliac crest is stripped down for only 1 cm without detaching the thigh muscle and tendon attachments. The outer cortex is then cut using an oscillating saw perpendicular to it, and the inner cortex is then cut 2–3 cm below the vascular pedicle. The posterior osteotomy is performed. The bone is then split between the inner and outer cortices with a large periosteal elevator. The inner cortex alone provides thin bony stock of approximately 5 mm thickness. The 1 cm height full-thickness rim of the iliac crest provides additional strength to the bone flap.

Deep Circumflex Iliac Artery Perforator Flap

One of the main disadvantages of the traditional iliac crest flap design is the obligatory inclusion of the full-thickness abdominal wall musculature if the skin paddle is needed. The soft tissue bulk is usually too large to be placed intraorally and may affect tongue mobility and oral function. The perforator anatomy of the DCIA that nourishes the skin paddle is well understood and allows harvest of a perforator flap without the muscle, thus reducing the flap bulk as well as providing greater freedom of movement of the skin paddle from the bone component to improve the inset.

For perforator flap harvest, the DCIA perforators should be located with a hand-held Doppler probe in a 4 × 6-cm rectangular area on the superior aspect of the

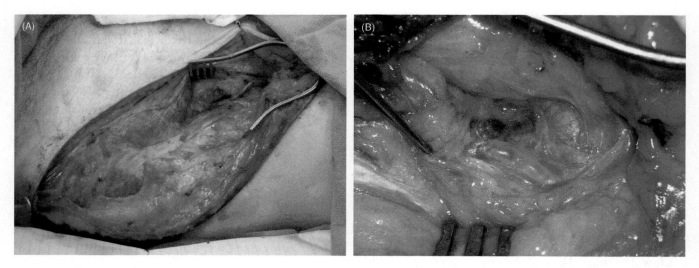

Figure 45.3 Once the skin incision is made, the spermatic cord in male or the round ligament in female patients is mobilized and retracted upward and medially to expose the inguinal floor and the origin of the deep circumflex iliac artery (DCIA). (A) Exposure of the inguinal ligament. (B) Exposure of the origin of the DCIA. The DCIV usually travels behind the external iliac artery to enter the external iliac vein.

iliac crest, 5 cm posterior to the ASIS (Figure 45.5), although the Doppler is not always accurate. Once the perforators are located and marked on the skin, the skin paddle should be centered on these. A superior to inferior suprafascial dissection through a superior skin paddle incision extending medially above the inguinal ligament allows identification of the DCIA perforators (Figure 45.6). There are, however, several perforators in the region that may arise from other source arteries, such as the intercostal, lumbar, and iliolumbar arteries. The DCIA perforators can be distinguished from the intercostal and lumbar perforators because they do not have an accompanying nerve. Distinction between the DCIA

and iliolumbar perforators can be made by spreading the external oblique muscle fibers at the base of the perforator. DCIA perforators have an anterior origin, whereas the iliolumbar perforators have a posterior course. Once the DCIA perforator is isolated and found to be of sufficient caliber, the lower skin incision of the skin island can then be performed. If no perforator is found, then the skin paddle can be based on the superficial circumflex iliac artery instead. The perforators are marked on the skin surface with a 5-0 Prolene suture and the flap design is recentered if necessary. The external oblique fascia is then incised around the perforators (Figure 45.6) and intramuscular dissection is performed to trace the perforator

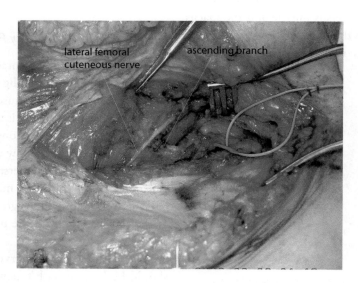

Figure 45.4. The internal oblique and transversus abdominis muscles are divided from the inguinal ligament to expose the vascular pedicle and the ascending branch near the anterior superior iliac spine (ASIS).

HEAD AND NECK SURGERY

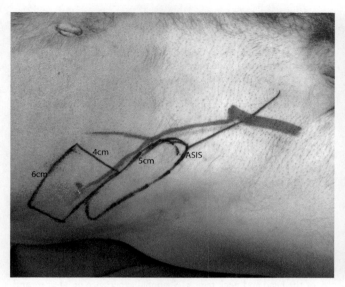

Figure 45.5. The deep circumflex iliac artery (DCIA) perforator flap: design of the skin paddle. The perforators are located using hand-held Doppler in a 6 ×4 cm rectangular area 5 cm lateral to the anterior superior iliac spine (ASIS).

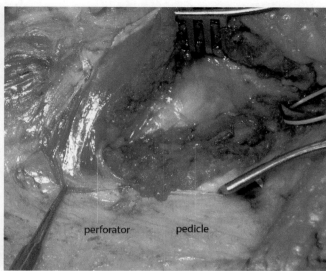

Figure 45.7. The perforator is traced back to the main vascular pedicle. The muscles are divided above the pedicle.

back to its main pedicle (Figure 45.7). The ascending branch is then divided (Figure 45.6). Once the perforator dissection to the DCIA has been completed, the abdominal muscle and fascia between the skin perforator and external iliac vessels are divided. The iliacus muscle below the vascular pedicle is also divided. The inner cortex only of the iliac crest can be harvested as described earlier to minimize donor site morbidity. The DCIA perforator flap has minimal soft tissue bulk, and the skin paddle can be inset with ease. Osteotomies can be performed to contour the flap to match the mandibular defect (Figure 45.8).

DONOR SITE CARE

With the conventional iliac crest flap, removal of the wing of the ilium creates a disruption of the lateral abdominal wall and the thigh muscle attachments. Careful closure is important to reduce the risk of abdominal hernia and gait

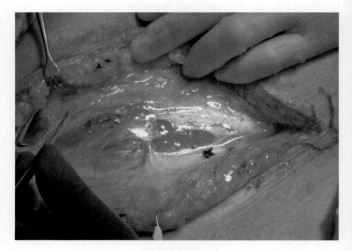

Figure 45.6. Only the superior skin incision is made initially, and suprafascial dissection proceeds inferiorly to identify the cutaneous perforators. Then the external oblique fascia is incised and intramuscular dissection performed to free the perforator.

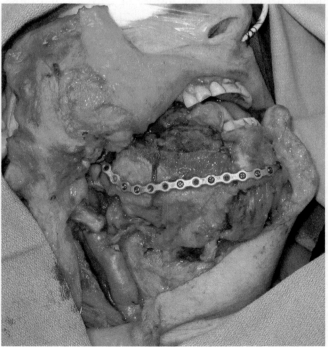

Figure 45.8. Osteotomies can be performed to further contour the flap. The inner cortex faces intraorally.

disturbance. It is essential to repair the transversus muscle to the iliacus or the remaining iliac bone. It may be helpful to drill several holes in the cut edge of the ilium to reattach the transversus muscle. In patients with significant abdominal wall laxity and weakness, mesh repair may be indicated. The second layer of closure involves suturing the external oblique muscle to the upper thigh muscles and tendons. Flexion of the ipsilateral knee is helpful to relieve tension in the closure. Closure should be done with strong permanent sutures such as no. 1 Prolene. With the inner cortex flap, the abdominal muscle and fascia are sewn to the fascia of the thigh muscle attachments and the periosteum. Early ambulation with assistance is encouraged, with the avoidance of straining movements that may disrupt the donor site repair.

CONCLUSION

The iliac crest flap, particularly with a modified approach to flap harvest that includes the split iliac crest based on the inner cortex to preserve the thigh muscle attachments and the DCIA perforator flap with preservation of the bulky abdominal wall musculature and greater freedom of movement of the skin paddle, remains an important option for reconstruction of mandibulectomy defects secondary to the free fibula flap. It is usually reserved for patients who are not fibular flap candidates, such as those with peripheral vascular disease, peroneal magnum, history of fractures, and those with previous bilateral fibular flaps. This flap is best suited for posterior mandibulectomy defects that do not require osteotomies on the flap. Anterior defects and extensive angle-to-angle defects that require multiple osteotomies are not good candidates for this flap unless bilateral iliac crest flaps are used. The pedicle artery is usually about 1.5 mm in diameter, making it less ideal for head and neck reconstruction.

REFERENCES

1. Taylor GI, Townsend P, Corlett R. Superiority of the deep circumflex iliac vessels as the supply for free groin flaps: clinical work. *Plast Reconstr Surg* 1979;64:745.
2. Taylor GI, Townsend P, Corlett R. Superiority of the deep circumflex iliac vessels as the supply for free groin flaps: experimental work. *Plast Reconstr Surg* 1979;64:595.
3. Sanders R, Mayou BJ. A new vascularized bone graft transferred by microvascular anastomosis as a free flap. *Br J Surg* 1979;66:787.
4. Urken ML, Vickery C, Weinberg H, et al. The internal oblique-iliac crest osseomyocutaneous microvascular free flap in head and neck reconstruction. *J Reconstr Microsurg* 1989;5:203.
5. Urken ML, Weinberg H, Vickery C, et al. The internal oblique-iliac crest free flap in composite defects of the oral cavity involving bone, skin, and mucosa. *Laryngoscope* 1991;101:257.
6. Pohlenz P, Klatt J, Schön G, Blessmann M, Li L, Schmelzle R. Microvascular free flaps in head and neck surgery: complications and outcome of 1000 flaps. *Int J Oral Maxillofac Surg* 2012;41:739.
7. Zhang C, Sun J, Zhu H, et al. Microsurgical free flap reconstructions of the head and neck region: Shanghai experience of 34 years and 4640 flaps. *Int J Oral Maxillofac Surg* 2015;44:675.
8. Schultz BD, Sosin M, Nam A, et al. Classification of mandible defects and algorithm for microvascular reconstruction. *Plast Reconstr Surg* 2015;135:743.
9. Jung HD, Nam W, Cha IH, Kim HJ. Reconstruction of combined oral mucosa-mandibular defects using the vascularized myoosseous iliac crest free flap. *Asian Pac J Cancer Prev* 2012;13:4137.
10. Brown JS. Deep circumflex iliac artery free flap with internal oblique muscle as a new method of immediate reconstruction of maxillectomy defect. *Head Neck* 1996;18:412.
11. Costa H, Zenha H, Sequeira H, et al. Microsurgical reconstruction of the maxilla: Algorithm and concepts. *J Plast Reconstr Aesthet Surg* 2015;68:89.
12. Safak, T., Klebuc, M. J., Mavili, E., et al. A new design of the iliac crest microsurgical free flap without including the "obligatory" muscle cuff. Plast. *Reconstr Surg* 1997;100:1703.
13. Kimata, Y., Uchiyama, K., Sakuraba, M., et al. Deep circumflex iliac perforator flap with iliac crest for mandibular reconstruction. *Br J Plast Surg* 2001;54:487.
14. Bergeron L, Tang M, Morris SF. The anatomical basis of the deep circumflex iliac artery perforator flap with iliac crest. *Plast Reconstr Surg* 2007;120:252–258.
15. Shenaq, S. M. Refinements in mandibular reconstruction. *Clin Plast Surg* 1992;19:809.
16. Ramasastry SS, Granick MS, Futrell JW. Clinical anatomy of the internal oblique muscle. *J Reconstr Microsurg* 1986;2:117.

46.

SCAPULAR OSSEOUS FREE FLAP

Alexander F. Mericli and Patrick B. Garvey

INTRODUCTION

The scapular osseous free flap is one variation of the numerous flaps that can be designed based on the subscapular vascular tree. Other variants include the latissimus dorsi muscular or musculocutaneous flap, the serratus anterior muscle flap, and the scapular or parascapular fasciocutaneous flap, as well as several perforator-based alternatives. The scapular flap is a useful option in situations where a fibula flap is not an option, and it is therefore an indispensable component of the reconstructive surgeon's armamentarium.

INDICATIONS AND ASSESSMENT OF THE DEFECT

The scapular osseous free flap is described for reconstruction of a variety of defects. It is most commonly used when vascularized bone is required in combination with a large soft tissue defect. The scapular flap is frequently considered a second-line option, to be employed in situations where other osseous flaps—such as the free fibula flap or the iliac crest flap—are not available for harvesting due to obesity, peripheral vascular disease, prior lower extremity trauma, or past surgery. The bone stock is best used without osteotomies due to its lacking a segmental blood supply. It can be osteotomized when there is a robust soft tissue cuff around the bone. However, the fibula free flap is the best choice when multiple osteotomies are required. The potential advantage of the scapula flap over the fibula is the large associated skin paddle, as well as the potential of a multicomponent chimeric flap (two skin paddles, muscle, bone) based on a single set of microanastomoses. The lateral border of the scapula is favored for its greater

diameter when compared with the medial segment (3 cm vs. 1.5 cm thick).

Most of the available literature discusses the use of the scapula for reconstruction of the head and neck. In terms of mandible reconstruction, a potential 14–16 cm long segment is available from the lateral scapula and is, therefore, sufficient to support a hemi-mandible reconstruction.[1-8] Additionally, the bone is thick enough to support osseointegrated dental implants.[3] The scapula has also been described for reconstruction of the maxilla, palate, orbit, calvarium, lower extremity, and upper extremity.[9-16]

CONTRAINDICATIONS AND DISADVANTAGES

The main disadvantage of the scapular flap is the relative inaccessibly of the flap during head and neck tumor resection, which often necessitates repositioning the patient intraoperatively for harvest and then inset. The procedure is lengthy and therefore the patient must be in a medically optimal condition. In general, the maximal length of bone that can be harvested from the scapula is 14 cm, so if a greater amount of bone is required, the fibula flap is a superior option. Donor site morbidity is low, but weakness of the rotator cuff muscle group is possible. Therefore, this flap may not be appropriate for patients with shoulder instability or past rotator cuff repair. Of note, because of this possibility, when the lateral aspect of the scapula is harvested and the teres major, teres minor, and serratus muscles are detached, they should be reinserted to the remaining scapula using either suture anchors or permanent sutures and drill holes. Other disadvantages include scar widening and the potential for brachial plexopathy due to intraoperative arm abduction during flap harvesting.[17]

Additional contraindications include prior ipsilateral axillary dissection and/or past latissimus flap.

ANATOMY

The scapular flap is based on the branches of the circumflex scapular artery (Figure 46.1). The subscapular artery emerges from the axillary artery and divides into the thoracodorsal and circumflex scapular branches. The circumflex scapular artery then passes through the triangular space, which is formed by the borders of the teres major muscle inferiorly, teres minor muscle superiorly, and long head of the triceps muscle laterally. After having traveled through the triangular space, the circumflex scapular vessels emerge posteriorly and divide into two main branches: the transverse branch, which supplies the transversely-oriented scapular skin paddle, and the descending branch, which supplies the obliquely-oriented parascapular skin paddle.

The lateral border of the scapula bone is also supplied by an osseous branch of the descending branch of the circumflex scapular artery and can provide up to 14 cm of thick, straight, corticocancellous bone that can be osteotomized where needed.[4] If the tip of the scapula is included as well as a portion of the medial border, and the bone flap is designed in a V shape, up to 20 cm can be harvested. The free medial scapular osteofasciocutaneous flap has also been described.[17] This portion of the scapula is much thinner than the lateral aspect, thus limiting its utility. The tip of the scapula can be harvested on a separate blood supply, based on the angular artery, which is a branch of the thoracodorsal artery. Using this angular branch, an additional segment of bone can be harvested, either as a second bony portion of the flap or as an isolated tip-only scapular bone flap. In addition to supplying the tip, the angular artery also contributes vascularity to the lateral scapula border.[2,18.] Harvesting a scapula angle flap based on the angular artery is technically less challenging

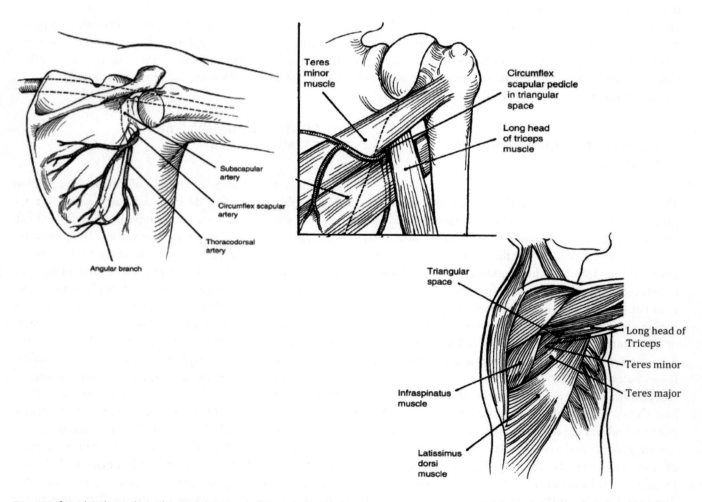

Figure 46.1. Associated vascular and muscular anatomy of the scapular flap. Note the triangular space, made up of the borders of the teres major, teres minor, and triceps muscles, through which travel the circumflex scapular vessels.

than harvesting a lateral scapula flap based on the osseous branch of the descending branch of the circumflex scapula artery, which represents an advantage of the scapula angle flap variant over the traditional scapula flap.

The mean pedicle length of the traditional scapular osseous flap, based on the circumflex scapular vessels, is 4–5 cm when only including the thoracodorsal artery; when the subscapular artery is included proximally, the pedicle length increases to 6–8 cm.[19] If the scapular bone flap is based on the angular artery, the pedicle length is increased significantly, up to 17 cm.[20,21]

ROOM SETUP

The patient can be placed in either the prone position or the lateral decubitus with the arm abducted. Decubitus is preferred because it allows for the possibility of a two-team approach, with simultaneous recipient site preparation and flap dissection. However, the need for repositioning is common. It is useful to turn the bed 180 degrees to allow full access to the head region if a mandible reconstruction is being performed. The use of an articulated, three-dimensional arm support, such as is commonly used in arthroscopic shoulder surgery, is strongly advised for the arm ipsilateral to the flap harvest, as this device allows for safe positioning and repositioning of the patient's arm in any desired position during the scapula flap harvest and inset.

PATIENT MARKINGS

The patient is marked in the upright position (Figure 46.2). The outline of the scapula should be drawn first. The circumflex scapular arterial pedicle travels through the triangular space, which is boundaried by the long head of the triceps laterally, the teres major inferiorly, and the teres major superiorly. The triangular space can be identified based on surface anatomy: an approximate location can be marked at the lateral border of the scapula, two-fifths the distance inferiorly on a line connecting the midportion of the scapula spine and its tip.[22] This can also be appreciated with manual palpation as a depression. A hand-held Doppler ultrasound pencil can be used to confirm that this is the location of the pedicle. If a cutaneous component is needed, the skin paddle dimensions and location are determined based on tissue laxity; a skin defect up to 10–12 cm in width can be closed primarily. The length of the skin

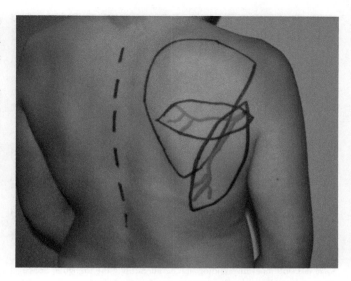

Figure 46.2. Preoperative markings for flap design. The patient is marked in the upright position with arms at the sides. The midline of the back is marked as is the outline of the scapula. The triangular space can be palpated as an indentation, nearly midway between the scapular spine and tip. The proposed skin component of the flap is provisionally outlined, with the width determined by reconstructive need and skin laxity. Either a longitudinal or transverse skin paddle (or both) can be designed. The paddle based on the descending branched should be designed to overlay with the lateral border of the scapula.

paddle can exceed 20 cm, if necessary. Beginning at the triangular space, the skin paddle should be placed along the axis of either the transverse or descending branches; this can be confirmed with a handheld Doppler. The proximal portion of each skin paddle should overlie the vicinity of the triangular space to ensure that it will receive a significant vascular contribution from the larger pedicle. If no soft tissue component is necessary, an incision can be designed directly over the lateral border of the scapula. For optimal pedicle orientation, typically the contralateral scapula is used for hemimandible reconstruction.

OPERATIVE TECHNIQUE

There are multiple permutations of scapular osseous flap design, allowing for many different chimeric flap combinations of bone (e.g., lateral scapula border, scapula tip, rib via the serratus muscle, medial scapula border), skin (transverse skin paddle, parascapular skin paddle, skin paddle directly overlying the latissimus muscle), and muscle (latissimus muscle, serratus anterior muscle).

We prefer harvesting the flap in a lateral to medial direction, to allow for immediate identification of the pedicle. The superior and lateral borders of the skin paddle are incised first, down to and through the deep investing fascia of

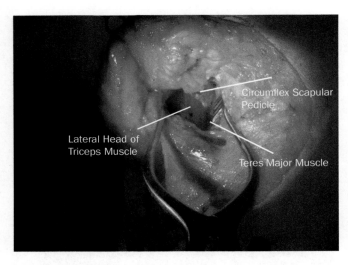

Figure 46.3. Intraoperative photograph demonstrating the triangular space and the circumflex scapular vessels.

the underlying musculature. The deltoid muscle is identified and retracted cephalad. The teres minor and triceps muscles are visualized; the teres minor is traced superiorly and will travel over the long head of the triceps to form one of the apices of the triangular space. This is where the circumflex scapular arterial pedicle will be identified exiting the triangular space. Self-retaining Weitlaner or Gelpy retractors are employed to open the triangular space, which in reality is less of a "space" and more aptly described as a closed confluence of muscles (Figure 46.3). Through the triangular space, dissection should be performed close to the muscular walls, at a distance from the vascular pedicle. Small branches to the teres minor and teres major muscle are clipped and divided. A template of both the bony and skin/soft tissue requirements of the flap should be made and transferred to the donor site. The bony template is laid over the lateral border of the scapula, sparing at least 1 cm of bone superiorly to avoid the glenoid fossa of the shoulder joint. The amount of bone harvested from the lateral border should not exceed 3–4 cm in width and 14 cm in length. If additional length is required, the scapula tip can be harvested; however, in this instance, the angular artery should also be included with the flap to ensure adequate bony perfusion.

The infraspinatus, teres major, and teres minor muscles overlying the medial border of the flap should be incised down to and through the periosteum of the underlying scapula. An osteotomy is then performed using a reciprocating or oscillating saw in order to free the lateral border of the scapula. The subscapularis muscle is attached to the deep surface of the scapula and must be divided. Inferiorly, toward the scapular tip, the serratus anterior muscle inserts onto the deep surface of the scapula as does the teres minor; both these muscle must also be divided in order to free the

bone flap. Placing a retractor on the tip of the scapula and retracting so as to "wing" the scapula can assist in exposure.

The circumflex scapular vessels are traced proximally and the branch point with the thoracodorsal vessel is identified. The incision can be extended into the axilla, or a separate axillary counter incision can be made to facilitate exposure. If neither the latissimus dorsi muscle nor the serratus anterior muscle is to be included with the flap, then the thoracodorsal vessels are clipped and ligated. The dissection is continued superiorly, and the pedicle can be divided at the subscapular artery level or even flush with the axillary artery. If the latissimus or serratus are included as components of the flap, then the teres major muscle must be divided in order to extricate the pedicle. After harvest of the flap, all detached muscles should be reinserted to the new scapular border with either suture anchors or permanent suture and drill holes.

If only the scapular tip is required, such as in reconstruction of the anterior mandible, palate, or hemi-maxilla, then the angular branch of the thoracodorsal artery can be used instead of the circumflex scapular (Figures 46.4 and 46.5). This design variation results in a significantly lengthened pedicle, up to 17 cm.[5,20,21] The angular branch originates from the thoracodorsal artery and lies within a submuscular fat pad deep to the latissimus dorsi and teres major muscles. An incision is made along the lateral border of the scapula, and the latissimus dorsi muscle is identified. The muscle is retracted and the underlying thoracodorsal vessels are traced proximally to the branch point with the circumflex scapular vessels. If only the scapular tip is needed and there is no chimeric design planned, then the circumflex scapular

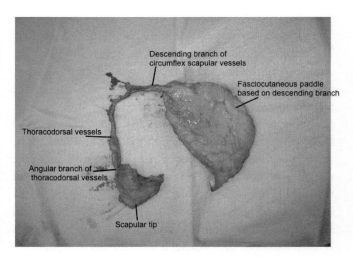

Figure 46.4. A chimeric scapular free flap with bone and fasciocutaneous components. The skin paddle is based on the descending branch, and the bone component consists of the scapular tip, which is supplied by the angular vessels via the thoracodorsal vessels.

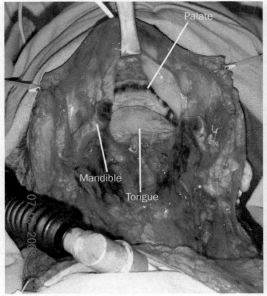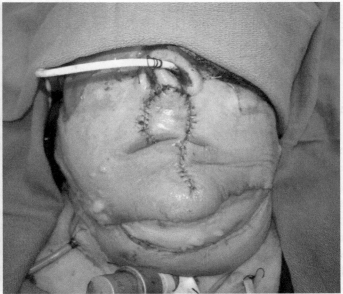

Figure 46.5. A 73-year-old patient with a locally aggressive squamous cell carcinoma invading the mandibular symphysis. A mandibulectomy of the anterior mandible was indicated (*left*). The defect was reconstructed with a free parascapular osseocutaneous flap. The scapular tip was used to reconstruct the anterior mandible, and a skin paddle was inset into the neck to minimize closure tension and serve as a monitoring segment (*right*).

vessels are divided in order to lengthen the pedicle. The thoracodorsal vessels are then traced distally and the branch to the serratus is identified. The angular artery arises from the thoracodorsal just proximal or just distal to the takeoff of the serratus branch. The angular vessels are then dissected through the fat pad deep to the latissimus and teres major muscles until it joins with the scapular tip periosteum. The periosteum is kept intact over the area of bone needed for the flap. The serratus, teres, and subscapularis muscles are divided as needed, and osteotomies are performed. Interestingly, there are reports of surgeons only using the angular vessels to supply both the scapular tip and lateral border of the scapula.[2,18]

If a large segment of bone is needed (up to 20 cm, including the lateral border of the scapula, scapular tip, and medial scapular border), then a bone flap can be harvested, based on both the circumflex scapular and angular arteries, as detailed earlier. This flap design will result in decreased maneuverability and pedicle length because the circumflex scapular artery must not be divided at its branch from the subscapular artery.[5]

A less commonly employed variant is to harvest a scapula flap incorporating the medial osseous border of the scapula. A medial osseous segment of the scapula cannot be reliably harvested as a bone-only flap. It must be incorporated into the design of a scapular flap, based off the transverse branch of the circumflex scapular vessels, and the paddle design must overlie the portion of bone to be removed.[17] The medial

bone is thinner and has been described for orbital or maxillary reconstruction. After incising the medial portion of the skin paddle, the trapezius muscle is identified and retracted superiorly. The dorsal thoracic fascia is to be kept continuous with the bone. As the skin paddle is undermined more laterally, the rhomboid muscle is divided on the medial aspect of the scapula, and the infraspinatus muscle is incised along the desired segment. The osteotomy is made, and the subscapularis and serratus anterior muscle on the deep surface of the bone are released. The remainder of the harvest progresses laterally toward the triangular space, progressing as already described. A medial osseous segment, 10–12 cm long and 2–3 cm wide is marked and osteotomies are made. The rhomboid, serratus, and subscapularis muscles are then reinserted to the remaining scapula using either permanent suture and drill holes or suture anchors. Utilizing the medial border of the scapula bone provides an additional 6 cm of pedicle length. Also, because the rotator cuff muscle are spared, shoulder dysfunction is minimized.

POSTOPERATIVE CONSIDERATIONS

Standard postoperative perfusion monitoring is recommended for this variant of free tissue transfer. If a bone-only flap is performed, an implantable Doppler probe should be used for monitoring. For most cases, a hospital stay of 5–7 days is sufficient. If the rotator cuff muscles were detached and reinserted, then shoulder motion should be restricted for 1 week and a shoulder immobilizer employed. Appropriate physical therapy is instituted 1 week after surgery to minimize shoulder stiffness.

CAVEATS

In most centers, the utility of the scapular/parascapular flap has been supplanted by the fibula flap and combined fibula/anterolateral thigh flaps, particularly for mandible reconstruction. However, flaps based off the subscapular system still have an important place in the reconstructive armamentarium. For example, many consider the scapular flap to be the first-line option for reconstruction of a hemimaxillectomy. The scapular flap is also particularly useful for obese patients, those with peripheral vascular disease, or those whose fibulae are unavailable from either prior surgery or injury. When harvested with a skin paddle, the scapular/parascapular flap provides a large surface area of thin, pliable, relatively hairless skin. An obliquely designed skin paddle can maximize the available width. The anterolateral thigh can provide a similar reconstruction, although the skin paddle is not quite as large and perforator anatomy can sometimes necessitate a muscular component to the flap, which may not be ideal. The most frequent disadvantageous outcome is a widened scar, owing to the location of the flap.

REFERENCES

1. Sevin K, Ustünsoy E, Kutlu N, Yormuk E. Hemimandibular reconstruction with bipedicled scapular osteocutaneous free flap. *Br J Oral Maxillofac Surg* 1993;31:104–107.
2. Coleman JJ 3rd, Sultan MR. The bipedicled osteocutaneous scapula flap: a new subscapular system free flap. *Plast Reconstr Surg* 1991;87:682–692.
3. Tahara S, Amatsu M, Sagara S. Dental implantation to free scapular bone flap used for mandibular reconstruction. *Auris Nasus Larynx* 1993;20:215–221.
4. Swartz WM, Banis JC, Newton ED, et al. The osteocutaneous scapular flap for mandibular and maxillary reconstruction. *Plast Reconstr Surg* 1986;77:530–545.
5. Hanasono MM, Skoracki RJ. The scapular tip osseous free flap as an alternative for anterior mandibular reconstruction. *Plast Reconstr Surg* 2010;125:164e–166e.
6. Kawahara H, Yamamoto Y, Minakawa H, et al. Facial contouring surgery with the scapular-osteo-adipo-fascial flap. *J Reconstr Microsurg* 1996;12:67–70.
7. Nakatsuka T, Harii K, Yamada A, et al. Surgical treatment of mandibular osteoradionecrosis: versatility of the scapular osteocutaneous flap. *Scand J Plast Reconstr Surg Hand Surg* 1996; 30:291–298.
8. Baker SR, Sullivan MJ. Osteocutaneous free scapular flap for one-stage mandibular reconstruction. *Arch Otolaryngol Head Neck Surg* 1988;114:267–277.
9. Kawamura K, Kawate K, Yajima H, et al. Vascularized scapular grafting for treatment of osteonecrosis of the humeral head. *J Reconstr Microsurg* 2008;24:559–564.
10. Kakibuchi M, Fujikawa M, Hosokawa K, et al. Functional reconstruction of maxilla with free latissimus dorsi-scapular osteomusculocutaneous flap. *Plast Reconstr Surg* 2002;109: 1238–1244.
11. Granick MS, Ramasastry SS, Newton ED, et al. Reconstruction of complex maxillectomy defects with the scapular-free flap. *Head Neck* 1990;12:377–385.
12. Asato H, Harii K, Yamada A, et al. Eye socket reconstruction with free-flap transfer. *Plast Reconstr Surg* 1993;92:1061–1067.
13. Futran ND, Haller JR. Considerations for free-flap reconstruction of the hard palate. *Arch Otolaryngol Head Neck Surg* 1999;125:665–669.
14. Sabino J, Franklin B, Patel K, et al. Revisiting the scapular flap: applications in extremity coverage for our U.S. combat casualties. *Plast Reconstr Surg* 2013;132:577e–585e.
15. Jaminet P, Pfau M, Greulich M. Reconstruction of the second metacarpal bone with a free vascularized scapular bone flap combined with nonvascularized free osteocartilagineous grafts from both second toes: a case report. *Microsurgery* 2011;31:146–149.
16. Hasan Z, Gore SM, Ch'ng S, et al. Options for configuring the scapular free flap in maxillary, mandibular, and calvarial reconstruction. *Plast Reconstr Surg* 2013;132:645–655.
17. Thoma A, Archibald S, Payk I, Young JE. The free medial scapular osteofasciocutaneous flap for head and neck reconstruction. *Br J Plast Surg* 1991;44:477–482.
18. Wagner AJ, Bayles SW. The angular branch: maximizing the scapular pedicle in head and neck reconstruction. *Arch Otolaryngol Head Neck Surg* 2008;134:1214–1217.
19. Leighton WD, Russell RC, Feller AM, et al. Experimental pretransfer expansion of free-flap donor sites: II. Physiology, histology, and clinical correlation. *Plast Reconstr Surg* 1988;82:76–87.
20. Seitz A, Papp S, Papp C, Maurer H. The anatomy of the angular branch of the thoracodorsal artery. *Cells Tissues Organs* 1999;164:227–236.
21. Seneviratne S, Duong C, Taylor GI. The angular branch of the thoracodorsal artery and its blood supply to the inferior angle of the scapula: an anatomical study. *Plast Reconstr Surg* 1999;104:85–88.
22. Zenn MR, Jones G. Scapular/parascapular flap. In: Zenn MR, Jones G, eds. *Reconstructive Surgery: Anatomy, Technique, and Clinical Applications*, 646–676. St. Louis, MO: Quality Medical Publishing, Inc., 2012.

47.

MICROTIA REPAIR

Melissa Kanack, Catherine Tsai, and Amanda Gosman

A variety of surgical techniques for auricular reconstruction for microtia have been described in the literature including autologous tissue, most commonly costal cartilage; porous polyethylene implants; and external prosthetics. Surgical construction of the auricle with autogenous tissues is a unique marrying of science and art. Although the surgeon's facility with both sculpture and design is imperative, the surgical result will be equally influenced by adherence to sound principles of plastic surgery and understanding anatomy. The surface anatomy of the fully developed external ear consists of the cartilaginous helix-antihelix, scapha, triangular fossa, conchal bowl, and tragus and anti-tragus, as well as the lobule, which does not have a cartilage component (Figure 47.1). The sensory nerves to the external ear include the occipital nerve, greater auricular nerve, auriculotemporal nerve (V3), and the auricular branch of the vagus nerve (Arnold's nerve). The vascular supply to the external ear is via the superficial temporal artery and postauricular artery, both branches of the external carotid artery.

ASSESSMENT OF THE DEFECT

The external ear develops from the first and second branchial arches, with the external auditory meatus arising from the first branchial groove. Microtia is thought to occur secondary to disruption of the stapedial artery in utero. It is also associated with teratogens and some genetic syndromes. Multiple grading systems exist to describe the severity of the auricular defect. Reconstruction is performed when there is adequate chest diameter and costal cartilage to construct the graft, and when the

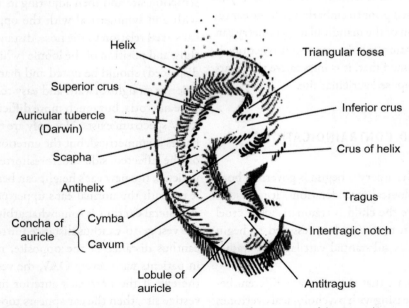

Figure 47.1. Normal external ear anatomy. This illustration demonstrates the normal surface anatomy of the external ear.

contralateral ear is a mature size, usually no earlier than 6 years of age.

The successful grafting of a well-sculpted cartilage framework is the foundation for sound ear reconstruction. By accomplishing this as the first surgical stage, the surgeon takes advantage of the optimal circulation and elasticity of the unviolated skin. Repositioning of vestige remnants is best postponed until after the first stage because resulting scars can inhibit circulation and restrict the skin's elasticity and ability to accommodate a three-dimensional framework. Secondary procedures, such as lobule rotation, tragus construction, and sulcus grafting, take place after sound healing of the "foundation."

Microtia may occur as an isolated finding or in conjunction with other associated anomalies or a genetic syndrome; reported data indicate that 20–60% of children with microtia have an associated anomaly or syndrome. The oculo-auricular-vertebral (OAV) spectrum is characterized by a wide variety of phenotypic findings. These include microtia, facial asymmetry, mandibular hypoplasia, macrostomia, microphthalmia, epibulbar dermoids, and pre-auricular and facial pits and tags, as well as renal, cardiac, and vertebral anomalies. Hemifacial macrosomia and Goldenhar syndrome are included within OAV. Microtia is also a finding in other craniofacial syndromes including Treacher-Collins and Nager syndromes. Assessment for any other anomalies and especially mandibular hypoplasia should be carefully performed during initial consultation for ear reconstruction. When both auricular construction and bony repairs are planned, careful, integrated timing is essential. For patients with significant mandibular hypoplasia that require mandibular distraction, this skeletal asymmetry should be addressed prior to embarking on the ear reconstruction. Correction of the mandibular asymmetry can provide a better foundation for the ear reconstruction. If the bony work is performed first, it is imperative that scars are peripheral to the proposed auricular site.

INDICATIONS AND CONTRAINDICATIONS

The patient age at which surgery is begun is governed both by physical and psychological considerations. It is best to initiate the repair before the child is traumatized by cruel teasing, but the surgeon must not be pressured to begin until rib growth provides substantial cartilage for framework fabrication.

Children become aware that their ears are different between ages 3 and 4, but teasing with psychological overtones does not become manifest until ages 7 to 10. Generally, there is substantial cartilage for the repair by age 6, by which time the child is aware of the problem, usually wants it resolved, and is surprisingly cooperative regarding the surgery. It is optimal to wait to start the reconstruction until the child is interested in having the appearance of the ear improved. If the opposite, normal ear is large and the child is small, the surgery may have to be postponed for several years. On the other hand, a large child with a small normal ear may permit surgery to begin by age 5½. Beginning surgery earlier than this merely invites technical handicaps and poor patient cooperation.

ROOM SETUP AND PATIENT MARKINGS

Prior to surgery, an x-ray film pattern tracing is made from the opposite normal ear, which is reversed and used to plan the new framework. For patients with bilateral microtia, the parent's or sibling's ear can be used for the tracing. This pattern is made several millimeters smaller in all dimensions to allow for the extra thickness that occurs when the cartilaginous framework is inserted under the skin. The framework includes the helical rim, and its inferior pole is extended to the level of the lobule to accommodate the earlobe on its transposition or to facilitate reconstruction of the earlobe when one does not exist. This is further defined when the ear is separated from the head with a skin graft.

The ear's location is determined preoperatively by positioning the reversed film pattern to the proposed construction site and then adjusting its position until it is level with and symmetrical with the opposite normal ear. The ear's axial relation to the nose, distance from the lateral canthus, and position of the lobule (which is usually superiorly displaced) should be noted and marked. The ear's new position is straightforward and easy to plan in a patient with pure microtia, but much more difficult to plan when severe OAV spectrum exists. Not only are the heights of the facial halves asymmetrical, but the anterior-posterior dimensions of the affected side are foreshortened as well. In these patients, the new ear's height can best be planned by lining it up with the normal ear's upper pole—its distance from the lateral canthus is somewhat arbitrary. In pure microtia, the vestige-to-canthus distance mirrors the helical root-to-canthus distance of the opposite, normal side. However, in patients with severe OAV, the vestige is much closer to the eye. If the new ear's anterior margin is placed at the vestige site, then the ear appears too close to the eye; if the measured distance of the normal side is used as a guide, then the ear appears too far back on the head. In these patients, it may be best to compromise by selecting a point halfway between these two positions.

OPERATIVE TECHNIQUE

HARVESTING THE RIB CARTILAGE

The rib cartilage graft is removed through a slightly oblique incision made just above the costal margin. Once the muscle has been divided, the film patterns are used to determine which cartilages will serve best for the framework (Figure 47.2).

To take advantage of the natural rib configuration, the cartilage is harvested from the side contralateral to the ear being constructed. The first free-floating rib's cartilage tapers favorably to form the helix; the synchondritic region of ribs six and seven provides an ample cartilage block to form the framework body.

To conserve anesthetic time, an assistant closes the chest wound while the surgeon fabricates the framework. Using this approach, the entire operation (rib harvest, framework fabrication, and its insertion beneath the auricular skin) routinely takes less than 4 hours. When

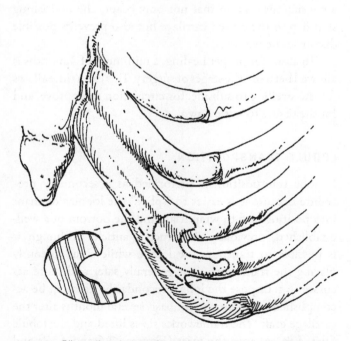

Figure 47.2. Rib cartilage harvest for ear framework fabrication. Film pattern is used as reference in harvesting synchondritic block of cartilage. Note that upper border of sixth cartilage is preserved; this helps to prevent subsequent chest deformity as the child grows. Entire "floating cartilage" is used to create helix.

grafting cartilage, intraoperative antibiotics are given as a prophylactic measure and continued for several days after the procedure. In subsequent stages of ear repair, only preoperative antibiotic prophylaxis is given, except when elevating and grafting the ear of an adolescent patient with intractable acne.

FRAMEWORK FABRICATION

The basic ear silhouette is carved from the synchondritic cartilage block. The film template is modified by cutting out the details of the scapha, antihelix, and triangular fossa. The cutout template can be used to transpose the surface anatomy onto the cartilage block and is marked with methylene blue as a stencil. The cartilage is then carved with careful consideration of the nuanced anatomy (Figure 47.1) at a back table set up with a bowl of saline, different types of scalpel blades, and a gouge. It is necessary to thin only little, if any, of the basic form for a small child's framework, but cartilage thinning is essential for an adult framework. When thinning is necessary, it is wise to preserve perichondrium on the lateral, outer aspect of the framework (notably the antihelical complex) to facilitate its adherence to and subsequent nourishment from surrounding tissues. The superior crus of the antihelix is carved so it gradually declines as it meets the helical ring. The inferior crus, on the other hand, is narrower, more projected, and has a greater vertical height as it abuts the rim. A small cartilage graft is used to augment the inferior crus if needed to obtain slight overcorrection of it projection. The triangular fossa is further defined by carving a 90-degree descent from the helical rim, which is carved full-thickness through the construct at the medial aspect of the fossa and then gradually becoming more superficial at the branch point of the crus. The scaphal groove is carved with preservation of the rim and terminates inferiorly, with an hourglass-shaped groove where the helix meets the lobule, using a narrow gouge or a no. 11 blade. The vertical wall of the conchal bowl descends at a 90-degree angle from the antihelix and extends superiorly to the level of the root of the helix. Above and below this point, the descent is much more gradual.

When creating the helix, the floating rib cartilage is thinned on its outer, convex surface to cause deliberate warping in a favorable direction (Figure 47.3). This allows the surgeon to produce the acute flexion necessary to create a helix, which is then fastened to the framework body with 0.28 mm threaded K-wires. For this purpose, the rim is attached by driving the K-wire through the anterior surface and withdrawing it from the posterior surface

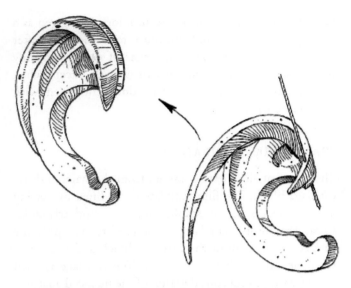

Figure 47.3. Carving helix from floating rib cartilage. To produce acute flexion necessary to create helix, cartilage is deliberately warped in a favorable direction by thinning it on the outer, convex surface.

so that it remains slightly buried anteriorly. The K-wire is then cut on the posterior surface flush with the cartilage. The K-wires are used at the three critical flexion points to stabilize the rim to the framework, starting anterior to the inferior crus and progressing to the superior pole of the helix and finally the posterior border of the framework to create a pleasuring curvature. Any additional stabilization is provided by 4-0 stainless steel suture which is mattressed through the rim and the framework, secured, and buried posteriorly (Figure 47.4). To aid in projection

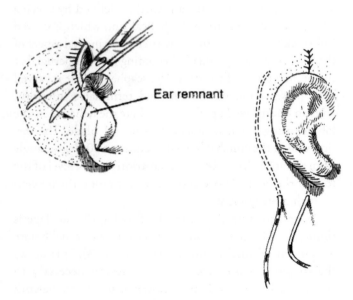

Figure 47.4. Ear framework fabrication with sculpted rib cartilage. Thinned helix is affixed to main sculptural block with k-wires.

and assist with the future elevation of the construct during stage 3, a block of cartilage is attached to the posterior aspect of the vertical wall of the conchal bowl with stainless steel wire.

THE CUTANEOUS POCKET AND SKIN COAPTATION

A cutaneous pocket is created with meticulous technique to provide an adequate recipient vascular covering for the framework. Because nearly 2 hours elapse during the rib harvest and framework fabrication, contamination risk is minimized by scrubbing the auricular region just before beginning the cutaneous dissection.

Using the template and preoperatively determined measurements, the ear's position is marked and a small vertical incision is made in the temporal scalp above the meridian of the planned pocket. On excising unusable vestigial cartilage, a thin skin "pocket" is developed; great care must be taken not to damage the subdermal vascular plexus. To recruit sufficient tension-free skin coverage, the dissection is carried well beyond the marked auricular outline (Figure 47.5).

Following any necessary adjustments either to the framework height or to the pocket adequacy, two small silicone drains are inserted beneath and behind the framework and then into a closed suction Hemovac. This creates a continuous suction that not only coapts the nourishing skin flap to the carved cartilage but also prevents possible disastrous hematomas.

To allow for proper healing, a minimum of 3 months is allowed between the stages of surgery. This extra time allows for the swelling to subside, for circulation to improve, and for the tissues to settle down.

LOBULE TRANSPOSITION

Earlobe transposition is performed as a secondary procedure because it is easier to "splice" the lobular remnant into position and to wrap it around the bottom of a well-established, previously constructed auricle. Although it is possible to transpose the lobule while simultaneously placing the framework, it is generally safer and more accurate to transpose the lobule secondarily. This can be accomplished on an outpatient basis several months after the cartilage graft. The framework's tip is lifted and the lobule filleted to enhance the inset (Figures 47.6 and 47.7) and facilitate the next procedure, in which the ear is separated from the head with a skin graft.

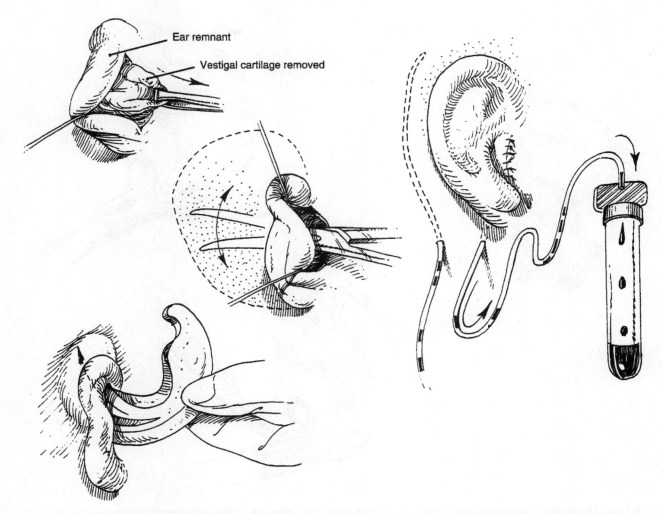

Figure 47.5. Cutaneous "pocket." Vestigial native cartilage is excised and skin pocket is created. To provide tension-free accommodation of framework, dissection is performed well beyond the proposed auricular position. Using two silicone catheters, skin is coapted to framework by means of Hemovac suction.

DETACHING AURICLE WITH SKIN GRAFT

In the next stage of the procedure, the ear is separated from the head with a skin graft and a sulcus is created to define the ear's posterosuperior margin. This improves the ear's appearance by eliminating a cryptotic appearance. This procedure can help adjust the projection by adjusting the position and support of the cartilage block that was placed behind the framework during stage 1. If additional support is needed, a portion of that cartilage graft can be placed under a small anteriorly based mastoid fascia flap. Frontal symmetry is achieved later during tragus construction, in which the contralateral ear can be set back while harvesting grafts for the tragus.

Beginning with an incision made several millimeters peripheral to its margin, the surgically constructed auricle is lifted from its bed, taking care to preserve connective tissue both on its cartilaginous undersurface and on the bony floor below (Figure 47.8).

The retroauricular scalp is then undermined and advanced toward the newly created sulcus and affixed to the fascia and periosteum with heavy sutures (Figure 47.8).

This not only decreases the size of the skin graft needed, but permits advancement of the hairline so that the graft is invisible from the lateral profile.

Because this graft is applied to the back of the ear and color match is not a significant issue, it is harvested it as medium-thickness split skin from the groin, with the resulting donor site hidden beneath the patient's bathing suit region.

TRAGUS CONSTRUCTION

In a single procedure, the tragus is constructed and the concha and the ear canal are further defined by inserting a

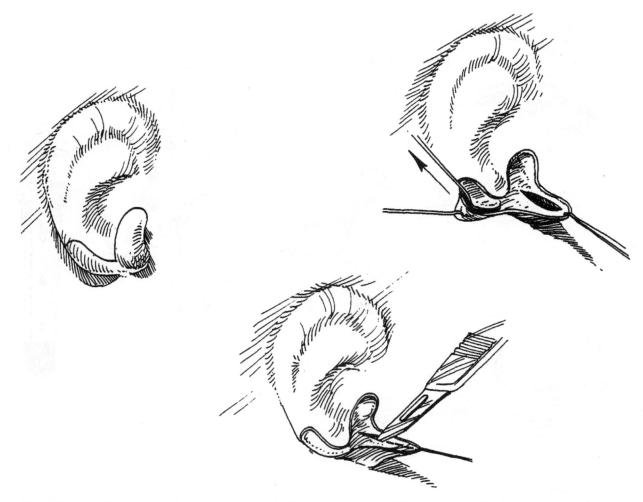

Figure 47.6. Earlobe transposition. By incising around lobule, it is mobilized as inferiorly based flap; incision is outlined at proposed superior inset margin. Skin overlying lower ear region is loosened so that it can be slid under elevated framework's lip to surface "floor" beneath it; lobule is filleted so that it can be wrapped around cartilaginous framework tip in two-layered closure (see Figure 47.7).

special, arched composite graft through a J-shaped incision in the conchal region. The main limb of the "J" is placed at the proposed posterior tragal margin; the crook of the "J" represents the intertragal notch (Figure 47.9). Extraneous soft tissues are excised from beneath the tragal flap to deepen the conchal floor. This excavated region looks quite like a meatus when the newly constructed tragus casts a shadow on it.

To create a realistic tragus with the best curvature, the composite graft is harvested from the anterolateral conchal surface of the normal ear. This technique is particularly ideal when a prominent concha exists because the donor site closure facilitates an otoplasty, which often is needed to attain frontal symmetry. If the concha is not prominent or the projection of both ears is not equal before tragus construction, the donor concha is reconstructed with a full-thickness skin graft. This is easily accomplished by

harvesting a small ellipse of skin from just in front of the retroauricular hairline.

BILATERAL MICROTIA

For optimal function and aesthetics in bilateral microtia, surgical procedures must be integrated so that one does not compromise the other. In these cases, the auricular construction should precede the middle ear surgery or placement of a bone-anchored hearing aid (BAHA) due to risk of infection and potential for compromise of blood flow to the skin flaps used for reconstruction. In bilateral microtia, cartilage grafting for each side is performed several months apart, and the second surgery is a combined with the lobule transposition on the existing framework. The subsequent stages are combined to reduce the overall number of anesthetic events. Simultaneous bilateral reconstruction necessitates

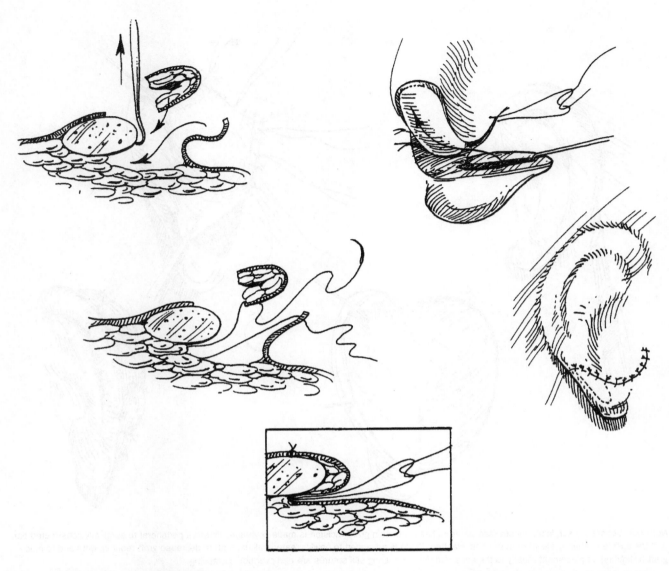

Figure 47.7. Earlobe transposition. Tip of cartilaginous framework is elevated from its soft tissue bed, and filleted earlobe is wrapped around it. In this repair, skin that overlaid cartilaginous tip is now shifted beneath it to surface the raw bed vacated by framework.

bilateral chest wounds with attendant splinting and risk for respiratory distress. Furthermore, the first auricular repair might be jeopardized on turning the head to do the second side if cartilage grafting is performed simultaneously.

To ensure that the gains of middle-ear surgery outweigh the risks and complications of the procedure itself, this surgery is typically reserved for bilateral microtia and selected unilateral cases in which there is high patient motivation and favorable radiologic evidence of middle-ear development. Then it must be thoughtfully planned in a "team approach" with an otologist who is competent and well-experienced in surgery for atresia. If BAHA are to be placed, this procedure is also performed after all stages of the ear reconstruction have been completed.

DRESSING AND POSTOPERATIVE CARE

The new ear's convolutions are packed with petroleum jelly (Vaseline) gauze and a bulky, noncompressive soft dressing is applied. Because the vacuum system provides both skin coaptation and hemostasis, pressure is unnecessary and contraindicated. Patients are admitted following the first stage of reconstruction. A postoperative chest radiograph is obtained in the postoperative acute care unit. Although the patient leaves the hospital after several days, the drains remain in place for 5–7 days, until the patient returns for the dressing and drain removal.

Postoperatively, the ear is checked 1 week after surgery and a lighter dressing with Xeroform gauze, Aquaphor, and

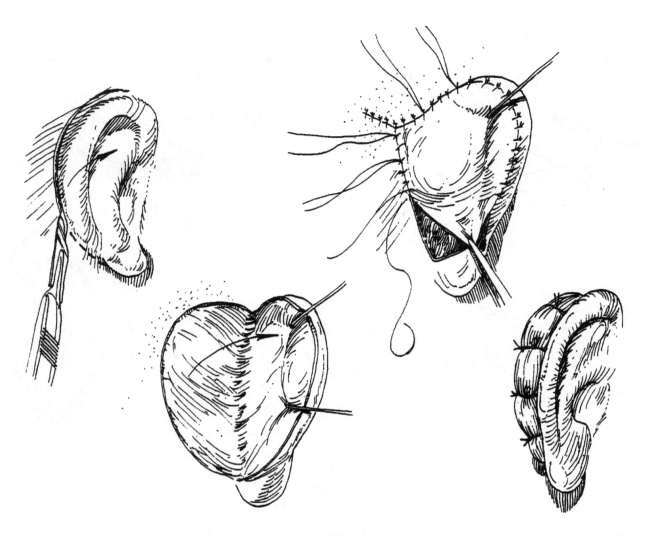

Figure 47.8. Separating surgically constructed ear from head with skin graft. Incision is made several millimeters peripheral to surgically constructed ear, and the auricle is sharply elevated from its fascial bed. Scalp is advanced to newly created sulcus, both to decrease graft requirements and to hide graft by limiting its placement mostly to the ear's undersurface. Long silk sutures are tied over bolus dressing.

Kerlix is applied every 2 days for the second postoperative week. At that time, the patient is allowed to resume school, but running and sports are restricted for 6 weeks after surgery while the chest wound heals.

CAVEATS

COMBINING SURGICAL STAGES

There are rare circumstances in which it may be appropriate to combine stages of ear reconstruction. In some instances, the surgeon may be able to combine upper-ear resurfacing with either lobule transposition or tragus construction. However, combining lifting an ear with constructing a tragus or lifting an ear with any major anterior resurfacing

procedure risks compromise of the reconstruction. The former perilously surrounds the auricle with incisions and undermining, whereas the latter dangerously "skeletonizes" the ear. It may also be feasible to simultaneously elevate the ear and transpose the lobule if the original earlobe vestige is short because its small wound closure will not compromise the ear's anterior circulation.

CONCLUSION

Successful ear reconstruction for patients with microtia requires a thorough understanding of the complex three-dimensional anatomy of the external ear, careful evaluation of each individual patient's defect, and thoughtful surgical planning and timing. Though techniques continue to

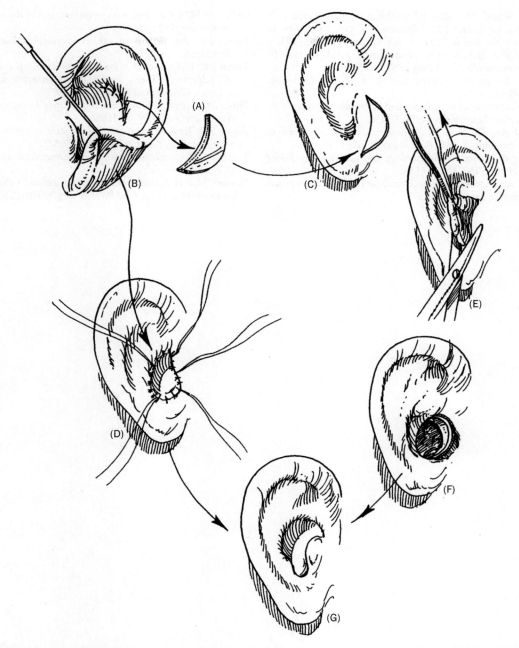

Figure 47.9. Tragus construction and conchal excavation. Harvested from opposite, normal ear's conchal region (A), a chondrocutaneous composite graft is placed under thin, J-shaped flap (C) to create tragus (F,G). Before surfacing floor of tragal region with a full-thickness skin graft (D), harvested from behind opposite earlobe (B), extraneous soft tissues are excised to deepen region (E).

evolve, a staged procedure with autogenous costal cartilage grafting as described in this chapter remains a mainstay of ear reconstruction for both pediatric and adult patients.

SELECTED READINGS

Baluch N, Nagata S, Park C, et al. Auricular reconstruction for microtia: A review of available methods. *Plast Surg* 2014;22(1):39–43.

Beahm EK, Walton RL. Auricular reconstruction for microtia: part I. Anatomy, embryology, and clinical evaluation. *Plast Reconstr Surg* 2002;109(7):2473–2484.

Brent B. Auricular repair with autogenous rib cartilage grafts: two decades of experience with 600 cases. *Plast Reconstr Surg* 1992;90:355.

Brent B. Technical advances in ear reconstruction with autogenous rib cartilage grafts: personal experience with 1200 cases. *Plast Reconstr Surg* 1999;104:319.

Brent B. The correction of microtia with autogenous cartilage grafts. I. The classic deformity. *Plast Reconstr Surg* 1980;66:1.

Brent B. The correction of microtia with autogenous cartilage grafts. II. Atypical and complex deformities. *Plast Reconstr Surg* 1980;66:13.

Broadbent TR, Woolf RM. Bilateral microtia: a team approach to the middle ear. In: Tanzer RC, Edgerton MT, eds. *Symposium on Reconstruction of the Auricle*. St. Louis: CV Mosby, 1974:168–173.

Gibson T, Davis WB. The distortion of autogenous cartilage grafts: its cause and prevention. *Br J Plast Surg* 1957;10:257.

Kirkham HLD. The use of preserved cartilage in ear reconstruction. *Ann Surg* 1940;111:896.

Knize DM. The influence of periosteum and calcitonin on onlay bone graft survival. *Plast Reconstr Surg* 1974;53:190.

Lauritzen C, Munro IR, Ross RB. Classification and treatment of hemifacial microsomia. *Scand J Plast Reconstr Surg* 1985;19:33.

Luquetti DV, et al. Microtia: epidemiology and genetics. *Am J Med Genetics Part A* 2012;158(1):124–139.

Song Y, Song Y. An improved one-stage total ear reconstruction procedure. *Plast Reconstr Surg* 1983;71:615.

Steffenson WH. Comments on reconstruction of the external ear. *Plast Reconstr Surg* 1955;16:194.

Tanzer RC. An analysis of ear reconstruction. *Plast Reconstr Surg* 1963;31:16.

Tanzer RC. Discussion of silastic framework complications. In: Tanzer RC, Edgerton MT, eds. *Symposium on Reconstruction of the Auricle*. St. Louis: CV Mosby, 1974:87–88.

Tanzer RC. Microtia: a long-term follow-up of 44 reconstructed auricles. *Plast Reconstr Surg* 1978;61:161.

Tanzer RC. Total reconstruction of the auricle: the evolution of a plan treatment. *Plast Reconstr Surg* 1971;47:523.

Tanzer RC. Total reconstruction of the external ear. *Plast Reconstr Surg* 1959;23:1.

Thorne CH, et al. Auricular reconstruction: indications for autogenous and prosthetic techniques. *Plast Reconstr Surg* 2001;107(5): 1241–1252.

48

OTOPLASTY FOR PROTRUDING EARS, CRYPTOTIA, OR STAHL'S EAR

David W. Furnas

ASSESSMENT OF THE PROTRUDING EAR

AURICULAR PROTRUSION IN THE NEONATE

If the neonate with protruding ears, mildly constricted ears, a Stahl's ear, or even cryptotia is seen by the plastic surgeon during the neonate's first days of life, the timing is auspicious.[1–19] By initiating immediate steps to mold the ear with tapes and splints, complete correction of the problem without surgery is a realistic expectation (Figure 48.1). The urgency and the effectiveness of early nonsurgical treatment of such ears is not yet widely appreciated by those responsible for primary medical care of neonates. It is the plastic surgeon's task to heighten awareness of such treatment. (*Note*: The term "ear" in this chapter is used as a synonym for the external ear, pinna, or auricle.)

AURICULAR PROTRUSION IN CHILDREN AND ADULTS

The first step in assessing the patient for otoplasty is determination of the anatomic causes of protrusion of the ear:

1. An underdeveloped or flat anthelix (Figure 48.2)

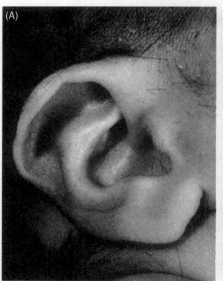
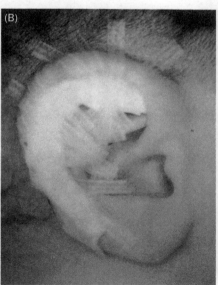
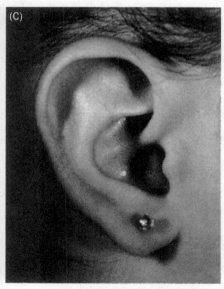

Figure 48.1. Nonsurgical treatment of prominent ears in neonatal period. (A) Prominent ears with "lopped" superior poles in 2-week-old infant. Molding with copper wire armature padded with silicone tubing held in scaphoid fossa with Steri-Strips was carried out for 1 week (see Figure 48.15F). (B) Molding was continued with rolled Microfoam tape armature (no metal core). (C) Appearance at 4 months of age. Correction was stable after 2 months of taping.

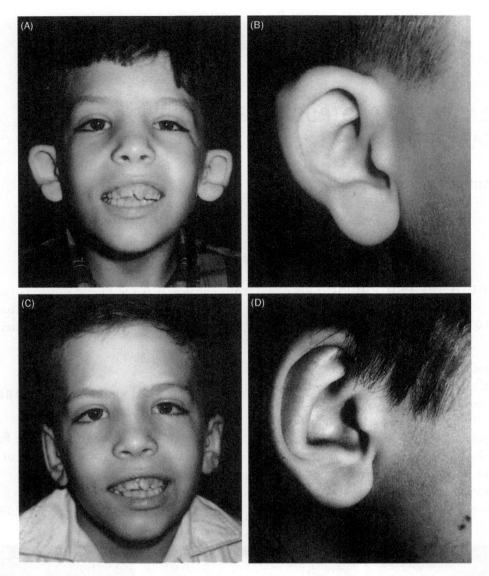

Figure 48.2. Mustardé sutures. (A,B) Preoperative views of 10-year-old with absent anthelix root and superior crus, which caused prominence of each ear. Repositioning with Mustardé sutures corrected prominence and mild overhang of rim of helix. (C,D) Postoperative view.

2. An overdeveloped, deep concha (Figure 48.3)

3. A combination of both of these features (Figures 48.4 and 48.5)

   Contributing features that accentuate auricular protrusion are:

1. Prominence of the mastoid process

2. Protrusion of the lower auricular pole (cauda helicis, lobule, and cavum concha)

3. A prominent, tipped upper auricular pole

COMPLEX AURICULAR DEFORMITIES THAT ARE ACCOMPANIED BY PROTRUSION

Auricular protrusion may be one element of a more complex auricular deformity, such as a constricted ear (Figures 48.6 and 48.7), Stahl's ear (third crus) (Figure 48.8), macrotia, or a syndromic facial deformity (Figure 48.9).

Certain anatomic parts may tend to be recalcitrant to correction and require special surgical maneuvers. These features are identified by a detailed manual "rehearsal" of the otoplasty, so that such problems do not appear by surprise at operation. When pressing the central pinna into its corrected position, the examiner is alert to persistent

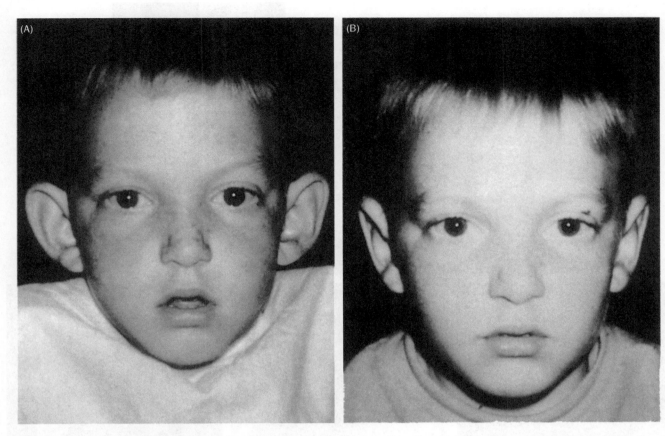

Figure 48.3. Concha-mastoid sutures. (A) Preoperative view. Boy, age 10, in whom auricular prominence was caused by excessively deep conchal cups. Treatment was bilateral concha-mastoid sutures. B, postoperative view.

protrusion of the upper or lower pole, to thick immobile auricular cartilage, or to cartilage that is so flabby that it bunches, rather than folds, when manipulated. Forewarned, the surgeon is prepared to deal with these problems during surgery.

The dimensions and projection of the ears are measured. Both ears are photographed and their morphology is recorded. (Two full-face photos are taken in case the patient's eyes blink during one.) The position of the ears relative to other facial features is noted. The morphology of the other facial features, the skull, and the oral cavity is surveyed.

AURICULAR ANATOMY
AND PROTRUDING EARS

SURGICAL PERSPECTIVE
OF AURICULAR ANATOMY

The anterior (lateral) surface of the ear is the traditional reference plane for the anatomic nomenclature of the ear

(Figures 48.10, 48.11 and 48.12). However, many steps in an otoplasty, such as placing cartilage sutures, removing soft tissue, or trimming cartilage, may be performed on the posterior (medial) surface of the ear. From a posterior perspective, the concha and the fossae are viewed as eminences and the crura are seen as grooves.

On cursory inspection, the shape of the cartilage framework appears to duplicate the visible ear. However, on closer examination, the auricular cartilage proves to be an incomplete skeleton with gaps, drop-offs, and irregularities in thickness, augmented with connective tissue and muscle. The surgeon must be skillful in integrating these hidden features and illusions into a thought model of the patient's auricular anatomy.

The qualities of the auricular cartilage as a material, and its biomechanical responses to external and internal forces, must be assessed not only preoperatively, but intraoperatively and, indeed, throughout the early postoperative period. Whether the auricular cartilage is made up of limber cartilage, stiff cartilage, or floppy cartilage is of prime importance in choosing the appropriate operative steps.

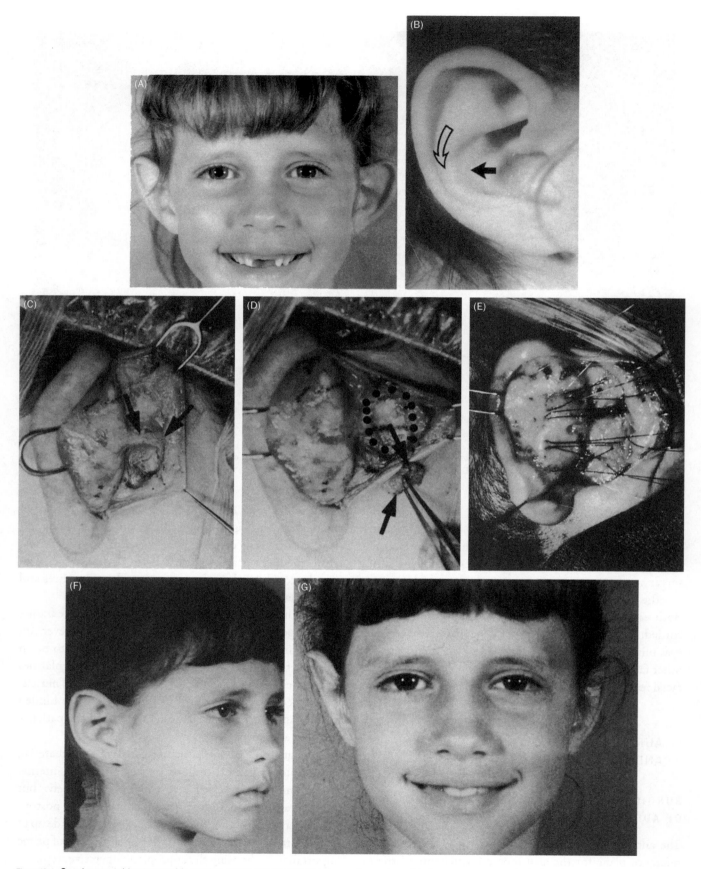

Figure 48.4. Concha-mastoid sutures with conchal nests and Mustardé sutures. A, conchae of both ears were excessively deep in this 7-year-old girl; in addition, anthelices were underdeveloped, more on left than right side. (B) Solid black arrow points to high posterior wall of right ear, and open arrow lies along underdeveloped root-superior crus of anthelix. (C) Left postauricular area exposed; arrow points to auricularis posterior. (D) Auricularis posterior and adjacent soft tissues have been excised to form conchal nest. Arrow points to excised soft tissue. (E) Sutures ready for tying in similar patient. Note heavy blue concha-mastoid sutures and clear, light Mustardé sutures. (F,G) Result from bilateral concha-mastoid sutures, multiple Mustardé sutures on left, and single Mustardé suture on right.

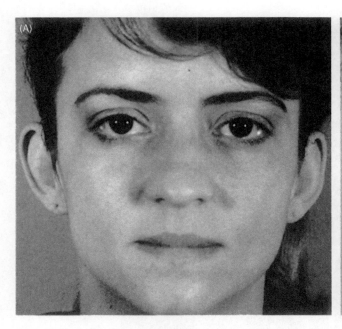
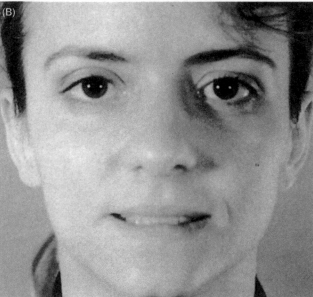

Figure 48.5. Fossa-fascia sutures, Mustardé sutures (including cauda helicis), and concha-mastoid sutures. (A) Preoperative view of 28-year-old woman with prominent ears, in which upper poles were resistant to repositioning. (B) Postoperative view of patient after bilateral placement of Mustardé sutures (including cauda helicis-concha suture), concha-mastoid sutures, fossa-fascia sutures (scaphoid fossa to deep temporal fascia), and simultaneous tip rhinoplasty.

THE ANTHELIX

The anthelix normally forms an asymmetrical "Y," in which the gently rolled or folded crest of the root of the anthelix continues upward as the superior crus. The inferior crus branches forward from the root as a folded ridge. The root of the inferior crus of the anthelix sharply defines the rim of the concha. The inferior crus also forms the wall that separates the concha from the triangular fossa. The root and superior crus of the anthelix form the anterior wall of the scaphoid fossa; the helix forms the posterior wall. The triangular fossa dips within the "Y" arms of the superior and inferior crura.

The corrugated contours of these auricular crests and valleys provide a pillar effect, which stabilizes the pinna. The vertical walls of the conchal cup are translated to a semihorizontal plane as the concha merges with the folded crest of the anthelix. The scapha-helix is nearly parallel to the plane of the temporal surface of the head. If the roll of the anthelix and its crest are effaced and flat, rather than rolled or folded, the steep pitch of the conchal wall continues into the unformed anthelix and scapha and ends at the helix with little interruption. This places the scapha-helix complex nearly perpendicular to the temporal plane of the head, and the ear appears unaesthetically prominent. Such an ear also lacks the stability provided by the pillar effect and thus allows the superior auricular pole to protrude.

THE CONCHA

The concha is an irregular hemispherical bowl with a defined rim. The normal scapha-helix surrounds the posterior part of the bowl as the brim of an inverted hat would surround the crown. The pitch at which the scapha-helix projects from the conchal cup is determined by:

1. The acuteness of the fold of the crest of the anthelix

2. The height of the posterior wall of the conchal bowl

3. The completeness of the partial sphere formed by the concha

If the posterior wall of the concha is excessively high and the concha is excessively spherical, then the angle and the distance between the plane of the scapha-helix and the plane of the temporal surface of the head will be excessive. This increased depth and extra spherical bulk are additive in causing auricular protrusion. Usually, such protrusion is evenly distributed around the posterior conchal wall. However, the cephalad part of the concha can protrude disproportionately, which is another cause for a protruding upper pole. Similarly, the caudal part of the concha can project disproportionately and cause a protruding lower auricular pole. These features require special attention in the operating room.

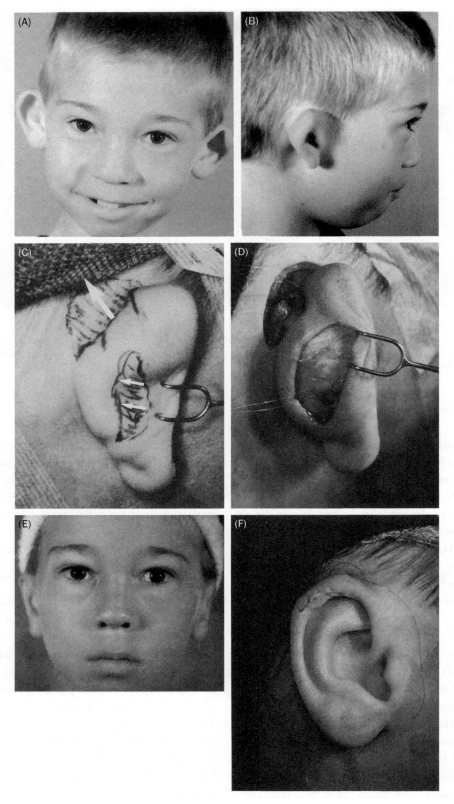

Figure 48.6. Constricted prominent ear treated with fossa-fascia and conchamastoid sutures and trimming of overhanging helix rim (9-year-old boy with mosaic deletion of chromosome 18-p). (A,B) Constricted prominent ears, preoperative views. (C) Incision patterns. Large white arrow shows direction of force to be applied with fossa-fascia sutures; small arrows show direction of force of Mustardé sutures. (D) Sutures in place, ready to tie. (E) Postoperative full face view. (F) Postoperative lateral view shows suture repair of excised area of helix. Upward displacement of fossa-fascia sutures obliterated superior auricular sulcus.

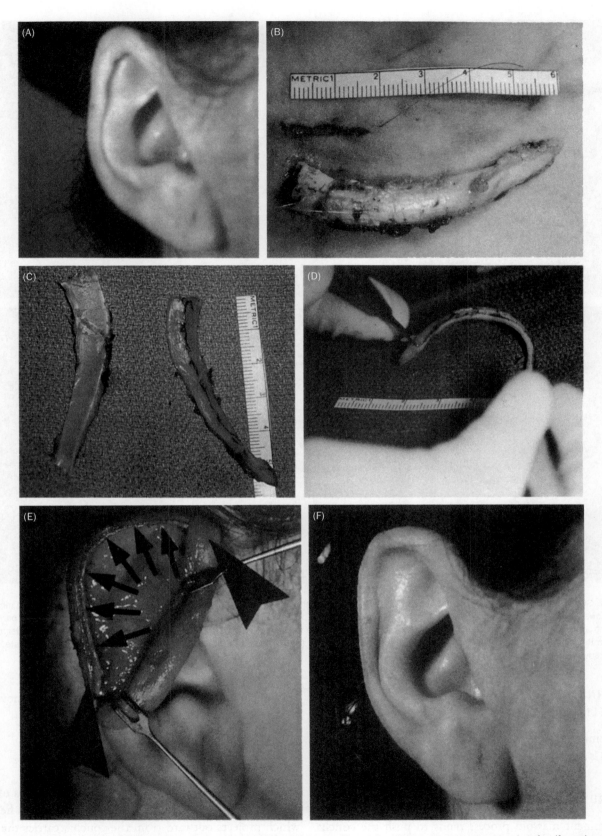

Figure 48.7. Constricted prominent ears treated with augmentation of auricular framework with costal cartilage and conservative trimming of malformed auricular cartilage. (A) Constricted prominent right ear with pixie shape (similar to left ear) in 49-year-old woman. (B) Right ninth (approximately) costal cartilage removed through 16 mm incision, retaining perichondrium on cartilage. (C) Cartilage graft split in half, one for each ear. (D) Medullary cartilage removed, leaving cortex with attached perichondrium, which converted stiff costal cartilage into limber, flexible graft. (E) Auricular framework exposed via postauricular incision. Graft secured to auricular cartilage with multiple sutures (*small arrows*), paying special attention to attaching it to crus of helix (*large arrow*). (F) View of right ear at 1 year postoperatively.

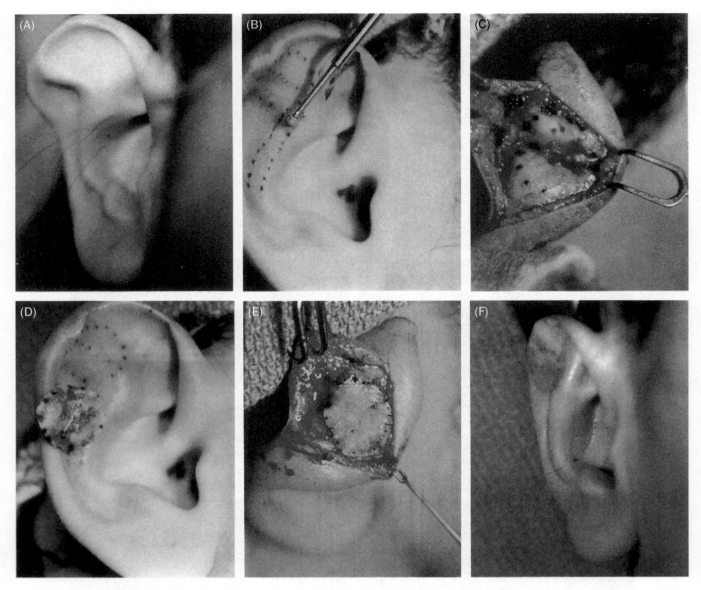

Figure 48.8. Stahl's ear with soft, floppy cartilage and third crus. (A) A 10-year-old Hispanic girl with Stahl's ear. (B) Diameter line of dotted 12 mm circle shows crest of third crus. Path of subcutaneous tunnel for abrasion of crest of anthelix is plotted with parallel dotted lines; diamond burr will be introduced from caudal direction. (C) Tattooed dots of 12 mm circle viewed posteriorly. (D) Excised circle is inverted and turned 90 degrees for illustration; third crus will become part of scaphoid fossa and anthelix. (E) Cartilage graft repositioned and sutured in place. (F) Immediate postoperative appearance.

COMBINATION OF PROTRUDING ANTHELIX AND CONCHA

The combined effect of an effaced anthelix and a deep concha is also additive, causing a severe auricular protrusion.

PROTRUDING MASTOID PROCESS

A prominent mastoid process tends to push the concha forward, causing auricular prominence. I have seen marked auricular protrusion caused by a dermoid cyst in the recess between the mastoid process and the concha. Removal of the cyst corrected the problem.

PROTRUDING CAUDA HELICIS

The cauda helicis is bound to the fibrofatty tissues of the earlobe by a network of connective tissue. A cauda helicis, which projects outward from the concha, carries the earlobe with it, causing it to protrude. This contributes to prominence of the lower pole.

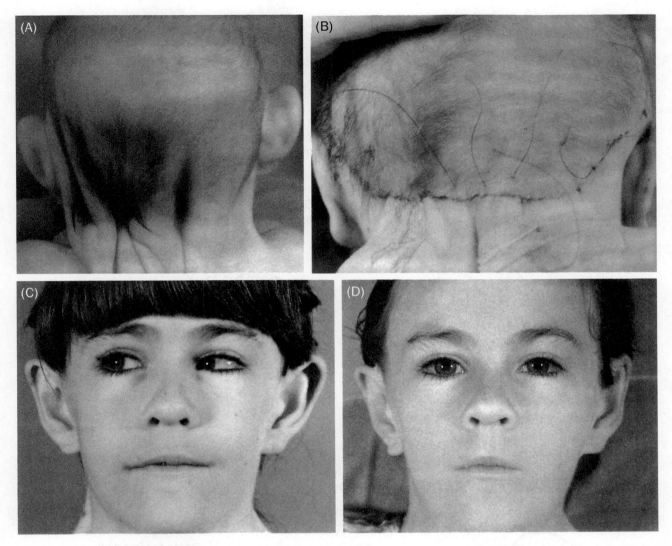

Figure 48.9. Prominent ears with true macrotia in Turner's syndrome. (A) Prominent ears and webbing of neck in girl with Turner's syndrome. (B) Prominent ears treated with Mustardé sutures and concha-mastoid sutures; webbing of neck treated by skin-scalp excision and advancement flaps at age 4 months. (C) Age 7, patient shows recurrence of auricular prominence and macrotia. (D) Prominent ears treated with repeat concha-mastoid sutures and Mustardé sutures. Macrotia was not treated.

PROTRUDING EARLOBE

Some earlobes are not only large and pendulous but are also prominent because of the structure and form of the dense, interlacing connective tissue fibers that shape the earlobe, independent of the cauda helicis.

CONGENITAL AURICULAR DEFECTS ASSOCIATED WITH PROMINENT EARS

CONSTRICTED EAR

Protrusion of the constricted ear (Figures 48.6 and 48.7) is the result of a helix that is diminished in diameter,

causing deformity of the related auricular structures. In its mild form, the features are auricular prominence, an abbreviated long auricular axis, and an overhanging helix eave. The spectrum of constricted ears is one of progressing severity stopping short of microtia (see further discussion in the later section on otoplasty for prominent constricted ears).

STAHL'S EAR

The major deformity in Stahl's ear (Figure 48.8) is a ridge (third crus) that traverses the midscaphoid fossa from the inferior crus of the anthelix to the superoposterior helix. The ear is also prominent. Stahl's ear is common among

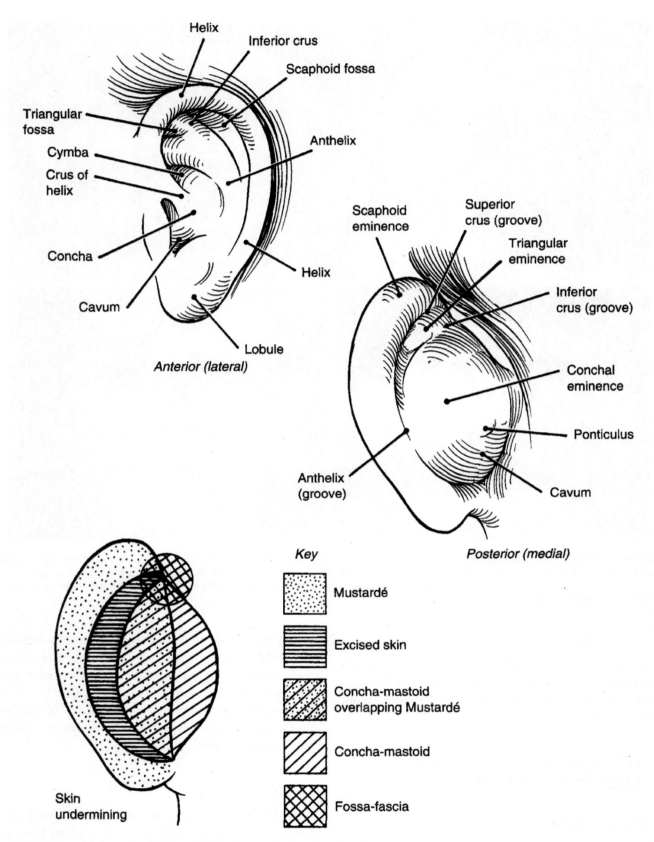

Figure 48.10. Surface anatomy of auricle (*top, middle*) and areas of skin undermining (*bottom*).

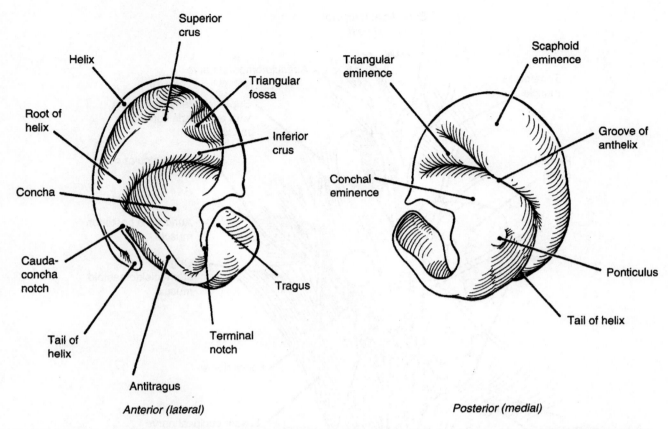

Figure 48.11. Anatomy of auricular cartilage, anterior (lateral) and posterior (medial) surfaces. Although anterior landmarks are most familiar, posterior auricular landmarks are of special importance in otoplasty.

Japanese people and rare among Caucasian people. The few treated on our service have been Caucasian or Hispanic with soft, flabby cartilage (see later discussion on otoplasty for Stahl's ear [third crus]).

CRYPTOTIA

Cryptotia (Figure 48.13) is common among Japanese people but rare among other groups. The upper anterior pole of a cryptotic ear retracts into a subcutaneous, skin-lined pocket, where it hides. Light traction on the ear everts the pocket and brings the hidden structures into view. Cryptotic ears may be prominent, but prominence of the ear is not necessarily part of the condition (treatment is discussed later).

MACROTIA

1. *Congenital.* True congenital macrotia, in which the vertical and transverse axes of the ear exceed normal limits, is rare. Macrotic ears are commonly also

protruding ears. Congenital macrotia is seen as an independent unilateral or bilateral finding, or it can by seen as part of Turner's syndrome (Figure 48.9) or other congenital conditions.

2. *Acquired.* Macrotia is also a secondary effect of involvement of auricular tissues with neurofibromatosis, lepromatous leprosy, mycosis fungoides, and other medical conditions. The gravitational effect of aging increases the vertical diameter of the soft tissues of the ear, but the dimensions of the auricular cartilage are unchanged. Auricular protrusion is not necessarily a characteristic of acquired macrotia.

ASSESSMENT OF AURICULAR CARTILAGE IN THE PROMINENT EAR

The texture, thickness, pliability, and mobility of the auricular cartilage are thoroughly evaluated by manipulation.

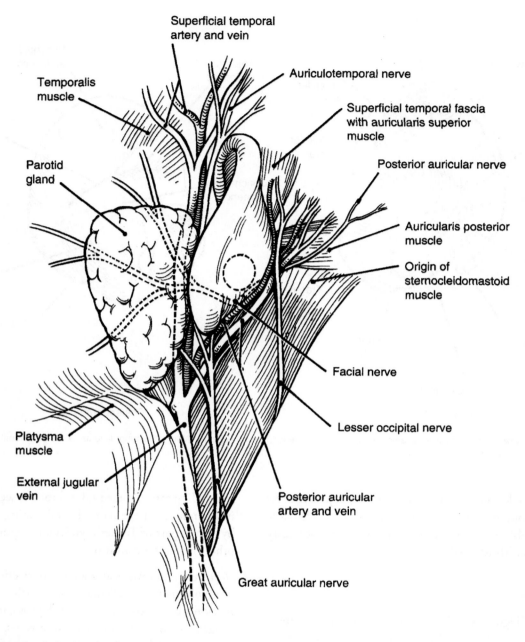

Figure 48.12. Anatomy of auricular vessels, nerves, and muscles.

The character of the cartilage influences the surgical method that will be most effective.

LIMBER CARTILAGE

Most commonly, the ear is composed of limber cartilage, which is of medium thickness and resilience and responds well to manipulation by the examiner; this cartilage should also respond well to any of the common otoplasty techniques. If the examiner accentuates the roll of the anthelix with his or her fingers, she does not meet excessive resistance. However, the roll has a stabilizing pillar effect, and the cartilage does not tend to shift axes or bunch up.

STIFF CARTILAGE

Not infrequently, protruding ears have stiff cartilage, particularly the ear with very deep conchae (Figure 48.14). Such cartilage is heavy, thick, and resistant to manual shaping and positioning. The strategy of the otoplasty and the postoperative management must be designed to surmount these problems.

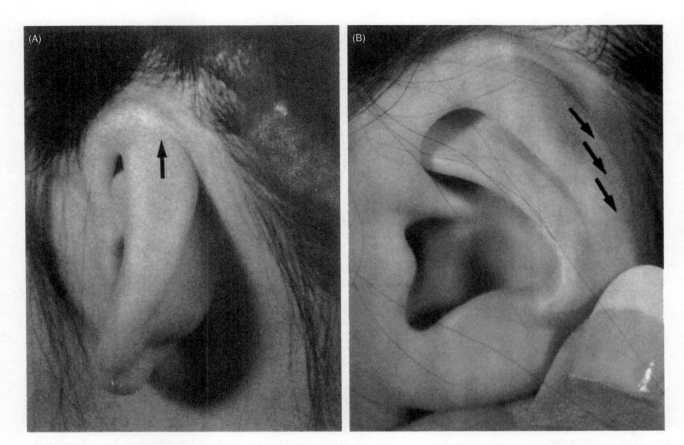

Figure 48.13. Cryptotia. (A) A 7-year-old Korean girl with cryptotia; anterosuperior auricular structures hidden in temporal pocket (arrow points to fold at entry of pocket). (B) Finger traction completely inverts pocket with almost no trace of fold, and superoanterior structures of ear come into view. Treatment is planned with postauricular skin expansion.

FLOPPY CARTILAGE

Rarely, the surgeon encounters floppy cartilage (Figure 48.15). This soft, malleable, flabby cartilage is unstable when reshaped by techniques that are effective in other ears, and special surgical steps are needed to obtain a stable result.

Scarred Cartilage

In the event of a revision of an otoplasty or treatment of previously injured ear, the mobility of the cartilage is inhibited by the layers of scar in which it is typically encased (Figure 48.16). Any cracks or sharp folds in the cartilage are vulnerable to fracture, and anatomic landmarks may be deceptive, so special care is exercised.

ASSESSMENT FOR OTHER RELEVANT PHYSICAL FEATURES

The presence of auricular asymmetry or malposition, facial asymmetry, chronic otitis, diminished auditory acuity,

deficient activity of facial musculature, branchial remnants, or evidence of previous operative procedures is noted to aid in identifying a syndromic pattern, a surgical contraindication, or a need for special preparations (such as special preoperative studies, endoscopic tracheal intubation, or intraoperative facial nerve monitoring).

INDICATIONS FOR OTOPLASTY

Protruding ears may be a source of psychological distress in either sex at any age. Most often, the patient will be a child brought in by parents who have been prompted by the child's sensitivity to taunts from other children. Playmates may invoke names from an ample inventory of cartoon characters and animal species to undermine the child's confidence. McGregor speaks of the "exquisite cruelty of young children toward the child who happens to look different." These pediatric patients are highly motivated and cooperative. A truly gratifying psychologic response to a well-performed otoplasty is the rule. These children do not

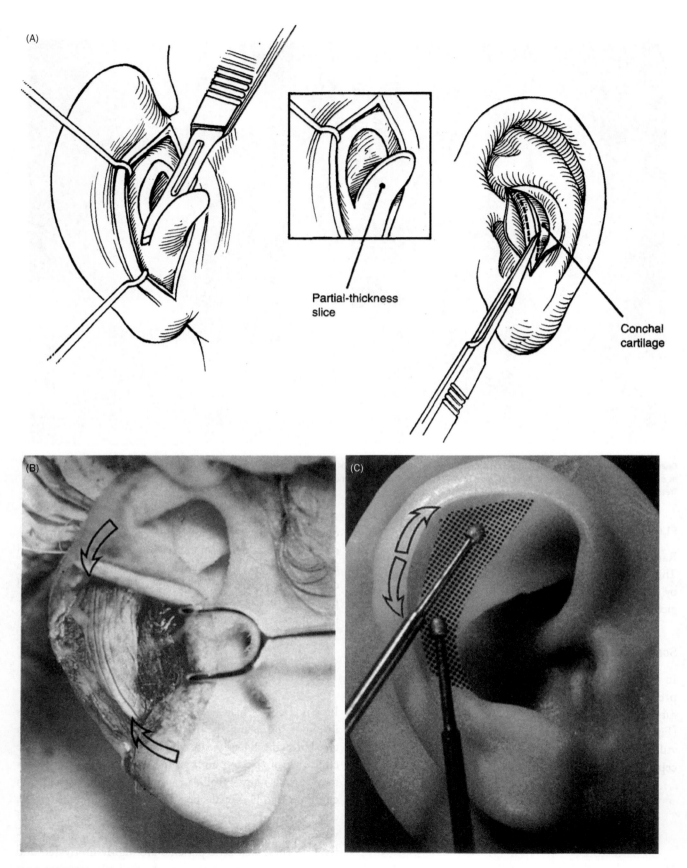

Figure 48.14. Stiff, heavy cartilage. (A) If cartilage is not limber and is resistant to force of sutures, surgeon can choose from among additional steps that provide compliance. To reduce deep concha, cartilage may be excised from either posterior (partial-thickness or full-thickness) approach or anterior approach. Folding of anthelix is enhanced by Stenstrom scoring; convexity of cartilage is produced by scoring one side of cartilage, which releases interlocked stresses that curl cartilage in opposite direction. (B) Stenstrom scoring has just been performed with no. 15 blade (*in line with arrows*) to augment camber of underdeveloped anthelix. (C) Abrasion of anthelix is performed with unmounted, discarded diamond burr (Midas B3D or B2D) via subcutaneous tunnel (acrylic ear model).

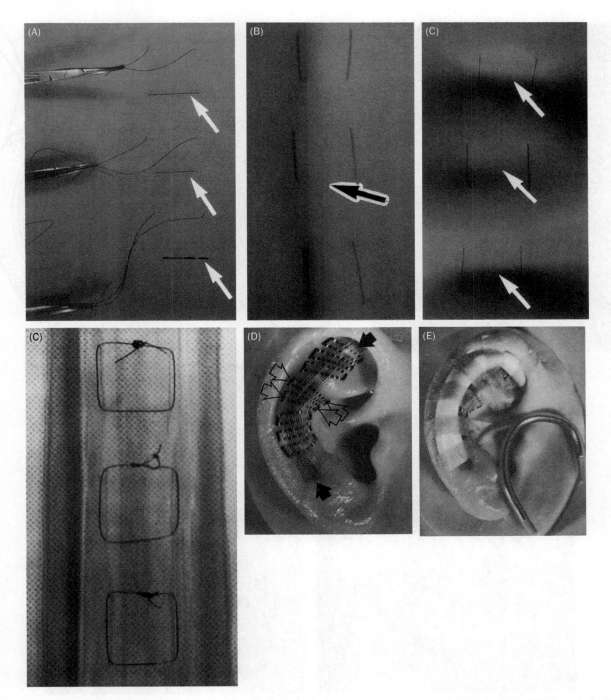

Figure 48.15. Soft, floppy cartilage. (A) Mattress sutures placed in Mustardé fashion in sheet latex (model for posterior surface of floppy auricular cartilage). White arrows point to transverse ("bowstring") component of mattress suture. Bowstrings compress longitudinal limbs of mattress sutures on anterior surface of latex. (B) Mattress sutures viewed from anterior surface after tightening. Longitudinal limbs of mattress sutures compress latex into "anthelix ridge." (C) Same model as Figure 48.14B after latex has been subjected to movement, but sutures themselves have not been disturbed. Longitudinal "anthelix ridge" has capsized into undulating series of transverse ridges, each oriented in manner of "third crus." (D) Similar model of "anthelix"; using flexible 10-mil ethylacetate sheeting in mattress sutures creates longitudinal ridge. Material is limber but not floppy; camber of "anthelix" has created semirigid pillar. (E) Surgical means of preventing anthelix ridge from capsizing. *Black arrows* indicate lines of scoring of lateral surface of ridge. *Open arrows* point to mattress sutures, which are greatly increased in number (acrylic model of ear). (F) External means of maintaining longitudinal anthelix ridge and preventing formation of transverse ridges. Soft roll of Microfoam tape secured with Steri-Strips maintains integrity of scaphoid fossa. Just in front of acrylic ear is armature of copper wire encased in soft silastic tubing, which could be used instead of Microfoam tape, if more rigid molding were needed. (Techniques in photo use same principles as nonsurgical treatment of prominent ears in neonates; see Figure 48.1).

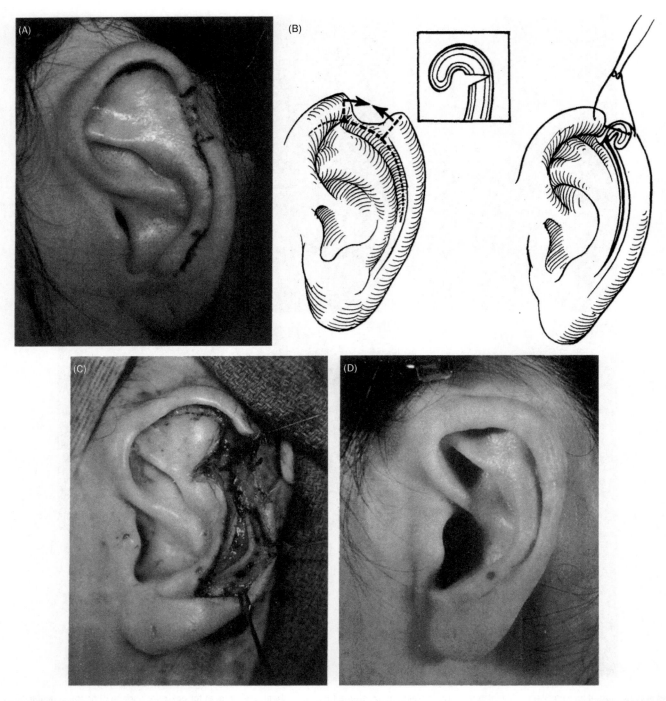

Figure 48.16. Reduction otoplasty of large prominent ears with iatrogenic defects using Antia-Buch excisions and advancement flaps. (A) Left ear after three previous otoplasties for prominent ears. Among cartilage deformities, large notch in cartilage of helix and scaphoid fossa (as marked) was most notable. A similar, slightly less severe defect was present on right. Ears were still prominent and vertical axis was quite long. (B) Diagram of modification of Antia-Buch excisions and advancement flaps. (C) Flaps elevated at surgery and excisions begun. (D) Postoperative view.

seek perfection in their otoplasty, but the surgeon must be aware that some parents may have unrealistic expectations. A frank discussion about the operation and what it can achieve is in order, including the negative side effects and the risks of surgery and anesthesia. Adolescent and adult patients often give a history of embarrassment about their prominent ears since childhood years, but circumstances have precluded corrective surgery. These patients also are likely to be highly satisfied with the results of surgery.

Asymmetrical features of the ears should be called to the attention of the patient and parents, and a distinction should be made between the features that are likely to be improved by surgery and those that will stay the same. The postoperative evaluation of the otoplasty by patient, family, and friends is inevitably more detailed than any preoperative evaluation.

CONTRAINDICATIONS FOR OTOPLASTY

The surgeon must be alert for the occasional adult who magnifies the severity of a small defect or who sees serious deformity in ears that are judged to be near-normal by others. Time is spent carefully listening to each patient (and parent) preoperatively and in soliciting and answering the patient's (and parents') questions. Dealing with concerns and expectations preoperatively reinforces the probability that a technically excellent otoplasty will be viewed with satisfaction and gratitude postoperatively. Ethnic and cultural considerations sometimes enter the algorithm. Prominent ears are the norm among Celtic people, and in Japan, prominent ears are said to denote intelligence. However, it usually does not take long for children to conform to the cultural values of their adopted country.

An important step in gaining patient satisfaction is development of an individual surgical strategy that will provide an excellent result for that patient. This starts with careful assessment of the defect, as previously discussed. Chronic conditions, such as otitis media, otitis externa, scalp infections, or acne, must be dealt with well in advance of surgery. A simple surgical wound infection can lead to an ear-threatening chondritis.

ROOM SETUP AND PREPARATION

GENERAL ANESTHESIA FOR PEDIATRIC CASES

After induction of anesthesia, the endotracheal tube is placed in the midline and is secured with a circummandibular or transmaxillary alveolar suture of 1-0 or 1 polypropylene (Prolene). The table is turned 180 degrees. An intravenous injection of a cephalosporin or other appropriate intraoperative antibiotic is given. The hair is shampooed with chlorhexidine gluconate (Hibiclens), rinsed, and blotted dry. The face, neck, and ears and nearby anesthesia and monitor tubing are prepared with aqueous povidone-iodine (Betadine). A head drape is placed with both ears exposed. Adhesive solution (Mastisol) is applied to the face, and a series of 1-in. Steri-Strips is placed to hold the head towels securely to the face and neck. Steri-Strips are placed over the eyes. The body sheet is made of crystal-clear plastic and provides visibility of the entire anesthesia apparatus. After markings have been placed, the postauricular areas are injected with 0.5% lidocaine solution with epinephrine 1:200,000 for hemostasis.

LOCAL ANESTHESIA FOR OLDER CHILDREN AND ADULTS

Children vary immensely in their suitability for local anesthesia. Occasionally, a mature 10-year-old with high motivation and uncomplicated prominent ears is a candidate for local anesthesia without premedication. A parent reads a favorite story or plays a favorite audiotape for the child during the procedure. A thick coat of eutectic mixture of lidocaine and procaine (EMLA) cream is applied to the postauricular area 2 or 3 hours in advance. Oral azithromycin (Zithromax) is given 2–3 hours before surgery in children. In adults, ciprofloxacin (Cipro) is given 1 hour before surgery. The posterior surface and retroauricular surface of each ear is slowly infiltrated with buffered 1% lidocaine (Xylocaine) solution with epinephrine 1:100,000 by means of a 27- or 30-gauge needle. This is followed by infiltration with bupivacaine (Marcaine), 0.25% solution, with epinephrine 1:100,000. Lidocaine or bupivacaine are reinforced during the procedure if needed to stay within the range of the recommended dosage.

AIDS IN VISUALIZATION

Attention to fine detail can determine the difference between a good and an excellent result. High-powered loupes (4.5×, 11- to 13-inch working distance) and a coaxial headlamp add immeasurably to the surgeon's ability to evaluate anatomy and to conduct the operative steps.

PATIENT MARKINGS

Manipulations are carried out as on the planning visit. Markings are made with gentian violet stain to indicate the crests of the anthelix and to indicate the sites of all sutures that are planned. A set of instant (Polaroid) photographs of the marked ears is made for use in the operating room, along with the other preoperative photographs. In the operating room, the skin markings are reinforced after facial preparation has been completed. The marks are not tattooed; rather, judgments for suture placement or other manipulation are made by intraoperative manipulation and testing and by careful observation of the anatomy of the posterior surface of the auricular cartilage manipulation. The gentian violet lines and suture marks serve more for rehearsal than for intraoperative guidance.

OPERATIVE TECHNIQUE

TYPICAL SUTURE OTOPLASTY (PROTRUDING EAR WITH LIMBER CARTILAGE)

Incision and Dissection

Incision or excision of postauricular skin (Figure 48.10). The posterior surface of the auricular cartilage is exposed by excising the premarked crescent of skin and subcutaneous tissue. The crescent is made wide enough to remove redundant skin and long enough to provide for necessary exposure at the upper or lower pole of the base of the ear. Hemostasis is maintained with bipolar cautery; monocular cautery is avoided because it inflicts damage if it touches cartilage.

Postauricular dissection. Postauricular landmarks are, of course, the reverse of the named anterior landmarks. Posteriorly, "crests" of crura are valleys, and fossae are projections. The surgeon embraces this perception as the dissection proceeds. The posterior surface of the auricular cartilage is exposed widely. Scissors-spreading dissection with a very fine, sharp-on-sharp iris scissor is combined with scalpel dissection. Both intrinsic and extrinsic auricular muscles tend to insert directly into cartilage with no obvious intervening perichondrium, putting the insertion sites at risk for nicking. Nicks in the cartilage are studiously avoided. If the intrinsic muscles and fibrous bands are bulky and obstructive, they are removed, paying particular attention to the valleys of the anthelix if Mustardé sutures are planned. The auricularis posterior muscle, with its paired bellies and its accompanying postauricular ligament, serves as a landmark. Just deep to the conchal insertion of the auricularis posterior muscle is a palpable protrusion of cartilage, the ponticulus, which provides anchorage for the postauricular ligament.

Dissection is then extended peripherally on the concha and the scapha-helix almost to the free edge of the helix. The helix rim is completely exposed if trimming or manipulation of the rim is planned. The surgeon anticipates the site where the cauda helicis diverges from the concha. The cauda

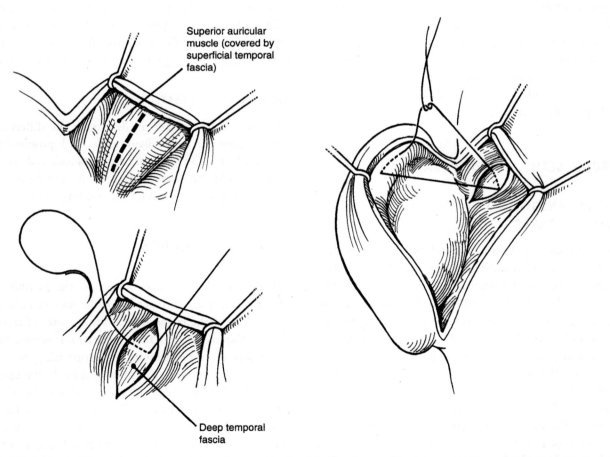

Figure 48.17. Fossa-fascia (F-F) sutures reduce prominence of upper pole of auricle. Deep temporal fascia is exposed by spreading fibers of auricularis superior and superficial temporal fascia. Sutures pass from deep temporal fascia to cartilage of scaphoid fossa or triangular fossa.

is exposed with precision, preserving its attachments to the fibrofat and skin of the earlobe. A well-attached cauda is an aid in positioning the ear lobe. The apex of the angle between the cauda and the concha is the site of entry for a tunnel if one is to be made on the anterior surface of the anthelix (see section on Stenstrom scoring) (Figure 48.14). If a conchal nest is to be made for concha-mastoid (C-M) sutures, dissection and soft tissue excision are extended as later described. If a prominent upper pole of the auricular cartilage is to be brought closer to the head with separate fossa-fascia (F-F) sutures (Figure 48.17), the local skin and scalp are elevated from the superficial temporal fascia and perichondrium of the helix root (otobasion superius) in preparation for the steps described later.

Mustardé Sutures (Concha-Fossa Sutures)

The surgeon uses Mustardé sutures to create an anthelix roll and crest when the cause of protrusion is deficiency or absence of the anthelix (Figures 48.2, 48.18 and 48.19). These sutures create or augment the roll of the anthelix by approximating the scaphoid fossa closer to the concha.

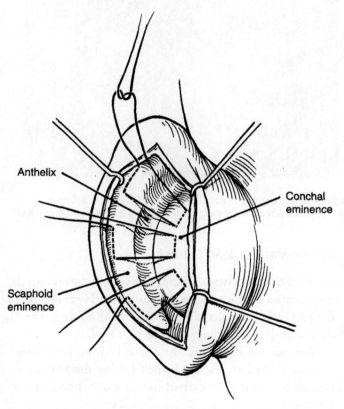

Anthelix

Conchal eminence

Scaphoid eminence

Figure 48.18. Mustardé (scapha-concha) sutures produce or increase anthelix fold where fold is absent or underdeveloped. Sutures "bowstring" from scaphoid fossa or triangular fossa to posterior conchal wall. In Kaye's modification, sutures are placed from anterior approach through tiny incisions.

A series of horizontal mattress sutures is placed in a row that centers on the "crest" (valley, viewed from posteriorly) of the anthelix. After surgical preparation has been completed, the surgeon shapes the ear with his or her fingers, forming the contours of the anthelix. (This step should be rehearsed at leisure preoperatively.)

Incision and dissection. These are carried out as previously described. Excess muscle and connective tissue are cleared from the area of the anthelix fold. The ear is manipulated and the suture sites are verified.

Placement of sutures. I favor tapered needles (e.g., Ethicon RB-1, C-1, or SH) because they have less tendency to split cartilage. I currently use 5-0 or 6-0 blue monofilament polypropylene because clear polypropylene is not supplied with these tapered needles. At the time of this writing, no suture has been visible through the anterior skin. Clear monofilament polypropylene sutures are available on a variety of cutting needles (e.g., Ethicon P-4, PS-2), which also give very satisfactory service. The first mattress suture penetrates the full thickness of the cartilage of the (potential) scaphoid fossa. The bite is wide enough for secure engagement of the cartilage but not so wide as to bend the cartilage on any axis other than the crest of the anthelix. The second bite engages a full thickness of the corresponding conchal cartilage. With each bite, before the needle is passed completely through the cartilage, the anterior auricular skin is checked to see that the suture did not penetrate or catch the anterior skin or subcutaneous tissue. The suture path is completed, and the suture is tentatively tightened. The resulting fold and adjacent contour changes are judged.

Final positioning of sutures. Mustardé sutures are pulled just tight enough to create the desired anthelix roll and to allow for a small amount of postoperative settling. The final position of the ear is judged by examining the full face with both ears in view, placing the table low enough to provide good perspective. An effort is made to place the fold so that the rim of the helix is barely visible outside the new anthelix crest.

Once the correct anthelix roll has been achieved, the mattress sutures do not coapt the cartilage surface to surface, but only bring the surfaces closer together. A double bowstring of suture spans the intervening gap. If the axis and curve of the anthelix appear correct, a surgeon's throw is laid, and the suture ends are clamped and set aside. After the complete series of sutures has been placed, the position of the ear is rechecked, and the sutures are readjusted, knotted, and cut. In some cases, it is more convenient to place, knot, and cut sutures individually.

Anterior approach for folding anthelix. An alternative to the posterior approach is placement of a series of tiny

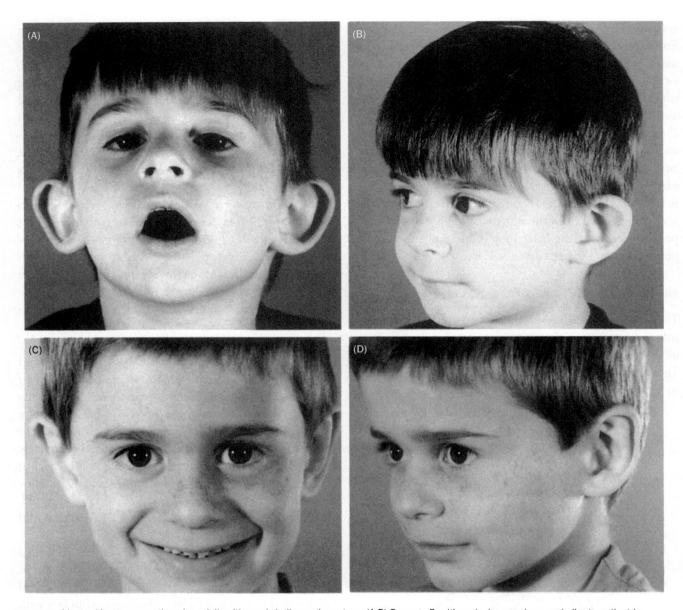

Figure 48.19. Mustardé sutures continued caudally with cauda-helix-concha suture. (A,B) Boy, age 5, with auricular prominence similar to patient in Figure 48.2. (C,D) Postoperative view after placement of Mustardé sutures in which caudal-most suture fixed cauda helicis to posterior wall of concha.

incisions anteriorly, through which the mattress sutures are passed through the cartilage, and subcutaneously. The knots are cut anteriorly beneath the skin.

Modifications. The most superoanterior Mustardé suture may be more effective if it is placed from the triangular fossa (rather than the concha) to the scaphoid fossa, enhancing the superior crus of the anthelix. The remaining sutures pass from the scaphoid fossa to the concha. Sometimes an additional suture is added, which passes from the cauda helix to the posterior conchal wall. This suture tends to reinforce the anthelix roll and to influence the position of the earlobe (see section on lobe sutures). Special steps are needed when the auricular cartilage is soft and floppy or when it is thick and stiff.

Concha-Mastoid (C-M) Sutures

C-M sutures are mattress sutures that correct the excessively deep concha (Figures 48.3 and 48.20). They lower or flatten the protruding concha, diminishing the distance between the conchal rim and the mastoid area.

Incision and dissection. The initial incision and dissection are started as described; then further dissection and soft-tissue excision are carried out to aid in lowering the concha.

Excavation of conchal nest. Bulky postauricular soft tissue is incised and folded posteriorly or excised to create a nest to accommodate the repositioned conchal cup

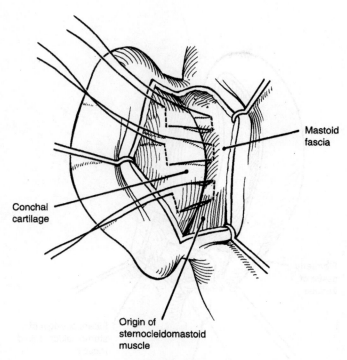

Mastoid
fascia

Conchal
cartilage

Origin of
sternocleidomastoid
muscle

Figure 48.20. Concha-mastoid (C-M) sutures and conchal "nest." Sutures reduce excessive conchal projection, passing from conchal cartilage to mastoid fascia and to aponeurotic fibers of origin of sternocleido-mastoid muscle. Sutures flatten conchal bowl against mastoid process. Removal of excess soft tissues provides easier identification of mastoid fascia and contributes to reduction of conchal projection.

(Figure 48.4). The mastoid skin and subcutaneous tissue are widely elevated from the auricularis posterior muscle, the sternocleidomastoid origin, the intervening fatty areolar tissue, and the investing mastoid fascia. Branches of the postauricular vessels and the great auricular nerve are identified. The surgeon presses the concha against the exposed mastoid surface to judge which soft tissues must be excised to provide the concave nest, which is designed to reflect the shape of the concha in size and orientation. The targeted oval of tissue is outlined with methylene blue. The tissue is excised, including the auricularis posterior, the fatty areolar tissues, the outer layers of mastoid fascia, and any intervening neurovascular structures that cannot be readily pushed aside. Alternatively, the oval is incised along its anterior, superior, and inferior edges and folded back, hinged on the posterior edge. Sufficient layers of mastoid fascia, sternocleidomastoid aponeurosis, and periosteum are retained on the floor of the nest to provide reliable anchorage for the C-M sutures. If these tissues are excised *too* thoroughly, the remaining mastoid periosteum is too thin to provide reliable anchorage. Advantages of removing bulky postauricular soft tissues are that (1) the conchal height is naturally reduced when the new postauricular surfaces are apposed, (2) the suture

force needed to reposition the conchal cartilage is diminished, and (3) the needles can be passed through the strongest fascial layers of mastoid fascia and sternocleidomastoid origin under direct vision, unobscured by bulky overlying soft tissue.

Once the anchorage provided by the postauricular soft tissues has been freed, the ear loses positional stability. Care must be taken to maintain orientation.

Placement of sutures. C-M sutures approximate the posterior wall of the concha to the mastoid fascia. This flattens the protruding concha and reduces the projection of the ear. The sutures pass from the posterior conchal wall to the mastoid periosteum and fascia. Because the C-M sutures bear more force than the Mustardé sutures, 4-0 or 5-0 sutures are employed. The materials and needles are otherwise the same as the Mustardé sutures. The surgeon holds the ear in its new position to judge the correct placement of the sutures. If the cartilage bite is placed too high on the wall of the conchal cup, the mattress suture will flatten the cup against the mastoid process excessively. If the cartilage bite is too low on the conchal wall, the suture will be ineffective. Alignment of the sutures is important. A mastoid bite that is too far posterior will elongate the concha transversely. A mastoid bite that is too far anterior may flatten or even kink the external auditory canal. Superior-inferior alignment must also be taken into account because loss of ligamentous and muscular support makes it possible to displace the ear vertically.

Once the correct sites have been determined, four or five 4-0 or 5-0 monofilament sutures are placed according to the markings and the anatomic landmarks. The first bite of the needle engages the full thickness of the conchal cartilage. The second bite of the needle engages the mastoid fascia or the aponeurotic origin of the sternocleidomastoid muscle. The sutures are tightened, seating the conchal cup in its nest and compressing the protruding side walls so that the conchal bowl is shallower and wider.

Tying the C-M sutures. Each suture is tied with the first throw of a surgeon's knot, and the effect is evaluated by a full frontal view of the face and both ears. If the conchal position is satisfactory, the sutures are tied and cut. If extra holding power is needed during the initial placement of trial sutures, surgeon's knots with triple throws or figure-of-eight mattress sutures are incorporated. Figure-of-eight sutures are more stable in holding their position after the first throw, but they may have a greater tendency to erode cartilage if pulled up tightly; thus, tension must be judged carefully.

The elasticity of the conchal cartilage transmits a continuous force to the sutures during the period of healing and maturation. Therefore, the bites of tissue must be of ample thickness and breadth, and the tension under which they are tied must give approximation without strangulation. If the position of the ear appears incorrect once the sutures have been tied and cut, strategic placement of another suture or two will usually correct the problem. If the problem persists, it may be necessary to remove and replace some or all of the sutures. If a particularly severe protrusion of the concha is corrected, a natural side effect is to lose the smooth transitional curve from conchal floor to posterior wall and instead to have a crease at the transition.

Fossa-Fascia (F-F) Suture for the Prominent Upper Pole

Sometimes the upper pole of a prominent ear is exaggerated in its protrusion and is difficult to correct with the usual combination of Mustardé and C-M sutures (Figures 48.5 and 48.17). This is usually the case in the constricted ear. Occasionally, a sharply protruding upper pole will be the patient's sole aesthetic problem. In such cases, the anchorage point selected is in the borderland of the mastoid fascia and the deep temporal fascia. For greatest effectiveness, the use of the deep temporal fascia itself gives the best result. Direct suturing of the cartilage of the triangular fossa, or the scaphoid fossa to the deep temporal fascia, provides excellent control over the upper auricular pole.

Dissection. Ample elevation of the skin and scalp on both sides of the superior auricular sulcus is carried out, exposing the cartilage of the anterior-most part of the scaphoid fossa and of the triangular fossa. On the medial side of the sulcus, the superficial temporal fascia is exposed. The ear is manipulated to judge the best sites for suture placement. The superficial temporal fascia is then windowed to expose the deep temporal fascia by scissors-spreading dissection in a vertical direction, avoiding injury to the branches of the superficial temporal and postauricular vessels.

Placement of sutures. Using the techniques just described, mattress sutures are placed from the deep temporal fascia to the cartilage. One or two carefully placed sutures are usually all that are needed since there is little resistance for the sutures to overcome.

A side effect is an inconspicuous effacement or elevation of the superior auricular sulcus.

Prominent Earlobes

It is not unusual for prominent earlobes to persist after a prominent auricle has been repositioned (Figure 48.21). Several techniques have proved useful.

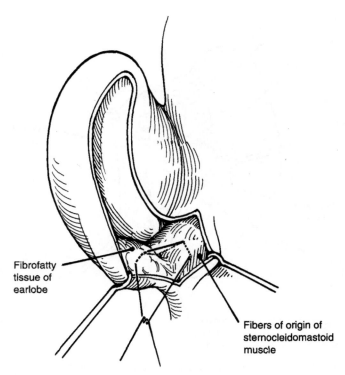

Fibrofatty tissue of earlobe

Fibers of origin of sternocleidomastoid muscle

Figure 48.21. Lobe sutures diminish prominence of projecting earlobe.

Patterned lobe reattachment. The crescentic pattern of postauricular skin excision is extended inferiorly into the postauricular sulcus. The pattern is widened in a dumbbell shape within the posterior sulcus of the earlobe. Thus, mirrored patterns of skin are removed from the medial surface of the lobe and from the mastoid. Skin closure reduces the prominence of the earlobe. A side effect is encroachment of the closure area on the earring area of the lobe. Medial placement of the lobe can be enhanced by placing mattress sutures from the fibrofatty tissue of the lobe to the conchal cartilage, or to the aponeurotic fibers of the insertion of the sternocleidomastoid muscle.

Percutaneous lobe anchoring sutures. One or more 2 mm punctures are made in the lateral surface of the earlobe, and, using fine-tipped scissors, the skin is undermined around each puncture to minimize dimpling of the lobe. A 7-0 polypropylene suture on a P-6 needle is passed through the puncture and then beneath the surface of the posterior skin of the lobe so that it emerges from the postauricular wound. Then an anchoring bite is placed through conchal cartilage, after which the path of the suture is reversed so that it emerges through the puncture wound. The to-and-fro paths of the needle are directed so that they are separated by ample fibrofat before they converge on the puncture. The suture is then tied so that the fibrofat incorporated in the suture is drawn toward the conchal anchorage point, thus drawing the prominent lobe into an inconspicuous position. The skin edges of the puncture are manipulated to avoid dermal penetration by the needle and resultant dimpling. The suture is cut on the knot, and the puncture is closed with 7-0 polypropylene. An alternative is to reverse the process, starting the first pass of the suture at the conchal cartilage, emerging from the puncture wound of the lobe, and then reentering the puncture wound, passing the suture beneath the skin of the lobe, and emerging near the concha. The knot is then placed on the conchal cartilage. A heavier suture can be used for this alternate variation, but judging the correct tension for tying the suture is more difficult.

Combined Sites of Suture Placement

The steps in a suture otoplasty are selected to deal with the particular clinical problem. The sutures discussed can be used in any combination. The sequence of steps is planned for ease of suture placement and for the ability to evaluate the position of the ear as the steps proceed. Often, the conchal bites of the different types of sutures intermingle. When this is the case, the sutures are kept separated by group to avoid entanglement. The Mustardé sutures are held anteriorly in a single mosquito clamp, the C-M sutures are held posteriorly in another clamp, and F-F sutures are held caudad in another. The C-M sutures are tied first; then the Mustardé sutures are tied, checking the changing position of the ears as these steps proceed. Finally, the F-F and lobe sutures are tied.

OTOPLASTY AND STIFF, HEAVY AURICULAR CARTILAGE

If the cartilage of the protruding ears is stiff and heavy, the force required to move the unmodified auricle may provoke erosion of the sutures through the cartilage, causing relapse of the otoplasty. C-M sutures bear more tension than the other types of sutures, and several modifications are designed to ameliorate the possibility of excess tension.

Conchal Thinning: Partial-Thickness Cartilage Excision, Posterior Approach

The accessible areas of the floor of the conchal cartilage are thinned with a scalpel, a Nagata-Hoshi gouge, or a looped Gillette Techmatic blade, if available (Figures 48.14 and 48.22). Great care is taken to avoid sharp edges or fractures at conspicuous sites. The trimming is continued from the conchal floor to the conchal walls, thinning the junction area between floor and walls. The trimming is continued as far forward as feasible on both the inferior and superior conchal walls. This step alone may reduce the "spring" of the concha sufficiently. The diminished conchal volume adds to the ease of conchal reduction. A side effect is a sharper angle or furrow at the transition zone, between the conchal walls and the floor.

FULL-THICKNESS CONCHAL CARTILAGE EXCISION

Posterior approach. For stiffer, thicker cartilage, full-thickness excision of conchal cartilage may be indicated (Figure 48.22). From a posterior approach, cartilage is removed from the floor and from the junction zone of the side walls. The farther forward the excision extends on the conchal bowl, the more thoroughly the spring of the concha is nullified.

Anterior approach. The popularity of auricular cartilage grafts in nasal reconstruction has made the anterior approach (Figure 48.23) to conchal cartilage familiar to all plastic surgeons. A full-thickness crescent of skin and cartilage, centered on the posterior wall but incorporating the entire posterior 180 degrees of the concha, cancels the resistance of the stiff cartilage. The cartilage crescent is designed for accurate approximation of the cut edges of cartilage with absorbable sutures. The crescent of excised skin is narrower than that of the crescent of cartilage. This provides for ease of skin closure, at the same time removing sufficient skin to avoid redundancy. A side effect is an anterior concha scar, which, with careful placement, is inconspicuous. Occasionally, the slope of the conchal bowl makes the scar difficult to hide. Also, scars can "bowstring" within any concavity.

Stenstrom Anthelix Scoring, Abrading, and Thinning

When heavy cartilage resists the effect of Mustardé sutures, release of Gibson's interlocked stresses by scoring or abrading the crests of the anthelix causes the anthelix to curl in the correct direction, as observed by Stenstrom (Figure 48.14). Access to the anthelix crest is gained by dissecting an anterior subcutaneous tunnel, which starts at the apex of the angle between the cauda helicis and the concha and continues subcutaneously along the crest of the anthelix. Careful scissors-spreading dissection with a fine sharp-on-sharp iris scissor is directed along the crest of the root and superior crus of the anthelix. To abrade the anthelix, a discarded Midas B3D or B2D diamond burr is used. Sufficient abrasion is produced to gain the desired release,

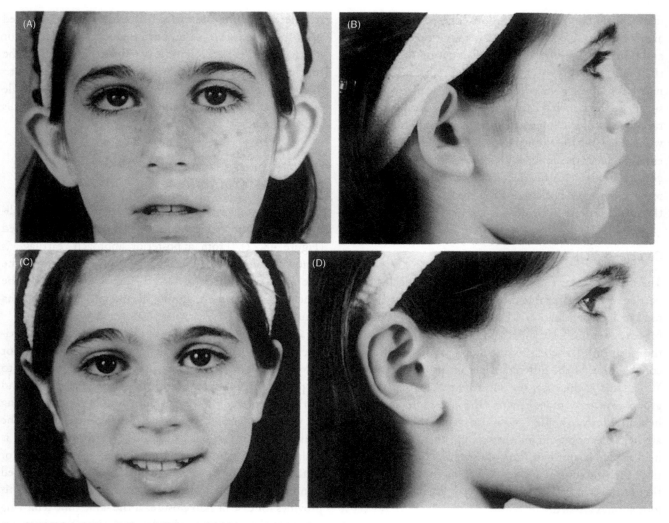

Figure 48.22. Heavy, thick auricular cartilage; partial-thickness excision of posterior conchal cartilage and Stenstrom scoring of anthelix. (A,B) Preoperative views. Ears of 9-year-old girl were repositioned with concha-mastoid (C-M) sutures after concha was thinned. Mustardé sutures were placed after Stenstrom scoring of each anthelix. Right ear was 10–15% larger than left. Earlobe sutures were placed from fibrofatty tissue of lobe to posteromedial conchal wall. (C,D) Postoperative views.

but care is taken to avoid excessive abrasion with the possibility of fracture and a sharp edge.

Posterior Groove of Anthelix

Direct thinning of posterior surface of thick cartilage of the anthelix is another method of reducing the resistance to formation of an anthelix fold and of controlling the line of the fold. Removing cartilage from the posterior surface is counter to the "Gibson effect," but this is readily overcome by Mustardé sutures. The cartilage excision must be done over a wide enough swath, leaving sufficient thickness so that a sharp fold or fracture will not result. Such a complication would significantly degrade the result.

OTOPLASTY FOR PROMINENT EARS WITH SOFT, FLOPPY AURICULAR CARTILAGE

Prominent ears with soft, floppy cartilage are uncommon in the child or adult (Figures 48.15 and 48.24). Such ears often have an incomplete helix rim and usually have both a deficient anthelix and a deep concha. Some present as a Stahl's ear (discussed later). A standard suture otoplasty for prominent ears with soft, floppy cartilage can be a treacherous procedure. Once the key sutures are placed, the correction may appear to be excellent, and then, within a matter of minutes, the position of the cartilage changes and what was at first a satisfactory anthelix roll lapses into a series of transverse undulations. In normal cartilage, the anthelix roll is formed by the compression

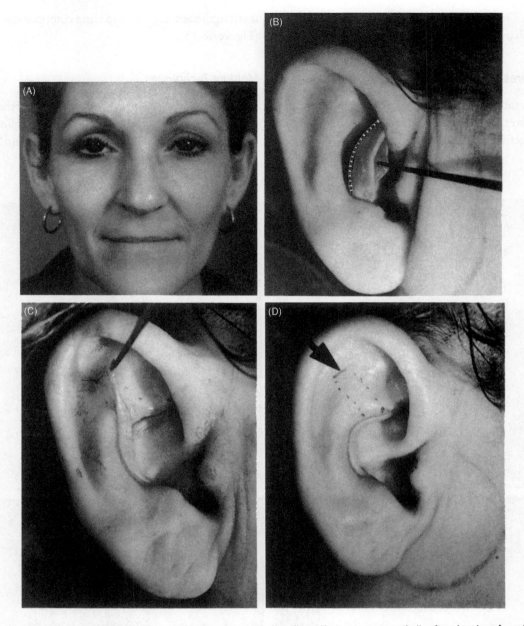

Figure 48.23. Heavy, thick auricular cartilage; anterior excision of excess conchal cartilage; Kaye sutures to anthelix after abrasion of crest. (A) A 46-year-old woman had prominent ears with stiff auricular cartilage. (B) After delivering conchal cartilage through anterior conchal rim incision, excess cartilage was excised (*dotted line*). (C) Lesser area of excess conchal skin was excised (held in forceps) to ensure easy skin closure. (D) Single Kaye suture was placed (*arrow and marks from surgical pen*) to enhance fold of superior crus. Combination of maneuvers left retroauricular area free for suture lines of routine rhytidectomy.

of the limbs of the mattress suture, which are parallel to the axis of the anthelix. The limbs of the suture that traverse the axis serve to maintain the compression of the axial limbs. If the cartilage is unduly flexible, compression and deformation can be exerted by the transverse limbs of the mattress sutures. This deformation takes the form of a transverse arch, such as a third crus, or a series of undulations. With some minor manipulation of the cartilage, the proper shape of the anthelix roll can

be retrieved, but this correction will most likely be only temporary.

Several steps are useful in correcting prominent ears with soft, floppy cartilage.

Stenstrom Scoring

Gentle scoring of the cartilage along the crest of the anthelix aids in giving stability to the roll of the anthelix

(Figure 48.8). Deep abrasion could fracture the soft cartilage, causing sharp edges and angles.

Multiple Sutures

If the mattress sutures are placed at very close intervals along the anthelix, so that the axial limbs of sutures are shorter and closer together, the axial compression of the cartilage is strengthened and the opposing compression is weakened (Figure 48.15).

Molding Techniques

After completion of scoring and suturing, further stability is provided by shaping the ear with a padded splint or a dental compound mold (Figures 48.1 and 48.24) and Steri-Strips.

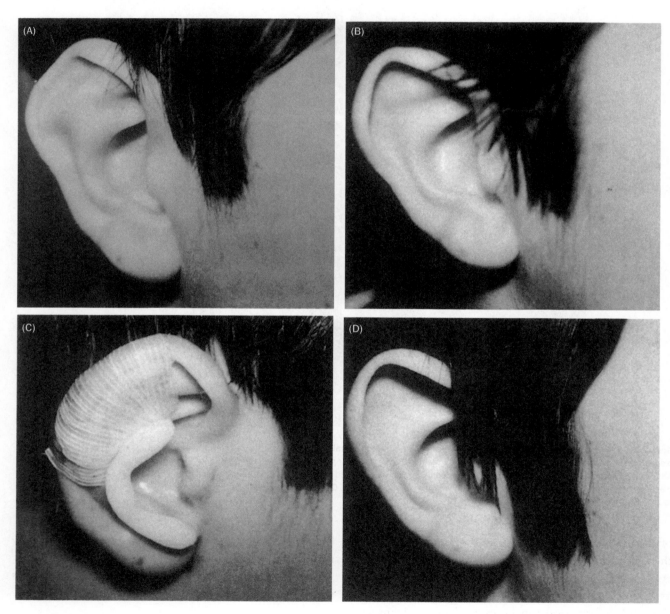

Figure 48.24. Soft, floppy cartilage; iatrogenic third crus corrected with repeat otoplasty and postoperative molding. (A) Preoperative view of 10-year-old boy with bilateral protruding ears with soft, floppy cartilage; right ear was more prominent than left. (B) Postoperative view. Third crus developed when soft cartilage shifted in position after dressing had been applied (see Figure 48.14). (C) Otoplasty repeated, employing Stenstrom scoring of anthelix, multiple Mustardé sutures, and postoperative molding of ear with bone wax. Visible C-shaped wax pattern is for illustration. True wax mold is hidden by Steri-Strips that hold wax in scaphoid fossa. (D) Postoperative view shows inconspicuous residual of third crus.

OTOPLASTY FOR THIRD CRUS (STAHL'S EAR)

Congenital Third Crus

Although Stahl is reported to have classified a series of related ear deformities, the term "Stahl's ear" has come to mean a third crus of the anthelix (Figure 48.8). This is an elevated fold that traverses the upper pole of the ear from the inferior crus to the upper helix rim and is associated with local deformation of the auricular cartilage. Sometimes the helix is pushed into a "pixie-ear" prominence. The superior crus may be deformed or absent, and the eave of the helix may be partially or totally absent.

The patients with Stahl's ear seen in our service have uniformly had associated prominence of the ears and soft, floppy cartilage. If identified in the neonate, Stahl's ear is corrected nonsurgically. In the ear with a small third crus, we have carried out otoplasty as described for ears with soft, floppy cartilage and have depended on molding to obliterate the third crus.

In the more severe case with a large, firm, immobile third crus, the crus itself is excised with a circular rim of cartilage. The circle is rotated 90 degrees and replaced so that the crus is aligned with the anthelix and is no longer conspicuous.

Iatrogenic Third Crus

I have iatrogenically induced formation of a third crus in the course of performing a suture otoplasty on a patient with soft, floppy cartilage and in nonsurgical treatment of a prominent ear in a neonate (Figure 48.24). Neonatal cartilage has physical characteristics reminiscent of the ear with soft and floppy cartilage and must be closely monitored during the course of nonsurgical treatment.

In both iatrogenic cases, the problem was corrected with ear-molding maneuvers.

OTOPLASTY FOR PROMINENT CONSTRICTED EAR

Tanzer observed a common thread in a series of apparently unrelated ear deformities. He noted that whether the ears had deformities that were mild or severe, they all shared the problem of a "purse-string" effect of diminished circumference of the helix. The growth and expansion of the helix, the scapha, and related structures were deformed by the inhibition of this unyielding circumferential obstacle. The spectrum of deformities included in the category "constricted ear" ranges from "almost microtia" to "almost normal."

Severe Constriction

Brent has wisely advised that if the constricted ear lacks more than 1.5 cm in height compared with the normal ear, correction of the problem requires replacement of the deformed framework with an autologous costal cartilage framework.

Moderate Constriction

An extraordinary number of operations have been described for treating moderate constriction of the ear. My experience has been disappointing with procedures that involve disassembling the auricular cartilage into flaps and grafts that expand the auricle when reassembled in a different form. The ear may look promising at first but then tends to deform as contraction of the healing skin overpowers the light framework.

The addition of costal cartilage to the native cartilage framework as an onlay, a splint, or a strut has proved a useful tool in moderately constricted ears (Figure 48.7). This would appear to be a useful adjunct, one that might bring success in the "disassembly" methods.

Mild Constriction

Prominence, "lopping" of the upper pole, and overhang of the skin and cartilage of the helix rim characterize mild constriction of the ear (Figure 48.6). The overhang of the helix is trimmed and closed, the prominence is corrected with Mustardé and C-M sutures, and the upper pole is positioned with F-F sutures. The resulting ear lacks the height of a normal ear, but the improved shape makes the ear inconspicuous.

CRYPTOTIA

In cryptotia, the anterosuperior pole of the auricle is hidden. It is invaginated forward and inward into a pocket of temporal skin (Figure 48.13). With gentle digital traction on the ear, the invaginated structures surface, completely everting the pocket of skin, which drapes around the framework with scarcely a trace of folding. If the digital traction is released, the ear retracts into the pocket again. Cryptotia is rare among Caucasian people but common among Japanese people. Numerous operations for cryptotia are described by many Japanese authors. Nonsurgical treatment in infants is described by Matsuo. Tissue expansion of the neighboring skin appears to be a promising method of correcting cryptotia in adults.

MACROTIA

True macrotia is rare (Figure 48.9). It is more obvious if the ear is prominent; the otoplasty methods already described apply in a mild macrotia. If the ear is so large as to be truly conspicuous, the Antia-Buch technique and its variations provide true reduction of the ear with minimal aesthetic compromise (Figure 48.16).

NONSURGICAL OTOPLASTIES IN NEONATES AND INFANTS

Matsuo reported successful nonsurgical treatment in neonates of all of the ear deformities mentioned herein, except macrotia (Figure 48.1). He described a molding device of malleable plastic material, which he secured to the ear with Steri-Strips. Commencement of treatment as early as possible is a key to success. Matsuo commonly begins treatment in the newborn nursery. In my limited experience, this method has proved excellent if commenced within the first 2 or 3 months of life. A molding armature formed with a core of thin solder or copper wire and padded with a wrapping of 3M Microfoam tape or plastic tubing is bent to fit the ear and shaped to press the deformed areas into a normal shape. The hair is clipped in a radius of about 2 inches around the ear. The ear, the scalp, and the armature are coated with Mastisol adhesive or tincture of benzoin. The armature is positioned on the ear and is secured with multiple ⅛- or ¼-inch Steri-Strips. The armature and the ear are secured to the periauricular skin and scalp with ¼- or ½-inch Steri-Strips. The ear of the neonate is delicate, and a pressure point could cause damage. Therefore, the ear is rechecked frequently and the armature is readjusted or replaced as needed. As the hair grows, clipping is repeated. When the ear begins to retain the desired shape, a roll of Microfoam tape without a metal core is used as a mold. Finally, the ear is held with tape alone until the new position is stable. The time needed for correction varies widely, from a few days to several months.

DRESSINGS

The ends of the subcuticular sutures are taped with Steri-Strips. Petroleum jelly (Vaseline) gauze is molded into the lateral contours of the ear and in the postauricular sulcus. The ears are covered with soft gauze pads. A long vertical Kerlix strip is placed over each eye, and the head is wrapped with a roll of Kerlix gauze, applying gentle, even pressure to both ears. Each vertical gauze strip is then tied tightly, compressing the head wrap to clear the visual fields. The head wrap is compressed lightly with circumferential paper tape. The wrap is taped to the skin at several points to minimize shifting.

POSTOPERATIVE CARE

The dressing is removed on the first postoperative day to check for any hematomas, pressure points, or shifts in position. The dressing is replaced by gauze pads held in place with a circumferential elastic surgical net or with an elastic headband. The position of the ears is rechecked at frequent intervals. Undesired features can be adjusted in the early postoperative period by molding the ears with the methods of nonsurgical treatment. Postoperative visits are scheduled frequently during the early postoperative phase so that prompt intercession with these conservative steps can be made, if necessary. I ask the patient to look in the mirror daily, to become familiar with the features of the newly positioned ears, and to note any change that should be called to my attention.

Preoperatively, I ask the patient or the parents to select several attractive elastic headbands for postoperative wear. The headband diminishes the force that is borne by any C-M sutures and helps to allay edema. Tennis sweatbands usually suffice. The use of two headbands at the same time may be helpful. Parents can purchase patterned elastic material from which to make customized headbands for their children. I ask my patients to wear the headband most of the time for 3 or 4 months, and then I ask them to wear the bands when they are in the privacy of home for another 3 or 4 months. If the patient is truly embarrassed or reluctant to use the headband, I don't insist on it, but objections are uncommon when the rationale is explained.

Any skin sutures are removed on about the fifth day. The subcuticular suture in the postauricular sulcus is left until the tenth day or later.

CAVEATS

1. Nonsurgical molding and splinting is an effective strategy for treatment of protruding ears during the neonatal period. Plastic surgeons need to promote awareness of this fact among pediatricians and primary care physicians.

2. Suture otoplasty customized to the patient's specific auricular problem is an effective strategy for treating prominent ears in children and adults.

3. Knowledge of auricular anatomy and the characteristics of auricular cartilage and skilled application of an effective array of surgical steps is the key to success in otoplasty.

4. Cut or fractured edges of cartilage cause unsightly subcutaneous ridges or bumps.

5. Always remove dressings the day after surgery. Vascular compromise or ear distortion from dressings that have shifted or hardened can cause major complications. Reapply dressings or a headband as often and for as long as needed.

SELECTED READINGS

Antia NH, Buch VI. Chondrocutaneous advancement flap for the marginal defect of the ear. *Plast Reconstr Surg* 1967;39:472–477.

Binder. Das morel'sche Ohr. *Arch Psychiatrie und Nervenkrankheiten* 1880;20:514–564.

Brent B. Reconstruction of the auricle (Chapter 30). In: McCarthy JG, ed. *Plastic Surgery*. Philadelphia: WB Saunders, 1990:2111.

Elliott RA. Otoplasty: a combined approach. *Clin Plast Surg* 1990;17:373–381.

Furnas DW. Suture Otoplasty Update. *Perspect Plast Surg* 1990;4:136–145.

Gault DT, Grippaudo FR, Tyler M. Ear reduction. *Br J Plast Surg* 1995;48:30–34.

Gibson T, Davis WB. The distortion of autogenous cartilage grafts: its cause and prevention. *Br J Plast Surg* 1958;10:257–274.

Hirose T, Tomono T, Matsuo K, et al. Cryptotia: our classification and treatment. *Br J Plast Surg* 1985;38:352–360.

Kaye BL. A simplified method for correcting the prominent ear. *Plast Reconstr Surg* 1967;40:44–48.

MacGregor FD. Ear deformities: social and psychological implications. *Clin Plast Surg* 1978;5:347–350.

Matsuo K. Study of cryptotia. I. Otoplasty for cryptotia. *J Jpn Plast Reconstr Surg* 1988;8:1233–1249.

Matsuo K, Hayashi R, Kiyono M, et al. Nonsurgical correction of congenital auricular deformities. *Clin Plast Surg* 1990;17:383–395.

Mustardé JC. Correction of prominent ears using buried mattress sutures. *Clin Plast Surg* 1978;5:459–464.

Mutimer KL, Mulliken JB. Correction of cryptotia using tissue expansion. *Plast Reconstr Surg* 1988;81:601–604.

Rogers BO. The role of physical anthropology in plastic surgery today. *Clin Plast Surg* 1974;1:439–498.

Stenstrom SJ, Heftner J. The Stenstrom otoplasty. *Clin Plast Surg* 1978;5:465–470.

Tan ST, Abramson DL, MacDonald DM, Mulliken JB. Molding therapy for infants with deformational auricular anomalies. *Ann Plast Surg* 1997;38:263–268.

Tanzer RC. The constricted (cup and lop) ear. *Plast Reconstr Surg* 1975;55:406–415.

Yamada A, Fukuda O. Evaluation of Stahl's ear, third crus of anti-helix. *Ann Plast Surg* 1980;4:511–515.

PART VIII.

CLEFT DEFORMITIES

49

CLEFT LIP REPAIR

Samuel Lance, Catherine Tsai, and Amanda Gosman

Cleft lip repair has undergone a myriad of changes throughout its surgical evolution. The goals of surgical treatment have also evolved to include not only the aesthetic and functional repair of the lip, but also correction of the cleft nasal deformity. Throughout the years of cleft lip repair, various surgical techniques have been described. For the unilateral cleft lip repair, the Millard rotation advancement technique continues as the most widely used technique. The current rotation advancement repair, including the technique described in this text, demonstrates several modifications from the original described cleft lip repair by Millard. The bilateral cleft lip repair has also seen significant changes over the years. The described technique in this text is based on principles promoted by Manchester[1] and further refined by Byrd[2] with several additional modifications. Additionally, the trend toward septorhinoplasty at the time of cleft lip repair has been shown to improve future nasal shape without negatively influencing nasal growth.[3,4] Achievement of a satisfactory lip repair requires a thorough analysis and understanding of the anatomic characteristics of each cleft lip deformity and application of principles directed toward functional correction of each unique cleft deformity.

CLEFT LIP ANATOMY

The first step in any cleft lip repair is evaluation of the specific characteristics of the anatomic defect. The interplay of intrinsic anatomic deficiency and extrinsic distortional forces are thought to contribute to the unique anatomic deformities noted in the cleft lip and nose. Analysis of cleft lip anatomy as described by Millard[5] and other authors[6,7] is summarized here.

Beginning with the deep structures of the unilateral cleft lip, one can note the anterior projection and rotation of the premaxilla relative to the hypoplastic and retro positioned maxilla of the cleft side. The cleft side medial lip elements are vertically shortened, with absence of a distinct philtral column but preservation of the non-cleft philtral column, cupid's bow peak, and valley of cupid's bow. The orbicularis muscle can be anatomically divided into its deep and superficial portions with discontinuity at the site of clefting. The deep portion of the orbicularis muscle is present but hypoplastic in both the medial and lateral lip. The superficial portion is noted to follow the cleft margin to insert laterally at the cleft side alar base and medially to the columellar base. The unilateral cleft nasal deformity is characterized by a hypoplastic, flared cleft side lower lateral cartilage creating an obtuse angle of the lateral segment and widening of the alar base. The medial crus is caudally displaced into the shortened columella with displacement of the columellar base toward the non-cleft side. The base of the caudal septum and anterior nasal spine are displaced toward the non-cleft side with compensatory bowing of the septum into the cleft side further leading to loss in nasal projection and distortion of the columella.

Anatomic variants of the bilateral cleft lip are similar to the unilateral cleft lip, but philtral columns and cupid's bow peaks are absent. The bilateral cleft lip nasal deformity is characterized by splayed, dislocated bilateral medial crural footplates leading to columellar shortening and lateral displacement of both alar bases. There is flattening of the lateral segment of both lower lateral cartilages leading to alar flaring and poor delineation of the alar facial groove.

CLASSIFICATION

Cleft lip deformities can be classified as complete, with no intervening lip tissue, or incomplete. Tissue crossing the incomplete cleft lip without intervening orbicularis muscle is classified as a Simonart's band. A microform cleft lip demonstrates intact overlying skin with discontinuity of the orbicularis musculature.

INDICATIONS FOR SURGERY

Any patient with cleft lip should be considered for cleft lip repair. The process of evaluation and planning is provided by a multidisciplinary team to assess the appropriateness of intervention. Although timing of intervention and indications for further surgery such as cleft palate repair may vary between patients, cleft lip repair can be considered even in patients with severe developmental delays. The social benefits of a repaired cleft lip can often justify intervention even in the setting of associated severe developmental delay.

CONTRAINDICATIONS TO SURGERY

Relatively few contraindications exist to cleft lip repair. Relative contraindications to repair include poor weight gain, signs of malnutrition, active intraoral infection, upper airway inflammatory conditions, or signs of associated airway compromise, as in the Pierre Robin sequence. An absolute contraindication for cleft lip repair is any condition prohibiting general anesthesia or significantly increasing the risk of general anesthesia.

PREOPERATIVE TREATMENTS AND CONSIDERATIONS

Patients with cleft lip with or without cleft palate are to be evaluated as early as possible to begin the multidisciplinary process of preparation for surgery. Diagnosis can occur as early as the first trimester of pregnancy via screening ultrasound, although the condition is most commonly diagnosed at birth. Prenatal diagnosis allows for early discussion with a dysmorphology specialist and preparation of parents for future discussions regarding management of the cleft. Care in the neonatal period is focused on management of acute issues such as airway or cardiac anomalies, prematurity, and nutrition. Infants with both cleft lip and palate demonstrate poor feeding due to a loss in the normal oral mechanisms needed to produce negative pressure and oral seal for suckling. As a result, many fall below goal weight for gestational age and require close observation by a physician for appropriate growth and nutrition. Cleft lip patients should undergo regular weight evaluations and feeding via a squeeze bottle with high-calorie formulas to ensure optimization of nutritional support.

ASSOCIATED ANOMALIES

Appropriate preoperative evaluation of patients with facial clefts includes a comprehensive evaluation by a multidisciplinary team comprising pediatric dysmorphologists, pediatricians, and surgeons. Although isolated cleft palate is more closely associated with a syndromic diagnosis,[8] the presence of a cleft lip is found in connection with several syndromes. Even in the absence of a clear syndromic diagnosis, each patient should undergo a thorough evaluation for associated anomalies. Associated anomalies are seen in as many as 50% of patients with cleft lip and palate and in 11% of patients with isolated cleft lip.[9,10] These anomalies can include central nervous system malformation, congenital cardiac anomalies, vertebral abnormalities, and feeding difficulties leading to poor nutrition. Anomalies identified in the initial examination should be investigated by an appropriate specialist prior to intervention for repair of the facial cleft. Sound physiologic condition for anesthesia should be confirmed prior to proceeding with elective repair of the cleft lip.

TIMING OF INTERVENTION

Timing of intervention for cleft lip repair remains in constant debate among practitioners. This variability centers on the competing elements of improved speech and limitations in facial growth. Current perspectives in cleft repair have identified a significant difficulty in correcting disordered speech when compared to surgical correction of midface deficiency. As a result, modern perspectives tend toward cleft lip repair at 3 months of age with subsequent palate repair at 10–12 months of age. The surgical timing protocol utilized by the senior author for treatment of cleft lip with or without cleft palate has been outlined in Table 49.1. Perhaps more importantly than timing of surgical intervention is the early timing required for successful nasoalveolar molding (NAM). NAM relies on the pliability of neonatal nasal cartilage and mobility of the alveolar and premaxillary segments if a cleft of the alveolus is present. A nasal hook and palatal splint are used to achieve this molding. Figure 49.1A,B demonstrate the initial deformity and subsequent molding appliance, respectively, with the final result

TABLE 49.1 TIMING OF SURGICAL INTERVENTION FOR CLEFT LIP WITH OR WITHOUT CLEFT PALATE

Neonatal	Nasoalveolar molding (NAM)
4 months	Primary lip and nasal repair, soft palate repair, +/− gingivoperiosteoplasty
6–12 months	Palatoplasty, +/− ventilation tube placement
5 years	+/− Lip and nasal revision, +/− surgery for VPI
7–11 years	Alveolar bone grafting, +/− Abbe
Skeletal maturity	+/− Orthognathic surgery, secondary rhinoplasty

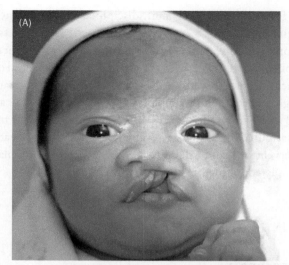

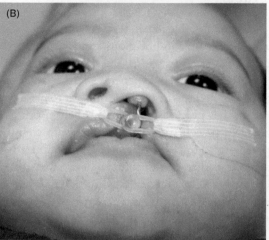

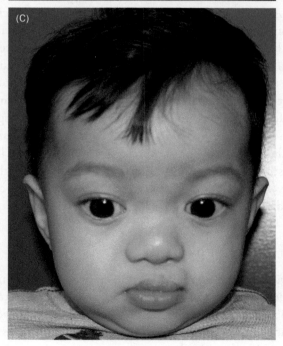

Figure 49.1. Unilateral complete cleft lip. (A) Preoperative with nasoalveolar molding (NAM) in place; (B) preoperative without NAM in place; (C) 1-year postoperative.

after repair demonstrated in Figure 49.1C. Consistent use of NAM has been shown to result in improved preoperative and postoperative nasal form, reduced need for revisional nasal surgeries, and increased ease of achieving a tension free surgical repair.[11-13] NAM ideally begins in the first 2 weeks of life and continues until the time of cleft lip repair at 3 months of age. The timing of 3–4 months of age for cleft lip repair falls in the generally accepted timeframe for cleft lip repair, although this timing may vary significantly between treatment centers and surgeons. Recent analysis of cleft lip repairs by the senior author has demonstrated an independent association between early cleft lip repair and future skeletal malocclusion requiring orthognathic intervention. These findings were noted to be independent of cleft palate repair timing. The senior author's protocol has adjusted the age of cleft lip repair to 4 months of age in order to improve the possibility of future maxillary growth.

Following NAM, alignment of the alveolar segments in a unilateral cleft may be sufficient to allow for primary gingivoperiosteoplasty at the time of cleft lip repair. Primary gingivoperiosteoplasty following NAM with good alignment of the alveolar segments has the additional benefit of reducing the need for secondary alveolar bone grafting to 40%.[14] Cleft palate repair is typically performed between 8 and 10 months of age, coinciding with the emergence of consonant-vowel sounds. Realignment of the anatomic structures need for velar closure before 12 months of age has been shown to significantly reduce the presence of compensatory articulation mechanisms and improve the development of normal speech.[15-17] To achieve early anatomic orientation of the velar musculature, some surgeons, including the senior author, will perform closure of the soft palate and intervelarveloplasty at the time of cleft lip repair when clefts of the lip and palate are both present. As studied by the senior author, this early reorientation of the velar musculature can improve speech outcomes, most notably in patients with bilateral cleft lip and palate. Final hard palate closure is then completed at 10–12 months of age.

Patients begin yearly multidisciplinary team evaluation beginning at 14–18 months of age. Each visit consists of a comprehensive evaluation including speech assessments. Should patients demonstrate persistent velopharyngeal dysfunction, anatomic studies are performed, and, if indicated, surgical correction is completed typically between the ages of 3 and 5 years. Patients are thus followed with yearly multidisciplinary craniofacial evaluations, with orthognathic intervention and definitive osseous septorhinoplasty completed following skeletal maturity.

INTRAOPERATIVE PREPARATION

ANESTHESIA

The pediatric cleft lip repair requires the use of a general anesthetic to avoid complications and airway compromise associated with local regional anesthesia and sedation in this age group. The risks of general anesthesia in the infantile period, including the negative impacts to neurologic development, has previously been identified in primates and evaluated in several studies of human neurocognitive development.[18-21] However, recent large randomized control trials have failed to demonstrate a clear, independent risk association between a single episode of general anesthesia in infancy and future neurodevelopment.[22] Nevertheless, long anesthetic times and multiple episodes of anesthesia are to be avoided if possible during the infantile period.

Airway control during cleft lip repair is generally maintained using an oral Rae endotracheal tube. The endotracheal tube is positioned in the midline and secured to the chin in such a way as to avoid undue tension on the lateral lip segments or interference with the lip closure. A cotton gauze throat pack can be placed in the retropharynx to further protect the airway from inadvertent aspiration of secretions or blood during the surgical procedure. Additional anesthesia is obtained via injection of local anesthetic into the surgical field and bilateral infraorbital nerve blocks following marking of the lip cardinal points (as discussed further in the operative details).

ANTIBIOTIC PROPHYLAXIS

Review of the current literature indicates no definitive evidence supporting or negating the use of perioperative antibiotics for cleft lip repair. Literature does, however, clearly support the use of preoperative antibiotics for septorhinoplasty, lending support to the practice of preoperative antibiotic prophylaxis in the setting of cleft lip repair

with extensive intraoral dissection and primary rhinoplasty as described in the techniques described herein.[23,24] Further support for preoperative antibiotic prophylaxis is also provided from studies of cleft palate repair and subsequent fistula formation.[25,26] Prophylaxis with preoperative third-generation cephalosporin is sufficient to provide coverage of expected nasal and oral floral and should be provided prior to incision.

PATIENT POSITIONING AND OPERATIVE SETUP

Once general anesthesia is achieved and the airway is secured, the patient bed can be rotated 90 degrees in the direction of the scrub table, leaving sufficient room for positioning of the operator at the head of the table while allowing for positioning of the scrub tech on the opposing side of the patient in relation to the anesthesiologist. The areas lateral to the head are left clear to allow for positioning of the surgical assistant to either side of the patient during surgery. The patient is positioned on the center of the bed with the top of the head positioned at the uppermost extent of the head rest. A 3–4 cm shoulder roll is positioned below the patient and the head maintained on a circular pillow. These adjuncts respectively provide mild extension of the neck with stabilization of the head from lateral movement. The eyes are lubricated and protected with taping over each eyelid, keeping the area of the nasal dorsum and nasolabial folds clear of tape to enhance surgical visualization of these structures. The entire face, mouth, and intraoral cavity are then prepared with iodine-based solution. A head drape is utilized to cover the patient from occiput to forehead, leaving the bilateral eyes free for reference during surgery. Two additional towels are placed over the chin and endotracheal tube followed by a U-draping. A single cotton sponge is moistened and packed into the retropharynx to further secure the airway. The surgeon is positioned at the head of the bed with the assistant at either side.

ASSESSMENT OF THE DEFECT

Each cleft demonstrates unique characteristics that should be evaluated prior to surgical intervention. These include the rotation and anterior projection of the premaxillary segment, width of the alveolar cleft or clefts in bilateral cases, fullness of the dry vermilion along the premaxillary segment, displacement of the caudal septum in unilateral cases, columellar length, fullness of dry vermilion along the lateral lip, and height of the lateral segments. These anatomic variants provide an indication of the cleft severity and will assist with surgical planning.

UNILATERAL CLEFT LIP AND CLEFT NASAL REPAIR

OPERATIVE TECHNIQUE

Marking

The anatomic structures and cutaneous landmarks to be reconstructed are all present but must be identified and realigned. Most of the cutaneous and vermilion landmarks can be identified by their relationship to the surrounding structures. Precise marking of the cardinal points on the lip and tattooing of these points with methylene blue is performed prior to the injection of local anesthetic to avoid distortion during identification of the cutaneous landmarks.

Identification and marking of the unilateral cleft lip as depicted in Figure 49.2 is as follows. The first anatomic structure to be marked is the "red line" or the junction of the wet nonkeratinized mucosa and dry keratinized vermilion on the cleft and non-cleft side. This is the first landmark identified, as it will assist in the identification of the cupid's bow peaks. The areas of the greatest vertical height of the dry vermillion correspond to the cutaneous peaks of cupid's bow. This is proceeded by marking the philtral column on the non-cleft side from the base of the nose superiorly to

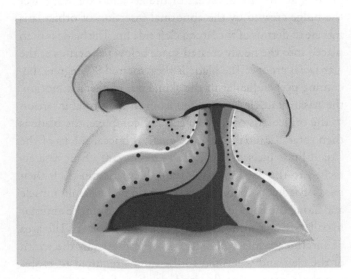

Figure 49.2. Cardinal markings of the unilateral cleft lip with identification of the redline in both medial and lateral cleft lip elements, the vermilion–cutaneous junction above the white roll bilaterally, the cupid's bow peak on the noncleft side, the valley of cupid's bow, the new cupid's bow peak on the medial and lateral cleft sides, and the rotation flap of the medial cleft lip.

its inferior junction at the white roll where it is easiest to identify cupid's bow peak on the non-cleft side. The location of this marking is confirmed by measuring the area of the greatest height of the dry vermillion. The peak marking is made just above and below the white roll in order to plan suture placement and preserve the three-dimensional topography of the white roll. Suture placement within the white roll can result in effacement of the three-dimensional contour of the white roll. The trough of cupid's bow is then marked at the midline, and this is confirmed by the relationship of the philtral trough and the labial frenulum which help to accurately identify the midline. The distance from the cupid's bow on the non-cleft side to the trough of cupid's bow is measured. This distance is then translated to the cleft side medial lip elements along the white roll thus identifying the new cupid's bow peak position on the medial cleft side. This marking usually correlates to the end of the white roll and should include a well-formed three-dimensional white roll.

The point of the newly identified cupid's bow peak on the medial cleft side is then utilized as the base for marking of the rotation flap using a curvilinear question mark-type incision extending from the new mark of cupid's bow peak to just beneath the labial columellar junction, taking care not to extend beyond the philtral column on the non-cleft side. The columellar or C-flap is identified by marking the skin along the cutaneous-vermilion junction lateral to the new cupid's bow peak on the non-cleft side. The vermilion and mucosa inferior to this marking will become the medial mucosal or M-flap.

The cardinal points of the cleft side lateral lip elements are then marked. The position of cupid's bow peak on the lateral cleft side is identified by examining the dry vermilion and placing marks above and below the white roll perpendicular to the region where the dry vermilion has the greatest vertical height. In most patients, an area of fullness and light reflection at the white roll can be visualized at the location of the cupid's bow peak. The advancement flap is marked as a curvilinear line from the new cupid's bow peak up to the alar base on the skin parallel to the lateral lip margin. The vermilion and mucosa medial to this line will become the lateral or L-flap.

After the cupid's bow peak on the cleft side lateral elements has been identified, a dry vermillion triangular flap, as originally described by Noordoff,[27] is then designed to augment the diminutive vermillion on the non-cleft side, as shown in Figure 49.3. To mark the triangular flap, the deficient dry vermillion is measured as the vertical distance from the white roll to the red line at the new cupid's bow peak on the medial side of the cleft. This distance is translated to the

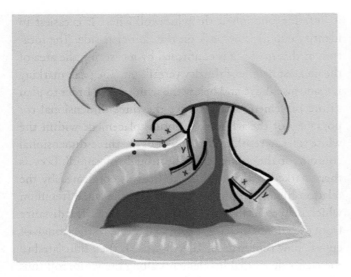

Figure 49.3. Unilateral cleft lip incisions with markings of the dry vermilion triangular flap.

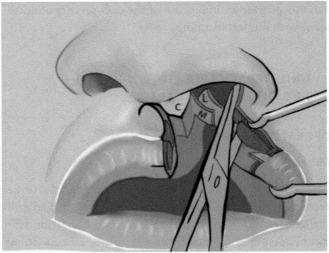

Figure 49.4. Unilateral cleft lip flap elevation demonstrating completed cutaneous incisions, elevation of the M- and L-flaps, separation of he orbicularis muscle from dermis and nasalis muscle at the alar facial groove, and release of the accessory chain of alar cartilage from the piriform rim.

superior dry vermillion beneath the new cupid's bow peak on the lateral side of the cleft and marked. A laterally based triangular dry vermillion flap is designed inferior to this mark with a base that extends inferiorly to the red line and a length that is equivalent to the distance from the cupid's bow peak to the midline trough. A back cut for inset of the triangular flap is then marked on the medial lip element along the red line from the cupid bow's peak to the midline trough. All lip anatomic structures and cardinal points are then tattooed with methylene blue using a 25-gauge hypodermic needle.

Once satisfactory marking has been obtained, 0.25% Marcaine containing 1:200,000 epinephrine solution is infiltrated into the lip, gingiva, nose, and anterior septum along the piriform aperture and as an infraorbital block bilaterally. A throat pack is placed while the local anesthetic is taking effect.

Dissection

Dissection of the lateral and medial lip as depicted in Figure 49.4 is initiated with the cleft side lateral lip elements. The lip is firmly grasped between the thumb and index finger with a single-ply, dry gauze and rotated to anatomic position. A no. 67 Beaver blade is then used to make the cutaneous incisions through the dermis and dry vermillion on the lateral lip segment or advancement flap. The no. 67 Beaver blade is used to cut the triangular flap, and care is taken to include portions of the orbicularis muscle within the base of the triangular flap by beveling away from the triangular flap during the incision. The L-flap of mucosa is then elevated from the lateral lip. This is achieved by inserting a no. 11 blade into the skin incision at the nasal sill of the cleft side ala full-thickness

in the lip mucosa of the lateral lip. The lateral lip mucosal flap is elevated from the lateral lip segment, taking care to leave the orbicularis muscle in the advancement flap. As this incision reaches the level of the triangular flap, the blade is then rotated 90 degrees to allow for inclusion of musculature deep surface of the triangular flap only.

The no. 11 blade is then used to separate the dermis from the underlying orbicularis muscle of the lateral cleft side lip. The release of dermis from muscle is performed beginning at the lateral aspect of the ala and extending over the bulge created by the abnormal insertion of orbicularis muscle to dermis of the lateral cleft side lip. The blade is then placed into the newly created space below the dermis at the alar-facial groove. The blade is then rotated 90 degrees, becoming perpendicular to the skin, and, in a single motion, the nasalis muscle is separated from its abnormal insertion to the orbicularis oris. With this cut complete, the blade is then rotated caudally and the gingival buccal sulcus of the lateral lip is incised, leaving a 1–2 mm cuff of mucosa attached to the fixed gingiva. The orbicularis muscle is then released from its abnormal insertion along the nasalis muscle and along the anterior maxilla. Dissection over the anterior maxillary is performed in a supraperiosteal plane. The area of anterior maxillary dissection is determined by the width of the cleft and is limited to the extent required to mobilize the advancement flap and alar base for a tension-free closure. In wide clefts that require more extensive dissection, the antero-lateral release extends to the adipose tissue surrounding the infraorbital neurovascular bundle. Care is taken to ensure that the infraorbital neurovascular bundle is protected during this dissection. Adequacy of the orbicularis oris release is confirmed by ensuring complete, independent mobilization of the cleft side lateral orbicularis muscle.

The accessory chain of cartilage along the cleft side lateral ala is then released from its abnormal insertion on the cleft side piriform aperture. This is performed using tenotomy scissors to incise full-thickness, releasing mucosa and accessory cartilage along the piriform aperture up to the level of the inferior turbinate. This allows for adequate mobilization of the cleft side alar-mucosal complex.

Dissection of the non-cleft side is begun with incision through the skin of the rotation flap and along the vermillion cutaneous junction using a no. 67 Beaver blade. The no. 11 blade is then passed into the apex of the rotation flap and carried down to the level of the periosteum. The rotation flap is then cut full-thickness through the orbicularis muscle and medial lip mucosa in a curvilinear manner, taking care to bevel away from the rotation flap including all of the orbicularis muscle in the rotation flap and leaving a mucosa-only M-flap. The no. 11 blade is then brought through the gingival buccal sulcus to complete the incision, leaving a 2 mm cuff of mucosa attached to the fixed gingiva. At this point, mobility of the rotation flap is examined. If additional release of the orbicularis muscle is needed for adequate rotation, the no. 11 blade can be inserted just beneath the dermis at the apex of the rotation cut, releasing the muscle without disturbing the overlying dermis. The cupid bow's peaks should be at the same horizontal level after adequate muscle release and rotation. Release of the C-flap from the base of the M-flap is then completed by inserting the no. 11 blade along the vermillion cutaneous junction incision at the base of the M-flap and incising a thin mucosa-only M-flap. The backcut incision is also made along the wet–dry junction of the medial lip to allow for inset of the triangular flap.

Nasal Reconstruction

Nasal dissection is begun with release of the medial crural footplates from the caudal septum and mobilization of the caudal septum from the anterior maxillary spine. This is performed using tenotomy scissors to identify the caudal septum and dissect between the medial crural footplates and caudal septum bilaterally. Using a caudal elevator, the septal mucosa is then elevated from both sides of the caudal septum along its insertion to the anterior nasal spine. The caudal septum is then incised, including mucosa of the cleft side along the anterior nasal spine to allow for mobilization of the cleft side septal mucosa and the septal cartilage as a composite.

Once the caudal septum is adequately mobilized, the abnormal cleft side lower lateral cartilage is then reoriented into anatomic position. An infracartilaginous incision is made through the nasal mucosa along the caudal aspect of the lower lateral cartilage on the cleft side. Tenotomy scissors are then used to sharply dissect in a supraperichondrial plane over the upper and lower lateral cartilages. After adequate release of the lower lateral cartilage is achieved, a modified Tajima suture[28] is utilized to elevate the cleft side alar cartilage at the level of the medial crus, as shown in Figure 49.5. This is performed using a 3-0 Vicryl suture extending full-thickness through the nasal mucosa and non-cleft side upper lateral cartilage at the junction of upper lateral cartilage and septal cartilage. The suture is then passed through the subcutaneous pocket created during elevation of the nasal skin and brought full-thickness through the cleft side lower lateral cartilage at the junction of the middle and lateral crus. The suture is then passed back through the lower lateral cartilage in a horizontal mattress fashion and passed into the subcutaneous pocket and back through the upper lateral cartilage adjacent to the point of entry. This is gently tied to ensure elevation of the lower lateral cartilage without overcorrection or excessive posterior displacement. Additional full-thickness interdomal sutures are then placed using 3-0 Vicryl suture, allowing for refinement of the nasal tip.

With redirection of the cleft lower lateral cartilage complete, attention is then directed to closure of the anterior nasal floor. The lateral cleft side nasal mucosa and the L-flap are sutured to the previously elevated caudal septal

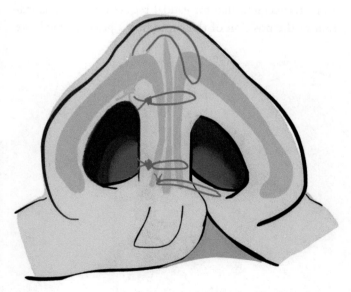

Figure 49.5. Unilateral cleft lip nasal correction with a Tajima suture, interdomal suturing caudal septal repositioning, and closure of the nasal floor defect using a lateral mucosal flap and medial mucosal/cartilaginous flap of caudal septum.

mucosal-cartilaginous composite using interrupted 4-0 chromic gut suture. This allows for repositioning of the caudal septum into the midline.

Lip Reconstruction

Mucosal closure of the lip is begun with inset of the M-flap across the alveolar cleft to augment the labial sulcus. This is performed using interrupted 5-0 chromic gut suture. The oral mucosa is then approximated beginning by placing a 4-0 chromic gut suture at the mucosal apex of the advancement and rotation flap. The advancement flap mucosa is closed along the gingival buccal sulcus using interrupted 4-0 chromic gut suture directed medially to allow for gradual, medial advancement of the advancement flap. The medial gingival buccal sulcus is then closed with interrupted 4-0 chromic gut suture. The mucosal closure of the advancement and rotation flaps is partially completed, but final closure of the most inferior portion of the lip is delayed until after the muscle reconstruction is complete.

The muscular closure is initiated from cranial to caudal. A small double hook is placed in the cleft nostril for cephalad retraction, and the splayed medial crural footplates are approximated to one another using buried 4-0 clear nylon suture, leading to elongation of the columella. This is followed by placement of an alar cinch stitch from the non-cleft side medial crural footplate to the nasalis muscle of the cleft side ala. The alar cinch suture should be tightened only sufficiently to equalize the alar base width. Small hooks are placed in the rotation and advancement flap for caudal retraction and equalization of the position of the cupid bow's peaks to facilitate the orbicularis closure. The muscular closure, as shown in Figure 49.6A, is performed by placing a suture from the superior medial tip of the advancement flap into the muscular back cut of the rotation flap. Additional sutures are similarly placed between the orbicularis of the rotation and advancement flaps using buried 4-0 clear nylon suture. The superficial portion of the orbicularis muscle is then separated from the deep portion just above the level of the white roll to allow for slight overcorrection in the rotation of the new cleft cupid's bow peak. At the completion of muscular closure, a slight overcorrection in length of the cleft side philtral column should be present as compared to the non-cleft side.

Skin closure is then performed using interrupted 6-0 black nylon suture beginning with precise approximation above and below the white roll, as shown in Figure 49.6B. The C-flap is inset vertically, lengthening the columella. The triangular vermilion flap is inset, and the remaining upper lip mucosa is then closed using interrupted horizontal mattress 5-0 chromic suture. The infracartilaginous incisions are also closed using interrupted 5-0 chromic suture. A 3-0 Vicryl suture is placed through the vestibular lining of the lateral nasal mucosa and plicated cutaneously through the alar groove. Silicone nasal conformers are then sized and placed to stent the bilateral nasal apertures. The stent is gently secured across the cartilaginous portion of the septum using a nylon suture. The throat pack is removed and antibiotic ointment is placed on the lip.

Long-term results using the preceding technique in treatment of the unilateral cleft lip and nasal deformity are demonstrated in Figure 49.7A–C. Sustained correction of the nasal deformity can be appreciated in these images.

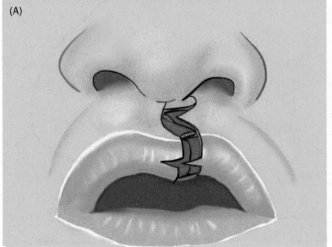
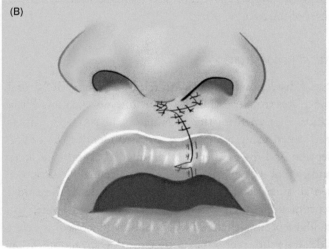

Figure 49.6. (A) Unilateral cleft lip muscular repair demonstrating medial advancement of the lateral orbicularis oris muscle above the caudally displaced rotation flap musculature. (B) The C-flap and triangular flap are inset with final skin closure.

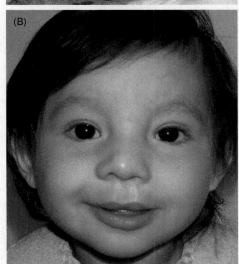

(A)

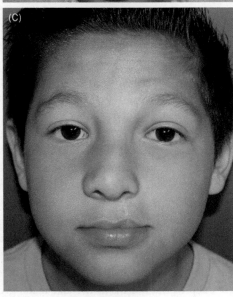

(B)

(C)

Figure 49.7. Unilateral incomplete cleft lip. (A) Preoperative; (B) 1 year postoperative; (C) 9 years postoperative.

BILATERAL CLEFT LIP AND CLEFT NASAL REPAIR

OPERATIVE TECHNIQUE

Markings

As with the unilateral repair, success of the bilateral cleft lip repair relies on appropriate marking of all cardinal points prior to infiltration of local anesthetic. Markings of the bilateral cleft lip repair are depicted in Figure 49.8. Marking is initiated by identifying the junction of the wet nonkeratinized mucosa and dry keratinized vermilion or red line along the prolabial segment and on both lateral lip segments. The prolabial midline at the white roll is then marked. The width of the columellar base is measured, and half of this distance is marked on either side of the white roll midline so that the width of the prolabial flap is the same as the columellar width. Marks identifying the new cupid bow's peaks are placed above and below the white roll to identify the width of the prolabial flap. Vertical lines are then placed from the cupid bow's peaks of the prolabial flap to the medial crural footplates at the columellar base. A triangular flap of dry vermillion is designed caudal to the cupid's bow with the apex at the red line. The triangular flap facilitates the inclusion of the prolabial white roll and prolabial dry vermilion into the prolabial flap. The fork flaps are identified by marking on the cutaneous side of the vermilion cutaneous junction along the lateral aspect of the prolabium.

The new cupid's bow peak on each side of the lateral lip elements is then identified as the point on the white roll that corresponds to the greatest vertical height of the

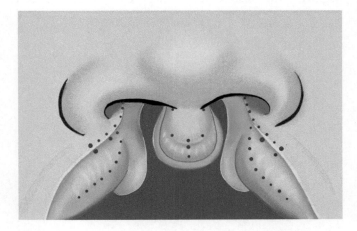

Figure 49.8. Cardinal markings of the bilateral cleft lip with identification of the redline of the lateral lips and prolabium, columellar base width, vermilion–cutaneous junction, and position of greatest dry vermilion of the lateral lips.

dry vermilion when measuring from the white roll to the red line. This new peak is marked above and below the white roll. A tubercle flap of the profundus portion of the orbicularis is designed by marking the dry vermilion medial to the peak. The tubercle flap ends at the point where the dry vermilion disappears and is marked below the white roll so that it does not include any cutaneous elements. The dry vermilion of these tubercle flaps will be eventually joined at the midline with the dry vermilion triangular flap from the prolabial segment. The cutaneous advancement flaps are marked along the curvilinear margin of the lateral lip elements from the new cupid's bow peak to the alar base, carefully excluding the white roll and any mucosa. The L-flap is the mucosal flap medial to this cutaneous incision. Once these markings are performed, all cardinal points are tattooed with methylene blue using a 25-gauge hypodermic needle.

The lip and nose are then infiltrated with local anesthetic using 0.25% Marcaine containing 1:200,000 epinephrine. Infiltration is performed into the prolabium and bilateral lateral lips, in a supraperichondrial plane over the bilateral upper lateral and lower lateral nasal cartilages, and as bilateral infraorbital nerve blocks.

Incision and Dissection

Incision begins with the prolabial segment and is demonstrated along with the lateral lip incisions in Figure 49.9. Incision is made using a no. 67 Beaver blade along the vertical markings of the prolabial segment, extending through the white roll. Care is taken to ensure retention of the white roll markings in the prolabial flap during incision. The triangular dry vermilion flap is then incised from the prolabial segment. The bilateral forked flaps and M-flaps are then

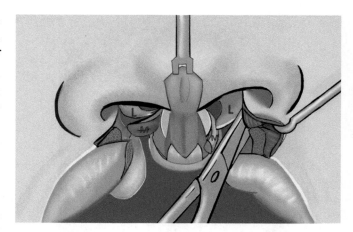

Figure 49.10. Bilateral cleft lip flap elevation demonstrating completed cutaneous incisions, elevation of the prolabial cutaneous flap, M-flap elevation, L-flap elevation, separation of the nasalis muscle from the orbicularis muscle at the alar facial groove, and release of the accessory chain of alar cartilage from the piriform rim.

incised with the no. 67 Beaver blade. The prolabial skin flaps are then incised full-thickness through the mucosa with a no. 11 blade scalpel to separate the M- and forked flaps from the central mucosal flap as shown in Figure 49.10. The prolabial skin flap is then separated from the central mucosal flap and is elevated superiorly to the level of the medial crural footplates. Excess subcutaneous tissue is excised from the inferiorly based central prolabial mucosal flap. The medial crural footplates are then separated from the caudal septum using blunt dissection and tenotomy scissors. The M-flap is mobilized to span across the alveolar cleft, and the fork flaps are mobilized to the junction of the caudal septal mucosa and preserved for possible use in the nasal sill if the cleft is wide.

Incision of the lateral lip elements begins with incision of the white roll and vermilion/cutaneous junction using a no. 67 Beaver blade. The incision is made taking care to exclude the white roll along the lip and the tubercle flap medial to cupid bow's peak. The Beaver blade is then used to incise the lateral advancement flaps superiorly to the base of the nose. The L-flaps are then created by passing a no. 11 blade full-thickness through the lateral lip mucosa beginning at the cephalad-most portion of the cutaneous incision and separating mucosa only in the L-flaps, leaving the orbicularis muscle with the lateral lip elements as shown in Figure 49.10. Following elevation of the L-flaps, the no. 11 blade is inserted just deep to the dermis of the lateral lip, separating dermis from the underlying bulge of orbicularis oris muscle along the lateral lip. The no. 11 blade is then placed just deep to the dermis at the alar facial groove and directed inferiorly, separating nasalis from orbicularis oris. Care is taken to leave a curvilinear cuff of nasalis along

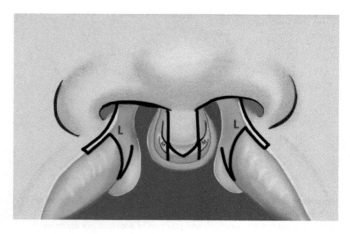

Figure 49.9. Bilateral cleft lip incisions with identification of M- and L-flaps.

the undersurface of the lateral alar rim to provide fullness to the lateral ala. The no. 11 blade is then used to separate orbicularis from the anterior maxilla in a pre-periosteal plane and complete the incision of the gingivobuccal sulcus, leaving a 1–2 mm cuff of mucosa attached to the fixed gingiva.

Tenotomy scissors are utilized to continue dissection of the nasalis muscle from the orbicularis muscle along the lateral ala to provide independent mobility of the lateral ala and lateral lip. Dissection is carried in a supraperiosteal plane along the maxilla, releasing the orbicularis oris muscle from the maxilla as much as is necessary until the lip demonstrates adequate medial advancement or the adipose tissue surrounding the infraorbital neurovascular bundle is identified. The tenotomy scissors are then directed medially to release the lateral ala and accessory cartilage chain from the piriform aperture, incising full-thickness through mucosa along the piriform rim up to the level of the inferior turbinate, as shown in Figure 49.10. Release is confirmed by complete medial mobilization of the lateral ala and mucosa as a composite flap.

Nasal Reconstruction

Once dissection of the prolabial flap, lateral lip, and ala is completed, attention is directed to the correction of the displaced bilateral lower lateral cartilages. Infracartilaginous incisions are placed bilaterally extending just through nasal mucosa. Dissection is then performed in a supraperichondrial plane above the bilateral lower lateral and upper lateral cartilages, as well as release of the interdomal fibrous connections. After adequate release of the lower lateral cartilages is achieved, bilateral modified Tajima sutures are placed to elevate the alar cartilages at the junction of the middle and lateral crus, as shown in Figure 49.11. This is performed using a 3-0 Vicryl bilaterally, as described earlier in the unilateral repair. Interdomal sutures are also placed as described in the unilateral repair. Columellar lengthening is achieved by approximation of the splayed medial crural footplates in a cephalad position onto the caudal septum utilizing a buried, 4-0 clear nylon suture. The L-flaps are then rotated to create the anterior nasal floor and sutured to the caudal septal mucosa, and the M-flaps are sutured to the lateral alveolar segment with a 5-0 chromic to augment the labial sulcus.

Lip Reconstruction

The first element addressed in reconstruction of the lip is creation of the central, gingival buccal sulcus. The central

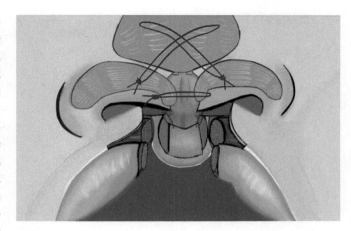

Figure 49.11. Bilateral cleft lip nasal correction with bilateral Tajima sutures, interdomal suturing, and medial repositioning of the splayed bilateral medial crural footplates. Inset of the prolabial mucosal flap at the columellar base.

flap of prolabial mucosa is secured to the periosteum at the columellar base using 5-0 chromic suture, as shown in Figure 49.11. Closure of the lateral lip mucosa is initiated at the midline along the cranial-most portion of the bilateral lateral lip mucosa to create the new labial portion of the gingival buccal sulcus. This is performed using interrupted 4-0 chromic suture. The central closure of the lip mucosa is then secured to the caudal septum with 4-0 chromic suture in a three-point fixation pattern including bilateral labial mucosa and caudal septum. The caudal septum is thus identified as the nexus point for fixation of the new gingival buccal sulcus at the junction of prolabial mucosa and lip mucosa at the midline. The lateral labial mucosa is then approximated to the edge of mucosal lining of the sulcus from lateral to medial. This completes creation of the gingivobuccal sulcus. The remaining labial mucosa is then partially approximated at the midline extending from the sulcus using interrupted horizontal mattress 4-0 chromic sutures.

The muscular repair is then performed in a cranial to caudal direction starting with an alar cinch suture of the nasalis muscle, as shown in Figure 49.12. Interrupted, buried 4-0 clear nylon sutures are placed into the orbicularis muscle perpendicular to the maxillary plane. The muscle is thus approximated to the level of the white roll. At this point, the profundus portion of orbicularis muscle on the tubercle flap is gently separated from the superficial portion of orbicularis. The profundus muscle is approximated, creating a prominent prolabial tubercle. At completion of the muscular closure, the skin edges should be appropriately aligned to provide a tension free closure of the lateral skin to the skin of the prolabial segment as will be described shortly.

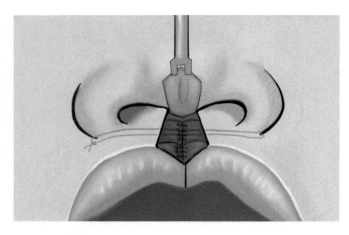

Figure 49.12. Bilateral cleft lip muscular repair demonstrating separation of the superficial and deep portions of the orbicularis oris muscle, midline muscular, and vermilion redundancy leading to creation of a central tubercle and narrowing of the alar base using an alar cinch stitch.

Skin closure shown in Figure 49.13 begins by securing the central underlying dermis of the prolabial skin flap to the midline muscular repair utilizing a single 6-0 Vicryl suture creating a philtral dimple. The prolabial segment white roll is then approximated to the lateral lip white roll using interrupted 6-0 nylon suture. This is followed by a half-buried three-point 4-0 chromic suture at the apex of the prolabial triangular dry vermilion flap to the dry vermilion of the bilateral tubercle flaps. The remaining dry vermilion is then closed using interrupted horizontal mattress 5-0 chromic sutures at the midline. The skin incisions are then closed along the philtral columns using interrupted 6-0 nylon suture. Finally, the infracartilaginous nasal incisions are closed using interrupted 5-0 chromic sutures, and the fork flaps are trimmed or used to augment

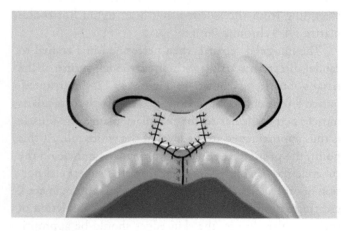

Figure 49.13. Bilateral cleft lip skin and vermilion closure. Inclusion of the prolabial white roll and prolabial dry vermilion in this closure is depicted. Vermilion closure with interrupted horizontal mattress suture is also depicted.

the nasal sill. Appropriately sized silicone nasal stents are then placed bilaterally and secured using a single transseptal nylon suture at the level of the cartilaginous septum.

The technique just described can produce reliable correction of the bilateral cleft lip and nose, as demonstrated in Figures 49.14A–D. These images highlight the incorporation of the prolabial dry vermilion and prominent central wet vermilion characteristic of this repair.

POSTOPERATIVE CARE

Although discussions regarding criteria for inpatient versus outpatient admission following cleft lip repair are ongoing,[29–31] traditional practice is for overnight admission with cardiorespiratory monitoring and hydration support using intravenous fluids if needed.[32] Bilateral soft elbow immobilizers are placed prior to extubation and used continuously for 6 weeks postoperatively to prevent self-injury to the lip repair. Oral intake is initiated in the recovery room using a standard cleft palate bottle or squeeze bottle with a soft nipple. Breast-feeding is permitted after cleft lip repair. Parents are instructed concerning care of the nasal stents and lip sutures, with twice daily cleaning using dilute peroxide followed by bacitracin ointment to the incision. Discharge criteria include adequate oral intake to allow for cessation of intravenous fluids and pain control with oral medication only. Patients are evaluated at 1 week postoperatively for skin suture removal and again at 3 weeks postoperatively for removal of the nasal stents. At the 6-week visit, restraints are discontinued, and, if a palatal cleft is present, planning for repair of the cleft palate is begun.

COMPLICATIONS

Analyses of postoperative complications has yielded a wide range in the literature from as low as 1% to as high as 13%.[33–35] In a recent large database analysis of postoperative complications, the overall complication rate appears to be approximately 4% with a readmission rates of approximately 4%.[36] Pulmonary complications comprise the largest subset of early postoperative complications, followed by wound infection and dehiscence. As expected, patients with preoperative associated congenital malformations, cardiac risk factors, or poor nutrition are most likely to suffer postoperative complications. Patients with these risk factors should be monitored closely in the

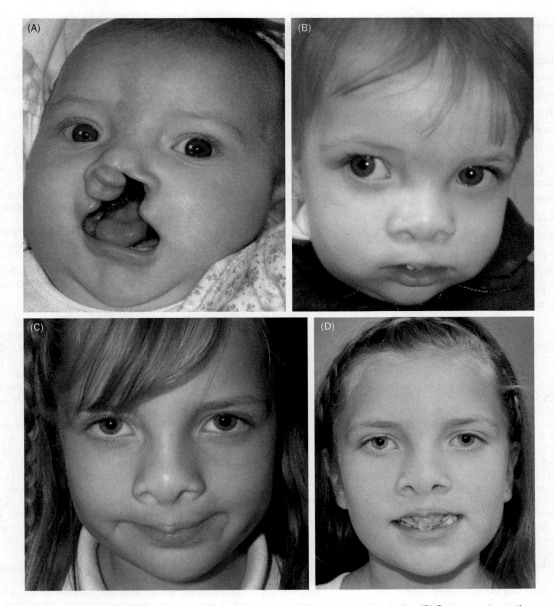

Figure 49.14. Bilateral complete cleft lip. (A) preoperative; (B) 1 year postoperative; (C) 6 years postoperative; (D) 8 years postoperative.

immediate and early postoperative period to mitigate the risk of potentially life-threatening complications.

Hypertrophic scarring is usually noted within the first 6 months following repair, with the lowest incidence in Caucasian ethnicity and highest incidence in Hispanic and Asian ethnicities.[37] In an attempt to decrease inflammatory response and improve wound healing, we recommend the use of permanent sutures for skin closure and removal of these sutures in 5–7 days. Additionally, postoperative massage, silicone taping, or gel and protective sunscreen are adjuncts to improve scar quality and appearance. Should hypertrophic scarring present, we recommend early management with Kenalog injections and continued massage.

FOLLOW-UP

A multidisciplinary team of specialists ensuring appropriate preoperative evaluation and postoperative follow-up should follow all patients with cleft lip and cleft of the alveolus or palate. The burden of care following cleft surgery is significant. Without structured, regular multidisciplinary team evaluations, many parents are overwhelmed by the demands of postoperative care, leading to delays in management and inadequate communication between the various treatment teams. The benefits of multidisciplinary team care and surgical outcomes have been reviewed extensively within the greatest data provided by the

European experience. Analyses of cleft outcomes continue to identify optimization of surgical outcomes through the consolidation of cleft centers into centralized, high-volume centers.[38] The criteria outlined by the American Cleft Palate and Craniofacial Association identifies basic standards for approved cleft palate and craniofacial teams, with high-volume centers defined by a minimum of 50 new patients evaluated per year and at least 10 operative, primary cleft lip or palate cases performed by at least one surgeon per year.[39] Investigations in the European literature[40] and by the senior author reveal similar trends in improved surgical outcomes when cleft repairs are performed by craniofacial, subspecialty-trained surgeons with a high volume of practice. As cleft outcomes are standardized, documentation at each visit can allow for critical analysis of surgical performance and early identification of areas for improvement.

REFERENCES

1. Manchester WM. The repair of bilateral cleft lip and palate. *Br J Surg* 1965;52(11):878–882.
2. Byrd HS, Ha RY, Khosla RK, Gosman AA. Bilateral cleft lip and nasal repair. *Plast Reconstr Surg* 2008;122(4):1181–1190.
3. Gawrych E, Janiszewska-Olszowska J. Primary correction of nasal septal deformity in unilateral clefts during lip repair-a long-term study. *Cleft Palate Craniofac J* 2011;48(3):293–300.
4. Salyer KE, Genecov ER, Genecov DG. Unilateral cleft lip-nose repair: a 33-year experience. *J Craniofac Surg* 2003;14(4):549–558.
5. Millard DR. *Cleft Craft: The Evolution of Its Surgery.* 1st ed. Boston: Little, Brown, 1976.
6. Fara M. Anatomy and arteriography of cleft lips in stillborn children. *Plast Reconstr Surg* 1968;42(1):29–36.
7. Nicolau PJ. The orbicularis oris muscle: a functional approach to its repair in the cleft lip. *Br J Plast Surg* 1983;36(2):141–153.
8. Jones MC. Facial clefting. Etiology and developmental pathogenesis. *Clin Plast Surg* 1993;20(4):599–606.
9. Natsume N, Niimi T, Furukawa H, et al. Survey of congenital anomalies associated with cleft lip and/or palate in 701,181 Japanese people. *Oral Surg Oral Med Oral Pathol Oral Radiol Endod* 2001;91(2):157–161.
10. Shaw GM, Carmichael SL, Yang W, Harris JA, Lammer EJ. Congenital malformations in births with orofacial clefts among 3.6 million California births, 1983-1997. *Am J Med Genet A* 2004;125A(3):250–256.
11. Cutting C, Grayson B, Brecht L, Santiago P, Wood R, Kwon S. Presurgical columellar elongation and primary retrograde nasal reconstruction in one-stage bilateral cleft lip and nose repair. *Plast Reconstr Surg* 1998;101(3):630–639.
12. Grayson BH, Cutting CB. Presurgical nasoalveolar orthopedic molding in primary correction of the nose, lip, and alveolus of infants born with unilateral and bilateral clefts. *Cleft Palate Craniofac J* 2001;38(3):193–198.
13. Liou EJ, Subramanian M, Chen PK, Huang CS. The progressive changes of nasal symmetry and growth after nasoalveolar molding: a three-year follow-up study. *Plast Reconstr Surg* 2004;114(4):858–864.
14. Santiago PE, Grayson BH, Cutting CB, Gianoutsos MP, Brecht LE, Kwon SM. Reduced need for alveolar bone grafting by presurgical

15. orthopedics and primary gingivoperiosteoplasty. *Cleft Palate Craniofac J* 1998;35(1):77–80.
15. Dorf DS, Curtin JW. Early cleft palate repair and speech outcome. *Plast Reconstr Surg* 1982;70(1):74–81.
16. Haapanen ML, Rantala SL. Correlation between the age at repair and speech outcome in patients with isolated cleft palate. *Scand J Plast Reconstr Surg Hand Surg* 1992;26(1):71–78.
17. Randall P, LaRossa DD, Fakhraee SM, Cohen MA. Cleft palate closure at 3 to 7 months of age: a preliminary report. *Plast Reconstr Surg* 1983;71(5):624–628.
18. Davidson AJ. Anesthesia and neurotoxicity to the developing brain: the clinical relevance. *Paediatr Anaesth* 2011;21(7):716–721.
19. Flick RP, Katusic SK, Colligan RC, et al. Cognitive and behavioral outcomes after early exposure to anesthesia and surgery. *Pediatrics* 2011;128(5):e1053–e1061.
20. Ing C, DiMaggio C, Whitehouse A, et al. Long-term differences in language and cognitive function after childhood exposure to anesthesia. *Pediatrics* 2012;130(3):e476–e85.
21. Brambrink AM, Back SA, Riddle A, et al. Isoflurane-induced apoptosis of oligodendrocytes in the neonatal primate brain. *Ann Neurol* 2012;72(4):525–535.
22. Davidson AJ, Disma N, de Graaff JC, et al. Neurodevelopmental outcome at 2 years of age after general anaesthesia and awake-regional anaesthesia in infancy (GAS): an international multicentre, randomised controlled trial. *Lancet* 2016;387(10015):239–250.
23. Lindeboom JA, Frenken JW, Tuk JG, Kroon FH. A randomized prospective controlled trial of antibiotic prophylaxis in intraoral bone-grafting procedures: preoperative single-dose penicillin versus preoperative single-dose clindamycin. *Int J Oral Maxillofac Surg* 2006;35(5):433–436.
24. Rajan GP, Fergie N, Fischer U, Romer M, Radivojevic V, Hee GK. Antibiotic prophylaxis in septorhinoplasty? A prospective, randomized study. *Plast Reconstr Surg* 2005;116(7):1995–1998.
25. Aznar ML, Schonmeyr B, Echaniz G, Nebeker L, Wendby L, Campbell A. Role of postoperative antimicrobials in cleft palate surgery: prospective, double-blind, randomized, placebo-controlled clinical study in India. *Plast Reconstr Surg* 2015;136(1):59e–66e.
26. Rottgers SA, Camison L, Mai R, et al. Antibiotic use in primary palatoplasty: a survey of practice patterns, assessment of efficacy, and proposed guidelines for use. *Plast Reconstr Surg* 2016;137(2):574–582.
27. Noordhoff MS. Reconstruction of vermilion in unilateral and bilateral cleft lips. *Plast Reconstr Surg* 1984;73(1):52–61.
28. Tajima S, Maruyama M. Reverse-U incision for secondary repair of cleft lip nose. *Plast Reconstr Surg* 1977;60(2):256–261.
29. Al-Thunyan AM, Aldekhayel SA, Al-Meshal O, Al-Qattan MM. Ambulatory cleft lip repair. *Plast Reconstr Surg* 2009;124(6):2048–2053.
30. Albert MG, Babchenko OO, Lalikos JF, Rothkopf DM. Inpatient versus outpatient cleft lip repair and alveolar bone grafting: a cost analysis. *Ann Plast Surg* 2014;73 Suppl 2:S126–S129.
31. Paine KM, Tahiri Y, Wes A, Fischer JP, Paliga JT, Taylor JA. Patient risk factors for ambulatory cleft lip repair: an outcome and cost analysis. *Plast Reconstr Surg* 2014;134(2):275e–82e.
32. Onyekwelu O, Seaward J, Beale V. Should we give routine postoperative intravenous fluids after cleft surgery? *Cleft Palate Craniofac J* 2016;53(2):e18–e22.
33. Fillies T, Homann C, Meyer U, Reich A, Joos U, Werkmeister R. Perioperative complications in infant cleft repair. *Head Face Med* 2007;3:9.
34. Hopper RA, Lewis C, Umbdenstock R, Garrison MM, Starr JR. Discharge practices, readmission, and serious medical complications following primary cleft lip repair in 23 US children's hospitals. *Plast Reconstr Surg* 2009;123(5):1553–1559.
35. Wilhelmsen HR, Musgrave RH. Complications of cleft lip surgery. *Cleft Palate J* 1966;3:223–231.

36. Paine KM, Tahiri Y, Wes AM, et al. An assessment of 30-day complications in primary cleft lip repair: a review of the 2012 ACS NSQIP Pediatric. *Cleft Palate Craniofac J* 2016;53(3):283–289.

37. Soltani AM, Francis CS, Motamed A, et al. Hypertrophic scarring in cleft lip repair: a comparison of incidence among ethnic groups. *Clin Epidemiol* 2012;4:187–191.

38. Shaw WC, Semb G, Nelson P, et al. The Eurocleft project 1996–2000: overview. *J Craniomaxillofac Surg* 2001;29(3):131–140; discussion 41–42.

39. Association ACP-C. Parameters for evaluation and treatment of patients with cleft lip/palate or other craniofacial anomalies. In: Sally Peterson-Falzone PD, ed. 2009 ed. The American Cleft Palate-Craniofacial Association (ACPA) 2009.

40. Shaw WC, Dahl E, Asher-McDade C, et al. A six-center international study of treatment outcome in patients with clefts of the lip and palate: Part 5. General discussion and conclusions. *Cleft Palate Craniofac J* 1992;29(5):413–418.

50.

CLEFT PALATE REPAIR

Catharine B. Garland and Joseph E. Losee

A cleft of the palate prevents the normal production of speech and language, which is essential to normal development and social interactions. Cleft palate repair is aimed at reconstructing the normal anatomic relationship of the tissues and muscles to allow for normal speech production. Prior to discussing the repair, however, it is essential to understand the normal anatomy and function of the dynamic structures of the palate. The history of cleft palate repair has evolved from techniques that simply closed the mucosal layers to those that return the musculature of the palate to its normal anatomic position. A variety of techniques remain in common use today; however this chapter will focus on our preferred method of repair, the Furlow palatoplasty.[1-4]

RELEVANT ANATOMY AND ASSESSMENT OF THE DEFECT

The primary palate comprises all structures anterior to the incisive foramen (the premaxilla). The secondary palate consists of the bony palate posterior to the incisive foramen as well as the structures of the soft palate. The soft palate contains five paired muscles: the levator veli palatini, tensor veli palatini, palatoglossus, palatopharyngeus, and muscularis uvulae. During normal speech, the soft palate elevates and contacts the posterior pharynx. In the normal palate (Figure 50.1A), the levator veli palatini muscle crosses midline in the middle 50% of the soft palate. This muscle originates from the posteromedial aspect of the Eustachian tube and meets its partner in the midline to create a *transverse* muscular sling. In addition to supporting the soft palate at rest, the levator veli palatini powers the elevation of the palate during speech by exerting pull in an upward, backward, and lateral direction.[5] The palatopharyngeus and palatoglossus originate in the midline of the soft palate,

oral to the levator veli palatini muscle. These muscles then travel posterior and inferior in the posterior tonsillar pillars and anterior tonsillar pillars, respectively. The tensor veli palatini muscle originates from the greater wing of the sphenoid bone and travels around the hook of the hamulus. It meets its counterpart in the anterior 25% of the soft palate in the form of a fibrous aponeurosis. The muscularis uvulae is a paired midline structure in the posterior 25% of the soft palate, extending from the tensor veli palatini aponeurosis anteriorly to the uvula posteriorly.

In the cleft palate, the paths of the soft palate muscles are disrupted (Figure 50.1B). Rather than uniting in the midline, the levator veli palatini travels in a *sagittal* direction from posterior to anterior. The levator veli palatini has three abnormal attachments in a cleft palate: to the posterior edge of the hard palate, to the aponeurosis of the tensor veli palatini, and, laterally, to the superior pharyngeal constrictor (Figure 50.2). In this position, the levator veli palatini cannot exert its usual upward, backward, and lateral pull to elevate the palate.[5]

In its mildest form, a cleft palate may present as a submucous cleft of the palate. No defect or clefting of the mucosa is present in these cases; however, the musculature of the soft palate takes on an abnormal anatomic relationship. This is classically characterized by a bifid uvula, a zona pellucida within the soft palate, and a notch at the posterior border of the hard palate.[6] However, even when these three signs are not present, an occult submucous cleft palate may be diagnosed by noting the vaulting V-shaped pattern of the velum when it elevates with speech or with a gag. This V-shaped pattern denotes the abnormal course of the levator veli palatini muscles as they course from the skull base toward an abnormal insertion on the posterior border of the hard palate.

Overt clefts of the hard and soft palate may be classified by multiple systems, which range from simple to complex.[7]

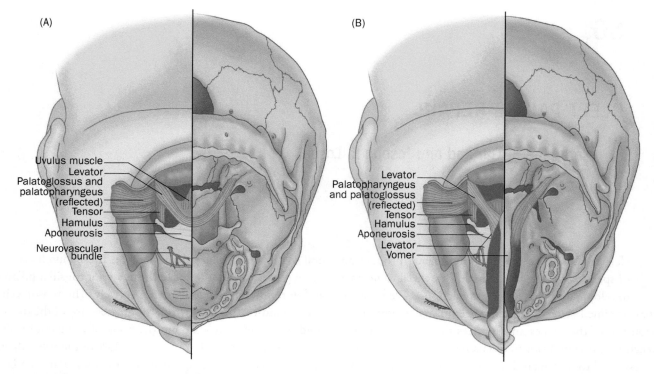

Figure 50.1. (A) Normal palatal anatomy. (B) Anatomy of the cleft palate. From Losee JE, Smith DM. Cleft palate repair. In Butler C, ed. *Head and Neck Reconstruction with DVD: A Volume in the Procedures in Reconstructive Surgery Series.* Philadelphia: Saunders Ltd.; 2008:271–294, figure 50.12.1.

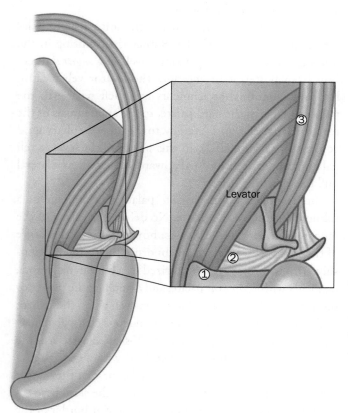

Figure 50.2. Three abnormal insertions of the levator veli palatini muscle: (1) hard palate, (2) tensor aponeurosis, (3) superior constrictor. From Losee JE, Smith DM. Cleft palate repair. In Butler C, ed. *Head and Neck Reconstruction with DVD: A Volume in the Procedures in Reconstructive Surgery Series.* Philadelphia: Saunders Ltd.; 2008:271–294, figure 50.12.3.

The Veau classification is simple and intuitive and will be used throughout this chapter. In this classification scheme, a Veau I cleft refers to a cleft of the soft palate only, Veau II is a cleft of the hard and soft palates, Veau III is a complete unilateral cleft of the alveolus and palate, and Veau IV is complete bilateral cleft of the alveolus and palate.

INDICATIONS

Any child with a cleft of the hard or soft palate is considered a candidate for repair. Repair separates the nasal from the oral cavity, preventing nasal regurgitation of liquid and food. Furthermore, cleft palate repair may help improve Eustachian tube function. In addition to these functions, the primary purpose of repair is to allow for the development of normal speech and language. Therefore, repair is commonly performed between 9 and 12 months of age in most centers, to coincide with the onset of speech.[3]

CONTRAINDICATIONS

Patients with additional medical comorbidities may not be candidates for cleft palate repair, such as infants with severe cardiopulmonary disorders unable to tolerate general anesthesia or with significant neurologic disorders that prevent the ability to feed or engage in speech. This reinforces the importance of having all cleft patients evaluated by a cleft center, as they are best equipped to make this determination as a team. In cases of compromised infants, it is not uncommon to perform repair at an older age than the usual 9–12 months. Patients with Pierre Robin sequence or other airway compromise may also require a delay in repair, as repair of the cleft may narrow the airway further.

PREOPERATIVE CONSIDERATIONS

Prior to surgery, the surgeon and cleft team must assess patient comorbidities, the status of the airway, and the need for any additional airway evaluation. Feeding history and weight gain should be monitored from birth. Infants with palatal clefts are unable to generate adequate negative pressure to breast feed and typically require specialized bottles, such as the Haberman or Pigeon feeders. Our practice is to try to wean patients from the bottle to a sippy cup prior to cleft palate repair. Hemoglobin is often checked prior to surgery as infants will typically reach their hemoglobin nadir between 8 and 12 weeks of age, and iron-deficiency anemia can peak between 12 and 24 months of age.

ROOM SETUP AND PREPARATION

General anesthesia is required. After mask induction and intravenous line placement, intubation is performed with an oral Rae endotracheal tube. The bend of the oral Rae tube must be at the lip in order to prevent compression of the tube during surgery and to facilitate the use of the Dingman mouth retractor. The bed may be rotated either 90 or 180 degrees according to surgeon preference. Care is taken to pad the patient, including all leads and lines, and the eyes are taped shut. The head is placed on a small gel donut with either a small shoulder roll or in slight Trendelenburg positioning. Data from a recent publication by the authors[8] support the preoperative use of a single dose of ampicillin-sulbactam (Unasyn).

The surgeon should wear loupes and a headlight to optimize intraoral visualization. After preparation with Betadine and placement of sterile drapes, the Dingman mouth gag is placed. An appropriately sized blade for the patient is selected to optimize tongue retraction while not touching the back of the oropharynx. Two silk sutures are placed in the anterior tongue to assist with tongue positioning under the mouth gag. In addition, two dental

rolls, one on either side of the endotracheal tube, are placed at the 90-degree bend in the Dingman blade, to prevent compression of the tube. A 10-French suction catheter is placed through one of the nares to rest within the posterior oropharynx and is used to suction any escaping anesthetic gases and also to prevent any blood or irrigation fluid from accumulating in the field during the operation. With this suction tube in place, a throat pack is not necessary. Local anesthetic is infiltrated using 0.25% bupivacaine to assist with pain management. Epinephrine (10 μg/mL) is infiltrated in the palate to optimize hemostasis during the operation. During the operation, we recommend releasing the Dingman retractor to relieve pressure on the tongue for 10 minutes every hour, thereby reducing the potential for postoperative tongue swelling.

OPERATIVE TECHNIQUE

All commonly used techniques for palate repair employ the same principles: closure of the nasal lining, closure of the oral lining, and alignment and repair of the soft palate musculature. The specifics of the closure technique may be separated into how the hard palate is repaired and how the soft palate is repaired. This is commonly determined by the cleft anatomy and surgeon preference. In this chapter, we describe in detail our preferred techniques for soft and hard palate repair.

The soft palate repair is routinely performed using a Furlow double-opposing Z-plasty. The Furlow palatoplasty technique described herein may be used for any type of Veau cleft or submucous cleft, or for secondary palatal lengthening. The Furlow palatoplasty lengthens the soft palate, overlaps and repositions the soft palate musculature to create a functional levator veli palatini sling, and narrows the caliber of the velopharyngeal port by the secondary "pharyngoplasty effect" resulting from the nasal lining Z-plasty.[1,2]

For Veau II, III, or IV clefts, the hard palate repair consists of a combination of either unipedicled or bipedicled hard palate flaps, reliant upon the greater palatine artery located in the posterior hard palate with or without the vascular pedicle at the incisive foramen, respectively. Bipedicled flaps are employed in the classic von Langenbeck repair, while unipedicled flaps require the division of the anterior pedicle and are the basis of the V-Y pushback (or Veau-Wardill-Kilner)[9] or two-flap palatoplasty proposed by Bardach (Figure 50.3).[10,11] The hard palate repair is combined with vomer flaps for nasal lining closure.

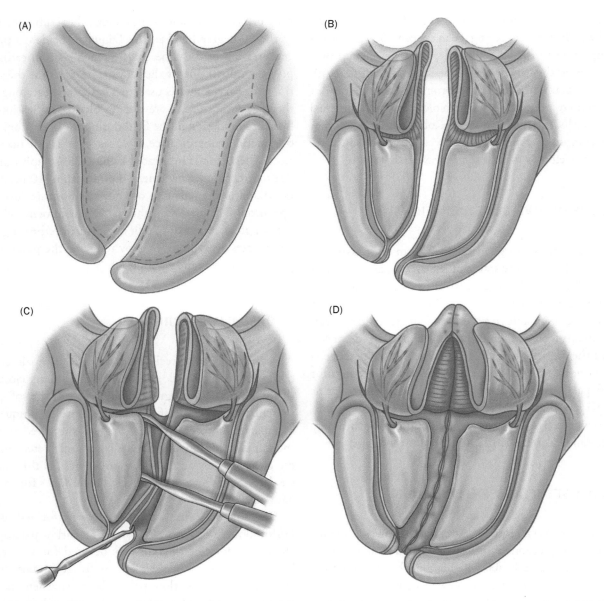

Figure 50.3. Bardach two-flap palatoplasty. (A) Design of bilateral unipedicled hard palate mucoperiosteal flaps by anteriorly connecting the hard palate lateral relaxing incisions and the medial cleft margin incisions. (B) Creation and dissection of bilateral unipedicled hard palate mucoperiosteal flaps with circumferential dissection of the greater palatine neurovascular pedicles. (C) Dissection of the nasal lining from the nasal side of the hard palate and release of the levator muscle from the posterior edge of the hard palate and the tensor aponeurosis, and swept free from the superior constrictor. (D) Following radical release of the levator muscle, the nasal lining is closed and an intravelar veloplasty is performed. (E) The oral mucosa of the velum is closed and the mucoperiosteal flaps of the hard palate are closed with horizontal mattress sutures. From Losee JE, Smith DM. Cleft palate repair. In Butler C, ed. *Head and Neck Reconstruction with DVD: A Volume in the Procedures in Reconstructive Surgery Series*. Philadelphia: Saunders Ltd.; 2008:271–294, figure 50.12.28.

HARD PALATE FLAP DESIGN AND MARKINGS

Veau II Clefts

For wider clefts, unipedicled flaps will connect the lateral relaxing incision to the medial cleft margin anteriorly and therefore allow for increased flap mobility. This design can also facilitate a true V-to-Y "push-back" of the hard palate. Bipedicled flaps, on the other hand, require less dissection and leave behind a smaller area of exposed hard palate. This, theoretically, may cause less maxillary growth restriction. In narrow or highly vaulted clefts, the hard palate flaps may be dissected free from the medial margin and closed, without the need for lateral relaxing incisions along the alveolus. The disadvantages of bipedicled flaps are less flap mobility, occasionally more tension at midline, and an inability to close wider anterior defects.

Veau III Clefts

A combination of either unipedicled (Figure 50.3) and/ or bipedicled flaps may be used. Most commonly, we design a bipedicled flap on the major segment with a unipedicled flap on the minor segment (Figure 50.5). This allows the minor segment to be rotated over to span the cleft, close the anterior hard palate near the alveolus, and offset the nasal and oral incisions. If more mobility of the hard palate flaps is needed, two unipedicled flaps are used.

Veau IV Clefts

Two unipedicled flaps are typically used to mobilize the hard palate flaps. Both flaps are inset to the premaxillary segment (Figure 50.4). This helps to close the defect at the incisive foramen under minimal tension. If the premaxillae is positioned too far anteriorly at the time of palatoplasty (e.g., with inadequate presurgical infant orthopedics) to allow for complete nasal and oral lining closure of the anterior hard palate, serious consideration is given to a primary premaxillary set-back.[12] This repositioning of the premaxillae facilitates the closure of the entire hard palate and lingual alveolar defects.

SOFT PALATE FLAP DESIGN AND MARKINGS

In a Furlow double-opposing Z-plasty, there are two oral and two nasal flaps. The anteriorly based flaps (one oral and one nasal) are mucosa-only flaps, while the posteriorly based flaps (one oral and one nasal) are myomucosal flaps,

each containing the ipsilateral levator veli palatini muscle. The posteriorly based oral flap may be designed on either the right or left side, although the authors design it on the left side by convention. The markings begin with the velar lateral relaxing incisions, which extend from the maxillary tuberosity toward the mandibular retromolar trigone, at the junction of the horizontally positioned palate and the vertically positioned lateral pharyngeal wall and cheek. Anteriorly, these lateral relaxing incisions extend along the junction of the hard palate and attached gingiva of the alveolus. Next, the medial margin of the cleft is marked, "cheating" slightly on the oral side in order to maintain adequate tissue for nasal lining closure. The medial edges of the uvula are also marked where they will be stripped of mucosa.

Four points are then marked that determine the Z-plasty. The base of the uvula, at the junction of the uvula and soft palate, is marked. Following this, the "normal" junction of the hard and soft palate (if no cleft were present), is found at a line drawn between the right and left maxillary tuberosities. The location of the hamulus on each side is noted. These four points determine the Z-plasty angle, which is usually approximately 60–90 degrees (Figure 50.5).

The left-sided posteriorly based oral myomucosal flap is formed by connecting the hard–soft palate junction to the left hamulus point. The right-sided anteriorly based oral mucosal flap is marked connecting the base of the

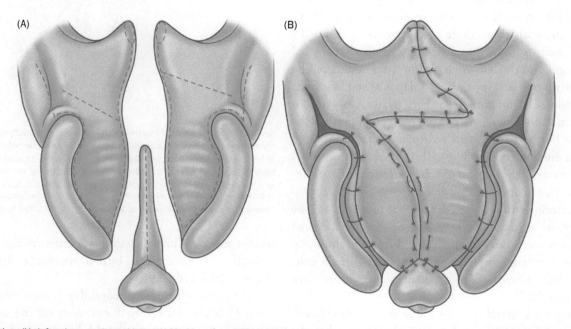

Figure 50.4. Veau IV cleft palate repair markings. (A) Markings for a bilateral cleft palate repair utilizing bilateral hard palate unipedicled mucoperiosteal flaps, bilateral vomer flaps, and a double-opposing Z-plasty repair of the soft palate. (B) Closure of the bilateral cleft palate. From Losee JE, Smith DM. Cleft palate repair. In Butler C, ed. *Head and Neck Reconstruction with DVD: A Volume in the Procedures in Reconstructive Surgery Series.* Philadelphia: Saunders Ltd.; 2008:271–294, figure 50.12.30 A,D.

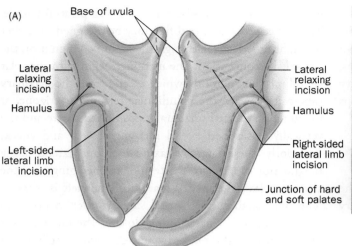

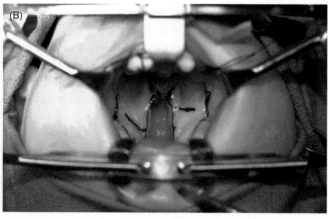

Figure 50.5. Veau III cleft palate repair markings. (A) Hard palate is marked with a unipedicled flap on the minor segment and a bipedicled flap on the major segment. The following points are noted for marking the soft palate double-opposing Z-plasty repair: velar relaxing incisions, the hamulus, junction of the hard and soft palate medially, the base of the uvulae. These points are used to design the right- and left-sided Z-plasty limbs. (B) Intraoperative markings for the double-opposing Z-plasty repair. From Losee JE, Smith DM. Cleft palate repair. In Butler C, ed. *Head and Neck Reconstruction with DVD: A Volume in the Procedures in Reconstructive Surgery Series.* Philadelphia: Saunders Ltd.; 2008:271–294, figure 50.12.8.

uvula to the right hamulus point. A bridge of oral mucosa is preserved between the lateral relaxing incisions and the Z-plasty limbs. After the markings are made, local anesthetic and epinephrine is infiltrated. The Dingman retractor is relaxed for 5–7 minutes to allow adequate effect prior to incision.

INCISIONS AND ORAL FLAP ELEVATION

The uvula is demucosalized medially with curved scissors, and the tip of each uvula is subsequently tagged with a suture to facilitate accurate alignment later. A no. 15 blade is used to make the incision along the left medial cleft margin and the left-sided oral myomucosal flap. The posteriorly based oral myomucosal flap is raised first from the anteromedial junction of the hard palate. Curved scissors are used to dissect the levator muscle away from the posterior border of the hard palate and separate it from the nasal mucosa (Figure 50.6). This dissection continues laterally to free the rest of the levator from the posterior hard palate and the tensor aponeurosis. It also proceeds posteriorly to separate the levator muscle from the nasal mucosa all the way to the base of the uvula. At the lateral-most extent, the levator is freed from its abnormal attachments to the superior constrictor muscle as it exits the skull base, allowing it to rotate medially without tension (Figure 50.7).

Through the lateral relaxing incision (described later), the tendon of the tensor veli palatini is visualized at the hamulus and divided to allow complete release of the

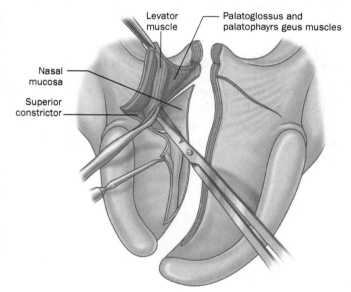

Figure 50.6. After incising the mucosa of the left-sided posteriorly based oral myomucosal flap, scissors are used to dissect in the plane between the left-sided levator muscle and the nasal mucosa. The levator muscle is released from the posterior edge of the hard palate medially, the tensor aponeurosis, and the superior constrictor laterally. From Losee JE, Smith DM. Cleft palate repair. In Butler C, ed. *Head and Neck Reconstruction with DVD: A Volume in the Procedures in Reconstructive Surgery Series.* Philadelphia: Saunders Ltd.; 2008:271–294, figure 50.12.11.

levator muscle. The soft palate musculature may then be radically retropositioned into a transverse orientation (Figures 50.8 and 50.9).

The right-sided oral mucosal flap is then incised with a no. 15 blade and elevated anteriorly off the underlying muscle. The submucosa should be dissected with the mucosal flap to maintain thickness and vascularity. The

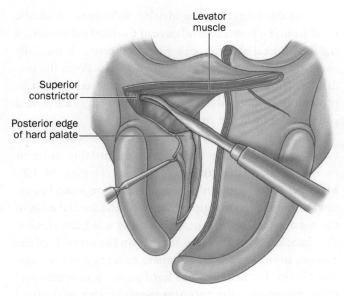

Figure 50.7. The levator muscle radically transposed from its abnormal anterior orientation to an anatomically correct horizontal location and swept free from the abnormal connections with the superior constrictor laterally. Levator muscle (*gold*), superior constrictor (*orange*). From Losee JE, Smith DM. Cleft palate repair. In Butler C, ed. *Head and Neck Reconstruction with DVD: A Volume in the Procedures in Reconstructive Surgery Series*. Philadelphia: Saunders Ltd.; 2008:271–294, figure 50.12.12.

underlying palatopharyngeus and palatoglossus muscles are kept together with the deeper levator veli palatini muscle and nasal mucosa. Care must be taken not to "button-hole" the anterior flap as dissection proceeds toward the posterior edge of the hard palate (Figure 50.10).

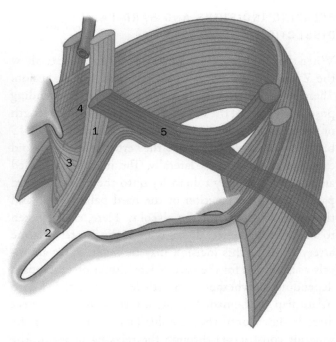

Figure 50.9. (*Left*) The abnormal orientation and attachments of the clefted levator muscle. (1) The incision noted by the dotted line releases the levator muscle from (2) the posterior edge of the hard palate, (3) the tensor aponeurosis, (4) the superior constrictor. (*Right*) Complete release of the levator muscle and radical reposition to the anatomic horizontal orientation in the middle 50% of the velum (5). From Losee JE, Smith DM. Cleft palate repair. In Butler C, ed. *Head and Neck Reconstruction with DVD: A Volume in the Procedures in Reconstructive Surgery Series*. Philadelphia: Saunders Ltd.; 2008:271–294, figure 50.12.15.

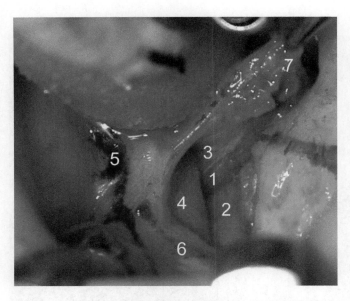

Figure 50.8. Intraoperative photographs of posteriorly based oral myomucosal flap dissection. (1) Levator muscle, (2) nasal mucosa, (3) cut tensor aponeurosis, (4) superior constrictor muscle, (5) uncut lateral velar relaxing incision, (6) posterior edge of the hard palate, (7) forceps retracting and retrepositioning the left-sided, posteriorly based oral myomucosal flap. From Losee JE, Smith DM. Cleft palate repair. In Butler C, ed. *Head and Neck Reconstruction with DVD: A Volume in the Procedures in Reconstructive Surgery Series*. Philadelphia: Saunders Ltd.; 2008:271–294, figure 50.12.14B.

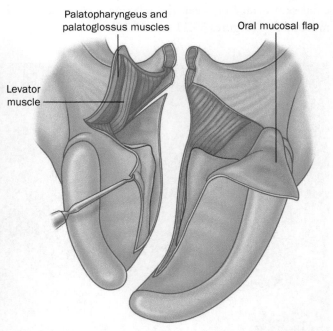

Figure 50.10. The incision for the right-sided, anteriorly based oral mucosa flap is made from the junction of the uvular base and soft palate medially, to the hamulus laterally. The right-sided oral mucosa flap is elevated, leaving the palatopharyngeus and palatoglossus muscles (*purple*) down and uninjured. From Losee JE, Smith DM. Cleft palate repair. In Butler C, ed. *Head and Neck Reconstruction with DVD: A Volume in the Procedures in Reconstructive Surgery Series*. Philadelphia: Saunders Ltd.; 2008:271–294, figure 50.12.17.

RELAXING INCISIONS AND HARD PALATE DISSECTION

When the cleft is wide, relaxing incisions are made to allow the Z-plasty flaps to transpose without undue tension. These are made from the maxillary tuberosity, extending posteriorly toward the retromolar trigone, with the length of the relaxing incision relative to the need. The no. 15 blade is positioned parallel to the vertical cheek to avoid exposing the buccal fat laterally. The incision is carried around the maxillary tuberosity onto the posterior hard palate, along the junction of the hard palate tissue and the attached gingiva of the alveolus. Here, care is taken to angle the blade laterally away from the greater palatine artery pedicle. This incision may be made as far anteriorly as is needed for the hard palate dissection and repair, depending on whether a unipedicled or bipedicled hard palate flap is planned. Scissors are then used to dissect directly down onto the hamulus (staying medial to the superior constrictor) through the relaxing incision. The dissection proceeds by spreading in the direction of the incision medially to the hamulus and superior constrictor muscle to enter the space of Ernst. The dissection plane of the relaxing incision then joins with the dissection plane of the soft palate. The tendon of the tensor veli palatini muscle is identified and divided medial to the hamulus. During this dissection, care is taken to preserve the mucosal skin bridge between the relaxing incision and oral mucosal flap (Figures 50.11 and 50.12).

From this lateral relaxing incision, soft tissue can also be freed from the posterolateral edge of the hard palate using a small periosteal elevator. This dissection proceeds medially along the posterior edge of the hard palate. From the medial border of the hard palate, the same dissection can also proceed laterally until the entire posterior edge of the hard palate is free from soft tissue.

Along the anterior hard palate, the Blair elevator is placed in the lateral relaxing incision anterior to the greater palatine artery pedicle (Figure 50.12). Mucoperiosteal flaps are elevated in a subperiosteal plane toward the medial margin of the cleft. The medial edge of the hard palate is then incised if it has not been already. This incision is again placed slightly on the oral side of the mucosa in order to leave adequate nasal mucosa for closure. From this incision, the hard palate mucoperiosteal flap is raised from the posterior medial corner of the hard palate. This is elevated anteriorly, then laterally, to meet the area of prior dissection. As the hard palate dissection is completed, care is taken to preserve the vascular pedicle. *An important point must be emphasized here.* The pedicle must be dissected circumferentially, freeing it of soft tissue and periosteal attachments to the anterior and posterior hard palate, in order to achieve adequate mobilization of the tissues. This is a slow and tedious dissection made with a tiny periosteal elevator. Rarely, even when this dissection is complete, there remains inadequate mobilization to achieve a tension-free closure. At

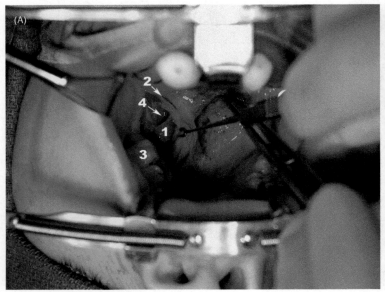
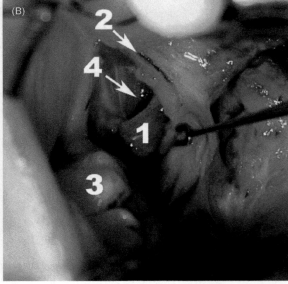

Figure 50.11. Intraoperative image of the tensor aponeurosis exposure through the left-sided lateral velar relaxing incision (A) in the field and (B) close up. (1) tensor aponeurosis as it courses medially around the hamulus, (2) lateral velar relaxing incision, (3) maxillary tuberosity, (4) space of Ernst, just medial to the superior constrictor. From Losee JE, Smith DM. Cleft palate repair. In Butler C, ed. *Head and Neck Reconstruction with DVD: A Volume in the Procedures in Reconstructive Surgery Series.* Philadelphia: Saunders Ltd.; 2008:271–294, figure 50.12.19A,B.

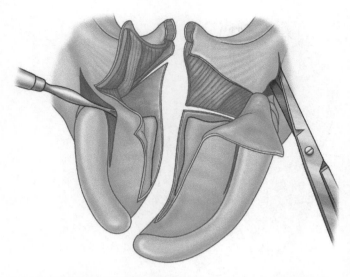

Figure 50.12. Bilateral relaxing incisions are made and the nasal flaps are created. The right side demonstrates scissor dissection to the space of Ernst for release of the tensor aponeurosis. On the left, the Blair elevator is placed into the lateral relaxing incision of the hard palate and elevation of the hard palate mucoperiosteal flaps. The left-sided, anteriorly based nasal mucosa flap is cut at about 60 degrees. The right-sided, posteriorly based nasal myomucosal flap is made at 60–90 degrees, leaving several millimeters of nasal mucosa along the posterior edge of the hard palate to facilitate nasal lining closure. From Losee JE, Smith DM. Cleft palate repair. In Butler C, ed. *Head and Neck Reconstruction with DVD: A Volume in the Procedures in Reconstructive Surgery Series.* Philadelphia: Saunders Ltd.; 2008:271–294, figure 50.12.20.

this time, an osteotomy may be made in the posterior aspect of the foramina to release the pedicle fully so that it may be mobilized medially.

The nasal mucosa is then separated from the hard palate. In a subperiosteal plane, a nasal mucoperiosteal flap is elevated from the medial cleft margin. The entire medial cleft margin is released. This dissection is then extended around the posterior edge of the hard palate to free the nasal mucosa of the soft palate from its attachment to the hard palate. In very wide clefts, this nasal lining dissection can be continued laterally, at the junction of the hard palate and below the hamulus at the pterygoid plate. Elevation of the nasal lining laterally, in this region, allows for medial mobilization of the nasal lining to facilitate a tension free closure. Some have advocated a relaxing incision in this area to facilitate the process.

NASAL FLAP INCISIONS

Once the hard palate flaps are elevated, the soft palate Z-plasty flaps are completed on the nasal side (Figure 50.12). The left-sided anteriorly based nasal mucosal flap is cut from medially at the base of the uvula toward the hamulus, where the levator can now be seen to exit the skull base. It is important to make this incision all the way laterally to

where the levator muscle exits the skull base because this will ultimately receive the opposite levator muscle, allowing them to be completely overlapped.

The right-sided posteriorly based nasal myomucosal flap is then dissected. The attachments of the levator veli palatini to the posterior edge of the hard palate are released medially if they have not already been during the hard palate dissection. They are also released from the anterior 5 mm of nasal mucosa in order to leave a larger rim of nasal mucosa along the posterior edge of the hard palate on the right side for closure. The muscle is dissected laterally and freed from the tensor aponeurosis and superior constrictor muscles. Through the right-sided lateral relaxing incision, the tensor aponeurosis is divided just medial to the hamulus. Once the muscle is swept posteriorly off the nasal lining, the nasal lining is cut. This incision is made from the hard–soft palate junction medially toward the hamulus laterally.

There are two important points to be emphasized here. First, leave approximately 5 mm of nasal lining cuff along the posterior edge of the hard palate; this facilitates the nasal lining repair. Second, this incision is made *only as long as is necessary* to allow the tip of the right-sided myomucosal flap to reach the contralateral skull base at the apex of nasal mucosa defect. Again, this allows for the levator muscles to be completely overlapped. Limiting the length of this incision results in a smaller nasal lining defect that needs to be filled by the left-sided anteriorly based nasal mucosal flap. Any remaining attachments of the right-sided levator to the surrounding mucosa or musculature are released in order to facilitate posterior rotation of this nasal myomucosal flap.

VOMER FLAPS FOR VEAU III AND VEAU IV CLEFTS

Vomer flaps are employed in Veau III and Veau IV clefts to assist with a two-layer closure and reduce tension on the nasal closure. In a Veau III cleft, the incision is marked along the junction of the hard palate–vomer mucoperiosteum on the unaffected side. In a subperiosteal plane, the vomer mucoperiosteum is elevated on the cleft side, turned over, and inset to the nasal mucosal flap on that side using a running 4-0 Vicryl suture.

In Veau IV clefts, the vomer is incised in the midline, and mucoperiosteal flaps are elevated on both sides. These are both turned over to be inset to the ipsilateral nasal mucosal flaps bilaterally (Figure 50.13). The vomer flap can extend posteriorly if needed to help close the anterior nasal lining (along the junction of the hard–soft palate) without tension.

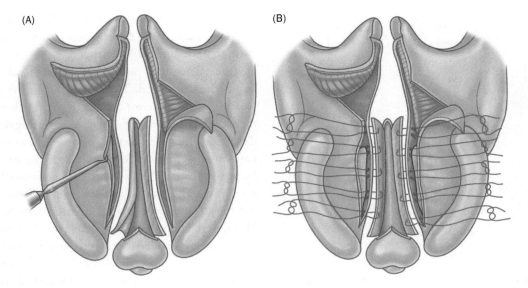

Figure 50.13. Vomer flaps for nasal lining closure in a Veau IV cleft palate. (A) Incision and elevation of vomer mucoperiosteal flaps. (B) Closure of the bilateral cleft palate nasal lining by repairing each vomer flap to the ipsilateral nasal lining. From Losee JE, Smith DM. Cleft palate repair. In Butler C, ed. *Head and Neck Reconstruction with DVD: A Volume in the Procedures in Reconstructive Surgery Series.* Philadelphia: Saunders Ltd.; 2008:271–294, figure 50.12.30B,C.

NASAL FLAP INSET AND CLOSURE

A nasopharyngeal (NP) airway of appropriate size is placed through one nostril prior to closure of the nasal lining flaps. This NP airway is left in place for several hours after surgery while the tongue is monitored for swelling (see the section on postoperative care).

The right-sided posteriorly based nasal myomucosal flap is inset first. The corner of this flap is inset to the corner of the nasal lining where the left levator veli palatini muscle leaves the skull base. This radically transposes the right-sided musculature so that it is now oriented in a transverse position (Figure 50.14). The tip of the left-sided anteriorly based nasal mucosal flap is then inset to the nasal mucosa at the apex on the right side. After the tips of the flaps are inset, the reconstruction of the uvula commences. The sutures placed at the tip of each uvula are reapproximated, and the uvula is subsequently closed with 1 mm sutures on both the nasal and oral sides. The Z-plasty limbs are repeatedly bisected with interrupted sutures until the nasal lining closure is complete. Care is taken to place sutures through the mucosa only, *not* through the muscle.

When there is undue tension at the junction of the hard and soft palate, or at the left anterior mucosal flap, one of several strategies may be used to reinforce the closure. These strategies may be used either in an attempt to prevent fistula formation, or to reduce the risk of contracture of the soft palate with scar formation. We occasionally place a layer of ultra-thin acellular dermal matrix

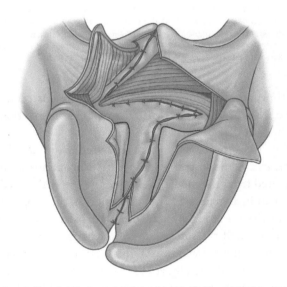

Figure 50.14. Nasal-side closure. Levator muscle (*gold*), palatopharyngeus and palatoglossus muscles (*purple*), superior constrictor (*orange*). From Losee JE, Smith DM. Cleft palate repair. In Butler C, ed. *Head and Neck Reconstruction with DVD: A Volume in the Procedures in Reconstructive Surgery Series.* Philadelphia: Saunders Ltd.; 2008:271–294, figure 50.12.24.

to cover the nasal lining anteriorly.[13] The acellular dermal matrix does not contact or overlay any of the muscle, nor is it sewn to the levator sling. It covers only the anterior 25% of the soft palate and hard palate as needed. In the bilateral cleft palate, the acellular dermal matrix extends anteriorly to reinforce the repair at the junction of the primary and secondary palates.[4] Other techniques to reinforce a compromised nasal lining closure, include the use of the buccal fat pad[14] and/or a buccal myomucosal flap.[15]

The buccal fat is harvested through the lateral relaxing incision and passed underneath the lateral tissue bridge to augment the anterior soft palate nasal lining repair. Often it will extend enough anteriorly to also reinforce the hard-soft palate junction and fill some of the relaxing incisions along the lateral hard palate. The buccal myomucosal flap technique is a useful adjunct for adding additional tissue to either the nasal or oral lining in the case of very wide clefts, or in revision cleft surgery.[16]

ORAL FLAP INSET AND CLOSURE

After the nasal repair is completed, the left-sided posteriorly based oral myomucosal flap is inset to the corner on the right side. This stitch incorporates a small bite of mucosa with a robust bite of deeper lateral tissue on the right. This completes the anatomic realignment of the levator sling, with the levator veli palatini muscles now overlapping each other. The tip of the right-sided anteriorly based oral mucosal flap is then inset into the left-sided mucosal defect. The limbs of the Z-plasty are closed with multiple bisecting sutures. The hard palate–soft palate junction and oral mucosa anteriorly are closed with horizontal mattress sutures to evert these tissues (Figure 50.15). When unipedicled hard palate flaps are used, the anterior tip of the flap is secured to the alveolar gingiva to close the anterior fistula using horizontal mattress or circumdental Vicryl sutures.

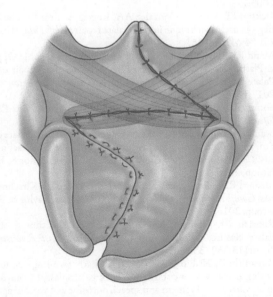

Figure 50.15. Repair of the oral side flaps and overlapping of the levator muscles under "functional tension." From Losee JE, Smith DM. Cleft palate repair. In Butler C, ed. *Head and Neck Reconstruction with DVD: A Volume in the Procedures in Reconstructive Surgery Series.* Philadelphia: Saunders Ltd.; 2008:271–294, figure 50.12.27.

ALTERNATIVE TECHNIQUES

STRAIGHT-LINE REPAIR WITH INTRAVELAR VELOPLASTY

Intravelar veloplasty (IVVP) was first introduced by Kriens in 1969, to re-establish a muscular sling in the soft palate.[11] Many IVVP operations do not adequately release *all* the abnormal attachments of the levator veli palatini muscle, however. It is our experience that the muscle then often ends up scarring back toward the posterior edge of the hard palate and reassumes a pathologic sagittal orientation. This is compounded by the inevitable shortening of the soft palate resulting from the scarring of the straight-line incision. Radical IVVP is necessary to release the levator from the hard palate, tensor, and superior constrictor muscles (Figure 50.3C,D). Sommerlad's technique, for example, includes a radical muscle dissection and retropositioning to accomplish this goal with a straight-line repair.[17,18]

TWO-STAGE PALATOPLASTY

Due to the potential for maxillary growth restriction with hard palate dissection at a young age, some surgeons prefer to separate the hard and soft palate repairs.[19] Rohrich and Gosman advocate an early cleft lip and soft palate repair at 3–6 months of age, followed by hard palate repair at 15–18 months.[20] Yamanishi et al. in Japan have endorsed performing soft palate Furlow repair at 12 months and hard palate repair at 18 months.[21] This demonstrated less maxillary growth restriction in their cohort, as compared with a one-stage V-Y pushback operation at 12 months of age.

Although uncommon, we occasionally perform a two-stage palatoplasty for excessively wide defects greater than 2 cm in width at the junction of the hard and soft palates. In our two-stage technique, we perform a straight-line palatal adhesion without any muscular dissection or repair. This is essentially a definitive hard palate repair at the first stage, with a staged reconstruction of the soft palate. In the second stage, a minimum of 3 months later, a conversion Furlow palatoplasty is performed for definitive repair of the velum, similar to repairing a submucous cleft palate.

POSTOPERATIVE CARE

After completing the cleft palate repair, hemostasis is again assessed, and Bovie electrocautery is commonly employed along the borders of the relaxing incisions to ensure hemostasis. Long-acting local anesthetic, such as bupivacaine, is injected. The oropharynx is irrigated and suctioned through the existing nasal catheter. This catheter is then placed deep into the esophagus or stomach to suction any residual fluid there. The catheter is left in the posterior oropharynx for the anesthetist to use to suction the oral airway upon awakening. This obviates the need for them to pass another suction orally and risk injury to the palate repair.

The NP airway is taped into place at the completion of the operation and left in place for several hours postoperatively. The patient is recovered in the postanesthetic care unit and transferred to a ward with continuous pulse oximetry monitoring and intravenous fluids. If there is no evidence of tongue or floor of mouth swelling, the NP airway can be removed on afternoon rounds or in the morning of the first postoperative day. The use of the NP airway has replaced the need for postoperatively retained tongue stitches. If there is untoward tongue or floor of mouth swelling, the patient can be moved to a monitored bed, sat upright in a mist tent, and the patient's airway will be maintained around the region of swelling by the NP airway.

Elbow restraints are placed in the operating room and used for the first 1–2 weeks after surgery. Clear liquids may be offered by an open or sippy cup immediately after recovering from surgery. This is transitioned to a full liquid diet at 48 hours for the remainder of the first week. The patients are discharged from the hospital when they have taken adequate oral intake to maintain hydration. Patients follow-up in clinic in 1–2 weeks and are cleared for a regular diet at 2 weeks if they are healing adequately. A full cleft team visit, including speech assessment, is performed 3 months after surgery.

CAVEATS

In our hands, this technique has excellent success in maintaining velopharyngeal competence and a low fistula rate.[13] Palatoplasty may contribute to maxillary growth restriction, and the degree to which technique and timing of palatoplasty restrict growth remains a source of controversy. The anatomic basis for the Furlow palatoplasty in lengthening the palate and repositioning the muscles, and timing of surgery at or just before 1 year of age has allowed us to optimize speech outcomes. Normal speech is essential to normal development and social interactions.

REFERENCES

1. Furlow LT Jr. Cleft palate repair by double opposing z-plasty. *Plast Reconstr Surg* 1986;78:724–736.
2. Furlow LT Jr. Cleft palate repair by double opposing z-plasty. *Oper Tech Plast Reconstr Surg* 1995;2:223–232.
3. Kaye A, Kirschner RE. The Furlow double-opposing Z-plasty repair for cleft palate. In: Losee JE, Kirschner RE, eds. *Comprehensive Cleft Care*. Vol 2. CRC Press: Taylor & Francis Group, 2016.
4. Losee JE, Smith DM. Cleft palate repair. In: Butler C, ed. *Head and Neck Reconstruction with DVD: A Volume in the Procedures in Reconstructive Surgery Series*. Philadelphia: Saunders Ltd., 2008.
5. Huang MH, Lee ST, Rajendran K. Anatomic basis of cleft palate and velopharyngeal surgery: implications from a fresh cadaveric study. *Plast Reconstr Surg* 1998;101:613–627.
6. Gosain AK, Lanier ST. Submucous cleft palate. In: Losee JE, Kirschner RE, eds. *Comprehensive Cleft Care*. Vol 2. CRC Press: Taylor & Francis Group, 2016.
7. Koch H, Grzonka M, Koch I. Cleft malformation of lip, alveolus, hard and soft palate, and nose (LAHSN)—a critical view of the terminology, the diagnosis and gradation as a basis for documentation and therapy. *Br J Oral Maxillofac Surg* 1995;33:51–58.
8. Rottgers SA, Camison L, Mai R, et al. Antibiotic use in primary palatoplasty: a survey of practice patterns, assessment of efficacy, and proposed guidelines for use. *Plast Reconstr Surg* 2016;137:574–582.
9. Millard DR Jr. *Cleft Craft*. Vol 3. Boston: Little, Brown, 1980.
10. Bardach J. Two-flap palatoplasty: Bardach's technique. *Oper Tech Plast Reconstr Surg* 1995;2:211–214.
11. Bardach J, Salyer K, eds. *Surgical Techniques in Cleft Lip and Palate*. St. Louis: Mosby-Year Book, 1991.
12. Vyas RM, Kim DC, Padwa BL, Mulliken JB. Primary premaxillary setback and repair of bilateral complete cleft lip: Indications, technique and outcomes. *Cleft Palate Craniofac J* 2016;53:302–308.
13. Losee JE, Smith DM, Afifi AM, et al. A successful algorithm for limiting postoperative fistulae following palatal procedures in the patient with orofacial clefting. *Plast Reconstr Surg* 2008;122:544–554.
14. Levi B, Kasten SJ, Buchman SR. Utilization of the buccal fat pad flap for congenital cleft palate repair. *Plast Reconstr Surg* 2009;123:1018–1021.
15. Jackson IT, Moreira-Gonzalez AA, Rogers A, Beal BJ. The buccal flap—a useful technique in cleft palate repair? *Cleft Palate Craniofac J* 2004;41:144–151.
16. Mann RJ, Martin MD, Eichhorn MG, et al. The Double Opposing Z-Plasty Plus or Minus Buccal Flap Approach for Repair of Cleft Palate: A Review of 505 Consecutive Cases. *Plast Reconstr Surg* 2017;139(3):735e–744e.
17. Sommerlad BC. A technique for cleft palate repair. *Plast Reconstr Surg* 2003;112:1542–1548.
18. Sommerlad BC. Cleft palate repair with minimal hard palate dissection and radical muscle reconstruction. In: Losee JE, Kirschner RE, eds. *Comprehensive Cleft Care*. Vol 2. CRC Press: Taylor & Francis Group, 2016.
19. Menard RM. Two-stage palate repair. In: Losee JE, Kirschner RE, eds. *Comprehensive Cleft Care*. Vol 2. CRC Press: Taylor & Francis Group, 2016.
20. Rohrich RJ, Gosman AA. An update on the timing of hard palate closure: a critical long-term analysis. *Plast Reconstr Surg* 2004;113:350–352.
21. Yamanishi T, Nishio J, Sako M, et al. Early two-stage double opposing Z-plasty or one stage push-back palatoplasty? Comparisons in maxillary development and speech outcome at 4 years of age. *Ann Plastic Surg* 2011;66:148–153.

51.

PHARYNGEAL FLAP

Raj Yvas, Lauren D. Patty, and Donald S. Mowlds

ASSESSMENT OF THE DEFECT

Closure of the velopharyngeal sphincter is necessary for the correct phonation of vowels and most consonants. Sphincter closure relies primarily on the contraction of the levator veli palatini, as well as the tensor veli palatini, palatoglossus, palatopharyngeus, musculus uvulae, salpingopharyngeus, and superior pharyngeal constrictor muscles. Contraction produces medial movement of the lateral pharyngeal walls and posterosuperior movement of the velum, or soft palate. Sphincter closure preferentially guides airflow into the oral cavity while also controlling air pressure, allowing the lips and tongue to produce intelligible speech.[1] Dysfunction of the velopharyngeal sphincter allows excess air passage into the nasal cavity, resulting in hypernasality, reduction in speech volume, facial grimacing, decreased intraoral pressure on oral consonant phonation, and nasal air emission.[2] Velopharyngeal dysfunction can be further divided into insufficiency versus incompetence based on underlying abnormality. Velopharyngeal insufficiency results from inadequate tissues or mechanical restriction of an unrepaired cleft palate or after palatoplasty from a short or hypodynamic velum.[3] Insufficiency can also be secondary to the palatopharyngeal disproportion seen in velocardiofacial syndrome and other anatomic conditions (i.e., velar dysplasia, adenotonsillectomy, etc.); recent studies demonstrate up to 30% of patients who undergo cleft palate repair require surgery for velopharyngeal insufficiency.[4] Velopharyngeal incompetence occurs secondary to neuromotor dysfunction.

Proper evaluation of velopharyngeal dysfunction is essential in determining the most appropriate corrective procedure. Specifically, velar and lateral wall movements are evaluated. Surgeons rely on a handful of established and new diagnostic modalities as well as perceptual speech analysis by cleft-trained speech-language pathologists. Videonasoendoscopy remains a primary modality for assessing the upper vocal tract during speech. It allows direct visualization of the mobility of the posterior and lateral walls of the pharynx, the size and pattern of the velopharyngeal aperture during sphincter closure, the function and location of the levator muscle, and the length of the soft palate.[1] It is performed predominantly in two dimensions; however, recent advances have allowed for three-dimensional imaging. Multiview speech videofluoroscopy utilizes serial radiographs in lateral and anteroposterior views to provide two-dimensional imaging of dynamic sphincter motion. Downsides to this imaging modality include radiation exposure and difficulty identifying patterns of velopharyngeal closure. Nasometry measures air escaping through the nose during phonation. It alone is not an accurate indicator of velopharyngeal sphincter dysfunction, but comparing pre- and postoperative nasal air emission values is useful when assessing postsurgical outcomes. Recently, magnetic resonance imaging (MRI) has been proposed as a tool to assess static and dynamic velopharyngeal anatomy, providing high-quality images that allow for visualization of velar muscle insertion sites.[4] Two- and three-dimensional MRI can provide enhanced visual information but are currently too costly to justify regular use.

INDICATIONS

The primary indication for a pharyngeal flap is velopharyngeal insufficiency resulting from a large anteroposterior central gap during closure of the velum and pharynx. It is considered when phonation is no longer improved with speech therapy, or in cases of iatrogenic defects (i.e., post-tonsillectomy/

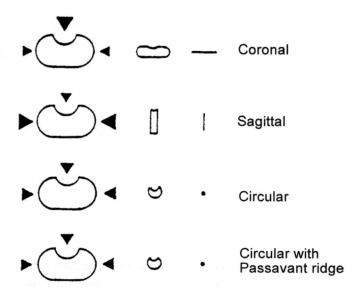

Coronal

Sagittal

Circular

Circular with Passavant ridge

Figure 51.1. Velopharyngeal closure patterns.[8]

-adenoidectomy/-tumor resection). The pharyngeal flap creates a static central obstruction while maintaining two patent lateral airway openings (lateral ports). The procedure is most effective in patients with limited anteroposterior wall mobility but intact lateral wall motion such that the lateral ports can close during phonation of oral consonants (Figure 51.1).[5–7]

CONTRAINDICATIONS

Relative contraindications to the pharyngeal flap procedure are general contraindications to surgery/general anesthesia, known or suspected airway obstruction, obstructive sleep apnea, adenotonsillar hypertrophy, poor lateral wall motion, and retrognathia. Those with suspected sleep apnea or history of retrognathia require upper airway assessment and polysomnography to evaluate the extent of airway obstruction; in retrognathic patients with significant upper airway obstruction, delaying allows additional time for mandibular growth. In patients with adenotonsillar hypertrophy, adenotonsillectomy should be performed 6 weeks prior to pharyngeal flap procedure.[5–6,9]

Medialized internal carotid arteries (visualized on MRI or seen as pharyngeal pulsations during videonasoendoscopy) require extra care during pharyngeal flap elevation to avoid iatrogenic vessel injury. Aberrant internal carotid anatomy is a common feature of velocardiofacial syndrome (22q11.2 chromosome deletion), warranting close

evaluation in these patients and subsequent adjustments to surgical planning.[5]

PATIENT POSITION AND ROOM SETUP

Once in the operating room, the patient is placed in a supine position and intubated with an oral right-angle endotracheal (RAE) tube that is secured to the lower lip/chin midline. The patient's head is placed on a Mayfield horseshoe headrest, which is then adjusted to allow mild extension of the neck. Hyperextension is avoided in patients with known cervical spine instability. The sterile surgical field is then established.

MARKINGS

Lateral flap borders are drawn parallel to the posterior tonsillar pillars. The inferior flap border should be at approximately mid-tonsillar level. Appropriate flap length is verified by measuring the distance between the posterior pharyngeal wall and the posterior margin of the soft palate. Flap width varies according to patient anatomy and velar closure pattern.

OPERATIVE TECHNIQUE

The pharyngeal flap was first described by Schoenborn in 1875 as an inferiorly based flap; he later modified this technique to a superiorly pedicled flap, enabling enhanced soft palate mobility. Today, superiorly based pharyngeal flaps predominate.[4–5,10] Traditionally, the procedure is performed under direct visualization; however, recent cadaveric studies by Smartt et al. have proposed utilization of robotic surgical systems for superior pharyngeal flap surgery to enhance ergonomics and surgical field exposure.[11]

SUPERIOR FLAP

The Dingman mouth retractor is inserted and a throat pack is placed and accounted for. Incisional markings are infiltrated with 25% bupivacaine with 1:200,000 units epinephrine, and 10–15 minutes are counted prior to incision for optimal vasoconstriction. Incisions are made along markings through mucosa and muscle down to prevertebral fascia. Flap elevation proceeds in the prevertebral fascial plane in an inferior to superior direction until reaching the nasopharynx. A red rubber catheter is placed in each nostril and passed through the nasopharynx into the mouth to establish the patency of each lateral port. Flap elevation and hemostasis are achieved with the use of needle-point monopolar electrocautery; however, bleeding is typically minimal in this relatively avascular plane. If the patient has medialized internal carotid arteries, elevation is only performed by blunt dissection. Primary closure of the posterior wall donor site is with interrupted 3-0 Vicryl sutures. Occasionally the donor site is too large to close primarily; it can be closed from inferior to superior as far as possible with the remainder left to heal by secondary intention.

The raw side of the pharyngeal flap is lined with velar nasal mucosa to minimize risk of contracture and tubing of the flap. The soft palate is split longitudinally at the midline, and nasal mucosa is raised on each side creating two flaps based on the distal edge of the soft palate. These flaps hinge posteriorly so the nasal surface of the velum lines the raw surface of the pharyngeal flap. The lined pharyngeal flap is then mobilized as superiorly as possible and sutured to the palatal musculature/oral velar mucosa of the soft palate with interrupted 3-0 Vicryl sutures. The palatal nasal mucosal flaps are hinged along posterior border and sutured to the raw surface of the pharyngeal flap using interrupted 4-0 chromic sutures to provide full lining for the flap. This is followed by closure of the oral mucosa of the palate using 3-0 Vicryl sutures. The red rubber catheters are removed, the throat packing is removed, and the stomach suctioned. A tongue stitch is placed to address possible obstruction during extubation and the early postoperative period. If there is additional concern for obstruction, a nasopharyngeal airway can be placed with care and direct visualization while in the operating suite and secured to the nose with tape (Figure 51.2).

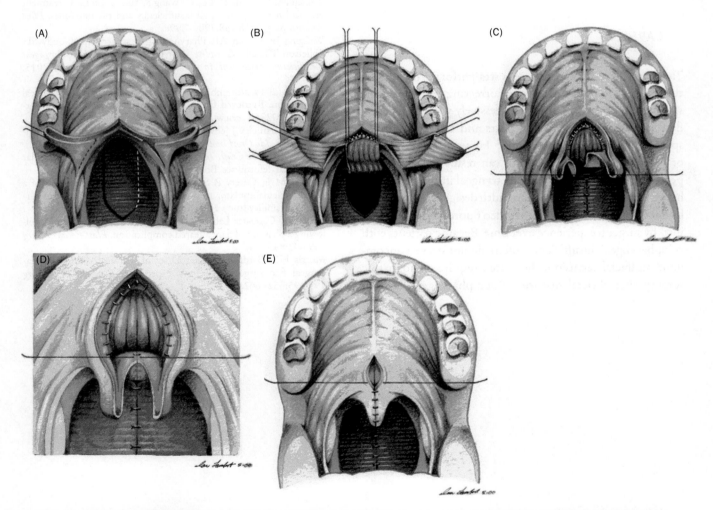

Figure 51.2. (A) Splitting of the palate at midline. (B) Attachment of pharyngeal flap to soft palate; nasal mucosa flaps elevated and hinged posteriorly. (C,D) Inset of nasal mucosal flaps to raw surface of pharyngeal flap. (E) Closure of the oral palate in standard fashion.[8]

POSTOPERATIVE CARE AND FOLLOW-UP EVALUATION

The patient is admitted overnight for observation. Intravenous ampicillin/sulbactam is administered at the time of surgery. Clear liquid diet is initiated the same day as surgery, followed by full liquids the day after surgery, then advanced to a soft diet the next day, which is continued for 1 month. The use of straws is prohibited. Intravenous maintenance fluids are continued until adequate oral intake is achieved. When placed, the nasopharyngeal airway is removed the morning after surgery; if it comes out before then, it should not be reinserted. Patients are typically discharged on postoperative day 2 after demonstrating no airway issues and adequate diet intake. The patient follows-up in clinic 2 weeks postoperatively. Speech evaluation and therapy is resumed 6 weeks after surgery to improve any residual speech abnormalities.

CAVEATS

The pharyngeal flap procedure is straightforward and relatively simple to perform, but overcorrecting velopharyngeal sphincter dysfunction with an excessively wide pharyngeal flap narrows the lateral nasal ports and causes hyponasal speech and airway obstruction.[12] However, narrow flaps or postoperative flap dehiscence can result in large lateral ports leading to persistent velopharyngeal insufficiency and hypernasality.[13] Pharyngeal flap width design is best inferred by data from nasoendoscopy or video fluoroscopy and modified by surgeon experience over time. Because patients with velopharyngeal insufficiency often demonstrate concomitant midfacial retrusion, they often require orthognathic surgery after skeletal maturity. Prior pharyngeal flap can limit the extent of midface sagittal movement, with larger movements (>9 mm) possibly requiring midfacial distraction prior to definitive occlusal surgery.

REFERENCES

1. Perry JL, Kuechn DP. Anatomy and physiology of the velopharynx. In: Losee JE, Kirschner RE, eds. *Comprehensive Cleft Care.* 2nd ed. Boca Raton, Fla: CRC Press, 2015:475–492.
2. Davis DJ, Sagnall AD. Velopharyngeal incompetence. In: McCarthy JG, ed. *Plastic Surgery.* Vol. 4. Philadelphia: Saunders, 1990:2903.
3. Kummer AW. Disorders of resonance and airflow secondary to cleft palate and/or velopharyngeal dysfunction. *Semin Speech Lang* 2011;32:141–149.
4. Naran S, Ford M, Losee JE. What's new in cleft palate and velopharyngeal dysfunction management? *Plast Reconstr Surg* 2017;139:1343e–1355e.
5. Forrest CR, Klaiman PM, Mason AC. Posterior pharyngeal flaps. In: Losee JE, Kirschner RE, eds. *Comprehensive Cleft Care.* New York: McGraw-Hill Medical, 2009:649–664.
6. Yamaguchi K, Lonic D, Lee C, Wang S, Yun C, Lo L. A treatment protocol for velopharyngeal insufficiency and the outcomes. *Plast Reconstr Surg* 2016;138:290e–299e.
7. Willging JP, Cohen AP. Pharyngeal flap surgery. In: Goudy SL, Tollefson TT, eds. *Complete Cleft Care: Cleft and Velopharyngeal Insufficiency Treatment in Children.* New York: Thieme, 2015: 169–176.
8. Patel PK. (2014, November 4). Surgical treatment of velopharyngeal dysfunction. Retrieved from https://emedicine.medscape.com/article/1279928-overview
9. Raol N, Hartnick CJ (eds.). Surgery for pediatric velopharyngeal insufficiency. *Adv Otorhinolaryngol* 2015;76:50–57.
10. Millard DR. *Cleft Craft: The Evolution of Its Surgery.* Vol. 3. Alveolar and palatal deformities. Boston: Little, Brown, 1980.
11. Smartt JM Jr, Gerety P, Serletti JM, Taylor JA. Application of a robotic telemanipulator to perform posterior pharyngeal flap surgery: a feasibility study. *Plast Reconstr Surg* 2013;131:841–845.
12. Sirois M, Caouette-Laberge L, Spier S, et al. Sleep apnea following a pharyngeal flap: a feared complication. *Plast Reconstr Surg* 1994;93:943–947.
13. Morris HL, Bardach J, Jones D, et al. Clinical results of pharyngeal flap surgery: the Iowa experience. *Plast Reconstr Surg* 1995;95:652–662.

52.

SPHINCTER PHARYNGOPLASTY FOR VELOPHARYNGEAL DYSFUNCTION

Donald S. Mowlds and Raj M. Vyas

ASSESSMENT OF THE DEFECT

Velopharyngeal insufficiency (VPI) results from an inability to completely isolate air escape via the nasal and oral cavities during speech production. It results from a structural or neuromuscular defect involving the pharyngeal walls or the velum at the level of the nasopharynx. Insufficient velopharyngeal closure allows nasal air escape and hypernasal speech, resulting in affected speech ranging from minor disruptions to unintelligibility. Up to 30% of children develop VPI after palatoplasty.[1]

The surgical correction of VPI seeks to augment the deficient aspect of the velopharyngeal apparatus. The sphincter pharyngoplasty was first described in 1950 by Hynes, who advocated for the elevation of bilateral salpingopharyngeus myomucosal flaps with transverse mobilization and inset.[2,3] Several variations have been subsequently popularized and include elevation of laterally based palatopharyngeus myomucosal flaps from the posterior tonsillar pillars.[4,5] The objective of the sphincter pharyngoplasty is to narrow the velopharyngeal gap transversely by addressing lateral pharyngeal wall motion when there is adequate coronal velopharyngeal closure.

INDICATIONS AND PATIENT SELECTION

SPEECH AND VELOPHARYNGEAL ASSESSMENT

A multidisciplinary team approach is ideal for the evaluation and management of patients with VPI. Specifically, the surgeon and speech pathologist work closely to match the gap size and velopharyngeal closure pattern to the appropriate intervention. In patients demonstrating symptoms of VPI (hypernasality, nasal emission, facial grimacing, compensatory misarticulations), diagnostic modalities include video-recorded standard perceptual speech, nasoendoscopy, nasometry, and/or fluoroscopy. Speech evaluations are obtained and reviewed by the multispecialty team consisting of a medical geneticist, speech pathologist, otolaryngologist, pulmonologist, plastic surgeon, and social worker.[6] Optimal visualization of velopharyngeal sphincter function is accomplished with video nasoendoscopy.[7] This modality permits direct visualization of the position and function of the levator musculature, the adequacy of closure, length of the soft palate, and the degree of lateral pharyngeal wall motion. However, an important limitation to video nasoendoscopy is its tolerability in young children who must cooperate with speech sampling and the inability to directly measure gap size as the scale changes with scope position.[8] Interestingly, recent advances in this technology have allowed for three-dimensional modeling of the velopharyngeal sphincter during speech using coronal, sagittal, and axial planes, thus increasing its diagnostic value. Two-dimensional dynamic visualization of the velopharyngeal sphincter motion during speech is obtained using multiview speech videofluoroscopy. Velar motion, adenoid size, cranial base angle, and lateral pharyngeal wall motion are easily ascertained. Furthermore, accurate size measurements are made possible using a ratio of selected distance markings and pixels, delivering reliable quantitative data regarding closure patterns and gap dimension.[9]

The objective of sphincter pharyngoplasty is to narrow the central aspect of the velopharyngeal orifice without creating lateral airway ports. This procedure results in less airway morbidity than the pharyngeal flap and is reserved for patients who demonstrate a large-gap, coronal pattern of velopharyngeal closure on nasoendoscopy.

It is often incorrectly assumed that younger patients undergoing surgical correction of VPI achieve better long-term speech outcomes. As a matter of fact, the timing of VPI surgery does not affect the length of postoperative speech therapy required to achieve normalization of velopharyngeal function.[3,10]

PATIENT PREPARATION

AIRWAY EVALUATION

Proper preoperative evaluation of the patient's airway is paramount to surgical planning. Enlarged tonsillar tissue impedes proper placement of the myomucosal flaps and obscures the plane of dissection, increasing the technical difficulty of the procedure. In a similar fashion, friable and enlarged adenoids can interfere with flap inset, potentially compromising the outcome. As such, patient may require tonsillectomy/adenoidectomy 3 months prior to sphincter pharyngoplasty. An interval nasoendoscopy and/or fluoroscopic speech evaluations is done to reassess the velopharyngeal closure pattern and gap size in order to confirm that the treatment plan does not require adjustment. It is important to convey to parents that the symptoms of velopharyngeal dysfunction are likely to worsen following tonsillectomy/adenoidectomy and that pharyngoplasty should be postponed for at least 3 months following this procedure. Additionally, it is recommended that the surgeon communicate the plan with the otolaryngologist so that he or she is aware of the importance of preserving posterior tonsillar tissue.

SUBSPECIALTY EVALUATIONS

Patients should be managed within a multidisciplinary craniofacial team setting that includes, at a minimum, medical genetics, speech pathology, otolaryngology, plastic surgery, and social work. Providers evaluate the patient in tandem and collectively formulate a treatment plan that addresses the patient's needs and the family's expectations. At this stage, diagnostic results must be rigorously reviewed in order to determine the most prudent course of action. The speech pathologist is the captain of the team; it is crucial to first differentiate abnormal speech resulting from velopharyngeal sphincter dysfunction versus abnormal speech that can benefit from behavioral speech therapy alone.

CONTRAINDICATIONS

Sphincter pharyngoplasty is not immediately performed in patients without a clear diagnostic picture or those whose closure pattern improves with speech therapy. In patients with preexisting obstructive sleep apnea, pharyngoplasty is deferred until the tonsils and adenoids are evaluated for hypertrophy. Patients with insufficient or damaged posterior tonsillar tissue due to previous tonsillectomy are not candidates for a sphincter pharyngoplasty procedure and may instead be better suited by a wide pharyngeal flap. The sphincter pharyngoplasty is almost exclusively reserved for patients with markedly impaired or absent lateral pharyngeal wall motion. Midline or medialized internal carotid vasculature represents a relative contraindication and caution is advised. To this effect, the posterior pharyngeal wall is carefully examined during nasendoscopy for anomalous pulsations indicative of medially displaced internal carotid arteries. When apparent or suspected, a magnetic resonance arteriogram is obtained to assess the feasibility of safely performing a sphincter pharyngoplasty. Finally, sphincter pharyngoplasty is of little benefit in patients with known neuromuscular deficits causing an adynamic palate.

PATIENT POSITIONING AND ROOM SETUP

The patient is positioned supine with slight Trendelenburg table position. The head is placed on a horseshoe headrest to allow for manipulation and slight hyperextension. It is important to avoid extreme hyperextension as cervical spine anomalies are common in the cleft population. Specifically, a superiorly positioned odontoid process may compress the spinal cord against the foramen magnum. Such anomalies are occasionally evident on preoperative speech videofluoroscopy, and attention should be paid to this end. The bed is rotated 180 degrees to the anesthesia setup so that the surgeon may stand at the head of the bed. The surgeon's assistant may stand to either side of the patient. The patient's face and neck are prepped and draped using a povidone iodine-based solution. A head wrap is fashioned to allow for sterile manipulation of the head and neck. A surgical headlight is employed as well as a lighted suction irrigator.

ANESTHESIA

General anesthesia is required with midline endotracheal intubation using an oral right angle endotracheal (RAE) tube. During the preoperative discussion with the anesthesiologist, the surgeon should request an awake extubation as a precaution given the potential for iatrogenic obstruction of the nasopharynx. A tongue stitch may be placed prior to the conclusion of the case and used for retraction in the event that the patient obstructs.

PLANNING AND PATIENT MARKINGS

Loupe magnification (2.5–3.5×) and a headlight assist with visualization and atraumatic manipulation of the tissues. A Dingman mouth gag and throat pack are placed. Adequacy of ventilation is confirmed with the anesthesiologist once the Dingman is expanded and the nasopharynx is visualized. The posterior pharyngeal wall is inspected for aberrant pulsations. The posterior tonsillar pillars are examined to confirm adequacy of volume for construction of the sphincter pharyngoplasty. A red rubber catheter is passed transnasally and sutured to the uvula, and the velum is reflected into the nasopharynx to achieve exposure of the posterior pharyngeal wall (Figure 52.1).

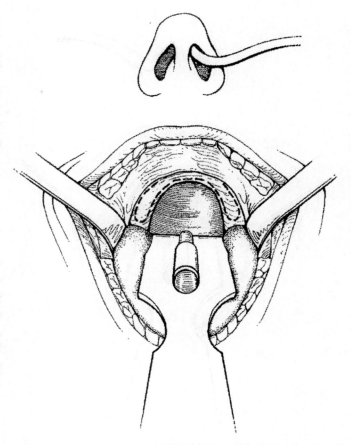

Figure 52.2. Proposed incisions (*dashed lines*).

Silk stay sutures are placed at the caudal aspect of each posterior tonsillar pillar.

The transverse incision line is drawn on the posterior pharyngeal wall corresponding to the atlas, which is easily palpated with the index finger. This typically corresponds to the height of attempted velopharyngeal closure, which is documented using the preoperative speech video fluoroscopy. Often, this line corresponds to the junction of the adenoid pad with the posterior pharyngeal wall. If so, a 2–3 mm cuff of nonlymphoid tissue should be left for suture placement.

Lines of incision are plotted with indelible ink on both the anterior and, with the aid of a retractor, the posterior aspects of the posterior tonsillar pillars, identifying the proposed myomucosal flaps (Figure 52.2). Local anesthetic is infiltrated for hemostatic purposes.

OPERATIVE TECHNIQUE

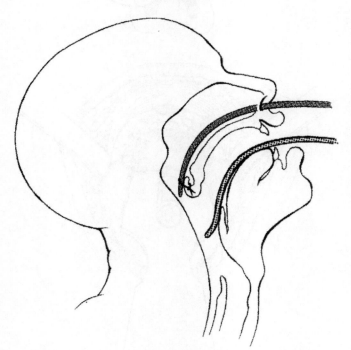

Figure 52.1. Lateral view of the positioning. The neck has been slightly hyperextended and the catheter has been passed transnasally and attached to uvula. A Dingman mouth gag is used for proper visualization of the nasopharynx.

Beginning on the left and then repeating the same maneuver on the right, the posterior tonsillar pillar is raised as a myomucosal flap, based superiorly (Figure 52.3). Dissection

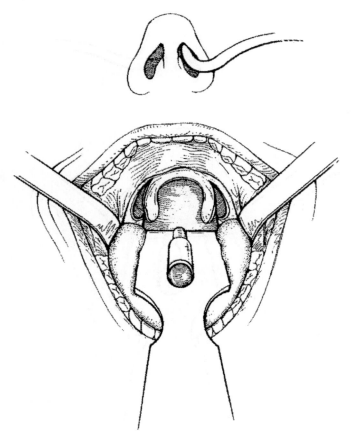

Figure 52.3. Elevation of both tonsillar pillar flaps.

proceeds deep until the prevertebral fascia is reached. The lateral palatopharyngeus myomucosal flaps are elevated to the height of attempted velopharyngeal closure as documented on the preoperative speech videofluoroscopy. Their length mirrors the transverse width of the site of inset.

The posterior pharyngeal wall is incised transversely at the proposed area of insertion. The incision is extended laterally to join the cephalad incision of the myomucosal flaps. The continuous cut extends from the superior end of the posterior limb of one lateral flap to the other and allows the lateral flaps to be transposed and fully inset. Care must be taken to ensure that only the mucosa is cut and the underlying pharyngeal musculature is left intact. Inadvertent division of the underlying superior pharyngeal constrictor can cause inferior migration of the sphincter pharyngoplasty, which compromises the long-term result.

The superiorly based lateral palatopharyngeus myomucosal flaps are transposed 90 degrees and inset into the posterior pharyngeal wall mucosa. Beginning on the left, the superior mucosal margin is sutured to the superior margin of the posterior pharyngeal wall mucosa. The inferior mucosal margin of the left flap is sutured to the superior mucosa of the right flap, overlapping the two flaps. The inferior mucosal margin

of the right flap is sutured to the inferior mucosa of the posterior pharyngeal wall incision. The red rubber catheter is removed and the sutures secured from superior to inferior. The tissues are approximated without tension, and the donor sites are closed (Figure 52.4). All suturing is undertaken with 3-0 Vicryl (Ethicon, Somerville, NJ). Following construction of the sphincter pharyngoplasty, an orogastric tube is placed to evacuate any gastric contents.

At the conclusion of the case, the central orifice of the sphincter pharyngoplasty port should be about 1 cm in diameter. A "tight" sphincter pharyngoplasty port usually measures about 0.5 cm in diameter, and a "loose" sphincter pharyngoplasty port usually measures about 1.5 cm in diameter.

Over the years, the literature has been replete with adaptations and refinements to the original technique described by Hynes. More recently, augmentation of the muscle sphincter with the longus capitis muscle, cerclage of the entire sphincter pharyngoplasty using polypropylene suture, and placement of the pharyngoplasty higher in the pharynx have been proposed. These highlight an advantage of the pharyngoplasty in that it provides the surgeon with flexibility to tailor the procedure to the degree of augmentation required.

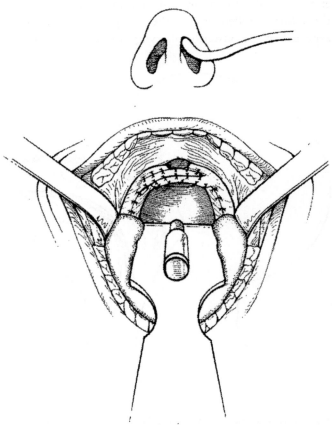

Figure 52.4. Completed pharyngoplasty. Note that flaps are overlapped, sutured to each other and posterior pharyngeal wall.

CLEFT DEFORMITIES

POSTOPERATIVE CARE

Following sphincter pharyngoplasty, the patient is monitored overnight in a setting with continuous pulse oximetry and a nursing ratio sufficient to detect any impending airway compromise. Patients are offered a clear liquid diet immediately following surgery, advanced to full liquids on the first postoperative day, and ultimately transitioned to a soft diet, which is continued for 1 month. Parents are counseled to avoid bottles or straws. An age-appropriate diet is resumed once examination demonstrates satisfactory healing. Speech evaluation and therapy is resumed 6 weeks postoperatively. If symptomatic VPI persists or if nasal airway obstructive symptoms become evident, repeat diagnostic nasendoscopy and/or fluoroscopic evaluation are performed. If indicated, the sphincter pharyngoplasty can be revised.

Success is determined by acceptable perceptual oral resonance, adequate velopharyngeal closure on endoscopy and fluoroscopy, and the absence of upper airway obstruction or sleep apnea. Symptoms of velopharyngeal dysfunction may be diminished by surgery, but residual articulation errors and learned habits can persist and must be addressed through behavioral speech therapy.

CAVEATS

PERSISTENT VELOPHARYNGEAL DYSFUNCTION

Persistent VPI symptoms result from dehiscence of the inset myomucosal flaps or from inadequate closure of a wide velopharyngeal gap. Of note, patients with DiGeorge syndrome have a higher likelihood of revision. Options for revision include sphincter augmentation with fat, cartilage, injectables, or the addition of posterior pharyngeal wall muscle. Low inset of the sphincter pharyngoplasty causes persistent VPI in up to 50% of patients. In general, if the entire sphincter is visualized on intraoral exam, then inferior positioning of the flaps might be an issue.[11,12]

AIRWAY DYSFUNCTION: ACUTE OBSTRUCTIVE SLEEP APNEA

Similar to the posterior pharyngeal flap, acute iatrogenic obstructive sleep apnea represents a significant morbidity associated with sphincter pharyngoplasty. Risk factors for the development of postoperative obstructive sleep apnea include (1) microretrognathia, (2) a history of perinatal respiratory dysfunction, (3) young age at sphincter pharyngoplasty surgery, and possibly (4) upper respiratory tract infections.

Occasionally, obstructive sleep apnea may be severe enough to precipitate hospitalization and treatment with continuous positive airway pressure (CPAP) and steroids. There is often an adaptation period during which the patient becomes accustomed to the diminished patency of the velopharyngeal sphincter. The sphincter area at rest increases with resolution of perioperative edema and progression of postoperative wound contraction. If symptoms persist, polysomnography should be obtained.

Another common theme among patients affected by obstructive sleep apnea is young age at treatment. It is hypothesized that the low pulmonary functional residual capacity in small children may place them at greater risk for hypoxia from shorter durations of apnea than adults.[13]

MICRORETROGNATHIA

The predisposition of patients with microretrognathia (with or without Pierre Robin sequence) toward obstructive sleep apnea after velopharyngeal narrowing procedures, including sphincter pharyngoplasty, indicates that in these patients the upper airway remains compromised well after birth. Thus, infants displaying significant improvement or resolution of symptoms shortly after birth might still have a compromised yet well-compensated airway. Caution in these patients is advised, as overt obstructive sleep apnea may not manifest itself until the time of velopharyngeal surgery. Such children maintain a patent airway when awake but develop obstructive sleep apnea with the relaxation of pharyngeal muscular tone during sleep.

Recognition of the presence of congenital anomalies may provide important predictive information regarding the potential for airway complications after velopharyngeal surgery.

DEHISCENCE

There are several anatomic and technical reasons for dehiscence. First, there is a learning curve whereby results improve with surgeon experience. Second, dehiscence may relate to tonsillectomy or adenoidectomy. A large adenoid pad can preclude high enough positioning of the palatopharyngeus flaps. For this reason, tonsillectomy or adenoidectomy is performed liberally in preparation for definitive velopharyngeal management. This eliminates the possibility of lymphoid port obstruction and the technical difficulties associated with placement of sutures in friable adenoid tissue. Previous tonsillectomy, however, may result in atrophy and scarring of the palatopharyngeus muscle, which threatens the integrity of the pharyngoplasty. Third, patients with Pierre Robin sequence often lack sufficient posterior tonsillar pillar tissue with which to construct the sphincter with tension-free inset. Excessive tension can jeopardize the integrity of the pharyngoplasty.

Fourth, adequate release of the lateral border of the myomucosal flap must be achieved, as tethering in this location will preclude tension-free closure.

REFERENCES

1. Naran S, Ford M, Losee JE. What's new in cleft palate and velopharyngeal dysfunction management? *Plast Reconstr Surg* 2017;139(6):1343e–1355e.
2. Boss EF, Sie KCY. Sphincter pharyngoplasty. In Goudy SL, Tollefson TT, eds. *Complete Cleft Care: Cleft and Velopharyngeal Insufficiency Treatment in Children.* New York: Thieme, 2015:177–186.
3. Marsh JL. Sphincter pharyngoplasty. In Losee JE, Kirschner RE, eds. *Comprehensive Cleft Care.* New York: McGraw-Hill Medical, 2009:665–671.
4. Cheng N, Zhao M, Qi K, Deng H, Fang Z, Song R. A modified procedure for velopharyngeal sphincteroplasty in primary cleft palate repair and secondary velopharyngeal incompetence treatment and its preliminary results. *J Plast Reconstr Aesthet Surg* 2006;59:817–825.
5. Abdel-Aziz M. Palatopharyngeal sling: a new technique in treatment of velopharyngeal insufficiency. *Int J Pediatr Otorhinolaryngol* 2008;72:173–177.
6. D'Antonio LL. Evaluation and management of velopharyngeal dysfunction: a speech pathologist's viewpoint. In: Lehman JA, ed. *Cleft Palate Surgery.* Hagerstown, MD: JB Lippincott, 1992:86–111.
7. D'Antonio LL, Muntz HR, Marsh JL, et al. Practical application of flexible fiberoptic nasopharyngoscopy for evaluating velopharyngeal function. *Plast Reconstr Surg* 1988;82:611–618.
8. de Stadler M, Hersh C. Nasometry, videofluoroscopy, and the speech pathologist's evaluation and treatment. *Adv Otorhinolaryngol* 2015;76:7–17.
9. Gilleard O, Sommerlad B, Sell D, Ghanem A, Birch M. Nasendoscopy: an analysis of measurement uncertainties. *Cleft Palate Craniofac J* 2013;50:351–357.
10. Pensler JM, Reich DS. A comparison of speech results after the pharyngeal flap and the dynamic sphincteroplasty procedures. *Ann Plast Surg* 1991;26:441–443.
11. Riski JE, Ruff GL, Georgiade GS, Barwick WJ. Evaluation of failed sphincter pharyngoplasties. *Ann Plast Surg* 1992;28:545.
12. Witt PD, Marsh JL, Grames LM, Muntz HR. Revision of the failed sphincter pharyngoplasty: an outcome assessment. *Plast Reconstr Surg* 1995;96:126–138.
13. Witt PD, Marsh JL, Muntz HR, et al. Nasal airway obstruction as a complication of sphincter pharyngoplasty. *Cleft Palate Craniofac J* 1996;33:183–189.

53.

CLEFT NASAL DEFORMITY

Jennifer L. McGrath and Arun K. Gosain

ASSESSMENT OF THE DEFECT: INDICATIONS

As in nasal reconstruction of any etiology, the laminar structure of the cleft nose must be appreciated. While much attention is paid to the structural aspects of the bony and cartilaginous support of the nose, the skin and soft tissue outer layer as well as the inner lining are vital to all surgical approaches to the cleft nasal deformity.

Focusing on unilateral complete cleft lip and palate, the hallmark of the unilateral deformity is asymmetry. The characteristic features of the tip, alar lower lateral cartilages (LLC), alar base, septum, and columella are listed in Table 53.1 for both unilateral and bilateral cleft lip (BCL). Appreciating the anatomic disturbances of unilateral and BCL facilitates an understanding of the resultant deformity. For example, the discontinuity of the orbicularis oris contributes to caudal septal deviation as well as alar flattening and lateral displacement of the alar base. The bilateral cleft nasal deformity is different from that of the unilateral presentation. Whereas asymmetry is a primary hurdle in the unilateral deformity, a symmetric, widened, and flattened nasal tip defines the BCL nose.

In older and more cooperative patients, a functional/airway assessment is important to identify potential points of nasal airway obstruction, particularly for secondary rhinoplasty. A thorough history from family members may indicate disordered breathing in young patients.

There are several opportunities to address the cleft nasal deformity along the timeline of cleft care. This includes:

• Presurgical nasoalveolar molding

• Primary rhinoplasty synchronous with cleft lip repair

TABLE 53.1 CHARACTERISTIC FEATURES OF THE UNILATERAL AND BILATERAL CLEFT NASAL DEFORMITY

	Unilateral deformity	Bilateral deformity
Tip	Asymmetric More projected on non-cleft side Poorly defined	Symmetric Flattened and wide Poorly defined
Alar cartilages	Cleft LLC wider than non-cleft LLC Cleft LLC flattened	Flattened, buckled Splaying of medial crura Subluxated from upper lateral cartilages Flared laterally
Alar base	Cleft alar base inferiorly, laterally, and posteriorly displaced Widened cleft nostril compared to non-cleft nostril	Bilateral alar base laterally and posteriorly displaced Wide, horizontally oriented nostrils bilaterally
Septum	Caudal septum deviated towards non-cleft side Mid and dorsal septum bow toward cleft side May be dislocated from vomerine groove	Straight, midline Inferiorly displaced compared to alar base
Columella	Base deviated toward non-cleft side Shorter on cleft side than non-cleft side	Shortened, attached to prolabium Midline, symmetric

LLC, lower lateral cartilages.

- School-aged or intermediate rhinoplasty
- Alveolar reconstruction/bone grafting
- Secondary or definitive cleft rhinoplasty in late adolescence or adulthood

While nasoalveolar molding (NAM) is not universally practiced or accessible, the literature suggests the use of NAM prior to primary cleft lip repair improves short- and long-term appearance of the cleft nasal deformity.[1,2] While differences in outcomes have been reported when comparing its use in unilateral and BCL nasal deformities, there is evidence for its benefit in both populations. Benefits to the nose include elongation of the columella, improvement in nasal symmetry, and narrowing of the alar base. The disadvantages of NAM include its increased cost and the burden placed on families regarding compliance and frequent office visits.

Insufficient bony support from the cleft piriform aperture contributes to alar base asymmetry in an anterior-posterior dimension. Alveolar bone grafting may affect the cleft nasal deformity by closing nasolabial fistulae and elevating the deficient bony support of the nasal sill in an anterior direction. Changes in the cleft side nostril after alveolar reconstruction have also been characterized, including increased width and decreased height.[3] However, patients should be aware that augmentation of the alar base following alveolar bone graft may recede over time due to resorption of the bone graft. Resorption is more likely in the nonstressed component of the bone graft, which is that part used to augment the inferior maxilla and alar base.

CONTRAINDICATIONS

Absolute contraindications to cleft rhinoplasty are uncommon and limited to active or recent infection and unstable soft tissue envelope or lining. Oronasal fistulae should be closed prior to rhinoplasty to reduce the risk of contamination. It is also generally practiced that definitive rhinoplasty be delayed until after orthognathic treatment in cleft patients with maxillary hypoplasia. Relative contraindications such as those related to growth will depend on the nature of the procedure and the severity of the deformity. Septal maneuvers and nasal osteotomies are usually delayed in the growing child; however, it is likely that these concerns are not evidence-based.[4] Definitive

rhinoplasty is often delayed until late adolescence when facial growth is complete. In this age group, the ability of the patient to participate in decision-making and informed consent is important as well.

ROOM SETUP

The patient is positioned supine with the head at the superior extent of the operating table. An oral right angle endotracheal (RAE) tube is ideal for endotracheal intubation as it is out of the operative field and can be positioned in the midline so as not to cause distortion. A shoulder roll is placed to lift the shoulders and give gentle neck extension to level the operative field, and a gel or foam donut is placed under the occiput for stability. Sterile preparation can be achieved with ophthalmic Betadine and should include the entire face, neck, and shoulders. Cartilage graft donor sites should be considered, even if not expected, and prepped into the field accordingly. A standard head drape allows visualization of the entire face. Local anesthesia with epinephrine is used for infiltration and hemostasis. Cocaine, epinephrine, or oxymetazoline-soaked cottonoids can be placed in the nasal cavity for vasoconstriction as well. Display of preoperative photographs may be helpful for reference, especially for secondary rhinoplasty.

PATIENT MARKINGS

PRIMARY UNILATERAL CLEFT RHINOPLASTY

The choice of incisions may depend on the requirements of an individual patient. Release of the fibrofatty tissue and repositioning of the LLCs can often be approached in a closed manner from medially and laterally without additional incisions. Alternatively, a semi-open approach can be used for direct visualization via a rim incision or a reverse-U incision. If utilizing a reverse-U incision as initially described by Tajima,[5] the non-cleft nostril serves as a guide for the external portion of the rim incision. While supporting the cleft side alar base in a more anatomic and symmetric position, the incision is marked by mimicking the shape and height of the non-cleft nostril. The apex of this incision crosses onto the external alar rim skin, with the medial and lateral aspects crossing back into the nostril along the membranous septum and inner aspect of the ala, respectively.

PRIMARY BILATERAL CLEFT RHINOPLASTY

While external incisions were used historically, most modern primary approaches to the bilateral cleft nose do not use visible incisions. Mulliken describes a semi-open approach using bilateral rim incisions.[6] Incisions are marked by first elevating the alar dome cartilages into a reasonable anatomic position. The rim incisions are marked in a hidden location along the inside of the rim or extended slightly onto the external rim in a reverse-U pattern. These may be extended onto the inner aspect of the columella as well. Mulliken's mantra of "the columella is in the nose" emphasizes that the columella is only deceptively short in the BCL nasal deformity owing to the abnormal position of the alar cartilages. Therefore, recruiting skin from nonanatomic locations to reconstruct and lengthen the columella is not necessary. Cutting prefers a retrograde approach to the tip when nasoalveolar molding has been adequate. A prolabium-columella-medial crura composite flap is elevated from inferior to superior. No additional external incisions are used. If NAM has not been adequate, the Cutting and Mulliken approaches have been combined, adding bilateral marginal rim or reverse-U incision extensions to the composite flap.[7]

SECONDARY CLEFT RHINOPLASTY

An open rhinoplasty approach is most often used with a transcolumellar incision, incision along membranous septum, and bilateral rims to deglove the nose. The columellar incision is designed in the mid-columella with a stair-step or gull wing to reduce scar contracture and conceal the scar. Rim incisions are designed along the inner aspect of the nostril. If nostril overhang is to be corrected, a reverse-U incision can be made that extends onto the rim skin as described above, usually by 2–3 mm.

Costal cartilage grafts are most often designed from the fifth or sixth rib. After palpation of the sternomanubrial joint to locate the second rib, ribs are counted inferiorly until the preferred donor site is identified. In female patients, the inframammary crease can be used to camouflage the donor site incision, with care taken not to extend the incision too far medially as to become visible in clothing or a swimsuit. The length of the incision varies by surgeon, typically between 3 and 5 cm.

OPERATIVE TECHNIQUES

PRIMARY CLEFT RHINOPLASTY

The decision to address the cleft nasal deformity at the time of cleft lip repair varies by surgeon. Historically, concerns regarding interference with nasal growth and iatrogenic trauma caused by primary cleft rhinoplasty at the time of lip repair led most surgeons to delay specific treatment of the cleft nasal deformity. As techniques have evolved over the past several decades, the literature suggests that primary rhinoplasty does not interfere with nasal growth.[4] Many surgeons argue that preservation of an unscarred nose for definitive rhinoplasty would lead to improved outcomes. However, long-term follow-up reveals that primary cleft rhinoplasty improves the overall nasal form and simplifies the approach for secondary rhinoplasty.[1,8]

Unilateral Primary Cleft Rhinoplasty

Most commonly, primary cleft rhinoplasty at the time of cleft lip repair includes reconstruction of the nasal floor, narrowing of the alar base, dissection of the fibrofatty soft tissue from the lower lateral cartilages, and repositioning of the lower lateral cartilages. The primary unilateral cleft rhinoplasty is synchronous with the lip repair.

In the McComb technique, no additional incisions are used. With the lip repair open and tissue planes dissected in the greater and lesser segments, nasal dissection can be performed from medial and lateral approaches. Using a blunt-tipped dissecting scissor or hemostat, the lower lateral cartilages are dissected from the overlying skin to allow independent movement.[9] McComb described bringing this dissection superiorly to the nasion, but most surgeons limit this dissection to the lower third.[10] The nasal floor is repaired in layers as lip approximation begins. Including a muscular closure in the base of the nasal floor repair obliterates dead space and reconstructs the anatomic continuity of the superior orbicularis oris. The nasal sill skin is approximated, narrowing the cleft-side alar base. An alar base stitch precisely positions the lesser segment alar base width. Following lip closure, attention is turned to repositioning the tip and cleft-side ala. Suspension sutures are then placed to define the new intercrural angle. Using a probing forceps to identify the desired location of elevation, a mattress suture is passed from this position on the inner aspect of the dome to the contralateral dome. Straight needles may be used for precision. The needles are drawn through the skin of the dome and passed back through the same hole while adjusting the subdermal course slightly to secure the mattress stitch. Bolsters or pledgets may also be used. A second mattress suture placed in a similar manner can be used laterally at the alar groove to appose the lateral wall of the vestibule. In rotation-advancement cleft lip repair techniques, the C-flap is rotated posteriorly, lengthening the cleft side columella. The nasal floor is reconstructed with mucosal flaps from the medial and lateral segments and/or the inferior turbinate.

Tajima described a reverse-U nasal rim incision to access the LLCs and address nostril asymmetry.[5] Dissection is carried out over the LLCs and lower third of the nose. The cleft-side LLC is then suspended to the non-cleft side upper lateral cartilage as the primary elevating vector. Additional suspension sutures are placed across the cleft and non-cleft side medial crura as well as from the cleft side lateral crust to the ipsilateral upper lateral cartilage. The distal aspect of the reverse-U flap is then advanced to the inner aspect of the nostril rim to reconstruct and define the soft triangle.

In the senior author's technique the C-flap is extended toward the nasal dome by incising the membranous septum and raising a chondrocutaneous flap consisting of the columellar skin and medial crus on the affected side (Figure 53.1A). Laterally, the L-flap is extended using an intranasal incision at the level of the pyriform aperture (Figure 53.1B). This allows direct access to the excess fibrofatty tissue that is consistently found in the cleft alar vestibule, which, if left undissected, can lead to vestibular thickening and decreased nasal airflow in the cleft nostril. Fibrofatty tissue that remains on the dome cartilage may prevent adequate approximation and suspension of the medial crura and predispose to relapse. From the nostril base, the lateral crus is dissected on its superficial surface, releasing it from the overlying fibrofatty tissue as well as any attachment to the lateral pyriform that may prevent medialization of the lateral crus. The lateral and medial dissections join at the alar dome to completely free the cleft alar cartilage from the overlying tissues. The majority of patients with complete cleft lip present with significant deviation of the caudal septum to the non-cleft side, and the senior author prefers to medialize the caudal septum at the time of primary lip and nose repair. Utilizing the cephalic extension of the C-flap in the membranous septum in continuity with the mucoperichondrial flap elevated to close the nostril floor, the caudal septum is exposed (Figure 53.1C). The caudal septum is detached from the anterior nasal spine to its point of maximum inflection and reflected medially to a more central position

(Figure 53.1D). The septum does not need to be fixed in its new position as there is no bony attachment in the midline to which it can be fixed. The repositioned soft tissues, along with the nasal stent placed following cleft repair, will stabilize the caudal septum in the midline (Figure 53.2). A trans-septal Prolene suture is placed to secure the stent during the first week, after which the suture is cut and the family is taught to clean the stent and replace it using alar Steri-Strips. We recommend use of the stent for the first 3 months following primary cleft rhinoplasty.

Bilateral Primary Cleft Rhinoplasty

Many approaches to the primary repair of the BCL nasal deformity have been presented over the years. Original descriptions, including that by McComb in 1975, were often multistaged, staging columellar lengthening and definitive primary nasal repair. Today, synchronous repair has become common place. Mulliken and Cutting have popularized two approaches to the primary repair of the BCL nasal deformity. Mulliken advocates a single-stage approach via bilateral rim incisions to access the dome cartilages.[6] Complete dissection of the cartilages free from the fibrofatty tissue and lateral piriform allows alar movement and repositioning. Interdomal sutures are placed to oppose the medial crura, defining the genu of the dome and narrowing the nasal tip. Sutures are then used to suspend the subluxated lower lateral cartilages to each ipsilateral upper lateral cartilage. The alar bases are narrowed using bilateral cinch sutures. Any redundant soft tissue at the alar base or vestibule can be addressed with direct excision and closure.

Access to presurgical orthopedics benefits the columella.[11] Rather than reconstructing or lengthening the columella via flaps, the Cutting approach advocates presurgical nasoalveolar molding to gradually stretch or lengthen the columella as well as the nasal lining. At the time of lip repair, an open approach is used to elevate the medial crura, columella, and prolabium as a single flap. Interdomal sutures similar to those described earlier define the tip and appose the medial crura. The lower lateral cartilages can be suspended to the upper lateral cartilages using suspension sutures over pledgets or mattress sutures. The columellar–labial angle is defined with a suture. As described earlier, the Cutting and Mulliken techniques may be combined by extending incisions bilaterally along the rims. This allows enhanced access to the alar cartilages for suture suspension as described above. Reverse-U incisions also lengthen the columella.

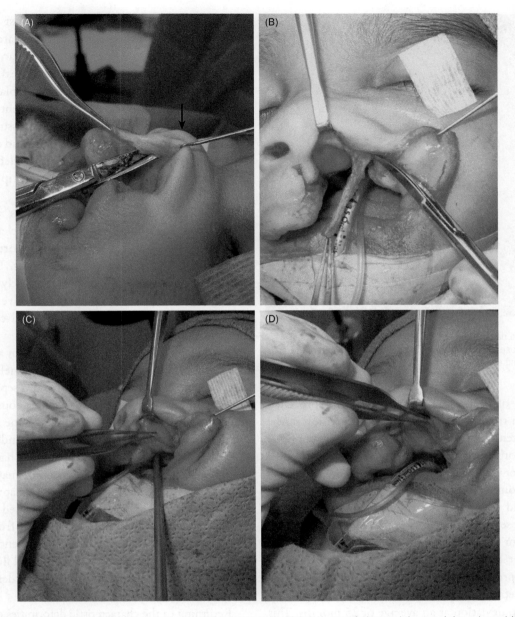

Figure 53.1. Primary cleft rhinoplasty. (A) Medial approach to nasal dissection. The C-flap is extended toward the nasal dome (*arrow*) by incising the membranous septum and raising a chondrocutaneous flap. (B) Lateral approach to nasal dissection. The L-flap is extended using an intranasal incision at the level of the pyriform aperture, allowing direct access to the excess fibrofatty tissue in the alar vestibule. Dissection of the lateral crus on is superficial surface will join the medial dissection for complete release of the cleft alar cartilage. (C) Mucoperichondrial flap is elevated to expose the caudal septum. (D) The caudal septum is centralized from its initial deviation to the noncleft side, allowing it to rest in a midline position.

INTERMEDIATE (SCHOOL-AGED) RHINOPLASTY

Intermediate rhinoplasty, performed on school-aged children, is an eclectic set of techniques used to improve the appearance of the cleft lip nasal deformity in the growing child. It is often employed in the early school-aged group to minimize obvious differences to peers as children become more aware, usually around first grade. While there is no set technique, intermediate rhinoplasty can include tip work with alar cartilage repositioning, caudal septoplasty, correction of nostril asymmetry with reverse-U incisions, alar base repositioning, and scar revisions. It is often limited to the soft tissues due to concerns over nasal growth disturbance with septal manipulation, but this concern may be unfounded.[12] Grafts are avoided if at all possible to save material for structural support in adolescence.

The senior author reported a series of intermediate rhinoplasty performed with absorbable plates for columellar

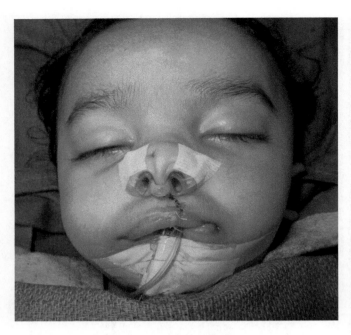

Figure 53.2. Silicone nasal stents are placed at the conclusion of the primary lip and nose repair, helping to retain the centralization of the caudal septum and elevation of the alar dome.

strut support of the nasal tip.[13] The nose is approached using an open rhinoplasty with a stair-step incision in the columella, extending to an alar rim incision (Figure 53.3, *top left*). A resorbable plate is cut to use as a columellar strut (*top right*). Hot water contouring of the plate in situ allows precise positioning of the strut and nasal tip, improving projection and tip support without the donor site cost of harvesting septal cartilage in a growing child (*bottom left*). Final trim of the redundant skin of the alar rim and a nasal bolster to support the repositioned alar cartilage complete the procedure (bottom right). Long-term results have shown retained improvements in nostril height, tip height, and tip deviation at an average of 25 months. This technique spares harvest of septal cartilage in the growing child, minimizing impact on nasal growth and leaving the septal cartilage should it be needed during the definitive secondary cleft rhinoplasty.

DEFINITIVE SECONDARY CLEFT RHINOPLASTY

Definitive secondary cleft rhinoplasty techniques can differ considerably as the residual deformity is quite variable from case to case. Definitive secondary cleft rhinoplasty is considered toward completion of facial skeletal growth at age 16 years or later. Unlike school-aged/intermediate rhinoplasty, nasal osteotomies and septal cartilage resection can be performed without concern for impairment of nasal growth. A cookie cutter approach

cannot be used; instead each patient must be addressed as a unique case. Photographs with standard rhinoplasty views are essential to creating a surgical plan that must be delineated preoperatively to achieve success. Thinking of the nose in layers, secondary cleft rhinoplasty routinely deals with all three layers. While most attention is paid to the structural support, an adequate soft tissue envelope as well as vestibular lining is essential to a good outcome. For example, columellar length in a bilateral cleft rhinoplasty may limit the ability to project the nasal tip to a satisfactory position.

Secondary cleft rhinoplasty maneuvers are similar to those of aesthetic rhinoplasty. The focus of cleft rhinoplasty is constructing a stable cartilaginous support to the nose, often requiring the use of cartilage grafts. However, the complexity is far greater than that routinely encountered in aesthetic rhinoplasty. Most cleft noses have been entered previously, increasing the scar burden and complexity of dissection.

Secondary rhinoplasty requires an open approach due to the scope of maneuvers. A midcolumellar approach allows direct visualization of the alar and septal cartilages. Incisions are extended along the membranous septum and along the rims bilaterally. The skin envelope is elevated as the dissection is carried out over the tip and dorsum in a subperichondrial plane. If the patient has had primary or intermediate rhinoplasty, this dissection may be difficult and tedious. Once the upper and lower lateral cartilages have been exposed, the septum is approached from the anterior septal angle. The septum is released from the upper lateral cartilages, and the interdomal ligament between the medial crura is incised. Mucoperichondrial flaps are raised along the septum bilaterally and the septal deformity is directly visualized.

Returning to the characteristic deformities of Table 53.1, the potential components of secondary cleft rhinoplasty are numerous. Tip refinement is a priority of this procedure. Standard maneuvers include columellar strut grafts, suture manipulation of the dome and tip-defining points, and tip grafts. Septal cartilage may be useful for creating a straight columellar strut; however, septal cartilage may not be adequate for all graft applications, and therefore rib cartilage may be necessary. A columellar strut increases symmetry and provides tip support and projection. Interdomal and transdomal sutures may be used to restore tip symmetry and definition. Tip grafts can also be used to increase projection and definition.

The lower lateral cartilages may be shaped by cephalic trim. Suture techniques can be used to refine the lower lateral cartilages. However, they often lack structural integrity

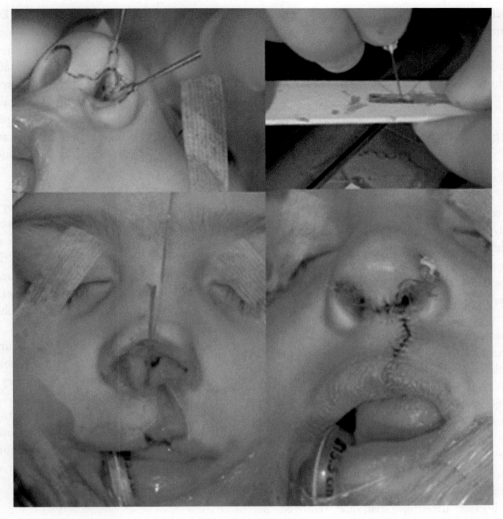

Figure 53.3. Intermediate cleft rhinoplasty. An intermediate cleft rhinoplasty and revision cheiloplasty performed on a 7-year-old girl. The nose is approached using an open rhinoplasty with a stair-step incision in the columella, extending to an alar rim incision (*top left*). A resorbable plate is cut to use as a columellar strut (*top right*), improving projection and tip support without the donor site cost of harvesting septal cartilage in a growing child (*bottom left*). Final trim of the redundant skin of the alar rim and nasal bolster to support the repositioned alar cartilage complete the procedure (*bottom right*).

and are prone to collapse. Lateral crural strut grafts can provide additional support or length to the alar cartilages, and alar batten grafts can prevent airway collapse and alar retraction. The tripod concept for tip projection and rotation should be considered when altering the lateral crura. The lower lateral cartilages may be advanced medially by V-Y advancement from the lateral vestibule. If the alar deformity is severe, such as notching or severe retraction, composite chondrocutaneous grafts from the ear may be needed.

A wide alar base can be addressed by direct excision. Alar base cinch sutures can also be used to narrow the alar base width. In unilateral cases, this may be suspended to the anterior nasal spine. An asymmetric alar base can also be addressed by local rotation or advancement techniques.

The septal deformity is the other primary component in cleft rhinoplasty. Creating a midline and symmetric dorsum as well as a functional nasal airway is the goal. Septal deviation is treated with submucous resection, taking care to leave an adequate L strut. Dorsal reduction, if needed, may be best performed prior to submucous resection so as not to inadvertently narrow the dorsal strut. A 12–15 mm L-strut is typical. Manipulation of the L-strut with cartilage scoring techniques centralizes the septum. Septal cartilage can be used for spreader or other necessary grafts. Spreader grafts have several purposes. They help support the new position of the septum, improve the patency of the internal nasal valve, and correct asymmetry in the dorsal aesthetic lines.[9] Nasal osteotomies may be used to address a broad dorsum or residual asymmetry of the bony vault.

The columella itself is difficult to improve in secondary rhinoplasty. Interdomal sutures that increase projection and medial crus length will increase columellar length minimally. Reverse-U incisions may also give the appearance of increasing columellar length and symmetry.

POSTOPERATIVE CONSIDERATIONS

The senior author places silicone nasal stents at the completion of primary cleft rhinoplasty (Figure 53.2). Nasal stents help prevent cicatricial contracture and nasal stenosis during the postoperative period. At the first postop visit, the stent is removed and cleaned and families are educated on nasal stent care, including removal of the stents, cleaning of the nares and stent, reinsertion of the stents, and securing the stents with skin adhesive and wound closure strips. Parents continue nasal stenting ideally for 3–6 months postoperatively if tolerated. Most patients tolerate nasal stenting well.

External and internal nasal splints may be used in secondary rhinoplasty as in aesthetic rhinoplasty. The goal of postoperative splinting is to provide stability to the reconstructed construct during early healing as well as to maximize graft take. Internal nasal splints are used for the first 7–10 days to support the septoplasty. External nasal splints stabilize and protect the bony vault and dorsum following osteotomies. These are typically discontinued after 7–10 days as well. The use of composite grafts necessitates postoperative bolster dressings that are removed at 7–10 days.

Postoperative home care includes head of bed elevation and ice packs to reduce postoperative edema, pain control with or without narcotics depending on the scope of the surgery, and local wound care with gentle cleansing and antibiotic ointment to the intranasal incisions twice daily. After splint removal, adjuncts such as oxymetazoline and pseudoephedrine may alleviate postoperative congestion.

About 2–4 weeks after primary cleft rhinoplasty, the senior author recommends initiating scar massage to the inner aspect of the alar rim using a cotton-tip applicator. An anterior vector is used with gentle force to help soften scar while maintaining projection of the dome. Scar massage is not used in rhinoplasty requiring structural grafts.

CAVEATS

NAM has been shown to positively impact the short- and long-term appearance of the cleft lip nasal deformity.

However, access to NAM is not universal. Even for patients with access to a NAM practitioner, the cost as well as the time required for office visits is often a barrier to treatment. Appliances must be modified regularly and refabricated as the infant grows. Successful NAM outcomes require a high degree of compliance. While NAM is typically well-tolerated by infants and families, daily taping can be burdensome to parents. Infants may not tolerate the device or may develop skin or mucosal irritation due to the device and taping.

Some advocate that the more severe the deformity, the more aggressive the surgeon must be when the patient is younger. While it is reasonable to concern oneself with inhibiting facial and nasal growth or introducing scar, it must also be appreciated that the same facial and nasal growth will contribute to worsening the deformity. Features such as septal deviation and tip asymmetry will become accentuated as the child grows into adolescence.

Recognize that certain iatrogenic features are very difficult to treat, such as nasal stenosis or a loss of soft tissue. Minimize risk to the prolabium in primary repair and the columella in secondary repair.

Long-term outcomes are difficult to study objectively. Individual surgeons must continuously assess their outcomes. All major advances in technique have resulted from surgeons continuing to hone their approach after looking critically at their own results.

REFERENCES

1. Garfinkle JS, King TW, Grayson BH, Brecht LE, Cutting CB. A 12-year anthropometric evaluation of the nose in bilateral cleft lip-cleft palate patients following nasoalveolar molding and cutting bilateral cleft lip and nose reconstruction. Plast Reconstr Surg 2011;127(4):1659–1667. Epub 2011/04/05. doi: 10.1097/PRS.0b013e31820a64d7. PubMed PMID: 21460673.
2. Nazarian Mobin SS, Karatsonyi A, Vidar EN, Gamer S, Groper J, Hammoudeh JA, Urata MM. Is presurgical nasoalveolar molding therapy more effective in unilateral or bilateral cleft lip-cleft palate patients? Plast Reconstr Surg 2011;127(3):1263–1269. Epub 2010/11/23. doi: 10.1097/PRS.0b013e318205f3ac. PubMed PMID: 21088643.
3. Wu Y, Wang G, Yang Y, Zhang Y. Influence of alveolar-bone grafting on the nasal profile: unilateral cleft lips, alveoli, and palates. J Craniofacial Surg 2010;21(6):1904–1907. Epub 2010/12/02. doi: 10.1097/SCS.0b013e3181f4b18b. PubMed PMID: 21119452.
4. Henry C, Samson T, Mackay D. Evidence-based medicine: the cleft lip nasal deformity. Plast Reconstr Surg 2014;133(5):1276–1288. Epub 2014/04/30. doi: 10.1097/prs.0000000000000096. PubMed PMID: 24776558.
5. Tajima S, Maruyama M. Reverse-U incision for secondary repair of cleft lip nose. Plast Reconstr Surg 1977;60(2):256–261. Epub 1977/08/01. PubMed PMID: 887664.

6. Mulliken JB. Primary repair of bilateral cleft lip and nasal deformity. Plast Reconstr Surg 2001;108(1):181–194; examination,95–96. Epub 2001/06/23. PubMed PMID: 11420522.

7. Morovic CG, Cutting C. Combining the Cutting and Mulliken methods for primary repair of the bilateral cleft lip nose. Plast Reconstr Surg 2005;116(6):1613–1619; discussion 20–22. Epub 2005/11/04. PubMed PMID: 16267421.

8. Haddock NT, McRae MH, Cutting CB. Long-term effect of primary cleft rhinoplasty on secondary cleft rhinoplasty in patients with unilateral cleft lip-cleft palate. Plast Reconstr Surg 2012;129(3): 740–748. Epub 2012/03/01. doi: 10.1097/PRS.0b013e3182402e8e. PubMed PMID: 22373979.

9. Fisher MD, Fisher DM, Marcus JR. Correction of the cleft nasal deformity: from infancy to maturity. Clin Plast Surg 2014;41(2): 283–299. Epub 2014/03/13. doi: 10.1016/j.cps.2014.01.002. PubMed PMID: 24607195.

10. McComb H. Treatment of the unilateral cleft lip nose. Plast Reconstr Surg 1975;55(5):596–601. Epub 1975/05/01. PubMed PMID: 1144536.

11. Grayson BH, Cutting CB. Presurgical nasoalveolar orthopedic molding in primary correction of the nose, lip, and alveolus of infants born with unilateral and bilateral clefts. Cleft Palate-Craniofacial J. 2001;38(3):193–198. Epub 2001/06/02. doi: 10.1597/1545-1569(2001)038<0193:pnomip>2.0.co;2. PubMed PMID: 11386426.

12. Ortiz-Monasterio F, Olmedo A. Corrective rhinoplasty before puberty: a long-term follow-up. Plast Reconstr Surg 1981;68(3): 381–391. Epub 1981/09/01. PubMed PMID: 7267813.

13. McDaniel JM, Alleyne B, Gosain AK. Secondary cleft nasoplasty at primary school age: quantitative evaluation of the efficacy of resorbable plates. Plast Reconstr Surg 2013;132(4):933–943. Epub 2013/10/01. doi: 10.1097/PRS.0b013e3182a053f1. PubMed PMID: 24076684.

PART IX.

MAXILLOFACIAL SURGERY

54.

MANDIBLE FRACTURES

Yeshaswini Thelekkat and Warren Schubert

The mandible is a strong solitary bone, unique in its shape, the only movable bone in the facial skeleton (other than the auditory ossicles) and the second most commonly fractured (next to the nasal bones). The mandible constitutes a major part of a person's appearance and expression of personality. It is also involved in the basic human functions of food intake, speech, and basic psychosexual function. The mandible supports the mandibular teeth, which occlude with the teeth in the maxilla and enable the act of mastication.

The primary objective of treating mandibular fractures is to restore the anatomic contours and premorbid occlusion. It is important to understand the concept of occlusion, which is of utmost importance when trying to restore the premorbid condition. Proper knowledge of the relevant surgical anatomy, correct understanding of the biomechanics of the bone involved, and sound concepts of bone healing are paramount in the successful treatment of fractures. With technological advancements in the field of imaging and instrumentation, today's surgeon has a plethora of surgical options to choose from.

It is useful to first understand the dentitions of the adult (Figure 54.1) and the child (Figure 54.2) and also understand concept of occlusion before delving into the scenario of restoration for the "eye can see only what the mind knows."

It should be borne in mind that the maxilla and mandible of a child will invariably house the tooth buds of the permanent teeth apical to the deciduous teeth, making the placement of (plates and screws) almost impossible without posing a threat to these tooth buds (Figure 54.3). The inferior border of the mandible remains the only choice for placing hardware in a pediatric skeleton without the risk of injury to the tooth buds.

OCCLUSION

No single word has greater significance in any discussion of the fracture of the jaws than does the term Occlusion
—Erich and Austin[1]

A valuable diagnostic guide to detect fractures, *occlusion* also dictates the final treatment of fractures of the jaws jaw not jaws?. It is useful for the surgeon to be aware of the normal dental relationship in order to successfully reestablish the premorbid occlusion. "Occlusion" encompasses a vast area in itself, and it is beyond the scope of this chapter to offer a complete review. This chapter will highlight those issues most relevant for the surgeon treating fractures of the jaw.

"Occlusion" refers to the contact relationships between the maxillary and the mandibular teeth as they approach each other during function or at rest. In trauma surgery, it is mandatory to restore the patient's premorbid occlusion. For all practical purposes, when working on the jaws jaw, the trauma surgeon should get the teeth into maximal intercuspation, ensuring the condyles are seated in their fossae. Digital palpation in the preauricular region of the condylar head and support superiorly at the angle region are usually sufficient to ensure proper seating of the condyle. This, along with anatomical realignment, and a careful assessment of the patient's pre-morbid wear facets will reestablish the premorbid occlusion.

Normally, the maxillary incisors overlap the mandibular incisors vertically for about 3–5 mm, which is the *overbite*, and horizontally for 2–4 mm, which is the *overjet* (Figure 54.4). An excessive overbite or deep impingement overbite may prevent one from having enough room to apply mandibular arch bars without having the maxillary incisors hitting the lower arch bar and preventing the teeth to come into proper contact (Figure 54.5).

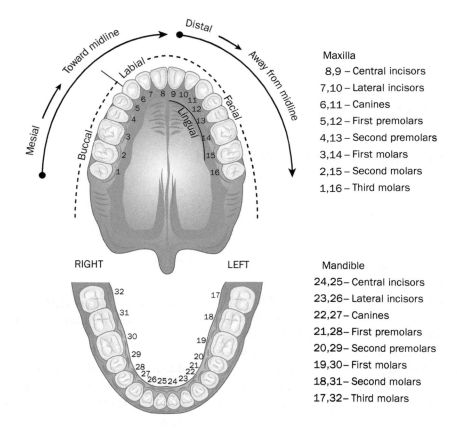

Maxilla

8,9 – Central incisors
7,10 – Lateral incisors
6,11 – Canines
5,12 – First premolars
4,13 – Second premolars
3,14 – First molars
2,15 – Second molars
1,16 – Third molars

Mandible

24,25– Central incisors
23,26– Lateral incisors
22,27– Canines
21,28– First premolars
20,29– Second premolars
19,30– First molars
18,31– Second molars
17,32– Third molars

Figure 54.1. Adult dentition with tooth numbering and dental terminology.

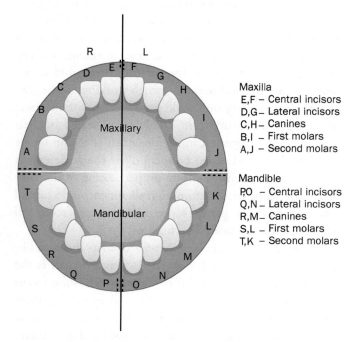

Maxilla

E,F – Central incisors
D,G – Lateral incisors
C,H – Canines
B,I – First molars
A,J – Second molars

Mandible

P,O – Central incisors
Q,N – Lateral incisors
R,M – Canines
S,L – First molars
T,K – Second molars

Figure 54.2. Deciduous teeth and their lettering system used for pediatric patients.

SURGICAL ANATOMY

Despite being the largest and strongest bone in the facial skeleton, the mandible is fractured twice as often than as the midface.[2,3] The energy required to fracture the mandible is in the order of 44.6–74.4 kg/m, which is about the same required to fracture the zygoma[3,4] and four times as much required to fracture the maxilla.[5] The osteology of the mandible, the presence (and absence) of dentition, foramen, and the various muscle attachments contribute factors to produce inherent areas of weakness (and strengths).

The body contains a superior alveolar process that houses the tooth roots and the basal bone below. The external cortex is particularly strong to bear osteosynthetic hardware (an average of 3–4 mm thick). In the anterior symphyseal region, the thickest cortex is at the inferior border of the symphysis and at the angle, along the upper part of the external oblique ridge.[6] It is likely that the relative strength of various

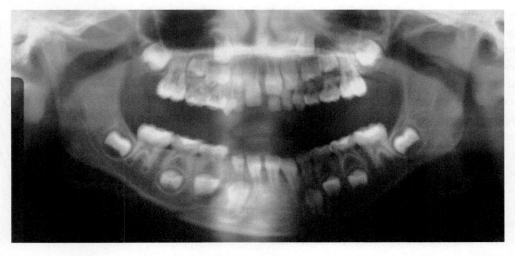

Figure 54.3. Orthopantomogram (OPG) of a child showing the permanent tooth buds relative to the deciduous teeth and a right mandibular body fracture.

regions of the mandible is somewhat proportional to the bony cross-sectional area of the mandible. The bony cross-sectional area between the symphysis and posterior body is fairly consistent and represents the thickest portions of the mandible. This cross-sectional area significantly decreases as one ascends cephalad up the ramus, until reaching the subcondylar portion or subcondylar neck, where the area is approximately one-fourth of the cross-sectional area compared to the span between the symphysis and posterior body.[7] The thickness of the bone in the tooth-bearing portions of the mandible is variable. The anatomy of the tooth roots restricts placement of hardware in this region, preventing the use of bicortical screws and limiting the length of monocortical drill bits and screws. In a dentate mandible, the presence of teeth makes the socket a weak zone, especially in the presence of impacted teeth. In children, however, the elasticity and resilience

of the young bone offsets the disadvantage of the multiple unerupted teeth.[3]

The neurovascular bundle is another important anatomical structure that needs to be respected in fracture treatment. The inferior alveolar nerve runs a concave course within the mandibular canal, and, from posterior to anterior, it runs closer to the outer cortex and inferior border. The distance between the canal and the outer cortex averages 4 mm in the premolar region increasing to 5–9 mm in the molar region. The mental foramen lies approximately at the middle of the distance between the alveolar crest and inferior border of the mandible along a vertical line at/

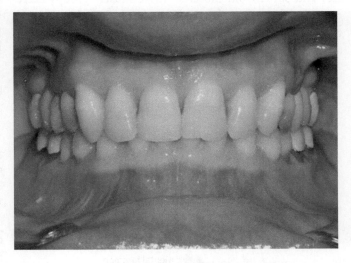

Figure 54.5. Clinical picture shows a deep bite (excessive overbite) where the maxillary incisors are almost closing over on the mandibular incisors and there is minimal overjet. This is also referred to as a *deep impingement overbite*. This kind of an abnormal scenario would make it very difficult to place an arch bar on the mandibular teeth as there is not adequate room, and the maxillary incisors would hit the mandibular arch bar, preventing a complete closure of the jaw.

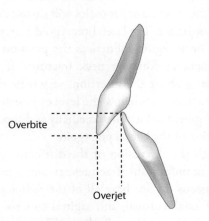

Overbite

Overjet

Figure 54.4. Illustration of overbite and overjet.

between/below the apices of the first or second premolar.[6] There may be some ethnic variability in the relative location of the mental foramen, with a study suggesting that in African Americans the foramen lies slightly more posterior (distal) to the second premolar relative to Caucasians.[8]

A mistake commonly made is the perception that the inferior alveolar nerve runs along a horizontal level to its exit point at the mental foramen. It generally runs inferior (caudad) to the foramen and often extends a few millimeter anterior (mesial) before curving superior (cephalad) and posterior (distal), and finally exiting at the mental foramen. This is referred to as the anterior loop (Figure 54.6).

Since the mental and incisive nerves are each covered with an epineurium within the anterior loop, damage at the relevant region might cause dysesthesia not only at the anterior teeth but also at the lower lip and chin.[9]

The relative position of the nerve to the mental foramen is important to remember when considering the use of bicortical screw placement or the use of lag screw fixation. Under these circumstances, bi-cortical screw hole or an osteotomy for a sliding genioplasty should be considered at least 5 mm caudad to the mental foramen to avoid injury to the inferior alveolar nerve.

The mandible is enveloped by strong muscle groups and an adequate soft tissue cover that enable the mandible to undergo proper functional loading, which is very essential for the normal growth of the mandible. The muscle groups can be categorized into masticatory muscles and suprahyoid muscles. These muscle groups exert opposing forces on a fractured mandible. The direction of the force of the trauma, the direction of the fracture line, and the muscle pull all influence the degree of fracture

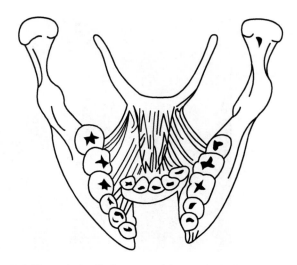

Figure 54.7. The posterior displacement of the symphysis due to a bilateral parasymphyseal fractures as a result of the pull of the genioglossus. Since this portion of the mandible represents the anterior attachment of the tongue, there is a significant risk of airway compromise, as the tongue falls posteriorly when the patient is supine.

displacement. The most common scenario is that the muscles of mastication pull the posterior fracture segment superiorly and the suprahyoid muscles pull the anterior segment inferiorly.[10]

A rare problem of concern is the possibility of bilateral mandibular fractures causing a flail central segment that supports the tongue (Figure 54.7). This may result in loss of the anterior support of the tongue and airway problems, especially when the patient is supine. This is more common in atrophic edentulous bilateral fractured patients and in gunshot patients who have avulsed and lost their symphyseal support.

FAVORABLE AND UNFAVORABLE FRACTURES

The direction of the fracture line is crucial in determining whether the masticatory muscles will distract or splint the proximal segment. The lateral pterygoid insertion into the condylar neck region influences the position of the condyle segment in condylar neck fractures. If the fracture line traverses above the insertion, very little displacement occurs. Fracture lines below the level of insertion cause the condyle segment to be pulled medially and anteriorly owing to the action of the lateral pterygoid.

Though the discussion of the distinction between favorable and unfavorable fractures remains a popular topic, most surgeons do not have all of the radiologic views required of axial, coronal, and sagittal cuts to determine if a fracture is favorable in all planes. The safest assumption

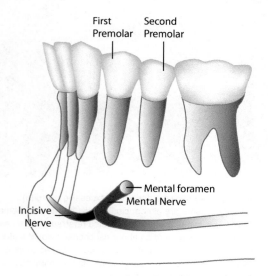

First Premolar   Second Premolar

Mental foramen
Mental Nerve
Incisive Nerve

Figure 54.6. The position of the mental foramen and the anterior loop.

for the surgeon when determining the amount of fixation required is to treat all fractures as if they are unfavorable. When examining mandibular angle fractures, most are indeed unfavorable in their pattern.

BIOMECHANICS OF THE MANDIBLE

Unique in its shape, the mandible can be compared to a cantilevered beam suspended at two points represented by the temporomandibular joint (TMJ). Once the mandible is loaded, although the load is distributed along the entire length of the mandible, owing to the topographical irregularities such as foramen, convexity, ridges, concavity, differences in cross-sectional areas, and the like, the distribution is uneven.

The mandible has tensile forces acting on the superior or alveolar process and compressive forces acting on the inferior or the basal process between the symphysis and the angle region. Because of the uneven force distribution, there is a neutral zone in between that is the most protected and least mobile. This coincides with the location of the mandibular canal and path of the alveolar nerve.[11]

More than 75% of the fractures occur at the tension zone, with the exception of comminuted intracapsular fractures of the condylar head which are purely compression in origin.[12–13] The condylar process has a slender neck before giving rise to the condylar head. This change in direction and the minimal cross-sectional area makes this area the most susceptible to fracture in the mandible.[2,14,15]

Upon loading the mandible anteriorly, the fracture segments tend to splay apart at the superior border (Figure 54.8). In the anterior zone, between the mental foramen, in addition to tensile and compressive forces are torsional forces. In a fractured mandible, it is important to neutralize these tensile, compressive, and torsional forces to achieve a functionally stable reduction. The hardware selected should be able to restore the tension and compressive zones of the mandible.

DIAGNOSIS

A good history and clinical examination is the basis of any diagnosis. Unless maxillofacial injuries pose a threat to airway, they are almost always a part of the Advanced Trauma Life Support (ATLS) secondary survey. The role of history-taking cannot be underestimated. Information about the mode of injury will suggest possible concomitant injuries. A detailed history from the patient should be taken. A thorough maxillofacial examination is critical when suspecting a facial fracture prior to ordering any imaging.

CLINICAL EXAMINATION

In addition to pain and swelling, deranged occlusion is usually seen in patients with fractures of the mandible. In this situation, bimanual palpation of the occlusal segments should be done to check for mobility and pain. The inferior body of the mandible should be palpated to check for step deformities. The mandible should be checked for its range of motion. Edema and pain often restricts

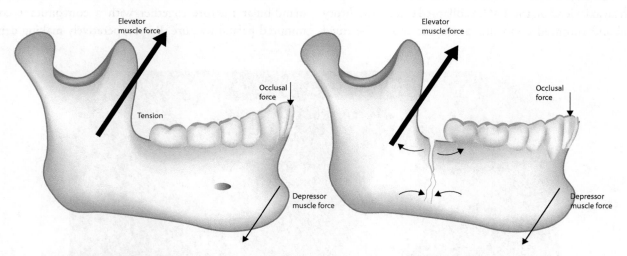

Figure 54.8. The superior tensile and inferior compressive force distribution on the mandible, opening of the tensile border upon loading with an occlusal force in a fractured mandible.

maximal mouth opening. Limited lateral excursions are noted usually toward the side of fracture in the case of a subcondylar fracture.

Clinical hallmarks of a mandibular fracture are:

- Pain on palpation or with mastication
- Deranged occlusion or inability to completely occlude
- Numbness of the mental nerve distribution
- A break or tear in the gingiva
- Deviation on mouth opening
- Definite step-deformity inferior border
- Sublingual ecchymosis (Coleman's sign, often noted the day after the trauma)

A tear in the gingiva can often be found that highlights the location of the mandible fracture. Sublingual ecchymosis (Coleman's sign) is usually indicative of a fracture of the mandibular arch. The finding of sublingual ecchymosis often does not appear acutely and may not be seen until the next day. Neurosensory disturbances are noted when the fracture passes through the inferior alveolar nerve which presents in the region supplied by the mental nerve. This should be documented prior to any surgical intervention. When the patient is in acute pain, numbness in the mental nerve distribution may not be realized by the patient until tested.

The proximity of the mandibular condyles and mandibular fossa to the external auditory canal should always be considered with the need to check the tympanic membrane. In cases where patients have had a sufficient impact with an axial load on the TMJ, a collapsed external auditory canal and ruptured tympanic membrane should be ruled out and consideration of decompression of a collapsed external canal considered.

RADIOLOGICAL EXAMINATION

Mandible fractures can be adequately diagnosed using plain films, keeping the important principle in mind that ideal imaging should be obtained in two planes, at right angles to each other. The commonly used films are an *orthopantomogram* (OPG, also known as a pantomogram, and sometimes referred to as a Panorex, after the company that made OPG radiologic machines; Figure 54.9) and a postero-anterior view of the mandible (PA mandible, Figure 54.10). If a subcondylar fracture is suspected, a Towne's view has been found to be extremely useful in assessing the displacement of the subcondylar fracture.

In the event that computed tomography (CT) is deemed necessary, the surgeon should ask for both the axial cuts and reformatted coronal and sagittal cuts, which may also allow a three-dimensional assessment of the fracture. Our studies comparing CT to the orthopantomogram found that the CT is more accurate in detecting mandibular fractures.[16,17]

Another view that can be particularly helpful intraoperatively, especially for symphyseal and parasymphyseal fractures is an occlusal view. This view can help confirm that there is no splaying of the mandible due to a failed reduction of the lingual cortex.

DENTAL MODELS

Dental impressions and the use of dental models can be very useful in complex cases, especially where there is a mandibular fracture together with a concomitant comminuted palatal fracture. By preoperatively making dental

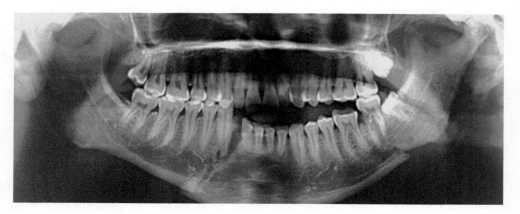

Figure 54.9. Orthopantomogram showing right parasymphysis and left angle fracture.

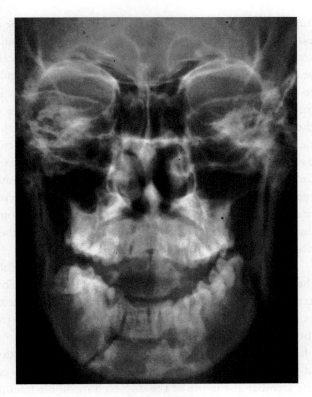

Figure 54.10. Posteroanterior view of the mandible showing left parasymphysis and right angle fracture.

impressions and pouring models, determining the most likely premorbid occlusion with the use an articulator is easy, allowing one to make a palatal splint and even dental splints. In some cases, a lingual splint can help with the reduction and stabilization of the mandible.

Lingual splints secured with circummandibular wiring are usually adequate in pediatric mandible fractures. Not only do these fractures heal quickly, but the patient also has tooth buds of the secondary dentition, making open reduction and internal fixation (ORIF) with screws a significant challenge.

TREATMENT CONSIDERATIONS

As with any other fracture, considerations for the treatment of mandible fractures include observation and careful follow-up with no surgical intervention, closed treatment with maxillo-mandibular fixation (MMF) alone or with ORIF. Proper treatment recommendations for various fractures remain controversial and may vary in different parts of the world depending on available technologies and social economic situations. Furthermore, several different modalities can often be

used in the management of mandibular trauma, often with equally good results.

It is important to select the appropriate fixation technique to not only ensure adequate anatomic reduction of the fractures, but also to maintain the alignment with stability during healing to ensure bony union. As seen earlier, the nature of the mandible and the functional load that it is subjected to requires adequately strong hardware to maintain stability of the fragments during healing.

INDICATIONS FOR TREATMENT OF MANDIBULAR FRACTURES

Indications for no surgical intervention or open versus closed treatment of mandibular fractures can vary with different schools of thought and practice (Box 54.1). With advances in skill sets and technology, the decision to treat fractures, either open or closed, remains subjective.

BOX 54.1 INDICATIONS FOR TREATMENT OF MANDIBULAR FRACTURES

Indications for No Surgical Intervention

Intracapsular fractures of the condyle

Minimally displaced fractures of the subcondyle where the occlusion is normal

Nondisplaced ramus fractures

Indications for Closed Treatment

Simple, nondisplaced isolated patterns of mandibular fracture

Nondisplaced pediatric fractures

Most condyle fractures

Situations where economics of hardware placement or adequate safe anesthesia can be challenging

Indications for Open Treatment

Closed techniques are unable to obtain or maintain an accurate reduction

Patient's desire to be able to mobilize mandible without postoperative MMF

Noncompliant patient/those unable to comply

Bilateral subcondylar fractures

Complex or comminuted fractures

Complications such as infection or nonunion

Defect type fractures

Fractures of the atrophic mandible

NO SURGICAL INTERVENTION

Indications for no surgical intervention include condylar intracapsular fractures, some subcondylar fractures where the occlusion is normal, and nondisplaced ramus fractures. These indications are likely to raise controversy in many circles. A large consensus is likely to exist for intracapsular fractures of the condyle considering the fact that uneventful healing is otherwise possible and intervention may result in further problems. The pterygomassetric sling of the ramus often provides adequate stability for undisplaced ramal fractures so that arch bars or an internal fixation are often not needed for a compliant patient willing to stick to a soft diet for a period of time.

MAXILLO-MANDIBULAR FIXATION

The goals of MMF are to stabilize the fractured segments and attain and maintain the premorbid occlusion. MMF is an important intermediary step in trauma care where intermaxillary traction is applied between the jaws to attain and maintain the pre-injury occlusion while performing ORIF. Although most patients would prefer to have their mandible swing open postoperatively for reasons of speech and diet, in some cases, continued MMF may be required postoperatively with limited opening.

There are *tooth-borne* and *bone-borne* devices that can be used to attain MMF. The most commonly used tooth-borne device is the arch bar. The arch bar is used to temporarily stabilize the fracture fragments during ORIF. It can also act as a tension band in some simple fractures and to stabilize the fractured alveolar process and luxated teeth, and it is

imperative in the closed treatment of certain fractures. In early years, MMF between the maxillary and mandibular arch bars was achieved with wire fixation. In more recent years, more surgeons are using elastics (short rubber bands) to achieve MMF. These have the advantage of being easier for patients, family, and healthcare workers to remove in the event of an emergency. Furthermore, a combative patient in the postoperative wake-up period may loosen arch bars when MMF is due to wire fixation. In contrast, during times of these extreme efforts to open a patient's mouth, the elastics may have some "give," but later when the patient is awake and cooperative again, elastics allow some mandibular excursions, significant enough to restore their occlusion.

If arch bars are used in a case of ORIF of the mandible, the surgeon may benefit from first performing the incision, exposing the fracture, and somewhat reducing the fracture prior to the placement of the mandibular arch bar. The tradition of placing the arch bar prior to making the incision often results in the arch bar preventing a proper reduction of the fractured segments, with the surgeon having to cut the arch bar at the site of the displaced mandible fracture to achieve a fracture reduction and proper occlusion in displaced fractures. Once cut, the structural integrity and stability offered by the arch bar is compromised.

In cases of multiple mandibular fractures, more commonly occurring with an anterior mandible with a bilateral condylar neck fracture combination, arch bars and MMF tend to increase the posterior flare at the angles, lingually inclining the molar segment and causing a lingual open bite (Figure 54.11).

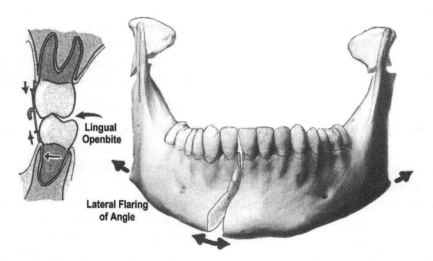

Lingual Openbite

Lateral Flaring of Angle

Figure 54.11. Maxillo-mandibular fixation (MMF) on the buccal side of a mandible with multiple fractures, combined with the forces of masticatory muscles, may cause a rotation of the fragments with a lingual open bite. In cases where there are multiple fractures, especially on opposing sides of the mandible, simultaneous reduction of the fractures is essential to prevent lingual cortical gaping. When combined with bilateral condyle fractures, open reduction and internal fixation (ORIF) of one of the condyle fractures should be given a higher priority to eliminate flaring during the application of MMF.

ORIF of the mandible should be performed by placing the patient in MMF intraoperatively after fracture exposure and reduction. Following plate fixation of the fractures, it is important to take the patient out of MMF and recheck the occlusion by opening and closing the jaw to make sure that, in the process of MMF and plating, premorbid "reduction" and fixation was not falsely achieved by distracting the condyle out of the fossa.

Other tooth-borne devices that can be used include Ernst ligatures, Ivy (eyelet) loops, or interdental wires (embrasure wires) using 22-gauge wire (Figure 54.12). The use of these time-saving "shortcuts" may be considered for temporary stabilization of simple fractures or for intraoperative MMF until a proper ORIF has been achieved. Interdental wiring with larger gauge wire is not recommended as a means of postoperative MMF as the wires can be difficult to remove.

Bone-borne devices, such as MMF screws and arch bar-type devices that are screwed into the mandibular and

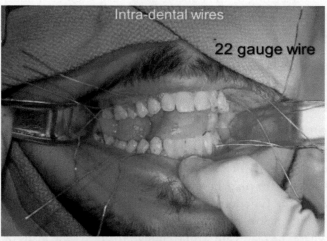

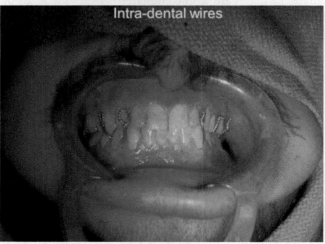

Figure 54.12. The use of intradental wires for maxillo-mandibular fixation.

maxillary bone, are now available that drastically reduce the application time of arch bars and diminish the risk of prick injuries. Downsides of these techniques include the risk of injury to the tooth roots, inability of some brands to serve as a tension band, the possibility of lateral rotation of the segments when wires are overtightened, and relative cost of the devices. From a cost standpoint, the savings in anesthesia time may justify the cost of the device, depending on the medical economics of the region and institution. It should be noted that if left on for an extended period of time, the mechanism of achieving occlusion with these devices is different from that with arch bars. With arch bars, one is pulling the teeth together to achieve MMF while with the bone-borne devices, one is pushing the maxillary-mandibular segments together to achieve occlusion.

CLOSED TREATMENT WITH MMF

There are some fractures that will heal uneventfully with simple immobilization of the jaws such as simple, undisplaced isolated fractures of the mandible, some subcondylar fractures, and most nondisplaced pediatric fractures. In these cases, MMF can be a modality of treatment by itself. The jaws will need to be immobilized for a period of 3–4 weeks with a limited soft diet for another 2–3 weeks for adequate healing.[18] Patient compliance is of utmost importance with this modality of treatment.

A key to the success of arch bar placement as a stand-alone treatment is adequate postoperative follow-up and management. One should consider seeing the patient at least at weekly intervals to monitor compliance and, when necessary, replace the elastics. Guidelines vary for every different fracture pattern, but consideration should be made to begin removal of many, if not most of the elastics by the third week and begin some movement, possibly with or without guiding elastics. Movement and adequate range of motion exercises should be monitored, with guidelines for self- or supervised therapy. The goal for an adult should be to achieve an interincisal distance of 45 mm. Particular care should be considered in children to make sure adequate range of motion is achieved early enough (after 10 days) to avoid TMJ ankylosis.

In simple undisplaced fractures of the edentulous mandible with good bone height, closed treatment may be considered in a willing patient. The patient's dentures can be used as *Gunning splint* to anchor arch bars (or using some other wire technique). The dentures are secured in the mouth using a palatal screw for the upper and circummandibular wiring for the lower denture. The anterior teeth of the dentures can be removed to keep open a portal for feeding. The Gunning splint is not a good option for a fractured atrophic mandible, and the use of ORIF and a large reconstruction plate should be considered.

OPEN REDUCTION AND INTERNAL FIXATION

Some fractures unequivocally mandate the use of ORIF rather than closed treatment with MMF alone. These include complex and displaced fractures, comminuted, defect, infected fractures, and fractures of the atrophic mandible. Some patients who desire full range of motion immediately and those who cannot comply with a closed treatment philosophy are also candidates for ORIF. Various schools of thought have been put forward, and it is important for the surgeon to select the appropriate fixation method to ensure stability during healing.

It is important to understand the concepts of load-sharing and load-bearing and to know the relative and absolute indications for using one technique versus the other.

CONCEPTS OF LOAD-SHARING AND LOAD-BEARING

LOAD-SHARING

When there is enough bone stock with good bone buttressing, a smaller plate is enough to share the load with the bone.[19] This is the basis of the "load-sharing" principle. The sharing can be *ideal*, where the bone takes most of the load, or *intermediate*, where the load is shared equally between the plate and the bone. Miniplates used are low-profile and have to be passively adapted to the bone contour: "adaption osteosynthesis."

The plates are placed in the neutral zones (Figure 54.13). Significant moments of torsional forces were found anterior (mesial) to the canines, reaching a maximum in the symphyseal area, and, therefore, two parallel miniplates rather than one are required in this region. Near the angle there are two potential lines for miniplate fixation. One line lies on the buccal cortex and the other on the lingual side of anterior border ramus, twisting anteriorly to the area of the third molar to the buccal cortex. The screws used in this technique are monocortical. This offers only a functionally stable occlusion and allows "micro-movements" with "relative stability" between the fractured segments. The functional load is "shared" by the bone.

The use of lag screws offers a rigid internal fixation that stabilizes the fragments by compression (Figure 54.14). This is possible only in the presence of good bone buttressing and

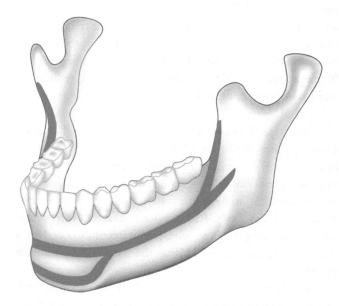

Figure 54.13. Illustration to show Champy's lines of osteosynthesis.

is load-sharing by the bone. If using a lag screw technique, the use of only a single horizontal lag screw in the symphyseal area is usually doomed to fail due to extreme torsional forces causing rotation in the area. Two parallel screws are required to counter the torsional forces anteriorly (Figure 54.15).

LOAD-BEARING

When the cross-sectional area of the available bone is minimal, the bone is inadequate for "sharing" the forces exerted on it. There is lack of adequate interfragmentary friction. The plate has to be strong enough to "bear" and resist the functional loads. Therefore, larger profile and stonger plates are required for a more absolute regidity, where the plates are strong enough to "bear" the loads of the forces on the mandible. The prefered screws used are bicortical and the surgery is more technically demanding.

Load-bearing is indicated in scenarios such as

1. *Deficient quanitity of bone*: Defect fractures, comminuted fractures, edentulous fractures

2. *Defective quality of bone*: Infected fractures

3. *Noncompliant patient* who refuses to adhere to postop care required following load-sharing osteosynthesis

In the first scenario of deficient quantity of bone, the bone stock is suboptimal and there is no bone buttressing. Hence, the entire load should be borne by the hardware itself.

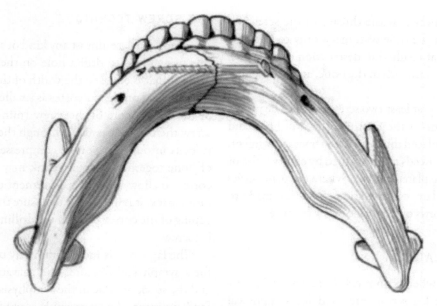

Figure 54.14. Lag screw with the fragments in compression with a perfect apposition of the lingual cortex.

While both conventional and locking screw reconstruction plates can be used, the locking plates have the added advantage of the screw heads being threaded into the plate hole to secure the plate, with a separate set of threads in the screw to capture the underlying bone. In addition, these plates do not require perfect bony adaptation and attain stabilization by internal splinting.

In the second senario of infected fractures, failure of miniplate fixation often occurs or there is poor quality infected bone at the fracture site. The use of a larger plate that gives a more rigid stability and spans the infected area and avoiding the use of screws in the infected area is desirable. In some cases, debridement of infected bone may be advised, resulting in a defect-type scenario.

PRINCIPLES OF PLATING

As a general rule, all fractured segments should be exposed and reduced as well as possible prior to beginning plating. Adequate exposure for visualization of the important anatomy should be achieved without devascularization of more bone than necessary. Often lower drill speeds with adequate water irrigation are preferable. If too much heat is

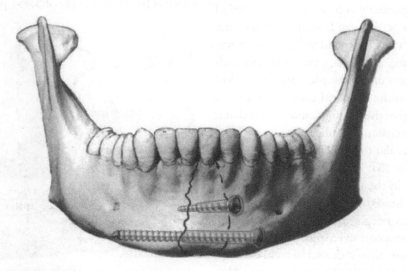

Figure 54.15. Anterior mandible fracture. Lag screw technique for fixation of symphyseal fracture. Obliquity of fracture allows superior screw to be placed from buccal to lingual cortices. Inferior screw engages buccal cortices.

produced, it may appear that the threads of the screw are engaging the bone at the time of surgery, only to find at a later date that the heat resulted in destruction of the bone, resorption of the screw threads in the bone, and a loosening of the hardware.

To achieve stability, at least two screws need to be placed in a plate on each side of the fracture. The drill holes and screws should not be placed too close to the fracture segment, and often the fracture needs to be spanned by empty holes or a designed span in the plate. For areas where the plate serves as a "load-bearing" plate, consideration should be made to place at least three screws on each side of the fracture.

COMPRESSION PLATING

The one technique where compression still plays an excellent role is when lag screws are used for symphyseal fractures. Techniques that advocate the use of compression of the bony segments through compression plating and drilling holes near the fracture site in an eccentric manner have fallen into disfavor due to higher complication rates.

LOCKING SCREW PLATES

Conventional larger plates require precise adaptation of the plate along the bony contour. This can be a challenging task, especially when reconstruction plates span the routine curvature of the anterior mandibular cortex. Locking plates were designed with threaded holes through which the screw head engages into the plate independently of the screw threads engaging in the bone. These plates offer two major advantages. First, they allow for a plate to be used even if it has not been perfectly contoured to the cortical surface of the bone. The screws can literally lock into the plate and mandibular bone independently, without any bony contact of the plate, and thus serve as an internal-external fixator. Small gaps under the plate also may allow better revascularization of the fractured cortical bone.[20,21]

The second advantage of the locking screw plate is that it offers stronger three-dimensional stability. The screw holes must be drilled perpendicular to the plate using drill guides that lock into the plate so that the screw threads perfectly engage the hole threads in the plate. Conventional screws (with nonlocking screw heads) can also be used with these locking screw plates when a degree of angulation is needed.

One caveat: if the surgeon overdrills the screw hole (making the drill hole wider than it should be) while using a locking screw plate, the screw will appear to be engaged because, with the final turns, the screw head will engage in the plate yet the threads may not be properly engaging the bone

LAG SCREW TECHNIQUE

A surgeon may use almost any kind of screw as a "lag" screw. The principle is to drill a hole on the near cortex using a drill bit that is equal to the width of the screw threads. The drill bit used on the far cortex is smaller, equal to the width of the central core of the screw (minus the threads). The screw then glides passively through the near cortex, and, as it locks into the far cortex, compresses the two fragments of bone together. A countersink may be used in the near cortex to allow for a flush placement of the screw into the near cortex. It is important to ensure that there is no lingual gaping of the cortex prior to the drilling of the holes for the lag screw.

The lag screw is most commonly used in the mandible for a symphyseal fracture. The curvature of the mandible and the stock of bone in the symphysis make it most suited for lag screws. If a coutersink is used to allow the screw head to be seated flush in the proximal cortex, it should be used with care not to remove too much of the cortex. If too much of the outer cortex is removed, the head of the screw may disappear into the spongeosal bone as the screw is tightened. If a countersink is performed, the special bit used for this procedure should be turned manually, and not with a power drill, which commonly results in too much cortical bone being removed.

TREATMENT CONSIDERATIONS BY FRACTURE LOCATION

Common locations for fractures are shown in Figure 54.16, which is based on a study of 5,451 patients. This frequency

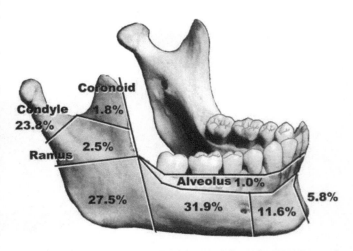

Figure 54.16. Mandibular fracture frequency. Frequency (percentage) of several types of mandibular fractures from several combined series (5,451 patients with 8,795 mandibular fractures).

of fracture site distribution may vary in different parts of the globe depending on the incidence of various etiologies.

ALVEOLAR PROCESS AND TEETH (DENTOALVEOLAR SEGMENT)

Fractures of the alveolar process and the teeth alone are uncommon, occurring as isolated injuries in only 1% of fractures of the mandible. They often go undiagnosed in the emergency room either due to the glaring urgency of other concomitant injuries or due to the lack of training in the evaluation of these injuries. The most probable causes for this to present as a stand-alone injury are interpersonal violence, sporting injuries, low-impact falls, and bike or motorcycle injuries. These injuries, whenever possible, should be addressed immediately to improve the prognosis of the involved teeth and restore function.

Periapical and occlusal films and OPG are useful in establishing a diagnosis of dentoalveolar fractures. The fracture can involve only a single tooth, a segment of teeth with the fracture line passing through the apices of the teeth involved, or a segment of teeth with the fracture line passing well below the apices of the teeth involved.

Management usually consists of mobilizing the segment digitally, verifying the occlusal relationship, then repositioning and stabilizing the segment using arch bars or composite splints under local anaesthesia, conscious sedation, or general anesthesia. While arch bars are very useful in stabilizing larger dentoalveolar segments, composite splints have been found to be more useful in stabilizing single, two, or three luxated teeth. When found in association with other fractures of the mandible, after the fractures of the mandible have been suitably addressed, the arch bars should be retained for 3–4 weeks to allow the segment to heal.

Fractures of the alveolar process in the pediatric age group are immobilized more often using composite splints than arch bars due to the morphology of the deciduous teeth and the different eruption status in the mixed dentition phase. Avulsed deciduous teeth are *not* replanted since this can disturb the position of the permanent tooth germ.

TEETH IN THE LINE OF FRACTURE

Fractures of the dentate mandible with the fracture line passing through the tooth socket are compound intraorally (see Box 54.2). Already prone to infection because of the portal of communication intraorally, teeth with preexisting dental disease further predispose the fracture to infection. There is fairly universal consensus on retaining healthy,

firm teeth in the line of fracture especially when they aid in fracture reduction or serve as the available occlusal stop. Salvaged teeth will often need dental treatment in addition to fracture management. In some cases, these teeth may be extracted after reducing and fixing the fracture.

Missing teeth due to acute trauma and/or extraction of teeth in a fracture site invariably converts the fracture to a defect situation, increasing the likelihood of morbidity. Teeth with advanced preexisting dental disease, loose or avulsed teeth, teeth associated with a nonviable alveolar segment, a tooth that obviously interferes with bony reduction, and teeth that have more than half of their bony sockets damaged in the fracture line are sure candidates for extraction. Teeth with fractured tooth roots should also be considered for removal.[22–24] Partially erupted third molars will often aid in attaining appropriate reduction of the segments especially at the superior border when using the Champy technique. In these situations, the health of the tooth should be assessed, and, if deemed necessary, the tooth may be extracted after attaining reduction and fixation.

SYMPHYSIS AND PARASYMPHYSIS

To combat the torsional forces that exist in addition to the tensile and compressive forces in the anterior mandible, ORIF is preferable to MMF alone for fractures of the symphysis and parasymphysis. Adhering to Champy's osteosynthetic lines, these fractures are best treated using a superior and inferior construct to counter the torsional forces.[25,26]

This can be in the form of two miniplates, two lag screws, a combination of either a superior plate and an inferior lag screw, or a superior arch bar and an inferior larger plate. The torsional forces are so great that use of a superior arch bar and an inferior miniplate offers adequate stability only in minimally displaced fractures of the symphysis. Another option to consider is the use of a three-dimensional plate such as a box or ladder plate, or a larger load sharing plate inferiorly. Whatever fixation is used, one key point especially important for these anterior fractures is to make sure that there is no gap on the lingual cortex, which will lead to lingual splaying. This is particularly important to consider when there are coexistent fractures at the angle or the condyles leading to a widening of the face at the angles.

Surgical access. Most simple and moderately displaced fractures of the anterior mandible can be accessed adequately through a transoral vestibular incision. A curvilinear incision is made extending anteriorly out into the lip mucosa, leaving 10–15 mm of mucosa attached to the gingiva to preserve the inferior labial sulcus. The underlying mentalis is then incised obliquely down to bone, leaving a good cuff of muscle to reattach after the procedure. Making a mucoperiosteal incision in the depth of the sulcus results in a scar that will markedly reduce the sulcus depth, making future removable prosthetic requirements difficult. The muco-periosteum is then degloved down to the inferior border to expose the fractures. To extend the incision posterior to the canines, the incision is curved superiorly to stay above the mental nerve and is about 5–6 mm away from the gingiva. During dissection, it is important to respect the mental nerve branches, and, if needed, skeletonization should be done to minimize traction trauma.[27] At the end of the case, it is important to reattach the mentalis muscle to its origin to prevent ptosis of the lip and chin. Suspension dressings may be used extraorally for added support for a few days after the procedure.

Complex fractures like comminuted and avulsive fractures will benefit from an extraoral approach. These fractures can be accessed either through the laceration (with suitable extension) or through a submental incision. The dissection is straightforward and is carried out to the inferior rim of the mandible. This allows the surgeon to visualize the lingual cortex and ensure its reduction.

Technique. Once the fractures are adequately exposed, the patient is placed into MMF and the fracture segments are reduced anatomically. If needed, two monocortical holes are drilled on either side of the fracture, and a bone clamp can be inserted to hold the segments in the reduced position during application of the hardware.

Miniplates. Two 2.0 mm miniplates are required to adhere to the load-sharing principle and counter the torsional forces. The mandible has a curvature anteriorly, and it is important to contour the plates passively onto the bony surface for adaptation osteosynthesis. The superior plate will serve as the tension band plate and has to be positioned below the root apices of the mandibular anterior teeth, or the drill bits and screws used must be short enough not to damage the root apices. The second plate should be placed closer to the inferior border and as far away from the superior plate as possible. The screws of the superior plate are monocortical, 4–6 mm long, and should be placed away from the tooth roots. Drill bits with stops should be used, if available, for the superior plate.

In simple, undisplaced fractures, the arch bars alone can serve as the tension band, and a single larger profile miniplate placed at the inferior border may suffice for functionally stable fixation. Another option for fixation is a three-dimensional type plate, also known as a *box plate* or *ladder-type plate.* This allows fixation with fairly minimal exposure, and the three-dimensional component helps protect the bone from extreme torsional forces in the symphyseal area.

In complex scenarios like comminuted fractures, load-bearing osteosynthesis will need to be considered. This can be obtained by an arch bar or a 2 mm miniplate as a superior tension band plate and a reconstruction plate on the inferior border. Many surgeons would consider slightly overbending the plates to try to avoid a splay of the lingual cortex.

Regardless of the technique used for symphyseal fractures, it is important to ensure that the lingual cortex is reduced appropriately before placing the plate and screws, especially when accompanied by condylar fractures. The reduction may benefit from manual compression at the mandibular angles applied by the assistant to eliminate the lingual gap, while the surgeon drills the hole to place the hardware for fixation.

Lag screws. Lag screws are best suited for simple fractures of the symphysis, either sagittal or oblique. They offer absolute rigidity with minimal hardware. However, their placement can be technically demanding. The symphysis is an area where the lag screw probably can be placed with relative ease, without the fear of injuring the inferior alveolar nerve. It can be challenging to place two parallel screws caudad enough so that both are below the branches of the inferior alveolar nerve branches serving the tooth roots.

In the parasymphysis, care should be taken that lag screws are placed caudad to the path of the inferior alveolar nerve. The authors have found that it is extremely difficult to place even one lag screw in the parasymphyseal area. The span of the screw in this area is quite long, and there is not adequate room for two parallel screws. There is not enough height of bone in the parasymphyseal area to confidently place two parallel screws below the inferior alveolar nerve.

BODY FRACTURES

Simple, undisplaced fractures of the dentate body can be treated by closed methods using arch bars and MMF. However, most patients would opt for ORIF to overcome the period of compulsive immobilization. The options of fixation are similar to those of the symphysis; however, unless there is an incredibly oblique fracture, a lag screw is not likely to be a viable option due to the presence of the tooth roots and the inferior alveolar nerve. It is important to consider the location of the tooth roots, the reduced distance between the roots and the inferior border of the mandible, and the presence of the inferior alveolar canal while performing ORIF in the body.

Surgical access. Most simple and minimally displaced fractures of the body can be accessed transorally through a vestibular incision, as described earlier. Behind the mental foramen, the incision should curve upward, if continuing from anterior, avoiding damage to the branches of the mental nerve. It is important to respect the mental nerve during dissection and hardware placement. The nerve and its branches can be skeletonized to minimize traction trauma.[27]

Displaced and comminuted fractures of the body may sometimes be best accessed by an extraoral submandibular approach. Importance should be given to the marginal mandibular branch of the facial nerve and the facial vessels. The skin incision is placed 3 cm away from the inferior border, the platysma is incised a little above the skin incision, and a subplatysmal dissection to the pterygomassetric sling usually preserves the marginal mandibular nerve.[27-30] Damage to the nerve results in a paralysis of the depressor muscles of the lip. The sling is then incised just above the inferior border so that the sling can be easily resutured afterward, and periosteum is incised at the inferior border to adequately expose the fracture.

Technique. The nature of the fracture (simple vs. comminuted) will dictate the exposure. Once exposed, the fracture fragments are appropriately reduced after placing the patient into MMF.

Miniplates. Simple fractures of the body are stabilized using a single 2 mm miniplate along the ideal osteosynthetic line for the body, above the inferior alveolar canal and below the tooth roots. The arch bars will serve as the tension band, and some surgeons may opt to retain the arch bars postoperatively during the initial healing phase.

Moderately displaced body fractures may require two miniplates. In this case, the superior plate should be positioned above the inferior alveolar nerve and the second plate below the inferior alveolar canal. The inferior plate has to be contoured very close to the bone surface to enable

adaptation osteosynthesis. When using an intraoral approach, it may be beneficial to use a transbuccal trochar for screw fixation to the inferior plate.

In some situations, when the surgeon feels the need to use stronger, more rigid hardware for additional stability or when there is fragmentation, a single reconstruction plate can be used as a load-bearing osteosynthesis. An extraoral approach usually makes these situations less challenging compared to a transoral approach. Emphasis on the use of a transbuccal trocar cannot be understated in the choice of a transoral approach.

Lag screws. Lag screws are seldom used for body fractures and are indicated only in simple sagittal or oblique fractures that have adequate bone buttressing. The screws can be placed toward the inferior border for bicortical engagement.

ANGLE FRACTURES

Management of angle fractures has seen the greatest trend for change in the past 20 years. The angle bound by the strong elevator muscles, if left untreated, poses a chance of distracting the ramal component. When coupled with the action of the depressors of the mandible, distraction of the ramus is even more likely.[31,32]

When the fracture occurs at the region of the third molar, there is no tooth distal to it in the proximal segment, and immobilization of fragments with an arch bar is not possible. These fractures are therefore managed by open reduction and internal fixation. Rigid fixation of these fractures had been advocated to prevent any movement of the segments during function.[33-35] Various studies have proved the adequacy of miniplate[36-39] fixation and relative rigidity in the management of simple fractures of the mandibular angle. A single superior border miniplate is preferred for treating simple, isolated mandibular angle fractures, as advocated by Maxine Champy.[37,40]

Angle fractures which require removal of the third molar present a form of mandibular defect. In such a case, caution should be exercised when considering the Champy technique. The molars comprise a significant percentage of the cross-sectional area in this part of the mandible, and, with their loss, the degree of potential load-sharing will be compromised due to lack of bone buttressing. This is ideally treated using two miniplates or a single reconstruction plate along the inferior border.

Surgical access. Fractures of the angle can be accessed intraorally or extraorally. The intraoral approach is advocated for simple fractures that can be treated with a single superior border plate or, in some situations, with two miniplates. The incision is placed in the vestibule, about 5 mm away from the gingiva and extends along the anterior border ramus. It can be extended into a crevicular incision, especially if the tooth in question is to be removed. It is important to use a transbuccal trocar to fix the inferior plate when using two miniplates transorally. The long buccal nerve must be salvaged as one moves up the anterior border.

Extraorally, the submandibular approach[27] is advocated for fractures of the angle that need rigid fixation with reconstruction plates or those that cannot be adequately accessed transorally. The approach is similar to that described for the body. It is important to resuture the pterygomassetric sling after closure of the periosteum at the end of the surgery.

Technique. The fractures are exposed as appropriate. The patient is placed in MMF. It is important to ensure that the proximal segment is seated correctly within the glenoid fossa before attempting to reduce the fragments, especially if it is a non–tooth-bearing fragment (Figure 54.17). If not seated properly, upon the release of MMF post-fixation, the "attained" occlusion will be lost once the patient is out of anesthesia.

Miniplates. Simple, isolated undisplaced or minimally displaced fractures of the angle can be successfully treated using a single 2 mm miniplate on the superior border along the ideal osteosynthetic lines of Champy (Figure 54.18). The plate can be a 4- or 6-hole with bar depending on the bone available for screw fixation or a straight plate that allows extra holes to span the fracture site. A 2–4 mm gap may be noted at the inferior border after superior border plating. This usually does not cause concern because the proximal segment eventually rotates antero-superiorly due to micro movements that occur between the segments during post-operative mandibular function and the gap closes.

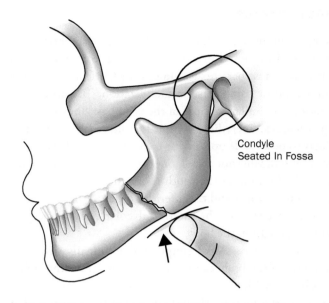

Condyle
Seated In Fossa

Figure 54.17. Digital pressure at the mandibular angle upward while externally palpating the condyle extraorally in the preauricular region.

Rigid or Load-Bearing Osteosynthesis

In the presence of coexisting fractures of the mandible, such as in the opposite condyle or symphysis, if it is decided to treat the second fracture by closed method or nonrigid fixation, then one should consider a more rigid fixation for the angle fracture, either by using another miniplate at the inferior border [41] or by using a load-bearing plate. Severely displaced angle fractures or those with fragmentation are indicated for rigid fixation using a larger load-bearing plate with at least three holes spanning on each side of the fracture (Figure 54.19). It is recommended to simplify the

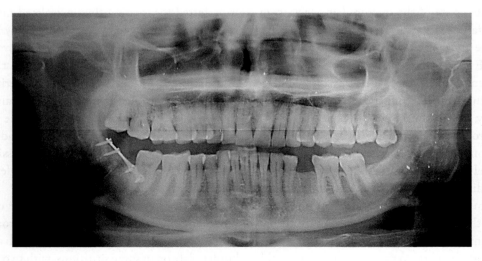

Figure 54.18. Orthopantomogram showing superior border plating with miniplate.

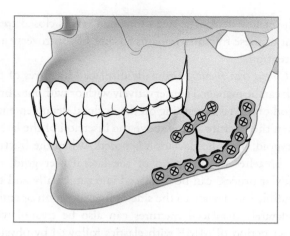

Figure 54.19. Diagram showing rigid fixation using 2.4 mm reconstruction plate after simplification with a superior miniplate.

fragments using miniplates to attain a structure on which the load-bearing plates can be contoured using a template.

RAMUS

Fractures of the ramus are rare, accounting for only 2.5% of the fractures of the mandible. Flanked by the masseter laterally, the medial pterygoid medially, and cradled by the pterygomassetric sling, fractures of the ramus are seldom displaced. Since it constitutes the nondentate segment of the mandible, occlusal discrepancy is rare when it occurs in isolation. These fractures can usually be managed nonsurgically with observation and soft diet. Some patients may benefit from immobilization with MMF in the acute period. Fractures extending low, just above the angle region, and/or displaced segments may require ORIF. The submandibular, intraoral, or retromandibular approach are options, depending on the fracture pattern, if ORIF is indicated. Mini-plate fixation is generally adequate.

CORONOID PROCESS

Fractures of the coronoid are rare and, when they occur, are rarely displaced. They can be managed conservatively with good results. Only rarely do they require open reduction and fixation.[42] The authors of this chapter have never had to treat a coronoid process fracture surgically, and it should be noted that patients who for other reasons have required a coronoid resection do well.

CONDYLAR PROCESS

The condylar process forms the main articulating component of the mandible and gains more importance because

of the complexity of the structures related to it and the role played by it during growth. The treatment is dictated by the patient's age, presence of other coexisting fractures (mandibular or maxillary), unilateral or bilateral nature of the condylar fracture, the degree of displacement of the process, and the surgeon's experience. The condyle is the second most commonly encountered fracture of the mandible (23.8%) owing to it being an area of natural weakness.

Fractures of the condylar process will be dealt with under the titles of condylar head (intracapsular or diacapitular fractures), condylar neck, and subcondylar fractures, adhering to Loukota et al.'s[43,44] classification. Although consensus has been reached for the nonsurgical management of fractures of the condylar process in children, their management in adults is still debated.

Surgical access. Access to the condylar process is commonly extraoral. Depending on the site of fracture and the preference of the surgeon, access can be accomplished either through the retromandibular incision, modified Risdon incision, preauricular incision, or, rarely, a modified endaural incision and intraorally (often endoscopically assisted). The retromandibular incision or the Hind's approach saves dissection time and is a more direct approach. The incision is placed 0.5 mm below the ear lobe parallel to and behind the posterior border of the mandible. The area of interest can be accessed either through a transparotid or retroparotid approach.[27] If transparotid is preferred, care must be taken to close the parotid fascia watertight to prevent a sialocele. Care should be taken to protect the facial nerve and, in particular, the marginal mandibular branch with the retromandibular and submandibular approaches.

With the preauricular approach, it is important to preserve the temporal or frontal branch of the facial nerve. The temporal branch should be protected if the surgeon stays deep to the superficial layer of the temporal fascia.[27] At the root of the zygoma, an incision is placed on the periosteum, that is then stripped lateral to the arch. Dissection proceeds inferiorly in the subperiosteal plane until the condylar neck is reached.

The transoral approach to the condylar neck is now being practiced by many surgeons with the aid of the endoscope. The incision is similar to that for the angle of mandible. Adequate visualization is then made possible using the endoscope. Special right-angled instruments are essential while trying to plate the condyle transorally. This leaves no external scar, and the facial nerve is protected. The endoscope can also be used together with the submandibular approach to better visualize the higher fractures. For some surgeons, it may be possible to achieve similar results using dental mirrors rather than an endoscope.

Condylar Head Fractures

Condylar head fractures are usually intracapsular injuries and may or may not include the articulating surface (Figure 54.20). The hematoma that occurs as a result of the injury tends to predispose the condyle toward ankylosis if the joint is left immobile for a prolonged period of time. Not only does the injury itself severely compromise the blood supply, the structure is too small to allow adequate hardware placement. These fractures are therefore best treated conservatively by most surgeons. When these fractures do not alter occlusion, the patient can be advised to eat a soft diet and encouraged to perform early limited function. In the event of a more significant injury, the hematoma in the articulating space can displace the condyle downward, causing an open bite posteriorly on the side of the fracture and deviation on opening to the opposite side. These patients may benefit with a short period of MMF of about 7–10 days or for a maximum of 2 weeks using elastics to tide over the acute phase of pain and discomfort while trying to maintain the occlusion and limited function. This should be followed by a period of physical therapy which will gradually increase mouth opening and help in performing greater range of lateral excursions. Early mobilization is of paramount importance in this fracture management to prevent the onset of ankylosis, especially in children.

Condylar Neck Fractures

When more than half of the fracture is superior to an imaginary line extending from the most inferior portion of the sigmoid notch perpendicular to the tangent of the ramus (line C–D in Figure 54.20), the fracture is referred to as a condylar neck fracture. The fracture can accordingly be

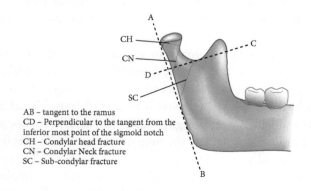

AB – tangent to the ramus
CD – Perpendicular to the tangent from the inferior most point of the sigmoid notch
CH – Condylar head fracture
CN – Condylar Neck fracture
SC – Sub-condylar fracture

Figure 54.20. Subclassifications of fractures of the condylar process, as proposed by Loukota et al.[50]

high- or low-neck. The need for open versus closed treatment of these fractures remains a point of controversy and contention.

Closed treatment. Minimally displaced fractures of the neck can be managed conservatively with or without a brief period of MMF depending on the occlusal derangement.[45] When the fracture line is above the insertion of the lateral pterygoid, often no deviation is noted. When the fracture line breaches the insertion of the lateral pterygoid, the condylar process can be displaced anteromedially and the mandible can deviate to the side of fracture upon opening. Moderately displaced fractures can also be treated with a brief period of MMF with elastics followed by physical therapy with guiding elastics to correct the deviation on opening.

Open treatment. If maintaining a stable occlusion becomes difficult in an extracapsular, low condylar neck fracture, or if the fracture is significantly displaced, ORIF can be contemplated.

Surgical access. The fracture site can be exposed using any of the incisions mentioned previously and is left to the comfort of the surgeon.

Technique. Once the fracture is exposed, the proximal segment has to be reduced to align the fracture. The mandibular fragment has to be distracted in the caudad direction to allow the displaced proximal fragment to be reduced into position. The assistant can distract the mandible manually if the displacement is not too great. More and prolonged distraction may be required for moderate to severe displacements, and this can be attained either by drilling a monocortical screw at the angle and placing a wire around the screw head or placing a wire through a hole drilled through the angle and using the wire to distract the mandible in the caudad direction. A spinal needle can be used to pierce the skin in the neck, inferior to the angle and thread this wire to a screw in the angle or loop the wire through the hole that has been drilled in the angle to allow for a better trajectory of pull in the caudad direction. By preserving the periosteum on lingual side of the subcondylar fracture, a downward traction at the angle of the mandible helps align the fracture segments by ligamentotaxis. This maneuver can also be accomplished by placing a bone clamp on the ramus of the mandible and pulling in a caudad direction. The proximal segment can be aligned by drilling the hole closest to the fracture in the proximal segment first to gain better control of the segment. The distal segment can then be distracted inferior and anterior to reestablish posterior height before inserting all the screws on the plate.

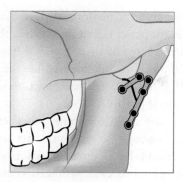

Figure 54.21. Fixation of screw into the proximal segment (A) and distracting the mandible manually to help align the proximal fragment (B); preferred placement of miniplates (C).

Miniplates. Biomechanical studies of the mandible have shown that torsional forces act in the functioning condyle.[46] Hence, the best stability of theses fractures is attained using two miniplates or a single larger plate.

If a single plate is used, a 2 mm large-profile miniplate is centered over the long axis of the condylar process. When the quantity of the bone allows for the placement of two miniplates, two are preferred over a single plate. The distal mandibular segment can be distracted inferiorly by using a bite block or fixing a bone clamp or a screw to the angle of the mandible on the side of fracture to help in distracting the mandible inferiorly to aid in reducing the displaced proximal segment. If there is inadequate room for a multihole anterior plate, a two-hole plate with bar or a continuous three-hole 2 mm miniplate may be used to serve as an antirotation plate (Figure 54.21). This also helps to stabilize the proximal fragment while a four-hole plate with bar or a five-hole plate can be adapted closely to the posterior border of the mandible.

Joos and Kleinheinz[47] list absolute indications for nonsurgical treatment of condylar fractures as including condylar neck fractures in children, high condylar neck fractures without dislocation, and intracapsular condylar fractures.

Subcondylar Fractures

When more than half of the fracture is inferior to the line extending from the most inferior portion of the sigmoid notch perpendicular to the tangent of the ramus, the fractures are said to be subcondylar (Figure 54.20). Their management remains controversial, with some favoring open reduction to correct the posterior ramal height and to ensure early mobilization with full range of movements.

As with the condylar neck, these fractures can be managed by observation and a soft diet, and closed treatment with MMF followed by physical therapy or ORIF.

Closed treatment. The condyle has been known to have regenerative abilities. In the very young patients, the regeneration that occurs is called *restitutional remodeling,* where a new condyle with normal morphology is recreated. In the adult, however, the remodeling potential is less robust and the regenerated condyle has an altered morphology and is referred to as *functional remodeling.* Functionally, the new condyle works just as well. This remodeling one of the main reasons[45] that these fractures heal well with closed treatment.[48–50] The degree of displacement and the dislocation of the condyle determines the choice of treatment.[50–55]

The absolute indications for ORIF are listed above.

Conservative treatment of minimally displaced subcondylar fractures (<10 degrees of displacement)[51] will involve MMF with guiding elastics and physical therapy. Guiding elastics are used to correct the deviation on opening. After 2 weeks, physical therapy should be included to improve mouth opening and the lateral excursions of the mandible. We recommend MMF with elastics rather than rigid wire fixation as invariably there is some amount of muscle wasting that occurs due to the rigid immobilization, and restitution of normal excursions takes a long time.[56] Moderately displaced subcondylar fractures (between 10 and 45 degree displacements)[51,57] are controversial to treat. If the occlusion can be attained and maintained stable after the release of the MMF, these fractures can also be managed with a brief period of MMF with elastics for 2 weeks before mobilizing the jaw freely. The condyle has proved to have great healing potential and undergoes excellent functional, skeletal, and dental remodeling. The reduced ramal height on the affected side is an adaptive mechanism to ensure optimal function.

Bilateral subcondylar fractures need special mention in terms of fracture reduction. When there is no articulation with the temporal bone to establish posterior vertical support, the patient may be able to bring the teeth into occlusion because of complex neuromuscular adaptations by the masticatory muscles. In the event that the patient is unable to bring the teeth into occlusion, one can also use the principle of a *hypomochlion,* where a spacer is placed between the posterior dentition, and the patient is placed into MMF.[58] The inferior distraction of the ramus may help to "upright" the displaced condylar process. These fractures benefit from ORIF of at least one of the fractures to establish the posterior vertical height, especially if associated with other fractures of the mandible and maxilla.[45,59,60]

Open treatment. When an attempt has been made to treat the fracture using a closed method and the occlusion is found to be deranged and unstable after the release of MMF, ORIF should be considered. The approach can be extraoral—either an extended submandibular, retromandibular, or transoral approach with endoscopic assistance. The reduction and plating is similar to that described under condylar neck fractures.

Severely displaced subcondylar fractures (>45 degrees of displacement)[51,57] are definite candidates for ORIF. These fractures will also have significant reduction in the ramal height on the affected side. These fractures are best fixed using either two miniplates, a three-dimensional plate, or a single heavy plate with bicortical fixation if the surgeon is experienced and comfortable with these techniques.

Surgical access. The fracture site can be exposed using any of the incisions mentioned previously and is left to the comfort of the surgeon.

Technique. The technique for fracture reduction is performed as explained previously. Low subcondylar fractures are easily visible and amenable to reduction.

Miniplates. Miniplates are commonly used to fix the condyle segment. Two four-hole, straight 2 mm miniplates are advocated as standard to rigidly fix the subcondylar fractures. This amount of rigidity is required to stabilize the proximal segment against the action of the masticatory muscles when in function. Alternatively, a single 2 mm compression plate can also be used.[61–64]

In some cases where the reduction cannot be achieved and malocclusion persists, a Le Fort I osteotomy may have to be considered to restore the patient's premorbid occlusion.

POSTOPERATIVE CARE

IMMEDIATE POSTOP

Fractures of the dentate mandible are usually compound intraorally and those further compounded by skin lacerations will benefit from adequate pre- and perioperative antibiotics with a spectrum that covers both oral and skin flora. It is important to protect the airway during emergence from anesthesia, and care should be taken to aspirate the stomach prior to extubation. Patients should be extubated only upon recovery of protective reflexes. Maintaining an elevated head position will help in resolving edema and in swallowing. Using elastics

(short rubber bands) to achieve MMF has the advantage of being easier for patients, family, and healthcare workers to remove in the event of an emergency. If wires are used, wire cutters should be available bedside for emergent release of MMF if needed. Adequate suction should also be present bedside, if possible.

If there is any question about whether the patient will be awake enough to maintain his or her airway, extubation should be deferred until the appropriate time. In cases of significant panfacial edema where the nasal airway may be compromised for a period of time, consideration should be made to leave the arch bars on but remove the elastics or wires of MMF, to be reapplied a within a few days after surgery, when the edema has improved and the patient is in a more reliable state to maintain an airway.

DIET AND NUTRITION

Clear fluids may be given once the patient has voluntary control of airway and swallowing reflexes. However, patients who have to be in MMF postoperatively tend to have an oral intake much less than adequate. It is important to maintain intravenous hydration until patients can train themselves to take in adequate oral fluids. Subsequently, they can advance to full fluids or blenderized foods. Those patients who are still unconscious or have a tracheostomy will need flexible feeding tubes to maintain their nutrition.

ORAL HYGIENE

Postoperative oral hygiene is of paramount importance to ensure the healing of intraoral wounds. Patients should be encouraged to use soft, pediatric brushes to clean their teeth gently as plaque begins to accumulate almost instantaneously. Gentle irrigation with saline or chlorhexidine mouthwashes using oral irrigators will help dislodge materia alba from the intraoral wound surfaces and sutures. When in MMF, it becomes even more difficult for patients to maintain hygiene as most teeth surfaces and mucosa become inaccessible to brushing. Oral irrigations and brushing the accessible areas are strongly encouraged. These patients will benefit from intermittent release of their MMF to clean their mouths once the occlusion has stabilized.

REHABILITATION

It is important to rehabilitate patients following treatment of fractures in terms of restoring muscular activity and teeth lost or damaged from trauma. People treated with MMF for condylar fractures may require physical therapy with isometric exercises against resistance and with guiding elastics. Minor occlusal discrepancies may have to be adjusted.

SPECIAL SITUATIONS REQUIRING LOAD-BEARING OSTEOSYNTHESIS

Load-bearing osteosynthesis is indicated where there is insufficient good bone to count on adequate stability for load-sharing. This could include an actual defect from significant avulsive trauma, a segmental defect in the mandible from tumor extirpation, or compromised bone following a dental extraction. In the case of an atrophic edentulous mandible, there is too little remaining bone to provide bone-sharing. In the case of an infected mandible with loose hardware, this is the equivalent of a defect as larger plates are needed to span and bypass the segments of infected or compromised bone. In the case of severe comminution, the segments offer so little stability that they need to be spanned in the same way that an actual defect is spanned.

DEFECT FRACTURES

These fractures typically exhibit loss of bone in the fractured area. Load-sharing techniques require adequate bone buttressing. When there is lack of bone buttressing (due to loss of bone), it becomes essential to place hardware strong enough to bear the entire mechanical load: 2.4 mm reconstruction or locking screw plates are placed spanning the defect with at least three holes on either side of the defect. Once stabilized, the need for grafting the defect using autogenous cancellous bone may be considered depending on the extent of the defect and the nature of the wound bed.

INFECTED FRACTURES

Mandibular fractures presenting late may be infected owing to the compound nature of these fractures and movements between the segments. Post treatment, fracture sites may become infected due to loose hardware, inappropriate fixation, and the presence of infected teeth in the vicinity of the fracture. In the past, some have advocated treating these fractures with antibiotics, MMF, and external fixators.[65] Those chronically infected will present with unhealthy

nonviable bone which will need debridement. An infected mandibular fracture treated with antibiotics alone as the primary treatment is generally inappropriate. Infection after a fracture or a fracture reduction suggests that a surgical intervention of some kind is required as it is either due to nonunion, failed hardware, a loose sequestrum of bone and/or hardware, or a periapical problem. If a tooth in the line of fracture is a cause for the infection, it will need to be extracted. This, along with debridement of the necrotic bone, presents a defect situation. The removal of infected edges of bone will also prevent bone buttressing. A more recent trend for these fractures is to avoid the use of external fixation and instead use internal fixation with load-bearing 2.4 mm reconstruction or locking screw plates to provide maximum stability. If needed, the bone defects will need to be grafted. The use of culture and sensitivity testing and suitable antibiotics is an important adjunct in treating infected fractures.[65-67]

COMMINUTION

According to Kazanjian, "the majority of non-united fractures are due to inadequate immobilization of comminuted fragments of bone, and subsequent infection, rather than to initial loss of bone."[68,69]

Stabilization of the bony fragments is identified as being most important for a reliable bony union, often with a load-bearing plate (Figure 54.22). ORIF is now advocated for comminuted fractures as it has been proved that stabilizing the fragments is most important for bony union and the sparse denudation of fragments that occurs in the process does not adversely affect the blood supply.[70-72]

Minimally displaced fractures with comminution may be treated by a closed method in a compliant patient. Displaced fractures with comminution are treated using load-bearing osteosynthesis to rigidly fix and stabilize the fracture. The hardware used is a large 2.4 mm conventional/locking reconstruction plate spanning the area of comminution, with at least three screws on either side of the defect. Simplifying the fracture using small adaptation plates to hold the segments together gives a more stable structure to work on while contouring the larger reconstruction plate. The adaption plates can be retained or removed if the surgeon feels the segments are adequately held together.

ATROPHIC MANDIBLE

Atrophic mandibles present a special challenge because of their minimal cross-sectional area of bone combined with

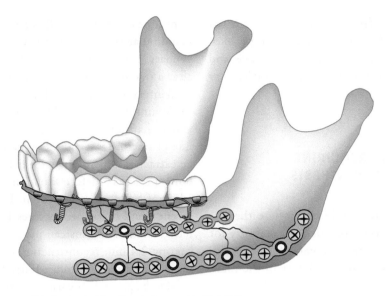

Figure 54.22. Comminuted fracture mandible fixed using load-bearing reconstruction plate.

their poor quality of bone. It is impossible to maintain stability between the fragments using a closed treatment method due to the pull of the masticatory muscles. These fractures should almost always be treated by ORIF. The plate applied across this fracture will therefore need be strong enough to bear all of the masticatory load during function and demands a load-bearing osteosynthesis.[73,74] Because of the poor quality of bone, the need to use a larger reconstruction place, the difficulty in achieving the proper contour of the mandible using a large plate, and the position of the alveolar nerve along the superior rim of the mandible, an extraoral apron incision in the submandibular area is recommended. Some fractures may also require the addition of autogenous bone or bone products to promote osseous union due to an otherwise deficit in the periosteal component.[75] Bilateral parasymphysis fracture in an atrophic mandible has been referred to as a "bucket handle fracture," and the anterior fragment can be posteriorly displaced due to the action of the genioglossus and cause airway interference due to the posterior movement of the tongue compromising the airway (Figure 54.23).

It should be noted that, in Figure 54.24, that the atrophic bone is so thin that the reconstruction plate is wider than the remaining bone in this patient. These patients should be warned that they cannot wear their previous dentures. If the patient is having difficulty fitting new dentures, the surgeon faces the challenging question of whether he or she would ever dare to remove this plate.

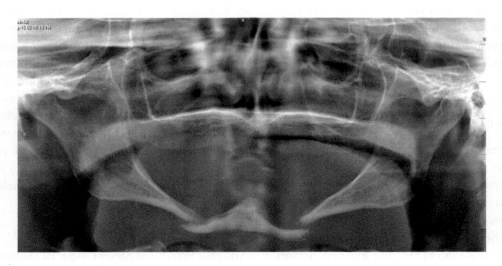

Figure 54.23. Orthopantomogram demonstrates a comminuted atrophic mandible with minimal bone height and bilateral fractured segments.

MAXILLOFACIAL SURGERY

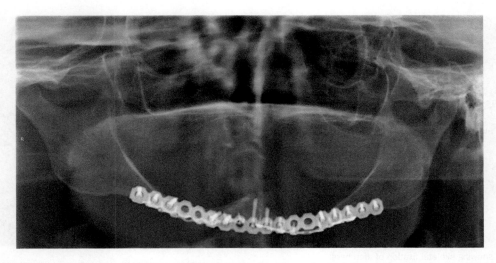

Figure 54.24. Orthopantomogram demonstrates the postop reduction of the previous figure. A miniplate was first placed on the inferior border of one of the fractures to allow better stability during the bending of a template and bending of the more important large reconstruction plate.

PEDIATRIC FRACTURES

Treatment of these fractures are unique for many reasons. The teeth are often in different stages of root resorption if the patient is in the mixed dentition stage. The pediatric skeleton has excellent osteogenic potential and heals very quickly, often without any intervention. Being in the growing stage, trauma itself can hamper growth, so treatment should not further impede growth. The pediatric bone is very resilient, accounting for the large number of greenstick fractures.[76] The fracture pattern of the mandible after the age of 10 years usually mimics that of the adult.[77] Minor discrepancies in occlusion are almost insignificant with maturation. The presence of the permanent tooth buds makes it difficult to consider using plates and screws

without injuring tooth buds. The shape of the deciduous dentition makes it hard to anchor arch bars.

Fractures of the dentate mandible can often be managed by observation alone, monomandibular fixation with occlusal/lingual splints (Figure 54.25), MMF (Figure 54.26), or ORIF. Needless to say, the nature of the fracture and the age of the patient will dictate the choice of treatment. Most pediatric fractures can be managed by manual reduction and fixation using an occlusal and/or lingual splint using circummandibular wires. Contrary to the belief that children may not tolerate MMF, when properly explained, some children tolerate it well. The dentition might mandate securing the superior arch with pyriform wiring and the lower arch with circummandibular wires (Figure 54.26). Techniques to accomplish this are demonstrated in Figures 54.27 and 54.28).

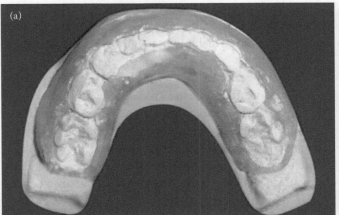
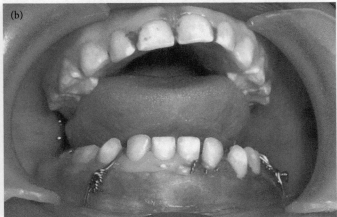

Figure 54.25. (A) Occlusal splint on both the lingual and labial sides of the teeth leaving the occlusal side open and (B) mono-mandibular fixation with circum-mandibular wiring.

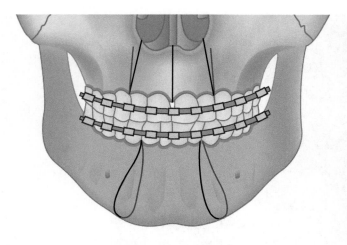

Figure 54.26. Diagram showing skeletal fixation of arch bars.

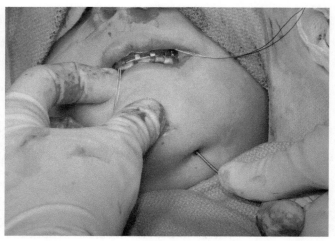

Figure 54.28. Placement of circummandibular wires. The photo shows an awl being used to puncture the skin to pull a wire on the buccal side and then push it around the inferior part of the mandible, feeding the wire cephalad on the lingual side. This wire is then fixated to the mandibular arch bar to hold it in the caudad position of a patient with deciduous dentition.

The duration of complete immobilization should be minimal (7–10 days) to prevent ankylosis. Some cases, however, may need ORIF to be stabilized. In such cases, care should be taken to place the plate at the inferior border, away from the tooth buds. If resorbable plates are not used, the surgeon must contemplate plate removal after the healing period to allow unrestricted growth. If the surgeon waits too long to remove the hardware, it will be incorporated by the growing bone.

Fractures of the condylar process commonly occur in the head of the condyle following an anterior trauma to the chin. This is contrary to adults, as the pediatric neck is usually short and stubby. Various studies have documented rapid, progressive restitutional remodeling resulting in the formation of a new condyle with normal morphology.[45,49,78,79]

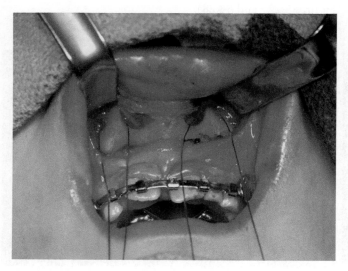

Figure 54.27. Piriform wires being placed in a pediatric patient to prevent the upper arch bar from slipping off of the teeth when the patient tries to open his mouth.

Closed treatment of fractures of the condylar process is the accepted treatment norm in children, with a very brief period of immobilization if necessary (7–10 days). This should be followed by aggressive physical therapy, if necessary, with guiding elastics used judiciously to prevent ankylosis.

COMPLICATIONS

Complications following mandibular fractures are not uncommon. Failure to seek treatment, nature of the primary injury, and inadequate treatment are the factors commonly contributing to the occurrence of complications. Immediate complications such as bleeding or soft tissue loss are dealt with during primary management. Of more concern are complications that arise after treatment of fractures. They include infection, malunion, nonunion, TMJ disorders, and nerve injury.

Infections may occur either in the early or late postoperative period. If in the soft tissue alone and acute, incision and drainage should be done and adequate antibiotics prescribed. Infections also occur most commonly from inadequate fixation, causing the segments to move and also when the screws loosen. This invariably requires retreatment with adequate debridement and fixation as discussed under infected fractures.

Malunion of mandible fractures commonly results from inadequate reduction and fixation or missed concomitant fractures. This presents as malocclusion with inability to function normally and, in some cases, as a facial deformity. Minor occlusal discrepancies can be corrected orthodontically. Surgical intervention in the form of osteotomies or refracturing may be required for more severe problems.[80]

Nonunions, though rare in the craniofacial skeleton, have been associated with mandibular fractures, most commonly at the mandibular body. Various factors contribute to nonhealing of a fracture, such as inadequate immobilization, anatomic location (body), teeth in the line of fracture, and the occurrence of late postsurgical infections.[81] Nonunion is more commonly associated with complex multiple fractures.[82] The treatment of nonunion generally consists of removing any infected teeth and bone, debriding the fracture, and reapplying rigid internal fixation with or without bone grafting.[82]

TMJ disorders are occasionally noted as a sequel to fractures of the condylar process. There can be damage to the surrounding soft tissues, especially the articular disk, causing potential growth disturbances, ankylosis, malocclusion, and iatrogenic injuries as a consequence of surgical treatment.

Sensory nerve injury is also a commonly encountered complication, especially in mandibular body fractures.[83] These injuries may be due to the trauma itself or iatrogenic due to surgical complications, improper placement of plates and screws, or the extraction of teeth, especially third molars, that may be in the line of fracture. Most of these nerve injuries are temporary in nature as they occur as a result of compression or stretching of the involved nerves. In markedly displaced fractures, however, complete transection of the nerve can occur, causing permanent neural dysfunction.[80]

CONCLUSION

As the second most commonly encountered fracture in the craniofacial skeleton, the horseshoe shape of the bone, the biomechanics of the bone, and role it has to play in esthetics, function, and occlusion makes the treatment of mandibular fractures challenging. The characteristics of the fracture will invariably determine the type of treatment. The skills and experience of the surgeon will also largely determine the choice of treatment option. It is mandatory to adhere to the principles of fracture fixation at all times—anatomical reduction, stable fixation, preservation of adequate blood supply, and early mobilization—as well as the circumstances of the patient regarding issues of maturity, compliance, health, nutrition, hygiene, immune status, and smoking history.

REFERENCES

1. Erich JB, Austin LT. *Traumatic Injuries of the Facial Bones.* Philadelphia: WB Saunders, 1944.
2. Gilmer TL. A case of fracture of the lower jaw with remarks on treatment. *Arch Dent* 1887;4:388.
3. Halazonetis JA. The weak regions of the mandible. *Br J Oral Surg* 1968;6(1):37–48.
4. Huelke DF. Location of mandibular fractures related to teeth and edentulous regions. *J Oral Surg Anesth Hosp Dent Serv* 1964;Sep 22:396–405.
5. Nahum AM. The biomechanics of maxillofacial trauma. *Clin Plast Surg* 1975;2(1):59–64.
6. Luce EA, Tubb TD, Moore AM. Review of 1,000 major facial fractures and associated injuries. *Plast Reconstr Surg* 1979;63(1): 26–30.
7. Harley F, Champy M, Terry BC. *Atlas of Craniomaxillofacial Osteosynthesis.* Stuttgart: Thieme, 1999;3–5.
8. Schubert W, Kobiena BJ, Pollock RA. The cross sectional area of the mandible. *J Oral Maxillofac Surg* 1997;55:689–692.
9. Cutright B, Quillopa N, Schubert W. An anthropometric analysis of the key foramina of maxillofacial surgery. *J Oral Maxillofac Surg* 2003;61:354–357.
10. Sun-Kyoung Yu, et al. Morphological assessment of the anterior loop of the mandibular canal in Koreans. *Anat Cell Biol* 2015;48(8):75–80.
11. Morrow BT, Samson TD, Schubert W, Mackay DR. Evidence-based medicine: mandible fractures. *Plast Reconstr Surg* 2014;134:1381.
12. Pauwels F. Bedeutung und kausale Erklarung der Spongiosaarchitektur in neuer Auffassung. *Arztl Wochenschr* 1948;3:379.
13. Huelke DF, Harger JH. Maxillofacial injuries: their nature and mechanisms of production. *J Oral Surg* 1969;27:451–60.
14. Huelke DF, Patrick LM. Mechanics in the production of mandible fractures: strain-gauge measurement of the impacts to the chin. *J Dent Res* 1964;43:437–446.
15. Shetty V, Atchison K, Belin T, Jiamming W. Clinician variability in characterizing mandibular fractures. *J Oral Maxillofac Surg* 2001;59:254–261.
16. Wilson IF, Lokeh A, Benjamin CI, et al. Contribution of conventional axial CT (non-helical), in conjunction with panoramic tomography (zonography), in evaluating mandibular fractures. *Ann Plast Surg* 2000;45:415–421.
17. Wilson IF, Lokeh A, Benjamin CI, et al. Prospective comparison of panoramic tomography (zonography) and helical computed tomography in the diagnosis and operative management of mandibular fractures. *Plast Reconstruct Surg* 2001;107:1369–1375.
18. Kelly J. *War Injuries to the Jaws and Related Structures.* Washington DC: US Government Printing Office, 1978.
19. Champy M, Pape H-D, Gerlach KL, et al. The Strasbourg miniplate osteosynthesis. In: Kruger E, Schilli W, eds. *Oral and Maxillofacial Traumatology*, Vol. 2. Chicago: Quintessence, 1986:19–43.
20. Haug RH, Street CC, Goltz M. Does plate adaptation affect stability? A biomechanical comparison of locking and non-locking plates. *J Oral Maxillofac Surg* 2002;60:1319.
21. Prein J, Rahn BA. Scientific and technical background. In: Prein J, ed. *Manual of Internal Fixation in the Cranio-Facial Skeleton: Techniques Recommended by the AO/ASIF Maxillofacial Group.* New York, Springer, 1998:9.
22. Ellis E, Moos KF, El-Attar A. 10 years of mandibular fractures: an analysis of 2,137 cases. *Oral Surg Oral Med Oral Pathol* 1985;59: 120–123.
23. Chuong R, Donoff RB, Guralnick WC, et al. A retrospective analysis of 327 mandibular fractures. *J Oral Maxillofac Surg* 1983;41:305.
24. Shetty V, Freymiller E. Teeth in the line of fracture: a review. *J Oral Maxillofac Surg* 1989;47:1303–1306.

25. Champy M, Lodde JP, Schmitt R, et al. Mandibular osteosynthesis by miniature screwed bone plates via a buccal approach. *J Oral Maxillofac Surg* 1978;6:14.

26. Chritah A, Lazow SK, Berger J. Transoral 2.0-mm miniplate fixation of mandibular fractures plus 2 weeks maxillomandibular fixation: A prospective study. *J Oral Maxillofac Surg* 2002;60:167–170.

27. Ellis 3rd E, Zide MF. Transoral approaches to the facial skeleton. Section 4. In: Ellis 3rd E, Zide MF, eds. *Surgical Approaches to the Facial Skeleton*. 2nd ed. Philadelphia, PA: Lippincott Williams & Wilkins, 2005:109–150.

28. Dingman RO, Grabb WC. Surgical anatomy of the mandibular ramus of the facial nerve based on the dissection of 100 facial halves. *Plast Reconst Surg* 1962;29(3):266–272.

29. Wang TM, Lin CL, Kuo KJ, Shih C. Surgical anatomy of mandibular ramus of the facial nerve in Chinese adults. *Acta Anat (Basel)* 1991;142:126–131.

30. Woltmann M, de Faveri R, Sgrott EA. Anatomosurgical study of the marginal mandibular branch of the facial nerve for submandibular surgical approach. *Brazilian Dental Journal* 2006;17(1):71–74.

31. Gerlach KL, Schwarz A. Bite forces in patients after treatment of mandibular angle fractures with miniplate osteosynthesis according to Champy. *Int J Oral Maxillofac Surg* 2002;31:345–348.

32. Tate GS, Ellis E, Throckmorton GS, et al. Bite forces in patients treated for mandibular anglefractures—implications for fixation recommendations. *J Oral Maxillofac Surg* 1994;52:734–736.

33. Spiessl B. New concepts in maxillofacial bone surgery. In: Spiessl B, ed. *Principles of Rigid Internal Fixation in Fractures of the Lower Jaw*. Berlin: Springer-Verlag, 1976.

34. Wald RM, Abemayor E, Zemplenyi J, et al. The transoral treatment of mandibular fractures using noncompression miniplates: a prospective study. *Ann Plast Surg* 1988;20:409–413.

35. Fox AJ, Kellman RM. Mandibular angle fractures: two-miniplate fixation and complications. *Arch Facial Plast Surg* 2003;5:464–469.

36. Cawood JI. Small plate osteosynthesis of mandibular fractures. *Br J Oral Maxillofac Surg* 1985;23:77–91.

37. Ellis E, Walker LR. Treatment of mandibular angle fractures using one non compression miniplate. *J Oral Maxillofac Surg* 1996;54:864–871.

38. Ewers R, Ha¨rle F. Biomechanics of the midface and mandibular fractures: Is a stable fixation necessary? In: Hjorting-Hansen E, ed. *Oral and Maxillofacial Surgery. Proceedings from the 8th International Conference on Oral and Maxillofacial Surgery*. Chicago: Quintessence, 1985:207–211.

39. Barry CP, Kearns GJ. Superior border plating technique in the management of isolated mandibular angle fractures: a retrospective study of 50 consecutive patients. *J Oral Maxillofac Surg* 2007;65:1544–1549.

40. Gear AJ, Apasova E, Schmitz JP, et al. Treatment modalities for mandibular angle fractures. *J Oral Maxillofac Surg* 2005;63:655–663.

41. Ellis E, Walker L. Treatment of mandibular angle fractures using two noncompression miniplates. *J Oral Maxillofac Surg* 1994;52:1032–1036.

42. Shen L, Li J, Li P, Long J, Tian W, Tang W. Mandibular coronoid fractures: treatment options. *Int J Oral Maxillofac Surg* 2013 Jun;42(6):721–726.

43. Loukota RA, Eckelt U, De Bont L, Rasse M. Sub-classification of fractures of the condylar process of the mandible. *Br J Oral Maxillofac Surg* 2005 Feb;43(1):72–73.

44. Cenzi R, Burlini D, Arduin L, Zollino I, Guidi R, Carinci F. Mandibular condyle fractures: evaluation of the Strasbourg Osteosynthesis Research Group classification. *J Craniofac Surg* 2009 Jan;20(1):24–28.

45. Ellis III E, Throckmorton GS. Treatment of mandibular condylar process fractures: biological considerations. *J Oral Maxillofac Surg* 2005;63:115–134.

46. Koolstra JH, van Eijden TM: Biomechanical analysis of jaw closing movements. *J Dent Res* 1995;74:1564.

47. Kleinheinz J, Anastassov GE, Joos U. Indications for treatment of subcondylar mandibular fractures. *J Craniomaxillofac Trauma* 1999 summer;5(2):17–23; discussion: 24–26.

48. Haug RH, Assael LA. Outcomes of open versus closed treatment of mandibular subcondylar fractures. *J Oral Maxillofac Surg* 2001;59:370–375.

49. Steisch-Scholz M, Schmidt S, Eckardt A. Condylar motion after open and closed treatment of mandibular condylar fractures. *J Oral Maxillofac Surg* 2005;63:1304–1309.

50. Throckmorton GS, Ellis E. Recovery of mandibular motion after closed and open treatment of unilateral mandibular condylar process fractures. *J Oral Maxillofac Surg* 2000;29:421–427.

51. Palmieri C, Ellis III E, Throckmorton G. Mandibular motion after closed and open treatment of unilateral mandibular condylar process fractures. *Oral Maxillofac Surg* 1999;57:764–775.

52. Ellis E, Throckmorton GS, Palmieri C. Open treatment of condylar process fractures: assessment of adequacy of repositioning and maintenance of stability. *J Oral Maxillofac Surg* 2000;58:27.

53. Ellis E 3rd, Simon P, Throckmorton GS. Occlusal results after open or closed treatment of fractures of the mandibular condylar process. *J Oral Maxillofac Surg* 2000;58:260.

54. Ellis E 3rd, Throckmorton G. Facial symmetry after closed and open treatment of fractures of the mandibular condylar process. *J Oral Maxillofac Surg* 2000;58:719.

55. Ellis E 3rd, Throckmorton GS. Bite forces after open or closed treatment of mandibular condylar process fractures. *J Oral Maxillofac Surg* 2001;59:389.

56. Bos RRM, Ward Booth RP, de Bont LGM. Mandibular condyle fractures: a consensus. *Br J Oral Maxillofac Surg* 1999;37:87–89.

57. Schneider M, Erasmus F, Gerlach KL, et al. Open reduction and internal fixation versus closed treatment and mandibulo-maxillary fixation of fractures of the mandibular condylar process: a randomized, prospective, multi-centre study with special evaluation of fracture level. *Br J Oral Maxillofac Surg* 2008;66:2537–2544.

58. Yeshaswini T, Shyammohan. Hypomochlion aided reduction for subcondylar fracture. *Kerala Dental Journal* 2014;3(1):16–17.

59. Ellis, E: Condylar process fractures of the mandible. *Facial Plast Surg* 2000;16:193.

60. Ellis III E, Dean J. Rigid fixation of mandibular condyle fractures. *Oral Surg Oral Med Oral Pathol* 1993;76:6–15.

61. Schon R, Gutwald R, Schramm A, Gellrich N C, Schmelzeisen R. Endoscopy-assisted open treatment of condylar fractures of the mandible: extraoral vs intraoral approach. *Int J Oral Maxillofac Surg* 2002;31:237–243.

62. Veras RB, Kriwalsky MS, Eckert AW, Schubert J, Maurer P. Long-term outcomes after treatment of condylar fracture by intraoral access: a functional and radiologic assessment. *J Oral Maxillofac Surg* 2007;65:1470–1476.

63. Champy M, Lodde JP. Mandibular synthesis. Placement of the synthesis as a function of mandibular stress (in French). *Rev Stomatol Chir Maxillofac* 1976;77:971–976.

64. Kokemueller H, Konstantinovic VS, Barth EL, et al. Endoscope-assisted trans-oral reduction and internal fixation versus closed treatment of mandibular condylar process fractures— A prospective double-center study. *J Oral Maxillofac Surg* 2012;70:384–95.

65. Alpert B, Kushner GM, Tiwana PS. Contemporary management of infected mandibular fractures. *Craniomaxillofac Trauma Reconstr* 2008 Nov;1(1):25–29.

66. Alpert B. Management of the complications of mandibular fracture treatment. *Oper Techn Plast Reconst Surg* 1998;5:325–333.

67. Benson P D, Marshall M, Engelstad M, Kushner G M, Alpert B. The use of immediate bone grafting in the reconstruction of clinically infected mandibular fractures: bone grafts in the presence of pus. *J Oral Maxillofac Surg* 2006;64:122–126.

68. Kazanjian VH. An outline of the treatment of extensive comminuted fractures of the mandible (based chiefly on experience gained during the last war). *Am J Orthod Oral Surg* 1942;28:265,

69. Kazanjian VH. Immobilization of wartime, compound, comminuted fractures of the mandible. *Am J Orthod Oral Surg* 1942;28:551.

70. Pistner H, Michel C, Kubler N, et al. Therapeutic concept in comminuted and defect fractures of the mandible. *Fortschr Kiefer Gesichtschir* 1996;41:157.

71. Kuriakose MA, Fardy M, Sirikumara M, et al. A comparative review of 266 mandibular fractures with internal fixation using rigid (AO/ASIF) plates or miniplates. *Br J Oral Maxillofac Surg* 1996;34:315.

72. Ellis E III, Muniz O, Anand K. Treatment considerations for comminuted mandibular fractures. *J Oral Maxillofac Surg* 2003;61:861–870.

73. Schilli W, Stoll P, Bahr W, et al. Mandibular fractures. In: Prein J, ed. *Manual of Internal Fixation in the Cranio-Facial Skeleton.* Berlin: Springer, 1998:87.

74. Ellis E, Price C. Treatment protocol for fractures of the atrophic mandible. *J Oral Maxillofac Surg* 2008;66:421.

75. Ellis E. An algorithm for the treatment of non-condylar mandibular fractures *J Oral Maxillofac Surg* 2014;72:939–949.

76. Kushner GM, Tiwana PS. Fractures of the growing mandible. *Atlas Oral Maxillofacial Surg Clin N Am* 2009;17:81–91.

77. Thoren H, Iizuka T, Halliikainen D, et al. Different patterns of mandibular fractures in children: An analysis of 220 fractures in 157 patients. *J Craniomaxillofac Surg* 1992;20:292–296.

78. Gilhous-Moe O. *Fractures of the Condyle in the Growth Period.* Stockholm: Scandinavian University Books, 1969.

79. Lund K. Mandibular growth and remodelling processes after condylar fracture. *Acta Odontal Scand* 1974;32(64):1–117.

80. Zweig BE. Complications of mandibular fractures. *Atlas Oral Maxillofacial Surg Clin N Am* 2009;17:93–101.

81. Haug RH, Schwimmer A. Fibrous union of the mandible: a review of 27 patients. *J Oral Maxillofac Surg* 1994;52:842.

82. Mathog RH, Toma V, Clayman L, Wolf S. Nonunion of the mandible: an analysis of contributing factors. *J Oral Maxillofac Surg* 2000;58:746.

83. Marchena JM, Padwa BL, Kaban LB. Sensory abnormalities associated with mandibular fractures: incidence and natural history. *J Oral Maxillofac Surg* 1998;56:822.

55.

APPROACH TO UPPER MAXILLOFACIAL FRACTURES

Daniel Murariu, Heather A. McMahon, and Kant Y. Lin

INTRODUCTION

When discussing fractures of the maxillofacial skeleton, the face is classically divided into the upper, midface, and lower regions. In this chapter, fractures of the upper face, specifically frontal sinus fractures, will be discussed.

Anatomically, the frontal region consists of the paired frontal sinuses. These structures are not present at birth and begin to develop in early childhood with radiographic evidence appearing between ages 5–7. They continue to undergo pneumatic expansion until approximately 18–20 years of age. The sinuses are 5–7 mL in volume and are lined by respiratory epithelium with mucin-secreting glands.[1] The mucosal lining has multiple invaginations along the channels of Brechet, which increases the difficulty of complete removal following injury, requiring burring of the bone.[2] The frontal sinus is divided asymmetrically by an intersinus septum, and each is drained by a frontonasal duct or nasofrontal outflow tract (NFOT).[3] This tract is usually located in the posteromedial floor of the sinus and drains into the frontal recess. The frontal recess is bordered by the agger nasi anteriorly, the middle turbinate medially, the ethmoid bulla posteriorly, and the lamina papyracea laterally.[4] The NFOT acts as the only egress for secretions from the frontal sinus. The lining of the sinus as well as the NFOT become clinically important when discussing fractures of this region because, when disrupted or obstructed, there is a high propensity to form a mucocele, as well as the potential for other infectious complications, such as meningitis.[5] The anterior and posterior tables form the borders of the sinus, with the posterior table forming the anterior aspect of the cranial vault. The dura is in close proximity to the posterior table and, along the caudal aspect, is thin and densely adherent.[6] The anterior table is generally twice the thickness of the posterior table and consists of thick cortical bone that can withstand approximately twice the force

of the other facial bones.[7,8] The blood supply of the frontal sinus consists of the supraorbital artery, and it is innervated by the ophthalmic division of the trigeminal nerve.[9]

Frontal sinus fractures represent approximately 5–15% of all craniomaxillofacial injuries. They occur most commonly as a result of high-energy trauma, such as motor vehicle accidents and assaults, and are most frequently seen in males in the second and third decades of life.[8,10] However, recent data suggest a growing number of frontal sinus fractures resulting from other etiologies, such as all-terrain vehicles and falls.[11] Because of the high energy required to fracture the frontal bone, these injuries are commonly seen in conjunction with cervical spine, intracranial, and other maxillofacial fractures.[2]

EVALUATION OF FRONTAL SINUS FRACTURES

Identification and evaluation of frontal sinus fractures typically rely upon physical exam and computed tomography (CT). On physical exam, one must be suspicious for frontal injury if any of the following are observed: periorbital ecchymosis, laceration, contour deformity, anesthesia in the distribution of the supraorbital nerve, subconjunctival hemorrhage, crepitus, tenderness, edema, or change in neurologic status.[3,12] The most commonly associated finding is forehead laceration, and one must have a high index of suspicion for fracture if a frontal laceration is present. Special attention must also be paid to whether there is any evidence of cerebrospinal fluid (CSF) leak as this represents a serious finding concerning for posterior table fracture and associated dural tear.[9,10]

On CT scan, thin slices of 5 mm or less are recommended for maximal diagnostic assistance, and reconstructions are often useful as well. Radiographic assessment should include particular attention to the integrity of the anterior table, posterior table, and, most importantly, to the patency of the NFOT. Obstruction of the NFOT has become increasingly recognized as one of the most important factors in predicting complication following frontal sinus fracture.[10,13] The three best indicators of tract injury include radiographic evidence of gross outflow tract obstruction, frontal sinus floor fracture, and anterior table medial wall fracture.[13]

CLASSIFICATION OF FRONTAL SINUS FRACTURES

Numerous classification systems have been proposed to describe and guide treatment for frontal sinus fractures. On the most basic level, fractures are first distinguished based on the degree of involvement of the anterior table, posterior table, or both. Attention is then turned to whether there is NFOT involvement and whether this has resulted

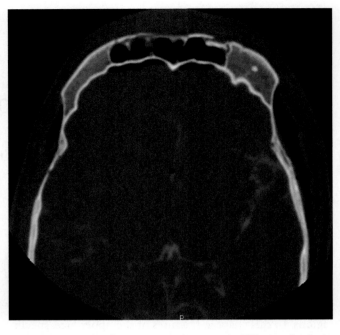

Figure 55.1. Image taken from a computed tomography (CT) scan of patient with a nondisplaced anterior table fracture managed nonoperatively.

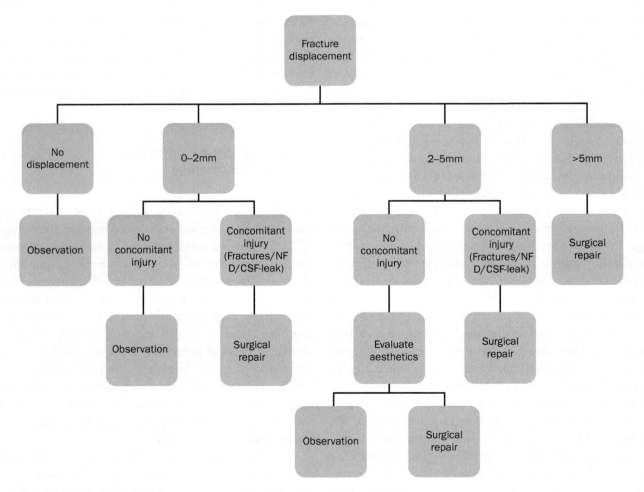

Figure 55.2. Fracture classification system based on degree of displacement, as described by Torre et al.[16]

in disruption or obstruction of outflow. Finally, the degree of displacement as well as comminution are also considered and weighed in the decision-making process regarding management.[9,10,14,15] Generally, the most common fracture pattern involves both the anterior and posterior table, with isolated anterior table fractures being less common and more often due to lower energy trauma. Isolated posterior table fractures do occur but are exceedingly rare.[14] When considering degree of displacement, the most widely accepted measure defines displacement as greater than one table width.

The multitude of proposed classification systems largely stem from the seminal article by Rohrich and Hollier who describe a classification system based upon fracture location. In their algorithm, fractures of the anterior table are divided into displaced and nondisplaced fractures. Nondisplaced anterior table fractures, as demonstrated in Figure 55.1, were managed nonoperatively, whereas displaced fractures were further evaluated to determine involvement of the NFOT.[9]

All displaced anterior table fractures met criteria for operative intervention, but treatment differed based on NFOT involvement. In their algorithm, fractures involving the anterior and posterior tables were again evaluated for degree of displacement, as well as presence of CSF leak. Nondisplaced fractures without CSF leak could be managed nonoperatively. All other fractures involving the anterior and posterior tables usually required some form of operative intervention, which varied based on displacement, CSF leak, and NFOT involvement.[9]

More recent articles, working off the model described by Rohrich and Hollier, further refine these recommendations. Manolidis proposes a classification system distinguishing fractures by type. They advocate for simple exploration and fracture reduction in all fractures, with more extensive operative intervention reserved for more complex fracture patterns.[15]

As shown in Figure 55.2, Torre et al. describe a system based on degree of displacement. In their experience, nondisplaced fractures, as well as minimally (0–2 mm) displaced fractures without associated injuries are safe to observe.[16] Any fracture associated with concomitant facial fracture, CSF leak, or NFOT involvement is managed surgically. Fractures with 0–2 mm of displacement with associated injuries are evaluated for aesthetic concerns to determine operative intervention. Any fracture with greater than 5 mm displacement automatically meets criteria for surgical repair.[16]

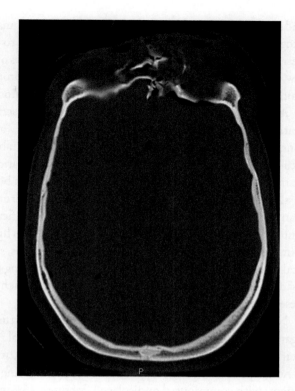

Figure 55.3. Image from a computed tomography (CT) scan of a patient with a displaced posterior table fracture, which ultimately required operative intervention.

Over time, these various classifications have continued to trend away from purely location-based criteria as the importance of a patent NFOT has become increasingly evident. A widely accepted algorithm by Rodriguez et al. heavily weighs NFOT injury when determining treatment. In their scheme, fractures are immediately segregated into those involving and those sparing the NFOT. Fractures without NFOT involvement can be safely observed. If the fracture involves the tract, further differentiation into obstructed and unobstructed groups is performed. Fractures involving the tract, but without obstruction may also be observed, as long as they are nondisplaced. Fractures demonstrating obstruction or lacking obstruction, but with displacement, meet criteria for surgical intervention.[10] Figure 55.3 demonstrates a displaced posterior table fracture, which, based on the preceding classification systems, would meet criteria for operative intervention.

NONOPERATIVE MANAGEMENT OF FRONTAL SINUS FRACTURES

As illustrated in the previous section, appropriate workup, injury identification, and fracture pattern are essential in guiding appropriate therapy. The general goals of managing these fractures is to return the bony contour to its pretraumatic conformation, preserve or reestablish sinus outflow, or eliminate the sinus cavity if maintenance of proper drainage is not possible to prevent infectious complications.[8]

As discussed earlier, Rohrich and Hollier describe treating nondisplaced anterior table fractures and nondisplaced fractures of the anterior and posterior tables without CSF leak nonoperatively.[9] These recommendations are mirrored by Torre et al., with the exception that in both classifications the presence of significant contour deformity is an indication for operative management.[9,16] Significant contour deformity is a major aesthetic concern, and, in light of improving endoscopic and percutaneous techniques, surgical intervention is increasingly feasible while avoiding the disadvantages associated with the traditional approach to these fractures, the coronal incision.[17–19]

Nonoperative management of posterior table fractures, regardless of displacement, is described by Choi et al.[2] In their series, 59 patients had posterior table fractures, with 32 nondisplaced and noncomminuted. In the remaining 27 patients with comminuted or displaced fractures, 96% were able to be treated without cranialization and 60% were managed nonoperatively without any significant complications. These data support the safety of a less aggressive surgical approach to these fractures and the possibility for even more patients to be managed nonoperatively. The caveat is that patients with open injuries, gross contamination, and higher degrees of comminution or displacement will likely still benefit from cranialization as they are at greater risk for infectious complications.[2]

Although many fractures are amenable to nonoperative treatment, these patients still require various interventions to promote healing and minimize complications. The literature traditionally recommends management with intravenous antibiotics and other supportive interventions, such as head of bed elevation and nasal decongestants.[20] However, reviews of more recent literature demonstrate only low-quality evidence available to address this issue.[21] Literature review reveals that the majority of practitioners used cefazolin or clindamycin when employing antibiotic therapy. Unfortunately, most studies only address antibiotic use in the operative population, but this evidence overall does not support the use of extended antibiotic therapy in this group and are only able to achieve a Grade C recommendation. A Grade C recommendation, according to the US Preventive Services Task Force, indicates that there is at least moderate certainty that the net benefit is small and the intervention should only be offered to selected patients depending on individual circumstances. Despite the evidence, 47% of practitioners are reported to use preoperative antibiotics, 94% use perioperative antibiotics, and 71% use postoperative antibiotics, with an average duration of 3–7 days.[21]

There appears to be some evidence supporting the use of perioperative antibiotics within 2 hours of a clean or clean-contaminated surgery involving mucosal incisions; however, beyond the perioperative period very little good data exist. In fact, some of the better evidence even indicates that pre- and postoperative antibiotics do not confer any advantage at reducing infection versus perioperative antibiotics alone. The exception is in cases of severe trauma involving multiple open facial fractures.[22] In light of the lack of evidence supporting prolonged use of antibiotics, particularly postoperatively, some groups are recommending standard perioperative antibiotics only, with extended courses reserved for patients at the highest risk of infection: operative delay, external CSF drainage devices (e.g., ICP monitor, lumbar drain), or concurrent soft tissue infection.[23]

SURGICAL MANAGEMENT OF FRONTAL SINUS FRACTURES

A number of different operative techniques and approaches are used in the surgical management of frontal sinus fractures. Historically, radical and disfiguring procedures were employed, such as ablation or exenteration. This procedure, first described by Reidel in 1898, involves removal of the anterior wall, mucosa, supraorbital rims, and proximal nasal bones.[9] Because of its significant cosmetic impact, the only remaining indication is in the setting of severe acute infection.[10] More commonly used approaches include obliteration, osteoneogenesis, and cranialization. Obliteration involves complete removal of the sinus mucosa, plugging the NFOT, and filling the sinus cavity with fat, muscle, bone, or alloplastic material.[10] In osteoneogenesis, the mucosa is removed by burring, the NFOT is sealed, and, while initially preserved, the cavity ultimately undergoes spontaneous obliteration via scar tissue and bone formation.[10] Cranialization involves removal of the posterior table and mucosa, incorporating the sinus space into the intracranial space.[2]

Open repair of frontal sinus fractures is typically done through a traditional coronal approach. In patients with receding hairlines and prominent forehead rhytids or large forehead lacerations, a direct approach may be considered if a more favorable scar would result. In those with male pattern balding, a more posterior coronal incision is typically done to conceal the scar within the hairline. When raising the coronal flaps, care must be taken to avoid injury to the pericranium, and we prefer elevating anteriorly based pericranial flaps as possible obliteration material.

Repair of any concomitant nasal or naso-orbital ethmoidal fractures should be done at the same time, with the goal of restoring nasal projection and nasofrontal contour. As long as the nasofrontal duct is intact and drainage is not disturbed, we typically do not remove the sinus membrane, although it is still debated and some authors will advocate for removal.[15]

In the case of displaced anterior table fracture only, we usually perform open reduction and fixation with titanium plates and screws. Because the frontal bone is a nonfunctional bone without significant load, absorbable plates and screws may also be used.[24] Similarly, in simple anterior table fractures, an endoscopic approach may be tried. Similar to a browlift approach with a central and two lateral hairline incisions, a 30-degree endoscope can be used to dissect in a subperiosteal plane. The anterior table can be elevated with the help of skin hooks via small stab incisions in the eyebrows. The fractures are then fixated using titanium plates inserted through the hairline incisions. The screws are placed through the stab incisions. K-wires may be used for added stabilization as necessary. Complex or severely comminuted fractures will often require an open approach.

Signs of obstruction of the frontal outflow tract are typically seen on coronal CT section and include frontal sinus fracture that is medial or involving the sinus floor, associated naso-orbito-ethmoidal (NOE) fractures, and frontal orbital fractures including the superior orbital wall. In order to prevent serious complications such as mucocele, brain abscess, or meningitis, the sinus must either be obliterated or the outflow restored. For obliteration of the frontal sinus, several methods are available. Our preferred method is removal of the frontal sinus mucosa and inner cortex of the frontal sinus wall with a rotating burr and complete obliteration of the frontonasal duct with the aforementioned pericranial flap by rotating it into the sinus. If performed carefully, fibrin glue is not necessary, but it may be used as an additional sealant. We prefer obliterating the sinus with a wide-based pericranial flap. The average frontal sinus measures about 35–40 cm³, but up to 200 cm³ has been reported.[24]

In order to avoid a forehead deformity, autologous fat can be used to fill any space not obliterated by the pericranial flap. Fat is easy to harvest, has minimal donor site morbidity, has (usually) ample donor site availability, and has favorable and predictable graft viability. It is our first choice for added volume material and maintaining a retrograde flow barrier for microbes from the nasal cavity into the neurocranium.

Other autogenous material include nonpedicled temporalis muscle and autogenous bone. The disadvantages of using nonpedicled temporalis muscle is potential hollowing at the donor site and trismus, as well as loss of volume as the nonvascularized muscle undergoes liquefactive necrosis and eventual replacement by fibrosis. Cancellous bone grafts have the advantage of promoting reossification through osteogenesis. Furthermore, compared to autologous fat, it can radiographically be distinguished from resorption, infection, and mucocele formation. Donor site morbidity from anterior iliac spine is typically minor, but, in our view, greater than for fat harvest.

Alloplastic materials have been used but are limited by potential complications. Although hydroxyapatite bone cement (Bone Source, Stryker, Dallas, TX) has been used to contour craniofacial defects and has osteoconductive properties resulting in gradual replacement by native bone without loss of volume, it is not recommended for use in the frontal sinus. Several authors have described material failure when it comes in contact with blood, CSF, or the moist conditions found in paranasal sinuses.[25] Furthermore, removal of hydroxyapatite can be difficult. Similarly, although calcium phosphate bone cement (Norion, Cupertino, CA) has favorable handling characteristics and is used in cranioplasty applications, its use in the frontal sinus is not recommended. The only alloplastic material with favorable results and recommended in frontal sinus obliteration is glass ionomer cement (Abmin Technologies, Turku, Finland). Though it has osteoconductive properties, in the frontal sinus it results in primarily fibroconnective tissue proliferation rather than bone. Nonetheless, resorption, inflammation, or foreign body reactions have not been reported.[26]

Long-term success depends on complete removal of the mucosa within the sinus and blockage of the duct to prevent nasal lining epithelium from regenerating into the sinus. While obliteration of frontal sinus mucosa in chronic sinusitis is technically easier, the same cannot be said about obliteration in acute fractures. Therefore, for anterior table fracture with sinus involvement or associated nasoethmoid type I or II fractures, some authors have advocated for an endoscopic approach for examination of the frontal sinus tract with removal of debris or bony spicules blocking the duct and irrigation with antibiotics, followed by rigid fixation.[24] While this may serve as an alternative for surgeons comfortable with an endoscopic approach, careful patient selection is paramount. In cases with associated NOE fractures, severe fracture, medial displacement of the middle segment, bony fragments, or lacerated mucosa can result in chronic frontal sinusitis, scarring, and/or blockage of the frontal recess and failure for adequate drainage of the sinus.

In severe head injuries involving the frontal sinus or anterior skull base, cranialization should be considered as the operation of choice. Our approach is the same as sinus obliteration with a pericranial flap, with the addition of performing removal of the posterior table either with a round burr or Kerrison rongeur. The brain will eventually expand in the extradural dead space. Given the likelihood of dural tear, underlying brain injury, or need for extended craniotomy, the neurosurgeon will perform this portion of the operation. Care should be taken to prevent injury to the cribriform plate, where dura is densely adherent, or to the sagittal sinus. If the intrasinus septum is intact and contralateral sinus is intact, it may be possible to preserve half the frontal sinus. To prevent forehead contour deformity, the anterior table is later reconstructed in the usual fashion.

COMPLICATIONS AND LONG-TERM SEQUELAE

In untreated or poorly treated frontal sinus fractures, complications and long-term sequelae may arise. Visual disturbances, meningitis, brain abscess, and even death have been reported as complications from frontal sinus infections and mucoceles. These complications may arise despite surgical intervention. In a case series of 50 patients with frontal sinus fractures who underwent operative repair, a 13.6% complication rate was reported, including meningitis, brain abscess, CSF leak, mucocele, and frontal osteomyelitis in a follow-up of maximum 90 weeks.[24] In a series of 43 patients treated surgically, the long-term complication rate was 16.3%, with headaches and continued pain as the most frequent complication.[27] In a series of 504 patients treated surgically, an overall 10.4% complication rate was seen.

Mucocele formation is typically seen years later with an insidious course as a result of regrowth of sinus mucosa. Patients typically present with an infection with a mass-like effect, including visual disturbances, nasal obstruction, or pain. Reoperation with obliteration of sinus mucosa and removal of hardware may be needed in cases of infection. In severe cases, removal of infected tissue may result in significant defect that may require vascularized free tissue transfer, such as a free fibula osteomyocutaneous flap.

Untreated or poorly reduced anterior table fractures with depression may result in forehead contour deformity. Correction using alloplastic materials or soft tissue fillers may be performed.

CONCLUSION

The extent of intervention for frontal sinus fractures depends on the extent and complexity of the fracture pattern. Non- or minimally displaced anterior table fractures with no frontonasal duct obstruction may be treated nonoperatively. Fractures that present with depression of the anterior table or duct obstruction should be reduced and obliterated if NFOT patency cannot be maintained. Severe fractures involving the posterior table, CSF leak, dural tear, or brain injury typically meet criteria for cranialization in conjunction with neurosurgery. However, there is evidence to support nonoperative management of this population as well, if significant comminution and gross contamination are not present.[2] Although alloplastic materials are available, our gold standard remains a large, anteriorly based pericranial flap with autologous fat graft or cancellous bone.

Complications, such as CSF leak, brain abscess, infection, or mucocele, may arise in the untreated or following treatment of frontal sinus fractures. Although still debated, we typically use perioperative antibiotics for noncomplicated fractures and a course of 7–10 days for complex fractures, such as those involving a dural tear or panfacial fractures.

REFERENCES

1. Stanley Jr RB. Management of frontal sinus fractures. *Facial Plast Surg* 1988;5:231–235.
2. Choi M, Li Y, Shapiro SA, et al. A 10-year review of frontal sinus fractures: clinical outcomes of conservative management of posterior table fractures. *Plast Reconst Surg* 2012;130:399–406.
3. Luce EA. Frontal sinus fracture: guidelines to management. *Plast Reconst Surg* 1987;80:500.
4. Saini AT, Govindarai S. Evaluation and decision making in frontal sinus surgery. *Otolaryngol Clin N Am* 2016;49:911–925.
5. Wallis A, Donald P. Frontal sinus fractures: a review of 72 cases. *Laryngoscope* 1988;98:593–598.
6. Manolidis S, Hollier Jr LH. Management of frontal sinus fractures. *Plast Reconst Surg* 2007;120:32S–48S.
7. Nahum AM. The biomechanics of maxillofacial trauma. *Clin Plast Surg* 1975;2:59–64.
8. Metzinger SE, Guerra AB, Garcia RE. et al. Frontal sinus fractures: management guidelines. *Facial Plast Surg* 2005;21:199–206.
9. Rohrich RR, Hollier LH. Management of frontal sinus fractures. Changing concepts. *Clin Plast Surg* 1992;19:219.
10. Rodriguez ED, Stanwix MG, Nam AJ, et al. Twenty-six-year experience treating frontal sinus fractures: a novel algorithm based on

anatomical fracture pattern and failure of conventional techniques. *Plast Reconst Surg* 2008;122:1850–1866.

11. Roden KS, Tong W, Surrusco M, et al. Changing characteristics of facial fractures treated at a regional, Level 1 Trauma Center, from 2005-2010: an assessment of patient demographics, referral patterns, etiology of injury, anatomic location, and clinical outcomes. *Ann Plast Surg* 2012;68:461–466.

12. Sataloff RT, Sariego J, Myers DL, et al. Surgical management of the frontal sinus. *Neurosurgery* 1984;15:593.

13. Stanwix MG. Critical computed tomographic diagnostic criteria for frontal sinus fractures. *J Oral Maxillofacial Surg* 2010;68:2714–2722.

14. Gerbino G, Roccia F, Benech A, et al. Analysis of 158 frontal sinus fractures: current surgical management and complications. *J Craniomaxillofacial Surg* 2000;28:133–139.

15. Manolidis S. Frontal sinus injuries: associated injuries and surgical management of 93 patients. *J Oral Maxillofacial Surg* 2004;62:882–891.

16. Dalla Torre D, Burtscher D, Kloss-Brandstatter A, et al. Management of frontal sinus fractures: treatment decision based on metric dislocation extent. *J Craniomaxillofacial Surg* 2014;42:1515–1519.

17. Molendijk J, van der Wal KG, Koudstaal MJ. et al. Surgical treatment of frontal sinus fractures: the simple percutaneous reduction revised. *Int J Oral Maxillofacial Surg* 2012;41:1192–1194.

18. Carter Jr KB, Poetker DM, Rhee JS. et al. Sinus preservation management for frontal sinus fractures in the endoscopic sinus surgery era: a systematic review. *Craniomaxillofacial Trauma Reconst* 2010;3:141–149.

19. Kellman R, Goyal P. Managing the frontal sinus in the endoscopic age: has the endoscope changed the algorithm? *Craniomaxillofacial Trauma Reconst* 2014;7:203–212.

20. Levine SB, Rowe LD, Keane WM, et al. Evaluation and treatment of frontal sinus fractures. *Otolaryngol Head Neck Surg* 1986;95:19–20.

21. Mundinger GS, Borsuk DE, Okhah Z, et al. Antibiotics and facial fractures: evidence-based recommendations compared with experience based practice. *Craniomaxillofacial Trauma Reconst* 2015;8:64–78.

22. Lauder A, Jalisi S, Siegel J, et al. Antibiotic prophylaxis in the management of complex midface and frontal sinus trauma. *Laryngoscope* 2010;120:1940–1950.

23. Bellamy JL, Molendijk J, Reddy SK, et al. Severe infectious complications following frontal sinus fracture: the impact of operative delay and perioperative antibiotic use. *Plast Reconst Surg* 2013;132:154–162

24. Bell RB, Dierks EJ, Brar P, et al. A protocol for the management of frontal sinus fractures emphasizing sinus preservation. *J Oral Maxillofacial Surg* 2007;65:825–839.

25. Freidman CD, Costantino PD, Synderman CH, et al. Reconstruction of the frontal sinus and frontofacial skeleton with hydroxyapatite cement. *Arch Facial Plast Surg* 2000;2:124–129.

26. Peltola MJ, Suonpaa JT, Maattanen HS, et al. Clinical follow-up method for frontal sinus obliteration with bioactive glass S53P4. *J Biomed Mater Res* 2001;58:54–60.

27. Sivori LA, 2nd, de Leeuw R, Morgan I, et al. Complications of frontal sinus fractures with emphasis on chronic craniofacial pain and its treatment: a review of 43 cases. *J Oral Maxillofacial Surg* 2010;68:2041–2046.

56.

RECONSTRUCTION OF ORBITAL DEFECTS

Marco F. Ellis and Mimis N. Cohen

INTRODUCTION

Surgical correction of periorbital defects is one of the most challenging procedures in facial reconstruction. The progress that has been seen in the treatment of orbital injuries and oncologic defects has evolved from the principles of exposure and segmental repositioning described by Paul Tessier to present-day vascularized composite allograft reconstruction. Thorough knowledge of the anatomy of the orbit is critical for the successful surgical management of these problems. The operative plan must be constructed on the basis of an accurate physical examination of the soft tissue, facial skeleton, and visual sensory system, combined with high-resolution cross-sectional imaging. Because of the unique geometry of the orbit, small errors in reconstruction can produce suboptimal functional and cosmetic results. The ultimate success or failure of the procedure depends on completing an accurate preoperative plan, reconstruction of the bony orbit, and correction of concomitant soft tissue malposition and shape.[1]

Conceptually, the orbit can be modeled as a pyramidal cone where the base refers to the bony rims (Figure 56.1). This model can be subdivided into three subunits: (1) the orbital rim, (2) the middle orbit, and (3) the posterior orbit.[2] Traumatic injuries of sufficient force to damage the orbit generally produce injuries to the orbital rim and middle section. The orbital rim (anterior orbit) is divided into three clinically separate sections: the zygoma and maxillary inferolaterally, the supraorbital section superiorly, and the nasoethmoidal section medially. Immediately posterior to the rim, the geometry of the orbit and the anatomic interrelationships between sections become more complex. The middle orbit contains four clinically distinct sections: the roof, the lateral wall, the floor, and the medial wall. The contour of the roof, as it extends posteriorly, exhibits a double superior curvature, both in the

medial-to-lateral plane and in the anterior-to-posterior plane. The lateral wall is the strongest portion of this section of the orbit and is composed of the orbital process of the zygoma and the greater wing of the sphenoid. The posterior section of the orbit is constructed of thicker bone.

The orbital floor, in contrast, is first concave, and then, just posterior to the globe, becomes convex, inclining upward at a 30-degree angle, creating (with the medial orbital wall) a postbulbar constriction of the orbit. This feature, combined with a medial inclination of the floor at approximately 45 degrees as one travels from lateral to medial, creates an "inferomedial bulge" as the orbital floor meets the vertical medial wall. The inferomedial bulge is a critical determinant of globe position; this unique feature of orbital architecture is often not corrected after injury. Posteriorly, the orbital floor is composed primarily of roof of maxillary sinus. This region, most frequently damaged in orbital floor fractures, is medial to the inferior orbital fissure in the area overlying the infraorbital groove.

The medial wall of the orbit is formed by the thin orbital plate of the ethmoid bone, which initially bulges inward just posterior to the globe. The medial wall is stronger and less likely to fracture than the orbital floor due to support from the honeycomb structure of the ethmoid air cells. An important landmark along the medial wall is the posterior ethmoid foramen and its accompanying posterior ethmoidal artery. This foramen is approximately 30–35 mm from the orbital rim and lies within the frontoethmoidal suture. It marks the boundary between the middle and posterior subunits and indicates the limit of safe dissection with the orbital apex, on average only 7 mm away. In addition, this foramen marks the location of the orbital keystone, the orbital process of the palatine bone. This vertical strut is frequently maintained in orbit fractures and serves as a posterior ledge of intact orbital bone along the medial orbital wall, which can facilitate support of implants.[3]

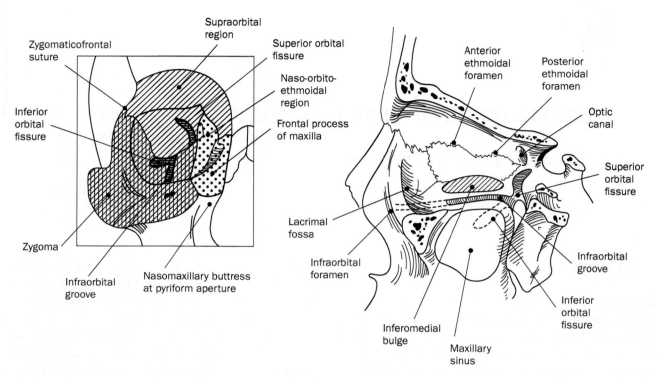

Figure 56.1. The orbit is divided into three sections: the orbit rim, middle orbit, and posterior orbit.

Dissection into the posterior orbit should be meticulously avoided. The orbital apex contains the optic nerve, ophthalmic artery, and proximal portions of the superior and inferior orbital fissures. In addition, the tendinous convergence of the extraocular muscles (annulus of Zinn) and motor branches are present. Immediately posterior to medial orbital rim is the nasolacrimal fossa.

The shape and volume of the bony orbit determine the position of the globe and periorbital contents; therefore, the accuracy with which the rim and walls of the orbit are reconstructed will determine the success of the correction. Since the volume of the orbit is 30–35 mL, small changes (approximately 10%) begin to cause a noticeable change in globe position. If the shape of the orbit is modeled as a cone, the volume is proportional to the cone length and the radius squared (Figure 56.2). Therefore, displacing the rim only a few millimeters increases the volume of the orbit significantly because, in the formula, the radius is squared. Displacing the inferomedial rim anteriorly in a laterally rotated zygoma or displacing the orbital floor in a blowout fracture increases the orbital volume but in a linear fashion. Volume alone is not the complete determinant of globe position or of the composite appearance of the orbital contents.[4,5]

In addition to the need to accurately restore the integrity of the facial skeleton, the surgeon must also be attentive to the complex interrelationships that exist between the bone, orbital soft tissue, and globe. The globe is suspended within soft tissue, supported by a sling of check ligaments stretched between the bony walls of the orbit, with the medial and lateral canthal ligaments forming the strongest

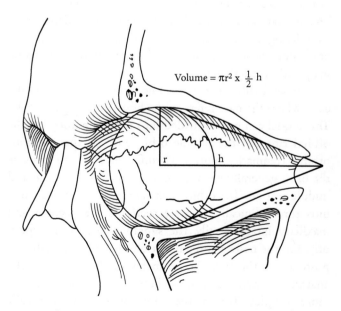

$$\text{Volume} = \pi r^2 \times \frac{1}{2} h$$

Figure 56.2. Orbital volume is directly related to the length of the orbit and the square of the orbital rim radius. This approximation does not account for subtle concavities of the floor and roof.

sites of attachment.[6] Orbital fractures may result in disruption of ligaments, which can result in displacement of intraconal and extraconal fat, disturbing the balance between bony volume and soft tissue contents and reducing the soft tissue support of the globe. *Dystopia* broadly defines any change in globe position whether in the vertical or anterior-posterior vector. Enophthalmos is associated with bony enlargement in volume, leading to the appearance of a retropositioned globe. This finding can be associated with inferior vertical dystopia, or hypoglobus, when the floor and ligamentous sling have been injured. Exophthalmos, an anteriorly projected globe, is a rare finding and is seen with a high-energy blow-in fracture of the orbital roof.

There is an additional distinction when describing the balance between periorbita and bony volume. Posttraumatic enophthalmos is a difficult functional and cosmetic defect to correct. These patients have both bony vault and soft tissue disturbances. Simple restoration of the bony orbital volume alone undercorrects the globe position. Generally, soft tissue follows the bone displacement, and its structure is recapitulated with bony reconstruction. In patients who have had delays in repair (>1–2 months), there develops an internal pattern of atrophy and scar that opposes correction to its original position. The precise mechanism of posttraumatic enophthalmos is usually multifactorial, and, regrettably, it is still incompletely understood.[7] Several theories have been advanced to account for the occurrence, including fat atrophy, soft tissue contracture, fibrosis, neurogenic influences, and loss of ligamentous support. This phenomenon becomes problematic when performing late orbital reconstruction, when merely restoring orbital volume alone with wall reconstruction undercorrects the globe position.[8] Definitive improvement may require overcorrection of the orbital walls with bone graft or alloplastic material.[9]

Comprehensive orbit reconstruction requires additional understanding of the complex interplay between the orbital rims and the periorbital soft tissues. Fractures caused by high-energy trauma can directly and indirectly injure the malar and temporal support system. Retaining ligaments are present that suspend surrounding skin, musculature, and fat pads (Figure 56.3). Improperly treated periorbital tissues predispose the patient to a prematurely aged appearance that can be difficult to correct. Soft tissue atrophy and scar deposition make attempts at correction difficult and require mid-face lift and fat transfer. The most frequent cause of this posttraumatic contour irregularity is iatrogenic and related to dissection needed for fracture identification, reduction, and fixation. In many acute orbital injuries, as well as in those with previous subperiosteal dissections where

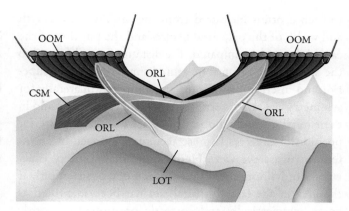

Figure 56.3. The periorbital retaining ligaments, orbitomalar ligament (OM), and lateral orbital thickening (LOT) define the boundaries of the bony orbit and soft tissue. Failure to reconstruct these attachments after wide dissection can predispose to malar soft tissue descent, lid malposition, and premature aging.

the soft tissue has not been repositioned properly onto the facial skeleton, the soft tissue of the cheek has migrated inferiorly and medially. This migration produces an effect that accentuates the deformity of posterior displacement of the malar eminence and shortens the distance between the nasolabial fold and the thickest part of the malar soft tissue. The orbitomalar ligament, lateral orbital thickening, and zygomaticomaxillary periosteum are well-defined structures that must be repositioned.

ASSESSMENT OF THE DEFECT

The operative plan must be based on an accurate physical examination and a complete radiographic evaluation of the orbit. The surgeon's exam must individually analyze the components of the soft tissue and the bone. Soft tissue analysis examines the position of the brows, the lids, and the medial and lateral canthi in three dimensions, relating the measurements to the contralateral side. The presence of a supratarsal sulcus deformity indicates that some pressure must be put along the inferior orbit directly behind the globe to force the superior orbital fat against the roof and thereby protrude it forward. Conversely, blepharoptosis can be a subtle sign suggesting an increase in orbital volume. The length and width of the palpebral fissure and the position and displacement of the various regions of soft tissue, such as the fat over the malar eminence or the zygomaticus major muscle, must be assessed and compared bilaterally.

The globe must be examined for its position in relation to the orbital rim, midline facial structures, and the lateral orbit. An imaginary midline should be drawn vertically through the nose and the distance to the pupil and to each canthus measured from the midline. The length and width of the palpebral fissures and the position of the canthi should be compared. The distance from the pupil to the lateral orbital rim is measured similarly, and the superior and inferior orbital rims are compared bilaterally for symmetry (i.e., both vertical height and projection) and in their relation to the globe. The relative anterior-posterior position of the eyes is most accurately assessed in an inferior, worm's eye view. Hertel exophthalmometry is accurate in defining the difference in globe position only if the area of the lateral orbital rim has been identified as being symmetrically and correctly positioned anteriorly and posteriorly and is symmetrical with the contralateral side. Neurologic examination may include infraorbital nerve anesthesia or paresthesia. Paralysis of the orbicularis oculi muscle or upper lip elevator muscles is seen rarely in blunt trauma. Any evidence of lacrimal system dysfunction should be documented.

The visual sensory system must be assessed, including, at minimum, the following: (1) visual acuity; (2) pupillary function, including specifically the presence or absence of a relative afferent pupillary defect; (3) ocular motility (if any diplopia or movement restriction is noted, perform a formal eye muscle evaluation to document any horizontal or vertical misalignment or muscle imbalance); (4) slit-lamp examination of the anterior segment to rule out a corneal perforation or hyphema; and (5) a dilated fundus examination to evaluate the optic nerve and retinal pathology. Consultation should be sought preoperatively from an ophthalmologist, who may recommended delayed reconstruction to allow adequate healing time for ocular pathology.

Imaging studies may include plain radiographs, but these rarely provide sufficient anatomic accuracy to assess rim position and size of the intraorbital defect. Helical computed tomography (CT) scans with axial slice thickness of less than 1 mm are ideal to delineate each fracture and minimize volume averaging.[10] Reformatted images in the coronal and sagittal planes, as well as three-dimensional reconstructions, provide additional information valuable to reduction and fixation.[11] The thin orbital floor sits in the craniofacial axial plane, so fracture characteristics are best analyzed in the coronal and sagittal planes. Axial plane images provide information about the inferior orbital rim and zygomatic arch.[12] Details regarding periorbita injury—such as rectus muscle entrapment or retrobulbar hematoma—can be visualized in the soft tissue windows. Three-dimensional CT scans are useful to compare rim position and symmetry but are seldom of value in the evaluation of the internal portion of the orbit. In addition, the CT scan should visualize adjacent cavities and structures, such as the brain, the anterior cranial fossa, the posterior orbit, all of the paranasal sinuses, zygomaticomaxillary and nasomaxillary buttresses, maxillary alveolus, and temporal bone.

From these simple measurements of orbital shape, globe, and soft tissue position and orbital volume, an idea forms of the changes in the position of the structures that must be accomplished for correction.

INDICATIONS FOR TREATMENT

Traumatic orbital defects span a spectrum of injuries from small, nondisplaced orbital floor or medial wall fractures to LeFort fracture patterns with involvement of all orbital walls. The most controversial topic in orbit fracture management is treatment of isolated orbital floor injuries. Multiwall fractures with associated dystopia, diplopia, and V2 paresthesia obviously require reconstruction. The question centers on how to manage small single-wall fractures without concomitant signs. Fractures without evidence of extraocular muscle entrapment may be observed for signs of enophthalmos that is cosmetically unacceptable to the patient. The orbital floor surface area measures approximately 5–6 cm² and the total orbital volume approximately 26–29 cm³. Traditionally, fracture surface area that measured more than half of the surface area met operative criteria. This area could be calculated by using the fracture dimensions measured on coronal and sagittal views. Multiple observational studies suggest that orbital floor fractures larger than 2 cm² and medial orbital wall fractures larger than 1 cm² begin to produce enophthalmos of more than 2 mm.[13] Volumetric analysis is a more complex measurement tool. While it has been suggested that 5–10% changes in volume can lead to enophthalmos, there is no simple radiographic tool to reliably measure the volume of the complex pyramidal orbit shape (Figure 56.4).[12] An additional criteria that can be used for borderline fractures is the shape of the inferior rectus. A large impact to the globe or inferior orbital rim can disrupt check ligaments around the inferior rectus muscle and extraconal fat leading to diplopia, delayed soft tissue displacement, and vertical dystopia. No size criteria exist for orbital roof or lateral orbital wall fractures due to the semi-rigid nature of the surrounding cavities (cranial base and temporalis, respectively). Absolute indications for reconstruction also include significant displacement of any orbital rim and isolated muscle entrapment seen in pediatric injuries.

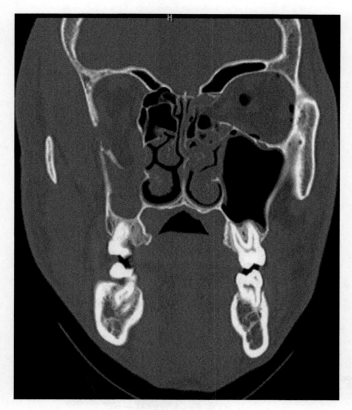

Figure 56.4. Computed tomography (CT) imaging demonstrating operative fractures in a patient with bilateral orbital fractures. The coronal image demonstrates significant periorbital herniation in the right orbital floor and left medial orbital wall.

CONTRAINDICATIONS

Surgical repair of a traumatic orbital injury should proceed without delay; however, there are contraindications to repair of the injury. The first and most obvious is the presence of a concurrent injury that requires acute medical or surgical treatment to stabilize the patient. In addition, the presence of a significant soft tissue, subperiosteal, or sinus infection, which has resulted from delay in the transport of the patient for definitive care, may preclude use of internal hardware. In this situation, drainage of the abscess or affected sinus and treatment with a course of intravenous antibiotics would be prudent before undertaking repair of the fracture. Treatment of retinal detachment as well as presence of hyphema may warrant delay for at least 10 days, with final clearance being provided at the discretion of the consulting ophthalmologist. On rare occasion, irreversible globe perforation or avulsion may require enucleation. The decision to proceed with orbital reconstruction may be postponed indefinitely until the type of rehabilitation is selected by a team of ocularists and oculoplastic surgeons.

ROOM SETUP

The patient should be positioned so that his or her head is freely accessible from all directions. It is a good idea to wire the endotracheal tube to a maxillary bicuspid tooth if uncrowned. Low- and high-speed drills should be available, as well as facial fracture instruments with a variety of periosteal elevators, rhinoplasty instruments for intranasal access, and a Bovie needle tip. In the case of elective osteotomies and tumor resection, bone graft instruments should include instruments for harvesting calvarial, rib, or iliac bone. Complex cases that require multiple surgical teams or a panfacial fracture should have a Foley catheter placed within the bladder. Several areas should be prepared for donor harvest; the combination of skull and hip is frequently used because different facial areas sometimes benefit from different bone harvest. Lacrimal instruments should be available for lacrimal intubation, including fine silicone tubes, lacrimal dilators, and lacrimal probes, when revisional surgery of the nasoethmoidal region is contemplated. Intravenous preoperative antibiotics and gentamicin or bacitracin irrigation is suggested. The patient should be typed and screened in the event of a transfusion in the perioperative period.

INCISION PLANNING

The use of local incisions and lacerations is possible, depending on their location and the need for access to the various orbital areas. Generally speaking, the most common pathology involves the orbital floor so lower eyelid incisions provide adequate exposure. The subciliary incision is the most traditional and simplest approach to the inferior orbital rim and orbital floor. However, several studies have shown that this approach carries the highest risk of lower eyelid malposition in the postoperative period. Several adjunctive maneuvers have been recommended to minimize complications, including use of a stair-stepped skin–muscle flap at the level of the inferior tarsal plate. Evidence from lower eyelid blepharoplasty has emphasized preservation of the pretarsal orbicularis to maintain muscular tone and involuntary blink. Additional supportive measures include mid-lid incision, mid-face suspension, and meticulous multilayered closure. In patients with decreased lid tone, such as elderly patients, a cutaneous midtarsal or inferior rim incision should be contemplated. The cutaneous scar from this incision is slightly more noticeable than that from a subciliary incision, but it is often not objectionable, especially in elderly patients in whom wrinkles are present, where lower lid tone is reduced, and the chance of an ectropion with a subciliary incision would be quite high.

The approach with the lowest likelihood of scleral show and lid retraction is a transconjunctival approach (Figure 56.5). After placement of a eye lubricant and a protective corneal shield, incision just anterior to the lower lid fornix minimizes injury to the capsulopalpebral fascia and lid retractors. Dissection onto the orbital rim can then proceed in two separate planes, retroseptal or preseptal. There are no studies to suggest one plane is statistically superior to the other; surgeon preference and experience dictate which approach is chosen. Preseptal dissection maintains integrity of the orbital septum, which simplifies orbital fat retraction during fracture reduction and reconstruction. However, it is a more time-consuming dissection to tease the orbicularis oris muscle from the orbital septum and enter the subperiosteal plane at the arcus marginalis.

Retroseptal dissection is preferred by most because it is technically easier and faster.

Simple fracture reduction can be performed from a transconjunctival incision that measures approximately 2.5 cm. However, fractures that involve a larger surface area of the orbit require incision extension along the medial or lateral orbital conjunctiva. This added exposure can prevent lower lid avulsion, chemosis, and muscle injury from excessive retraction. The most common option is a lateral canthotomy, where the external canthal skin is incised and a inferior conjunctival back cut is performed to disconnect contributions by the inferior retinaculum. A less disruptive alternative is to incise the conjunctiva behind the caruncle for a retrocaruncular approach (Figure 56.5). This added posterior to the lacrimal sac provides equally increased access to the orbit without the added inconvenience of reconstructing the lateral canthus at the procedure's end. The

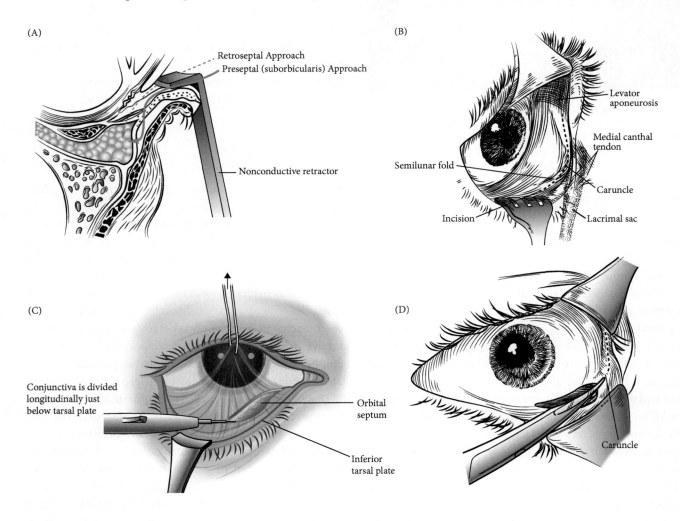

Figure 56.5. (A) A transconjunctival approach along the fornix and caruncle can provide large access to the orbital floor and medial orbital wall. (B) The dissection plane to the orbit can be either retroseptal or preseptal. (C) The pigmented caruncle is easily identified easily with the medial aspect of the upper and lower eyelid on stretch. (D) Incision from the fornix proceeds behind the caruncle and posterior to the lacrimal sac and canthal apparatus.

medial canthal apparatus and canalicular system are avoided in a retrocaruncular approach. This dissection plane proceeds posterior to Horner's muscle, and, with subperiosteal elevation of the inferior oblique muscle off the orbital floor, the entire orbital floor and medial wall can be visualized.

Additional periorbital incisions are available to provide access to the superior and lateral orbit. Complicated fractures involving the zygoma often require exposure of the lateral orbital rim and lateral orbit. A transconjunctival incision can provide exposure of the zygomaticosphenoid suture, but better access can be achieved with an external incision. Most surgeons prefer to incise the lateral 1–1.5 cm of a standard upper blepharoplasty incision. This area heals well without significant scarring and allows straightforward fixation of the zygomaticofrontal suture. The gingivobuccal sulcus incision is used whenever exposure of the lateral pyriform region, zygomatico-maxillary buttress, and anterior face of the maxilla is necessary. Complete orbital reconstruction, specifically access to the orbital roof and superior orbital rim, requires a coronal incision. This incision in combination with a lower eyelid incision provide 360-degree access with minimal morbidity. The degree to which a coronal incision is required depends on a CT scan analysis of the orbital roof, superior orbital rim, and nasoethmoidal area.

SURGICAL APPROACH

Previously, it was thought that the entire circumference of orbital soft tissue had to be dissected to achieve a change in globe position and that material should be wedged behind the globe in all locations to correct enophthalmos. Recently, these maneuvers have been found to be unnecessary; in fact, they may not achieve as normal a globe position as "anatomic reconstruction." They also have more chance of impairing visual function. We believe the anatomy of the deformity should precisely dictate the anatomy of the surgical correction.

Correction of posttraumatic orbital deformities is conceptualized in three steps:

- Gain surgical access with mobilization of soft tissue to delineate the fracture

- Reposition (with repair) the anterior and middle sections of the bony orbital rim and walls into their proper position

- Reattach the soft tissue to the bone at the proper location

The first step is to safely access the bony orbit and sweep the periorbita and extraocular musculature in a subperiosteal fashion. The area of mobilization must include an area slightly beyond the entire area of fracture. The second step restores the anatomic integrity of the facial skeleton. Reducing the periorbita, which can herniate into the surrounding paranasal sinuses, reestablishes intraorbital volume. After bony reconstruction, correction of the normal soft tissue preinjury contour is accomplished in the final step.

Generally, it is assumed that most patients have a normal volume of orbital soft tissue. Although CT analyses can determine fat atrophy, it is generally difficult to determine this in the acute setting. One should therefore aim to restore the bony volume of the orbit and then assess the resultant soft tissue position and volume.[14] As the bony reconstruction is accomplished, the soft tissue of the orbit is squeezed and molded toward its original configuration by the repositioning of the walls and the rim. To repair a more complex fracture, it is recommended to fixate the orbital rims first. Orbit implant placement is simplified when adjacent buttresses are in alignment. For each segment to be realigned, all of the peripheral buttress articulations must be visualized simultaneously. The major contributions of these buttresses are the zygoma, frontal bar/ superior orbital rim, and nasoethmoid region. This reduction and fixation may require viewing through several incisions.

One example of this algorithmic approach is the complex zygomaticomaxillary fracture. Generally, the position of the zygoma is first approximated by loosely fixating the zygomaticofrontal suture. The remainder of the bone can then be more accurately positioned and the accuracy of the positioning increased with each area of fixation. The bone is then minimally stabilized, viewing the alignment in the lateral orbit at the time the arch is mobilized medially, placing forward traction on the malar eminence, and stabilizing with plate and screw fixation. The inferior orbital rim is fixated first followed by the zygomaticomaxillary buttress. If the orbital floor meets reconstruction criteria, it is reconstructed last. It is important to achieve near perfect rim reduction. A mere 5 mm displacement of the rim can produce significant enophthalmos and lower lid malposition. The most common mistake currently made is that primary placement of the lateral and inferior orbital rims is too wide and too inferior, which greatly increases the volume of the cone. Revisional rim osteotomies are required in any patient with malposition and enophthalmos to significantly decrease the volume of the orbit.

Complex orbital injuries involving the orbital rim and corresponding wall should be analyzed in the same way before rigid fixation (Figure 56.6). The most difficult

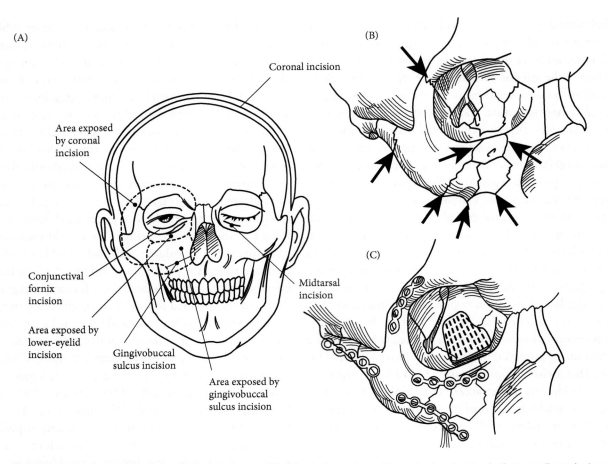

(A)

Coronal incision

Area exposed
by coronal
incision

Conjunctival
fornix
incision

Area exposed by
lower-eyelid
incision

Gingivobuccal
sulcus incision

Area exposed by
gingivobuccal
sulcus incision

Midtarsal
incision

(B)

(C)

Figure 56.6. Treatment of a complex orbitozygomatic fracture. A coronal incision in the scalp, an intraoral sulcus incision in the upper lip, and a lower eyelid incision will permit wide access to the orbit and periorbital sutures. The primary goal is to achieve fracture reduction that realigns bony discontinuity and achieves appropriate facial projection and symmetry. Fixation is often placed along the orbital rim, zygomatic arch, and lateral maxillary buttress. A thin titanium plate, porous polyethylene plate, or combination of the two can reconstruct the orbital floor.

reconstructions involve injuries displacing all four walls and all of the rim segments of the orbit. Recognition of the deformity in each area is thus critical, and the preinjury physical examination and CT scans provide a guide to the most appropriate procedure. Following rim repositioning, the inner walls of the orbit should be reconstructed. It is our belief that at least two inner walls of the orbit must be rigidly fixed. Generally, the roof and floor are the most amenable to rigid fixation. The roof is best approached with an intracranial correction, since a simultaneous intracranial exposure of the superior orbit is easily achieved with the necessary exposure for intracranial correction. Roof correction, if required, by grafting should be placed externally to the remaining sections of the roof. The correct orbital floor position is best identified by dissecting to intact bone in the posterior portion of the orbit. With either the roof or floor, bone graft or alloplastic material is placed from the posterior orbit to the anterior orbit, over the edges of the anatomically identified defect, and is rigidly fixed to guarantee this

position. While bone is preferred for the roof, alternatives are feasible for other orbital walls.[15] The choice of titanium, alloplastics, or bone depends on surgeon preference, the degree of sinus exposure, and the need for predictability in achieving a stable construct. New anatomic titanium implants are available and allow simultaneous rigid fixation of the medial wall and orbital floor. However, the medial wall and lateral wall can also be reconstructed by inlay grafting, in which bone is stacked into the defect and wedged against the floor reconstruction. In most cases, it is difficult to rigidly fix grafts in these two areas, but they should be considered for fixation when possible.

POSTOPERATIVE CARE

At the completion of internal orbital reconstruction, it is important to rule out impingement on the extraocular muscle system. Comparison should be made to the contralateral, unoperated eye position and the preoperative duction exam. Attention should be focused on the orbital wall that was reconstructed. For example, reduction and reconstruction of medial orbital wall fractures places the medial rectus muscle at risk. If it were compromised, expect to see the globe medially rotated and limited duction laterally. In cases of chronic enophthalmos correction, where fibrosis has penetrated the periorbita and extraocular muscles, there may be expected decreased range of motion after reconstruction. These patients require preoperative counseling of persistent diplopia and close ophthalmologic supervision.

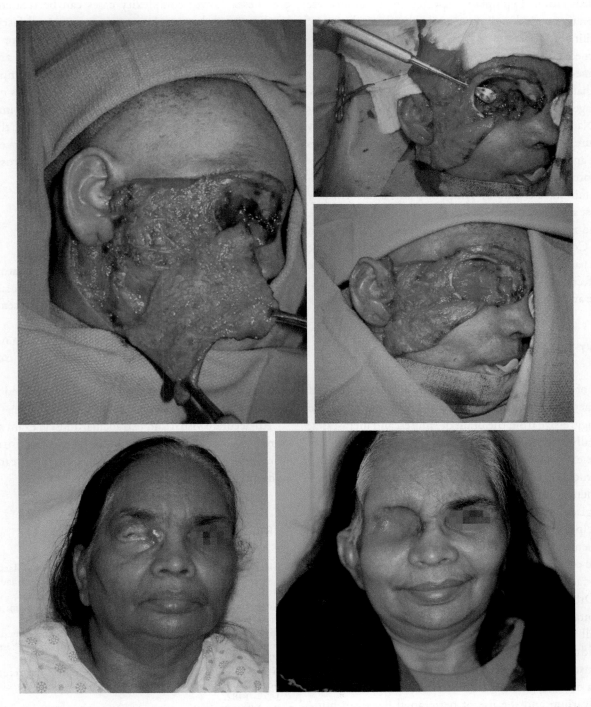

Figure 56.7. Exenteration reconstruction. A 72-year-old woman with invasive upper eyelid melanoma. A pedicled temporalis flap was tunneled through a lateral orbitotomy. A skin graft completed the reconstruction to provide an open cavity that is amenable to wearing a prosthesis.

Postoperatively, vision should be checked and monitored at least twice daily. Mobility of the eye is often reduced with swelling. Some surgeons believe that corticosteroids reduce swelling, but the drug must be given before the surgical incision to be maximally effective. Corticosteroids should be continued for 48 hours postoperatively. It is not known whether the incidence of infection is increased with the use of corticosteroids. Diplopia is expected in the immediate postoperative period and often resolves with resolution of the swelling.

Corneal integrity should be closely monitored in the immediate postoperative period. Check patients for lagophthalmos, which can exacerbate dry eye symptoms. Encourage use of lubricants (Lacri-Lube) and rewetting drops (Tears Naturale). The cornea should always be protected by lid closure and ointment. Conjunctival edema is sometimes marked and demands protection with antibiotic and sometimes corticosteroid ointments. Several adjuncts are available to minimize chemosis. Temporary lateral tarsorrhaphy and Frost sutures can be placed to support eyelid closure. Eye pads and nonallergenic tape can provide light compression as well. Corticosteroid-containing ointments should not be used in patients with high intraocular pressures or in those with infections. Ultimately, light massage of soft tissues and patience are required.

SOFT TISSUE RECONSTRUCTION

Lesions of the eyelids, globe, and periorbita can be classified as primary tumors of the orbit, secondary tumors that are locally aggressive from the brain or sinuses, and metastases. The locally advanced tumors and skin neoplasms can necessitate extensive resection. Oncologic management and reconstruction require collaboration by head and neck surgeons, neurosurgeons, ophthalmologists, plastic surgeons, radiologists, and medical oncologists. Tumor control is the first priority of surgery, but cosmetic and functional consequences must be taken into consideration. On occasion, eye conservation surgery is appropriate when there is limited radiographic and pathologic periorbital involvement. Orbital exenteration can be limited to the eyelids and orbital contents but can also involve extension into the skull base and paranasal sinuses.[16] Reconstruction must address each cavity in turn for optimal results. The orbit must be separated from the anterior skull base in the case of a orbitozygomatic craniotomy. Bone grafting with split calvarium and the use of pericranial flaps can minimize cerebrospinal fluid leak, abscess, and meningitis.

Similarly, maxillectomy complicates surgery as the goals now involve sinus obliteration and palate reconstruction. Closed-cavity reconstruction is the mainstay where a large bulky myocutaneous or fasciocutaneous flap can treat multiple areas. However, open-cavity reconstruction, where the contours of the orbit are maintained, provides the ideal aesthetic result for patients seeking a periorbital prosthesis. Lower complexity cases can be treated with local regional flaps, such as a temporoparietal fascia flap or temporalis muscle flap with skin graft (Figure 56.7). Larger defects are treated best with free tissue transfer using thigh- or abdomen-based flaps. After the completion of adjuvant radiation and chemotherapy, patients may be eligible for revision surgery to minimize bulk and improve symmetry. Anaplastologists serve a unique role at the end of the soft and bony reconstruction. Experience with osseointegrated implants and implant-based prostheses simplify the challenges of daily wear.

CAVEATS

The anatomy of the defect should dictate the anatomy of the repair. Complete examination, including an ocular evaluation with axial and coronal thin CT scans, is essential in completely defining the extent of the defect.

Orbital volume should be restored as close to normal as possible, including meticulous alignment of the orbital rim.

The soft tissue must be mobilized and reattached to the skeleton after surgery.

An accurate visual and extraocular muscle exam are required to track patient's success during the reconstructive process. Collaboration with an ophthalmologist can help guide adjunctive treatment.

REFERENCES

1. Manson PN, Iliff NT. Surgical anatomy of the orbit. In: Marsh J, ed. *Current Therapy in Plastic and Reconstructive Surgery.* Philadelphia: BC Decker, 1985:117.
2. Koorneef L. *Sectional Anatomy of the Orbit.* Amsterdam: Aeolus Press, 1981.
3. Manson PN, Ruas EJ, Iliff NT. Deep orbital reconstruction for correction of post-traumatic enophthalmos. *Clin Plast Surg* 1987;14(1):113.
4. Nam SM, Kim YB, Shin HS, Park ES. Orbital floor reconstruction considering orbital floor shape. *J Craniofac Surg* 2011;22:1479–1482.
5. Pearl RM. Surgical management of volumetric changes in the bony orbit. *Ann Plast Surg* 1987;19:349.

6. Manson PN, Clifford CM, Su CT, et al. Mechanisms of global support and posttraumatic enophthalmos: I. The anatomy of the ligament sling and its relation to intramuscular cone orbital fat. *Plast Reconstr Surg* 1986;77:193.

7. Chen CT, Huang F, Chen YR. Management of posttraumatic enophthalmos. *Chang Gung Med J* 2006;29:251–261.

8. Converse JM, Smith B. Enophthalmos and diplopia in fractures of the orbital floor. *Br J Plast Surg* 1957;9:265.

9. Grant MP, Iliff NT, Manson PN. Strategies for the treatment of enophthalmos. *Clin Plast Surg* 1997;24:539.

10. Gilbard SM. Management of orbital blowout fractures: the prognostic significant of computed tomography. *Adv Ophthalmic Plast Reconstr Surg* 1987;6:269–280.

11. Bite U, Jackson IT, Forbes GS, Gehring GE. Orbital volume measurements in enophthalmos using three dimensional CT imaging. *Plast Reconstr Surg* 1985;75:502.

12. Manson PN, Grivas A, Rosenbaum A, et al. Studies on enophthalmos: II. The measurement of orbital injuries and their treatment by quantitative computed tomography. *Plast Reconstr Surg* 1986;77:203.

13. Whitehouse RW, Batterbury M, Jackson A, et al. Prediction of enophthalmos by computed tomography after "blow out" orbital fracture. *Br J Ophthalmol* 1994;78:618.

14. Glassman RD, Manson PN, Vanderkolk CA, et al. Rigid fixation of internal orbital fractures. *Plast Reconstr Surg* 1990;86:1103.

15. Antonyshyn O, Gruss JS, Galbraith DJ, Hurwitz JJ. Complex orbital fractures: a critical analysis of immediate bone graft reconstruction. *Ann Plast Surg* 1989;22:220.

16. Weizman N, Horowitz G, Gil Z, Fliss DM. Surgical management of tumors involving the orbit. *JAMA Otolaryngol Head Neck Surg* 2013;139:841–846.

57

NASO-ORBITO-ETHMOIDAL COMPLEX INJURIES

Husain T. AlQattan, Ajani Nugent, and Seth Thaller

BACKGROUND

Management of naso-orbito-ethmoidal (NOE) fractures continues to be one of the most challenging problems encountered in the treatment of facial trauma. The NOE complex is located at the interface between the mid and upper third of the maxillofacial skeleton, at the junction of the bones between the nose, maxilla, orbits, and cranium. NOE fractures have substantial bony and soft tissue sequelae, including medial canthal disruption. Other complications can result in concomitant adjacent fractures; cerebrospinal fluid (CSF) leaks; and globe, nasolacrimal duct, and intracranial injuries. Early diagnosis and repair is paramount in order to obtain optimal functional and aesthetic results.

ANATOMY

As with any surgical endeavor, a comprehensive appreciation of the regional anatomy is paramount. The NOE complex represents an area where the nasal, lacrimal, ethmoidal, maxillary, and frontal bones meet. Two nasal bones are attached inferior to the frontal bone, medial to the frontal process of the maxilla, and anterior to the ethmoid bone. Nasal support is from the underlying perpendicular plate of the ethmoid, vomer, and the cartilaginous septum. Ethmoid labyrinth lies between the orbit and the nasal cavity. Superolaterally, the fovea ethmoidalis forms the ethmoid sinus roof. Cribriform plate forms the roof of the nasal cavity medially. These two structures separate the anterior cranial fossa from the NOE.

The superior border of the NOE region is the very dense frontal bone. It contains the frontal sinuses. Frontal sinus has a very thick anterior wall, a much thinner posterior wall, and it separates the anterior cranial fossa from sinus contents. The inferior border of the frontal sinus interfaces with the roof of the orbital cavity. The inferior boundary of the NOE region is formed by the frontal process of the maxilla representing the anteromedial orbital rim. It comprises the lacrimal, ethmoid, orbital surfaces of the frontal and maxillary bones thus forming the medial orbital wall. Here, the medial canthal tendon attaches. This area is critical in operative reduction and fixation of NOE fractures. This is the significant component to restore preinjury appearance.

The medial canthal tendon lies anterior to the lacrimal caruncle and has three limbs. The posterior limb runs behind the lacrimal sac, attaching to the posterior lacrimal crest, whereas the superior limb runs superiorly, attaching to the superior lacrimal crest. The anterior limb inserts into the lateral surface of the nasal bone. Then it attaches to the superior and posterior limbs before broadening out to merge with the tarsal plates and orbicularis oculi muscle. The "central fragment" is an area of bone along the medial orbital wall where the tendon is attached. The Markowitz classification system uses the degree of displacement and comminution of the "central fragment" to assess both the severity and predict the surgical method needed for fixation of NOE fractures. Intercanthal distance is normally 30–35 mm. This is equivalent to the width of the nasal base or half the interpupillary distance (60–70 mm).

Structural support of the face is provided by the horizontal and vertical buttresses. Superior horizontal buttresses include the frontal bone and superior orbital rims. Inferior orbital rims with a zygomaticomaxillary component form the horizontal buttress inferiorly. The medial vertical buttress comprises the frontal bone with the frontal process of the maxilla. Laterally, the vertical buttress consists of the frontal and zygomatic bone processes with the maxilla inferiorly. If compromised, these buttresses must be reduced appropriately. They form the basic foundation upon which complex NOE fractures are reconstructed.

Branches of both the internal and external carotid arteries supply the NOE complex. Main branches include the anterior and posterior ethmoidal arteries, while the maxillary, greater palatine, infraorbital, and sphenopalatine arteries are all branches of the external carotid artery. Sensation to the area is from the ophthalmic and maxillary divisions of the trigeminal nerve.

ASSESSMENT OF THE DEFECT

A high index of suspicion is required in any patient with midface trauma in order to avoid missing any NOE fractures. This is essential since delays in operative repair uniformly lead to compromised outcomes. High-velocity trauma to the central midface may result in NOE as well as other facial fractures. In addition, there is potential for injury to intracranial, ocular, and periocular structures. A thorough physical exam combined with thin section (1–2 mm) computed tomography (CT) scanning will identify these fractures and help develop a comprehensive management plan.

It is important to completely assess the relative integrity and position of the overlying soft tissue. While this may be compromised by the presence of swelling or bruising, it is crucial to pay particular attention to the medial canthus. Accordingly, the intercanthal distance, palpebral fissure dimensions, and medial canthal angle should be evaluated. Presence of a raccoon sign or periorbital ecchymosis can assist the examiner in determining the possibility of an orbital hematoma. Blunting of the normally acute medial canthal angle as well as an intercanthal distance of less than 35 mm can also be suggestive of NOE complex disruption. Additionally, loss of dorsal nasal projection and generalized dorsal nasal widening are also associated with these fractures. Palpation of the area is also crucial to a thorough evaluation. In addition to discerning general step-offs, palpation of the medial canthal tendon while maintaining lateral traction on the eyelids is essential for assessing canthal stability. This is known as the "bowstring" test.

Both the nasal dorsum and caudal septum should be palpated to assess the presence and quality of underlying cartilage support. Any deficiency suggests the need for primary bone or cartilage grafting. The nasal septum should be evaluated for a hematoma. With NOE fractures, the nasal pyramid is typically shifted posteriorly and slightly inferiorly, with a loss in nasal height, elevation of the nasal tip, an increase in the interorbital distance, flattening of the nasal dorsum, disappearance of caudal septal support, and

displacement of the canthi and lacrimal systems. Presence and location of any facial lacerations should be noted. They may provide additional sites of surgical access to the facial skeleton.

A comprehensive assessment of ocular integrity is also important to assess. In addition to documenting visual acuity and diplopia; sensory afferent/efferent defects, extraocular movement, and a funduscopic examination should be performed. Non-ophthalmologic practitioners should obtain an ophthalmology consult for detailed evaluation as well as preoperative risk assessment if surgical intervention is necessary.

While uncommon, CSF leaks should always be looked for, given the relative proximity to the intracranial cavity. This can result from dural tears, which can also result in parenchymal injury and/or intracranial hemorrhage. If a CSF leak is present, clinically it results in rhinorrhea. Therefore, intranasal evaluation for thin clear rhinorrhea is important.

CSF rhinorrhea can be diagnosed by detection of β-2 transferrin. Otherwise, a perfunctory bedside halo sign can be observed by placing the suspected fluid on filter paper. CSF will separate from the blood components, creating a "halo" around the central bloodstain. If a CSF leak is detected and/or suspected, neurosurgical consultation is mandatory.

Thin-cut CT scans (1–2 mm) are the gold standard for imaging NOE fractures. Axial images are helpful in evaluating the frontal sinus, lamina papyracea, ethmoid complex, globe position, presence/absence of an orbital hematoma, nasal bones, and septum. Coronal images clearly visualize the orbital roof and floor, globe position, rectus muscle entrapment, cribriform plate, nasofrontal recess, lamina papyracea, ethmoid complex, and the medial vertical maxillary buttress.

Intravenous contrast helps identify any CSF leaks or dural tears. Both bone and soft tissue windows are necessary. Plain radiographs are rarely helpful in these anatomically complex fracture patterns. Three-dimensional reconstruction can be used for a gross evaluation of the facial skeleton, but these often underestimate the details of these fractures. Intraoperative CT scanning is increasingly used to ensure precise reduction and fixation in complex facial fractures. This enables the surgeon to evaluate the repair and make appropriate maneuvers. This is in contrast to postoperative CT, which limits us to observation or a second-look operation. Additionally, computer-aided design and manufacturing technology uses preoperative CT scans to design custom-made implants if needed. This offers the advantage of creating the smallest sized implant to cover complex defects and also avoids impinging on surrounding structures.

CLASSIFICATION AS THE BASIS FOR OPERATIVE EXPOSURE

The Markowitz classification system is the most commonly used. It is simple and helps predict the appropriate operative repair. This divides NOE fractures into three groups based on the degree of comminution in the "central fragment" onto which the medial canthal tendon inserts.

I. Complete or incomplete fracture, single fragment (Figure 57.1)

    IA. Incomplete fracture, single fragment

    IB. Complete fracture, single fragment

    IC. Complete fracture, bilateral monoblack (Figure 57.2)

II. Comminuted fractures external to the canthal insertion (Figure 57.3)

III. Comminuted fractures extending within the canthal insertion (Figure 57.4)

As mentioned earlier, type I fractures can be further subcategorized. This subcategorization is done according to the relative location of the respective fracture patterns that create the single bony fragment that is characteristic of type I fractures. Type IA fractures are essentially "greenstick" fractures, in which the fracture itself is incomplete. These fracture patterns are displaced at the infraorbital and pyriform aperture. However, the frontal process of the maxilla and frontal bone articulation remains nondisplaced. For type IB fractures, this articulation is displaced unilaterally and requires stable fixation. In type IC fractures, the articulation is displaced bilaterally. A common feature of all type I fractures is the presence of a single, noncomminuted bony fragment with an intact medial canthal tendon.

Type II fractures are characterized by a comminuted bony fragment instead of a single bony fragment as described with type I fractures. Fracture and comminution with type II patterns are always medial to the central canthal-bearing segment. Therefore, the medial canthal tendon remains intact.

If the fracture results in comminution laterally or through the canthal-bearing segment, this will result in disruption to the medial canthal tendon. This feature is the hallmark distinction of type III fractures. Such fracture patterns are the most challenging to manage.

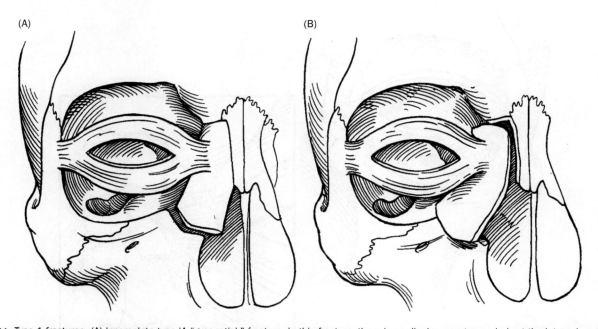

(A)   **(B)**

Figure 57.1. Type 1 fractures. (A) Incomplete type IA "greenstick" fracture. In this fracture, there is no displacement superiorly at the internal angular process of frontal bone; however, there is fracture with displacement at inferior orbital rim and pyriform aperture. (B) Complete type IB fracture. Complete fractures have inferior displacement at the internal angular process of the frontal bone and inferiorly at the inferior orbital rim and pyriform aperture. Fracture requires operative treatment at three locations. In incomplete fracture, displacement may be corrected by approaches to only inferior fractures.

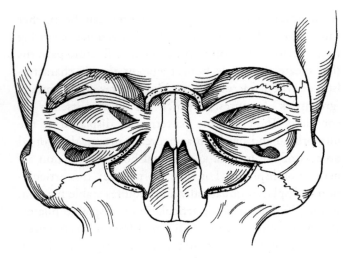

Figure 57.2. Monoblock NOE fracture (complete bilateral monoblock). Fracture results in one-piece bilateral fracture that isolates single bony fragment containing insertions of both medial canthi. Since bone continuity is retained across midline, telecanthus is not possible.

INDICATIONS

In our opinion, any displaced NOE fracture, regardless of pattern, should be reduced and rigidly fixated. Failing to recognize and surgically treat these fractures can result in suboptimal long-term aesthetic outcomes.

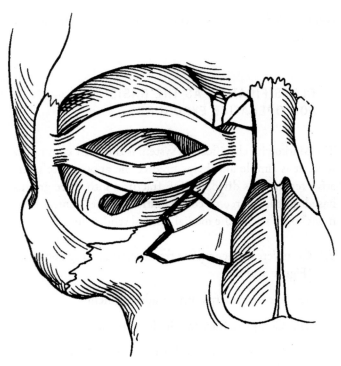

Figure 57.3. Type II complete fracture.

A stepwise approach beginning from the skull base (stable point) to the central facial skeleton is preferred. This creates a frame upon which the NOE complex

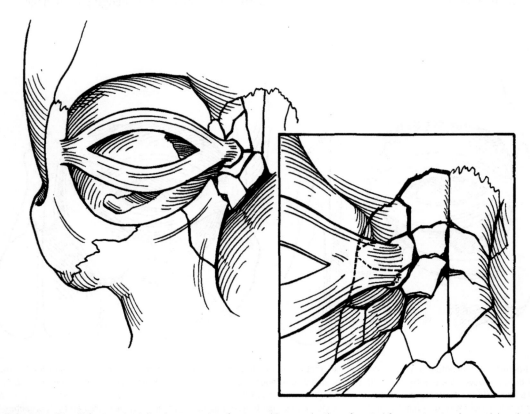

Figure 57.4. Type III fracture. Type III fracture is defined as complete fracture with comminution of central fragment or tendon avulsion. In these situations, transnasal reduction or canthal realignment is necessary in addition to reduction of bony frontal process of maxilla.

MAXILLOFACIAL SURGERY

repair attaches. Initially, the cranial base, frontal bone, and sinus should be reconstructed. This is followed by the orbital rims and medial vertical buttress. Then the nasal dorsum and projection are addressed. This may require bone grafting to restore preinjury frontonasal angle, nasal projection, and contour. Following this, the medial orbital wall and medial canthal tendons are realigned. They are held in position by transnasal wires and plating. Finally, the lacrimal duct is repaired if needed. Overlying soft tissue is managed with dermal sutures, bolsters, and splints.

CONTRAINDICATIONS

As with any surgical procedure, contraindications exist. Due to the force required to fracture, these patients often have concomitant traumatic injuries. They include, but are not limited to the cervical spine, ocular structures, neurologic system, musculoskeletal system, and/or the cardiovascular system. If any of the other traumatic injuries renders the patient medically unstable, proceeding with elective repair of the NOE should be delayed. Another contraindication to open reduction and internal fixation (ORIF) of NOE fractures is the presence of an acute local infection. An acute suppurative infection should be controlled prior to the placement of stabilizing hardware.

ROOM SETUP

NOE fractures should be managed in the operating room, with the patient under general anesthesia. Ideally, orotracheal- or tracheostomy-dependent ventilation should be established. Nasotracheal ventilation is suboptimal. However, if it can permit adequate manipulation and bony reduction, it can still be utilized. The surgical team should have unrestricted access to the patient's head. This is best facilitated by rotating the head of the bed 180 degrees from the anesthesia team and ventilator.

In addition to the reduction of the NOE fracture, frequently the nasal dorsum must also be addressed. If this is the case, the setup and surgical prep should also include potential graft harvest sites, such as rib or calvarium.

To maintain fixation after reduction, a low-profile mid-face 1.3 or 1.5 mm plate is utilized. If there is significant

comminution, multiple fragments might need to be wired. This can be performed with wires ranging from 26 to 30 gauge. Additionally, a 2-0 or 3-0 nonabsorbable suture should be present in the event that the canthal tendon must be repaired.

Finally, it would be ideal to have preoperative photographs and maxillofacial imaging with radiographs or plain films available for intraoperative review as well.

INCISION PLANNING

Some advocate using existing lacerations to obtain wide exposure for reduction and fixation of NOE fractures. Thorough reduction assessment is rarely completely facilitated via that technique. Several points of access must be established to permit a comprehensive assessment of reduction, these are outlined here.

1. A standard coronal incision starting posterior to or at the hairline provides optimal exposure to the upper third of the face. This encompasses the frontal bone, superior aspect of orbital rims, and the glabella region. Dissection starts subgalealy in the scalp. Then it transitions to a subperiosteal plane approximately 2 cm above the orbital rims. Laterally, the dissection is carried out immediately superficial to the deep aspect of the deep temporal fascia, overlying the temporalis muscle. The supraorbital and supratrochlear pedicles should be mobilized. Trochlea detachment should proceed carefully so as not to injure the muscle. Care is necessary when dissecting along the medial orbital wall to avoid inadvertent injury to the medial canthal tendon.

2. Access should also be obtained to the inferior orbital rim and orbital floor. This can be done via a lower lid incision, transconjunctival incision, or any method the surgeon is comfortable performing. During this exposure, extreme care should be taken not to disrupt the lacrimal drainage system. It could have already been compromised from the fracture itself.

3. Finally, exposure of the inferior aspect of the medial buttress (frontal process of the maxilla) can be facilitated via a sublabial incision in the gingivobuccal sulcus. This is crucial to adequately reduce comminuted fractures extending to the inferior attachment of the NOE buttress.

SURGICAL APPROACH

Surgeons must consider the fracture types critically when determining the appropriate surgical approach. Associated anatomic features play the most important role in determining which incisions to perform (Figure 57.5).

For incomplete type I fractures, fixation along the inferior orbital rim might be required. This can be achieved through several types of periorbital incisions. Also, these provide access to the orbital floor, which is often also fractured. If a complete type I fracture is present, fixation must be achieved superiorly as well, requiring access via a coronal incision.

Type II fractures mandate utilizing all of the three approaches described earlier. The most important step is to first reduce the central fragment. The complexity of this task is increased for the inexperienced surgeon due to difficulty in recognizing the transition from periosteum to tendon. It is crucial not to detach the tendon from the central fragment. If this occurs, the fracture then becomes a type III instead of a type II fracture. After exposure is obtained, small fenestrations are created via drilling through the central fragment. Transnasal wires are then used to position the fragment superior and posterior to the medial canthal ligament and lacrimal fossa. Care must be taken not to place the wires too anterior to the tendon insertion. This can result in lateral migration and postoperative telecanthus. Wires should then be tightened medially to reduce the central fragment.

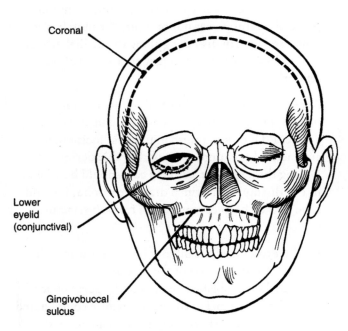

Figure 57.5. Three types of incisions required for complete exposure: coronal, lower eyelid, and gingivobuccal sulcus.

One must bear in mind that undercorrection occurs much more frequently than overcorrection (which can result in a narrowed intercanthal distance). Once the central fragment is positioned correctly, all other bony fragments are then fixated to it in order to recreate the NOE complex. Usually this is performed using a thin 1.3 mm plate (Figure 57.6).

A modification to the transnasal wiring technique for fixation of the medial canthal tendon has recently been described. This utilizes a wire with a barbed hook via a transcaruncular approach to "catch" the medial canthal tendon remnant and fix it to a miniplate placed on the medial orbital wall and/or frontal bone. This is advantageous as it can be used when there is significant comminution of the central fragment precluding transnasal wiring without bone grafting. It obviates the need for medial canthal tendon dissection.

NOE fractures frequently lead to septal injuries and loss of support to the nasal dorsum with resultant loss of projection. This requires septal repair and dorsum reconstruction to restore preinjury frontonasal angle and projection. Calvarial bone graft obtained from the parietal region is easily harvested via the coronal incision. This autogenous graft is contoured and stabilized with miniplate fixation.

Regional edema will be exacerbated by the bony and soft tissue dissections. To account for this, external compression bolsters should be placed intraoperatively. These can be made from Xeroform secured to the skin via sutures or wires that are passed through the central fragment reduction fenestrations. Intranasal septal splints may also be used to provide additional support for the nasal dorsum.

POSTOPERATIVE CARE

It is important to monitor for postoperative visual compromise. Most commonly, this can be effected by intraorbital bleeding. As such, no anticoagulants should be used postoperatively. If the patient requires anticoagulation, this should be considered a contraindication to proceeding with surgery. Head elevation is crucial to help with edema and drainage. Cold compresses also assist in minimizing postoperative edema and ecchymosis.

Restrictions to nose blowing are also important within the postoperative period. If a laceration is present over the fracture site, strong consideration should be given to continuing perioperative antibiotics for 48 hours. This is true for patients with an associated CSF leak as well. Modifications to the antibiotic regimen should be conducted to minimize microbial selection and colonization of the meninges.

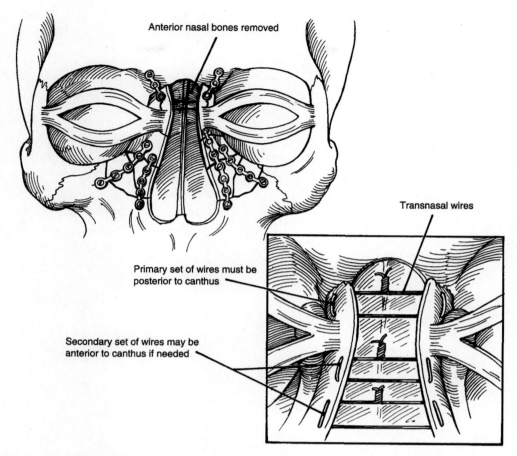

Anterior nasal bones removed

Transnasal wires

Primary set of wires must be posterior to canthus

Secondary set of wires may be anterior to canthus if needed

Figure 57.6. Strategy for reduction of unilateral type II comminuted fracture with large central fragment containing insertion of medial canthal tendon. Superior aspect of fracture is exposed via coronal incision. Fracture requires transnasal wiring; nasal bones may be temporarily removed to provide maximum exposure for frontal process reduction; 28-gauge transnasal wires are passed through drill holes placed superior and posterior to lacrimal fossa. Following replacement of nasal bones, screw may also be used to affix dorsal nasal bone graft if required. Following linking of all small fractures with wires, junctional rigid fixation is used to stabilize linked fragments to intact facial skeleton at periphery of nasoethmoidal segment. Because intercanthal soft tissue distance is rarely overcorrected, transnasal reduction should deliberately minimize distance between medial orbital rims. After closure of incisions, soft tissue bolsters are secured by two additional transnasal wires, one placed at time of canthal reduction superiorly and one inferiorly passed over pyriform aperture. Soft tissue reduction aids in preventing soft tissue thickening, which produces telecanthus, just as chronic edema produces scar tissue after surgery.

SUGGESTED READINGS

Converse JM, Smith B. Naso-orbital fractures and traumatic deformities of the medial canthus. *Plast Reconstr Surg* 1966;38:147.

Engelstad ME, Bastodkar P, Markiewicz MR. Medial canthopexy using transcaruncular barb and miniplate: technique and cadaver study. *Int J Oral Maxillofac Surg* 2012 Oct;41(10):1176–1185.

Gruss JS. Naso-ethmoid-orbital fractures: classification and role of primary bone grafting. *Plast Reconstr Surg* 1985;75:303.

Lauer G, Pinzer T. Transcaruncular-transnasal suture: a modification of medial canthopexy. *J Oral Maxillofac Surg* 2008 Oct;66(10):2178–2184.

Markowitz BL, Manson PN, Sargent L, et al. Management of the medial canthal tendon in nasoethmoid orbital fractures: the importance of the central fragment in clarification and treatment. *Plast Reconstr Surg* 1991;87:843.

Merville LC, Real JP. Fronto-orbital nasal dislocations: initial total reconstruction. *Scand J Plast Reconstr Surg* 1981;15:287.

Morrison AD, Gregoire CE. Management of fractures of the nasofrontal complex. *Oral Maxillofac Surg Clin North Am* 2013 Nov;25(4):637–648.

Paskert JP, Manson PN. The bimanual examination for assessing instability in naso-orbito-ethmoidal injuries. *Plast Reconstr Surg* 1989;83:165.

Pawar SS, Rhee JS. Frontal sinus and naso-orbital-ethmoid fractures. *JAMA Facial Plast Surg* 2014 Jul-Aug;16(4):284–289.

Potter JK, Muzaffar AR, Ellis E, Rohrich RJ, Hackney FL. Aesthetic management of the nasal component of naso-orbital ethmoid fractures. *Plast Reconstr Surg* 2006 Jan;117(1):10e–18e.

Rosenberger E, Kriet JD, Humphrey C. Management of nasoethmoid fractures. *Curr Opin Otolaryngol Head Neck Surg* 2013 Aug;21(4):410–416.

Stanc MF. Primary treatment of naso-ethmoid injuries with increased intercanthal distance. *Br J Plast Surg* 1970;23:8.

Tollefson TT, Strong EB. Nasoorbitoethmoid fractures treatment & management Medscape 2015. http://emedicine.medscape.com/article/869330-overview

Wolff J, Sándor GK, Pyysalo M, Miettinen A, Koivumäki AV, Kainulainen VT. Late reconstruction of orbital and naso-orbital deformities. *Oral Maxillofac Surg Clin North Am* 2013 Nov;25(4):683–695.

Zide B, McCarthy J. The medial canthus revisited—an anatomical basis for canthopexy. *Ann Plast Surg* 1983;9:1.

58.

ORTHOGNATHIC SURGERY

Ryan M. Moore and Raj M. Vyas

INTRODUCTION

Orthognathic surgery restores the skeletal function and facial disharmony affected by dentofacial deformities. Facial skeletal discrepancies are broadly characterized as maxillary or mandibular excess or deficiency in the anterior-posterior, transverse, or vertical dimensions. These skeletal deformities beget occlusal imbalance and masticatory dysfunction, compromise the patency of the airway, and distort the platform for the overlying soft tissues of the middle and lower thirds of the face. Dentofacial anomalies thereby affect facial function, aesthetics, and patient self-image. As such, surgical restoration of facial function and harmony must address the maxillary-to-mandibular occlusal relationship and dental compensations, as well as facial proportions and aesthetics.

PREOPERATIVE EVALUATION

Preoperative evaluation should include a complete history, with emphasis on pertinent medical, surgical, and dental factors. Inquire about obstructive sleep apnea and use of continuous positive airway pressure, temporomandibular joint disorders, history of cleft lip/palate repair, velopharyngeal insufficiency, and associated congenital anomalies and genetic syndromes, as well as any other previous surgery (e.g., uvulopalatopharyngoplasty, mandibular distraction osteogenesis, fistula repair, pharyngeal flap) and associated sequelae (e.g., scarring). Discuss dental history, including oral hygiene, dental caries, periodontal disease, dental extraction, orthodontia, and habits (e.g., tongue thrusting or thumb sucking).

Examination of the face is performed to evaluate aesthetics and skin quality. Facial proportions are assessed in lateral and frontal views for comparison with facial aesthetic ideals. In frontal view, the face can be divided into horizontal fifths by vertical lines drawn through the medial canthi, lateral canthi, and the most lateral surfaces of the face (Figure 58.1).[1] When viewed in profile or frontal view, the face can be divided into vertical thirds by horizontal lines drawn through the trichion (anteroinferior aspect of midsagittal hairline), glabella, subnasale, and menton (Figure 58.2). The lower third can be further subdivided by the stomion into an upper third and lower two-thirds.[1] Divergence from ideal proportions indicates the presence of underlying facial skeletal disharmony. Incisor show is the vertical height of the maxillary central incisor on display when the lips are in repose and while smiling. During repose, 2–3 mm of show is ideal in men while 4–6 mm may be attractive in women in the absence of mentalis strain. The entire maxillary central incisor should be visible with at most 2 mm of gingival show during full smile.[2,3]

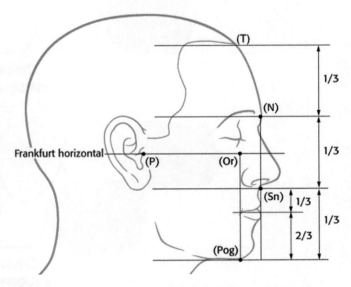

Figure 58.1. Vertical thirds. Adapted from Mast G, Ehrenfeld M, Bartlett S, Sugar A, eds. *Facial proportions.* In: *AO Surgery Reference.* The AO Foundation, Davos, Switzerland. April 10, 2013.

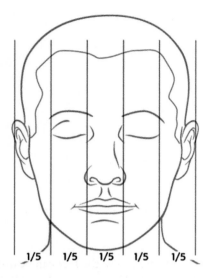

Figure 58.2. Horizontal fifths. Adapted from Mast G, Ehrenfeld M, Bartlett S, Sugar A, eds. Facial proportions. In: *AO Surgery Reference.* The AO Foundation, Davos, Switzerland, April 10, 2013.

A complete intraoral examination begins with an assessment of overall mucosal, periodontal, and dental health. Evaluate for dental caries and restorations. Assess for periodontal disease. Note the presence and type of any orthodontia (e.g., braces or Kobayashi hooks). Ascertain whether the third molars are present, as they lie along LeFort I and bilateral sagittal split osteotomy and fixation lines. Determine the occlusal pattern. Normal occlusion is defined as the relationship of the dental arches when the mesiobuccal cusp of the maxillary first molar occludes in the buccal groove of the mandibular first molar. Distortion of this relationship, or malocclusion, is characterized according to Angle's classification (Figure 58.3)[3–5]:

- *Class I*: Mesiobuccal cusp of the maxillary first molar occludes in the buccal groove of the mandibular first molar; however, teeth are malposed or malrotated.

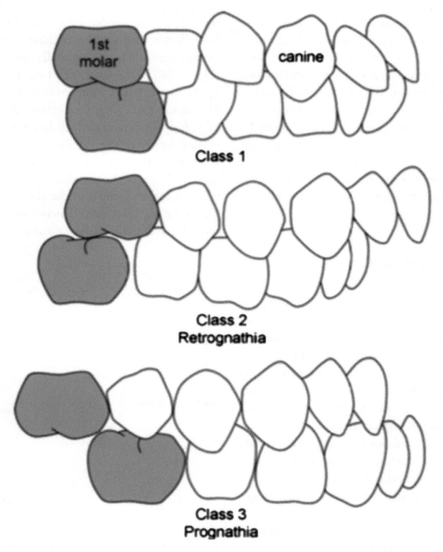

Figure 58.3. Angle's classification. Adapted from Hurst CA, Eppley BL, Havlik RJ, Sadove AM. Surgical cephalometrics: applications and developments. *Plast Reconstr Surg* 2007 Nov;120(6):92e–104e. Review.

- *Class II*: The mandibular first molar is distally positioned relative to the maxillary first molar.
  - Division I: Maxillary incisors proclined, resulting in excessive overjet
  - Division II: Central maxillary incisors retroclined, while the lateral maxillary incisors proclined, resulting in a deep overbite
- *Class III*: The mandibular first molar is mesially positioned relative to the maxillary first molar.

Centric occlusion (CO) refers to the occlusion of teeth in maximal intercuspation regardless of position of the condylar head within the glenoid fossa, as influenced by habit and dentition. In contrast, centric relation (CR) describes the occlusal relationship of the maxilla and mandible when the condylar head is in its most superior position within the glenoid fossa.[2]

Evaluate the degree of overjet and overbite (i.e., the horizontal and vertical overlap of the incisal edges of the maxillary and mandibular central incisors, respectively). Note the presence and type of an open bite (anterior or posterior) or crossbite (buccal or lingual). Characterize incisor inclination. The dentition are said to be *proclined* or *retroclined* when the anterior surface of the teeth are flared labially or lingually, respectively. Identify presence of crowding or edentulous spaces. Assess the occlusal plane of both the maxillary and mandibular arch, noting the degree of anterior-posterior curvature (curve of Spee) and transverse curvature (curve of Wilson). Evaluate for possible occlusal cant by asking the patient to bite down onto a tongue depressor. Canted occlusion is present if the tongue blade is positioned obliquely to a line drawn through the lateral canthi.[3]

Imaging is an essential component of the preoperative evaluation. Standard two-dimensional radiographs, including lateral, anteroposterior (AP), and panoramic views, are necessary to evaluate the facial skeletal and dental anatomy. Historically, preoperative planning for correction of dentofacial deformities would entail cephalometric analyses performed using lateral plain films. With technological advancement, three-dimensional volumetric studies, such as cone-beam computed tomography CT (CBCT) and multidetector row CT (MDCT), have supplanted traditional two-dimensional radiographs.[6-9] Furthermore, such studies require lower radiation dosage while providing a more detailed view of the skeletal structure, dentition, and overlying soft tissue. Importantly, CBCT must be performed with the head in the natural, upright position with the maxilla and mandible in CR.

Anesthesia evaluation determines whether the patient can safely undergo general anesthesia. Preoperative planning ensures a steady, controlled blood pressure intraoperatively and facilitates operative technique while enhancing patient safety. Additionally, nonsteroidal anti-inflammatories (NSAIDs) and aspirin should be held at least 1 week preoperatively. The following is a list of cephalometrics used in assessment.

- Cephalometrics[5,9-10]
- Landmarks
  - Skeletal (Figure 58.4)
    - Define the cranial base and reference points
      - S (sella): Center of the pituitary fossa
      - N (nasion): Junction of the nasal and frontal bones
      - Or (orbitale): Most inferior point of the inferior orbital rim
      - Po (porion): Most superior point of the external auditory meatus

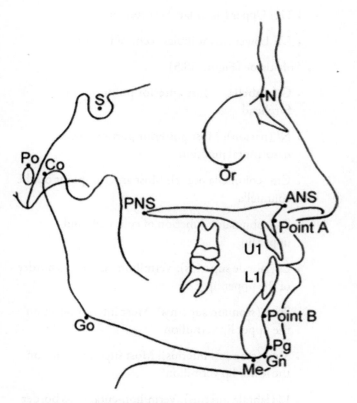

Figure 58.4. Skeletal and dental landmarks. Adapted from Hurst CA, Eppley BL, Havlik RJ, Sadove AM. Surgical cephalometrics: applications and developments. *Plast Reconstr Surg* 2007 Nov;120(6):92e–104e. Review.

- Define the maxilla
  - PNS (posterior nasal spine): Most posterior point of the hard palate
  - ANS (anterior nasal spine): Most anterosuperior point of the maxilla
  - Point A: Most posterior point along the curvature of the anterior maxillary contour
- Define the mandible
  - Point B: Most posterior point along the curvature of the anterior mandibular contour
  - Pg (pogonion): Most anterior point on the anterior mandibular contour
  - Me (menton): Most inferior point of the mandible
  - Go (gonion): Most inferoposterior point at the mandibular angle
  - Co (condylion): Most posterosuperior point of the condyle
- Dental (Figure 58.4)
  - U1: Upper (maxillary) central incisor
  - L1: Lower (mandibular) central incisor
- Soft-tissue (Figure 58.5)
  - G (glabella): Most anterior point on the forehead
  - N′ (nasion): Most posterior portion of the nasofrontal junction
  - Cm (columella point): Most anterior point on the columella
  - Sn (subnasale): Junction of columella and upper lip
  - Ls (labrale superius): Vermilion-cutaneous border of the upper lip
  - Stms (stomion superius): Most inferior point on the upper lip vermilion
  - Stmi (stomion inferius): Most superior point on the lower lip vermilion
  - Li (labrale inferius): Vermilion-cutaneous border of the lower lip
  - Pg′ (pogonion): Most anterior point of the chin

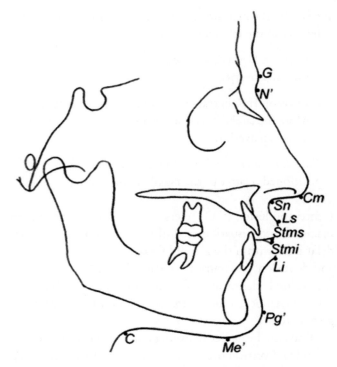

Figure 58.5. Soft tissue landmarks. Adapted from Hurst CA, Eppley BL, Havlik RJ, Sadove AM. Surgical cephalometrics: applications and developments. *Plast Reconstr Surg* 2007 Nov;120(6):92e–104e. Review.

  - Me′ (menton): Most inferior point of the chin
  - C (cervical point): Point at which the neck transitions from horizontal to vertical
- Planes (Figure 58.6)
  - Horizontal
  - Reference
    - S-N: Sella-nasion plane (SN)
      - Used to describe landmark positions and relationships of the maxilla and mandible to the anterior cranial base
    - Po-Or: Frankfort horizontal (FH)
      - Alternatively, may be used as a standard reference
      - Unlike SN, independent of the length or inclination of the anterior cranial base
    - Interrelationship of SN-FH: 7°
    - ANS-PNS: Palatal plane (PP)
    - Occlusal plane (OP): Between the occlusal surfaces of the first molars and incisal edges of the central incisors during maximum intercuspation
    - Go-Me: Mandibular plane (MP)

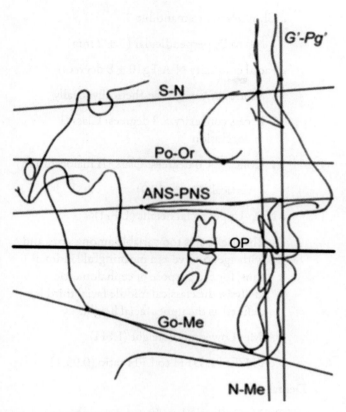

Figure 58.6. Cephalometric planes. Adapted from Hurst CA, Eppley BL, Havlik RJ, Sadove AM. Surgical cephalometrics: applications and developments. *Plast Reconstr Surg* 2007 Nov;120(6):92e–104e. Review.

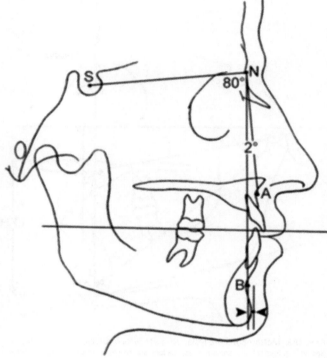

Figure 58.7. Steiner's analysis. Adapted from Hurst CA, Eppley BL, Havlik RJ, Sadove AM. Surgical cephalometrics: applications and developments. *Plast Reconstr Surg* 2007 Nov;120(6):92e–104e. Review.

- Vertical
  - N-Pg: Facial plane (FP)
  - N-A: Maxillary plane
- Dental
  - U1 axis: Maxillary incisor inclination: A line through the incisal edge and apex of the root of U1
  - L1 axis: Mandibular incisor inclination: A line through the incisal edge and apex of the root of L1
- Cephalometric analysis
  - Determine the relevant angles and measurements that relate the aforementioned landmarks and planes
  - Historically performed by hand, now done digitally with two-dimensional and three-dimensional software
  - Ideal angles and measurements are based on population normative data

- Surgical goals are based on aesthetic ideals and patient preferences
- Several analyses dating back as early as the mid-twentieth century, although Steiner's analysis guides most surgeons in their aim to satisfy treatment objectives (Figures 58.7 and 58.8)[11–14]
- Accuracy of cephalometrics is inversely proportional to asymmetry; errors are exacerbated even more for two-jaw surgery
- Skeletal
  - Sagittal
    - Maxilla relative to cranial base
      - SNA (82 ± 3 degrees)
      - NA-FH (90 ± 4 degrees)
    - Mandible relative to cranial base
      - SNB (79 ± 3 degrees)
      - MP-FH (24 ± 3 degrees)

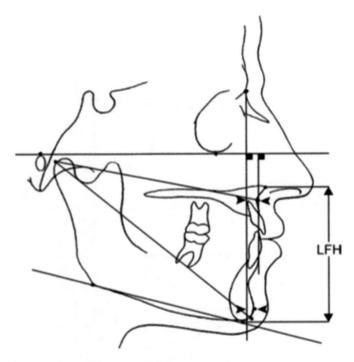

Figure 58.8. McNamara's analysis. Adapted from Hurst CA, Eppley BL, Havlik RJ, Sadove AM. Surgical cephalometrics: applications and developments. *Plast Reconstr Surg* 2007 Nov;120(6):92e–104e. Review.

- Maxillary depth relative to cranial base (FH)
  - A to N perpendicular (mean)
    - Male 1.1 mm
    - Female 0.4 mm
- Mandibular depth relative to cranial base (FH)
  - Pg to N perpendicular (mean)
    - Male −0.3 mm
    - Female −1.8 mm
- Maxilla relative to mandible
  - ANB = SNA-SNB (3 ± 2 degrees)
- Chin relative to cranial base
  - SNPg (80 ± 3 degrees)
    - >83 degrees prognathism
    - <77 degrees retrognathism
  - Facial angle NPg-FH (87 ± 4 degrees)
    - >91 degrees prognathism
    - <83 degrees retrognathism

- Chin relative to mandible
  - NB to Pg perpendicular (3 ± 2 mm)
- Facial convexity N-A-Pg (0 ± 8 degrees)
  - Subtle convexity is aesthetically ideally
  - Excess convexity > 8 degrees: Class II malocclusion
  - Concave < 0 degrees: Class III malocclusion
    - Vertical (Figure 58.9)
- N-A: Upper facial height (UFH)
  - The trichion is too variable among sexes and with age to serve as a meaningful landmark; thus, for the purpose of cephalometric analysis, the classical middle facial third is defined as the upper facial height.
- A-Me: Lower facial height (LFH)
- UFH/LFH: UFH to LFH ratio (0.95:1)
- Dental
  - OP-FH: Occlusal plane (8 ± 4 degrees)
  - Interincisal relationship
  - Overjet: Horizontal distance between the incisor tips (2 ± 1 mm)

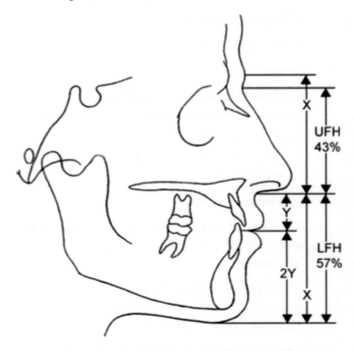

Figure 58.9. Vertical proportions. Adapted from Hurst CA, Eppley BL, Havlik RJ, Sadove AM. Surgical cephalometrics: applications and developments. *Plast Reconstr Surg* 2007 Nov;120(6):92e–104e. Review.

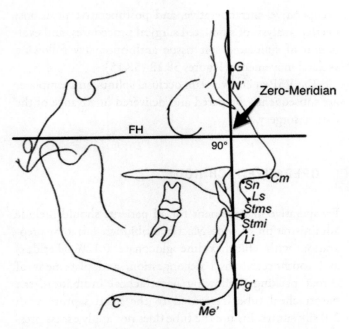

Figure 58.10. Zero meridian. Adapted from Hurst CA, Eppley BL, Havlik RJ, Sadove AM. Surgical cephalometrics: applications and developments. *Plast Reconstr Surg* 2007 Nov;120(6):92e–104e. Review.

- Overbite: Vertical distance between the incisor tips (2 ± 1 mm)

- Soft tissue

  - Facial convexity at Sn (G-Sn-Pg') (12 ± 4 degrees)

    - Excess convexity: Class II malocclusion

    - Concave: Class III malocclusion

  - Zero-Meridian (Gonzales-Ulloa line): Line perpendicular to FH through N'; ideal chin position occurs when Pg' falls along the Zero-Meridian (Figure 58.10)[15]

  - Facial Angles (e.g., Nasolabial angle: Measured at Sn (102 ± 8 degrees); more acute in males than in females) (Figure 58.11)[16]

OPERATIVE PLANNING

Following a complete preoperative evaluation, the surgeon should recognize the dentofacial deformities in need of surgical correction. Importantly, operative planning must account for maxillary-to-mandibular occlusal relationship and dental compensations, as well as for facial proportions in all dimensions (anterior-posterior, transverse, vertical).

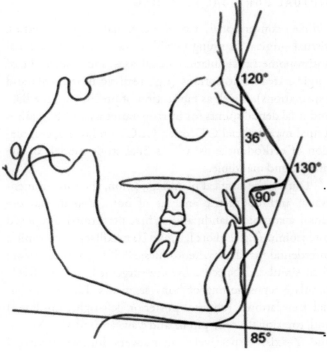

Figure 58.11. Facial angles. Adapted from Hurst CA, Eppley BL, Havlik RJ, Sadove AM. Surgical cephalometrics: applications and developments. *Plast Reconstr Surg* 2007 Nov;120(6):92e–104e. Review.

Common skeletal deformities and their management may be broadly categorized according to presence of maxillary or mandibular excess or deficiency. In general, maxillary excess is addressed by LeFort I impaction, while maxillary deficiency is addressed by LeFort I advancement. For surgical optimization of occlusion in cases of complex dentofacial deformities, especially with history of clefting, a segmental LeFort I procedure may be required. Furthermore, mandibular excess is corrected by mandibular setback via bilateral sagittal split osteotomies (BSSO) and/or maxillary advancement via LeFort I, while mandibular deficiency is corrected by mandibular advancement via BSSO.[17]

Following surgical correction of the maxillary-to-mandibular occlusal relationship, genioplasty may be used for aesthetic fine-tuning or correction of minor asymmetry.

In cases of two-jaw surgery, the maxilla is usually addressed before the mandible. (In special circumstances, such as muscle restriction or cases necessitating large surgical movements, the mandible may require initial correction.) To facilitate two-jaw surgery, intermediate and final occlusal guides (e.g., acrylic splints) should match the proposed operative sequence (e.g., intermediate: post-LeFort I; final: post-BSSO).

VIRTUAL SURGICAL PLANNING

Unlike conventional two-dimensional cephalometrics, virtual surgical planning (VSP) allows three-dimensional anthropometric simulation in all axes and evaluation of surgical treatment options (e.g., realistic movements and expectations) as well as fabrication of precise intermediate and final dental splints for intraoperative use. VSP requires a final maxillofacial CT (often CBCT) following completion of orthodontia, as well as final stone models of the maxilla and mandible.

During the surgical planning session, the three-dimensional anthropometric analysis of bony, dental, and occlusal anatomical landmarks is first performed. Proposed osteotomies (e.g., LeFort I, II, and III maxillary osteotomies; interdental maxillary osteotomies; BSSO; genioplasty) are then simulated. Specifically, the surgeon is able to freely simulate repositioning of bony segments through potential translational (anterior-posterior, left-right, up-down) and rotational (roll, pitch, and yaw around the X-, Y-, and Z-axis, respectively) maneuvers following virtual osteotomies.[9] Finally, the summarized movements from preoperative position to simulated postoperative position are reviewed, including a workflow summary with

preoperative, intraoperative, and postoperative positions; overlap analysis of simulated surgical procedures; and evaluation of simulated soft tissue anthropometry following skeletal movements (Figures 58.12–58.15).

The VSP operative plan, occlusal splints, and templates are subsequently prepared and delivered in advance of the date of surgery.

OPERATIVE TECHNIQUE

Preoperative management for all patients should include administration of prophylactic antibiotics, intraoral preparation with chlorhexidine gluconate 0.12% (Peridex) and toothbrush, nasal decongestion, and placement of throat packing. Following nasotracheal intubation, the nasotracheal tube is secured to the nasal septum with 2-0 silk suture. Ensure the tube does not apply excess pressure on the nasal columella, soft triangle, or tip. Place a nasogastric tube at the time of intubation so that the nasal mucosa is not violated by trying to pass a tube at the end of the operation. Corticosteroids are given to reduce postoperative swelling.

Point	Name	Anterior/Posterior	Left/Right	Up/Down
ANS	Anterior Nasal Spine	4.35mm Posterior	0.91mm Left	2.98mm Up
A	A Point	3.17mm Posterior	0.87mm Left	2.12mm Up
ISU1	Midline of Upper Incisor	0.00	2.50mm Left	3.00mm Up
U3L	Upper Left Canine	1.54mm Posterior	2.39mm Left	0.89mm Up
U6L	Upper Left Anterior Molar (mesiobuccal cusp)	2.41mm Posterior	1.08mm Left	0.02mm Up
U3R	Upper Right Canine	0.20mm Posterior	1.28mm Left	1.31mm Up
U6R	Upper Right Anterior Molar (mesiobuccal cusp)	0.11mm Posterior	0.37mm Left	0.13mm Up
ISL1	Midline of Lower Incisor	8.22mm Anterior	0.49mm Right	0.59mm Down
L6L	Lower Left Anterior Molar (mesiobuccal cusp)	8.75mm Anterior	0.08mm Left	1.87mm Down
L6R	Lower Right Anterior Molar (mesiobuccal cusp)	7.44mm Anterior	0.05mm Left	1.32mm Down
B	B Point	10.06mm Anterior	0.30mm Right	1.62mm Down
Pog.	Pogonion	10.46mm Anterior	0.39mm Right	1.59mm Down

Figure 58.12. Movement summary for simulated segmental LeFort 1 and BSSO.

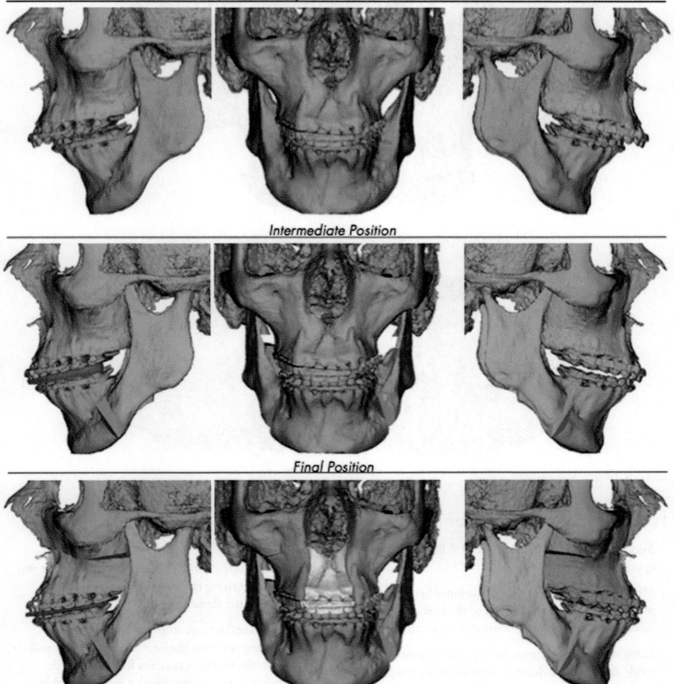

Figure 58.13. Virtual planning workflow for patient with vertical maxillary excess (mentalis strain and excess gingival show on smile) as well as increased occlusal plane angle and mandibular deficiency. Segmental interdental maxillary osteotomies between lateral incisors and canines were done to optimize postsurgical occlusion.

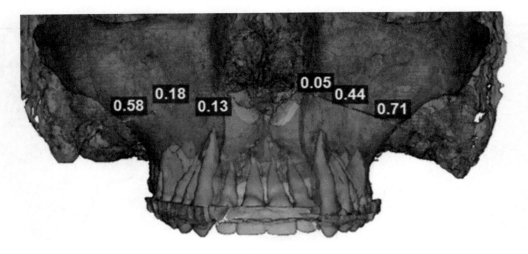

Measurements outlined in red indicate an overlap.

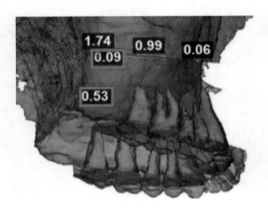

Figure 58.14. LeFort overlap analysis.

LEFORT I OSTEOTOMY TECHNIQUE

- Inject gingivobuccal incision with 1% lidocaine with epinephrine.

- Measure and record the vertical distance between the medial canthus and the bracket of the lateral incisor bilaterally; keep for post-osteotomy comparison.

- Using needle-tip electrocautery, incise the mucosa on cut mode and continue down to periosteum on coagulation mode. Leave an adequate cuff of mucosa to allow for easier closure. Minimize the length of the gingivobuccal incision as it risks devascularization of the maxillary segment, particularly in cleft patients.

- Use a Molt periosteal elevator to dissect superiorly in a subperiosteal plane to the level of the infraorbital nerve and posteriorly around the pterygomaxillary buttress. A Selden retractor or curved malleable may be placed within the pterygomaxillary junction to facilitate

dissection to the pterygoid plates. Dissect inferiorly as well to provide a suturing edge for closure.

- Dissect the nasal mucosa off the pyriform aperture and soft tissues overlying the anterior nasal spine with a curved or Cottle elevator.

- Begin the maxillary osteotomy by running the reciprocating saw from the lateral (zygomaticomaxillary) buttress to the pyriform aperture bilaterally while protecting the nasal mucosa with a small malleable. Maintain a perpendicular orientation of the blade relative to the maxilla.

- Complete the medial maxillary buttress osteotomy using a guarded osteotome bilaterally.

- After palpating the pterygoid through the mouth posteriorly, divide the pterygomaxillary junction using a Tessier-Kawamoto (curved) osteotome bilaterally. During the pterygoid osteotomy, ensure that the

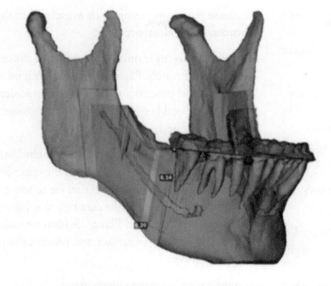
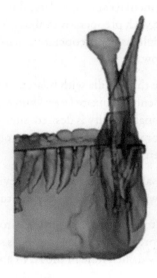

Measurements outlined in red indicate an overlap.

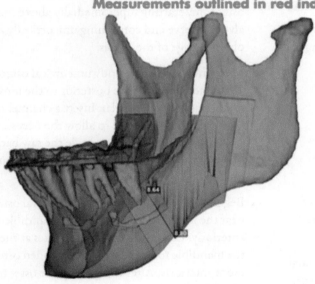
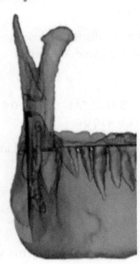

Figure 58.15. Bilateral sagittal split osteotomies (BSSO) overlap analysis.

osteotome is positioned sufficiently posterior to capture the entire pterygoid plate and avoid injuring the most distal molars.

- Separate the vomer from the anterior nasal spine using an olive osteotome. A finger in the mouth behind the posterior nasal spine helps protect against inadvertent injury to the nasotracheal tube.

- Within the thicker bone stock of the lateral maxillary buttress, insert a Smith's spreader to separate the posterior attachments of the maxilla with counterpressure on the anterior floating maxilla.

- Use a rongeur to remove bony spurs and interferences, particularly over the vomer and laterally as needed

depending on the direction of LeFort I movement (impaction requires more bone removal).

- Drill a hole in the anterior nasal spine and place a 24-gauge wire to obtain traction on the maxilla in order to confirm adequate mobility. Alternatively, utilize Rowe disimpaction forceps or place Tessier retractors behind the pterygoid plates bilaterally to help stretch restrictive soft tissues and mobilize the maxilla.

- Apply the intermediate or final occlusal splint and confirm occlusion with the condyles seated within the glenoid fossae (i.e., centric relation).

- Establish centric occlusion with 24- or 26-gauge wire placed around the maxillary and mandibular teeth.

- Measure the medial canthus to lateral incisor distances and compare with preoperative values. Adjust the maxillary height as per preoperative plan and the degree of incisor show.

- Rigidly fixate the maxilla with bilateral medial buttress step plates. Bend and fixate lateral buttress plates when additional stability is desired, such as for large movements or when segmental LeFort osteotomies are made between the maxillary dentition.

- Close the nasal mucosa if torn (e.g., previous history of cleft repair) with running 3-0 Vicryl suture.

- Place a 2-0 Prolene alar-cinch suture through bilateral alar bases to prevent alar widening. Pass suture through the previously drilled hole in the ANS and secure.

- Close the frenulum in V-Y fashion to lengthen the upper lip, if needed.

- Irrigate the maxilla, then close the mucosa in a single layer using 3-0 chromic suture.

BILATERAL SAGITTAL SPLIT OSTEOTOMY (BSSO) TECHNIQUE

- Infiltrate bilateral gingivobuccal incisions with 1% lidocaine with epinephrine.

- Place a bite block opposite the side of the planned initial osteotomy. Use a Sweetheart to retract the tongue.

- Use needle-tip electrocautery to incise the mandibular gingivobuccal sulcus on cut; dissect to periosteum on coagulation mode. Leave all muscle on the buccal side to reduce the possibility of intervening soft tissue during mandibulotomy. Take care to actively avoid injuring the lingual nerve in the retromolar region.

- A Molt periosteal elevator is used to dissect subperiosteally from the inferior border of the body of the mandible to the angle.

- Use an Obwegeser "J" stripper to fully free the inferior border of the mandible. Be careful to avoid the submandibular/retromandibular venous plexus.

- Utilize an Obwegeser toe-in retractor to retract mucosa while using a Molt elevator to expose the ramus, condyle, and coronoid process in a subperiosteal plane.

- Use a V-notch retractor to free the coronoid process from its soft tissue and temporalis attachments.

Release remaining temporalis muscle from the coronoid process using electrocautery.

- Insert a right-angle under the coronoid process to define the sigmoid notch. Place a Kocher clamp on a chain to the coronoid process and pull to the opposite side of the head of the bed (i.e., Kocher on left coronoid secured to right side of bed).

- Gently expose the lingual surface of mandibular ramus and coronoid process with a Freer elevator. Slide a nerve hook along the lingual surface to identify the mandibular foramen; take care to avoid injury to the inferior alveolar nerve. Place a Seldon or malleable retractor medially to retract and protect the inferior alveolar nerve.

- Use the reciprocating saw to make a unicortical osteotomy starting superomedially above the inferior alveolar nerve and continuing unicortically along the oblique ridge of the ramus.

- Make the mandibular body unicortical osteotomy along the buccal surface posterior to the most distal remaining (second) molar. Insert a channel retractor for access, turn it on its side to allow the necessary angle for the reciprocating saw, then angle the saw backward to perform the corticotomy along the inferior mandibular border.

- Beginning posteriorly, place a thin metal osteotome near the ramus to wedge open the mandible then travel anteriorly. Use small metal osteotomes at the angle of the mandible followed by larger wooden osteotomes more anteriorly. After completing the osteotomy, place a Smith's spreader or a large wooden osteotome into the space and turn it to lever the buccal mandible free.

- Monitor inferior alveolar nerve position before completing the osteotomy.

- Complete an identical procedure on the contralateral side.

- Place the intraoral splint and secure it with 26-gauge wire to the maxilla. Use 24- or 26-gauge wire to secure the centric occlusion in the splint.

- Use a 25-gauge needle to set a track for the transbuccal trocar incision that allows for rigid fixation of the mandible using lag screw technique (not true lag screws).

- Make a small oblique skin incision using a knife in line with and below the mandibular border.

- Pierce mucosa using a mosquito, then bluntly insert a transbuccal trocar and secure it into position.

- Use lag screw technique to rigidly fixate mandibular segments while avoiding the inferior alveolar nerve and maintaining the centric relation. Aggressively irrigate intraorally and extraorally to avoid thermal injury. The trans-trocar drill should move passively and not be torqued. Watch color on a rainbow drill to assess screw depth.

- After placing 2–3 screws, test the security of the screw fixation by attempting to separate the segments using a Freer elevator. If it does not separate, it is secure.

- Irrigate dissection area copiously.

- Close intraoral incisions using interrupted 3-0 chromic sutures.

- Close the trocar skin incision sites using 5-0 nylon suture.

- Remove the maxillary-mandibular fixation wires and test passive occlusion. If satisfied, apply heavy elastics to secure final occlusion in the final splint.

GENIOPLASTY TECHNIQUE

- Infiltrate anterior gingivobuccal sulcus with 1% lidocaine with epinephrine.

- Use needle-tip electrocautery to cut through mucosa; use coagulation to dissect to bone. Preserve a cuff of mentalis muscle bilaterally on the mandible to assist with mentalis closure.

- Use a Molt elevator to dissect subperiosteally to expose the mandibular symphysis, parasymphysis, and body. Dissect and expose the inferior border of the mandible while elevating soft tissues for later osteotomy. Dissect and preserve the mental nerve bilaterally.

- Use a sagittal saw to vertically mark the mandibular midline above and below the proposed genioplasty osteotomy site for later reference.

- Use a reciprocating saw to make a transverse osteotomy at least 5 mm below the mental foramen from the inferior cortex of the mandibular body toward the symphysis. Use a sagittal saw to complete the osteotomy centrally.

- Mobilize the genioplasty segment with osteotomes as needed. Slide the segment into desired position and ensure midlines are aligned.

- Fixate the genioplasty segment to the mandibular symphysis using a centrally placed titanium step plate; fixate additional hardware laterally as needed.

- Reapproximate the mentalis muscles precisely with 3-0 Vicryl mattress sutures bilaterally.

- Close the mucosa with interrupted 3-0 chromic sutures.

POSTOPERATIVE MANAGEMENT

Orthognathic procedures necessitate inpatient admission (typically 1–2 days) for airway monitoring, assessment of oral intake, and management of possible nausea or bleeding postoperatively. Head of bed position should be maintained at 30-degree elevation. Ice should be applied to the face for comfort and to reduce swelling; ensure cold compresses are used intermittently to prevent thermal injury while the face is expectedly numb. Antibiotic prophylaxis with ampicillin-sulbactam is continued for 1 week to cover for oronasal flora. Antiemetics are provided around the clock for 48 hours. The patient may begin taking oral fluids the evening of surgery and is advanced to a mechanical soft diet 2 days postoperatively. Most patients may be advanced to a regular diet after 2 months. Oral rinses using chlorhexidine gluconate 0.12% (Peridex) should be performed three times daily starting on postoperative day 1. Narcotic pain medication is substituted for NSAIDs after 24 hours.

Initial follow-up is scheduled 2 weeks after surgery. The final occlusal splint should remain in place for 1 month, with substitution of heavy elastics for light elastics at 2 weeks. Physical therapy consisting of tempormandibular joint (TMJ) range of motion exercises should begin after splint removal. Patients should follow-up with their orthodontist for final adjustments and retainer fabrication after splint removal or as needed.

CAVEATS

Often, the effect of underlying skeletal imbalance on overall facial asymmetry and morbidity is underappreciated. Orthognathic surgery restores facial function and harmony. Understanding of skeletal and soft tissue anthropometry and relational cephalometrics is fundamental to diagnosing and correcting orthognathic morbidity. VSP now facilitates more precise and accurate surgical planning; it is especially helpful in multisegmental movements requiring intermediate fixation. Perioperative care is multidisciplinary and requires significant patient/caretaker understanding and involvement.

REFERENCES

1. Facial proportions. In: Mast G, Ehrenfeld M, Bartlett S, Sugar A, eds. *AO Surgery Reference*. The AO Foundation, 10 Apr.2013. Web. 30 Nov. 2016.
2. Garri JI, Tuchman M, Urrego AF, Santangelo G. Orthognathic surgery. In: Thaller SR, Bradley JP, Garri JI, eds. *Craniofacial Surgery*. New York: Informa Healthcare USA, Inc., 2008:197–217.
3. Mackay DR, Henry CR. Facial evaluation in orthognathic surgery. In: Taub PJ, et al., eds. *Ferraro's Fundamentals of Maxillofacial Surgery*. New York: Springer Science + Business Media, 2015:323–330.
4. Angle EH. Classification of malocclusion. *D Cosmos* 1899;41:248.
5. Hurst CA, Eppley BL, Havlik RJ, Sadove AM. Surgical cephalometrics: applications and developments. *Plast Reconstr Surg* 2007 Nov;120(6):92e–104e. Review.
6. Kolokitha OE, Tipouzelis N. Cephalometric methods of prediction in orthognathic surgery. *J Oral Maxillofac Oral Surg* 2011;10: 236–245.
7. Kolokitha O E, Chatzistavrou E. Factors influencing the accuracy of cephalometric prediction of soft tissue profile changes following orthognathic surgery. *J Maxillofac Oral Surg* 2012;11(1):82–90.
8. Cutting C, Bookstein FL, Grayson B, et al. Three-dimensional computer-assisted design of craniofacial surgical procedures: optimization and interaction with cephalometric and CT-based models. *Plast Reconstr Surg* 1986;77:877–887.
9. Patel PK, Zhao L, Ferraro JW. Surgical Planning: 2D to three-dimensional. In: Taub PJ, et al., eds. *Ferraro's Fundamentals of Maxillofacial Surgery*. New York: Springer Science + Business Media, 2015:331–368.
10. Goldberg M. Cephalometrics. *Int J Orthod* 1973;11:111.
11. Steiner CC. The use of cephalometrics as an aid to planning and assessing orthodontic treatment. *Am J Orthod* 1960;46:721.
12. Steiner CC. Cephalometrics for you and me. *Am J Orthod* 1953;39:729.
13. Steiner CC. Cephalometrics in clinical practise. *Angle Orthod* 1959;29:8.
14. McNamara, JA, Jr. A method of cephalometric evaluation. *Am J Orthod* 1984;86:449.
15. Gonzalez-Ulloa M. Quantitative principles in cosmetic surgery of the face (profileplasty). *Plast Reconstr Surg* 1962;29:186–198.
16. Powell N, Humphreys B. *Proportions of the Aesthetic Face*. New York: Thieme-Stratton, 1984.
17. Cottrell DA, Edwards SP, Gotcher JE. Surgical correction of maxillofacial skeletal deformities. *J Oral Maxillofac Surg* 2012 Nov;70(11 Suppl 3):e107–e136.

59.

ZYGOMATICOMAXILLARY COMPLEX FRACTURES

Russell E. Ettinger and Steven R. Buchman

INTRODUCTION

The paired zygomatic bones occupy a central position within the craniofacial skeleton and contribute to several key structural buttresses of the midface. The zygoma's prominence and general convex contour place it at risk for injury during facial trauma. Fractures of the zygomatic bone are the second most common facial fracture after nasal bone fractures.[1] Etiologic factors implicated in isolated fractures of the zygoma include interpersonal violence, motor vehicle accidents, falls, gunshot wounds, and sports-related injuries.[2] Fractures involving the malar region are often termed *zygomaticomaxillary complex (ZMC) fractures,* referring to disruption of the zygomatic bone at its four key articulation points: the zygomaticomaxillary, zygomaticofrontal, zygomaticosphenoid, and zygomaticotemporal articulations.[3] The prominent position of the zygoma makes it a primary determinant of both malar projection and midfacial width. The zygomatic bone also defines the contour of the lateral orbital rim and provides an ancillary contribution to orbital volume through its intraorbital articulation with the greater wing of the sphenoid. The complex three-dimensional relations of the ZMC make appropriate reduction and fixation challenging. This results in relatively high rates of malreduction, malunion, and persistent facial asymmetry following injury.

Successful surgical reduction of ZMC fractures is highly contingent on a complete understanding of the intricate anatomy of the malar region. Historically, the ZMC has been incorrectly referred to as a "tripod structure," which originated from the description of the zygoma's three external sutures: zygomaticomaxillary, zygomaticofrontal, and zygomaticotemporal. The "tripod" description of the ZMC neglects its significant articulation with the sphenoid bone within the lateral orbital wall. More accurately, the ZMC is a "tetrapod" structure with four key points

of contact at the (1) zygomaticomaxillary articulation and inferior orbital rim, (2) zygomaticosphenoid articulation in the lateral orbital wall, (3) zygomaticofrontal articulation and the lateral orbital rim, and (4) zygomatic arch (Figure 59.1). Fractures of the ZMC complex can occur at any of these four articulation points, and each must be evaluated for both involvement and degree of comminution during initial radiographic assessment.

Beyond its four articulation points, the zygoma also contributes to two critical buttresses of the midface. Buttresses in the craniofacial skeleton represent thickened regions of bone which provide strength and rigidity to the midface in both the horizontal and vertical dimensions. Buttresses are not synonymous with the articulations points between the individual bones in the craniofacial skeleton.

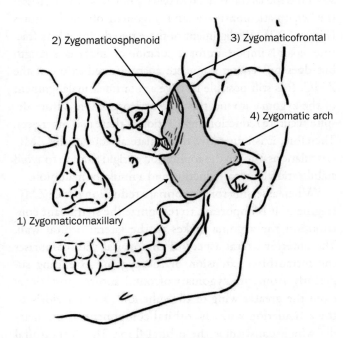

Figure 59.1. The four key articulation points of the zygomatic bone.

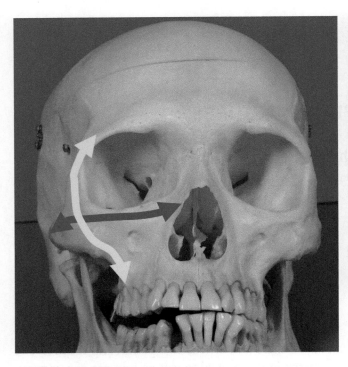

Figure 59.2. Craniofacial buttresses crossing the zygoma. Upper transverse maxillary buttress (blue) and the vertical maxillary buttress (*yellow*).

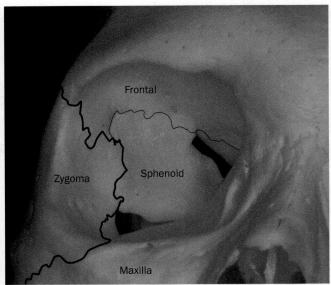

Figure 59.3. Intraorbital relationship of the zygoma and contribution to the lateral orbital wall.

Rather, buttresses represent confluent regions of thickened bone that traverse multiple facial bones and provide the structural integrity to maintain proper facial height, width, and projection. The first buttress traversing the ZMC is the upper transverse maxillary buttress, which crosses the zygomaticomaxillary and zygomaticotemporal sutures. The second is the lateral vertical maxillary buttress, which crosses the zygomaticomaxillary and zygomaticofrontal sutures (Figure 59.2).[4] Realignment of these two during ZMC fracture repair is important for restoration of midfacial strength but does not ensure complete anatomic reduction of the ZMC. It is still possible to have a rotational malalignment of the zygoma around the zygomaticosphenoid suture despite accurate reduction and fixation at these two buttresses. Therefore, it is imperative to evaluate all four of the ZMC articulations prior to the application of rigid fixation to avoid stabilization of a malreduction and a resultant malunion.

When assessing for appropriate reduction of the ZMC fragment, it is important to recognize the significant contribution the zygoma makes to the lateral orbital wall. The anterior-lateral aspect of the orbital wall comprises the intraorbital extension of the zygoma extending superiorly from the zygomaticofrontal suture, posteriorly from the greater wing of the sphenoid, and inferiorly to the articulation with the orbital component of the maxilla which constitutes the orbital floor. This intraorbital

relationship is important because it represents the longest articulation of the zygoma with the adjacent facial bones and constitutes articulations in the "x, y, and z" axes of rotation (Figure 59.3). The portion of the zygomatic bone contributing to the lateral orbital wall is also significantly thicker than the associated bones of the orbit. As a consequence, the zygomatic bone rarely demonstrates a significant degree comminution within the lateral orbital wall except in extremely high-energy injuries. These attributes make the lateral orbital wall the most important assessment point by which to judge the adequacy of ZMC reduction.

The zygomatic arch warrants special attention and understanding of its preinjury anatomy to avoid iatrogenic malreduction following injury. Though referred to as an "arch," its true structure is more linear than most appreciate. The central 75% of the arch maintains only a gentle convex curvature as it runs primarily in the anterior to posterior plane.[5] Only at its most rostral and caudal extents does the arch demonstrate significant curvature as it meets the body of the zygoma and the temporal bone, respectively (Figure 59.4). Failure to appreciate the linearity of the arch upon placement of stable fixation can result in arch malposition and unintended widening of the midface, which can be significantly disfiguring to the patient. Understanding the zygomatic arch's linearity is also paramount during manual reduction of isolated arch fractures without fixation to avoid over correction of the initial traumatic deformity.

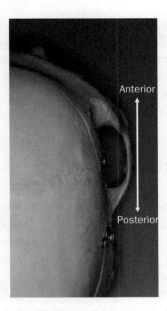

Figure 59.4. Zygomatic arch viewed from above. Note the linearity of the central segment.

ASSESSMENT OF THE DEFECT

As noted earlier, the prominence of the ZMC makes it extremely susceptible to injury. Therefore, a high index of suspicion should be maintained in any patient presenting with trauma to the midface region. Concomitant injuries to other facial bones are seen in up to 25% of ZMC fractures owing to the multiple points of articulation of the zygoma.[6] Assessment of midfacial trauma should consist of a thorough craniofacial exam in combination with dedicated thin-cut maxillofacial computed tomographic (CT) scanning in the axial, coronal, and sagittal planes. Three-dimensional reformats of the CT scans can also aid in diagnosis and surgical planning but often underplay the degree of comminution and displacement of fracture fragments.

Physical examination following facial trauma should be approached in a systematic fashion to avoid missing occult injuries. Starting with visual inspection, the examiner should evaluate overall facial proportion and note any asymmetry of the malar region. Often, soft tissue edema will be significant at the time of evaluation and can mask malar depression, which is a pathognomonic finding in displaced ZMC fractures. A decreased facial width may be seen in isolated zygomatic arch fractures as the arch is the primary contributor to facial width at the midface level. Examination for suspected ZMC fracture should also include orbital evaluation, with special attention to globe position relative to the uninjured side. Either enophthalmos or proptosis can

be seen with ZMC fractures depending on the vector of displacement of the zygoma. Inwardly displaced fractures may manifest as acute proptosis, whereas outwardly displaced fractures can result in enophthalmos secondary to increased orbital volume.[4] The examiner should be aware that intraorbital soft tissue edema following trauma can negate any increase in bony orbital volume, resulting in underappreciated enophthalmos during the initial examination of outwardly displaced fractures. Additional external findings including subconjunctival hemorrhage and periorbital and malar ecchymosis can be seen in ZMC fractures. For patients with significant bilateral facial injuries, evaluation of the patient's driver's license photograph can provide valuable baseline information about facial proportions prior to injury.

After visual inspection, gentle manual examination of the entire orbitomalar region should be performed. Systematically, the frontal bone, orbital rims, nasal dorsum, malar regions, and zygomatic arches are palpated for bony step-offs, instability, or point tenderness. Three of the four ZMC articulations, including the zygomaticomaxillary, zygomaticofrontal articulation, and zygomatic arch, are readily assessable during manual examination. Elicitation of crepitus, indicative of subcutaneous emphysema, is suggestive of an occult fracture with extension into the underlying maxillary sinus. Bilateral infraorbital nerve sensation should be evaluated during the course of head and neck examination. Paresthesias in the V2 distribution suggest traumatic injury to the infraorbital nerve, which may be secondary to fracture extension in the nerve foramen with concomitant compression injury to the nerve or stretch injury due to ZMC fracture displacement. Finally, palpation of the zygomatic arch should be completed both alone and with opening and closing of the mouth. Trismus is a common finding following ZMC fracture and can be caused by muscle spasm induced by the injury as well as by potential impingement of a depressed zygomatic arch on the temporalis muscle or the coronoid process.[7] A retropulsed ZMC fragment can also cause trismus via impingement of the coronoid process without depression of the zygomatic arch. Unrecognized ZMC fractures resulting in restriction of mandibular range of motion put the patient at risk for late sequelae, including ankylosis of the temporomandibular joint, and therefore require operative reduction and fixation.

A complete ocular and visual examination is mandatory during the evaluation of a suspected ZMC fracture. The ZMC contributes to a significant portion of the lateral orbital wall, and its disruption can have a direct impact on the globe and the periorbita. Baseline visual acuity should be tested and documented. Specific findings of globe trauma, such as hyphema or optic nerve injury demonstrated by the presence of a relative afferent pupillary defect, should prompt urgent ophthalmologic evaluation. Diplopia or double vision is frequently seen in patients with ZMC fractures and should raise suspicion for fracture involvement of the zygomaticosphenoid suture. Diplopia at the extremes of gaze is commonly seen secondary to periorbital edema, whereas diplopia at central gaze is a more concerning finding and suggests significant disruption of the normal orbital volume. Displaced bone fragments may also impinge on the extraocular muscles, resulting in entrapment and gaze restriction. Full extraocular motion must be verified for both eyes. The most commonly involved extraocular muscles in ZMC fractures are the inferior rectus and lateral rectus, which result in limited inferior and lateral gaze respectively. Recognition of entrapment is paramount, especially in pediatric patients who often develop "greenstick" fractures with concern for ensuing ischemia of the entrapped extraocular muscle. Patients with ZMC fractures involving the orbit may also present with manifestations of the "oculocardiac reflex" including bradycardia, dizziness, light-headedness, nausea, and hypotension. This reflex arc is initiated by compression or stretch of an extraocular muscle and is transmitted via parasympathetic fibers of the ophthalmic branch of the trigeminal nerve. The stimulus results in increased vasovagal tone to the cardiovascular and gastrointestinal end organ systems.[8] Cases of true entrapment or patients demonstrating symptoms of oculocardiac reflex warrant emergent operative reduction and decompression of the involved extraocular muscle.

Finally, evaluation of a dedicated thin-cut maxillofacial CT scan is essential for the evaluation of ZMC fractures. Review of CT imaging should be approached in a systematic fashion just as was done for the physical examination. Images should include cuts in axial, coronal, and sagittal planes to allow for complete characterization of the fracture pattern.[9] Each of the four articulation points of the ZMC must be evaluated for involvement, displacement, and degree of comminution. The zygomaticomaxillary articulation and zygomatic arch are best visualized on the axial images, whereas the zygomaticofrontal articulation is best viewed on the coronal images. The zygomaticosphenoid articulation should be assessed on review of the axial, coronal, and sagittal views given its articulations in the x, y, and z planes. The coronal and sagittal images are the best for diagnosing concurrent orbital floor fractures. Three-dimensional reformatted CT images are beneficial for determining the global orientation of a ZMC fracture fragment and for

characterizing the relationship of fractures traversing the orbital rim. However, three-dimensional reformatted CT images may underplay the degree of comminution and should not be considered as a substitute for a thorough systematic review of the axial, coronal, and sagittal images of a suspected ZMC fracture.

INDICATIONS FOR TREATMENT

The decision to pursue operative reduction is determined based on the degree of displacement of the ZMC at its four points of articulation and its impact on the appearance of the individual. Significant variation in fracture patterns can be seen with injury to the ZMC depending on the mechanism of injury. As a general rule, nondisplaced fractures of the ZMC typically do not require open reduction and fixation and can be followed closely for emergence of facial asymmetry once swelling has resolved around 2 weeks post-injury. Close follow-up is mandatory in patients considered for nonoperative management as the zygoma serves as the insertion site for the masseter muscle, which can exert a powerful displacement force on the zygoma. If there is displacement or comminution at any of the four articulation sites that either inhibits function or significantly alters appearance and symmetry, then surgical correction is indicated. Other special cases requiring operative reduction include restriction of mandibular movement as seen with fracture impingement on the coronoid process or temporalis muscle and outwardly displaced ZMC fractures resulting in early enophthalmos via disruption at the lateral orbital wall. Open reduction and internal fixation is typically deferred until 10–14 days after injury to ensure adequate resolution of soft tissue edema, which can hamper access and exposure of the fracture sites.[10] Urgent indications for operative reduction following injury include extraocular muscle entrapment with concern for muscle ischemia or systemic manifestations of the oculocardiac reflex.

CONTRAINDICATIONS

There are relatively few contraindications to operative reduction and internal fixation of ZMC fractures, which typically occurs in the delayed setting to allow for resolution of soft tissue edema. Contraindications to immediate operative reduction ZMC fractures in the acute setting do exist, however. All patients presenting with maxillofacial injury as a consequence of major trauma should undergo complete trauma workup to rule out concomitant injuries. Significant facial trauma can easily distract from other occult life-threatening injuries and should never preclude completion of primary and secondary surveys. A missed head injury or intraabdominal injury could have devastating consequences if a patient is taken emergently to the operating room to address facial fractures prior to completion of trauma workup. Outside of polytrauma, there are also specific contraindications for emergent operative fixation with isolated facial trauma. Significant ocular injury with evidence of hyphema, globe rupture, or optic nerve injury should take precedence over bony orbitozygomatic injuries, with the timing of operative repair to be dictated by the consulting ophthalmology team.

ROOM SETUP

Operative reduction and fixation of ZMC fractures necessitates general anesthesia and orotracheal intubation. It is prudent to secure the endotracheal (ET) tube to the anterior dentition with a large-diameter suture or a light-gauge wire to prevent inadvertent extubation with repositioning during the case. Following intubation, the patient's head should be positioned at the top edge of the bed to facilitate access to the head from either side and from behind. Anesthetic tubing and monitors should be secured so they do not restrict the head rotation or neck extension required to access the intraoral and external sites for ZMC exposure. Alternatively, the inhalational tubing can be placed into a sterile ultrasound probe cover and included in the sterile field, thus allowing the operator to have complete control of the ET tube and associated monitors. Head rotation and neck flexion/extension may be contraindicated in patients with associated cervical spine injuries, thereby making adequate fracture exposure challenging. Use of a neurosurgical horseshoe headrest in patients with cervical spine precautions may provide the surgical team a greater level of access to the head.

The entirety of the head should be prepped into the field for some cases, given the variable need for coronal access, harvest of calvarial bone grafts, or the use of a Gillies incision, which will be discussed in the following sections. Foley placement is indicated if the case time is expected to exceed 2 hours. Relevant imaging, including CT scans and three-dimensional reformats, should be displayed on intraoperative monitors or be readily accessible by the operative team to guide exposure, fracture mobilization, and ultimate reduction.

INCISION PLANNING

The ideal surgical access for any facial fracture should provide adequate exposure of fracture segments through inconspicuous incision points that minimize potential injury to vital craniofacial structures. Exposure of ZMC fractures abides by the same principles, with the caveat that open exposure may not be required to achieve adequate reduction in all instances. Minimally displaced ZMC fractures without comminution often have a preserved periosteal sleeve allowing the ZMC to remain in stable reduction following mobilization via closed or limited open approach. The type of access that will ultimately be required is determined preoperatively based on review of the maxillofacial CT scan and the patient's physical exam. Each of the four articulation points of the ZMC should be evaluated for fracture involvement, degree of displacement, and presence of comminution. If multiple articulation points are involved and demonstrate comminution or significant displacement, then open approach and rigid internal fixation is typically indicated.

UPPER BUCCAL SULCUS INCISION

The upper buccal sulcus provides wide exposure of the ZMC complex extending from the zygomaticomaxillary buttress inferomedially, to the infraorbital rim superiorly, and origin of the zygomatic arch laterally. Placement of the upper buccal sulcus should occur approximately 2–3 mm above the attached gingiva to preserve a cuff of tissue which will be utilized at the time of closure. Prior to making an incision, the location of the Stenson (parotid) duct ostia should be visualized adjacent to the maxillary second molar and kept well away from the planned incision line. Needle tip Bovie electrocautery is utilized to enter the submucosal plane and expose fibers of the buccinator muscle. The dissection plane is then immediately transitioned 90 degrees to parallel the occlusal surface of the teeth and carried down directly to the alveolar process of the maxilla. The periosteum is then incised with electrocautery, and a subperiosteal dissection is then carried out with a periosteal elevator. The wide access provided by this approach facilitates exposure of the infraorbital nerve under direct visualization during subperiosteal dissection, thus minimizing the chance of iatrogenic injury. Elevation of the soft tissues on either side of the infraorbital nerve can be carried out to the level of the infraorbital rim as needed, depending on the extent of fracture involvement, and can facilitate subsequent eyelid access by defining the proper plane of dissection for comminuted

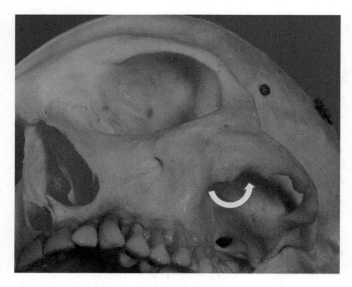

Figure 59.5. Zygomaticomaxillary complex (ZMC) fracture mobilization via upper buccal sulcus incision can be safely leveraged via placement of a blunt elevator behind the origin of the zygomatic arch.

rim fractures. Lateral isubperiosteal dissection via the upper buccal sulcus approach also provides exposure of the origin of the zygomatic arch and allows a blunt elevator to be placed behind the zygoma for initial mobilization and disimpaction (Figure 59.5).

LOWER EYELID

There are several transcutaneous lower lid incisions that can be utilized to provide access to the infraorbital rim and lateral orbit. External approaches include the subciliary, subtarsal, and infraorbital incisions, which provide wide exposure but result in a potentially conspicuous external scar and carry increased risk of lower lid malposition and ectropion. The transconjunctival approach obviates the shortcomings of external incisions, allowing simple and rapid access to the infraorbital rim with a lower risk of lid malposition and the benefit of a hidden scar although entropion and change in lid position is still possible. The transconjunctival approach can be carried out in its most direct form via a retroseptal approach which avoids dissection within the lid but results in periorbital fat herniation which can impair visualization. The preseptal approach requires dissection within the lid but maintains the integrity of the orbital septum, thereby preventing orbital fat herniation. In either case, corneal shields should be utilized when performing a transconjunctival approach. Traction sutures are placed into the gray line of the lid margin to facilitate retraction and lid eversion. An incision is made with Bovie electrocautery 2–3 mm below the tarsal plate in the palpebral

conjunctiva in the middle part of the lower eye lid, and dissection is carried out in a preseptal or postseptal plane to the level of the infraorbital rim. When the orbital rim is encountered, the periosteum is incised and subperiosteal dissection is carried out to expose the rim, orbital floor, and lateral orbital wall. The transconjunctival or subciliary transcutaneous approach can be extended via a lateral canthotomy to enhance exposure of the lateral orbital wall and the zygomaticofrontal articulation. Lateral canthotomy requires a canthal resuspension at the completion of the case with appropriate attention to resuspend the lateral canthus with a posterior lateral vector inside the lateral orbital rim to prevent canthal malposition. Intraorbital dissection of the lateral orbital wall should be sufficient to expose the zygomaticosphenoid articulation, which is a key anatomic landmark for proper ZMC reduction prior to the application of rigid fixation. The risk of lower lid malposition with either internal or external eyelid incisions can be reduced by placement of a temporary tarsorrhaphy suture to suspend the lower lid. This suture is placed lateral to the cornea and is passed through the external skin, through the gray lines of the lid margins and then back out through the external skin in a horizontal mattress fashion. The suture ends are tied over bolsters to prevent suture migration through the lid margin tissues. Use of an absorbable Monocryl (poliglecaprone 25) suture to perform temporary tarsorrhaphy obviates the need for suture removal as the tarsorrhaphy will release spontaneously as the suture dissolves.

UPPER EYELID

The zygomaticofrontal articulation can be accessed via a lower lid incision with lateral extension, as mentioned earlier, or via a separate upper lid "blepharoplasty"-type incision. A small incision is performed using a natural skin crease (the crow's foot) in the outer third of the upper eyelid, well above the lid margin and the lateral canthus. The lateral rim and zygomaticofrontal articulation is readily palpable owing to the thin soft tissue coverage in this region, and therefore dissection can be carried down directly through the orbicularis oculi muscle to the periosteum. The periosteum is then incised and a subperiosteal dissection is carried out to expose the zygomaticofrontal suture and superolateral orbital rim.

INDIRECT APPROACHES TO THE ZYGOMATIC ARCH

Indirect or limited access approaches to the zygomatic arch are utilized for isolated, nondisplaced, noncomminuted arch fractures with a preserved periosteal sleeve that can stabilize the fracture following reduction. The Gillies approach utilizes a 2 cm incision through the temporal hair-bearing scalp 2.5 cm anterior and superior to the apex of the helix. Incision placement should account for the course of the superficial temporal artery to prevent undue bleeding. Dissection is carried out down through the subcutaneous tissue and superficial temporal fascia to the level of the superficial portion of the deep temporal fascia investing the temporalis muscle. The superficial layer of the deep temporal fascia is opened to expose the temporalis muscle belly. A blunt elevator is then inserted in the intervening plane below the superficial layer of the deep temporal fascia and above the temporalis muscle. This plane is developed inferiorly to the level of the zygomatic arch. A disimpaction elevator can then be placed deep to the zygomatic arch to apply an outward force to reduce the arch. Adequate fracture reduction without overcorrection should be verified with manual palpation to ensure an appropriate linear contour to the arch. Drawbacks to the Gillies approach include an external scar and potential scar alopecia.

A transoral or Keen approach can also be utilized for isolated nondisplaced arch fractures. The approach is a limited 2 cm upper buccal sulcus incision made lateral to the maxillary second molar overlying the base of the zygoma. The oral mucosa is incised with needle-tip Bovie electrocautery, and the dissection is carried out directly down to the bone along the alveolar process of the maxilla. A periosteal elevator is then used to expose the base of the zygoma along the zygomaticomaxillary buttress so that a blunt elevator can be passed deep to the zygomatic arch to elevate the fracture. The coronoid process of the mandible maintains a close relationship to the deep surface of the zygomatic arch and can impinge upon the arch, impairing reduction. Distracting the mandible inferiorly to mobilize the coronoid away from the arch may facilitate placement of the periosteal elevator or digital pressure behind the arch for subsequent reduction. The transoral approach offers the most direct access to the zygomatic arch and obviates the need for an external incision. Digital palpation using this technique can assure maintenance of reduction via proprioception, which is not possible using the Gilles approach.

CORONAL INCISION

The degree of injury to the zygomatic arch is a key determinant of the type of surgical incisions required for adequate exposure of a ZMC fracture. If the zygomatic arch is minimally displaced with a preserved periosteal sleeve, then limited approaches such as the Gillies or Keen may

be utilized. If there is significant medial or lateral displacement, telescoping, comminution, or segmentation requiring ORIF, then exposure via a coronal incision is indicated. The coronal approach also provides access to the zygomaticofrontal articulation, the lateral zygomatic body, and even the infraorbital rim if preauricular extensions and intraorbital dissection are performed. Concomitant facial fractures may also necessitate the use of a coronal incision and should be accounted for during preoperative planning. The coronal incision should be designed over the vertex of the hair-bearing scalp and may be designed in a "zig-zag" or "wave" pattern. Ideally, incisions should be made at right angles to the direction of hair growth such that hair follicles will grow through the scar line and limit the degree of scar alopecia. For men, the design of the incision should also account for future androgenetic hair loss with age that may expose a poorly placed incision.

Initial skin incision is made through the skin, subcutaneous tissue, and galea down to the level of the loose areolar plane superficial to the pericranium. Anterior dissection can then be carried out in a subgaleal or subperiosteal plane at the discretion of the surgeon. The lateral extent of the coronal incision is carried out to the temporal fusion line, at which point the dissection is transitioned to a plane on top of the superficial layer of the deep temporal fascia. The superficial layer of the deep temporal fascia is incised 1 cm above the zygomatic arch to enter the temporal fat pad that invests the zygomatic arch between the superficial and deep layers of the deep temporal fascia. The temporal branch of the facial nerve lies in a superficial plane within the temporoparietal fascia and is protected during this deeper dissection to expose the arch (Figure 59.6). When

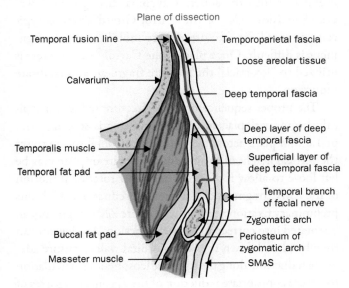

Figure 59.6. Approach to the zygomatic arch from a coronal incision.

the zygomatic arch is reached, the periosteum is incised, and subperiosteal dissection is utilized to fully expose the arch for subsequent reduction and fixation.

SURGICAL APPROACH

Selection of the appropriate access incisions should be based on preoperative assessment of the underlying fracture pattern, CT scan, and physical manifestations of the fracture, such as degree of perceptible deformity and asymmetry. In all instances, the minimal access required to adequately achieve exposure, reduction, and fixation of the ZMC should be selected. Complete subperiosteal dissection of the ZMC is unnecessary and should be avoided. Excessive dissection of fracture fragments disrupts periosteal blood supply, which is critical for subsequent fracture healing. Following exposure, the next key step is aggressive mobilization of the fracture fragment. Inadequate mobilization of the fracture will impair future attempts to maintain reduction across the four key articulation points of the ZMC during application of rigid fixation. Often the inferior pull of the masseter muscle may hinder adequate mobilization of the ZMC fragment. This can be overcome with chemical paralysis or partial release of the fibrous origin of the masseter muscle from the lateral body of the zygoma. Fracture mobilization can be achieved with slow, sustained, outward traction using a blunt elevator placed behind the body of the zygoma below the origin of the zygomatic arch (Figure 59.5). Alternatively, some surgeons choose to utilize a Carrol-Girard bone screw inserted through a cutaneous stab incision into the body of the zygoma or into the superior zygoma through the lower eyelid incision. Use of the Carrol-Girard screw is typically reserved for fractures where mobilization or alignment is difficult. Once placed, the Carrol-Girard screw is utilized to "joy-stick" the fracture fragment and facilitate reduction.

The proper sequence of ZMC fracture reduction typically begins with placement of a transosseous 26-gauge wire or 1.0 mm plate across the zygomaticofrontal suture to set the vertical height of the zygoma. The wire or plate may be left loose to allow for a small degree of rotational motion of the ZMC fragment for subsequent reduction. With this preliminary fixation achieved, the entire ZMC segment can be rotated into correct anatomic reduction. An elevator can then be placed down the lateral orbital wall to ensure adequate reduction along the zygomaticosphenoid articulation to ensure appropriate reduction of the zygoma in all axes of rotation. The zygomaticosphenoid is a broad articulation,

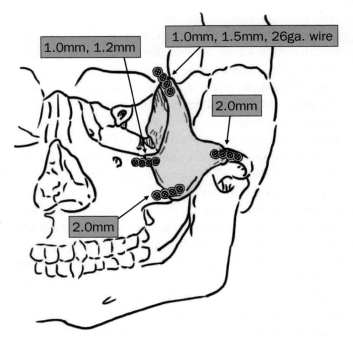

Figure 59.7. Plating guidelines for zygomaticomaxillary complex (ZMC) fracture stabilization.

and therefore any malreduction will manifest as irregularity of the lateral orbital wall. If the zygomaticosphenoid articulation is reduced, then attention can be turned to application of rigid fixation. Currently, there is no consensus on the strength/size of plates required at each fracture site to ensure true rigid fixation capable of withstanding the regional deforming forces of the soft tissue envelope and facial musculature. The surgeon must always weigh the benefits of thinner plates with less palpability against larger plates that require more dissection and risk palpability but offer improved stabilization for bony union. Current maxillofacial plating systems offer an assortment of plates in various shapes, sizes, thicknesses, and strengths which can be applied to fit the clinical fracture pattern. In general, the author's preferred plate sizes for ZMC stabilization can be found in Figure 59.7.

After placement of preliminary fixation at the zygomaticofrontal suture and verifying reduction at the lateral orbital wall, attention is then directed to the inferior orbital rim. Typically, a 1.0 mm plate is used to fixate the inferior orbital rim given the thinness of the overlying soft tissue of this region. To further prevent palpability, the plate can be placed just inside the inferior orbital rim within the orbit rather than externally along the external rim. The zygomaticomaxillary articulation is typically plated with a 2.0 mm plate to resist the deforming pull of the masseter muscle, which acts to collapse this articulation if not rigidly fixated. Palpability of the larger 2.0 mm plate at this articulation is less of a concern given the thick soft tissue envelope over the malar region. The zygomaticomaxillary articulation can demonstrate significant comminution in high-energy injuries. The surgeon should have a low threshold for bone grafting this region given the structural importance of zygomaticomaxillary articulation, which serves as the confluence of the upper transverse maxillary buttress and vertical maxillary buttress. Finally, attention is turned to the zygomatic arch, which is also plated with a stronger 2.0 mm plate. Contouring of the zygomatic arch plate should account for the natural anatomic shape of the arch, which is essentially linear over the middle 75% of its course (Figure 59.3). Iatrogenic overcorrection of the zygomatic arch leads to an unwonted increase in midfacial width and resultant facial deformity.

Following rigid fixation, attention should be directed to resuspension of the soft tissues of the midface. The elevated malar soft tissue periosteum is captured with polydioxanone (PDS) or Vicryl suture and suspended through drill holes in the inferior orbital rim or to plates in this region. Resuspension of the soft tissues prevents early midfacial descent and posttraumatic soft tissue ptosis. Malar resuspension also provides lower lid support and reduces the risk of lower lid retraction. When lateral canthotomy has been made as part of an extended lower lid access, then a lateral canthoplasty to the inner aspect of the lateral rim periosteum is performed with a permanent suture. If extensive intraorbital dissection was performed, then forced duction testing should be completed at the end of the case to verify unrestricted extraocular motion.

POSTOPERATIVE CARE

Depending on the severity of injury, patients undergoing ZMC fracture repair may be managed on an outpatient or inpatient basis. Patients requiring extensive intraorbital dissection should be monitored with visual checks for 24 hours. The patient's head should be kept elevated, and no pressure should be applied to the reconstruction site. There is no evidence-based indication for continuation of postoperative antibiotics, which remains at the discretion of the operating surgeon. Ophthalmic ointments should be applied copiously to the periorbital incisions and standard skin ointments utilized for skin or scalp incisions. An initial liquid diet advanced to a soft mechanical diet is typically instituted during the first 3 weeks to allow healing of intraoral incisions. Oral care with chlorhexidine gluconate or salt water rinses should be initiated until regular oral

hygiene can be resumed. Patients are placed on sinus precautions and instructed to sneeze with their mouth open and not blow their nose to prevent pneumatization of the subcutaneous tissues. External sutures used for incision closure are typically removed in 7–10 days.

CAVEATS

Preoperative planning is based on clinical assessment of the defect after edema resolution (10–14 days) and fracture pattern demonstrated on dedicated maxillofacial CT scan.

All four articulation points of the ZMC should be assessed for fracture involvement, degree of displacement, and comminution. Incision planning is based on fracture pattern and should involve the least amount of soft tissue dissection to adequately expose the involved fracture segments without extensive stripping of periosteum from uninvolved bone.

Outside of concomitant facial fractures, the presence of a displaced, comminuted zygomatic arch fracture is a primary indication for a coronal incision in repair of ZMC fractures. Inadequate fracture mobilization will severely impair subsequent attempts at appropriate reduction of the ZMC at all four of its articulation points.

The zygomaticosphenoid suture in the lateral orbital wall is the most reliable point by which to judge adequate ZMC reduction given its thick bone, resistance to comminution, and simultaneous articulations in the x, y, and z planes.

Soft tissue resuspension is required at the completion of fracture fixation to prevent late sequelae such as posttraumatic malar descent and lower lid and canthal malposition.

REFERENCES

1. English GM. *Otolaryngology: A Text Book*. Hagerstown, MD: Harper & Row, 1976.
2. Erdmann D, Follmar KE, DeBruijn M, et al. A retrospective analysis of facial fracture etiologies. *Ann Plastic Surg* 2008;60(4):398–403.
3. Meslemani D, Kellman RM. Zygomaticomaxillary complex fractures. *Arch Facial Plast Surg*, 2012;14(1):62–66.
4. Kelley P, Hopper R, Gruss JS. Evaluation and treatment of zygomatic fractures. *Plast Reconst Surg* 2007;120(7):5S–15S.
5. Gruss JS, Van Wyck L, Phillips JH, Antonyshyn O. The importance of the zygomatic arch in complex midfacial fracture repair and correction of posttraumatic orbitozygomatic deformities. *Plast Reconst Surg* 1990;85(6):878–890.
6. Ellis E, el-Attar A, Moos KF. Analysis of 2,067 cases of zygomatico-orbital fractures. *J Oral Maxillofacial Surg* 1985;43(6): 417–428.

7. Hollier LH, Thornton J, Pazmino P, Stal S. The management of orbitozygomatic fractures. *Plast Reconst Surg* 2003;111(7): 2386–2392.

8. Sires BS, Stanley RB, Levine LW. Oculocardiac reflex caused by orbital floor trapdoor fracture: an indication for urgent repair. *JAMA Ophthalmol* 1998;116(7): 955–956.

9. Manson PN, Markowitz B, Mirvis S, Dunham M, Yaremchuk M. Toward CT-based facial fracture treatment. *Plast Reconst Surg* 1990;85(2): 202–214.

10. Ellstrom CL, Evans GR. Evidence-based medicine: zygoma fractures. *Plast Reconst Surg* 2013;132(6): 1649–1657.

PART X.

BREAST AND TRUNK SURGERY

AXILLARY DISSECTION

Ashkaun Shaterian and Erin Lin

Evaluation of the axillary lymph node basin provides prognostic and therapeutic value for cancer patients. Complete lymph node removal was first advocated for the treatment of invasive breast cancer in the eighteenth century by Lorenz Heister.[1] In addition, William Halsted advocated complete lymph node removal in his radical mastectomy technique, where his publication of patient survival led to the foundation of axillary lymph node dissection (ALND). ALND has since become integrated in the treatment algorithm for breast cancer patients. ALND offers pathologic staging of cancer,[2] (2) therapeutic removal of clinically apparent axillary disease, and (3) the removal of lymph nodes with possible subclinical disease following sentinel lymph node biopsy (SLNB). ALND is largely described in the context of breast cancer but is utilized in the treatment of other malignant neoplasms (i.e., malignant melanoma, high-risk squamous cell carcinoma) that may drain to the axillary lymph node basin.

INDICATIONS

Axillary lymphadenectomy is indicated with the primary breast cancer operation (i.e., mastectomy, lumpectomy) in patients with (1) locally advanced breast cancer, (2) inflammatory breast cancer, or (3) some biopsy-proven metastatic disease in the axillary lymph nodes.[3] An ALND may also be indicated following an SLNB in a subset of breast cancer patients. A completion ALND can be indicated in patients undergoing SLNB, particularly those with multiple positive sentinel lymph nodes or patients with positive nodes that will not receive whole-breast irradiation (i.e., patients undergoing mastectomy, receiving partial breast irradiation, or refusing breast irradiation).[3]

An ALND is also indicated for a failed SLNB, an inadequate previous ALND with residual suspicious nodes, or an axillary recurrence following previous breast cancer treatment.[3]

The axillary lymph nodes drain structures in the upper extremity, shoulder, lower neck, breast, thorax, and lumbar area. As such, an axillary dissection may be necessary in the workup and treatment for a variety of histopathologic diagnoses, including malignant melanoma, squamous cell carcinoma, and others.[4,5]

CONTRAINDICATIONS

There are few absolute contraindications to performing an ALND. ALND is contraindicated in first-line axillary staging in early-stage breast cancer patients who have clinically negative nodes. Similarly, the utility of an axillary dissection in the presence of distant metastases remains controversial. Relative contraindications include preexisting ipsilateral upper extremity lymphedema, shoulder immobility, or comorbidities prohibiting operative procedures.

PREOPERATIVE EVALUATION

Preoperative assessment commences with a detailed history and physical exam. Examination should evaluate for breast disease and the presence of regional lymphadenopathy. The patient should not be paralyzed until the identification of large motor nerves during the dissection is accomplished. For patients undergoing general anesthesia, primary prophylaxis for prevention of deep venous thrombosis, such as sequential compression devices, should be employed. A preoperative antibiotic should be administered after arriving in the operating room and within 1 hour before the incision is made.

ANATOMY

The axillary space is a pyramidal-shaped region confined by an apex, base, and four walls. The apex of the axilla is the costoclavicular ligament. The base of the axilla comprises skin and axillary fascia near the fourth or fifth rib spaces. The anterior boundary of the axilla is formed by the pectoralis major, pectoralis minor, and subclavius muscles. The posterior boundary of the axilla is defined by the subscapularis, teres minor, and latissimus dorsi muscles. The lateral wall of the axilla is identified at the bicipital

groove of the humerus between the muscles insertions of the anterior and posterior walls. The medial border of the axilla spans the first four to five ribs spaces and is covered by the serratus anterior muscle.

The axillary space contains blood vessels, axillary lymphatic structures, and motor/sensory nerves that supply the upper extremity (Figure 60.1). The axillary artery and vein courses through the superior aspect of the axilla and are enclosed within the axillary sheath. The axillary vessels give off several branches that may be encountered during the dissection. These include the thoracoacromial artery, lateral thoracic artery, and the subscapular artery. The thoracodorsal artery is a branch from the subscapular artery and travels with the thoracodorsal nerve in its course to the latissimus dorsi muscle. The accompanying veins travel alongside these arteries and drain into the

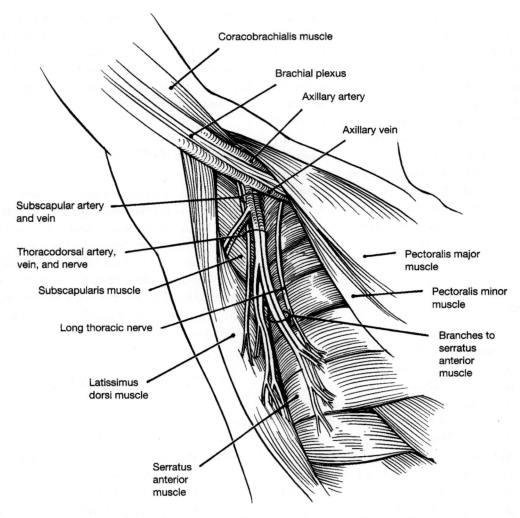

Figure 60.1. Anatomy. The axillary lymph nodes are confined to the pyramidal-shaped axillary space. The pectoralis major and minor muscles are located superomedially. The serratus anterior muscle is located medially, along with the long thoracic nerve coursing on its superficial surface. The latissimus dorsi muscle is located laterally, and the thoracodorsal neurovascular structures are identified on its deep surface. The axillary vessels and brachial plexus are located superiorly.

axillary vein. These vessels should be identified amid the axillary dissection and preserved unless grossly involved by tumor.

The axilla contains an average of 20–30 lymph nodes that are divided into three levels in relation to the pectoralis minor muscle.[2] Level I lymph nodes are inferior and lateral to the pectoralis minor muscle. Level II lymph nodes are posterior to the pectoralis minor muscle. Level III lymph nodes are medial to the pectoralis minor muscle. A level I and II lymph node dissection with a minimum of 10 lymph nodes is recommended in breast cancer patients requiring an ALND.[6] In some cases of malignant melanoma, the axillary lymphadenectomy will include lymph node levels I, II, and III.[7]

The brachial plexus is located along the superior aspect of the axilla. It provides several motor nerve branches, including the long thoracic nerve, thoracodorsal nerve, medial pectoral nerve, and lateral pectoral nerve. These nerves should be identified during the axillary dissection and preserved unless grossly involved by tumor. The long thoracic nerve travels superficial and lateral to the chest wall, located near the subscapularis muscle, and innervates the serratus anterior muscle. Injury can result in denervation and the protruding "winged" scapula deformity. The thoracodorsal nerve courses obliquely through the axilla to innervate the latissimus dorsi muscle, joining the thoracodorsal artery in its course to the latissimus dorsi muscle. Injury to the thoracodorsal nerve can lead to denervation of the latissimus dorsi muscle and weakness of internal rotation and shoulder adduction. The medial and lateral pectoral nerves traverse the axilla to innervate the

pectoralis major and minor muscles. Injury to these nerves can result in limited shoulder mobility and strength. Finally, the sensory nerves encountered in the dissection include the intercostobrachial nerves originating from the second and third intercostal nerves. These nerves traverse the axilla to supply the skin on the medial and posterior arm, axilla, and posterior axillary line. Injury may result in decreased sensation or hyperesthesias in their respective nerve distributions.

ROOM SETUP AND POSITIONING

The room is set up for a standard breast case. The patient is placed in the supine position with the ipsilateral arm abducted up to 90 degrees on an arm board (Figure 60.2). The ipsilateral thorax/chest wall should be positioned along the edge of the table for easy access. Patients with deeper axillas may benefit from a soft padded bump under the shoulder to raise the axilla. All boney prominences should be well padded. The ipsilateral chest, shoulder, axilla, and arm are prepped and draped into the surgical field. The arm board is draped with a Mayo stand cover. The arm can be covered with a free drape or draped into the field with a sleeve to allow for repositioning during the dissection if preferred. The surgeon is positioned below the patient's arm while the assistant is placed above the arm and near the patient's head. Neuromuscular blocking agents should be avoided to facilitate the identification and preservation of the motor nerves.

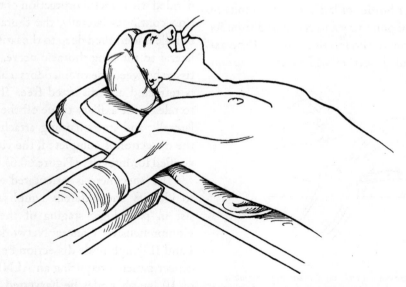

Figure 60.2. Patient positioning. The ipsilateral chest, neck, shoulder, axilla, and arm are prepped. The arm is abducted on an arm board and is covered with a sleeve to allow for repositioning. A small bump is placed under the ipsilateral axilla to improve visualization.

OPERATIVE TECHNIQUE

An ALND may be performed within the context of a modified radical mastectomy, in combination with a partial mastectomy for breast conservation, or as an individual procedure. Therefore, for patients undergoing standard modified radical mastectomy without reconstruction, the ALND can be performed through the long oblique mastectomy incision. For patients undergoing an ALND alone or with partial mastectomy, a curvilinear incision is made approximately 1-2 cm below the edge of the axillary hair line following the natural skin folds (Langer's lines), extending from the anterior to the posterior axillary fold (Figure 60.3). For patients undergoing a skin-sparing mastectomy with immediate reconstruction, the skin opening may be adequate to reach to axilla. Alternatively, a separate incision in the axilla can be utilized.

The ALND skin flaps are then elevated and the clavipectoral fascia is divided to expose the underlying fat pad and axillary lymph nodes within the fat. The next steps focus on identifying the boundaries of the axillary contents with the anterior border of the latissimus dorsi muscle laterally, the lateral aspect of the pectoralis muscle medially, the axillary vein superiorly, and the fourth or fifth rib inferiorly. Blunt dissection with finger palpation along the lateral border of the pectoralis major helps to isolate its edge easily. The pectoralis major muscle is then retracted medially, exposing the lateral border of the pectoralis minor muscle and allowing inspection of any enlarged Rotter nodes. Dissecting from the medial border of the pectoralis minor, the advential tissue is divided, carefully preserving the medial pectoral neurovascular bundle and the muscle fibers. Next, the anterior border of latissimus dorsi muscle is identified as the lateral boundary and is exposed from its insertion on the humerus to the inferior extent of the axillary dissection. Careful dissection will avoid disruption

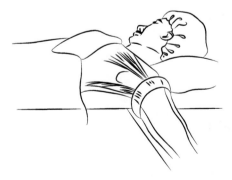

Figure 60.3. Axillary incision. A curvilinear incision is made approximately 1–2 cm below the edge of the axillary hair line following the natural skin folds extending from the anterior to the posterior axillary fold.

of the sensory nerves located superficial to and beyond the latissimus dorsi muscle. Similarly, the thoracodorsal nerve located laterally and the long thoracic nerve located medially must be identified and preserved. Next, the inferior border of the dissection is identified inferior to the axillary tail of the breast, often extending to the fourth or fifth rib. Finally, the superior border is delineated, and the axillary vein is approached. The axillary vein can be identified by following the latissimus dorsi muscle superiorly where the axillary vein emerges from its medial border.

Once the axillary space has been delineated, the axillary lymph node tissue is harvested (Figure 60.4). The pectoralis major and minor muscles are retracted medially to allow access to the level I and II lymph nodes (Figure 60.5). Positioning the arm into a 90-degree angle can help facilitate the dissection. The medial pectoral nerve will emerge just lateral to pectoralis minor and should be preserved. Lymphatic tissue on the chest wall is then retracted inferolaterally, and the dissection is continued along the inferior aspect of the axillary vein. The arm can be flexed and abducted to relax the pectoralis major muscle and allow better access to the apex. Superficial branches coursing inferior from the axillary vein are ligated carefully. The interpectoral space is palpated and any suspicious nodes should be removed if present. The pectoralis minor muscle can be delineated and retracted to facilitate exposure and removal of lymph nodes. As the dissection is continued, the long thoracic nerve is identified and preserved. It can be can be palpated as a "piano string" amid the fatty tissues where it is located deep in the axilla and superficial to the serratus anterior muscle along the rib cage. The tissue lateral and inferior to the long thoracic nerve can be divided with careful protection of the nerve. As the dissection continues laterally, the thoracodorsal neurovascular bundle is identified deep to the latissimus dorsi muscle and lateral to the long thoracic nerve. The remaining axillary tissue between the thoracodorsal and long thoracic nerves is retracted and dissected free. The dissection continues to release the axillary tissue off the latissimus dorsi muscle laterally and its remaining attachments inferiorly. Once the dissection is completed, the vital structures should be verified for integrity (Figure 60.6).

The specimen is orientated with a marking stitch to identify the different lymph node levels and to assist in pathologic staging of the tumor. The National Comprehensive Cancer Network recommends a level I and II lymph node dissection be performed in all breast cancer patients requiring an ALND and that a minimum of 10 lymph nodes be harvested.[6] In some cases of malignant melanoma, the axillary lymphadenectomy will

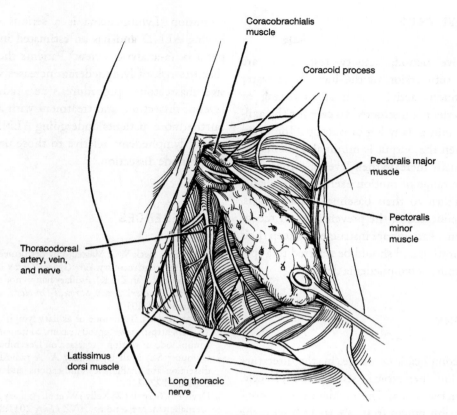

Figure 60.4. Dissection of axillary contents. Axillary contents are dissected along the pectoralis muscle, latissimus dorsi muscle, serratus muscle, and the axillary vein. Care must be taken to identify and preserve the thoracodorsal and long thoracic nerves.

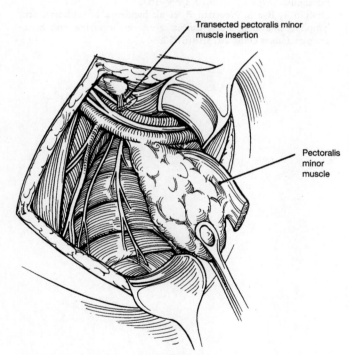

Figure 60.5. Dissection of axillary contents deep to pectoralis minor muscle. The pectoralis minor muscle can be retracted medially and the arm rotated anteriorly across chest to gain access to level II and III lymph nodes.

include levels I, II, and III, along with the fibrofatty tissues superficial and superior to the axillary vein.[7] The pocket is then irrigated and hemostasis is obtained. A single closed-suction drain is placed within the pocket to exit from a separate stab incision.

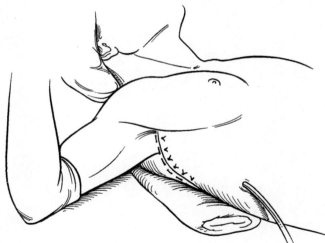

Figure 60.6. Completion of axillary dissection. Location of vital axillary structures once the axillary specimen has been removed.

AXILLARY DISSECTION

639

POSTOPERATIVE CARE

In the postoperative period, activity restrictions are cautioned to avoid submersion of the incision in water and to avoid strenuous activity such as exercising or heavy lifting. The patient is instructed to care for the axillary drain and maintain a daily log of outputs. The drain can be removed when the output is minimal. Patients are encouraged to gradually increase their level of activity and arm motion. Simple range of motion exercises will enable most patients to return to their baseline activity levels. Patients should be educated in the prevention and recognition of lymphedema. Patients are instructed to keep their arm elevated while resting and should be referred to a specialist should symptoms of lymphedema develop.

COMPLICATIONS

Rates of specific complications range in the literature and include infection, hematoma, seroma, lymphocele, lymphedema, and nerve injury. The incidence of postoperative wound infection ranges from 3% to 15% with the most common organisms representing gram-positive streptococcal or staphylococcal species.[3] The reported incidence of postoperative hematoma varies from 2% to 10% and that of major nerve injury less than 1%.[3] Disruption of the lymphatic system can lead to seroma formation, which can be prevented with use of drains or managed via percutaneous aspiration. Lymphedema is a serious complication following ALND and has an estimated incidence of 19.9% per a meta-analytic review.[8] Patients should be counseled that the risk of lymphedema increases with more aggressive mastectomy procedures (i.e., radical mastectomy), level of dissection, and treatment with axillary radiation.[3] Furthermore, patients undergoing ALND are at increased risk of lymphedema relative to those undergoing sentinel lymph node dissection.[3]

REFERENCES

1. Meyer KK, Beck WC. Mastectomy performed by Lawrence Heister in the eighteenth century. *Surg Gynecol Obstet* 1984;159(4):391–394.
2. Neuman HB, Van Zee KJ. Axillary lymph node dissection. In: Kuerer HM, eds. *Kuerer's Breast Surgical Oncology*, chapter 63. New York McGraw-Hill, 2010.
3. Margenthaler J. Technique of axillary lymph node dissection. Chen W (ed.). https://www.uptodate.com/contents/technique-of-axillary-lymph-node-dissection (Accessed on December 1, 2017)
4. Gumport SL, Lyall D, Zimany A. A radical axillary lymph node dissection for malignancy. Indications and technique. *Arch Surg* 1961;83: 227–230.
5. Davis PG, Serpell JW, Kelly JW, et al. Axillary lymph node dissection for malignant mela- noma. *ANZ J Surg* 2011;81(6):462–466.
6. Gradishar WJ, Anderson BO, Baiassanian R, et al. NCCN Guidelines insights: breast cancer, version 1.2017. *J Natl Compr Canc Netw* 2017;15(4):433–451.
7. Love TP, Delman KA. Management of regional lymph node basins in melanoma. *Ochsner J* 2010;10(2):99–107.
8. DiSipio T, Rye S, Newman B, et al. Incidence of unilateral arm lymphoedema after breast cancer: a systematic review and meta-analysis. *Lancet Oncol* 2013;14(6):500–515.

61.

AUGMENTATION MAMMOPLASTY

Sheri Slezak

Breast augmentation is the most frequently performed aesthetic surgical procedure in the United States,[1] and recent advances have provided more choices in implant selection and technique, such that high levels of patient satisfaction can be obtained. Yet data tell us that reoperation is distressingly frequent in augmentation mammoplasty. Careful analysis of the patient's anatomy and goals, with full education and participation of the patient, can lead to a positive experience for both patient and surgeon.

ASSESSMENT OF THE BREAST

The preoperative visit is the most important determinant of a successful outcome and satisfied patient and surgeon. Often, preoperative counseling takes longer than the operation itself. A fully informed patient who has realistic goals will be pleased with her outcome; a patient who "never knew that an implant could rupture" or who was "made smaller than I wanted" will not be happy in the coming years. Augmentation must be viewed as a long-term choice, and initial decisions will affect the patient's breasts for years to come. The patient may have a long list of wishes, and often some are contradictory: "a lift but no scars." The surgeon must educate the patient and ask her to prioritize her desires.

PHYSICAL EXAMINATION

A physical examination at the initial visit, including the patient's general health, history, medications, allergies, clotting history, and pregnancy history and plans, should be noted. Augmentation is an elective, cosmetic operation that is appropriate for healthy patients. Mammography should be up to date if the patient is older than 40 years of age.

Specific attention should be given to the following items:

1. *Existing breast size.* The patient's natural breast size can be assessed by cup size and a pinch test in the upper and lower poles. This is important because a patient with little native breast tissue will show the edges of the implant, and ripples will be easily palpable.

2. *Desired breast size.* Patients generally desire to "be a C and look completely natural." However, some wish to be a B or a D. Cup size is problematic because a C cup at one bra manufacturer is markedly different from another. Some women like loose versus tight band size, and some like full coverage versus demicups. It is unwise to promise a particular bra size.

3. *Height, weight, and hip size of the patient.* Larger implants will balance larger hips, but on a small-hipped, thin woman, large implants would not look natural. Taller women can have larger implants and still look proportional.

4. *Base diameter of breast.* A 300 mL implant will look small on a wide chest but large on a narrow chest where it has less platform to sit on and therefore more projection. Base diameter cannot be the only determinant of implant size since one patient may want to be a B cup, whereas another patient with the same base diameter may wish to be a D cup.

5. *Ptosis.* Ptosis is a common source of postoperative dissatisfaction. If the nipple is below the inframammary fold (IMF), augmentation alone will not achieve an aesthetically pleasing breast. Mastopexy with augmentation may be needed. If the patient has first-degree ptosis, augmentation alone will generally fill out this extra skin and the nipple-areolar

complex (NAC) will look higher without the scars of mastopexy. If ptosis is adequately discussed preoperatively, the patient will have realistic ideas of the shape of her postoperative breasts.

6. *Upper pole convexity/concavity.* Most small-breasted patients want upper pole cleavage, whereas others think that this looks unnatural and draws attention to the fact that they are augmented. Patients with involutional hypoplasia may totally lack upper pole fullness and thus the implant edge will be more evident here.

7. *Nipple size and location.* A very small nipple will not allow a periareolar approach. You generally need 3–4 cm of incision length. Areolas may be more lateral or medial than the patient desires, and this may not change.

8. *Breast and nipple asymmetries.* Breasts are always different in shape and size preoperatively; this is also true postoperatively. This difference should be pointed out to the patient to avoid unrealistic expectations of two perfectly identical breasts. Remember "they are sisters, not twins." Preoperative pictures are absolutely necessary to remind patients of their preoperative asymmetries.

9. *Inframammary fold position.* The distance from the nipple to the IMF is noted. The natural fold may be lowered at operation for larger implants or to disguise ptotic breasts. Some patients also have asymmetric folds. The placement of implants and the stretching of the skin usually lowers the fold by a centimeter or so. This is why incisions are best placed in or shortly below the natural fold.

10. *Presence of striae.* Striae are not changed by surgery. They may look a bit better initially as a result of stretching, but they are still present.

11. *Sternal intermammary width.* Patients often perceive that their breasts will touch in the middle after augmentation, but this is determined by whether they have breast tissue on top of their sternum. Many small-breasted women do not. Their distance will usually decrease, but they will only touch with push-up bras.

12. *Bony chest wall asymmetries.* If one shoulder is higher, if ribs are concave on one side, or if there is significant scoliosis, then implants may also look asymmetric, and differential sizes may be needed.

HOW TO CHOOSE A SIZE

The size of the implant to be placed is frequently a matter of long debate and repeated visits for sizing and discussion. Patients agonize over 25 mL. Generally most patients will fall into the 200–450 size range, and deviations from this should be carefully considered. Various experts debate whether the predominant factor in sizing should be patient desires, breast measurements, or implant volume. Various recommendations for sizing include rice measurements,[2] in-office implant sizing,[3] three-dimensional computer imaging, or the Tebbetts scale.[4] Reoperation for sizing is reported at 5–8% and causes excess cost and anguish for both patient and surgeon alike.[5,6]

Asking the patient the following questions is helpful: (1) Would you like to be a B, C, or D cup size? (2) Do you want people to notice your chest in clothes? In a bathing suit? (3) Do you mind if family and friends guess that you have implants?

I find that these patient comments correlate with these implant sizes:

200–250 mL implants (B cup size): "I want no one to know and I want to look completely natural."

300–400 mL implant (middle to full C cup size): "I want people to notice my figure in a bathing suit."

400–450 mL (full C or small D): "I want people to notice my chest, and I'm telling everyone."

I have the patient place 200 to 450 mL implants in a bra and look in a mirror in the office. Implants look a bit smaller when implanted under the skin than when trying them on, so add 25 mL to what they like. If the patient is torn between two sizes, the larger one is generally better. Remember that only people who like big breasts come in for breast augmentation. After the patient chooses a size, the surgeon must concur that her choice is realistic, achievable, and correlates with her verbally expressed desires and her anatomical measurements. Discuss discrepancies or concerns with the patient. Allowing the patient to participate in the selection of the implant size is very important—many women choose one size but wish postoperatively that they had chosen a larger one. I rest the responsibility of the selection with the patient. Postoperatively they say "I wish I had chosen one size larger," rather than "you made me too small."

At the end of the preoperative visit(s), a chart (Figure 61.1) should be filled out for each patient. This clear documentation avoids confusion on the day of surgery when the patient has been premedicated. Patients frequently request a larger or smaller implant on the day of

Patient Name: ______________________	
Saline________ mL inflated to ______ mL	
Silicone ________mL	
Manufacturer___________	
Shape:	round, anatomic
Texture:	smooth, textured
Location:	partial submuscular, subglandular, subfascial
Incision:	inframammary, areolar, axillary, periumbilical
Anesthesia:	general, local, regional

Figure 61.1. Patient chart, to be completed after preoperative visit(s).

surgery, so order a size above and a size below the chosen size. Always order three implants so that if a problem is found with one implant, you will have an adequate supply. Hospital consignment stocks can be lifesavers.

HOW TO CHOOSE AN INCISION

Many different incisions are possible, but two are predominantly used. The *inframammary* incision is hidden in the fold, and the patient will not see it as she looks down. It allows easy access to the submuscular position and is commonly used by 80% of surgeons.[7] However, this incision on a breast is recognized as an augment scar. The quality of the scar varies from barely perceptible to noticeable.

The *areolar* incision heals extremely well with a barely perceptible scar. A small areola may preclude this incision. Submuscular placement is deeper and more difficult unless the breast is very hypoplastic. The areolar incision may also transverse some breast ducts, which may carry bacteria. Implant infection and extrusion may cause nipple loss or fibrosis.

The *axillary* incision results in a scarless breast, but the axillary scar may be noticed in sleeveless clothing. Lower pole symmetry can be a problem since it is more difficult to visualize the lower pocket and muscle. *Umbilical* incisions offer a scarless breast but endoscopic instrumentation and expertise are needed. Implant manufacturers have not endorsed this approach and state in their package insert that "endoscopic placement or periumbilical approach in placement of the implant should not be used."[8,9]

HOW TO CHOOSE A POCKET LOCATION

Implants may be placed in the *submuscular* or *subglandular* position. Because the pectoralis does not usually extend down to the IMF, a submuscular implant is only covered by the muscle in the upper half of the breast. The lower pole is subcutaneous, so this is known as a *dual-plane* or *partial muscular* coverage. *Submuscular* placement has a lower incidence of capsular contracture and rippling, and mammograms are easier to read. Eighty percent of surgeons use this plane.[7] There is good superior pole fullness. The drawback of submuscular placement is more postoperative pain and breast deformity associated with pectoralis contractions; if the patient exercises frequently or dances in a bathing suit or leotard, this deformity can be noticeable.

Subglandular placement is the natural location of the breast. The implant fills out excess skin, as seen in postpartum atrophy and pseudoptosis. The implant ages more naturally with the patient's own breast tissue, and there is less incidence of a "double bubble" with time. Subglandular placement in the thin individual results in more rippling and a rubbery, palpable feel at the edges of the implant. Capsular contracture is more common in this position.[10]

Subfascial placement has been described, which places the implant behind the pectoralis fascia but above the muscle. Advocates say that it has more natural appearance and eliminates the visibility of muscle movement. They claim that implant position is controlled superiorly and capsular constracture is low, but evidence is limited at this point. Others find that the fascia of 0.5–1 mm thickness is not much different from the subglandular position.

Implant placement advantages and disadvantages are summarized in Table 61.1.

HOW TO CHOOSE AN IMPLANT TYPE, SHAPE, TEXTURE, AND PROJECTION

Implants are available in *saline* and *silicone*. The outer elastomer shells of both types are made of silicone; it is only the inner filling that is different. Saline implants are attractive because of the lack of a foreign substance, the immediate detection of rupture without magnetic resonance imaging (MRI), the lower cost, and the small incisions needed to

TABLE 61.1 PLACEMENT OF BREAST IMPLANTS

Submuscular	Subglandular
Less capsular contracture	Fills out excessive skin
Less noticeable rippling	Good projection, lower pole fullness
Less palpable implant edges	Less pain, faster recovery
Better delineation of breast tissue on mammogram	More capsular contracture; rippling; rubbery, palpable feel
Distortion with pectoralis function	Implant sits lower and ages naturally

place them. They are, however, firmer and more rubbery feeling, like a water balloon. Ripples may be palpable or visible. Silicone implants are softer and move more naturally. They have fewer wrinkles, but rupture is often silent. The US Food and Drug Administration (FDA) recommends following a silicone implant by MRI, starting at year 3 and then every other year. Silicone is FDA-approved for women over the age of 22 years.[11]

Shape may be round or anatomic. A profiled implant provides more lower pole projection with less upper pole fullness; this is more natural but not always desired. It can disguise mild ptosis. An anatomic implant has a risk of malrotation and requires a larger incision to insert. A round implant produces more upper pole fullness, as in a push-up bra. Most patients desire this. Round implants are generally softer than a form-stable implant.[12-14]

Texture may be smooth or rough. Textured implants were developed to decrease capsular contracture. Studies show that texturing may improve contracture in the subglandular position, but submuscular studies are more variable. Texturing can cause tissue to adhere to the implant, causing noticeable wrinkling. This wrinkling may increase with time, as the skin thins out. Texturing also seems to be a risk factor for ALCL. Most form-stable, anatomic implants are textured to prevent malrotation.[15,16]

Implants now come in a confusing array of moderate, moderate plus, high, and ultra-high *projection*. As the projection increases, the diameter decreases. This can be very advantageous to match the patient's breast diameter to her desired volume. However, the patient's skin and muscle will also shape the implant and change the package measurements.

INDICATIONS

The basic indications for breast implant surgery are a healthy patient with breast hypoplasia who is fully informed, has realistic goals and intrinsic motivation, and realizes that implants may not last a lifetime and that further surgery may be required.

FDA informational websites and the manufacturer implant package insert websites[8,9,11] may be given to each patient preoperatively to reinforce the verbal information that is given.

Interestingly, I have found that patients in gratuity jobs, such as waitresses, dancers, hairstylists, and bartenders, report actual economic benefits in increased tips after augmentation. Most women report increased confidence and

TABLE 61.2 COMPLICATIONS OF BREAST IMPLANTS

Rupture eventually: 100% chance
Asymmetry common preop and postop
Reoperations 25–36% at 10 years[6]
Capsular contracture 8–19% at 10 years[6,17,18]
Nipple numbness common initially but improves[19]
Wrinkling 2–7%[6,17]
Infection <1%
Hematoma <1%
Ptosis with aging
Visibility of edges
Mammogram changes
Implant malrotation 2–7%[6]
Scarring
Muscle deformity with movement
Risk of anaplastic large-cell lymphoma; rare[20]

pleasure in their appearance from a more balanced figure. Women with involutional hypoplasia after childbirth and breast-feeding often want to regain their old body image. Women in the entertainment industry often feel that a certain body image is a requirement of their profession. Whatever their motivation, these patients must learn the potential complications of implants. Then they can assess whether these complications will balance the benefits in their personal situation. Documentation of a discussion of the following complications in your chart with a copy for the patient will be invaluable (Table 61.2).

CONTRAINDICATIONS

I have declined to perform augmentation for patients who are extrinsically motivated by the desire to please a spouse, boyfriend, or parent. Patients with significant (second- or third-degree) ptosis are poor candidates for augmentation alone. Patients should not have an active infection at the time of surgery. A preop pregnancy test is necessary. Patients who choose extraordinarily large implants are prone to long-term complications and are not worth the risk. A patient who is unable to understand or accept the complications of implants after two visits is not a good candidate.

ROOM SETUP

Verification of the correct implants in the room should occur before the patient is anesthetized. The operating room table must have the break at the waist position, so that the patient may be elevated into the sitting position while asleep. This allows the evaluation of pockets and folds for symmetry.

I usually use a lighted retractor, or a head light should be available. For silicone implants, a Keller funnel may be used.[21] For saline implants, a closed fill system from an intravenous bag is used to fill the implants. Noninjectable saline, or saline in open containers on the table, may become contaminated with airborne microorganisms or fungus. Bovie extenders and lighted retractors help with full visualization of the pocket. Saline and silicone sizers should be available for preliminary pocket and symmetry evaluation. Operating room staff should be instructed that no one touches the implant except the surgeon.

PATIENT MARKINGS

The IMF is marked in the standing position (Figure 61.2). It is 0.5 cm higher in the supine patient. The breast is pushed superiorly, medially, and laterally to define the borders of the breast. In the severely hypoplastic patient, no IMF is present, so a fold is drawn 5–6 cm below the nipple.

For an inframammary incision, a 3–5 cm line is marked in the IMF. Two-thirds of this incision lies lateral to the breast midline.

For an areolar incision, a 3–4 cm incision is designed at the medial and inferior border of the nipple (Figure

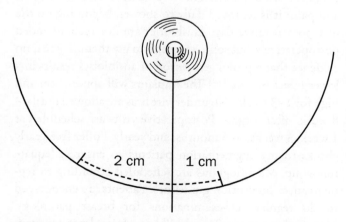

Figure 61.2. Patient markings for inframammary incision.

61.3), with the surgeon being cognizant that the fourth intercostal nerve enters at approximately the 7 o'clock position on the right and at the 5 o'clock position on the left. Some patients may have nipples that are too small for an areolar incision.

For an axillary incision, a natural skin crease in the lower axilla is chosen. Care is taken to keep the incision behind the anterior axillary fold.

OPERATIVE TECHNIQUE

Intravenous antibiotics are given 30–60 minutes before incision. Sequential compression devices are placed on the legs. General anesthesia is induced, and the patient is prepared and draped with arms at 90 degrees. Adhesive plastic sheeting may be used to secure the drapes or cover the breast or nipple.

The incision is marked and measured. The skin and subcutaneous fat are incised and the pectoralis muscle is identified. Dissection is continued above or below the muscle as planned. The pocket is dissected under direct vision. All bleeders are cauterized. Care is taken to look for intercostal perforators medially. Dissection must not cross the midline. Lateral and inferior dissection is reserved until pocket symmetry and implant placement are checked. Lateral dissection is done conservatively and bluntly to avoid division of the intercostal nerve to the nipple and lateral implant displacement.

If submuscular dissection is performed, the medial inferior muscle insertions from the 3 o'clock position to the 6 o'clock position are divided to lessen the deformation seen with pectoralis contraction and allow the implant to sit in the subcutaneous plane in the lower pole.

The pocket is irrigated with saline and Betadine, chlorpactin, or antibiotic solution. If Betadine is used, the pocket must be irrigated with saline before implant placement, as described in the manufacturer's package insert. Hemostasis is meticulously checked. Local anesthesia can be instilled or injected into the skin and muscle.

A sterile implant is opened after verifying the size and type. It is not allowed to touch the patient's skin or the drapes during preparation. For a silicone implant, it is soaked in antibiotic solution, and a Keller funnel may be used to insert the implant in the pocket without touching the skin. If placed by hand, the left hand holds tension on the implant while the right index finger is used to insert the implant edge in the cavity. After

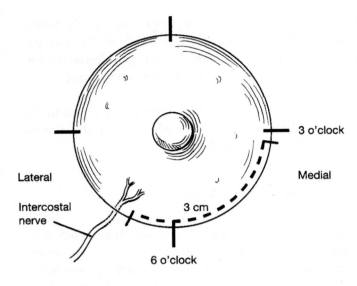

3 o'clock

Medial

Lateral

Intercostal
nerve

3 cm

6 o'clock

Figure 61.3. Patient markings for areolar incision.

approximately 50% of the implant is introduced, compression by the left hand can be used to displace the implant into the cavity. The implant is then smoothed and oriented in a flat position with palpation or a Yankauer suction tip.

For a saline implant, the fill valve is placed and the air in the implant is evacuated. The edges are rolled centrally, and the implant is placed into the pocket. It is unrolled and positioned with the finger. Filling to the desired size is quickly accomplished with the one-way closed-fill system using normal saline. Overfill of 25–50 mL (depending on implant size) is recommended by manufacturers to decrease wrinkling and fold failure of the device. Additional inflation beyond the maximum volume can also cause deflation.

The patient is brought into the upright position and the breasts are checked for symmetry. Additional lateral dissection may be performed with the finger to increase lateral fullness. Inferior dissection will drop the IMF.

For an anatomic implant, one should verify that the 6 o'clock position marker is in the correct position. For a saline implant, the fill valve is pulled and palpation will verify that the tab is in place. Substantial asymmetry requiring differently sized implants is generally recognized in the preop visits. Some degree of asymmetry will always be present, but generally the same size of implant is used on each side.

The incision is closed in three layers: deep fascia, deep dermis, and subcuticular closure. If excessive tension has been placed on the incision edges and they appear to be bruised, 1 mm of skin may be excised before closure.

OTHER APPROACHES

In the *areolar* approach, initial dissection can proceed through the breast tissue or a tunnel may be made inferior to the edge of the breast. The latter approach is easiest in the small-breasted patient and eliminates the potential contamination of breast ducts by bacteria. Submuscular augmentation by the areolar approach is more difficult but possible. The pectoralis is split centrally in the direction of its fibers; dissection then proceeds as described earlier.

In the *axillary* approach, the pectoralis muscle is identified superiorly. Dissection proceeds above or below the muscle, taking care not to extend the dissection lateral to the anterior axillary line. Inferior and medial dissection is carefully completed so that the pocket is bloodless and symmetrical pockets are obtained in the sitting position. An endoscope or lighted retractor is most helpful. Implant placement and filling are as described earlier. The incision is closed with deep absorbable suture and a subcutaneous skin closure.

POSTOPERATIVE CARE

The wound is dressed with glue and/or sterile gauze. I place the patient in a good support bra in the operating room to decrease motion. Some surgeons use a superior band routinely, but I have found that superior dressings or elastic wraps to lower the implants are unnecessary; gravity will lower the implants in 1–3 weeks. One often comes down earlier that the other, but they equalize over time. No drains are used. The patient can expect moderate pain for 1–5 days; submuscular and large implants will have more pain. Skin sutures—if used—are removed any time between day 7 and day 14; a subcuticular suture will leave no marks. A bra is worn day and night for 1 week to decrease motion and pain; it is removed daily to shower, beginning on the first postoperative day. Antibiotics are not recommended postoperatively, but some surgeons do use them. There is no evidence that a prolonged period of antibiotics results in a lower infection rate.[15,22] The implants will appear firm and high for 1–3 weeks. No underwire bras are allowed until 6–8 weeks after surgery. Postoperative visits are scheduled at 1 week, 3 weeks, 3–6 months, and yearly. I offer free yearly checks to my augmentation patients to ensure adequate follow-up. Mammograms are scheduled according to regular cancer prevention guidelines. Patients are encouraged to do regular self-examinations for breast pathology. Massage is taught at 2 weeks if smooth implants are used; textured implants are not massaged.

CAVEATS

The preoperative visit for the breast augmentation patient may take 30–60 minutes, but it is your best insurance for a happy postoperative patient. Documentation of your teaching will aid you should the patient be unhappy. FDA information, manufacturer booklets, and American Society of Plastic Surgeons literature may be valuable in helping the patient to give full informed consent. The possibility of future rupture and reoperation must be discussed. Patients should participate in all decision-making, including size, style, placement, and incisions. The vast majority of patients are very pleased with their new look. They report improved self esteem and less self-consciousness about their breasts. They feel that the benefits of breast augmentation outweigh the possible complications and are very happy with their decision.

REFERENCES

1. https://www.plasticsurgery.org/documents/News/Statistics/2015/plastic-surgery-statistics-full-report-2015.pdf
2. http://www.ricetest.com/rice-test-breast-implants.html
3. Hidalgo DA, Spector JA. Preoperative sizing in breast augmentation. *Plast Reconstr Surg* 2010;125:1781–1787.
4. Tebbetts JB, Adams, WP. Five critical decisions in breast augmentation in 5 minutes: the high five decision support process. Plast Reconstr Surg 2006;118:35S.
5. Choudry U, Kim N. Preoperative assessment preferences and reported reoperation rates for size change in primarybreast augmentation: a survey of ASPS members. *Plast Reconstr Surg* 2012;130:1352.
6. Spear S, Murphy DK. Natrelle round silicone brest implants core study results at 10 years. Plast Reconstr Surg 2014;133:1354.
7. Hidalgo DA, Sinno S. Current trends and controversies in breast augmentation. *Plast Reconstr Surg* 2016;137:1142.
8. http://www.mentorwwllc.com/Documents/MENTOR%C2%AE%20MEMORYSHAPE%C2%AE%20BREAST%20IMPLANTS%20102942-001%20Rev%20E.pdf
9. https://www.allergan.com/miscellaneous-pages/allergan-pdf-files/l034-03_silicone_dfu
10. Hidalgo DA, Spector JA. Breast augmentation CME. Plast Reconstr Surg 2014;133:567e.
11. http://www.fda.gov/MedicalDevices/ProductsandMedicalProcedures/ImplantsandProsthetics/BreastImplants/default.htm
12. Adams WP, Mallucci P. Breast augmentation. Plast Reconstr Surg 2012;130:597e.
13. Hedén P, Montemurro P, Adams WP, et al. Anatomical and round breast implants: how to select and indications for more. Plast Reconstr Surg 2015;136(2):263–272.
14. Hsia H, Thomson JG. Differences in breast shape preferences between plastic surgeons and patients seeking breast augmentation Plast Reconstr Surg 2003;112:312.
15. Lista F, Ahmad J. Evidence based medicine augmentation mammaplasty. Plast Reconstr Surg 2013;132:1684.
16. Davidge KM, Levine R, Brown MH. Comparative outcomes of smooth versus textured round gel implants in primary breast augmentation. Plast Reconstr Surg 2010 October;126:66.
17. Codner MA, Mejia JD, et al. A 15-year experience with primary breast augmenstation. Plast Reconstr Surg 2011;127:1300.
18. Headon H, Kasem A, Mokbel K. Capsular contracture after breast augmentation an update for clinical practice. Arch Plast Surg 2015;42:532.
19. Okwueze M, Spear M, et al. Effect of augmentation mammaplasty on breast sensation. Plast Reconstr Surg 2006;117:73.
20. Gidengil CA, Predmore Z, Mattke S, et al. Breast implant–associated anaplastic large cell lymphoma: a systematic review. *Plast Reconstr Surg* 2015 March;135(3):713–720.
21. Moyer HR, Ghazi B, Saunders N, Losken A. Contamination in smooth gel breast implant placement: testing a funnel versus digital insertion technique in a cadaver model. Aesthet Surg J 2012;32:194–199.
22. Khan UD. Breast augmentation, antibiotic prophylaxis, and infection: comparative analysis of 1,628 primary augmentation mammaplasties assessing the role and efficacy of antibiotics prophylaxis duration. Aesthetic Plast Surg. 2010;34(1):42–47.

62.

REDUCTION MAMMOPLASTY

M. Mark Mofid, Gehaan D'Souza, Benjamin E. Cohen, and Michael E. Ciaravino

Breast reduction is one of the more common plastic surgery operations performed in the United States. There were over 100,000 operations performed in 2015.[1] The etiology of breast hypertrophy is unclear and likely involves some combination of hormonal, genetic, and developmental factors. Patients with mammary hypertrophy complain of intertriginous infections, back and shoulder pain, shoulder notching, physical inactivity, dissatisfaction with breast appearance, poor sexual well-being, and poor psychological well-being.[2] The goals of breast reduction surgery are to reduce overall breast volume, maintain nipple-areola viability, and to achieve a shape that is aesthetically pleasing. Breast reduction improves patient satisfaction with breast appearance as well as physical and psychosocial well-being. Overall patient satisfaction is most strongly correlated with happiness with the appearance of the breasts.[3] A number of techniques have been developed that effectively meet these goals.

Rohrich et al. conducted a survey of 1,500 members of the American Society for Aesthetic Plastic Surgery to ascertain the type of breast reduction techniques used by the members and to assess physician satisfaction, physician-reported patient satisfaction, and complication rates associated with the applied techniques.[4] The inferior pedicle Wise pattern reduction mammoplasty is one of the most common breast reduction technique in the United States.[4] The description of an inferiorly based parenchymal flap was first described by Ribeiro and Backer in 1973.[5] It is shaped at the central part of the lower pole of the breast, in the portion to be resected in superior pedicle reduction mammoplasty, so as to provide good projection and maintain the conical shape of the breast. The breast flap then can be tailored as an autologous small implant and precisely anchored to the pectoralis muscle. This technique is used to decrease the size of the breast while reshaping the breast. The Wise pattern also preserves adequate vascularity,

sensation, and position of the nipple-areola complex. The disadvantages of the inferior pedicle technique are the potential tendency for the breast to "bottom-out" over time because of a lack of parenchymal support.

The vertical pattern breast reduction has been a common technique in Europe and is now becoming more prevalent in the United States as well.[4] Lejour introduced the vertical scar technique for breast reduction in the early 1990s. The horizontal scar in the inframammary fold is avoided with no adverse effect on the cosmetic shape of the breast.[6] As a standard procedure, this technique can be used on all breast types. Lejour showed that only the reduction technique is important in relation to breast shape. She noted that shape is not significantly influenced by suture technique, gland tissue, or skin tension. Lejour's method gives the operating surgeon the freedom to vary the technique by adapting it to each patient.[7] The vertical scar technique may lead to suboptimal scarring due to excessive pleating and decreased blood supply to the wound edges or to long vertical scars. Basetto et al. introduced a modification to Lejour's technique to avoid these issues.[7]

A third technique, partial breast amputation with free nipple-areola grafting, is useful in extremely large reductions (>1,500 g per side) or in patients with significant risk factors.

ASSESSMENT OF THE DEFECT

A thorough preoperative assessment is essential. During the initial consultation, a detailed medical history focusing on weight change and overall medical status is recorded. Smoking history should be determined during the assessment. Recommendations include smoking cessation for 10 weeks prior to surgery and 4 weeks after surgery. Nicotine levels should be checked prior to procedure if questions arise. Risk of deep venous thrombosis (including Caprini score) should be determined. Patients may require the use of pneumatic compression devices or chemoprophylaxis administered in the perioperative period.[8] A history of cardiopulmonary disease should also be obtained for assessment of patient ability to undergo general anesthesia.

Documentation regarding the process of breast development, previous or anticipated pregnancies, breast-feeding history, and oral contraceptive pill and hormone use should be obtained. Breast cancer history including any history of positive breast mass, family history of breast cancer, and positive breast biopsy history should be recorded. Mammograms are obtained if the patient's age or history warrants them. The American Cancer Society recommends women younger than 40 years with a family history of breast cancer or other risks factors and any woman older than 40 should have a mammogram prior a reduction mammoplasty. It is also recommended to obtain mammograms 6 months after surgery to serve as a baseline for future breast evaluation. The patient's motivations for seeking surgical care are addressed. Symptoms relating to breast weight, such as neck, back, and shoulder pain, are documented.

On physical examination, one should begin by calculating the body mass index [(weight in kilograms)/ (height in meters)^2]. A thorough breast exam should include examination of the breast for masses and axillary or supraclavicular adenopathy. This should include a bimanual examination to palpate for masses and to evaluate the consistency of the parenchyma. The overall size and shape of the breasts are noted including an assessment for breast symmetry, evidence of shoulder grooving from bra straps, and evidence of rashes or inframammary intertrigo. The skin is examined for elasticity, looseness, and striae.

Evaluation of breast ptosis is completed. Regnault ptosis scale describes the position of nipple in relation to the inframammary fold and breast glandular tissue.[9]

- *Grade I: Mild ptosis*: The nipple is at the level of the inframammary fold and above most of the lower breast tissue.

- *Grade II: Moderate ptosis*: The nipple is located below the inframammary fold but higher than most of the breast tissue.

- *Grade III: Advanced ptosis*: The nipple is below the inframammary fold and the level of maximum breast projection.

The position of the nipple-areola complex relative to the inframammary fold is assessed. Measurements are taken from the sternal notch to the nipple and from the nipple to the inframammary fold, indicating the degree of vertical correction that will be necessary. Other objective measurements that may help in preoperative evaluation include breast width, nipple-areola complex width, and nipple to sternal midline distances. These factors, coupled with the patient's ultimate size goals, will determine the amount of reduction required as well as the most appropriate method to use. While it is important to estimate the weight of reduction preoperatively, the ability to do so accurately comes only with surgical experience.

INFORMED CONSENT

Central to the discussion is location of scars postoperatively. Patients should understand the extent of scarring depending on the choice of operation and how these scars should be managed in the months after the operation. Patients should be made aware of asymmetries, chest wall irregularities, and breast skin quality. A discussion of common complications should follow including nipple loss, hematoma, seroma, problems with nipple sensation, and breast asymmetries. The patient must also understand that the incidental finding of a breast cancer is about 0.5–0.8%.[10] For a woman of child-bearing age, the question of lactation after a reduction mammoplasty must be noted. Studies show that 70% of patients can breast-feed after undergoing a reduction mammoplasty.[11]

INDICATIONS

The most common indication for breast reduction is relief of physical pain and discomfort associated with heavy, pendulous breasts. Patients frequently complain of chronic back and neck pain, headaches, shoulder pain, and deep bra-strap grooves. Upper extremity neuropathy and postural changes are also noted. Intertrigo and other dermatologic manifestations in the inframammary fold are common. Women with hypermastia are often limited in their ability to engage in physical activity or exercise, which may be a factor in the development of obesity commonly seen in these patients. Many have difficulty finding properly fitting clothes. The psychological impact of hypermastia is significant, and many patients are embarrassed and self-conscious about the size of their breasts. Reduction mammoplasty can eliminate or decrease these problems in most instances. Breast reduction may also be indicated to correct an asymmetry caused by unilateral hyperplasia or to achieve symmetry after unilateral breast reconstruction.

The specific reduction technique selected should depend on the patient's physical characteristics, her attitude toward the scars, and the judgment and experience of the surgeon. The inferior pedicle technique is the most widely used approach in reduction mammoplasty today. It is a reliable technique associated with a high degree of patient and surgeon satisfaction, and it can be used on virtually any size and shape of breast. The nipple-areola complex can be transposed over a considerable distance, and nipple-areola sensation and the ability to lactate are generally preserved. This technique is also effective in the correction of breast asymmetries and ptosis.

A variety of superior pedicle techniques have been described. The vertical mammoplasty popularized by Lejour is a superior pedicle technique that eliminates the need for a horizontal inframammary scar. It is based on the principles of wide skin undermining to promote skin retraction, overcorrection of the lift to produce better long-term results, and liposuction to facilitate breast shaping and tissue removal. While this technique can be used in breasts of all sizes, we find it best suited for small to moderate reductions. The absence of the inframammary incision is of particular benefit in patients with a propensity toward hypertrophic scarring or in those who are very concerned about the scars. The main disadvantage of this technique is that the final results are not obtained immediately, and patients and the surgeon must contend with somewhat deformed, wrinkled breasts for the first few postoperative months. It is essential that the patient clearly understand this before surgery to avoid an unpleasant surprise during the first dressing change.

Amputation with free nipple-areola graft is a rapid, effective reduction mammoplasty technique that is used when there is particular concern over patient safety or nipple-areola viability. Since it is applied as a graft, the nipple-areola complex may be elevated a significant distance, whereas transposition on a pedicle would be too long to be safe. It is also indicated in patients requiring massive reductions, as large volumes of glandular tissue may be resected without concern for preserving a vascular pedicle. Other indications include patients with a high degree of anesthetic risk or those who have had previous breast surgery that has potentially compromised pedicle vascularity. The disadvantages of this technique are loss of nipple-areola sensation, inability to breast-feed, and hypopigmentation of the nipple-areola complex, especially obvious in dark-skinned individuals. Hypopigmentation occurs because of the almost inevitable loss of some portion of the graft with subsequent secondary healing.

Regardless of the technique selected, it is essential that, during the consultation, the patient and surgeon thoroughly discuss the risks and benefits of the procedure, the patient's wishes, and the limitations based on her morphologic characteristics.

CONTRAINDICATIONS

The patient should meet the usual criteria for undergoing an elective surgical procedure. There is no specific age limit provided the patient is in reasonable health. Medical conditions, such as diabetes and hypertension, should be adequately controlled. Smokers must be informed of the increased risks of flap necrosis and problems with wound healing and must stop smoking at least a few weeks before surgery. Patients must be carefully evaluated to confirm that they are indeed candidates for breast reduction. It is not uncommon for a patient with severe breast ptosis to present requesting reduction when they actually require a mastopexy. A thorough breast examination should be performed on all patients, and mammograms should be obtained on those over 35 years of age or with a family history of breast cancer. Any suspicious findings should be addressed by a surgical oncologist before undertaking elective breast reduction.

ROOM SETUP

Breast reductions should be performed in a fully equipped operating room under general anesthesia. The anesthesiologist should be positioned at the patient's head. An electronically adjustable bed with the capacity to incline the back to an upright position is important. Thigh-high stockings and sequential compression devices are recommended. A Foley catheter is generally not required. A sterile ruler, a wire keyhole pattern, and a 38- or 42-mm Freeman "cookie cutter" areola marker are helpful for planning. A smoke evacuation Bovie cauterization unit will be used for the majority of the dissection and for hemostasis.

PATIENT MARKINGS: INFERIOR PEDICLE TECHNIQUE

Accurate preoperative marking is essential to obtaining a good surgical outcome. All planned incisions are determined and marked before surgery, eliminating the need for much improvisation and guesswork during the course of the procedure. Marking is usually performed in the preoperative holding area with the patient seated, facing the surgeon. A thick, felt-tip marking pen, a tape measure, and a wire keyhole pattern are used. The sternal notch and midclavicular points are identified and marked. A line is drawn from the midclavicular point through the nipple-areola complex, marking the breast meridian on each breast. The inframammary fold is marked. Next, the new nipple-areola position is determined using the inframammary fold as a landmark. The inframammary fold position is transposed onto the anterior surface of the breast and marked. A large obstetric caliper, if available, proves particularly useful for marking this point (Figure 62.1), which corresponds to the future nipple location. The periareolar marking is drawn with the help of keyhole wire. The circumference varies between 13 and 16 cm to match an areolar diameter of 4–4.5 cm.

We discourage basing nipple position on specific distances from the sternal notch or relative to the humerus because such approaches are unreliable. Particular caution should be taken to avoid placing the nipple too high, a common error which is extremely difficult to correct secondarily. The inframammary fold mark should end medially 3 or 4 cm from the xiphoid to avoid an easily visible, and potentially hypertrophic, scar. At the breast meridian, the inframammary mark is made 0.5–1.0 cm above the anatomic fold to avoid excess tension at the site of "T" closure. Laterally, the inframammary mark should follow the normal breast contour up onto the breast rather than continuing laterally in the fat fold. This helps to confine the resulting scar to the breast and improves final shape.

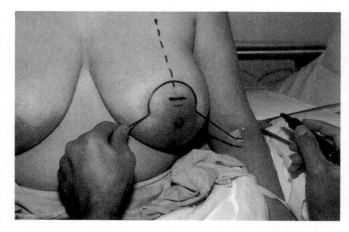

Figure 62.2. Marking for inferior pedicle technique. Wire keyhole pattern is outlined. Vertical limbs should measure 5–6 cm.

The lateral incision can be extended intraoperatively, if necessary, to have a smooth finish. The adjustable wire keyhole pattern is once again placed (Figure 62.2). The width of the keyhole is adjusted according to the characteristics of the breast and the amount of resection required. Lax, ptotic breasts may require widening of the keyhole vertical limbs to allow relatively more skin removal, while large, tense breasts may require limb narrowing to avoid tight skin closure. The width of the keyhole limbs can also be estimated by displacing the breast laterally and medially to mark each limb where it corresponds to the breast meridian. We want to err on the side of a conservative skin resection initially, since more skin can be resected intraoperatively. The height of the vertical limbs should measure 5–6 cm from the bottom of the keyhole circle. Lines are then drawn at right angles from the base of the vertical keyhole limbs to intersect with the inframammary fold laterally and medially (Figure 62.3). The remainder of the markings are made with the patient in

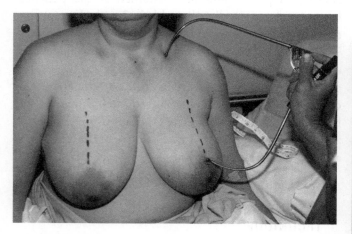

Figure 62.1. Marking for inferior pedicle technique. The breast meridian and inframammary fold are marked. Obstetric calipers are useful to transpose level of inframammary fold onto anterior surface of breasts, identifying the future location of the nipple-areola complex.

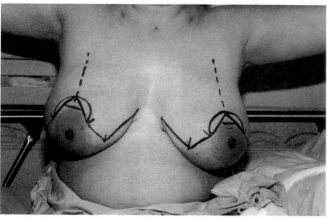

Figure 62.3. Marking for inferior pedicle technique. Completed preoperative markings.

BREAST AND TRUNK SURGERY

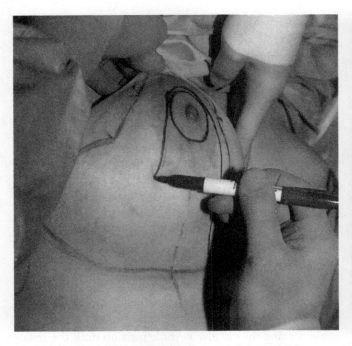

Figure 62.4. Marking for inferior pedicle technique. Inferior pedicle is marked with patient supine. Recommended pedicle width is 8–9 cm.

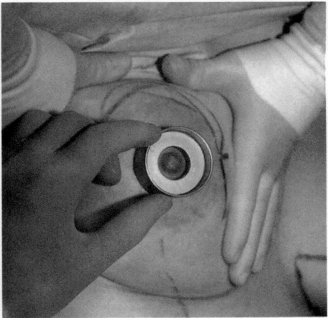

Figure 62.5. Technique for inferior pedicle breast reduction. A 38 or 42 mm "cookie cutter" is used to mark areola for reduction.

the supine position. The planned inferior pedicle is designed vertically below the nipple-areola complex (Figure 62.4). It should measure approximately 8–9 cm wide at the base and be centered on a line from the nipple to the inframammary fold. It extends 1 cm around and above the nipple-areola complex. The size of the actual pedicle is tailored to meet the tissue requirements of the case.

OPERATIVE TECHNIQUE: INFERIOR PEDICLE

Breast reduction is performed in the operating room under general anesthesia. The patient is positioned supine with the arms abducted 80 degrees. The arms should be sufficiently padded and secured to the arm boards with tape or Velcro fasteners to allow the bed to be inclined to a full upright position at various points during the case. The preoperative markings are reevaluated with a ruler and reinforced with a marking pen or scored lightly with a scalpel. The breasts are prepped and sterile drapes are applied. While the assistant holds the breast with the areola under moderate stretch, the surgeon applies a 38 or 42 mm stainless steel "cookie cutter" marking device to make an impression on the areola for reduction (Figure 62.5). The areola is then marked or incised to the dermis. The opposite breast is held under equal stretch by the same assistant to minimize areolar size discrepancies.

De-epithelialization of skin over the pedicle, including a 1 cm cuff around the upper border of the nipple-areola complex, is performed with the breast under tension (Figure 62.6). Good traction is the key to rapid de-epithelialization. A laparotomy pad clamped tightly around the base of the breast proves helpful if the breast is somewhat loose. The de-epithelialization is performed

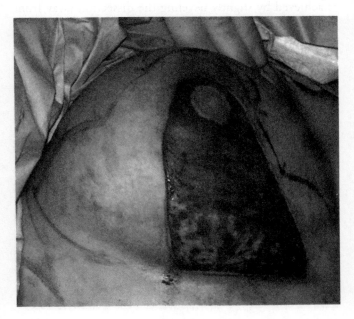

Figure 62.6. Technique for inferior pedicle breast reduction. Pedicle is de-epithelialized.

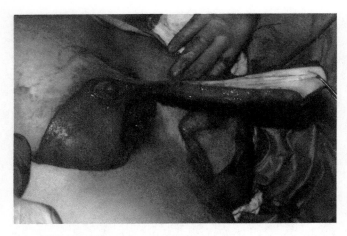

Figure 62.7. Technique for inferior pedicle breast reduction. Resection of medial breast wedge.

using either a scalpel with a no. 10 blade or a sharply curved Mayo scissor. The rationale for de-epithelialization is to facilitate healing in the event of minor skin slough at the line of closure, to preserve the subdermal vascular plexus, and to allow easier handling and orientation of the pedicle.

Resection of breast tissue should proceed systematically, although the exact sequence of steps may vary. In general, we begin with resection of the medial breast wedge (Figure 62.7). The skin along the medial border of the pedicle is incised through the dermis. Cutting electrocautery is used for dissection of the breast parenchyma. The most crucial principle of inferior pedicle breast reduction is to maintain a well-vascularized pedicle (Figure 62.8). This is achieved by slightly beveling the dissection away from the pedicle base, avoiding the common tendency to undermine the pedicle. The assistant should support the breast centrally on the chest wall while the surgeon protects the

pedicle with his or her nondominant hand. Dissection should extend almost to the level of the pectoralis fascia, leaving a thin layer of tissue over the fascia. The medial inframammary incision is made and dissection proceeds superiorly in the same plane. The superior flap incision is made and extended perpendicularly to the chest wall. The medial wedge of breast tissue is removed and weighed.

The lateral breast wedge is approached in essentially the same fashion. Again, caution must be taken to avoid undermining the pedicle. It is important to maintain a thin layer of breast tissue over the pectoralis muscle to preserve laterally based vessels and nerves. Excess adipose tissue may be excised from the lateral fat fold, although excision of axillary lymphatics should be avoided. In general, more tissue is removed laterally than medially.

The keyhole pattern is incised along the vertical limbs and extended through the proposed nipple-areola site to form a triangle at the apex of the keyhole pattern. We avoid making the circular keyhole incision until the resection has been completed, the skin temporarily closed, and the patient inspected in the seated position. This technique is helpful in obtaining symmetry of the nipple-areola complexes.

A superior flap composed of skin and subcutaneous and breast tissue is raised at approximately 2.0 cm in thickness with cutting electrocautery (Figure 62.9). Care must be taken to avoid upper breast hollowing. Leahy or Allis clamps applied to the edge of the flap and held by the assistant at 45 degrees toward the ceiling greatly facilitate uniform flap dissection. The superior flap should be raised and evenly thinned to the pectoral fascia. The remaining volume of breast tissue superior to the pedicle is resected. Care must again be taken to avoid undermining the pedicle, and a gentle "J" incision away from the base is recommended,

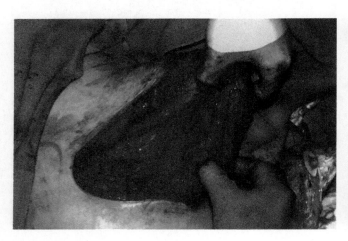

Figure 62.8. Technique for inferior pedicle breast reduction. Pedicle after resection of lateral and medial breast wedge.

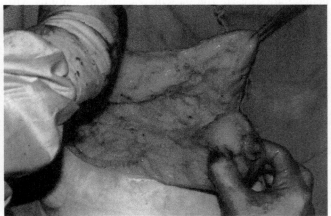

Figure 62.9. Technique for inferior pedicle breast reduction. Development of superior flap.

BREAST AND TRUNK SURGERY

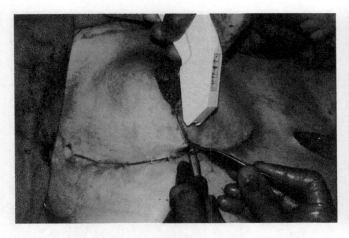

Figure 62.10. Technique for inferior pedicle breast reduction. Temporary closure for inspection of breasts in near-upright position.

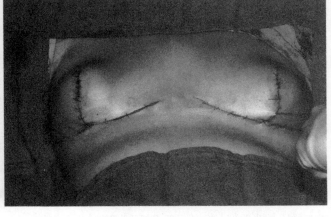

Figure 62.12. Technique for inferior pedicle breast reduction. Completed closure.

which preserves the maximum blood supply to the pedicle without undue bulk.

The contralateral breast is approached in the same manner. The two sides should be carefully inspected to ensure equal volume pedicles and flaps. The skin flaps are temporarily closed with 2-0 silk sutures or staples, and the patient is placed in a seated upright position (Figure 62.10). The breasts are compared for size, shape, and symmetry. Adjustments in the skin envelope and correction of dog-ears are made with "tailor tacking" sutures. The final location of the nipple-areola complex is checked, altered if necessary, and marked in this position. The patient is then lowered to

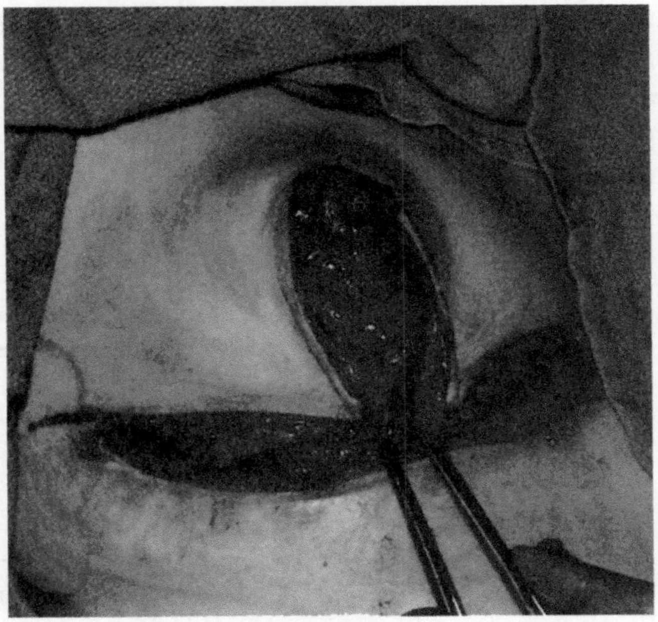

Figure 62.11. Technique for inferior pedicle breast reduction. Nipple-areola complex is brought through skin and sutured into position. Skin flaps are brought together with three-way stitch.

the supine position, the wounds reopened, and the marked adjustments are effected. Both sides are inspected for hemostasis and irrigated with saline. Suction drains are generally not used.

Prior to closing, it may be advantageous to give medial support to the pedicle with a few absorbable sutures. The flaps are approximated to each other and to the inframammary incision by placing a buried 2-0 Vicryl suture through the deep dermis and subcutaneous tissues as a three-way stitch, forming the junction of the "T" closure (Figure 62.11). The inframammary incision is closed in layers using buried interrupted 3-0 Vicryl sutures in the deep tissue and running 3-0 Monocryl subcuticular stitch in the skin. The vertical limb of the "T" closure is closed with interrupted 4-0 Vicryl, followed by a running 3-0 Monocryl subcuticular suture (Figure 62.12). The skin at the site of the nipple-areola complex is excised, and the nipple-areola complex is brought out and secured with 4-0 Vicryl in the deep dermis followed by a running 4-0 Monocryl subcuticular stitch. STERI-strips are applied to all incisions. Dressings consist of sterile 4 × 4 gauze fluffs secured with tape. Alternatively, a soft, loose-fitting surgical bra can be used.

PATIENT MARKINGS: LEJOUR VERTICAL MAMMAPLASTY

As with the inferior pedicle technique, marking is done preoperatively with the patient in a seated or standing upright position. With this technique, however, marking is performed free-hand rather than using a wire pattern (Figures 62.13, 62.14, and 62.15). First, the midline is marked from the sternal notch to the xiphoid process, and

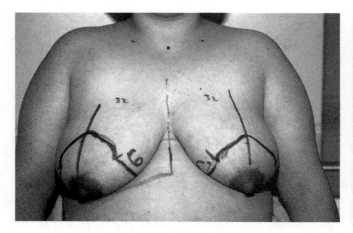

Figure 62.13. Marking for Lejour vertical mammoplasty. Midline and meridian of each breast are marked. Nipple position is determined as in inferior pedicle technique.

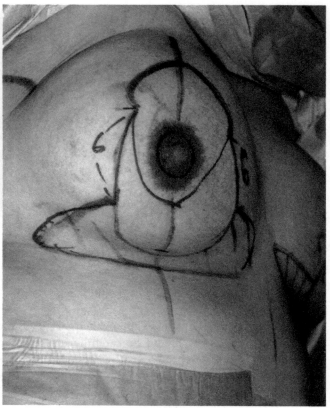

Figure 62.15. Marking for Lejour vertical mammoplasty. Inferior mark is 2–4 cm above inframammary fold.

the inframammary fold is marked bilaterally. The vertical breast meridian is determined on each side and is marked through each inframammary fold onto the abdomen. This generally measures 7–8 cm from the midline. The nipple position is then marked by palpating the tissue starting from the middle of the inframammary fold.

While displacing the breast superiorly and medially, the line through the inframammary fold, which corresponds to the breast meridian, is extended up onto the breast marking the lateral margin. Likewise, the breast is displaced superiorly and laterally to mark the medial margin. These vertical lines are joined inferiorly by a curvilinear line drawn 2–4 cm above the inframammary fold. Superiorly, these lines will connect with the periareolar outline, which is made 2 cm above the new nipple position and designed as a "mosque-dome" shape rather than as a

circle. The purpose of this variation is to produce a more circular areola with less tension once the skin is closed. This periareolar circumference should measure 14–16 cm. Exceeding these values may predispose to widening of the areola and the scars.

OPERATIVE TECHNIQUE: LEJOUR VERTICAL MAMMAPLASTY

The areola is marked so as to reduce its diameter to 38–42 mm. The skin around the areola, including that within the mosque-shaped outline above and 2–3 cm below the areola, is de-epithelialized (Figure 62.16). This is done before liposuction, since de-epithelialization is easier to perform while the breast is still firm.

A 1 cm incision is made just above the curved, inferior skin mark, and a moderate amount of local solution, consisting of 250 ml of 0.25% lidocaine and 1:400,000 epinephrine, is infiltrated throughout the breast. Liposuction is usually performed in conjunction with the Lejour vertical mammaplasty, although it is not required and is not limited to this breast reduction technique. The proposed

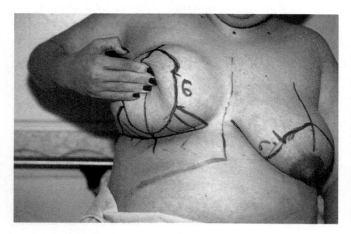

Figure 62.14. Marking for Lejour vertical mammoplasty. Breasts are displaced to mark 6 cm lateral and medial pillars. Periareolar outline is mosque-shaped and measures 14–16 cm.

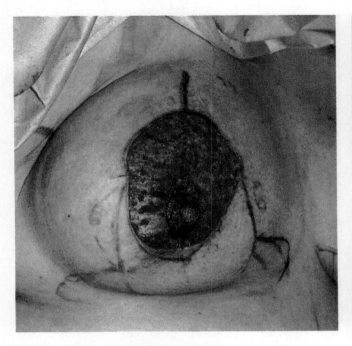

Figure 62.16. Technique for Lejour vertical mammoplasty. De-epithelialization.

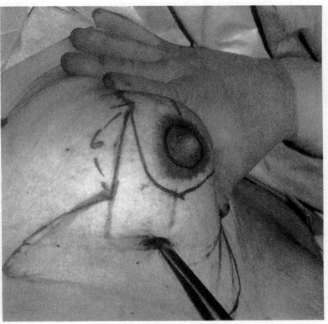

Figure 62.17. Technique for Lejour vertical mammoplasty. Liposuction of breast. Incision is placed above inferior mark, in portion of breast to be removed.

benefits of liposuction include easier breast shaping, softer feel, preservation of blood vessels and nerves, and a greater degree of breast reduction. It is difficult to determine pre-operatively how much fat contributes to the composition of the breast; therefore, liposuction is generally undertaken as a trial. A 6 mm blunt cannula is used to perform liposuction from all areas of the breast with the exception of that portion just behind the nipple (Figure 62.17). Liposuction is continued until no further yield is obtained or the aspirate becomes bloody.

Breast reduction begins by incising the skin around the nipple. Skin excision continues along the medial, lateral, and inferior markings (Figure 62.18). The entire excised flap is de-epithelialized and the skin is completely cut through in the area of the preoperative markings. The skin over the lower aspect of the breast is undermined in a subcutaneous plane, similar to a mastectomy. Cutting electrocautery or scissor dissection is recommended. The skin is then laterally and medially undermined. The breast glandular procedure is then mobilized in an epifascial plane. Undermining continues to the upper margin of the gland at the height of about the third intercostal space. It is essential to make these flaps relatively thin (i.e., less than a centimeter) to promote contraction of the excess skin, which is fundamental to the success of this procedure in the absence of the inframammary incision. Dissection is carried down to the level of the inframammary fold and continued superiorly over the pectoralis fascia, freeing

the lower portion of the breast. Centrally, this dissection continues under the nipple-areola complex to the upper limit of the breast. Next, two 6 cm vertical incisions (one medial, one lateral) are made from the inferior aspect of the future areola to the lower breast. These incisions are

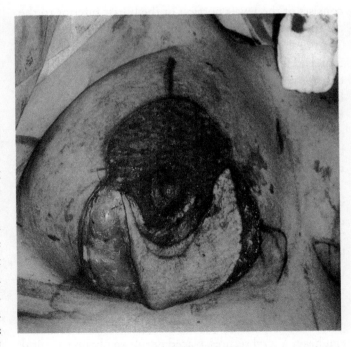

Figure 62.18. Technique for Lejour vertical mammoplasty. Lower aspect of breast is undermined, raising thin, inferior flaps.

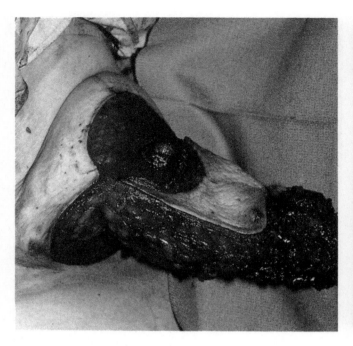

Figure 62.19. Technique for Lejour vertical mammoplasty. Breast tissue isolated for removal.

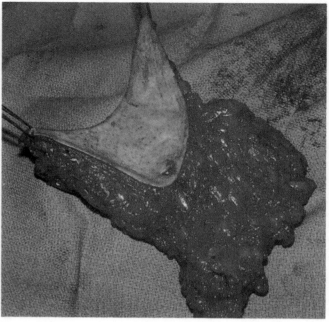

Figure 62.20. Technique for Lejour vertical mammoplasty. Specimen consisting of inferior aspect of breast, including lateral medial extensions.

carried down through the parenchyma to the chest wall, isolating the central portion of tissue to be removed (Figure 62.19) and creating 6 cm lateral and medial pillars of breast tissue, which will be sutured together. Inferior to the pillars, these vertical incisions diverge outward to allow the removal of the medial and lateral tissue of the lower breast. The breast tissue that is removed, therefore, consists of the lower portion of the breast inferior to the areola and its medial and lateral extensions (Figure 62.20). The skin between the areola and the lower incision is also removed with the specimen. In larger breasts, additional tissue is removed from behind the nipple-areola complex, being careful to preserve a pedicle of at least 2–3 cm in thickness. The tissue resection in the Lejour technique is somewhat analogous to removing the medial and lateral breast wedges, as well as the pedicle, in the inferior pedicle technique.

The breast is then elevated as high as possible on the chest wall by suturing the gland at the level of the upper areola to the pectoralis muscle with 2-0 Vicryl (Figure 62.21). This intentional overcorrection creates a temporary upper breast fullness, which will alleviate with time. The areola is sutured to its new position with buried 4-0 Vicryl interrupted sutures in the deep dermis. A drain is placed over the chest wall and brought through the incision. The lateral and medial breast pillars are approximated using several heavy Vicryl sutures, placed deeply to obtain a conical

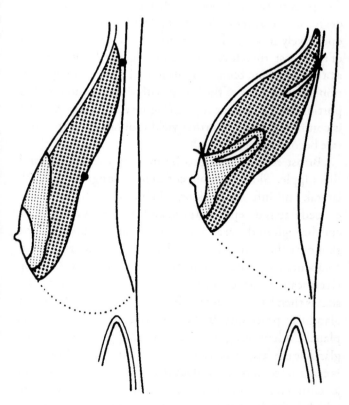

Figure 62.21. Technique for Lejour vertical mammoplasty. Superior fixation of breast. From Cohen M. *Mastery of Plastic Surgery.* Boston: Little, Brown, and Co., 1994:2152. Reprinted with permission.

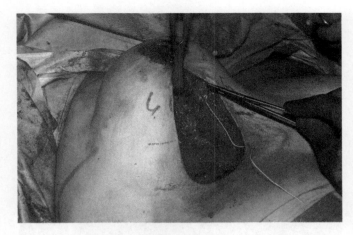

Figure 62.22. Technique for Lejour vertical mammoplasty. Coning of breast parenchyma.

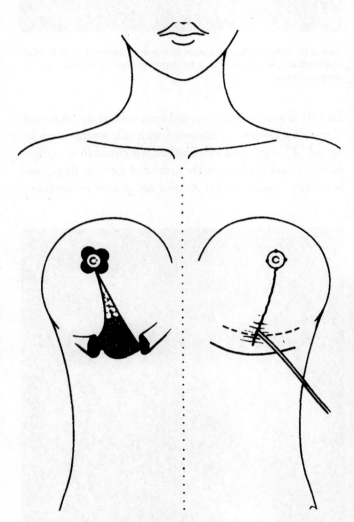

Figure 62.23. Technique for Lejour vertical mammoplasty. Layered closure with intentional wrinkling to reduce incision length. From Cohen M. *Mastery of Plastic Surgery*. Boston: Little, Brown, and Co., 1994:2152. Reprinted with permission.

shape, enhance projection, and eliminate skin tension (Figure 62.22).

After shaping the breast, the significant amount of excess skin is readily apparent. Although this excess can be corrected by excising the skin to create a horizontal inframammary scar, in most instances this can be managed with a vertical two-layer closure, which gathers the excess skin in pleats (Figure 62.23). As per Basetto et al., instead of placing the superior mastopexy suture it is recommend that the submammary fold being fixed using three H points.[7] The three H points serve as a pivot by which later sagging is avoided. The skin closure does not have a shaping function without tension. The vertical pleated suture is not forced but adjusted to the retraction ability of the patient's skin. Use of the vertical pleated suture is limited; in cases of longer incisions, it is combined with a horizontal submammary transverse pleated suture. A running 3-0 Vicryl subcutaneous suture is placed from the skin to the gland in a manner that wrinkles the skin, considerably reducing its length. This length is further reduced by placing a more superficial 4-0 Prolene subcuticular suture with very small bites. The wrinkled vertical incisions, although unappealing on the operating table, improve with time. A firm dressing is applied to the lower portion of the breast for support.

At the conclusion of the treatment, the breasts should appear full on top and flat, with wrinkled skin on the bottom (Figure 62.24). Provided that both the patient and the surgeon are fully aware of this, early postoperative anxiety and dissatisfaction are avoided.

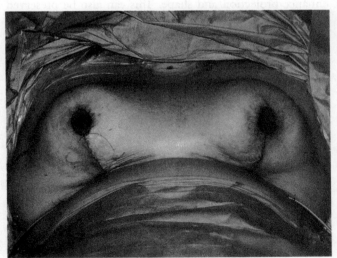

Figure 62.24. Technique for Lejour vertical mammoplasty. Completed closure. Note superior fullness; inferior flatness and wrinkling; drains.

PATIENT MARKINGS: AMPUTATION WITH FREE NIPPLE-AREOLA GRAFT

Preoperative marking for amputation and free nipple-areola grafting is similar to that used in the inferior pedicle technique. The breast meridian, inframammary fold, and approximate position of the nipple are determined and marked as described earlier. The keyhole pattern may be used. However, because the actual position of the nipple-areola complex is determined intraoperatively after shaping the breast mound, we prefer to modify this marking by designing the vertical limbs in the form of a triangle rather than committing to a specific location with the keyhole pattern (Figure 62.25). The decision to use the keyhole versus the triangle design depends on the surgeon's preference.

OPERATIVE TECHNIQUE: AMPUTATION WITH FREE-NIPPLE GRAFT

The technique of amputation with free nipple-areola grafting is safe, reliable, and relatively easy to perform. The breast is placed under moderate stretch, and the areola is marked with a 42 mm cookie cutter. The nipple-areola complex is then removed as a full-thickness graft and preserved in a moist saline gauze. The area within the keyhole or the triangle is de-epithelialized (Figure 62.26). Glandular resection is initiated by removing the lower portion of the breast caudal to the marking (Figures 62.27 and 62.28). An inferiorly based de-epithelialized pedicle of breast tissue can be preserved and tucked under the center of the breast to enhance projection and shape. This can also be preserved

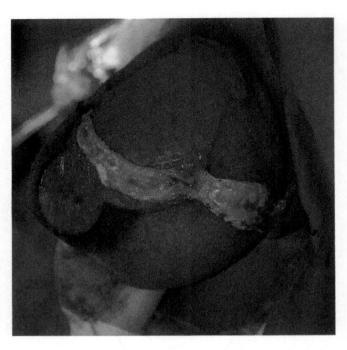

Figure 62.26. Technique for amputation with free nipple-areola graft. Nipple-areola complex is harvested as a full-thickness graft. Periareolar area is de-epithelialized.

initially to ensure that adequate breast volume is maintained. Temporary closure is performed with silk sutures as an inverted "T" (Figure 62.29). The bed is inclined to an upright position, and the breasts are inspected for size, shape, and symmetry. Tailor-tacking sutures are placed as necessary.

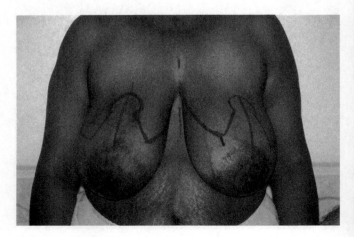

Figure 62.25. Marking for amputation with free nipple-areola graft. Keyhole pattern may be used, as depicted here. However, it may be advisable to begin with triangular pattern rather than keyhole so that nipple-areola position can be adjusted.

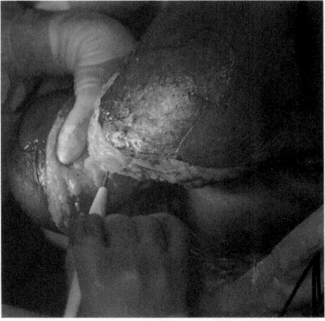

Figure 62.27. Technique for amputation with free nipple-areola graft. Glandular resection.

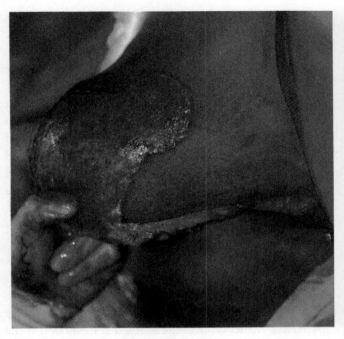

Figure 62.28. Technique for amputation with free nipple-areola graft. Glandular resection.

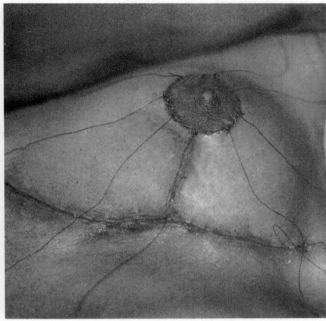

Figure 62.30. Technique for amputation with free nipple-areola graft. Thinned nipple-areola graft placed on de-epithelialized bed.

Final closure is performed in layers using buried absorbable sutures followed by a running 3-0 Prolene subcuticular pull-out suture. Nipple-areola graft position is selected in this position based on visual inspection and specific measurements. Ideally, the location of the nipple-areola grafts should correspond to the center of the breast mound and measure 5–6 cm

from their inferior border to the inframammary fold. The distance from the nipple to the clavicle and the sternal notch should be compared between the sides. After selecting the graft position, the site is marked using methylene blue and the 42 mm cookie cutter and then de-epithelialized. The undersurface of the nipple-areola grafts is thinned to the level of the dermis, and the grafts are placed on the recipient sites (Figure 62.30). The grafts are secured with a 4-0 silk tie-over bolster dressing made from glycerine-soaked cotton wrapped in Xeroform gauze (Figure 62.31). A protective 4 × 4 gauze fluff and tape dressing is applied.

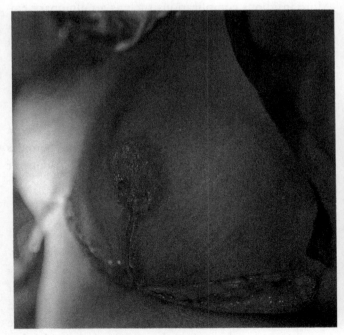

Figure 62.29. Technique for amputation with free nipple-areola graft. Temporary closure.

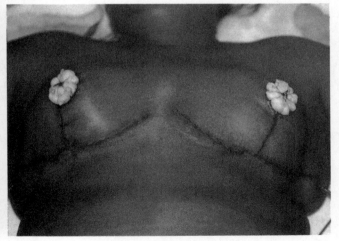

Figure 62.31. Technique for amputation with free nipple-areola graft. Nipple-areola grafts secured with tie-over bolsters.

POSTOPERATIVE CARE

Incisions should have Steri-Strips placed in the operating room. Kerlix should be laid over the breasts, and an adequately fitting surgical bra should be placed on the patient. Dressings should be removed on the first postoperative day. Lejour recommends wearing a support bra day and night for 2 months after her procedure. If drains are used, output is carefully recorded and the drains removed when the output is less than 30 mL in 24 hours. The patient is permitted to shower on postoperative day 1 if there are no drains; otherwise, the patient can shower when they have been removed. Patients should avoid heavy lifting and strenuous physical activity for at least 4 weeks following surgery.

CAVEATS

All patients should be thoroughly informed of the risks of reduction mammoplasty, including the potential for scarring, asymmetry, nipple-areola loss, and decreased sensation.

The reduction mammoplasty technique should be individualized according to the breast characteristics, the patient's medical status, and the surgeon's preference. Cases requiring massive volume reductions or nipple transposition over a significant distance may be more safely approached using amputation with free nipple-areola grafting rather than pedicle techniques.

Accurate preoperative marking is important; however, final breast shape and symmetry are achieved intraoperatively. After the initial tissue resection, the breasts are inspected in the upright position and adjustments are made with "tailor-tacking" sutures or staples.

Proper determination of the new nipple-areola complex location is essential. Nipple-areola complex malposition is difficult to correct secondarily.

Preserve nipple-areola viability by developing a well-perfused pedicle or dermal graft bed. Avoid the tendency to undermine the pedicle. If the pedicle nipple-areola complex viability is questionable at the end of treatment, it should be converted to a free graft.

COMPLICATIONS

NIPPLE NECROSIS

The breast must be monitored for nipple necrosis. A bluish nipple intraoperatively should warrant rewarming patient and monitoring of fluid status. If duskiness persists, the wound must be opened to monitor for hematoma. If nipple bluishness persists, the patient may benefit from fluorescein dye test and Wood's lamp monitoring. Finally, free nipple graft may be the only option if nipple duskiness continues. The grafting should be done on a well-vascularized breast parenchyma. Nipples showing signs of immediate tension should have sutures removed to rule out hematoma. If relief of tension does not improve blood flow, the patient should be taken back to the operating room for free nipple graft onto a well-vascularized bed. For patients whose nipple necrosis is not found until the late postoperative period, general wound care should be undertaken and nipple reconstruction thereafter.

WOUND HEALING

Wound healing is related to closure under tension. In the inverted T reduction mammoplasty, the T junction is the most common location for wound healing issues. The purse string closure is a frequent wound healing problem location in the vertical technique.

DEEP VENOUS THROMBOSIS/PULMONARY EMBOLUS

Patients needs to be evaluated for deep venous thrombosis (DVT) if they develop leg swelling. The best method for evaluation of DVT is a duplex ultrasound. More insidious complications such as a pulmonary embolus need to be evaluated by computed tomographic scan of the chest or ventilation/perfusion scan if contrast is contraindicated.

SEROMA

Seromas are a common long-term complication. If a seroma is suspected, needle aspiration is attempted. Seromas that are resistant to aspiration are managed by drains or reopening and closure of dead space.

HEMATOMA

Breast swelling with distensibility is most likely a hematoma. Hematomas occur immediately postoperatively or in the few weeks after operation. Bloody output from drains or a tight swollen breast should be drained at the time of the diagnosis in the operating room. Late hematomas must be evaluated and treated to avoid infection or fat necrosis.

BOTTOMING-OUT

Bottoming-out or pseudoptosis is characterized by an excess amount of breast tissue below the inframammary fold with a normal nipple position. This is most commonly a complication of a Wise pattern breast reduction.

NIPPLE PARESTHESIAS

Changes in nipple sensation should be discussed in the preoperative appointment. Early changes in sensation should be managed expectantly. Studies have shown contrasting findings on the relation of specific dermal pedicles correlating with nipple paresthesias.

REFERENCES

1. American Society of Plastic Surgeons. 2015 Cosmetic and Reconstructive Plastic Surgery Statistics. https://d2wirczt3b6wjm.cloudfront.net/News/Statistics/2015/plastic-surgery-statistics-full-report-2015.pdftrends.pdf. Accessed January 8, 2017.
2. Saariniemi K, Luukkala T, Kuokkanen H. The outcome of reduction mammoplasty is affected more by psychosocial factors than by changes in breast dimensions. *Scand J Surg* 2011;100:105–109.
3. Coriddi M, Nadeau M, Taghizadeh M. Analysis of satisfaction and well-being following breast reduction using a validated instrument: the Breast-Q. *Plast Reconstr Surg* 2013;132:285.
4. Rohrich RJ, Gosman AA, Brown SA, Tonadapu P, Foster B. Current preferences for breast reduction techniques: A survey of board-certified plastic surgeons 2002. *Plast Reconstr Surg* 2004;114:1724.
5. Ribeiro L, Backer E. Mastoplastia com pediculo de siguridad. *Rev Esp Cir Plast* 1973;16:223–227.
6. Lejour M. Vertical mammoplasty and liposuction of the breast. *Plast Reconstr Surg* 1994;94:100.
7. Hoffman A, Wuestner-Hofmann M, Bassetto F. Breast reduction: modified "Lejour technique" in 500 large breasts. *Plast Reconstr Surg* 2007;120:1095.
8. Young V, Watson M. Patient safety: the need for venous thromboembolism (VTE) prophylaxis in plastic surgery. *Aesthet Surg J* 2006;26:157.
9. Regnault, P. Breast ptosis: definition and treatment. *Clin Plast Surg* 1976;3:193.
10. Pitanguy I, Torres E, Salgado F, Pires Viana GA. Breast pathology and reduction mammoplasty. *Plast Reconstr Surg* 2005;115:729.
11. Brzozowski D, Niessen M, Evans HB, Hurst LN. Breast-feeding after inferior pedicle reduction mammoplasty. *Plast Reconstr Surg* 2000;105:530.

SELECTED READINGS

Courtiss EH, Goldwyn RM. Reduction mammoplasty by the inferior pedicle technique. *Plast Reconstr Surg* 1977; 59:500–507.

Gradinger GP. Reduction mammoplasty with nipple graft. In: Goldwyn RM, ed. *Reduction Mammoplasty*. Boston: Little, Brown, 1990: 513–529.

Lejour M. Vertical mammoplasty and liposuction of the breast. *Plast Reconstr Surg* 1994; 94:100–114.

Little JW, Spear SL, Romm S. Reduction mammoplasty and mastopexy. In: Smith JW, Aston SJ, eds. *Grabb and Smith's Plastic Surgery*. Boston: Little, Brown, 1991:1157–1185.

Maxwell GP, White DJ. Inferior pedicle technique of breast reduction. In: Jurkiewicz MJ, Culbertson JH, eds. *Operative Techniques in Plastic and Reconstructive Surgery*. Philadelphia: WB Saunders, 1996:170–175.

63.

MASTOPEXY

Bernard W. Chang and Nishant Bhatt

Breast ptosis or sagging is the most common reason for performing a mastopexy. Ptosis may be present as breast development occurs or may develop with aging. Many factors contribute to breast ptosis, including abnormal breast development, poor skin tone, postpartum involutional changes, changes in body weight, and gravitational factors, with increased stretching of the skin. Mastopexy may be performed to reshape the breast and restore more ideal proportions. Mastopexy may also be performed to attain symmetry for developmental abnormalities and for the contralateral breast in postmastectomy reconstruction. It is important to accurately assess the patient's expectations regarding the ultimate breast shape and volume and whether an implant may be sufficient or used to supplement a mastopexy.

PREOPERATIVE ASSESSMENT

When examining the breast, it is first important to know the ideal relationships of its various anatomic structures. In the ideal breast, the nipple position is usually located approximately 2 cm above the projection of the inframammary fold. Ideally, the majority of the breast tissue should be centered behind the nipple-areola complex, without a significant amount of skin from the nipple to the inframammary fold (the ideal in most cases is 7 cm). Measurements are determined and recorded after certain landmarks are established. These include the chest midline, sternal notch, inframammary fold, and breast meridians (lines drawn from the midclavicular points to the midportion of each breast and projected onto the inframammary fold, which usually is drawn through the mid–nipple-areola complex). Measurements are taken from the sternal notch to the nipples, the nipple to inframammary fold, and the nipple

to midline, as well as the breast width and diameter of the areola. The amount of breast tissue is assessed as well. In some cases, the nipple-areola complex may be medially or laterally displaced and may need to be centralized. Any degrees of asymmetry are noted with regard to measurements and breast size, and these are described to the patient as well. Asymmetry may be compensated for in the amount of skin excised from each side and positioning the nipple-areola complex at the same level.

DEGREES OF PTOSIS

Based on the preoperative assessment, each patient may be classified according to the degree of ptosis present, as described by Regnault:

- *Grade 1 (minor ptosis)*: The nipple lies at the level of the inframammary fold but above the lower contour of the gland and skin brassiere.

- *Grade 2 (moderate ptosis)*: The nipple lies below the level of the fold but remains above the lower contour of the breast and skin brassiere.

- *Grade 3 (major ptosis)*: The nipple lies below the level of the fold and at the lower contour of the breast and skin brassiere.

- *Pseudoptosis*: Characterized by a hypoplastic breast in which the full lower quadrants appear to have descended while the nipple remains above the inframammary fold.

- *Glandular ptosis*: Characterized by descent of the lower breast quadrants with retention of the nipple at its normal level (most common after breast reduction).

INDICATIONS

Patients with breast ptosis who desire a more ideal shape to the breast and who are willing to accept the necessary scars are candidates for mastopexy. Candidates generally include those with Grades 1–3 ptosis. Patients with pseudoptosis may benefit from augmentation mammaplasty as well. Patients with larger breasts may require some degree of reduction. Contralateral balancing procedures for developmental anomalies and postmastectomy reconstruction may require mastopexy, especially in the expander or implant reconstruction patient.

CONTRAINDICATIONS

Contraindications for mastopexy include patients who are unwilling to accept breast scars, patients with unrealistic expectations, and patients with other significant medical problems (i.e., cardiovascular disease, pulmonary disease). Patients with a history of heavy smoking also may be at increased risk for wound dehiscence or skin necrosis or other healing complications. Risks of altered sensitivity in the breast skin and nipples should also be discussed, and some patients may not elect to have surgery performed because of potential complications or scarring. Patients should also be reminded that ongoing aging processes may cause recurrence of ptosis.

ROOM SETUP

The patient is placed in the supine position with both arms on arm boards. The patient is centered on the table with the shoulders even. A urinary catheter is generally not necessary, and standard monitoring equipment is used. The operative table must allow the patient to be placed in the upright sitting position during the procedure. Local anesthesia with intravenous sedation may be sufficient for minor degrees of correction. For larger amounts of skin resection and flap elevation, general anesthesia is necessary.

PATIENT MARKINGS

Preoperative markings vary, depending on the degree of ptosis present. Markings are done in the standing upright position. All anatomic landmarks are identified and marked (breast midline, breast meridian, inframammary fold). In marking the inframammary fold, it is important to follow the lateral border of the breast up along the direction of the anterior axillary line. Frequently, in patients who are obese, the inframammary fold extends as a fold of skin and fat onto the back. This is not the proper line to follow, because a lateral dog-ear deformity may be produced. This lateral fold of tissue may be liposuctioned as part of the operative procedure to attain a better result.

After the basic anatomic landmarks are drawn, the new position of the nipple-areola complex is determined along the breast meridian. The projection of the inframammary fold onto the anterior breast is determined with calipers (or by palpation), and a mark is placed 2 cm above this level. This is the new center position for the nipple-areola complex. An additional mark is made 2 cm above this point and defines the upper margin of the repositioned nipple-areola complex. Using a malleable-wire Weiss pattern device, the outline for the new nipple-areola complex is drawn using the upper mark to align the top of the wire Weiss pattern. The degree of opening of the wire pattern may be adjusted depending on the degree of ptosis and proximity of the existing nipple-areola complex. When only minor degrees of nipple-areola elevation are necessary, the wire Weiss pattern may be placed so that the existing areola may be enveloped by the circular portion of the device. Because the circumference of the Weiss pattern stays constant, opening or closing the width of the device always results in a circle of constant diameter. Once the position of the nipple-areola complex is determined, it should not be altered intraoperatively since the most accurate assessment for attaining symmetry is in the standing upright position. The remainder of the markings are usually made in the supine position and are actually easier in the supine position if there is significant ptosis. Curvilinear lines are then drawn from the bottom edges of the circular nipple-areola marking to the inframammary fold. For minor degrees of ptosis, no additional horizontal incisions may be necessary. For larger degrees of ptosis, where the distance from the bottom of the nipple-areola markings to the inframammary fold is greater, a horizontal component of skin may need to be marked for excision. The lower border of the horizontal ellipse is determined by the inframammary crease, and the upper border is marked 5–6 cm below the bottom of the marked nipple-areola complex. The limbs of the horizontal ellipse are made approximately equal on the medial and lateral sides. Final adjustments in shape are made at the completion of the operation with the patient in the sitting upright position.

Alternative types of mastopexy patterns which limit the length of the incisions or degree of undermining have been described as well. The purpose of all of these different techniques remains the same: to tighten or readjust the skin envelope of the breast to reduce the amount of breast ptosis. Goulian described the dermal mastopexy technique, which was performed with minimal undermining and skin excision only. Benelli described a technique whereby the incisions are limited to the outer areola and a circumferential donut of tissue is removed from around the nipple-areola complex. Widening of the areola and flattening of the central breast is a pitfall of the Benelli technique. Regnault described a technique, called the B-technique, whereby the incisions are limited to the lateral portion of the inframammary fold, the nipple-areola complex, and a vertical component from the nipple-areola complex to the inframammary fold. Lejour described a technique for mild to significant ptosis using a vertical incision only and tightening the excess skin with a gathering suture along the vertical skin closure.

The short scar periareolar inferior pedicle (SPAIR) technique was described in 1998 by Hammond et al. for reduction mammoplasty. This technique was later applied and adapted to mastopexy. It involves a circumvertical skin resection pattern with an inferiorly based pedicle. This operation addresses the problem of recurrent upper pole concavity by direct suspension of the upper pole in the superior position. In the SPAIR mastopexy, the inframammary folds and breast meridians are marked in usual fashion. A transverse line connecting the inframammary folds is drawn, and a parallel line is drawn 4–6 cm above this line between the breasts. The top of the periareolar pattern is represented by an intersection between this line and the breast meridian. The inferior pedicle is 8 cm wide at the base and is bisected by the meridian; 8–9 cm limbs are drawn at the medial and lateral boundaries of the pedicle upward onto the breast, and the apex of the limbs are connected with a curvilinear line, paralleling the inframammary fold. This represents the bottom of the periareolar pattern. The inferior pedicle is drawn within the periareolar pattern with the apex of the pedicle 2 cm above the areolar border.

OPERATIVE TECHNIQUE

After completion of markings, the patient is brought to the operating room and placed in the supine position. Preoperative antibiotics are given. General anesthesia is usually indicated; however, in lesser degrees of ptosis, local anesthesia with intravenous sedation may be appropriate. The skin is then prepared and scored in the inframammary crease at the breast meridian. The existing nipple-areola complex is stretched and a circumferential incision is made between 38 and 42 mm. The remainder of the breast markings are incised with a scalpel and continued through the dermal layer

using the electrocautery. De-epithelialization of the marked areas is performed with curved Mayo scissors. The surrounding skin is then undermined so that the skin may be closed with minimal tension (usually 1–3 cm). The flaps are elevated at least 1 cm in thickness to avoid ischemia at the wound margins. The nipple is then elevated in the cephalad direction to the newly designated position determined preoperatively. Preliminary staple closure is performed, and the patient is placed in the upright sitting position. Additional skin is then removed as necessary to refine the completed shape. Excess skin is frequently removed from the medial and lateral portions of the breast to further create a rounded breast as opposed to a "boxy" shape. Final closure is performed with absorbable inverted dermal sutures, followed by a complete subcuticular closure and Steri-Strips or Dermabond. Drains are usually not necessary. Marcaine is usually placed into the incisions at the end of the case.

Conversely, in the SPAIR mastopexy, the areola is incised under stretch with a diameter of 42–44 mm. The aforementioned periareolar incisions are made, and the intervening skin is de-epithelialized. The dermis is incised at the superior aspect of the periareolar incision leaving a 5 mm cuff of dermis, which is to be used for the purse-string suture. Medially and superiorly, thin flaps are elevated and are beveled to be thicker as the dissection reaches the pectoralis fascia. The thickness at the level of the pectoralis fascia is between 3 and 6 cm. Once the pectoralis fascia is reached, further elevation is performed superiorly toward the clavicle and medially toward the internal mammary artery perforators. Laterally, uniform 2 cm flaps are elevated above the level of the breast capsule. With the patient sitting up at 60 degrees, three maneuvers are used to shape and auto-augment the upper pole of the breast while rounding out the medial breast. First, the leading edge of the superior flap is folded onto itself and tacked to the pectoralis fascia with two to three 3-0 monofilament sutures. Second, the medial flaps are plicated together to created a rounded medial contour to the breasts. The inferior pedicle is then tacked superiorly to the pectoralis fascia. With the medial and superior poles addressed, the inferior pole is contoured by tailor-tacking the medial and lateral skin of the lower pole together with staples. The skin within the staple line—which overlies the inferior pedicle—is marked, and the staples are removed. The intervening skin is de-epithelialized. A Gore-Tex suture on a straight needle is passed between the nipple-areola complex and the aforementioned 5 cm dermal cuff. The suture is cinched to set a diameter of 35–40 mm of the areola. Otherwise, final closure is performed in the usual manner. As in the Wise pattern mastopexy, drains are not necessary.

DRESSINGS AND POSTOPERATIVE CARE

Gauze dressings are applied to the breasts followed by a surgical bra. Mastopexy is usually performed in an outpatient setting, unless it is done in conjunction with other inpatient procedures. The patient is instructed to change the dressings on the second postoperative day and clean the suture lines with hydrogen peroxide. If a drain has been placed, the dressings and the drains are removed in the office on the second to third postoperative day. The patient is then allowed to get the incision lines wet. Skin flaps are inspected for signs of ischemia on the first postoperative visit. Sensory changes in the skin and nipples are noted as well. Follow-up visits are usually scheduled at 1 month, 6 months, and 1 year to assess the aesthetic outcome, scars, and any sensory changes in the skin.

CAVEATS

It is always important to assess the patient's needs as carefully as possible so that both patient and physician are satisfied with the outcome of surgery. This is especially true when performing a mastopexy. As plastic surgeons, we are often perceived as being able to produce the least amount of scarring. For patients with only moderate amounts of ptosis, the degree of scarring may not outweigh the benefits of improved appearance. Inform the patient, show pictures of different results and the types of scars, discuss risks and complications, and make sure the patient has realistic expectations before proceeding with surgery.

SELECTED READINGS

Benelli L. Technique de plastie mammaire: le "round bloc." *Rev Fr Chir Esthet* 1988;50:7.

Bostwick J. *Plastic and Reconstructive Breast Surgery*. St. Louis: Quality Medical, 1990.

Goulian D. Dermal mastopexy. In: Lewis JR, ed. *The Art of Aesthetic Plastic Surgery*. Boston: Little, Brown, 1989:873.

Hammond D. Short scar periareolar inferior pedicle reduction (SPAIR) mammaplasty. *Plast Reconstr Surg*. 1999 Mar;103(3):890–901.

Hammond D, Alfonso D, Khuthaila D. Mastopexy using the short scar periareolar inferior pedicle reduction technique. *Plast Reconstr Surg* 2008 May;121(5):1533–9.

Lejour M. *Vertical Mammaplasty and Liposuction*. St. Louis: Quality Medical, 1994.

Regnault P. Ptosis, asymmetry, tubular breast, and congenital anomalies. In: Owsley JQ, Peterson RA, eds. *Symposium on Aesthetic Surgery of the Breast*. St. Louis: CV Mosby, 1978.

64.

BREAST RECONSTRUCTION WITH IMPLANTS AND TISSUE EXPANDERS

Ruth J. Barta, Omotinuwe Adepoju, and Bruce Cunningham

The advantages of reconstructing breasts with implants were first described by Freeman. The introduction of tissue expansion in the 1980s has increased the versatility of this method and expanded its indications. Since then, additional advances in technique, implant design, acellular dermal matrix (ADM), and fat grafting have improved the aesthetic results even further. In the meantime, Noone and colleagues have provided the reassurance that immediate, prosthetic reconstruction does not interfere with local recurrence surveillance.

Over the past decade, the number of women choosing reconstruction with tissue expanders and implants has steadily increased, while the percentage of women having autologous reconstruction has plateaued or fallen off. According to the American Board of Plastic Surgeons database, in 2014, 81% of breast reconstruction was reported by plastic surgeons as implant- or tissue expander-based.

There are several aspects of prosthetic reconstruction that make it appealing to women. This method avoids long, complex operations; prolonged exposure to anesthetic agents; and extended hospitalizations that are associated with autogenous tissue reconstruction. Of greater significance, the choice of a prosthetic reconstruction avoids the risks, side effects, and prolonged recuperation following autogenous procedures. This is particularly true in bilateral cases, in which symmetry with an implant is less of a problem and where bilateral autologous reconstruction may pose substantial demands on the patient and the surgeon. The expander or implant option is very appealing for small-breasted women, older patients, those who are less motivated, and active women who are not able to spare the recuperative times required by autologous reconstruction. Women are now more aware of the options available to them, and the option of immediate reconstruction with tissue expanders and implants has made a major impact in the mass media market.

More effective screening measures, particularly genetic testing, has brought a much younger cohort of women with higher aesthetic concerns and goals to oncologic and plastic surgeons. These younger women are great candidates for nipple-sparing, immediate reconstruction with implants or tissue expanders. Many other women who are being more effectively staged have become candidates for nipple-sparing mastectomy and immediate reconstruction. Additionally, women may be aware that there are new techniques that are yielding significantly superior aesthetic results compared to those in the past.

Several major changes have increased the aesthetic outcomes and safety of breast reconstruction with tissue expanders and implants. As oncologic surgery has evolved, plastic surgeons are provided with much more skin resource to manage for the reconstruction than was available in the past. In the past, tissue expanders were required to create more skin; today, these devices should be regarded more as skin shaping or shape maintaining rather than as actually stretching devices.

Ten years ago, in addition to scant skin to work with, the surgeon was confronted with a long expansion process with the expander generally placed beneath the rectus fascia. This was done to protect the skin against pressure by creating an internal support system of a fibromuscular bra. The main limitation of the quality of the result was a lack of ability to create fullness in the lower pole. This resulted in many reconstructions that were too high on the chest and abnormally placed (Figure 64.1). Alternatively if the reconstruction was placed on top of the rectus fascia, the weight of the implant resulted in ptosis of the reconstruction, albeit with a fuller inferior pole (Figure 64.2).

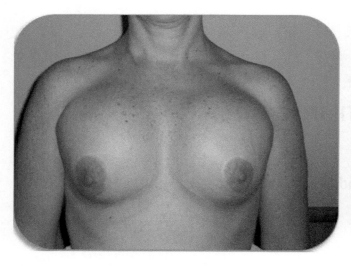

Figure 64.1. Superiorly displaced implant due to subpectoral/subrectus fascia placement. Notice lack of inferior pole fullness.

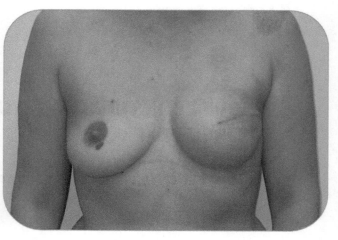

Figure 64.3. Implant reconstruction with acellular dermal matrix (ADM) support. Notice well-defined intramammary fold without superiorly displaced implant. The contralateral side can undergo a balancing procedure such as augmentation, mastopexy, or both.

The use of ADM overcame the constraints imposed by placing the reconstruction underneath the rectus fascia and allowed a great deal more flexibility for the surgeon to achieve a better aesthetic result (Figure 64.3). While some argue that the use of this foreign material has increased the risk of complications, the overall result has been so positive that use of a dermal support unit that recreates the anatomical fold and is attached to the pectoralis muscle has become the standard of care.

Advancements in the ability to evaluate the tissue in real-time intervals during the mastectomy and reconstruction has allowed plastic surgeons a much greater zone of safety when evaluating how much fluid to place in the tissue expander. Women want to get the result as quickly as possible, and, by safely evaluating the skin, significantly larger

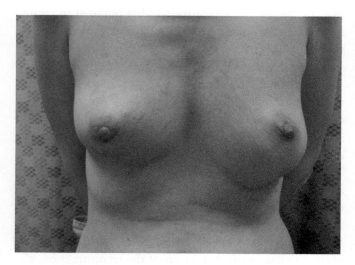

Figure 64.2. Loss of control of inframammary fold, on the right, due to supra rectus placement of the implant without inferior pole reinforcement.

volumes of saline can be placed on the table without causing skin necrosis. This allows the surgeon to maximize the skin resource available and often to send the patient home after surgery with the final result virtually achieved. The advantage of a tissue expander versus a direct implant is that, if the initial evaluation of the skin proves that perfusion is not adequate, fluid can be removed from the tissue expander on the first postoperative day.

Radiation is playing an increasingly common role in mastectomy and reconstruction. In many instances, the reconstructive plastic surgeon cannot know for sure the amount and location of radiation that patients may receive after surgery. Generally, there is a limited period of time after surgery before the radiation oncologist believes the patient should begin her treatments to obtain the best result. This increased pressure to complete the reconstruction before radiation begins has made the accurate perfusion evaluation more important, so that as much fluid as possible can be placed in the tissue expander during the initial operation. This more aggressive approach has allowed the reconstruction of mound volume and shape to be completed in time for the radiation to begin in a timely fashion.

Finally, the widespread use of fat grafting in breast reconstruction has significantly benefited patients having reconstruction with tissue expanders and implants. The final result can be enhanced by using fat grafting from the abdomen or the hips to camouflage irregularities due to lack of subcutaneous tissue and to increase the lower pole and the projection of the nipple. Fat grafting has also been shown to be of benefit in rescuing a failed reconstruction prior to replacement of a tissue expander, often allowing the patient to avoid an autologous flap. Fat appears to significantly improve the quality of the skin and soft tissue padding after radiation at the time of or before the second-stage operation is done. Fat grafting seems particularly beneficial in rejuvenating the radiated tissue during the interval between the cessation of radiation and the performance of the second-stage operation.

Our current preference among prosthetic reconstruction techniques is a minimum two-stage technique. This method includes placement of the tissue expander at the time of mastectomy and an initial expansion with a textured, saline-filled expander with an integrated valve system. This allows for smoother expansions with fewer complications or technical difficulties. The second stage is typically performed 3–6 months later and involves the permanent implant plus revision of the pocket when needed. An exception to the two-stage technique is the patient who is appropriate for immediate implant reconstruction. Size of the reconstructed breast is determined by a combination of preoperative discussion with the patient and what their natural breast footprint will accommodate.

INDICATIONS AND CONTRAINDICATIONS

Prosthetic reconstruction is indicated for the patient undergoing a mastectomy who desires an implant to reconstruct her breast. The size of the contralateral breast and the amount of skin excised at the time of mastectomy determines whether an implant alone or a staged approach with a tissue expander is required. This method is also indicated for select cases of subcutaneous mastectomy in which the breasts have multiple scars, thin subcutaneous tissue, or tight inframammary folds. Reconstruction with implants is also indicated for the patient who desires autologous tissue but is not a good candidate for reasons of obesity, scars, available tissue, or health.

It is well known that perioperative radiation therapy interferes with all types of breast reconstruction. Results are better when autologous tissue is used in these situations, and the complication rates are lower. Some may contend that prosthetic reconstruction is contraindicated when radiation therapy is used. We believe implant reconstruction can be successful in select patients with minimal radiation injury. These patients should be counseled on the diminished cosmetic results of a prosthetic reconstruction and the potential increased need for fat grafting or autogenous methods should the implant method fail.

ACELLULAR DERMAL MATRIX

ADM was introduced for immediate implant, breast reconstruction in 2005 by Breuing and Warren. In 2007, Bindingnavele described the two-stage technique using tissue expanders. Indications for its use is reconstructing the inframammary fold, better lower pole contour and projection, and lateral coverage of the implant while sparing the serratus anterior muscle. Most important, it allows greater initial expansion volumes by matching the size of the subpectoral implant pocket to the dermal pocket. With the acceptance of skin sparing mastectomy (SSM) and subsequently larger skin flaps, it is important to fill the pocket to a volume that the flaps will tolerate in order to preserve the soft tissue contour and minimize time and number of fills needed to reach the goal volume (Figure 64.4).

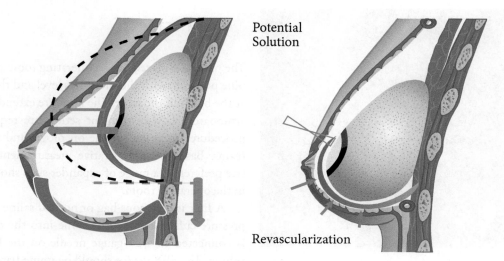

Potential Solution

Revascularization

Figure 64.4. The use of acellular dermal matrix (ADM) allows for expansion of the inferior pole while offering support for the implant once the pectoralis major has been released.

ASSESSMENT OF THE DEFECT AND PERFUSION

When performing an immediate reconstruction, it is important to assess the entire soft tissue envelope that will cover the prosthesis. The early recognition, correction, and management of ischemic skin and muscle flaps will help avoid serious problems later. The capillary refill in the skin flaps should be assessed. In cases of questionable viability, perfusion studies, such as SPY (Novadaq) or floruosine with Wood's lamp, should be performed to guide the surgeon on the margin of ischemic tissue. We prefer to use SPY (Novadaq) for our intraoperative assessment. Each kit contains 10 cc of indocyanine green. Each study can be performed with 3–5 cc of dye followed by a 10 cc normal saline flush. This allows for multiple studies during the operation. We assess perfusion at the start of the reconstructive part, to determine the margin of necrotic tissue and after intraoperative fill, and then before final closure, to determine if the fill volume is tolerated by the mastectomy flaps (Figure 64.5).

It is important to discuss with the oncologic surgeon the need to avoid using epinephrine in their injection fluid as this can induce vasospasm that will falsely lower perfusion scan readings. Indocyanine green has been shown to be renally safe but should be avoided in patients with known contrast allergies. In cases in which there is significant injury to the soft tissue envelope, it may be prudent to forego the immediate procedure and opt for a delayed reconstruction. Delayed prosthetic reconstruction is substantially less risky than immediate prosthetic reconstruction. Wound infection, implant extrusion, or other wound problems are rare in delayed cases.

PATIENT MARKINGS

When performing a prosthetic breast reconstruction, meticulous preoperative planning, assessment of the defect, and preoperative markings are essential to achieving an optimal aesthetic result. A careful assessment of the contralateral breast must be done and a decision made based on the need for any modification. We prefer not to alter a normal, aesthetically attractive breast and generally only modify those that will benefit from a reduction or mastopexy.

It is important to plan the incision with the oncologic surgeon so a safe and thorough extirpation can be performed while preserving as much breast skin as possible. In patients with breast cancer, the skin excision must encompass the biopsy site and areola and, when possible, facilitate access to the axilla. While we believe the skin-sparing concept is generally applicable to prosthetic reconstruction, the isolated periareolar incision is not helpful and is difficult to close except in those cases where a flap is used to replace the missing skin. When the opposite breast is being modified, the mastectomy incision should be designed whenever possible so that the resulting scars match those on the contralateral breast.

The patient should be marked in the upright position with her face forward and her arms at the sides. The midline, inframammary folds, and the lateral and medial borders of the breast are marked.

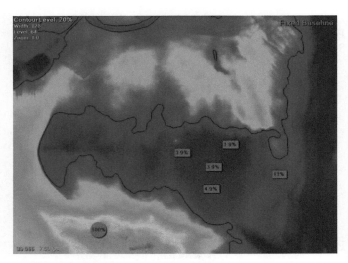

Figure 64.5. Indocyanine green imaging demonstrating poor perfusion to part of the mastectomy skin flap after on-table fill of the expander.

ROOM SETUP

The patient is placed on the operating room table in the supine position, with the shoulders level and the hips located at the break in the table. The arms are extended on padded armboards. Two instrument setups are required for this procedure, one each for the oncologic and reconstructive teams. Based on preoperative measurements and patient size preference, a range of expander sizes should be present in the operating room.

A liter intravenous bag of normal saline is used with a pressure cuff to help instill saline into the expander. This is connected to a 21-gauge needle on the field by sterile tubing. The SPY device should be immediately available at the start of the reconstructive portion.

OPERATIVE TECHNIQUE

THE FIRST STAGE

For both cosmetic and safety reasons, the tissue expander is placed subpectorally in the majority of cases. Direct to implant reconstruction is gaining popularity but is beyond the scope of this chapter. In immediate reconstruction, once hemostasis has been obtained and the soft tissue envelope assessed, the subpectoral pocket can be developed by elevating the lateral border of the pectoralis major muscle. This is accomplished with a fiberoptic or suction electrocautery unit or an endoscope and long right-angled retractors. The muscle is elevated laterally to medially by carefully releasing the origins of the muscle. The medial border of the pocket must precisely correspond to the preoperative markings; the pectoralis major muscle can be divided medially as far as the level of the pectoral fascia in this region. The fascia should be preserved to protect the prosthesis from migrating across the midline. The pocket is then developed cephalad nearly to the level of the clavicle; this dissection can be performed with blunt dissection once the subpectoral plane is developed. The inferior aspect of the pocket is developed by elevating the inferior border of the muscle and ultimately entering the subcutaneous or subfascial plane at the inferior most extent of the dissection. The dissection proceeds carefully in this plane to help create the inframammary fold, which must precisely correspond to the preoperative markings. Once the pocket has been created, its continuity is verified by sweeping a finger along the borders of the pocket; any constricting bands are transected under direct vision (Figure 64.6).

Once the pocket is adequately dissected, hemostasis is obtained with the electrocautery. The pocket is irrigated with triple antibiotic and all surgical debris is removed. Size of the ADM used is based on the size of the defect, available soft tissue envelope, and anticipated reconstructed breast size. We prefer to use shaped, perforated ADM as we believe this allows better egress of fluid and decreases seroma formation from between the ADM and vascularized skin flap. Reducing seroma in this plane facilitates better incorporation of the ADM. The ADM is anchored at the medial border of the chest wall at the most inferior, remaining attachment of pectoralis major. The inframammary fold is then recreated by anchoring the ADM to chest wall, at approximately the sixth rib, while incorporating dermis at the preoperatively marked fold. This can be performed using interrupted or running continuous sutures. The lateral breast margin is recreated by anchoring the ADM to the chest wall along the anterior lateral fold. Dermal bites are not taken along the lateral fold to avoid unwanted puckering or scaring. If the axillary pocket is significant, several dermal to chest wall sutures can be placed to diminish the dead space (Figure 64.7).

The selection of the appropriately size tissue expander is based on the width of the recreated breast footprint, keeping in mind patient size preference. The tissue expander is prepared by verifying that no leaks or surface defects are present. The expander is deflated and placed into the pocket after a final irrigation with triple antibiotic solution. The pectoralis major should drape over the expander and meet the superior edge of the ADM without undue tension. It is essential that the inferior edge of the device is placed precisely at or slightly below the level of

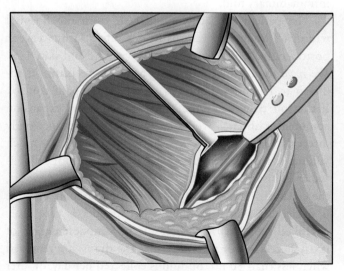

Figure 64.6. Release of the pectoralis major muscle along intramammary fold to create pocket for the expander.

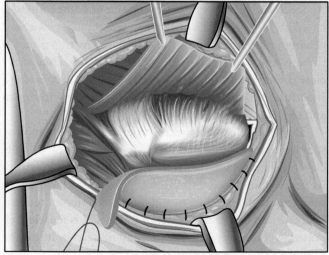

Figure 64.7. Sewing in the acellular dermal matrix (ADM) along intramammary fold to redefine fold and support inferior pole.

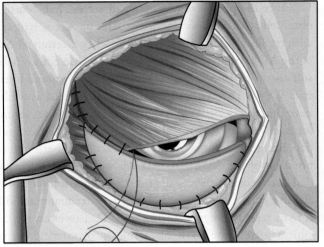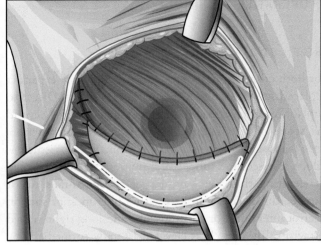

Figure 64.8. Placement of expander within new subpectoral pocket. The size of acellular dermal matrix (ADM) used to create the neopocket can be determined by amount of skin available after mastectomy.

the new inframammary fold and as far medial as possible (Figure 64.8). If the expander is equipped with tabs, these should be secured to the chest wall. A drain is placed in the implant pocket and brought out at the lateral skin edge. The subpectoral pocket is then closed by sewing the superior edge of the ADM to the inferior border of pectoralis major. Care should be taken to protect the expander. If there is any question of implant compromise, a few drops of methylene blue can be added to the expansion fluid to check for a leak. If there is any doubt, it is better to replace the expander at this stage. A second drain is placed in the subcutaneous pocket. A 20-gauge needle is inserted through the muscle or skin into the expander port under direct vision or magnetic guidance. Saline infusion is commenced, via a closed system, using a three-way stopcock and 60 cc syringe. The amount of saline infused is based on how much the pocket can accommodate without placing undue tension on the skin flaps. At this point, if there is any concern regarding the flaps, we temporarily close the pocket and check perfusion using SPY (Novadaq). If perfusion is questionable, some saline can be withdrawn and the flaps reassessed.

During immediate reconstruction, if a complete, submuscular pocket is required, it is created by initially elevating the pectoralis major muscle along the length of its fibers, approximately 1 cm from the lateral border. The subpectoral plane is entered and the dissection proceeds laterally toward the serratus anterior muscle. This muscle is elevated in continuity with the pectoral muscles by lifting the origins of the muscle off the respective ribs. Care must be taken to remain on the external surface of the ribs because

entry into the intercostal space may create pneumothorax. Once the muscle slips have been elevated off individual ribs, the surgeon can place a retractor into each of these tunnels and lift the muscle outward, exposing the attachments to the intercostal fascia and muscles. With careful dissection using the cautery, these attachments are divided, which completely elevates the serratus anterior muscle from the lateral chest wall. The lateral border of the pocket must conform to the preoperative markings. The remainder of the subpectoral pocket is developed in a similar fashion to the subpectoral-only technique, with the exception that the subcutaneous plane is not entered inferiorly. The inferior border of the pectoralis muscle is elevated in continuity with the rectus sheath or rectus muscle to the level of the inframammary fold.

The patient is usually discharged from the hospital within 48 hours and returns to our office within a week postoperatively for assessment of the wound and skin flaps. We have found that prescribing a muscle relaxant, in addition to narcotics, improves postoperative pain control. If the soft tissue envelope is viable, additional expansion commences about 3 weeks later and continues in weekly intervals until the desired volume is instilled. As much volume as tolerated is injected at each expansion; saline is typically instilled until the patient experiences discomfort, the expander feels tight to the examining surgeon, or there is noticeable skin blanching. The expander is ultimately overfilled by 10–20% to help create a modest degree of laxity necessary for a good result. The drains are removed when less than 30 mL of fluid is collected per day, or after 14 days, whichever comes first.

The expander is left in place for 3–6 months, or occasionally longer, to allow the overlying tissues to become supple. This period is variable and depends on factors such as adjuvant therapy, wound healing, and the duration of the active expansion process. Chemotherapy should not interfere with the expansion process; however, the second stage should be delayed until the patient's immunologic status returns to normal. Adjuvant radiation therapy should be deferred, if possible, until the active expansion process is completed. We prefer to complete the second-stage operation and wait 3 weeks prior to commencement of radiation. This reduces the burden of wound healing on irradiated skin. It is important to address skin necrosis early to protect the expander. If the wound edges become necrotic, we prefer to excise them and close the wound primarily, typically an office procedure. This ensures coverage of the device with well-vascularized tissue and minimizes the risk of device exposure. If the loss of soft tissue is extensive and the patient wishes to pursue reconstruction, the implant method may need to be abandoned and plans for autologous method commence.

THE SECOND STAGE

The preoperative planning and preparation is similar to the first stage. Several implant sizers and final implant sizes should be available based around the known volume at final expansion plus 60 cc to account for the volume displacement of the expander. The position of the implant, especially the level of the inframammary fold, must be carefully assessed. Any changes to the level of the fold must be carefully marked preoperatively. Consideration should be given at this point to adjusting the contralateral breast, including consideration of a mastopexy, reduction, augmentation, mastectomy, or revision of a previous procedure.

An incision is made and scar removed along some or all of the original mastectomy scar if no radiation has been used, or in the Infra-mammary fold or outside the zone of radiation damage. Fat grafting during post radiation period can improve the wound bed condition prior to the second stage procedure. With the electrocautery, the subcutaneous tissue and pectoralis muscle are divided until the expander capsule is encountered. A short flap is dissected over the capsule inferiorly, and the capsule is entered about 1–2 cm from the skin edge. This stepwise opening ensures that, should the skin incision open postoperatively, the implant is less likely to be exposed. The expander is removed by bluntly separating it from the capsule. It may be necessary

to remove some saline from the expander to facilitate its removal.

Capsulotomies or capsulectomies are performed where necessary, and a capsulorraphy or internal fold procedure is often required to further define the inframammary fold and implant pocket. Implant sizers are used to determine the best volume for the permanent implant. The breasts are inspected for symmetry in size, contour, and fold position, and the necessary adjustments are made. When the result is satisfactory, the pocket is irrigated with triple antibiotic solution and the final implant inserted. The wound is closed in layers, including muscle and skin, and then is covered with surgical glue and appropriately dressed. A nipple reconstruction can be performed at the same time the expander is replaced, but we prefer to delay it to a later stage.

The second stage is usually an outpatient procedure, and the patient is discharged soon after the treatment is concluded. Follow-up occurs at intervals 1, 3, and 7 weeks after surgery. We use absorbable sutures, so suture removal need not be addressed. Preneo dressing is removed at the 3-week visit.

TERTIARY STAGES

Adjuvant procedures such as fat grafting, nipple reconstruction, and contralateral balancing procedures can be performed at any time to improve the quality and symmetry of the reconstruction. The wide acceptance of fat grafting has contributed significantly to the final quality of reconstruction. The discussion of fat grafting is beyond the scope of this chapter and is addressed in chapter 16. Patients who have undergone radiation therapy are not candidates for nipple reconstruction due to poor healing potential and risk of exposing the implant should the nipple flaps fail. Three-dimensional tattooing may be an alternative option for these patients but still carries the risk of wound healing issues.

CAVEATS

A few salient points should prevent some common problems. It is essential that a reasonable preoperative plan is devised; the appropriate procedure must be chosen for the appropriate candidate. Careful pre- and intraoperative measurements are required to select the right size and shape of expander and implant. A decision on altering the contralateral breast must also be made. Once the plan is formulated, it must be coordinated with the oncologic surgeon's plan to ensure an adequate extirpation. We like to mark the premastectomy incision as a guide for the oncologic surgeon. The inframammary fold should be preserved whenever possible; if an error in positioning the fold is to be made, it should be more cephalad. It is easier to lower the fold than it is to raise it at the second stage.

The surgeon must exercise good judgment when filling the tissue expander during the first stage. If too much tension is placed on the skin, flap necrosis can result, which can jeopardize the reconstruction. If there is any question about undue tension on the skin from the volume of saline injected into the expander, simply remove some!

There are some cases where direct to implant reconstruction is an option. This requires healthy mastectomy flaps to minimizes risk of complications. Experience on the part of the oncologic and reconstructive surgeon improves consistency of healthy flaps and patient selection, respectively. There have been preliminary reports of prepectoral implant-based reconstruction, but there are not enough data available to warrant discussion at this time. Such an operation would eliminate the animation deformity and risk of lateral displacement of the implant with time.

Finally, if marginal skin necrosis develops in the postoperative course, we excise it immediately since this reduces the risk of device exposure. It is not wise to wait to see if the affected area will heal secondarily; this is usually not the case.

SELECTED READINGS

Alderman A, Gutowski K, Ahuja A, Gray D. Postmastecomy expander implant breast reconstruction guideline work group. ASPS clinical practice guideline summary on breast reconstruction with expanders and implants. *Plast Reconstr Surg* 2014;134:648e-655e

Evans GR, Schusterman MA, Kroll SS, Miller MJ, Reece GP, Robb GL, Ainslie N. Reconstruction and the radiated breast: is there a role for implants? *Plast Reconstr Surg* 1995;96:1111-1115

Freeman BS. Subcutaneous mastectomy for benign breast lesions with immediate or delayed Prosthetic replacement. *Plast Reconstr Surg* 1962;30:676–682.

McCarthy CM, Mehrara BJ, Riedel E, et al. Predicting complications following expander/implant breast reconstruction: an outcomes analysis based on preoperative clinical risk. *Plast Reconstr Surg* 2008;121: 1886-1892

Noone RB, Frazier TG, Hayward CZ, et al. Patient acceptance of immediate reconstruction following mastectomy. *Plast Reconstr Surg* 1982;9:632–638.

Noone RB, Murphy JB, Spear SL, et al. A 6-year experience with immediate reconstruction after mastectomy for cancer. *Plast Reconstr Surg* 1985;76:258–269.

Plastic Surgery Organization. http://www.plasticsurgery.org/Documents/news-resources/statistics/2014-statistics/plastic-surgery-statsitics-full-report.pdf

Sbitany H, Sandeen SN, Amalfi AN, Davenport MS, Langstein HN. Acellular dermis-assisted prosthetic breast reconstruction versus complete submuscular coverage: A head-to-head comparison of outcomes. *Plast Reconstr Surg* 2009;124:1735–1740

Spear SL, Onyewu C. Staged breast reconstruction with saline-filled implants in the irradiated breast: recent trends and therapeutic implications. *Plast Reconstr Surg* 2000;105: 930-942

Spear SL, Sher SR, Al-Attar A. Focus on technique: supporting the soft tissue envelope in breast reconstruction. *Plast Reconstru Surg* 2012;130 (5 Suppl 2): 89s-94s

Vardanian AJ, Clayton JL, Roostaeian J, et al. Comparison of implant-based immediate breast reconstruction with and without acellular dermal matrix. *Plast Reconstr Surg* 2011;128: 403e-410e

65.

BREAST RECONSTRUCTION WITH THE LATISSIMUS DORSI FLAP

Michael Klebuc, Elizabeth Killion, Jesse Selber, and Gregory R. D. Evans

The latissimus dorsi myocutaneous flap has enjoyed unparalleled utility and longevity. First described in 1896 by Tansini, the latissimus dorsi has evolved into a reliable, first-line method of breast reconstruction. Traditionally, musculocutaneous flap coverage is placed over an implant to yield a single-stage reconstruction. This hybrid of modalities amalgamates the benefits (ptosis, softness, adjustability) and drawbacks (capsular contracture, implant failure, back scar) of autogenous and implant reconstruction. Refined reconstructions can be achieved when these physical properties are recognized and advantageously controlled. This technique is well described; however, there are salient points that are worthy of reiteration. In addition, reconstruction of segmental mastectomy defects, use of expander implants, skin-sparing mastectomies, extended flaps, and laparoscopy-assisted harvesting represent current and evolving applications of this technique.

INDICATIONS

Breast reconstruction using the latissimus dorsi myocutaneous flap in conjunction with an implant is reliable and frequently yields a natural-appearing breast with ptosis and consistency that falls somewhere between an implant and a completely autogenous reconstruction. The latissimus dorsi breast reconstruction is well-suited to the patient with (1) multiple previous abdominal operations, (2) limited infraumbilical soft tissues, (3) an extensive pendulous pannus, or (4) previous abdominoplasty that limits the potential for transverse rectus abdominis myocutaneous (TRAM) flap reconstruction. The single-stage nature of this reconstruction is advantageous, and the technique is well-suited to patients with breasts of small to moderate size.

If future pregnancy is desired, the latissimus dorsi flap does not violate the anterior abdominal wall, although successful pregnancies have been reported after TRAM reconstruction. Recovery times are generally shorter than those seen with TRAM reconstructions because the effects of abdominal surgery are avoided. Because there are fewer random components to the latissimus dorsi flap, it may be more resistant to the effects of diabetes mellitus and smoking. However, the distal muscle and skin can succumb to these effects. The latissimus dorsi breast reconstruction can be used in previously irradiated patients, but caution must be used in those patients with extensive axillary treatment. The latissimus furnishes an important reserve option in the face of a failed autogenous TRAM or DIEP flap reconstruction. Fisher has demonstrated clinically and in a primate model that "reverse flow" through the retained serratus anterior branch of more proximally divided thoracodorsal vessels can sustain a latissimus dorsi flap. This vascular pattern enables use of the latissimus reconstruction after failed free TRAM flap breast reconstruction. Additionally, the latissimus represents an important reserve option after TRAM reconstruction if a second primary neoplasm develops in the contralateral breast. Frequently, it is difficult to achieve symmetry, especially in patients with ptosis, if an implant is used alone.

In robust patients with relatively small breasts, an extended latissimus dorsi myocutaneous flap can afford a pure autogenous reconstruction. A superior and inferior apron of subcutaneous tissue and fascia are harvested in conjunction with the desired skin island (up to 30 × 8 cm) and can consistently yield a breast volume of 300–400 mL, depending on the amount of back tissue, without an implant.

Greater versatility has been achieved by using the flap in concert with an expander and implant. Postoperatively, the volume of the prosthesis can be manipulated to refine

677

symmetry. This is performed through an adjacent port, which is later removed under local anesthesia.

The latissimus dorsi musculocutaneous flap has also been used in reconstruction of regional breast deformities arising after segmental mastectomy and radiation for stages I and II breast cancer. The flap can be used with a skin paddle or de-epithelialized and embedded. Frequently, the defects are limited, and the flap can be split to preserve a segment of muscle. Local recurrence rates of 2–6% have been reported after segmentectomy and radiation, necessitating careful postoperative oncologic surveillance. Preoperative and postoperative mammography (at 6 months) are essential to aid in differentiating malignant microcalcification from fat necrosis.

Finally, the latissimus dorsi flap provides a source of healthy, nonirradiated soft tissue to reconstruct chest wall defects after salvage mastectomy and neoadjuvant chemoradiotherapy for stage IV breast cancer.

CONTRAINDICATIONS

A disadvantage of the latissimus dorsi reconstruction is the frequent necessity of an implant to achieve the desired volume. Implants have their own inherent complications, including extrusion, migration, infection, and capsular contracture rates of 25–31%. Recent studies have reported long-term rupture rates of more than 50% in older silicone gel implants. Therefore, we believe it is essential in the preoperative assessment to stress that breast implants do not last indefinitely. They are devices and, like all appliances, eventually succumb to wear. Patients offered this reconstructive option should not be adverse to the possibility of future implant exchange or revision.

Assessment of motor function and inspection of the posterior axillary folds for symmetry are undertaken at the initial visit. Alterations in the normal appearance of the latissimus dorsi may indicate the need for alternative flap selection. Patients are asked to place their hands on their hips and push inward, while the physician looks for outward winging of the scapula and muscular contraction. Additionally, pushing off with the arms from a seated position evaluates the motor function of the latissimus dorsi muscle. The thoracodorsal artery and nerve lie in direct proximity, and denervation is associated with a high rate of vascular injury. The denervated muscle is thin and atrophic but can be transferred if the serratus branch is preserved. Preoperative evaluation by Doppler, magnetic resonance angiography, or arteriography may be indicated. Alternatively, the pedicle can be explored before

flap elevation. Functional loss from latissimus elevation is minimal; however, complaints have been reported in athletic patients participating in skiing, bowling, and weight lifting.

Loss of the latissimus dorsi can be problematic in patients with knee fusion or lower extremity weakness resulting from stroke or poliomyelitis. Here, the muscle may influence gait by elevating the hemipelvis, permitting easier circumduction. The latissimus dorsi plays an integral role in wheelchair transfers, and its loss may prove deleterious in paraplegic patients. Selection of alternative flaps may be indicated in these patients.

Additionally, a posterolateral thoracotomy scar is highly suggestive of damage to the intramuscular blood supply and a notable contraindication. Previous axillary lymph node dissection and irradiation are associated with higher complication rates but are not absolute contraindications for this technique.

PATIENT MARKINGS

The popularity of the conventional, horizontally oriented flap design has gradually waned. Although concealed under the bra strap, the scar tends to hypertrophy and widen and is a frequent source of dissatisfaction. Segmental mastectomy reconstructions, however, pose an exception to this principle. The skin island dimensions are frequently limited (reduced wound tension) and the resultant scar is narrower and well-camouflaged by most bathing suits and brassieres. Oblique and laterally oriented skin islands produce more cosmetically acceptable scars. The oblique design is well suited to the more Reubenesque patient. The skin island is designed to incorporate a fatty "backroll," which orients the scar along the lines of relaxed skin tension. Flap width typically measures 7–8 cm but can be extended to 12 cm when mandated. A "pinch test" verifies the ability to approximate the proposed wound before flap elevation. Flap lengths commonly measure from 20 to 30 cm.

The fatty billow is marked preoperatively in the standing position along with the location of the inframammary folds. A template is fashioned intraoperatively, corresponding to the skin defect. With the most apical posterior region of the axilla acting as a fulcrum, a pendulum created from the pattern and a heavy suture determine the exact position of the skin island and adequacy of its reach.

Segmental defects may require flaps composed predominantly of muscle and subcutaneous tissue, with limited or no skin island. Here, a small horizontal back incision hidden beneath the bra provides a good cosmetic result.

A fleur-de-lis (T-shaped) skin island with limbs 7–10 cm wide can be designed in an attempt to maximize the volume of available soft tissue. Closure produces an inverted T-shaped scar on the back. Excessively tight wound approximation results in necrosis of the trifurcation point. Additionally, an obliquely oriented skin island can be marked on the back with superior and inferior aprons of subcutaneous tissue extending to the borders of the muscle.

ROOM SETUP

Orienting the patient in the lateral decubitus position with the shoulder abducted provides unfettered access to the posterior thorax and axilla (Figure 65.1). The patient is placed on a deflatable beanbag extending from the trochanteric region to the inlet of the axilla. Care is taken to ensure the device does not extend beyond the spinous processes posteriorly. A shoulder roll is placed under the dependent axilla to guard against brachial plexus injuries, and the distal pulses are palpated to evaluate perfusion. The free arm is draped with an impervious stockinette to the midbrachium and supported on a padded Mayo stand. Alternatively, the entire arm is prepared, and the hand is wrapped with sterile towels fastened with penetrating towel clips. Draping the arm in this unencumbered fashion allows maximized surgical exposure and facilitates dissection high in the axilla.

A Foley catheter and sequential compression devices for deep venous thrombosis prophylaxis are standard. Great care is taken to liberally pad pressure points. A pillow is positioned between the knees, and the malleoli are covered with foam heel protectors. Resting the head on a foam donut protects against folding of the ear or undue pressure. The position of the dependent breast must be appraised to protect against pressure necrosis. A cloth tape restraint extending over the posterior iliac spine aids in securing the patient to the operating table. Direct contact with the skin is avoided to prevent development of tape burns. The lower extremities are covered with a thermal air blanket for temperature modulation. Additionally, collaboration with the anesthesia service with regard to electrocardiographic and line positioning often proves fruitful. The chest wall and axilla are prepared in the standard fashion, and the operative site is squared off with towels or adhesive 10 × 10 cm plastic drapes. Again, the drapes should not cover the spinous processes, which provide an important landmark. The free arm is drawn through the aperture of a disposable laparotomy sheet, which provides adequate exposure

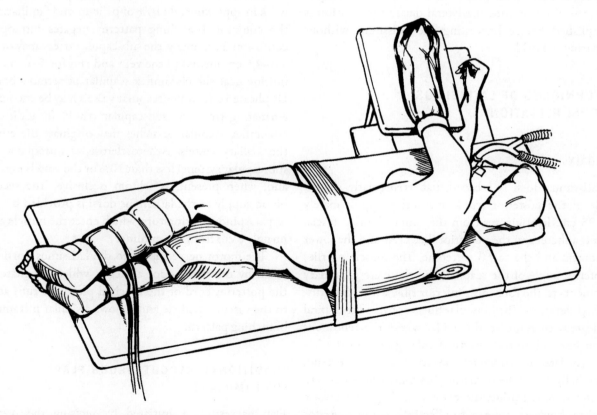

Figure 65.1. Room setup. Patient in lateral decubitus position supported by deflatable bean bag. Arm is draped independently and spinous processes are exposed.

of the operative site. Special equipment requests frequently include a lighted retractor and disposable surgical clips, which tend to decrease surgical time.

Several key issues emerge when repositioning the patient into a supine orientation for flap insetting. Sterility of the operative field is maintained by covering the flap and anterior chest wound with an adhesive, occlusive, polyurethane dressing. The beanbag is removed, and the upper extremities are secured to foam-reinforced armboards with cast padding or soft cotton gauze roll. The shoulders should not be abducted more than 80–85 degrees, since hyperextension can lead to brachial plexopathy. The patient's trochanteric region should lie over the table break, and the ability to adjust the table into the sitting position should be verified before further skin cleansing. Draping the chest with both breasts exposed enables intraoperative comparison for symmetry.

The room setup is significantly altered for immediate, bilateral reconstructions. In this situation, the patient can be placed in the prone position and a two-team approach is used when possible. The mastectomy and reconstruction can also be done simultaneously, with the patient in the lateral position when the general surgery team is agreeable. Alternately, the mastectomy can be undertaken with the patient, widely prepared, in a semidecubitus position. Full rotation into the lateral decubitus position is accomplished before harvesting the latissimus without repreparing the field.

TECHNIQUES OF LATISSIMUS DORSI ELEVATION

ANATOMY

The latissimus dorsi is a broad, flat, triangularly shaped muscle of the posterior trunk, measuring approximately 25 × 35 cm. It originates from the thoracolumbar fascia, which is adherent to the posterior iliac crest and the lower six thoracic and the sacral vertebrae. The muscle overlies the inferior angle of the scapula, and there are secondary attachments to the four most inferior ribs, which can frustrate flap elevation. The muscular fibers converge and spiral 180 degrees en route to the axilla, where the tendinous portion inserts into the intertubercular groove of the humerus. The latissimus dorsi muscle serves to adduct, extend, and medially rotate the humerus. The muscle also serves to draw the scapula toward the chest wall. Regional muscle synergism, however, appears to effectively compensate for the absent latissimus dorsi muscle.

The latissimus dorsi is classified as a type V muscle flap because it contains a dominant pedicle in association with multiple secondary pedicles. The thoracodorsal artery and vein are the principal blood supply to the latissimus dorsi muscle and are terminal branches of the subscapular system (Figure 65.2). The subscapular vessels originate from the third portion of the axillary artery and vein. They run for approximately 5 cm and then divide, forming the circumflex scapular and thoracodorsal vessels. The thoracodorsal vessels course along the posterior axilla and liberate a series (one to three) of branches to the serratus anterior muscle, before penetrating the deep surface of the latissimus dorsi muscle 8.7 cm distal to the origin of the subscapular vessels and 2 cm medial to the muscular border. The thoracodorsal vessels have an average length of 9.2 cm and a mean diameter of 2.7 mm (artery) and 3.4 mm (vein). In approximately 85% of patients, the thoracodorsal artery divides into a transverse and lateral branch after penetrating the muscle. The transverse branch charts a medial course 3.5 cm below the superior border. The lateral branch runs parallel to the lateral border, 2 cm from the free margin. The most frequent intramuscular variation is the absence of the transverse branch, however, the lateral branch is invariably present.

Variability exists within the subscapular, vascular network in approximately 10% of patients and familiarity with the common branching patterns negates intraoperative confusion. Proximally, the subscapular artery may originate 4.0–4.5 cm medial to the vein and run for 5–6 cm before uniting near the circumflex scapular or serratus branches. Duplicated circumflex scapular vessels may be encountered, emanating from the subscapular trunk. In addition, the circumflex scapular branches may originate directly from the axillary vessels. Atherosclerosis is infrequent in the subscapular system (less than 10% of the vessels examined) and, when present, is seldom occlusive. The secondary blood supply to the latissimus dorsi is provided by a series of paraspinous perforators, which enter the muscle approximately 8 cm from the midline.

The motor nerve supply to the latissimus dorsi is provided by the thoracodorsal nerve, which originates from the posterior cord of the brachial plexus. It runs adjacent to the vascular pedicle and follows a similar intramuscular branching pattern.

TRADITIONAL MYOCUTANEOUS FLAP WITH IMPLANT

Flap harvesting is initiated by incising the previously designed skin island. The dissection through the fibrofatty

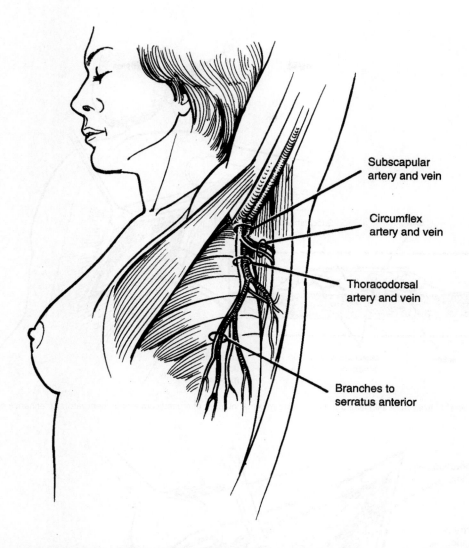

Figure 65.2. Vascular anatomy. Type V muscle flap with principal blood supply provided by thoracodorsal artery and vein. Secondary pedicles originate from paraspinous perforators. Adequate flow can be provided by serratus branch after proximal thoracodorsal vessels are ligated.

tissues of the back is beveled away from the skin island to incorporate the maximal number of musculocutaneous perforators (Figure 65.3). After reaching the muscle, attention is directed to elevating thick skin and subcutaneous tissue from the medial and lateral back. Elevation of the back flaps is carried out in the fibroareolar layer of tissue directly above the muscle fascia. The dissection extends inferiorly and medially until the thoracolumbar fascia is visualized. Flap elevation in the caudal direction is facilitated by using a lighted retractor and cautery extension. The dissection in this region can typically be carried to a point 5 to 7 cm above the posterior iliac spine. Laterally, skin flap elevation is terminated when the free lateral border of the muscle is encountered. The superior extent of the dissection is extended to the inferior angle of the scapula. The dissection can be safely continued toward the axilla as the pedicle runs deep to the muscle.

Elevation of the deep surface is approached by means of the free, lateral border in the middle third of the muscle (Figure 65.4). This zone of relative safety is

bordered between the muscle's secondary origin from the lower four ribs inferiorly and serratus anterior insertion and vascular pedicle superiorly. An avascular plane, bridged by fine areolar tissue, is present in this zone, permitting rapid dissection. Definition of this plane and gentle traction greatly facilitate separation of the latissimus dorsi from the adjacent serratus anterior and confluence of the external oblique, serratus posterior inferior, and latissimus from the inferior four ribs. After freeing the distal two thirds of the lateral border, the inferior origin of the muscle is incised through the thoracodorsal fascia and reflected. The deep dissection progresses expediently in a caudad-to-cephalad direction along the relatively avascular plane.

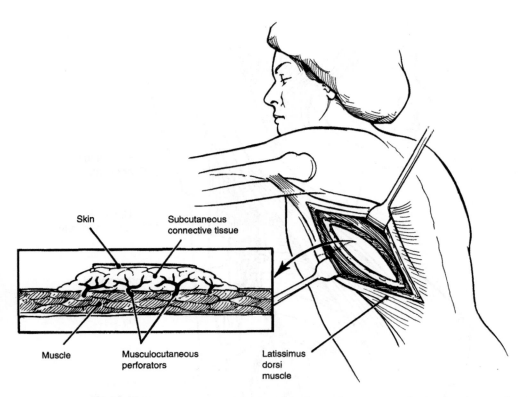

Skin

Subcutaneous
connective tissue

Muscle

Musculocutaneous
perforators

Latissimus
dorsi
muscle

Figure 65.3. Dissection is beveled away from skin island to incorporate maximal number of musculocutaneous perforators to enhance cutaneous perfusion.

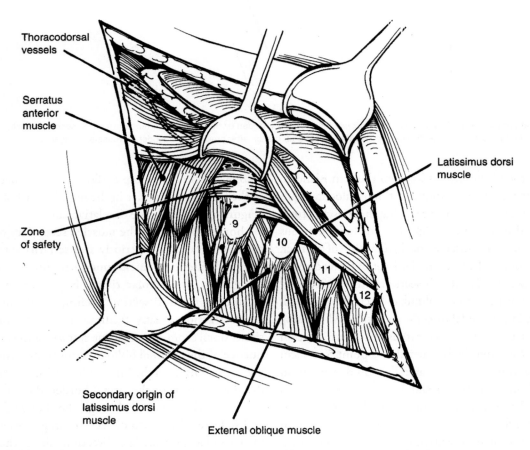

Thoracodorsal
vessels

Serratus
anterior
muscle

Zone
of safety

Latissimus dorsi
muscle

9

10

11

12

Secondary origin of
latissimus dorsi
muscle

External oblique muscle

Figure 65.4. Approaching deep surface from middle third of lateral free border provides easy access to avascular plane.

Large musculocutaneous perforators, which are encountered emanating from the paraspinous and posterior intercostal systems, should be carefully ligated with ties or surgical clips. This is imperative as ligatures dislodged during flap transposition and cauterized vessels are subject to episodes of postoperative hypertension, which can produce extensive bleeding and hematoma formation. As the inferior angle of the scapula is approached, the plane of dissection may become progressively obscured. This ambiguity results from the coalescence of connective tissues from the serratus anterior, teres major, and rhomboideus muscles with the latissimus dorsi (Figure 65.5). To prevent inadvertent elevation of these associated muscles, attention is often better redirected to the superior border of the muscle. The dissection is resumed in the interval between the inferior angle of the scapula and spinous processes, where the tissue plane is more distinct.

With its origins completely divided and the muscle reflected, the dissection is continued toward the axilla.

The thoracodorsal, neurovascular bundle will be identified entering the posterior surface of the muscle approximately 10 cm below the humeral insertion or at the midaxillary point with the arm abducted 90 degrees. The serratus anterior branches are often visualized initially and herald the proximity of the dominant vessels. Scissors dissection with the aid of loupe magnification is now begun to define the vascular anatomy and isolate the thoracodorsal nerve, which can be segmentally excised and ligated (Figure 65.6). A finger can now be passed around the muscle near its insertion to safeguard the underlying pedicle, and the origin of the muscle is divided to enhance the flap's mobility, when required (Figure 65.7).

A subcutaneous tunnel is created high in the axilla, connecting the back and mastectomy wounds, through which the flap is transposed. A high axillary pivot point provides soft-tissue fill and reduces the anterior chest wall hollowing characteristic of mastectomy. The flap is delivered through the tunnel using a gentle pushing action, since pulling

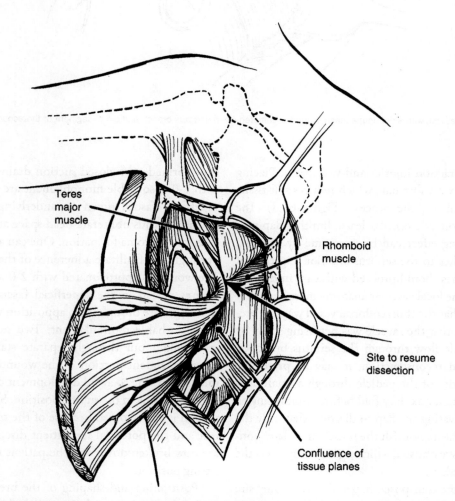

Figure 65.5. Coalescence of tissue planes may develop where latissimus dorsi interfaces with teres major and serratus anterior. Redirecting dissection to superomedial border, between spinous processes and scapula, may aid in re-establishing plane of dissection.

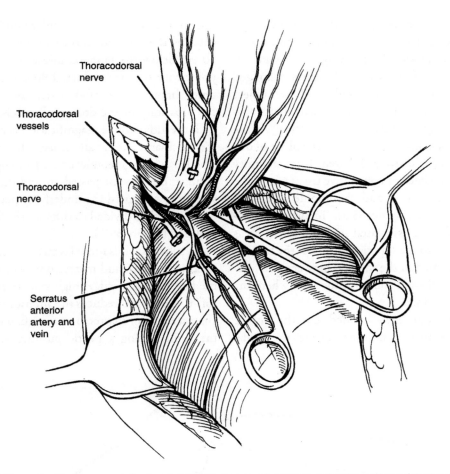

Thoracodorsal
nerve

Thoracodorsal
vessels

Thoracodorsal
nerve

Serratus
anterior
artery and
vein

Figure 65.6. Scissors dissection, with aid of loupe magnification, is initiated when serratus branch and distal segment of thoracodorsal vessels come into view.

tends to produce traction injuries and vasospasm. Placing the flap in a sterile x-ray film bag, which reduces soft tissue resistance, can facilitate the process (Figure 65.8). The pedicle may function as a vascular leash, limiting flap mobility. This tethering effect can be overcome by dividing the vascular branches to the serratus anterior. Ligation of the serratus branches should proceed with care in delayed reconstructions. The local vascular anatomy must be clearly defined to ensure that the thoracodorsal vessel was not previously ligated and that the muscle was perfusing solely by means of retrograde flow through the serratus branches. In cases of delayed reconstruction, it may be preferable to verify the integrity of the pedicle through a small incision along the posterior axillary fold before committing to flap dissection. Elevating the flap to discover that only the paraspinous perforators nourish the muscle mandates conversion to a free tissue transfer, which significantly alters the tempo of the procedure.

At this point, the transposed flap and mastectomy site are covered with a large, transparent, adhesive, polyurethane dressing and a layered closure of the back incision is performed over closed suction drains. Quilting sutures with 2-0 absorbable monofilament are used to secure the superficial fascial down to underlying serratus or teres fascia, and thus obliterate dead space and decrease the incidence of seroma formation. One can also consider use of fibrin glue to facilitate adherence of the two tissue planes. The wound is approximated with 2-0 and 3-0 absorbable sutures placed in the superficial fascia and dermis. The skin edges are brought into apposition with a subcuticular 4-0 absorbable monofilament. Two no. 15 Blake drains are brought out through separate stab incisions at the most dependent portion of the wound and exit near the midaxillary line to avoid development of pressure necrosis while reclining in the supine position. Staple closure of the wound is also avoided because of the pressure necrosis effect and the potential for patient discomfort. The drapes are now broken down and the patient reoriented into the sitting position.

Positioning and shaping of the breast mound is now initiated, drawing on the surgeon's skill and artistry. The breast mound is a composite of the residual skin envelope

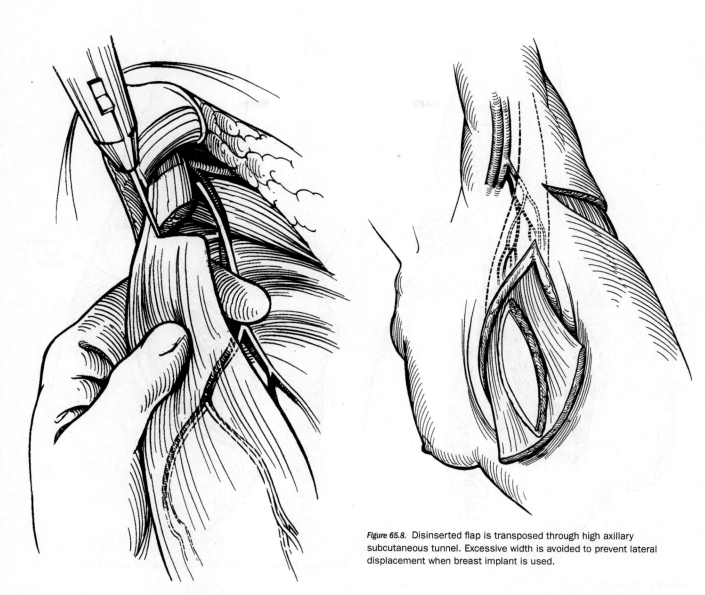

Figure 65.7. Humeral insertion is freed with pedicle protected by interposed digits.

Figure 65.8. Disinserted flap is transposed through high axillary subcutaneous tunnel. Excessive width is avoided to prevent lateral displacement when breast implant is used.

provided by the mastectomy flaps in conjunction with a subpectoral implant and myocutaneous flap. Proper implant selection is rarely described but essential to achieving symmetry and projection. The base of the unoperated breast is measured and an implant of corresponding width is selected. Preoperative sizing of the contralateral breast with prefabricated templates (issued by various manufacturers) aids in selecting the appropriate shape. A wall chart displaying implant widths, volumes, and projection, in conjunction with intraoperative sizers and access to a large inventory, also simplifies the process. Anatomic profile implants may prove beneficial for patients requesting greater upper-pole fullness.

A subpectoral pocket is created and the lateral aspect of the dissection is limited to prevent migration of the implant toward the axilla. An implant sizer is placed in the subpectoral pocket and covered with the latissimus flap, which is temporarily fixed into position with staples (Figure 65.9). The sizer is inflated with saline until the desired volume and projection is achieved. The sizer is now exchanged for a permanent implant of equal volume, and care is taken to ensure complete muscular coverage of the implant (Figure 65.10). It is important to close the lateral aspects of the defect to prevent migration of the latissimus dorsi muscle and implant. Several medial and lateral sutures anchoring the latissimus to the pectoralis major may aid in this regard. Further flexibility can be achieved by substituting an expander implant. The volume of the device can be adjusted postoperatively by means of an adjacent filling port, which is easily removed under local anesthesia in the clinic.

Extensive excision of the pectoralis major may leave insufficient residual muscle to cover an implant. In this

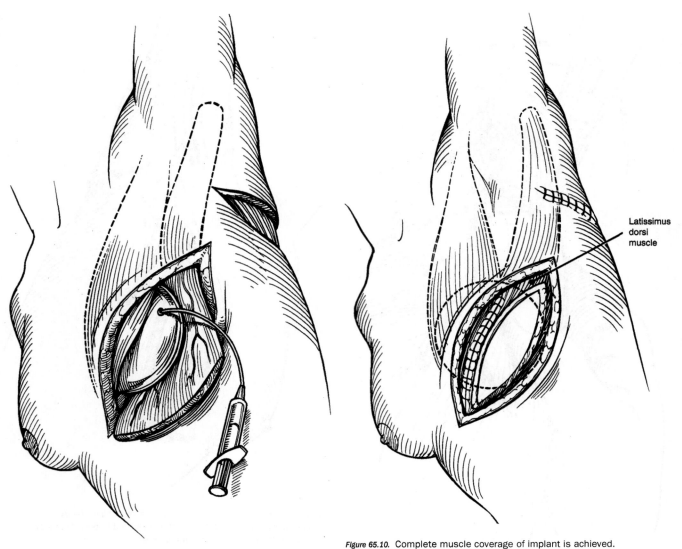

Figure 65.9. Sizer-implant is positioned in subpectoral pocket before temporary staple closure and volume trials.

Figure 65.10. Complete muscle coverage of implant is achieved.

Latissimus
dorsi
muscle

situation, the implant is placed in a subcutaneous position and enshrouded with latissimus muscle.

Careful consideration should be given to the location of the inframammary fold. The most exact result is achieved in immediate reconstruction when the structure has not been violated during the resection. Repositioning is accomplished by suture plication of the mastectomy flap to the fascia of the chest wall or rib periosteum, with the patient in the sitting position if required (Figure 65.11). In delayed reconstruction, using the skin-island in an oblique, inferolateral orientation without regard for the mastectomy incision produces a soft-tissue sling with greater ptosis and a regular, contoured inframammary fold. Frequently, a sizable portion of the re-elevated inferior mastectomy flap is excised and replaced by flap skin. The residual inferior mastectomy flap typically heals well, despite having its random

pattern blood supply traversed by the old mastectomy scar. The fold is marked on the chest wall, and the excess skin is de-epithelialized. If the preoperative markings have become obscured, the position of the fold is determined by measuring its location on the opposite breast with respect to the umbilicus. Suturing the dermis of the flap to the de-epithelialized chest wall skin provides good purchase and produces a well-defined inframammary fold. The implant is completely covered with muscle, and the skin is closed in a layered fashion over a closed suction drain. Alternately, a rim of inferior skin is preserved, abutting the inframammary fold after re-elevating the mastectomy flaps. This tissue cuff provides a site for suture fixation and a limited transition between the flap skin and inframammary fold, which is hidden beneath the inferior pole of the breast. One or two Blake drains are placed through separate stab incisions at the most dependent region of the wound. The

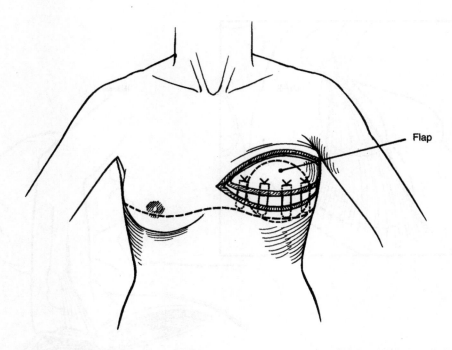

Flap

Figure 65.11. Symmetry of inframammary folds can be achieved with plication sutures (3-0 absorbable monofilament) if mastectomy flap was excessively developed in caudal direction. Defining inframammary fold flap is sutured to de-epithelialized chest wall skin (Ryan technique); cuff of inferior mastectomy flap is preserved to facilitate insetting.

latissimus dorsi's flap position is secured to the chest wall with 3-0 absorbable sutures, and the skin island is inset with 3-0 absorbable sutures in the dermis, followed by a running subcuticular absorbable monofilament.

EXTENDED LATISSIMUS DORSI RECONSTRUCTION

A purely autogenous reconstruction, with volumes ranging from 300 to 400 mL, can be achieved with the latissimus dorsi by extending the quantity of fibrofatty tissue contained within the flap. A general impression of the volume of soft tissue available can be calculated using specified formulas; however, in practice, this may be less useful. Thin skin and subcutaneous back flaps are elevated in a natural plane between the immediate layer of subcutaneous tissue and the deeper more dense fibrofatty tissue. The deep fibrous layer is elevated in continuity with the latissimus muscle and can be extended beyond the borders of the muscle. Skin islands up to 8 × 30 cm can be elevated, and fleur-delis-shaped skin paddles provide large surface areas while facilitating wound approximation. Closure of the incision produces a sizeable T-shaped scar. The remainder of the procedure progresses as described in the section on general technique. Again, closure of the lateral defect is critical to properly shape the breast and to prevent lateral migration of the muscle.

LAPAROSCOPY-ASSISTED LATISSIMUS MUSCLE FLAP

Laparoscopic assistance enables the elevation of a latissimus dorsi muscle flap through the existing mastectomy incision and avoids additional back scars. Using this technique, a pure muscle flap can be mobilized to provide coverage over a breast implant after skin-sparing mastectomy or to furnish a sizeable quantity of functional muscle for reconstructing chest wall abnormalities (Poland's syndrome). The latissimus muscle is approached through a limited posterior-axillary incision. Aided by a C-shaped lighted retractor, approximately half of the dissection can be performed using the conventional technique (Figure 65.12). When direct vision becomes limited, laparoscopic assistance is initiated. An optical trochar is advanced between the latissimus dorsi muscle and fibrofatty tissue to produce a series of adjacent subcutaneous tunnels. A balloon dissector is introduced into the cavities and insufflated. This further separates the skin and subcutaneous tissue from the underlying muscle and creates an optical cavity. Balloon dissection proceeds in a relatively bloodless fashion as the musculocutaneous perforators are spared. These perforators are clipped or divided with cautery scissors under endoscopic guidance (Figure 65.13). These maneuvers are then repeated along the deep surface of the muscle, which is less adherent and yields rapidly to this technique. The muscle is now transposed and inset as described in the conventional technique.

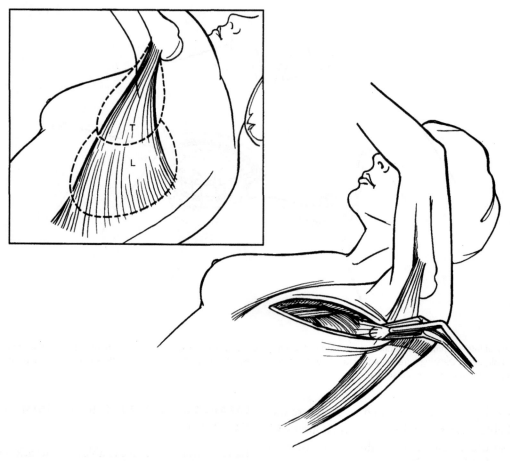

Figure 65.12. Endoscopically assisted muscle harvesting. (L) C-shaped, lighted retractor and endoscopic instrumentation are used after completing initial 40–50% of dissection with traditional technique (T).

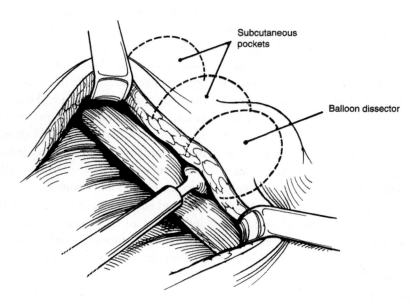

Figure 65.13. Endoscopically assisted muscle harvesting. (A) Subcutaneous tunnels are created with optical trochar. (B) Subcutaneous tunnels are extended into larger caverns, using balloon dissector. (C) Video screen image of residual connective tissue septa and musculocutaneous perforators being divided with endoscopic cautery scissors.

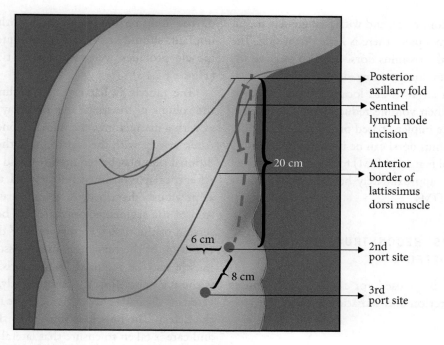

Figure 65.14. Port sites for robotic assisted latissimus dorsi muscle flap harvest.

ROBOT-ASSISTED LATISSIMUS DORSI FLAP

The patient is placed in similar position to traditional flap harvest. An incision approximately 5 cm long is made in the axilla, or an existing sentinel lymph node biopsy or mastectomy incision is used. Dissection using Bovie cautery continues down to the muscle, dissecting the anterior muscle edge free. The neurovascular pedicle is then identified. Dissection continues anteriorly to allow for port placement. Ports are placed through the skin along the anterior border of the muscle at approximately 7 cm, 14 cm, and 21 cm from the posterior axillary fold (Figure 65.14). A 0-degree endoscope is introduced through this port to allow for visualization of the final port, which is located four finger breadths or 8 cm distal to the camera port. The robot is positioned on the dorsal side of the patient and the arms are brought over the patient and parallel to the floor (Figure 65.15). The robot is docked and insufflation is maintained at 10 mm Hg. Marionette sutures are used to suspend the muscle to the skin during dissection of the deep surface of the muscle. These are then released for dissection of the superficial portion of the muscle. The submuscular dissection is performed first because otherwise the dissected muscle would be pushed down against the chest wall secondary to insufflation, which greatly decreases the optic window. The inferior border of the muscle is divided using monopolar scissors, and the muscle is transposed anteriorly. To decrease animation and improve mobility, the

posterior 75% of the humeral insertion is divided. The port sites are then used for drain placement.

In delayed-immediate breast reconstruction, patients receive a tissue expander at the time of mastectomy. If radiation is required, the expander is deflated to optimize external beam delivery, then re-expanded. Often, re-expansion volume is adequate, but the skin is of poor quality for a lasting implant reconstruction. The robotically harvested latissimus dorsi flap is a perfect solution. The muscle protects the thin skin and permits the surgeon to aggressively remove a radiation-induced capsule. There is

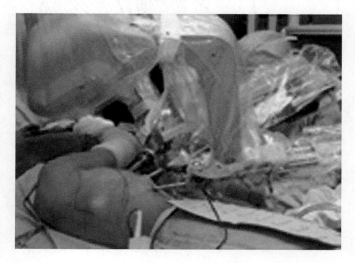

Figure 65.15. Positioning for robotic assisted latissimus dorsi muscle flap harvest.

virtually no visible donor site, and with a single-day hospitalization and minimal pain, there is little down side. The robotically harvested latissimus dorsi can also be used for upper-outer quadrant lumpectomy defects which are either too large or in an awkward location for local tissue rearrangement or when volume reduction is undesirable. Finally, in immediate implant-based breast reconstruction, a muscle-only latissimus dorsi can be used interchangeably with acellular dermal matrix (ADM) for lower-pole or total implant coverage at approximately half the cost of most comparable-sized ADMs.

LATISSIMUS DORSI RECONSTRUCTION OF SEGMENTAL DEFECTS

The latissimus has been used for regional deformities after segmental resection and radiation therapy. Because

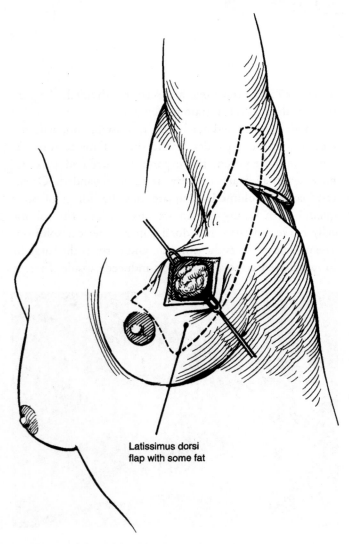

Figure 65.16. Latissimus dorsi muscle flap and subcutaneous island utilized to reconstruct lumpectomy defect.

of the long-term effects of radiotherapy, the use of implants should be avoided. Consequently, the latissimus muscle provides well-vascularized tissue for defect fill (Figure 65.16).

The muscle is harvested as outlined earlier. Because the volume of the tissue required may not be as extensive as with a mastectomy, the muscle alone is frequently used. Alternatively, with the expansion of the breast volume, additional skin may be required to avoid breast flap necrosis. After the flap is outlined and elevated, the muscle is rotated as previously described. A lateral breast incision or extension of the segmentectomy site can be performed for insertion of the tissue. Preservation of the nipple is critical. Elevation of the remaining breast tissue off the pectoralis muscle may be required for the latissimus muscle to lie without a step deformity. Alternatively, the skin can be elevated off the native breast tissue as the muscle is placed into the defect. The muscle is sutured to the remaining tissue, and care is taken to ensure that lateral migration does not occur. A lateral fullness may be present as a result of the rotation of the muscle. The wounds are closed with dermal 3-0 absorbable suture and 4-0 absorbable monofilament for skin approximation.

THORACODORSAL ARTERY PERFORATOR FLAP AND MUSCLE-SPARING LATISSIMUS FLAP

In select patients, such as the young, high-level athletes, or bilateral cases, one may want to avoid the donor site morbidity of harvesting the entire latissimus. A perforator flap based on a consistent vessel that branches from the descending branch of the thoracodorsal artery, approximately 9–14 cm inferior from the posterior axillary line and 2–5 cm medial from the lateral edge of the muscle is a reliable option. The perforator is located using a Doppler device. A skin paddle is then marked overlying the perforator, extending 3 cm anterior to the perforator location. The length of the paddle can extend for 21 cm and the width is determined by the pinch test. The skin paddle can be oriented obliquely or transversely, depending on the patient's skin laxity, but is centered over the muscle (Figure 65.17). An incision is then made around the skin paddle, and dissection using Bovie cautery in a beveled fashion down to the muscle is performed in a similar fashion to the traditional latissimus flap. The fasciocutaneous flap is then raised in a medial to lateral fashion, working expeditiously at the medial aspect and then slowing as one approaches the perforator. If the perforator is less than 0.5 mm, it is advantageous to take a 2 cm cuff of muscle

DRESSINGS

Suitable dressings range from the simple application of antibiotic ointment to fluffed cotton gauze with a loosely applied, circumferential, elastic bandage. Foam tape is intermittently applied in an arching fashion over the upper pole of the reconstructed breast to prevent upward and lateral migration of the implant. Seven to ten days postoperatively, the patient is placed in a cotton sports bra without an underwire.

POSTOPERATIVE CARE

Physical examination provides adequate postoperative evaluation of the latissimus dorsi flap, which is typically robust and well perfused. Patients receive perioperative intravenous antibiotic therapy and are continued on oral antibiotic therapy for 5–7 days. Seroma formation in the posterior thoracic wound is a common complication resulting from premature drain removal. Leaving the posterior drains in place for approximately 2 weeks, or until drainage is less than 30 mL in 24 hours for 2 consecutive days, has significantly reduced the rate of seroma formation. Gentle, active range of motion exercises, including circumduction of the shoulder and finger-walking the shoulder into abduction against a wall, are begun on the third postoperative day.

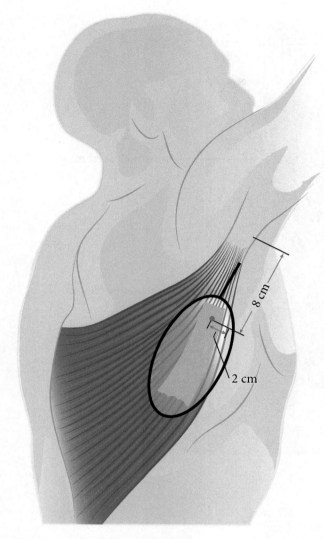

Figure 65.17. Cutaneous landmarks for TAP flap perforator.

CAVEATS

Evaluate the local vascular anatomy preoperatively if the patient has a denervated latissimus, or explore the thoracodorsal pedicle before flap elevation.

Orienting the skin paddle in the oblique or lateral position improves the aesthetics of the back incision.

Skin islands of more than 8 cm in width may prove difficult to close. Evaluate with a pinch test before incising.

An avascular plane exists between the secondary muscle origin from the lower four ribs and the serratus anterior insertion. The deep dissection is facilitated by approaching the muscle in this zone of relative safety.

Paraspinous musculocutaneous perforators must be ligated to guard against postoperative hematoma formation.

Intraoperative sizers are useful to evaluate proper implant size.

Debride contused or compromised edges from the mastectomy flaps before inserting. Designing the skin island

to protect the pedicle. All nondominant perforators are clipped to allow for full rotation of the flap (Figure 65.18). The anterior edge of the muscle can also be released for further mobilization, if needed (Figure 65.19). The skin paddle can be secured down to fascia with braided suture prior to passing the flap into the breast pocket to prevent shearing.

MUSCLE-SPARING

A muscle-sparing technique may also be utilized for those less experienced in dissection of perforators, where a 2 cm strip of lateral muscle is harvested and thus included the descending branch of the thoracodorsal artery. This is, in theory, a safer, more efficient operation with minimal donor site morbidity (Figures 65.20 & 65.21).

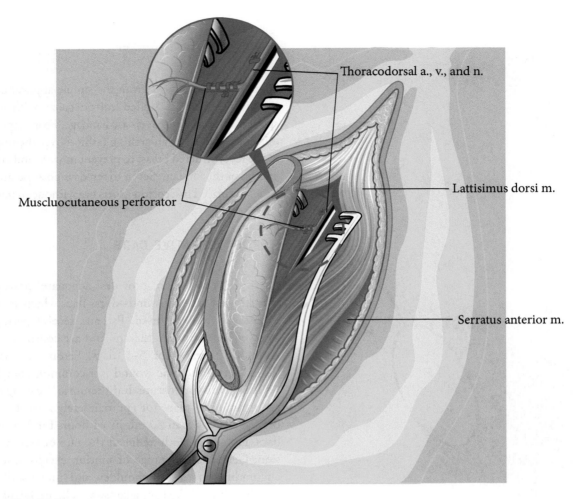

Thoracodorsal a., v., and n.

Lattisimus dorsi m.

Muscluocutaneous perforator

Serratus anterior m.

Figure 65.18. Main TAP flap perforator skeletonized

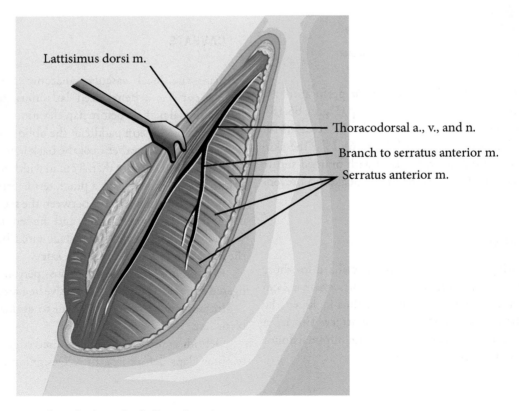

Lattisimus dorsi m.

Thoracodorsal a., v., and n.

Branch to serratus anterior m.

Serratus anterior m.

Figure 65.19. Lateral border of muscle elevated to facilitate dissection.

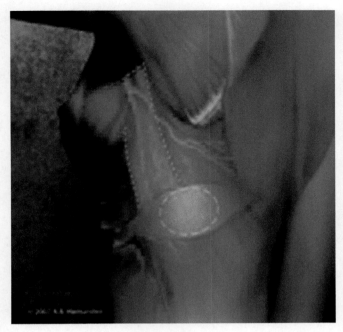

Figure 65.20. Muscle sparing flap design: Lateral border of latissimus dorsi muscle with associated intra-muscular lateral branch of the thoracodorsal artery and skin island.

slightly larger than predicted by a pattern permits this flexibility. If uncertainty persists, indocyanine green angiography can be used to evaluate skin viability.

Delaying the removal of closed suction drains from the back for approximately 14 days, or until the output is less

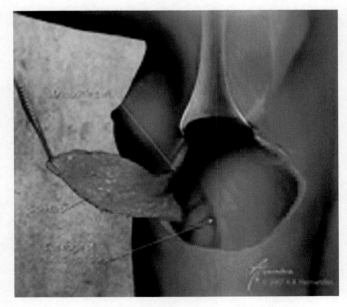

Figure 65.21. Muscle sparing flap elevated on lateral muscular pedicle.

than 30 mL in 24 hours for 2 consecutive days, will greatly reduce seroma formation.

SELECTED READINGS

Bailey S, Oni G, Guevara R, Wong C, Saint-Cyr M. Latissimus dorsi donor-site morbidity: the combination of quilting and fibrin sealant reduce length of drain placement and seroma rate. *Ann Plast Surg* 2012;68: 555–558.

Bartlett SP, May JW, Yaremchuk MJ. The latissimus dorsi muscle: a fresh cadaver study of the primary neurovascular pedicle. *Plast Reconstr Surg* 1981;67:631–636.

Beekman WH, Feitz R, Hage JJ, et al. Life span of silicone gelfilled mammary prostheses. *Plast Reconstr Surg* 1997;100:1723–1726.

Bostwick J III. Partial breast reconstruction using a latissimus dorsi flap. *Perspect Plast Surg* 1996;10:109–111.

Carlson GW, Bostwick J III, Styblo TM, et al. Skin-sparing mastectomy: oncologic and reconstructive considerations. *Ann Surg* 1997;225:570–575.

Chen L, Hartrampf CR, Bennett GK. Successful pregnancies following TRAM flap surgery. *Plast Reconstr Surg* 1993;91:69–71.

Fisher J, Bostwick J III, Powell RW. Latissimus dorsi blood supply after thoracodorsal vessel division: the serratus collateral. *Plast Reconstr Surg* 1983;72:502.

Germann G, Steinau HU. Breast reconstruction with the extended latissimus dorsi flap. *Plast Reconstr Surg* 1996;97:519–526.

Hokin J, Inoue T, Sasake K, et al. Breast reconstruction without an implant: results and complications using an extended latissimus dorsi flap. *Plast Reconstr Surg* 1987;79:58.

Kim JT. Latissimus dorsi perforator flap. *Clin Plast Surg* 2003;30: 403–431.

Kroll S, Schusterman MA, Reece GP, et al. Breast reconstruction with myocutaneous flaps in previously irradiated patients. *Plast Reconstr Surg* 1994;93:460–469.

Kroll S, Schusterman MA, Tadjalli HE. Risk of recurrence after treatment of early breast cancer with skin-sparing mastectomy. *Ann Surg Oncol* 1997;4:193–197.

Laitung JFG, Peck F. Shoulder function following the loss of the latissimus dorsi muscle. *Br J Plast Surg* 1985;38:375.

Lejour M, Alemanno P, De Mey A, et al. Analysis of 56 breast reconstructions using the latissimus dorsi flap. *Ann Chir Plast Esthet* 1985;30:7.

Marshall DR, Anstee EJ, Stapleton MJ. Soft tissue reconstruction of the breast using an extended composite latissimus dorsi myocutaneous flap. *Br J Plast Surg* 1984;37:361.

Masuoka T, Fujikawa M, Yamamoto H, et al. Breast reconstruction after mastectomy without additional scarring: application of endoscopic latissimus dorsi muscle harvest. *Ann Plast Surg* 1998;40:123–127.

Moore TS, Farrell LD. Latissimus dorsi myocutaneous flap for breast reconstruction: long-term results. *Plast Reconstr Surg* 1991; 89:667–672.

Schaverien M, Wong C, Saint-Cyr M. Thoracodorsal artery perforator flap and latissimus dorsi myocutaneous flap—anatomical study of the constant skin paddle perforator locations. *J Plast Reconstr Aesth Surg* 2010;63:2123–2127.

Schwabegger A, Harpf C, Rainer C. Muscle-sparing latissimus dorsi myocutaneous flap with maintenance of muscle innervation, function and aesthetic appearance of the donor site. *Plast Reconstr Surg* 111: 1407, 2003.

Selber J. Robotic latissimus dorsi muscle harvest. *Plast Reconstr Surg* 2011;128, 88e–90e.

Selber J, Baumann D, Holsinger F. Robotic latissimus dorsi muscle harvest: a case series. *Plast Reconstr Surg* 2012;129:1305–1312.

Slavin SA, Love SM, Sandowski N. Reconstruction of the radiated partial mastectomy defect with autogenous tissue. *Plast Reconstr Surg* 1992;90:854–856.

Slavin SA, Schnitt SJ, Duba RB, et al. Skin-sparing mastectomy and immediate reconstruction: oncologic risks and aesthetic results in patients with early-stage breast cancer. *Plast Reconstr Surg* 1998;102:49–62.

Tobin GR, Schusterman BA, Peterson GH, et al. The intramuscular neurovascular anatomy of the latissimus dorsi muscle: the basis for splitting the flap. *Plast Reconstr Surg* 1981;67:637–641.

Wolf LE, Biggs TM. Aesthetic refinements in the use of the latissimus dorsi flap in breast reconstruction. *Plast Reconstr Surg* 1982;69: 788–793.

66.

BREAST RECONSTRUCTION WITH THE TRAM FLAP

Windy A. Olaya

Breast reconstruction with the transverse rectus abdominis myocutaneous (TRAM) flap offers a completely autogenous tissue reconstruction for women requesting either a delayed or immediate breast restoration. The donor site scar on the lower abdomen is hidden by most clothing styles. The success of the reconstruction depends on attention to detail in preserving an adequate blood supply when designing the TRAM skin paddle and during selection of perforators from the rectus muscle to the skin island. The flap can be harvested as a pedicle flap based on the superior epigastric vessels, including one or both rectus muscles, depending on the volume of tissue required.

ASSESSMENT OF THE DEFECT

Breast skin deficit and mound volume needs are assessed before reconstruction. For patients with a healed mastectomy site, the flap provides adequate skin to reconstruct the skin brassiere, as well as fatty tissue for breast volume. For an immediate reconstruction after a skin-sparing or nipple-sparing mastectomy, the TRAM skin is de-epithelialized with the TRAM subcutaneous fat buried under the mastectomy flaps. During immediate reconstruction, both the oncologic and reconstructive surgeons can operate simultaneously, continuously communicating during the surgical procedure about the incisions and mastectomy defect. The match between the tissue volume of the patient's abdominal TRAM flap and her desired breast size determines the eventual aesthetic success of the reconstruction. A thicker pannus for a smaller breast reconstruction often requires a secondary revision for symmetry, while a thin patient with a larger breast may need implant augmentation of the TRAM flap or reduction of the opposite breast.

INDICATIONS

Breast reconstruction is indicated for women who feel that the chest wall defect from a mastectomy that is treated with the use of an external prosthesis restricts their lifestyle or negatively affects their self-image. For these women, who are in good health and who agree to the donor defect and postoperative recovery, a TRAM flap provides an excellent autogenous breast reconstruction. The TRAM flap breast reconstruction is particularly attractive for women with previous radiation to the chest wall who are at an increased risk of developing a capsular contracture with an implant reconstruction.

CONTRAINDICATIONS

Strategically located postoperative scars can interfere with the blood supply of the TRAM flap. The skin paddle available for reconstruction is reduced by scars either vertically or horizontally across the TRAM flap (i.e., lower midline, appendectomy). The significance of these scars depends on the volume of tissue needed for the breast mound. Contraindications to the pedicle TRAM flap include prior ipsilateral subcostal and paramedian incisions, with a chevron incision disrupting both rectus pedicles. Although there are reports of TRAM flaps used after abdominoplasty procedures, such flaps are risky because the perforators to the skin and subcutaneous tissue from the pedicle have been surgically divided. Previous abdominal liposuction may also disrupt major perforators. Breast reconstruction with the TRAM flap is a major abdominal wall operation. Hartrampf has outlined medical conditions he believes are contraindications to a successful TRAM reconstruction, including severe cardiovascular disease, chronic pulmonary disease, uncontrolled hypertension, morbid obesity, and insulin-dependent diabetes. Smoking, moderate obesity, autoimmune disease, and non–insulin-dependent diabetes increase the risk of complications but are not contraindications.

ROOM SETUP

The patient is positioned supine on the operating room table. The table is positioned so that the back can be elevated intraoperatively, with the patient flexing at the hips, to assess symmetry while shaping the breast mounds. The patient's head is securely stabilized by the anesthesia team to prevent neck injury while the patient is upright. The arms are secured with gauze wraps on armboards at about 75–80 degrees out from the table. Care is taken to ensure that the level of the armboards is slightly below the level of the shoulders to prevent stretching of the brachial plexus while the patient is in the sitting position. Because of the large body surface area exposed and the need to maintain the patient's body temperature during the surgical procedure, the room is heated before the patient's arrival and a Bair hugger warmer should be placed on the lower body. Placement of two or more grounding pads for electrocautery allows two surgeons to work simultaneously. Sequential compression devices (SCDs) are recommended during the surgical procedure and postoperatively.

PATIENT MARKINGS

The lower abdominal transverse rectus abdominis is the usual design of the TRAM flap and is centered in the infraumbilical region (Figure 66.1). The mound begins just above the umbilicus and ends in the suprapubic crease. This leaves the least objectionable scar and provides the longest leash for the pedicle TRAM flap.

The arterial perforators can be assessed with a hand-held Doppler and marked. The superior skin margin of the abdominal flap is drawn as a line curving from the upper limit of the umbilicus toward each anterior superior iliac spine and designed around the best arterial perforators. If the upper incision is placed below the umbilicus, then the upper perforators may be missed in the flap. There is better vascularity of the flap the more centered the flap is around the umbilicus. The inferior skin margin of the flap is drawn from the suprapubic crease

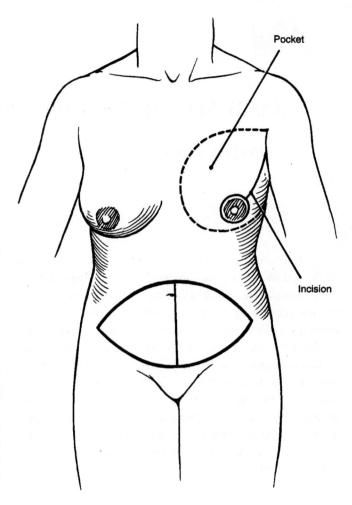

Figure 66.1. Preoperative markings for transverse rectus abdominis myocutaneous (TRAM) abdominal flap and breast pocket.

laterally along the natural skin fold, curving upward to meet the upper line previously drawn. The distance between the two lines is designed to equal the width of the normal breast but is limited by the amount of skin that

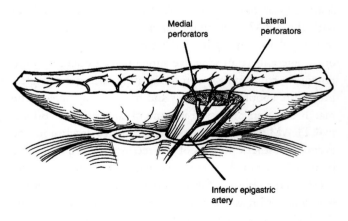

Figure 66.2.

can be closed after flap harvest; sometimes this can only be determined after the patient is under general anesthesia and the abdominal wall is completely relaxed. By varying the position where the superior and inferior lines intersect, the lateral extent of the donor site scar can be placed above or below the anterior iliac spine, depending on patient preference.

OPERATIVE TECHNIQUE

The superior incision is made first and the flap is elevated to the subcostal margin. After the flap has been raised, the upper abdominal flap is advanced toward the planned lower skin incision with the bed slightly flexed to ensure adequate length for closure. Then the inferior portion of the incision is made on the flap. The flap is elevated laterally to the lateral row of perforators on the side of the muscle pedicle. On the opposite side, the perforators are sacrificed and the flap dissection is carried across the midline at the anterior rectus fascial level to the medial perforators of the flap. The fascia is divided laterally just lateral to the perforators, and the inferior epigastric vessels are identified and ligated after preservation of an adequate length for microvascular rescue, if required (Figure 66.3). After dividing the fascia just medial to

the medial row of perforators, it is the surgeon's choice whether to take the full width of muscle for the pedicle or to split the muscle laterally or medially, or both. The goal for each patient is to perform a safe and reliable TRAM flap, while minimizing harm to the integrity of the abdominal wall. Dividing the rectus muscle distally above the arcuate line helps preserve the integrity of the lower abdomen. After elevation of the upper abdominal flap, it is helpful to use transcutaneous Doppler to aid in marking the superior epigastric vessels on the upper abdominal wall. Then, either the fascia can be split off-center to this or a strip of fascia can be preserved over the vascular pedicle. If a muscle-splitting dissection is performed, this dissection is continued to the subcostal margin. A tunnel is created in the medial inframammary fold and onto the xiphoid process to minimize disruption of the important inframammary fold landmark. The single pedicle flap is then usually rotated 90 or 180 degrees into the breast pocket (Figures 66.4 and 66.5). The flap can be designed either as a contralaterally or ipsilaterally based flap.

Abdominal wall closure is facilitated by preserving as much anterior rectus fascia as possible, but not at the expense of jeopardizing flap vascularity. The abdominal wall closure is especially important because the risk of hernia following pedicled TRAM is the highest among

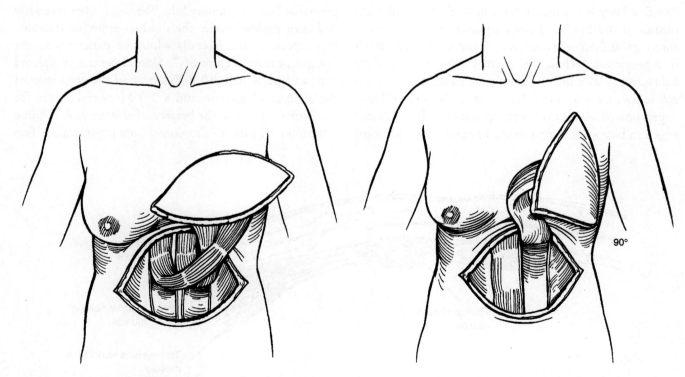

Figure 66.3. Medial and lateral perforating vessels from rectus muscle to skin paddle.

Figure 66.4. Contralateral transverse rectus abdominis myocutaneous (TRAM) flap placement, rotated 180 degrees (double pedicle).

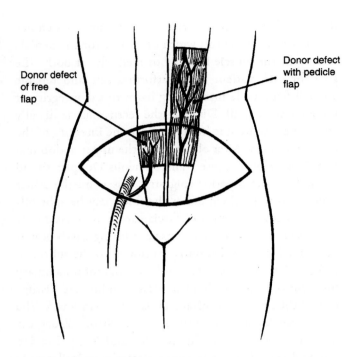

Figure 66.5. Ipsilateral transverse rectus abdominis myocutaneous (TRAM) flap placement, rotated 90 degrees (single pedicle).

abdominally based breast reconstructions. Usually the anterior abdominal wall is closed primarily (Figure 66.6). Occasionally, an interposition piece of mesh is necessary. The fascial defect is closed with a two-layer closure. The first layer is performed with multiple figure-of-eight sutures of 0-0 Ethibond from xiphoid to pubis. Then a running 0-0 Prolene is used as a second layer of closure. It is important to include the internal oblique, particularly below the arcuate line, where it can retract deep and lateral to the external oblique layer. The fascia can be directly approximated, or, if extra laxity is present, the lateral fascial edge can be approximated to the linea alba for additional

strength. If the sutures tear against the fascia, an overlay of Marlex mesh is placed over the lower abdominal closure and is secured with 2-0 Prolene, after the second layer is closed. The second layer of the closure begins at the subcostal margin and continues in a running fashion to the pubis with a 3-0 Prolene suture. In the epigastric and lower suprapubic area, the fascia is imbricated to prevent a bulge in these two areas relative to the new tight lower abdominal wall (Figure 66.7).

When shaping the breast, there is an element of surgeon's preference in positioning the TRAM flap on the chest wall. A pedicled TRAM reconstruction is usually placed ipsilaterally in either a 90-degree counterclockwise or 180-degree clockwise position. The choice depends both on the stress or stretch of the pedicle and the shaping of the breast. A horizontally positioned TRAM flap can be coned inferiorly to increase central projection. For the bilateral breast reconstruction, the TRAM flap is often placed in the ipsilateral breast pocket to prevent compression of a dorsal pedicle. In the immediate reconstruction after a skin-sparing mastectomy, the flap is tacked circumferentially to the chest wall with 3-0 polydioxanone (PDS) sutures and examined for symmetry in an upright position (head of the table is elevated), then trimmed as needed to conform the flap to the mastectomy flaps and breast shape. In the delayed reconstruction, usually the lower mastectomy flap is removed to within 1–2 cm of the premarked inframammary fold. The flap is inset inferiorly and then molded under the residual upper mastectomy flap superiorly and laterally while the patient is in the upright position Figure 66.7. Skin closure is completed with an interrupted 2-0 PDS suture in the deep layer of the abdominal incision and a 3-0 Monocryl suture for the dermal closure of the breast and abdomen. A running 4-0 Monocryl subcuticular skin closure is performed. Two

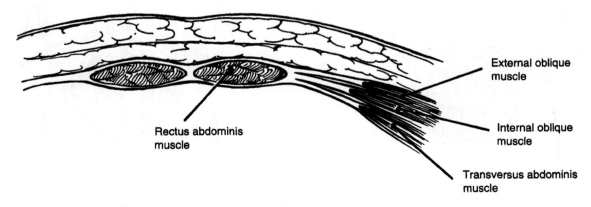

Figure 66.6. Donor defect of abdomen with free flap harvest (L) and single pedicle harvest (R).

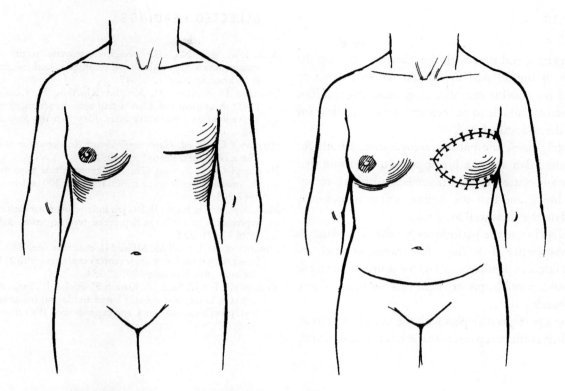

Figure 66.7. Abdominal wall closure. Inset of cross-section of internal oblique and external oblique layers.

drains are placed under the abdominal flap and one drain in each breast.

POSTOPERATIVE CARE

After surgery, the patient is kept well hydrated and in a warm room to discourage vasoconstriction. A nasogastric tube, which was placed intraoperatively, is usually removed at the end of the surgery. The patient's diet is slowly advanced over 3–4 days, beginning with clear liquids on the first postoperative day. On the afternoon of the first postoperative day, the patient is assisted in sitting on the side of the bed or in a chair. Ambulation begins the second postoperative day, and the Foley catheter is removed that day. SCDs are used until ambulation. Excellent pain control is achieved with a patient-controlled analgesic pump, from which the patient is weaned by the third or fourth postoperative day. The patient is discharged on the fourth or fifth day after surgery.

If a pedicle TRAM flap becomes congested on the operating table, the inferior epigastric vessels can be anastomosed to the thoracodorsal system to supercharge the flap. If the congestion occurs in the early postoperative period, within 6–8 hours after surgery, the patient can be taken back to surgery in an attempt to decompress or reposition the flap. If a smaller area of the TRAM flap or the mastectomy flap develops congestion and demarcates in the first 3 or 4 days, the flap can be definitely debrided in surgery before hospital discharge.

A surgical delay can also be used to increase flap viability when perfusion is a concern preoperatively. The inferior epigastric vessels are ligated on the flap side prior to the pedicled TRAM flap reconstruction. The periumbilical perforators on the opposite side of the flap should also be ligated via a periumbilical incision. The pedicled TRAM should be performed 1–2 weeks after the inferior epigastric ligation. Note that if the inferior epigastric vessels are ligated, then there is no ability to supercharge the flap or for a microvascular salvage if the superior epigastric vessels are inadequate.

Drains are removed when output is less than 30 mL each for 24 hours. No special dressings are required. Steri-Strips or antibiotic ointment is placed on the incisions. Either no breast support garment or a loose surgical bra can be used for the chest wall area for the first 1–2 weeks. And abdominal binder is used for 2–3 weeks. Nipple reconstruction is usually delayed for 3 months to allow the edema of the surgical site to resolve and to ensure that the reconstruction is symmetrical before committing to nipple placement.

CAVEATS

Before surgery, spend time with the patient discussing the complexity of the TRAM flap breast reconstruction to prepare her for possible complications, including flap loss, and the need for an adequate recovery period to allow for healing of the abdominal wall.

Accurately mark the patient preoperatively, both for the abdominal flap and the breast pocket, to ensure that the proper amount of TRAM tissue is available to reconstruct the breast and that the reconstruction is optimally positioned on the chest wall for symmetry.

Carefully choose the perforators for the skin island to maintain vascularity of the flap while leaving as much anterior wall fascia as possible to allow for primary closure of the fascia and, possibly, preservation of a continuous strip of rectus muscle.

Develop a postoperative plan with the nursing staff to assist the patient in effective pain control and timely ambulation.

SELECTED READINGS

Buck DW, Fine NA. The pedicled transverse rectus abdominis myocutaneous flap: indications, techniques, and outcomes. *Plast Reconstru Surg* 2009; 124:1047

Erdmann D, Sundin BM, Moquin KJ, Youg H, Georgiade GS. Delay in unipedicled TRAM flap reconstruction of the breast: a review of 76 consecutive cases. *Plast Reconstr Surg* 2002;110: 762–767

Hartrampf CR Jr, ed. *Hartrampf's Breast Reconstruction With Living Tissue.* New York: Raven Press, 1991.

Hartrampf CR Jr, Bennett GK. Autogenous tissue reconstruction in the mastectomy patient: a critical review of 300 patients. *Ann Surg* 1987;205:508.

Marck KW, van der Biezen JJ, Dol JA. Internal mammary artery and vein supercharge in a TRAM flap breast reconstruction. *Microsurgery* 1996;17:371–374

Schusterman MA, Kroll SS, Miller MJ, et al. The free TRAM flap for breast reconstruction: a single center's experience with 211 consecutive cases. *Ann Plast Surg* 1994;32:234.

Shubinets V, Fox JP, Sarik JR, Kovach SJ, Fischer JP. Surgically treated hernia following abdominally based autologous breast reconstruction: prevalence, outcomes, and expenditures. *Plast Reconstru Surg* 2015;137:749

67.

NIPPLE-AREOLA RECONSTRUCTION

Mark W. Clemens and Bradley P. Bengtson

ASSESSMENT OF THE DEFECT

In striving to achieve the best aesthetic and functional results in any reconstructive procedure, a number of factors must be recognized and carefully evaluated. The two most important are (1) the study of the *normal anatomy,* including the meticulously accurate, *three-dimensional evaluation of the defect,* and (2) reconstruction of the defect, keeping the types of tissue and three-dimensional framework in mind. The best or ideal autogenous reconstruction outcome with the least accompanying morbidity is accomplished by replacing exactly the tissue that is taken, to the millimeter, with the same tissue that is resected and accomplishing this with the greatest amount of preservation of normal anatomy at the donor site. Today, reconstruction to this degree is not yet technically possible. With the future advent and use of cultured tissues in conjunction with matrix frameworks, the prefabrication of all types of tissues may bring us closer to optimizing results and minimizing morbidity. The reconstructive surgeon can, however, maximize results by being an avid student of the "normal," or the patient's contralateral, anatomy and choosing a reconstructive method that best matches and replaces all of the tissues that are absent. This is true in all reconstructions, be they mandibular, nasal, or nipple-areolar, all of which should focus on replacing lining, bone, or soft tissues and skin surface when appropriate. Thus, the most successful nipple-areola reconstructions (NARs) include consideration of all structures present: the nipple substance and projection, areola, outer surface, and color.

The final stage in breast reconstruction is the creation of a nipple-areola complex (NAC). Many features, including pigmentation, position, projection, texture, and size, all contribute to this hallmark structure in a well-reconstructed breast.

ANATOMY

To reconstruct any body structure, the surgeon must study the normal anatomic shape and form along with its most common variants. If a unilateral reconstruction is being performed, that "normal anatomy" becomes the patient's contralateral side, unless that structure is to be altered. Many common variations of nipple and areolar tissue have been described. The patient's wishes and concerns also play a major role in the decision making.

Normal nipple position is typically 16–21 cm from the sternal notch or midclavicular line and generally 9–11 cm from the midpoint of the sternum. The distance from the inframammary fold to the mid-nipple position varies greatly based on breast size, but is approximately 8–10 cm with the skin on stretch. Average areolar diameter is 42–45 mm and nipple diameter is 8 mm (range, 5–10 mm) with a projection of 4–6 mm, unstimulated. The areola itself projects from the breast mound a few millimeters and contains a variable number of Montgomery glands. Color varies widely and depends on race and parity and is usually darker and more roughly textured than the surrounding skin. Innervation to the nipple is variable. Most commonly, the anterior and lateral branches of the third through fifth intercostal nerves serve as the source of sensory innervation to the NAC. Ninety-three percent of patients will have nipple sensation arising from the deep branch of the fourth intercostal lateral cutaneous nerve. These branches enter the NAC medially. Hence, in centrally located tumors, a medial peri-areolar incision is discouraged.[1] Blood supply to the NAC is primarily from branches of the internal thoracic artery but augmented by branches from the anterior intercostal and lateral thoracic arteries. In an ideal breast, the horizontal access is determined by transposition of the inframammary fold. This marks the superior margin of the

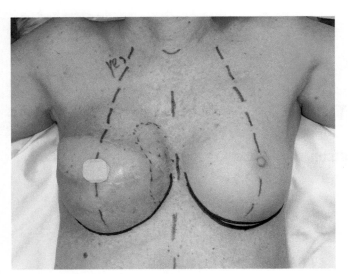

Figure 67.1. The use of a flesh-colored circular Band-Aid to mark the nipple can be tremendously helpful. Not only does it allow the surgeon to approximate the aesthetic result of the nipple-areolar complex (NAC) location, but it also allows the patient to appreciate its proposed location. We recommend placing the Band-Aid a few days prior to surgery so the patient can get accustomed to the positioning and comment on whether it suits her.

new NAC and should also correlate with the point of maximal projection. The vertical access is of greater debate and various methods have been proposed. Regardless of the specific measurements, the unifying concept is that both nipples should be symmetric in relation to fixed anatomic landmarks including the midline, sternal notch, and the mid-clavicular line and at or just above the maximum projection of the breast (Figure 67.1).

INDICATIONS

In previous years, the nipple and areola were either not emphasized or were thought to be unimportant after completion of reconstruction of the breast mound and thus were often not reconstructed. However, as breast reconstructive techniques have dramatically improved and evolved, NAR is being performed much more commonly. This is a reflection of both the level of sophistication of the techniques used and the quality of reconstructions that are being obtained. Most patients and plastic surgeons now do not consider a breast reconstruction complete until the NAR is completed. Patient wishes and insurance reimbursement may be active issues; however, because of the limited amount of surgical time typically involved, quick recovery, and low complication rate, nearly all patients should be offered NAR. The nipple and areola are the focal point of the breast, and reconstruction is indicated in all patients.

CONTRAINDICATIONS

The main contraindication for NAR is active progression of an underlying disease process. In this instance, NAR should certainly be delayed (or not performed) until the patient is in remission. If the flap or tissue used in the breast reconstruction has undergone radiation, this may be considered a relative contraindication to NAR; however, with adequate education and involvement of the patient in the decision process, NAR may be performed if there are minimal skin changes present, usually a minimum of 6–8 weeks after radiation therapy. The final "contraindication" is patient choice, and some patients do not elect to undergo the procedure.

TIMING

Most NAR procedures are best performed after the breast mound reconstruction. We most commonly perform the NAR 6 months after the breast reconstruction, usually in conjunction with any breast mound revision that may be required and 1 month after completion of the patient's chemotherapy, if required. Postoperative changes occur in all breasts, and it is more difficult to attempt to move a NAC once completed than to reconstruct it in the correct location once these changes have occurred. Complications also cannot be predicted with 100% accuracy, and if fat or skin necrosis develops postoperatively, nipple position may be affected. This does not mean immediate nipple reconstruction should never be considered. If a skin-sparing mastectomy is done, the reconstruction chosen is very predictable, and there is nothing being done to surgically alter the contralateral breast, an immediate NAR may be considered (i.e., a latissimus dorsi and implant reconstruction where the breast volume can be very closely matched or a free transverse rectus abdominis myocutaneous [TRAM] flap in conjunction with a skin-sparing mastectomy). As discussed, NAR is not a time-consuming procedure to perform, and, because of its profound effect on the completed breast appearance, we feel it is often best delayed until the final breast volume and contour are stable.

ROOM SETUP

Setup and equipment required for NAR are minimal. Surgery may be performed in an office procedure room, if necessary. We perform the procedure with sterile technique, preparing both of the patient's breasts and squaring off with towels only, versus full and complete draping, unless additional procedures are being performed. Antibiotics are not routinely administered unless there are additional procedures or the patient has an underlying implant.

The anesthetic drug routinely used is lidocaine with epinephrine, and the instruments are a measuring tape, nipple marker, no. 15 blade scalpel, Adson forceps, needle driver, and skin hooks. Bipolar cautery is also available for all cases.

PATIENT MARKING

Along with the choice of the method of reconstruction, the marking and positioning of the NAC is the most critical part of this procedure. Marking of a patient depends on a variety of factors, including (1) unilateral versus bilateral reconstruction; (2) individual patient anatomy of the reconstructed and "normal" breast, if present; (3) patient positioning; and (4) surgeon and patient preference of nipple position.

Ideally, the nipple is located in the exact position as on the normal or contralateral side, or, if the procedure is bilateral, position is based on normal breast dimensions and anatomy, and temporary methods to determine position are very helpful. Figure 67.1. However, this may vary if the breast mounds are not of equal shape or size.

Choosing the proper nipple position is done in the sitting or standing position, often with the patient in front of a full-length mirror, so patient and surgeon can interact and decide on position. A mark is made on the breast in the most ideal location visually from the patient's and surgeon's standpoint, and then confirmed with measurements. In unilateral reconstructions, the nipple and areola may be measured out on the reconstructed side. Electrocardiographic (EKG) stickers also work well to temporarily mark nipple position. Reference marks in the sternal notch, midclavicular line, and midline are chosen and rechecked. Shoulders are checked for symmetry. Any asymmetries, such as sternal angulation or soft tissues from a TRAM pedicle, are taken into consideration in proper positioning of the midline. Three-dimensional imaging with technologies such as Canfield Vectra can be very helpful. After the measurements are made and the nipple and areola are drawn in, the patient is asked for feedback on the positioning. If the general aesthetic position of the nipple and areola does not correspond to the measurements, the measurements should be rechecked. If they still do not correspond (i.e., "it just doesn't look right"), then the breast mounds are not symmetric. In this instance, the surgeon and patient need to decide which should take priority: the numerical measurement or the general look or "gestalt" of the nipple and areola position. This situation, particularly, is seen in skin-sparing–type mastectomies. In general, if there is a discrepancy, the optimal nipple position is the one that looks the most symmetric, regardless of the position indicated by the numerical markings. In bilateral reconstructions, nipple position is first determined by temporary markers, and then position is confirmed by comparing breast measurements. In rare instances, minor variation in nipple position may be altered slightly secondary to an underlying scar, although another type of reconstruction, such as the tab flap, may be chosen if scars may affect tissue viability. Four to six weeks after NAR and complete healing, nipple tattooing is performed.

OPERATIVE TECHNIQUE

One caveat is that when the breast mound is being reconstructed, an additional diameter of 1.0–1.5 cm of tissue is added to the nipple and areolar region in preparation for the tissue required for NAR. This is especially useful in skin-sparing mastectomies in which the nipple and areolar tissue is the only tissue removed at mastectomy. For instance, if the original areolar diameter was 4.0 cm and the biopsy scar was placed directly in the areola, and thus a 5.0-cm skin defect is present, the surgeon may bring in a 6.0–6.5-cm skin paddle. The normal areola also usually projects higher than the breast mound and adding additional tissue helps to reduce flattening or underprojection that may occur with nipple reconstruction.[2] Table 67.1 outlines the options, when considering composite tissue transfer for nipple reconstruction.

Nearly 100 types and variants of NAR, along with a dozen sources for the replacement of nipple tissue, have been described (Table 67.1). These may be categorized into autogenous or alloplastic, or by site as local, regional, or distant. Most commonly, nipple reconstruction with local tissue (i.e., breast skin) or tissue brought in for the original breast mound reconstruction is utilized. Tattooing alone does not provide texture, additional tissue redundancy, or projection of the normal areola, and if an excellent breast mound has been accomplished. The procedure that yields the "best" NAR for each patient's tissue requirements should be entertained There are, however, always tradeoffs of donor site morbidity. Tissue from the lateral breast or abdomen may be used, but it may have insufficient diameter or cause a donor-site deformity. Medial thigh skin just below the thigh crease has been advocated by many surgeons.

TABLE 67.1 **MOST COMMON SOURCES FOR NIPPLE-AREOLA RECONSTRUCTION**

Tissue		Method/Source	Site
Areola	Local	Local skin/tattooing	Local tissue
	Distant	Skin grafts	Contralateral areola
			Dog ear/lateral skin (breast)
			Dog ear/lateral skin (abdomen)
			Proximal thigh
			Medial thigh below skin crease
			Labia
Nipple	Local	Local tissue/breast skin or flap skin	Local tissue
	Distant	Other sites	Contralateral nipple
			Toe pulp
			Ear lobe
			Cartilage
			Dermal fat grafts
	Allograft		
	Alloplast		

The types of NAR described herein will include (1) nipple sharing, (2) the skate flap, and (3) the star flap, the (4) CV flap, and the (5) quadrapod flap. These all have some advantages and disadvantages, and each method is described and presented.

NAC RECONSTRUCTION: TISSUE TRANSFER

NIPPLE-SHARING

Free nipple grafts have withstood the test of time. Proposed as one of the initial composite tissue transfer options, it is the only one still widely in use today. Apprehensions regarding donor nipple sensitivity, projection loss, and donor nipple cosmesis are weighed against the feasibility of a tissue flap in radiated and thinned skin. Most recent studies show that although theoretic donor site morbidity exists, in reality, most are rare and clinically unnoticed. Although nipple sharing can be widely applied, patients in whom a

flap confers a higher risk of complications and/or those with large nipples are optimal candidates.

The technique is described as follows[3]:

1. Using the fixed anatomic structures mentioned earlier, mark the distances to the existing nipple. Then mirror these measurements onto the recipient breast. Do not rely solely on measurement; make sure it appears symmetric when the patient is upright. Err to a medial location as opposed to a lateral one.

2. Place a traction suture on the distal tip of the donor nipple.

3. Mark approximately 50% of the height of the nipple; at least 50% should be left in the donor nipple, so err distal on the nipple.

4. Use a no. 11 blade to incise at the waist of the nipple and make a straight cut across.

5. De-epithelialize the recipient skin.

6. Use an interrupted suture to anchor the nipple in place (some authors recommend suture-less healing to minimize scar[4]).

7. The donor nipple can be closed using a purse-string suture to maximize projection.

8. A nipple protector is placed over the recipient nipple.

An alternative closure method is described in Figure 67.2.

Regardless of technique, global comments can be made with respect to both the donor site and the newly reconstructed nipple. The donor nipple will inevitably be smaller.[10] This makes nipple-sharing more aesthetic in patients with a larger NAC and a less preferred option in patients with a small NAC. The recipient nipple will also be small given that it is but a portion of the donor nipple. Again, this can be appropriate if the donor nipple is redundant and large, but is a clear disadvantage in patients with small nipples. Loss of nipple sensation has also been implicated in donor site morbidity. The most recent studies show that objective measurements of pressure needed to

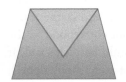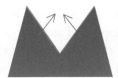

Figure 67.2. The inverted triangle is the excised portion that becomes the new nipple. The donor nipple is then closed by bringing the two peaks together.

induce perception are decreased but are statistically insignificant in human perception.[9,10] Other studies have shown up to 50% of patients with subjective complaints of decreased sensation.[11] Lee et al. proposed harvesting the superior portion of the nipple to maintain the lateral cutaneous nerve of the fourth intercostal intact for sensation.[5] The most significant *long-term* concern is maintaining nipple projection. A loss in nipple projection of up to 32% has been reported. In the same study, they note that although initial postoperative projection may be up to 3 mm greater in the flap subgroup, that projection at 1 year was within 1 mm of the nipple-sharing subgroup. More importantly, patient satisfaction with projection was comparable in *both* subgroups. Figure 67.3 highlights the pre- and

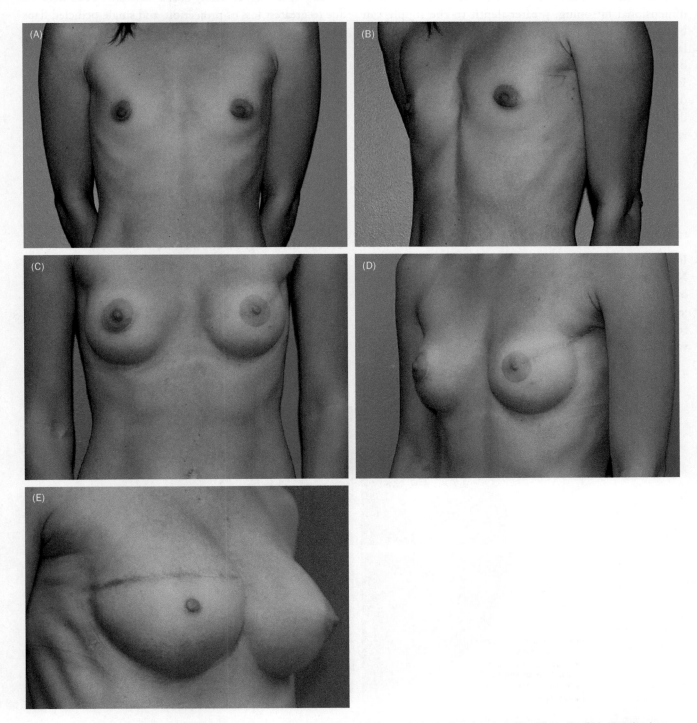

Figure 67.3. (A,B) Preoperative images. (C,D) Postoperative images in a patient status post nipple sharing procedure after 18 months. Note that the donor site is well-healed with minimal scaring. Projection, although decreased from preop, is symmetric postoperatively. (E) A free nipple graft prior to tattooing.

postoperative images of a patient status post nipple-sharing for nipple reconstruction.

Flaps require well-perfused, thick skin flaps; therefore, nipple-sharing is a good option in patients with a tight skin pocket, thin skin flaps, re-do nipple reconstructions, or post radiation.[9] It also allows for immediate reconstruction since the harvest can be done at the same time as the breast reconstruction. With advances in three-dimensional tattooing, greater depth to the nipple can be created, along with color matching of the contralateral areola.[6] Overall, concerns for donor site morbidity have brought flap techniques into the forefront. However, recent literature conveys that the proposed risk of donor site morbidity is minimal in actuality,[7] and the degree of patient satisfaction supports its use in NAC reconstruction.[9-11]

NAC RECONSTRUCTION: TISSUE FLAPS

INTRODUCTION

Innumerable options exist for flap reconstruction of the NAC. These flaps vary based on number of pedicles, degree of tissue dissection and elevation, and overall expected projection. Surgical planning should include special attention to existing scars, tissue integrity, desired projection, and the vascularity to the skin pedicle.[8]

Some principles should be kept in mind when considering any flap reconstruction for the NAC. First, the estimated *long-term* projection should match the contralateral side. Keeping this in mind, expect the long-term nipple projection to be less than what you see at the completion of the case.[12-14] Different flaps lose projection to varying degrees, but no flap can boast 100% projection retention. Broadly speaking, centrally based flaps have been rejected due to greatest loss of projection, and single-pedicled flaps have fallen out of favor due to decreased vascularity when compared to multipedicled flaps.[14] Figure 67.4 reviews which flaps may be appropriate based on patient specific criteria.

SKATE FLAP

A dermal flap with two "wings" was first introduced by Hartrampf[9] and then modified by Little and Spear to become the skate flap.[10] Many modifications have been proposed since, but the original skate flap continues to be an excellent option for nipple reconstruction. The skin defect can then be grafted, which we will discuss later in this section.

The steps in designing the skate flap are as follows:

1. Mark the nipple based on the location of contralateral nipple and its relation to the fixed sternal notch—approximately 1 cm in width.

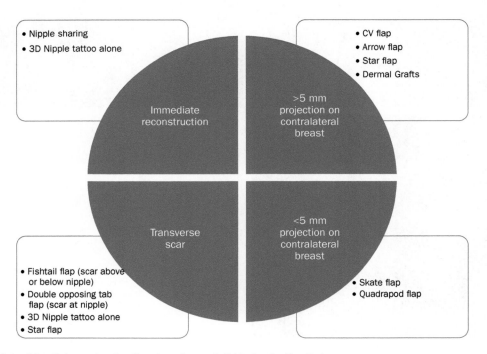

Figure 67.4. Diagram of possible nipple construction flaps based on an individual patient's criteria.

2. Center the areolar marking around the nipple using a 38–42 mm sizer.

3. At the superior edge of the nipple, draw a transverse line.

4. Draw a line perpendicular to the transverse line, extending from each side of the nipple down. Each side inferior to the line will become a flap—approximately 2 cm in length (Figure 67.5A).

5. De-epithelialize the skin above the line (Figure 67.5B).

6. Raise subdermal flaps until the edge is parallel lines (Figure 67.5C).

7. Dissect the central pillar until the drawn nipple *including the deep fat*. This will become the central pillar of the nipple. Approximate the dermis with one interrupted suture in the midline where the central pillar was dissected (Figure 67.5D).

8. Wrap each flap around the raised teardrop perpendicular to the breast.

9. Suture each wing of the flap to the other, down the midline of the nipple, most often with 4-0 absorbable monofilament suture (Figure 67.5E).

10. Close the central pillar by fixating the apical skin of the nipple to the midline of the flaps (Figure 67.5E).

11. Skin graft the residual defect (Figure 67.5F). Figure 67.5G demonstrates 2 weeks postoperative.

The skate flap should be designed to orient the flaps *away* from the scar. The scar should not be included in the flaps since vascularity needs to be optimal. Furthermore, the flap itself can be oriented vertically or transversely, allowing for modification based on the orientation of the scar. Modifications to the skate flap include primary closure of the flap site. This, however, limits the size of the flap wings, which then minimizes projection.[11] Hammond et al. described closure of the skin defect around the nipple using a purse-string suture. This could potentially distort the areola, creating an ovoid shape, as opposed to circular. Both of these modifications also require autologous tissue, which is not always the case.[12] We harvest a full-thickness graft from previous scar, usually in the abdomen, most commonly from the TRAM closure. This allows the scar to be ellipse-shaped (the maximal height of this ellipse becomes the location of the skin graft) and revised. Given the advances and accuracy in tattoo technology, the use of a full-thickness skin graft for the areola is an optimal option with low donor site morbidity and excellent cosmetic outcome. Therefore, modifications to avoid the additional grafting are not worthwhile.

Goal projection of the postoperative nipple height should be *at least* twice that of the contralateral nipple. Authors have debated the degree of postoperative projection loss and when the process settles.[13] Few et al. suggested a 50% decrease in nipple projection in both TRAM and implant reconstruction patients with an average follow-up of 730 days. Zhong et al. reviewed implant reconstruction patients exclusively and report a much greater loss in projection.[19,20] Overall, you can expect at least a 50% decrease in projection within 2 years of reconstruction. Thus, it is key to account for this loss when planning for the initial NAC reconstruction.

CV FLAP

The CV flap is one of the most commonly employed flap techniques for nipple reconstruction. This flap is based on two lateral V flaps extending from a central C flap. The V flaps can be closed primarily and the central C portion becomes the nipple itself. This technique avoids the need for donor site grafting, which is often necessary for the skate flap, as illustrated in Figure 67.6.

As with all nipple reconstruction, the center of the NAC should be marked preoperatively and confirmed with the patient. The base of the nipple is the starting point of the two V flaps. The width of this base will be the diameter of the future nipple and also the diameter of the C drawn across from it. The two V flaps extend from this centered base. The height of the V flap will determine nipple height at the end of the case. As with all of these flap reconstructions, projection loss of approximately 50% can be expected, and therefore initial measurements should be made to accommodate for that loss.[14]

As with the star flap, subdermal flaps are raised, becoming thicker as you move toward the center. A small portion of the base can be mobilized to include subcutaneous fat. This is to allow tension free projection of the reconstructed nipple. Each V flap is rotated toward the C flap, and the C flap is then sutured over the top of the nipple to secure the apex. Again, similarly to the star flap, the remaining incisions are closed primarily. Figure 67.7 shows the elevated C and V flaps, as well as the flap rotation, and the final appearance.

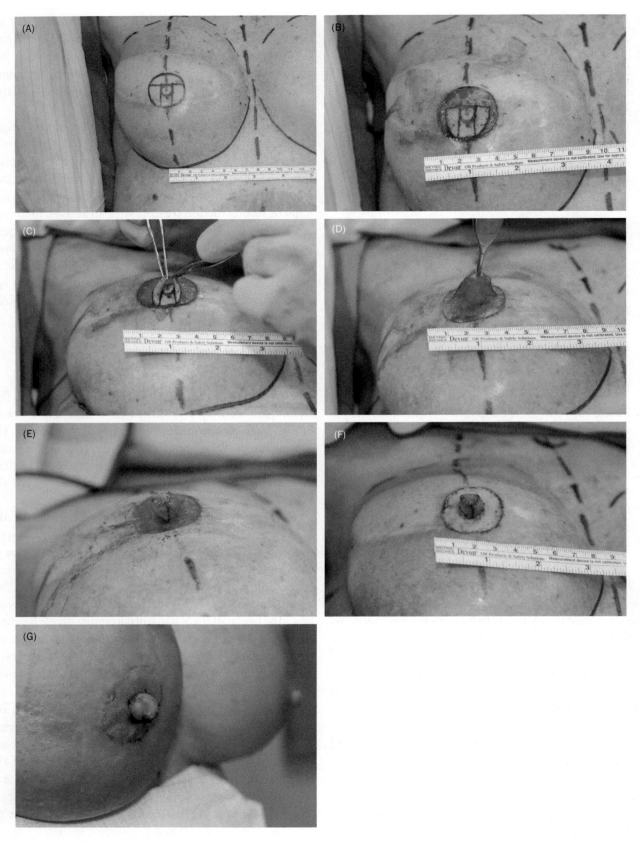

Figure 67.5. Patient example demonstrating step-by-step approach to a skate flap nipple construction. The skate flap is designed at the maximal projection of the breast mound (A) and partially de-epithelialized (B). Subdermal flaps are elevated (C), and a central pillar is raised including the deep fat. The dermis is then approximated in the midline. (D) Medial and lateral wings are then reflected on each other and sutured in place (E), and the central pillar is closed with suture. (E) Finally, the residual defect is skin-grafted (F), and the final result is shown at 2 weeks postoperative (G).

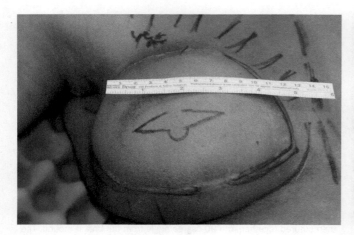

Figure 67.6. Patient illustrates the preoperative markings for a CV flap.

STAR FLAP

A modification of the skate flap, the star flap design is illustrated in Figures 67.8 and 67.9. Many modifications have been proposed, but certain key principles are ubiquitous. The star flap can be oriented in *any* direction, although a superiorly based flap allows for the most natural projection. Second, the flap can in fact be oriented along a scar,[15] expecting sufficient subdermal blood supply,[16] as long as the scar is greater than 6 weeks old.[17]

The design of the flap begins with marking the center of the nipple. The x-axis should measure 150% of the length desired in nipple projection. This accounts for the approximate 50% loss in projection that should stabilize by 2 months postoperatively. The y-axis should measure the desired diameter of the reconstructed nipple.[23]

The skin is incised except for the base. Subdermal flaps are elevated, getting thicker as you move centrally toward the base. The base itself is elevated just enough to allow the nipple to stand erect sans tension. The "wings" should be thick dermal flaps, including subcutaneous fat closer to the center of the star. Both wings are wrapped: the right wing wrapped toward the left, and the left wing wrapped toward the right. One wing will sit toward the base of the nipple and the other will gently overlap and sit above.[23] Deep dermal sutures of a 4-0 absorbable material are used. These flaps can be approximated using 5-0 plain gut suture. The "cap," or the smaller inverted triangle, is then brought over the top and sutured in place. The remaining incisions can then be closed primarily. Long-term nipple projection is relatively well maintained, with projected loss around 50%, similar to the projected loss in the skate flap.[22] It is important to distinguish, however, that the skate flap requires grafting of the donor site whereas with the star flap, the incisions can be closed primarily.

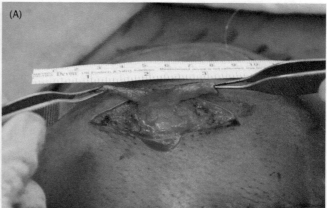

(A)

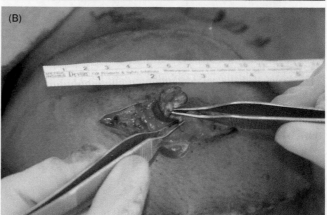

(B)

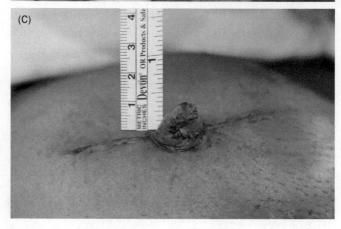

(C)

Figure 67.7. (A) The elevated C and V flaps including dermis and, centrally, subcutaneous fat. (B) Each of the V flaps fold inwards. Note that the height of the V flaps determines the projection. (C) The reconstructed nipple after the C and V flaps are secured in place, and primary closure of the donor sites.

The arrow flap is another modification of the skate flap, constructed similarly to the star flap. Figure 67.9 illustrates the markings for the arrow flap. This flap has similar benefits to the star flap in that the donor site can be closed primarily, and long-term nipple projection is approximately 45%.[18] The arrow flap also has its "wings" raised to include subdermal fat, allowing the flaps to be thicker. It is

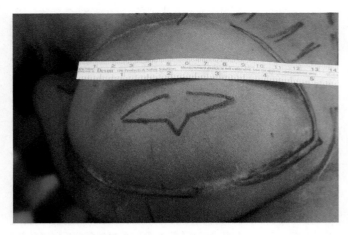

Figure 67.8. Patient illustrates the preoperative markings for a star flap (A).

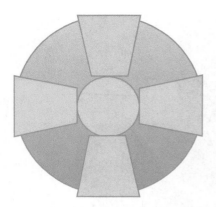

Figure 67.10. The blue portions are excised. The trapezoidal portions are then sutured together, at a 90-degree angle from the breast mound. The new island of tissue surrounding the nipple can then be grafted.

otherwise constructed very similarly to the star flap, with each wing folding laterally and a "cap" to create the apex of the nipple.[19]

QUADRAPOD FLAP

This flap is one of many "pullout flaps." These flaps are prone to loss of projection since scar contracture over time pulls the central mound back toward the breast. These pullout flaps have one vascular pedicle: the central tissue that is to become the nipple and contribute most significantly to projection. Since this tissue cannot be undermined, it is tethered to the underlying dermis and therefore will retract along with scar contracture.[14] (We discuss bipedicled flaps later.) These flaps, in contrast, have laterally based pedicles where the central projection is undermined tissue with no tethering to the subcutaneous tissue below.[9] As such, they can be manipulated to allow for greater projection.

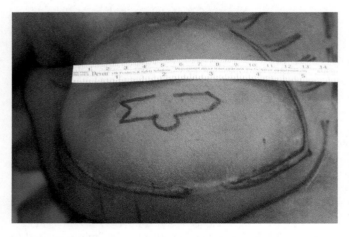

Figure 67.9. Patient illustrates the preoperative markings for the arrow flap.

Little et al. originally described the quadrapod flap with four trapezoidal flaps surrounding a central disk. Refer to Figures 67.10 and 67.11 for a schematic representation. Once the skin between the trapezoids is de-epithelialized, the edges are sutured together, 90 degrees from the breast mound. This creates a projection of the central disk, which is now the nipple. The areola can be grafted either from redundant areola in the contralateral breast or from full-thickness grafts from the upper thigh or posterior ear.[20]

ADJUNCTS FOR NIPPLE PROJECTION

Despite the numerous techniques for nipple reconstruction, no single technique is immune to projection loss. Various adjuncts have been described in augmenting nipple projection. The most commonly employed is a *dermal graft*, which is applied as a strut over which the flap can be secured. This dermal graft can be harvested from numerous locations including the tissue flap itself or excess from the full-thickness graft[21] (Figure 67.11). Other autografts, such as auricular cartilage[22] and costal cartilage,[23] have also been described. Although the techniques are well described and long-term projection is at least that of with a flap alone,[27] no study has shown a statistically significant increase in projection with the use of a dermal graft.

The use of allografts such as AlloDerm (LifeCell Corp., Branchburg, NJ)[24] has also been described. Essentially, a small piece of AlloDerm is rolled with the dermal side facing outward. Its shape is secured using a Vicryl suture. The AlloDerm is then placed in the center of the nipple and the dermal flaps are wrapped around it.[30] Projection at 12 months postoperatively was

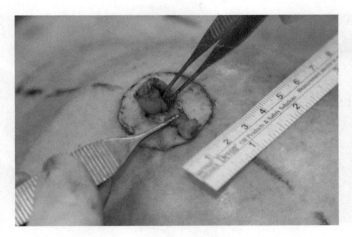

Figure 67.11. Insertion of a dermal graft to improve the projection of a nipple construction.

comparable to projection from other studies without the graft.[21,26,30]

Fat grafting is used to mask tissue loss in multiple forums, including nipple reconstruction. It is susceptible to the same complications, including fat loss over time. Multiple injections can be performed, but failure after multiple attempts should prompt pursuit of another therapy. It is to be noted that patients who do best with fat grafting are ones in whom the skin envelop for the nipple is lax, allowing for increased volume. Patients with tight skin pockets for the nipple will not retain the grafted fat in long-term follow-up.[25]

The use of dermal fillers for postoperative augmentation of nipple projection is useful for numerous reasons. First, multiple injections can be used until desired projection is achieved. Furthermore, dermal fillers can be used regardless of the type of reconstruction. Although

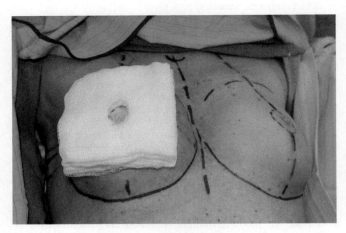

Figure 67.12. Sterile dressings are cut with an opening to protect projection of the nipple. Antibiotic ointment is applied daily for 1–2 weeks until the completion of healing.

a relatively new adjunct in nipple reconstruction, various dermal fillers are available, and subsequent injections can be administered until the desired result is achieved.[26]

Overall, multiple adjuncts are available when a patient's nipple reconstruction has left them dissatisfied with projection. Some are employed at the time of surgery, and some are available for use postoperatively. Each case should be evaluated individually for the cause of failure, and the appropriate adjunct should be matched with the most fitting type of reconstruction.

POSTOPERATIVE CARE

Postoperative care after NAR is straightforward. Sterile dressings are applied for 48 hours, and antibiotic ointment is applied to the nipple area itself (Figure 67.12). Steri-Strips are placed along the donor site regions at the base of the nipple. A cut 10 cc syringe may be used if protection is desired. Healing usually proceeds without complications within 1 week. Patients are allowed to shower, avoiding direct water pressure to the nipple area, 48 hours after surgery. If partial skin loss occurs, which is unusual, antibiotic ointment is applied.

TATTOOING

The use of tattoos as a surgical adjunct in reconstructive surgery has been available for many decades, with the first application in NAC reconstruction described in 1975 by Rees et al.[27] Spear later established intradermal nipple tattooing as not only a viable option, but also possibly the gold standard in achieving color match and the most realistic appearance.[28] Figure 67.13 shows the use of intraoperative tattooing in NAC reconstruction. Four to six weeks after NAR and complete healing, nipple tattooing is performed. A color is chosen by the patient, with some direction concerning the most common colors used by patients for bilateral reconstructions. For unilateral reconstructions, a tattoo pigment is chosen that is slightly darker than the patient's normal areolar color. A no. 14 or 18 Permark needle is then used. The patient is placed on multivitamin supplementation with iron, because the pigment is iron-based and could theoretically be absorbed if the patient is iron-deficient. The patient is also informed that secondary touch-up tattooing is usually required because it is difficult to obtain a completely uniform pigment color at one sitting.

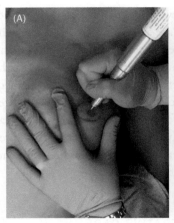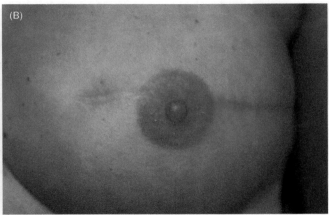

Figure 67.13. By applying shading and shadowing (A), nipple tattooing alone can give a three-dimensional look to the breast mound without actually creating a nipple (B).

Although standard tattooing techniques have achieved satisfactory results, newer techniques employed by professional tattoo artists use three-dimensional tattooing to achieve the most realistic results. Shadowing techniques allow for the optimal appearance of a projected nipple within the surrounding areola. Tattooing of meibomian glands creates a realistic and more natural appearing areola.[13] Tattooing should be considered as adjunct in all nipple reconstruction to optimize the natural appearance of the NAC post reconstruction.

CONCLUSION

The NAC is the epicenter of the breast, and, despite numerous flap techniques all with their own pros and cons, projection and patient satisfaction are the main criteria in judging outcome. The surgeon should appreciate a patient's specific perception of what is natural and desired. One should be familiar with multiple methods and be able to apply each one based on which option is most appropriate. One should also be aware of the adjunctive tools available both at the time of surgery and postoperatively to optimize the natural appearance of the reconstructed NAC.

CAVEATS

Look at the scar location when choosing the type and placement of the nipple reconstruction. Pick the method that best matches the contralateral nipple and areola, depending on tissue characteristics and patient desires, as well as surgeon goals, preferences, and experience.

Bring in additional tissue during the reconstruction of the original breast mound to account for the tissue requirements of the nipple reconstruction.

If you are fortunate enough to have completed a beautiful breast mound reconstruction, do what it takes to make the best nipple and areola possible.

Patients who smoke should be strongly advised to stop prior to this procedure.

Maximize the use of the new technology of nipple tattooing with permanent cosmetics.

NOTES

1 Tamer, M. (2012). *Principles and techniques in oncoplastic breast cancer surgery* (p. 10). Singapore: World Scientific Publ.
2 Nahabedian, M. (2009). Nipple-Areola Reconstruction. In Nahabedian, M (ed.) *Cosmetic and reconstructive breast surgery* (p. 208). Edinburgh: Saunders.
3 Spear, S.L. Schaffner, A.D. Jespersen, M.R. Goldstein, J.A. Donor-site morbidity and patient satisfaction using a composite nipple graft for unilateral nipple reconstruction in the radiated and nonradiated breast. *Plast Reconstr Surg.* 2011;127:1437–1446.
4 [11] Haslik, W. (2014). Objective and subjective evaluation of donor-site morbidity after nipple sharing for nipple areola reconstruction. *Journal of Plastic, Reconstructive & Aesthetic Surgery, 68*(2), 168–174.
5 Lee, T., Noh, H., Kim, E., & Eom, J. (2012). Reducing Donor Site Morbidity When Reconstructing the Nipple Using a Composite Nipple Graft. *Archives of Plastic Surgery, 39*(4), 384–389.
6 Halvorson, E. (2014). Three-Dimensional Nipple Tattooing: A New Technique with Superior Results. *Plastic and Reconstructive Surgery, 133*(5), 1073–1075.
7 Zenn MR, Garofalo JA. Unilateral nipple reconstruction with nipple sharing: Time for a second look. *Plast Reconstr Surg.* 2009;123:1648–1653.22.
8 Shestak, K. (2006). Revision of Nipple Areola Reconstruction. In *Reoparative Plastic Surgery of the Breast* (pp. 455–468). Philadelphia: Lippincott Williams and Wilkins.
9 Hartrampf, C. A Dermal-Fat Flap for Nipple Reconstruction. *Plastic and Reconstructive Surgery* 1984; 73(6), 982–986.

10 Little JW. Nipple-areolar reconstruction. *Clin Plast Surg* 1984; 11:351–364

11 Bogue, D., Mungara, A., Thompson, M., & Cederna, P. (2003). Modified Technique for Nipple-Areolar Reconstruction: A Case Series. *Plastic and Reconstructive Surgery, 112*(5), 1274–1278.

12 Zhong, T., Antony, A., & Cordeiro, P. (2009). Surgical Outcomes and Nipple Projection Using the Modified Skate Flap for Nipple-Areolar Reconstruction in a Series of 422 Implant Reconstructions. *Annals of Plastic Surgery, 62*(5), 591–595.

13 Few, J. (1999). Long-term predictacble nipple projection following reconstruction. Plastic and Reconstructive Surgery, 104 (5), 1221–1324.

14 Losken, A., Mackay, G., & Bostwick, J. (2001). Nipple Reconstruction Using the C-V Flap Technique: A Long-Term Evaluation. *Plastic and Reconstructive Surgery, 108*(2), 361–369.

15 Gurunluoglu, R., Shafighi, M., Williams, S., & Kimm, G. (2012). Incorporation of a Preexisting Scar in the Star-Flap Technique for Nipple Reconstruction. *Annals of Plastic Surgery, 68*(1), 17–21.

16 Shestak, K., Gabriel, A., Landecker, A., Peters, S., Shestak, A., & Kim, J. (2002). Assessment of Long-Term Nipple Projection: A Comparison of Three Techniques. *Plastic and Reconstructive Surgery, 110*(3), 780–786.

17 Eskenazi, L. (1993). A One-Stage Nipple Reconstruction with the "Modified Star" Flap and Immediate Tattoo. *Plastic and Reconstructive Surgery, 92*(4), 671–680.

18 Rubino, C., Dessy, L., & Posadinu, A. (2003). A modified technique for nipple reconstruction: The "arrow flap". *British Journal of Plastic Surgery, 53*, 247–251.

19 Farace, F., Bulla, A., Puddu, A., & Rubino, C. (2010). The arrow flap for nipple reconstruction: Long term results. *Journal of Plastic, Reconstructive & Aesthetic Surgery*, (63), E756-E757.

20 Little, J. One-Stage Reconstruction of a Projecting Nipple: The Quadrapod Flap. *Plastic and Reconstructive Surgery* 1983; *71*(1), 126–33.

21 Eo, S., Kim, S., & Lio, A. (2007). Nipple Reconstruction With C-V Flap Using Dermofat Graft. *Annals of Plastic Surgery, 58*(2), 137–140.

22 Tanabe, H., Tai, Y., Kiyokawa, K., & Yamauchi, T. (1997). Nipple-Areola Reconstruction with a Dermal-Fat Flap and Rolled Auricular Cartilage. *Plastic & Reconstructive Surgery, 100*(2), 431–438.

23 Cheng, M., Rodriguez, E., Smartt, J., & Cardenas-Mejia, A. (2007). Nipple Reconstruction Using the Modified Top Hat Flap With Banked Costal Cartilage Graft. *Annals of Plastic Surgery, 59*(6), 621–628.

24 Garramone, C., & Lam, B. (2007). Use of AlloDerm in Primary Nipple Reconstruction to Improve Long-Term Nipple Projection. *Plastic and Reconstructive Surgery, 119*(6), 1663–1668.

25 Bernard, R., & Beran, S. (2003). Autologous Fat Graft in Nipple Reconstruction. *Plastic and Reconstructive Surgery, 112*(4), 964–968.

26 Garramone, C., & Lam, B. (2007). Use of AlloDerm in Primary Nipple Reconstruction to Improve Long-Term Nipple Projection. *Plastic and Reconstructive Surgery, 119*(6), 1663–1668.

27 Rees, T. (1975). Reconstruction of the breast areola by intradermal tattooing and transfer. Case report. *Plastic and Reconstructive Surgery, 55*(5), 620–621.

28 Spear, S., & Arias, J. (1995). Long-Term Experience with Nipple-Areola Tattooing. *Annals of Plastic Surgery, 35*(3), 232–236.

REFERENCES

1. Tamer M. *Principles and Techniques in Oncoplastic Breast Cancer Surgery.* Singapore: World Scientific, 2012:10.

2. Nahabedian M. Nipple-areola reconstruction. In: *Cosmetic and Reconstructive Breast Surgery.* Edinburgh: Saunders, 2009:208.

3. Spear, SL Schaffner, AD Jespersen, MR Goldstein, JA. Donor-site morbidity and patient satisfaction using a composite nipple graft for unilateral nipple reconstruction in the radiated and nonradiated breast. *Plast Reconstr Surg.* 2011;127:1437–1446.

4. Haslik W. Objective and subjective evaluation of donor-site morbidity after nipple sharing for nipple areola reconstruction. *J Plast Reconstr Aesthet Surg* 2014;68(2):168–174.

5. Lee T, Noh H, Kim E, Eom J. Reducing donor site morbidity when reconstructing the nipple using a composite nipple graft. *Arch Plast Surg* 2012;39(4):384–384.

6. Halvorson E. Three-dimensional nipple tattooing: a new technique with superior results. *Plast Reconstr Surg* 133(5):1073–1075.

7. Zenn MR, Garofalo JA. Unilateral nipple reconstruction with nipple sharing: Time for a second look. *Plast Reconstr Surg.* 2009;123:1648–1653.

8. Shestak K. Revision of nipple areola reconstruction. In Nahabedian, M (ed.) *Reoparative Plastic Surgery of the Breast.* Philadelphia: Lippincott Williams and Wilkins, 2006:455–468.

9. Hartrampf C. A dermal-fat flap for nipple reconstruction. *Plast Reconstr Surg* 1984;73(6):982–986.

10. Little JW. Nipple-areolar reconstruction. *Clin Plast Surg* 1984;11: 351–364

11. Bogue D, Mungara A, Thompson M, Cederna P. Modified technique for nipple-areolar reconstruction: a case series. *Plast Reconstr Surg* 2003;112(5):1274–1278.

12. Zhong T, Antony A, Cordeiro P. Surgical outcomes and nipple projection using the modified skate flap for nipple-areolar reconstruction in a series of 422 implant reconstructions. *Ann Plast Surg* 2009;62(5):591–595.

13. Few J. Long-term predictacble nipple projection following reconstruction. Plast Reconstr Surg 1999;104(5):1221–1324.

14. Losken A, Mackay G, Bostwick J. Nipple reconstruction using the C-V flap technique: a long-term evaluation. *Plast Reconstr Surg* 2001;108(2):361–369.

15. Gurunluoglu R, Shafighi M, Williams S, Kimm G. Incorporation of a preexisting scar in the star-flap technique for nipple reconstruction. *Ann Plast Surg* 2012;68(1):17–21.

16. Shestak K, Gabriel A, Landecker A, Peters S, Shestak A, Kim J. Assessment of long-term nipple projection: a comparison of three techniques. *Plast Reconstr Surg* 2002;110(3):780–786.

17. Eskenazi L. A one-stage nipple reconstruction with the "modified star" flap and immediate tattoo. *Plast Reconstr Surg* 1993;92(4): 671–680.

18. Rubino C, Dessy L, Posadinu A. A modified technique for nipple reconstruction: the "arrow flap." *Br J Plast Surg* 2003;53: 247–251.

19. Farace F, Bulla A, Puddu A, Rubino C. The arrow flap for nipple reconstruction: Long term results. *J Plast Reconstr Aesthet Surg* 2010;63:E756–E757.

20. Little J. One-stage reconstruction of a projecting nipple: the quadrapod flap. *Plast Reconstr Surg* 1983;71(1):126–33.

21. Eo S, Kim S, Lio A. Nipple reconstruction with C-V flap using dermofat graft. *Ann Plast Surg* 2007;58(2):137–140.

22. Tanabe H, Tai Y, Kiyokawa K, Yamauchi T. Nipple-areola reconstruction with a dermal-fat flap and rolled auricular cartilage. *Plast Reconstr Surg* 1997;100(2):431–438.

23. Cheng M, Rodriguez E, Smartt J, Cardenas-Mejia A. Nipple reconstruction using the modified top hat flap with banked costal cartilage graft. *Ann Plast Surg* 2007;59(6):621–628.

24. Garramone C, Lam B. Use of AlloDerm in primary nipple reconstruction to improve long-term nipple projection. *Plast Reconstr Surg* 2007;119(6):1663–1668.

25. Bernard R, Beran S. Autologous fat graft in nipple reconstruction. *Plast Reconstr Surg* 2003;112(4):964–968.

26. Garramone C, Lam B. Use of AlloDerm in primary nipple reconstruction to improve long-term nipple projection. *Plast Reconstr Surg* 2007;119(6):1663–1668.

27. Rees T. Reconstruction of the breast areola by intradermal tattooing and transfer. Case report. *Plast Reconstr Surg* 1975;55(5):620–621.

28. Spear S, Arias J. Long-term experience with nipple-areola tattooing. *Ann Plast Surg* 1995;35(3):232–236.

SELECTED READINGS

Anton MA, Eskenazi LB, Hartrampt CR Jr. Nipple reconstruction with local flaps: star and wrap flaps. *Perspect Plast Surg* 1991;5:67–78.

Becker H. The use of intradermal tattoo to enhance the final result of nipple-areola reconstruction. *Plast Reconstr Surg* 1986;77:673.

Bostwick J. *Plastic and Reconstructive Breast Surgery*. St. Louis: Quality Medical, 1990.

Grotting JC, ed. *Reoperative Aesthetic and Reconstructive Plastic Surgery*. St. Louis: Quality Medical, 1995:1136–1143.

Hartrampf CR, Culbertson JH. A dermal-fat flap for nipple reconstruction. *Plast Reconstr Surg* 1984;73:982.

Kroll S, Hamilton S. Nipple reconstruction with the double-opposing tab flap. *Plast Reconstr Surg* 1989;84:520.

Kroll S. Nipple reconstruction with the double-opposing tab flap. *Plast Reconstr Surg* 1999;104:511.

Little JW. Nipple-areolar reconstruction. In: Habal MB, et al., eds. *Advances in Plastic and Reconstructive Surgery*, Vol 3. Chicago: Mosby-Year Book, 1987:43.

Little JW. Nipple-areola reconstruction. *Clin Plast Surg* 1984:11:351.

Penn J. Breast reduction. *Br J Plast Surg* 1978;7:357.

Ramirez MA. Normal size and shape of the breast and elaboration of a natural pattern. *Aesth Plast Surg* 1978;2:383.

Rees TD. Reconstruction of the breast areola by intradermal tattooing and transfer: case report. *Plast Reconstr Surg* 1975;55:620.

Spear SL, Convit R, Little JW. Intradermal tattoo as an adjunct to nipple areola reconstruction. *Plast Reconstr Surg* 1989;83:907.

68

GYNECOMASTIA

Jonathan T. Unkart, Ahmed Suliman, and Anne M. Wallace

INTRODUCTION

Gynecomastia is defined as enlargement of the male breast caused by the development and proliferation of female breast tissue. The etiology relates to an increased estrogen-to-androgen ratio. The proliferation itself is benign and, as such, is often underestimated. However, a myriad of pathologic conditions and agents may give rise to gynecomastia, and it is necessary for anyone treating this process to have a full understanding of its pathogenesis.

ASSESSMENT OF THE DEFECT

The incidence of gynecomastia is trimodal, occurring in infancy, adolescence, and middle-age.[1,2] However, male breast proliferation can occur at any time when an imbalance deviates from the patient's normal androgen-to-estrogen ratio. This may result from increased estrogen, decreased androgen, receptor defects, or an altered sensitivity of the breast to estrogen. Therefore, when gynecomastia is encountered, a systematic analysis of the possible pathogenesis should be considered. Some of the more common drugs, tumors, and conditions associated with gynecomastia are presented in Table 68.1.

DIAGNOSIS

The diagnosis and cause of new-onset gynecomastia must be made only after careful evaluation of the affected patient. It should not be assumed that the breast proliferation is idiopathic and benign. A comprehensive history and physical exam are required.

HISTORY AND PHYSICAL EXAM

Typically, gynecomastia presents as a bilateral asymmetric breast enlargement with a disc-like mass below the nipple.[3] Gynecomastia occurs in two phases. The initial florid phase is defined by stromal and glandular tissue hypertrophy in the breast. The second phase is the fibrous phase. This stage is characterized by the replacement of adipose tissue by dense collagenous tissue present between the ducts.[4] While often asymptomatic, patients may complain of tenderness. Careful attention should be paid to signs and symptoms related to (1) liver dysfunction and cirrhosis[5]; (2) testicular insufficiency suggested by impotence/decreased libido, with testicular exam for size and masses and evaluation of secondary sexual characteristics[6,7]; (3) abdominal exam for abnormal masses; and (4) extensive medication review including prescribed drugs as well as recreational drugs (i.e., marijuana and alcohol). It is essential to exclude neoplasia.[8]

A proper breast exam is critical. With the patient supine, the breast is held between two fingers on either side of the nipple. Gently, the fingers are brought together while the examiner feels for a disk of tissue below the nipple-areola complex (NAC). Gynecomastia must be distinguished from pseudogynecomastia and breast cancer. With pseudogynecomastia, the breast has enlarged due to increased fat deposition as opposed to increased glandular tissue. The examiner can distinguish the two by comparing the tissue palpated at the enlarged breast with the subcutaneous fat present in the axillary fold. With pseudogynecomastia, patients are often obese with enlarged and nontender breasts. Breast cancer, on exam, typically has more discrete borders and is, typically, harder than gynecomastia.

The age of the patient dictates the clinical workup. In the mid to late puberty patient without any other abnormalities, gynecomastia usually resolves within 6 months. The patient

TABLE 68.1 PATHOLOGIC CAUSES OF GYNECOMASTIA

Drugs

Hormones: estrogens, gonadotropins, aromatizable androgens, antiandrogens (cyproterone), flutamide, growth hormones

Chemotherapeutic agents: alkylating agents

Antibiotics/antituberculous agents: isoniazid, ketoconazole, metronidazole, minocycline

Cardiovascular agents: calcium channel blockers, angiotensin converting enzyme (ACE) inhibitors (captopril, enalapril), antihypertensives (methyldopa, reserpine, Aldomet), digitalis, amiodarone, spironolactone

Antiulcer agents: cimetidine, omeprazole, ranitidine

Central nervous system agents: diazepam, tricyclic antidepressants, phenytoin, diethylpropion, haloperidol

Drugs of abuse: alcohol, marijuana, heroin, methadone, amphetamines, anabolic steroids

Other: auranofin, clomiphene, etretinate, penicillamine, sulindac, theophylline, methotrexate, vitamin E

Neoplasms

Tumors of steroid-producing cells

a. Testicular: germ cell, Leydig cell, Sertoli cell

b. Adrenal: hyperplasia, carcinoma, or adenoma

Tumors with paraneoplastic production of human chorionic gonadotropin

a. Giant cell carcinoma of the lung

b. Pancreatic cancer

c. Gastric cancer

d. Transitional cell carcinoma of the bladder

Other Urologic Disorders

Primary or secondary hypogonadism

Androgen-insensitivity syndromes

Chromosomal abnormalities (Klinefelter's)

Enzymatic testicular defect

Hermaphroditism

Other Associated Medical Conditions

Cirrhosis of the liver

Hyperthyroidism

Renal failure

Malnutrition

Idiopathic

Source: From References 6, 7, 30–51.

can be reassured and seen at 6 months for follow-up. However, if the testes are small and firm and the penile and scrotal development are abnormal, a karyotype should be performed.

In the adult population, one should evaluate for hepatic, renal, and thyroid function. If these are normal, the patient should return in 6 months for re-evaluation. If symptoms remain unchanged, then one should initiate an endocrine workup. This workup up consists of evaluating levels of human chorionic gonadotropin (HCG), testosterone, estradiol, luteinizing hormone (LH), and follicle stimulating hormone (FSH). Low testosterone levels may signal primary or secondary hypogonadism and will be differentiated by high or low levels of LH and FSH, respectively. Elevated estradiol or HCG levels warrant testicular ultrasound imaging. If no testicular lesion is seen, computed tomographic (CT) scanning of the chest and abdomen should be ordered to rule out adrenal mass or an extragonadal germ cell tumor. If all these values are found to be normal, testicular ultrasound should still be considered. The sign of gynecomastia may be the only hint of an underlying testicular tumor.

DIFFERENTIATION FROM MALE BREAST CANCER

Male breast cancer is an important consideration when evaluating a patient for gynecomastia. Although rare, conditions associated with an increased risk of male breast cancer include (1) testicular abnormalities, such as undescended testis and orchitis; (2) family history of female breast cancer; (3) previous chest wall radiation; and (4) Klinefelter's syndrome.[9–15] All solid and complex cystic masses warrant biopsy. Tissue samples may initially be attempted with fine needle aspiration (FNA).[16] If inadequate tissue is obtained, a core needle biopsy or open biopsy will be required.

ROLE OF RADIOLOGY

Controversy exists as to whether all men with diffuse breast enlargement or those with a palpable central mass need to under mammography. Three mammographic patterns of gynecomastia have been observed: glandular, dendritic, and nodular. On ultrasound, gynecomastia is seen as a diffuse or focal process. Regardless of imaging findings, gynecomastia may be diagnosed on clinical exam on the basis of patient's symptoms.[17,18] Mammography may be of benefit only to guide percutaneous biopsy of a suspicious mass.

TREATMENT OF GYNECOMASTIA

The treatment of gynecomastia can be divided into medical and surgical approaches. The simplest treatment is often removal of all agents that may be causing gynecomastia or treating the disease process leading to its development. For those cases occurring during puberty, spontaneous regression is the norm.

MEDICAL TREATMENT

Once breast cancer has been ruled out and the possible offending agents have been removed, a trial of medical therapy is possible. Various classes of medications have been tried with varying success in the treatment of gynecomastia. Altering estrogen levels is the most common form of medical treatment. Clomiphene and tamoxifen, both antiestrogens, have been used and found to be effective, particularly in alleviating pain. With clomiphene, approximately 50% of patients achieve partial reduction in breast size and about 20% note complete resolution.[19] With tamoxifen, up to 80% of patients report partial or complete resolution.[20,21] Danazol, a synthetic derivative of testosterone, inhibits secretion of LH and FSH resulting in a decrease in estrogen synthesis. With danazol, a complete resolution of breast enlargement has been reported up to 23% of cases, but the treatment is often limited secondary to weight gain.[22]

If medical therapy is unsuccessful, the patient should be referred to a surgeon for surgical correction.

SURGICAL MANAGEMENT

INDICATIONS

The surgical management of gynecomastia has evolved over the past few decades in that minimal scars and "no" visible sequela of surgery should now be the norm. Past surgeries involving scars across the chest left men with significant cosmetic deformities. Of note, many young adult men still have slight gynecomastia from puberty, and this is emotionally bothersome to them. The surgeon should be mindful that even the smallest amount of tissue protuberance can be very troublesome to a young man. Thus, surgery may be warranted for even the smallest deformity.

CONTRAINDICATIONS

There are relatively few contraindications to pursuing surgical management for gynecomastia after a trial of conservative therapy or medical management. Relative contraindications to surgical management include patient comorbidities that increase the risk of complications related to anesthesia or increase risk of bleeding (i.e., anticoagulants). Active breast cancer is an absolute contraindication to surgical therapy. Additionally, if the patient has unrealistic expectations related to the cosmetic or psychological outcome, then surgical management should be deferred.

ROOM SETUP

After appropriate anesthetic selection with either laryngeal mask or endotracheal intubation, the patient should be placed supine with both arms out. No paralysis is necessary. Tumescent solution should be prepared on the back table consisting of 1 L of normal saline with one 50 mL bottle of 1% lidocaine and one vial of 1:1,000 epinephrine, bringing the final liter's concentration of epinephrine to 1:1,000,000. Ensure you have all parts of your commercial power-assisted liposuction unit, including the liposuction cannula and canister. For postoperative care, have ready a gynecomastia "vest" or surgical bra for postoperative compression.

OPERATIVE TECHNIQUE

SURGICAL TREATMENT WITH LITTLE OR NO PTOSIS

The majority of young males with persistent gynecomastia after puberty fall into this category. Other older males who have suffered gynecomastia secondary to tumor may also present with minimal ptosis. For these patients, the use of tissue suction has been shown to be highly successful, especially when some form of periareolar glandular excision is included. This author (AMW) almost always utilizes power-assisted liposuction and a modification of the pull-through technique.[23-28] Since most gynecomastia presents as a combination of both lipodystrophy and glandular breast enlargement, this technique is very feasible. Liposuction alone will often not relieve the "pointing" of the NAC and will lead to a suboptimal result. Please see Figures 68.1 through 68.4 for technique and results.

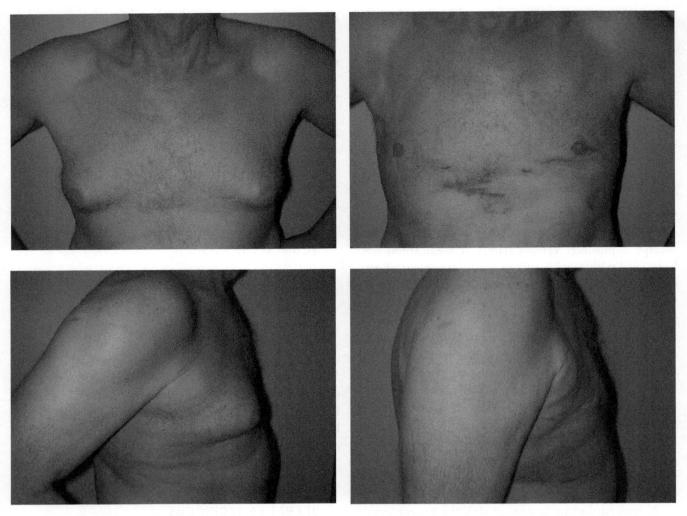

Figure 68.1. Preoperative and postoperative anterior/lateral views of middle-age male with moderate gynecomastia secondary to prostate cancer medications treated with liposuction and pull-through technique.

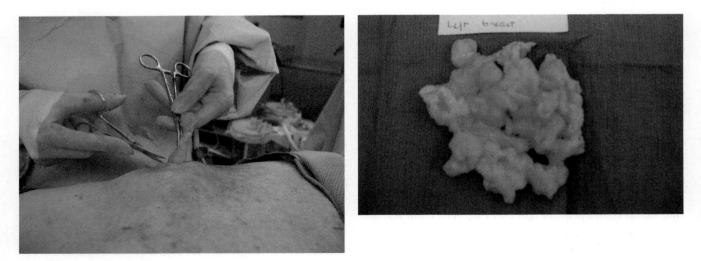

Figure 68.2. Intraoperative example of pull-through technique. This is done after completion of liposuction. The mound of tissue that can be removed is also demonstrated.

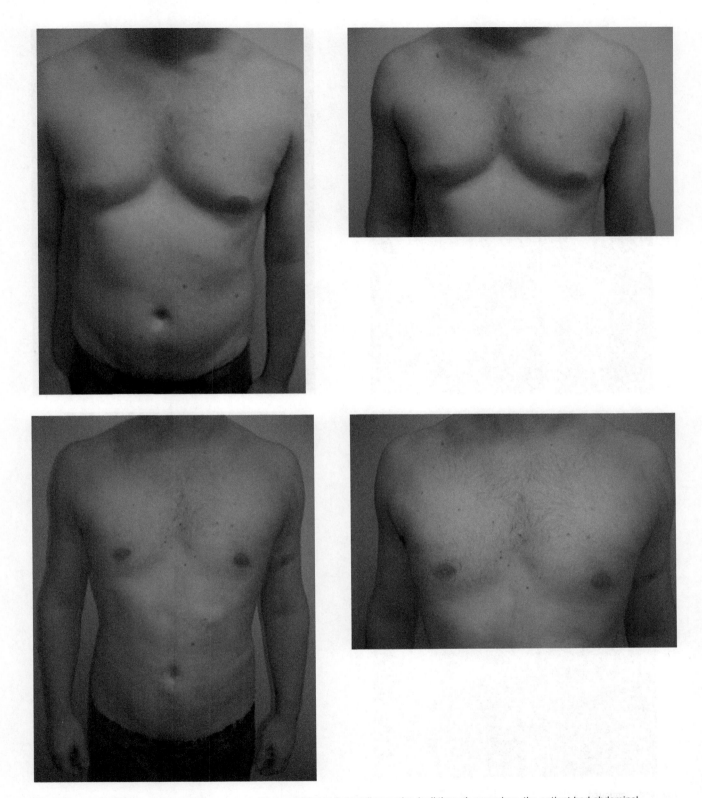

Figure 68.3. Preoperative 32-year-old man with gynecomastia. In addition to breast liposuction/pull-through procedure, the patient had abdominal liposuction.

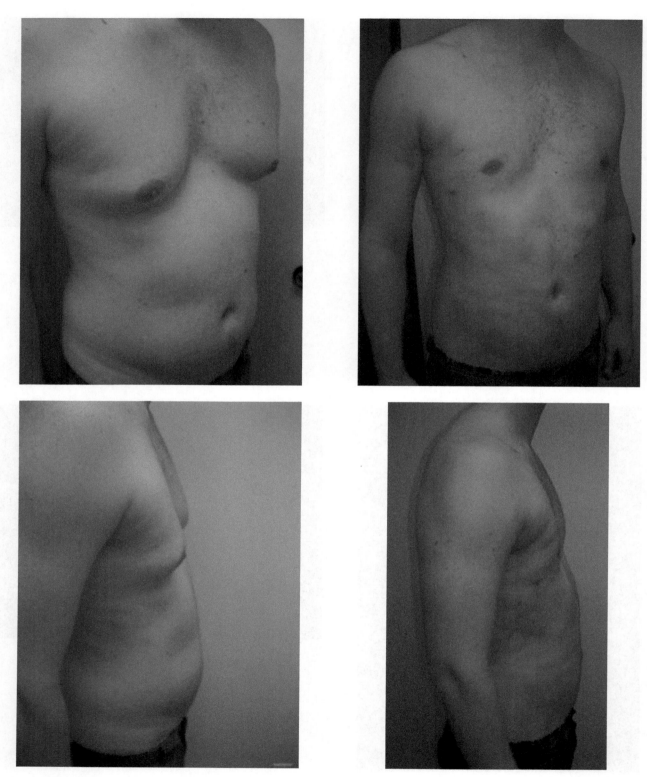

Figure 68.3. Continued

TECHNIQUE

Areas to be suctioned are marked preoperatively. Either general or local anesthesia can be used, depending on the patient's desires. Two small incisions are made inside the areola. If necessary, an inframammary or axillary incision can be added. The breast is infused with a tumescent solution previously prepared. After appropriate time for the hemostatic effect to take place, liposuction

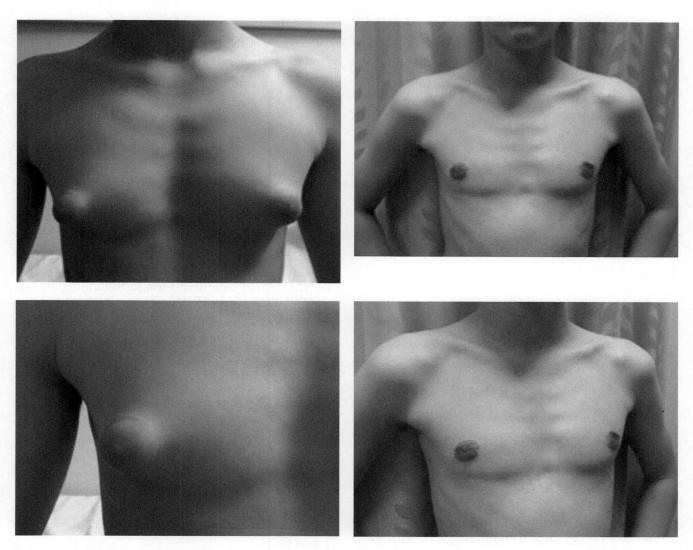

Figure 68.4. A 14-year-old boy with 2-year history of gynecomastia and history significant for patient being bullied at school. Preoperative and postoperative photos.

is begun. We use a combination of ultrasound-assisted liposuction with standard syringe liposuction. The ultrasound-assisted cannula can be hollow or solid. The solid-tip cannula is gently passed through a given area of the breast, taking care not to burn the surrounding skin. Once the fat is emulsified, the syringe cannula is inserted and used to extract the fat. Because the breast is a combination of fat, parenchyma, and supporting ligaments, it is often necessary to be very persistent in a given area until the breast tissue "releases" from the supporting ligaments. The key to breast liposuction is patience and persistence. The procedure should continue in each zone marked preoperatively until satisfactory contour is achieved. Finally, liposuction under the NAC is performed.

Once liposuction is complete, there will be an element of glandular tissue remaining that cannot be suctioned: the amount varies, depending on the severity of disease. I perform a modification of the pull-through technique. Through the same two incisions made on either side of the areola, a small hemostat is placed under the NAC, approximately 1 cm below the skin, so as not to leave the areola devoid of supporting tissue. The glandular tissue is easily pulled through these incisions, because it has already been released from fat and supporting ligaments by the previous liposuction. Tenotomy scissors are used to gently dissect the glandular tissue away from the breast both superficially and deep. This procedure is continued until the proper contour is achieved. Usually this sharp dissection is necessary only around the areola, but it can be carried further in the breast if necessary. A core of glandular tissue is then removed en bloc and may be sent to pathology. The surgeon must continually roll the breast within his or her fingers to gauge the extent of tissue excision. The natural male breast has approximately 1 cm of tissue remaining. Typically, we will leave a 10 mm flat Jackson-Pratt drain in the lateral space for approximately 1 week.

Postoperative care consists of the patient wearing a gynecomastia "vest" continuously for 3 weeks and as necessary thereafter. Hematoma and seroma formation are potential complications that must be addressed quickly to avoid contour deformities. Temporary nipple numbness is possible, but generally resolves within the first year postoperatively.

SURGICAL TREATMENT OF GYNECOMASTIA WITH EXTENSIVE HYPERTROPHY OR PTOSIS

CASE OF PSEUDOGYNECOMASTIA

Older patients may present with a mixed gynecomastia and pseudogynecomastia picture. The pseudogynecomastia is often improved with weight loss; however, there is an excess of skin and although the fatty deposits will improve, the fibrous glandular tissue usually has minimal improvement. After weight loss, we typically perform surgery in a two-staged fashion. The first stage is liposuction of the chest (previously described). After 3–6 months of compression therapy that allows the skin envelope has settled, the patient is brought back for a second procedure to address the excess skin. The excess skin is usually managed via skin amputation and an inferior pedicle approach.

TECHNIQUE

The first-stage liposuction is similar to that described in the previous section. The second stage involves a bilateral breast reduction using an inframammary fold incision and an inferior dermoglandular pedicle (Figure 68.5).

Preoperatively, the amount of excess breast tissue and skin are marked in addition to the typical anatomical landmarks (inframammary fold, midline, and sternal notch). The new NAC is marked 20 cm from the sternal notch or at the lateral border of the pectoralis major muscle. Intraoperatively, we start by making an incision encompassing the inframammary fold, including the whole width of the excess tissue. We then draw a dermal glandular pedicle including the NAC that was inferiorly based and approximately 10 cm wide. Next, we make incisions along our ellipse and dermoglandular pedicle. We de-epithelialize the dermoglandular pedicle leaving the NAC intact. We then continue to make our elliptical incision and excise all the excess breast tissue. We elevate the superior subcutaneous mastectomy flaps up into the clavicle. Next, we tailor-tack the end of skin and bury the dermoglandular pedicle containing the NAC. The patient is sat up, and we confirm the locations of the new NACs. We cut the ellipse of skin out and then deliver our NAC through this defect. After closing deep Scarpa's fascia, placing deep dermal sutures and closing the skin, the NAC is fixed using deep 3-0 absorbable monofilament interrupted sutures and half-buried 4-0 Prolene sutures to inset the NAC. Steri-Strips are placed on the incisions and a compression dressing applied.

CASE OF LARGE PTOTIC BREASTS

Hormonal anti-androgen treatment for prostate cancer remains a significant component of treatment for prostate cancer. Given the commonality of prostate cancer, there is a significant proportion of antiandrogen associated gynecomastia. These patients tend to develop large and very dense breast tissue that is not amenable to liposuction. In these cases, we almost always perform subcutaneous mastectomies with bilateral free nipple grafting[29] (Figure 68.6).

Technique

The patient's standard anatomical landmarks including the sternal notch, sternum, and inframammary folds are identified. The new NAC position is marked at the junction of the pectoralis major and rectus fascia. We draw out elliptical incision markings to perform a standard subcutaneous mastectomy. Additionally, we outline a 3 cm diameter NAC for position of the final graft. Intraoperatively, we start with excising the NAC and placing it in saline until grafting. Next, we make our elliptical incision and use electrocautery to elevate flaps superiorly to the level of the clavicle, medially to the level of the sternum, inferiorly to the level of the inframammary fold, and laterally to the serratus muscle. We irrigate the breast cavity, obtain hemostasis, and place our subcutaneous drains. We perform a layered closure and then confirm the new position

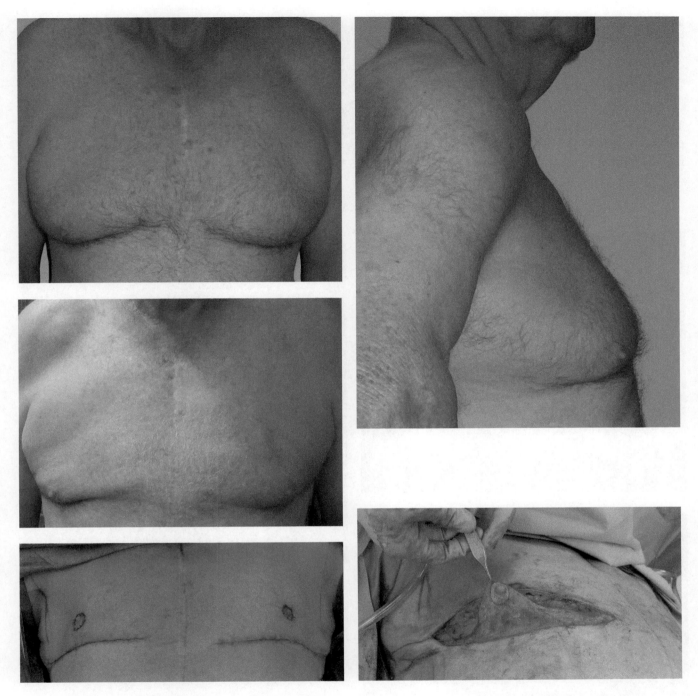

Figure 68.5. (A) A 71-year-old man who experienced significant weight loss after undergoing coronary artery bypass grafting (CABG). He had residual pseudogynecomastia despite adequate weight loss. He underwent staged bilateral liposuction followed by bilateral breast reduction with an inferior dermoglandular pedicle with 1-year interval. (B) Preoperative pseudogynecomastia. (C) Post first-stage liposuction. (D,E) Intraoperative inferior dermoglandular pedicle. The dermal glandular pedicle, which included the nipple areolar complex, was inferiorly based and 10 cm wide.

of the NAC. We typically draw a 3 cm circle around the area at the junction of the lateral pectoralis major border and sit the patient up to confirm adequate placement. We deepithelialize a 3 cm oval-shaped area along the new nipple position. We obtain our previously removed NAC out of the saline and suture it, typically with 3-0 Prolene, into the de-epithelialized area. We place Xeroform, mineral oil, and a cotton ball bolster over the graft. Steri-Strips are placed along all incision lines, followed by a compression bra. Nipple sensation is lost with this technique, and it is important to discuss this risk with the patient preoperatively.

CAVEATS

The care of the patient with gynecomastia is complex in that the proper diagnosis is as important as the surgical treatment. Attention should always be given to the possibility of breast cancer or underlying causative pathology. Once surgical treatment for gynecomastia is established, the degree of hypertrophy and skin excess dictates the method. The majority of patients are satisfactorily treated with liposuction and minor excisional procedures. More severe cases of gynecomastia require reduction techniques. Whichever procedure is chosen, the natural male breast contours should always be remembered and contouring should be performed carefully and meticulously.

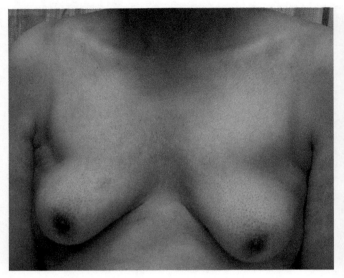
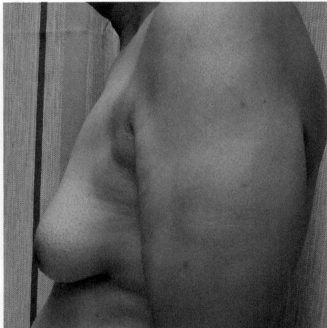
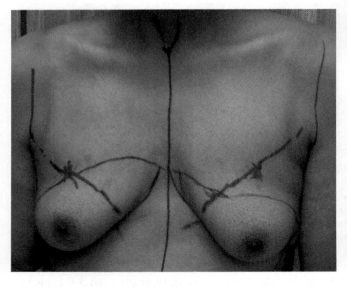
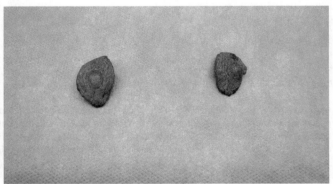

Figure 68.6. A 66-year-old male with a history of prostate cancer and bilateral antiandrogen-induced gynecomastia with grade 3 ptosis. After his prostatectomy (stage 4 prostate cancer), he underwent adjuvant treatment with prednisone and abiraterone, which resulted in persistently enlarging breasts. He underwent bilateral subcutaneous mastectomies and free nipple grafting. (A,B) Preoperative images. (C) Preoperative markings: using the pinch test, elliptical marking were made incorporating the excess breast tissue and skin to be resected. (D–F) Intraoperatively, the full thickness NACs were excised and saved until the end of the case. Subcutaneous mastectomies were performed excising all breast tissue and redundant skin. (G) Specimens: Right breast, 443 g; left breast, 380 g.

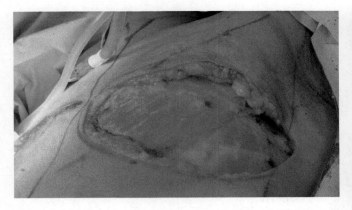
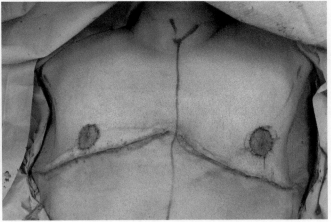
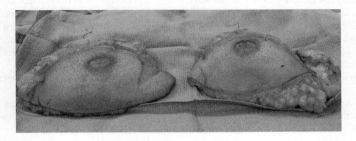

Figure 68.6. Continued

REFERENCES

1. Gikas P, Mokbel K. Management of gynaecomastia: an update. *Int J Clin Pract* 2007;61:1209–1215.
2. Braunstein GD. Gynecomastia. *N Engl J Med* 1993;328:490–495.
3. Andersen JA, Gram JB. Male breast at autopsy. *Acta Pathologica Microbiologica Scandinavica Series A:Pathology* 2009;90A:191–197.
4. Wilson JD, Aiman J, MacDonald PC. The pathogenesis of gynecomastia. *Adv Intern Med* 1980;25:1–32.
5. Testosterone treatment of men with alcoholic cirrhosis: a double-blind study. The Copenhagen Study Group for Liver Diseases. *Hepatology* 1986;6:807–813.
6. Castro-Magana M, Angulo M, Uy J. Male hypogonadism with gynecomastia caused by late-onset deficiency of testicular 17-ketosteroid reductase. *N Engl J Med* 1993;328:1297–1301.
7. Cavanah SF, Dons RF. Partial 3 beta-hydroxysteroid dehydrogenase deficiency presenting as new-onset gynecomastia in a eugonadal adult male. *Metabolism* 1993;42:65–68.
8. Deepinder F, Braunstein GD. Drug-induced gynecomastia: an evidence-based review. *Expert Opin Drug Saf* 2012;11:779–795.
9. Mabuchi K, Bross DS, Kessler, II. Risk factors for male breast cancer. *J Natl Cancer Inst* 1985;74:371–375.
10. Scheike O, Visfeldt J, Petersen B. Male breast cancer. *Acta Pathologica Microbiologica Scandinavica Section A Pathology* 2009;81A:352–358.
11. Hultborn R, Hanson C, Kopf I, et al. Prevalence of Klinefelter's syndrome in male breast cancer patients. *Anticancer Res* 1997;17:4293–4297.
12. Olsson H, Ranstam J. Head trauma and exposure to prolactin-elevating drugs as risk factors for male breast cancer. *J Natl Cancer Inst* 1988;80:679–683.
13. Thomas DB. Breast cancer in men. *Epidemiol Rev* 1993;15:220–231.
14. Thomas DB, Jimenez LM, McTiernan A, et al. Breast cancer in men: risk factors with hormonal implications. *Am J Epidemiol* 1992;135:734–748.
15. Wooster R, Bignell G, Lancaster J, et al. Identification of the breast cancer susceptibility gene BRCA2. *Nature* 1995;378:789–792.
16. Das DK, Junaid TA, Mathews SB, et al. Fine needle aspiration cytology diagnosis of male breast lesions. A study of 185 cases. *Acta Cytol* 1995;39:870–876.
17. Munoz Carrasco R, Alvarez Benito M, Munoz Gomariz E, et al. Mammography and ultrasound in the evaluation of male breast disease. *Eur Radiol* 2010;20:2797–2805.
18. Cooper RA, Gunter BA, Ramamurthy L. Mammography in men. *Radiology* 1994;191:651–656.
19. Plourde PV, Kulin HE, Santner SJ. Clomiphene in the treatment of adolescent gynecomastia. Clinical and endocrine studies. *Am J Dis Child* 1983;137:1080–1082.
20. Lawrence SE, Faught KA, Vethamuthu J, Lawson ML. Beneficial effects of raloxifene and tamoxifen in the treatment of pubertal gynecomastia. *J Pediatr* 2004;145:71–76.
21. McDermott MT, Hofeldt FD, Kidd GS. Tamoxifen therapy for painful idiopathic gynecomastia. *South Med J* 1990;83:1283–1285.
22. Jones DJ, Holt SD, Surtees P, et al. A comparison of danazol and placebo in the treatment of adult idiopathic gynaecomastia: results of a prospective study in 55 patients. *Ann R Coll Surg Engl* 1990;72:296–298.
23. Morselli PG. "Pull-through": a new technique for breast reduction in gynecomastia. *Plast Reconstr Surg* 1996;97:450–454.
24. Lista F, Ahmad J. Power-assisted liposuction and the pull-through technique for the treatment of gynecomastia. *Plast Reconstr Surg* 2008;121:740–747.
25. Stark GB, Grandel S, Spilker G. Tissue suction of the male and female breast. *Aesthetic Plast Surg* 1992;16:317–324.

26. Rosenberg GJ. A new cannula for suction removal of parenchymal tissue of gynecomastia. *Plast Reconstr Surg* 1994;94:548–551.

27. Hammond DC, Arnold JF, Simon AM, Capraro PA. Combined use of ultrasonic liposuction with the pull-through technique for the treatment of gynecomastia. *Plast Reconstr Surg* 2003;112:891–895.

28. Morselli PG, Morellini A. Breast reshaping in gynecomastia by the "pull-through technique": considerations after 15 years. *Eur J Plast Surg* 2011;35:365–371.

29. Murphy TP, Ehrlichman RJ, Seckel BR. Nipple placement in simple mastectomy with free nipple grafting for severe gynecomastia. *Plast Reconstr Surg* 1994;94:818–823.

30. Carvajal A, Martin Arias LH. Gynecomastia and sexual disorders after the administration of omeprazole. *Am J Gastroenterol* 1995;90:1028–1029.

31. Boyd IW. Adverse Drug Reactions Advisory Committee. Gynaecomastia in association with calcium antagonists. *Med J Aust* 1994;161:328.

32. Cespedes RD, Caballero RL, Peretsman SJ, Thompson IM, Jr. Cryptic presentations of germ cell tumors. *J Am Coll Surg* 1994;178:261–265.

33. Davies JP, Price-Thomas JM. Gynaecomastia in association with minocycline. *Br J Clin Pract* 1995;49:179.

34. Forst T, Beyer J, Cordes U, et al. Gynaecomastia in a patient with a hCG producing giant cell carcinoma of the lung. Case report. *Exp Clin Endocrinol Diabetes* 1995;103:28–32.

35. Gana BM, Windsor PM, Lang S, et al. Leydig cell tumour. *Br J Urol* 1995;75:676–678.

36. Jacobs U, Klein B, Klehr HU. Cumulative side effects of cyclosporine and Ca antagonists: hypergalactinemia, mastadenoma, and gynecomastia. *Transplant Proc* 1994;26:3122.

37. Lanigan D, Choa RG, Evans J. A feminizing adrenocortical carcinoma presenting with gynaecomastia. *Postgrad Med J* 1993;69:481–483.

38. Lemack GE, Poppas DP, Vaughan ED, Jr. Urologic causes of gynecomastia: approach to diagnosis and management. *Urology* 1995;45:313–319.

39. Lindquist M, Edwards IR. Endocrine adverse effects of omeprazole. *BMJ* 1992;305:451–452.

40. Llop R, Gomez-Farran F, Figueras A, et al. Gynecomastia associated with enalapril and diazepam. *Ann Pharmacother* 1994;28:671–672.

41. Malozowski S, Stadel BV. Prepubertal gynecomastia during growth hormone therapy. *J Pediatr* 1995;126:659–661.

42. Matoska J, Ondrus D, Talerman A. Malignant granulosa cell tumor of the testis associated with gynecomastia and long survival. *Cancer* 1992;69:1769–1772.

43. Nagi DK, Jones WG, Belchetz PE. Gynaecomastia caused by a primary mediastinal seminoma. *Clin Endocrinol (Oxf)* 1994;40:545–548;discussion:548–549.

44. Neild D. Gynaecomastia in bodybuilders. *Br J Clin Pract* 1995;49:172.

45. Nishiyama T, Washiyama K, Tanikawa T, et al. Gynecomastia and ectopic human chorionic gonadotropin production by transitional cell carcinoma of the bladder. *Urol Int* 1992;48:463–465.

46. Otto C, Richter WO. Unilateral gynecomastia induced by treatment with diltiazem. *Arch Intern Med* 1994;154:351.

47. Pope HG, Jr., Katz DL. Psychiatric and medical effects of anabolic-androgenic steroid use. A controlled study of 160 athletes. *Arch Gen Psychiatry* 1994;51:375–382.

48. Roberts HJ. Vitamin E and gynecomastia. *Hosp Pract (Off Ed)* 1994;29:12.

49. Thomas E, Leroux JL, Blotman F. Gynecomastia in patients with rheumatoid arthritis treated with methotrexate. *J Rheumatol* 1994;21:1777–1778.

50. Volpi R, Maccarini PA, Boni S, et al. Case report: finasteride-induced gynecomastia in a 62-year-old man. *Am J Med Sci* 1995;309:322–325.

51. Bowman JD, Kim H, Bustamante JJ. Drug-induced gynecomastia. *Pharmacotherapy* 2012;32:1123–1140.

69

CHEST WALL RECONSTRUCTION

Gregory P. Reece and Daniel Goldberg

Before undertaking a chest wall reconstruction, several issues must be considered. The patient's overall medical condition must be assessed and cardiopulmonary function optimized if the patient is determined to be a surgical candidate. The extent of malignant disease and the presence of pulmonary and mediastinal radiation-induced injury should be assessed by history and physical examination, pulmonary function tests, and computed tomography of the chest. Patients with a history of previous ipsilateral chest wall surgery or high-dose radiation therapy to the chest wall or axilla may not be candidates for some types of reconstruction, such as the latissimus dorsi flap. Under these circumstances, another flap option should be considered. A biopsy must be done for suspicious lesions, including infected chest wall ulcers, to determine the presence of malignant neoplasms. From this information, the potential size of the chest wall skeletal defect should be estimated to determine whether vital organs will be exposed or removed after chest wall resection and whether a chest wall prosthesis will be required. The surgeon should also determine whether the patient will have to be repositioned during surgery. For example, sternal resections are usually performed with the patient in the supine position. If the latissimus dorsi flap is considered for wound closure, the reconstructive surgeon will have to reposition the patient to harvest the latissimus flap; another flap that does not require repositioning may be a better option.

Only after these issues have been addressed can the reconstructive surgeon select the best method of chest wall reconstruction. In this chapter, we review some of the commonly used flaps for chest wall reconstruction. These flaps include the latissimus dorsi, rectus abdominis, and pectoralis major myocutaneous flaps and the omental flap. Although the University of Texas M. D. Anderson Cancer Center is well known for the use of microsurgery in cancer patients, it is our opinion, as well as the opinion

of other authors, that a free flap chest wall reconstruction is seldom indicated.

LATISSIMUS DORSI MYOCUTANEOUS FLAP

ASSESSMENT OF THE DEFECT

After the chest wall resection, the reconstructive and thoracic surgeons must determine whether a chest wall prosthesis, such as Marlex mesh with or without methyl methacrylate, will be required to protect exposed vital organs and to avoid postoperative pulmonary insufficiency. As a general rule, a prosthesis is not required to prevent pulmonary insufficiency when fewer than three or four ribs have been removed. For skeletal defects of more than four ribs and for patients who have undergone sternectomy, a prosthesis is useful to prevent paradoxical chest wall movement, to decrease ventilator dependence and hospital stay, and to maintain an aesthetic chest wall contour. Nevertheless, the exact size of the skeletal chest wall defect that requires a prosthesis to avoid pulmonary insufficiency remains unknown, and each case must be considered individually.

The soft tissue closure is planned by determining the size and shape of the soft tissue defect. If the patient has not received previous radiation therapy, the soft tissue around the defect can often be undermined and advanced to decrease the size of the defect and thus decrease the size of the latissimus dorsi skin island required. For chest wall defects located in irradiated tissue, this maneuver is usually not possible, and the skin island must be designed to fill either the entire defect or the defect closed with the latissimus dorsi muscle and a skin graft. If the myocutaneous flap is to be used, a template of the defect can be made to transfer the design to the latissimus dorsi skin island on the back.

If the patient is undergoing chest wall resection for an extensive breast cancer, the breast and chest wall can often be reconstructed simultaneously using an extended latissimus dorsi myocutaneous flap. The decision to perform such a reconstruction should be determined preoperatively after consulting with the oncologic surgeon and medical and radiation oncologists. Factors to consider include the size of the breast to be reconstructed, the amount of chest wall skin to be resected, the availability of sufficient skin and subcutaneous tissue to create the needed breast size and to close the skin defect, the extent of the patient's disease, probability of recurrence, and the need for postoperative adjuvant therapy. Because many of these patients have such advanced disease and because the presence of the reconstructed breast may compromise the adequacy of such treatments as radiation therapy, the decision to perform a breast reconstruction should be postponed until all adjuvant therapy has been completed and the patient is free of disease.

INDICATIONS

The latissimus dorsi myocutaneous flap is indicated on any chest wall defect located within its arc of rotation. This flap is usually used for lateral and anterior defects; however, sternal defects located in the upper two thirds of the sternum also may be closed with this flap.

CONTRAINDICATIONS

The most common contraindication for a latissimus dorsi myocutaneous flap is a history of previous chest wall surgery on the ipsilateral side. A posterolateral thoracotomy performed on the same side as the chest wall defect for related or unrelated reasons is usually considered an absolute contraindication for a latissimus dorsi myocutaneous flap. Although many thoracic surgeons now try to preserve this muscle when possible, a thoracotomy through this approach usually involves transection of the muscle in its midportion for better exposure. The thoracodorsal blood vessels, the dominant blood supply to this flap, are sometimes injured or divided in patients who require an axillary dissection for other reasons. Because the nerve is intimately associated with the vascular pedicle, a functional latissimus dorsi muscle is generally considered evidence that the vascular pedicle to the latissimus dorsi muscle is still intact. Latissimus dorsi muscle function may be assessed preoperatively by having the patient press down with the elbow against the examiner's hand while palpating the muscle.

Nevertheless, the operative report from the axillary dissection should always be carefully reviewed before considering this flap option.

Relative contraindications for a latissimus dorsi myocutaneous flap include a history of high-dose radiation therapy delivered to the area of the flap or to the ipsilateral axilla, massive ipsilateral upper extremity lymphedema, and massive chest wall defects that involve the base of the flap. A well-healed incision from a previous chest tube placed through the anterior margin of the latissimus dorsi muscle flap is not a contraindication to performing a latissimus dorsi myocutaneous flap.

ROOM SETUP

In most cases, the patient is positioned in a lateral decubitus position for flap dissection. This position permits tumor resection and immediate reconstruction of most anterior, lateral, posterior, and some sternal chest wall defects without repositioning the patient. Patients who require sternal resection in the supine position must have the wound closed with sterile dressings and their position changed to the lateral decubitus position for wound closure with a latissimus dorsi flap. All patients positioned in the lateral decubitus position should have an axillary roll in place and the head properly secured to avoid brachial plexus injuries. Also, the ipsilateral arm should be prepared and draped in a fashion that permits manipulation of the arm to easily dissect the vascular pedicle.

PATIENT MARKINGS

The latissimus dorsi muscle originates from the iliac crest, the external surface of the external oblique muscle, the thoracolumbar fascia, and the spines of the lower six vertebrae posteriorly. The muscle inserts on the lesser tubercle and intertubercular groove of the humerus. The midportion of the superior border of the muscle passes over the tip of the scapula. Also, the muscle is attached to the serratus anterior muscle and several ribs on their posterior surface.

The blood supply to this flap arises predominantly from the thoracodorsal artery and vein and the terminal branches of the subscapular artery and vein. As the thoracodorsal vessels enter the proximal part of the muscle, they divide into an upper horizontal branch that traverses along the superior border of the muscle and a lower oblique branch that runs along the anterior oblique border of the muscle. Other vascular contributions that must be divided when elevating the latissimus dorsi flap come from the posterior branches of the intercostal vessels and paraspinous perforating vessels.

The landmarks of the latissimus dorsi myocutaneous flap may be marked preoperatively with the patient standing but are more frequently marked intraoperatively after the defect has been created. To avoid a split-thickness skin graft closure of the donor site, the skin island should be designed so that the island's width is no more than 10 cm and so that the skin island is positioned over the proximal two-thirds of the flap, where the perforators coming from the muscle to the skin are more numerous (Figure 69.1). Because the blood supply to the distal end (origin) of the latissimus dorsi muscle arises from paraspinal perforators, skin islands located over the distal end of the muscle are usually unreliable. However, if the latissimus dorsi flap is designed to incorporate the entire thoracodorsal-scapular arterial system, as much as half of the skin of the back can be taken for repair of a massive chest wall defect.

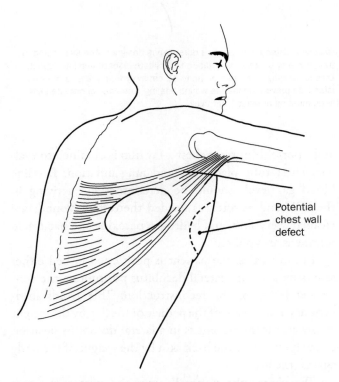

Figure 69.1. Skin island of flap should be designed over latissimus dorsi muscle after first determining size of chest wall defect and distance of defect from insertion of latissimus dorsi muscle. Skin island design is facilitated by making template of defect with sterile glove paper and transferring it to appropriate location over the muscle. Skin island should be designed no wider than 10 cm to avoid problems closing donor site primarily.

SURGICAL TECHNIQUE

With the patient prepared and draped in a sterile fashion, the skin is incised in an oblique line from the posterior axillary fold to and along the perimeter of the skin island. The incision is beveled away from the skin island for 1–2 cm as the dissection proceeds toward the muscle. The skin overlying the muscle is then elevated proximally toward the insertion and distally to the origin, so that the only skin remaining on the muscle is the skin island. To prevent avulsion of the skin island, the skin may be sutured to the muscle fascia with interrupted sutures circumferentially.

The muscle is then elevated from its bed, beginning at the anterior-lateral border of the muscle near the origin of the serratus anterior muscle and proceeding toward the scapular tip. Upon completing this portion, the dissection turns distally toward the spine and posterior iliac crest. All large posterior branches of the intercostal blood vessels and paraspinous perforating vessels entering the latissimus dorsi muscle are divided between clamps and ligated with 3-0 silk suture. Care must be taken to avoid inadvertent elevation of the serratus anterior muscle near the spine. After the distal end of the muscle is elevated, the flap is elevated proximally toward the vascular pedicle with care not to injure the long thoracic nerve. A subcutaneous tunnel is created between the axilla and the chest wall defect. The flap is temporarily passed through this is tunnel to check the position of the skin island. If the skin island will not inset easily into the defect, the flap is returned back through the tunnel, and the serratus branch of the thoracodorsal vessels is divided. The vascular pedicle may be dissected back to the axillary vessels, if necessary, to improve the reach of the muscle (Figure 69.2). If this maneuver is still unsuccessful, the insertion of the muscle must be divided, and the muscle must be advanced as much as possible without excessive tension on the vascular pedicle. Once the full length of the vascular pedicle has been used, the flap should be sutured to the chest wall to avoid tension on the pedicle from a gravitational shift of the flap when the patient stands.

If a simultaneous breast reconstruction is planned, an extended latissimus dorsi flap should be designed. Although a fleur-de-lis skin pattern has been described for this procedure, closure and healing of the donor site has been problematic in our experience. The donor site incision frequently heals poorly where the three limbs of the incision come together, which often results in skin necrosis and dehiscence; this is especially true for patients who smoke. Alternatively, the extended latissimus dorsi myocutaneous flap can be harvested with an elliptically shaped skin island, using the same dimensions for the skin island as for a conventional

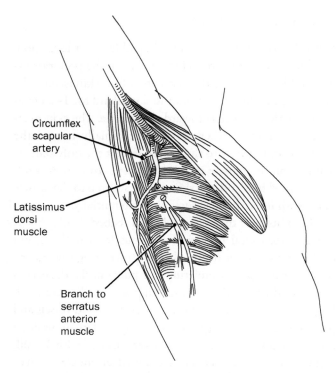

Figure 69.2. Branch to serratus anterior muscle and circumflex scapular artery is dissected, clamped, and ligated, which effectively frees vascular pedicle of flap for easier flap rotation. Dissection is most easily accomplished from anterior and undersurface of flap.

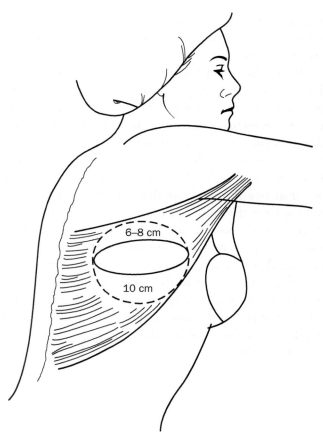

Figure 69.3. Extended latissimus dorsi flap is designed with skin island in transverse or diagonal orientation to facilitate inset of flap into defect. Dissection may be performed up to 10 cm away from margins of skin island. To prevent donor site wound healing problems, donor site skin flaps must be at least 1 cm thick.

latissimus dorsi myocutaneous flap. The difference between the two procedures is in the way the skin island is dissected. Instead of tapering away from the skin island for only 1 or 2 cm before reaching the muscle, the surgeon dissects away from the skin island for approximately 10 cm below the lower border of the skin island incision and for 6–8 cm above the superior border of the skin island (Figure 69.3). The remaining skin over the latissimus dorsi muscle should be at least 1 cm thick to prevent wound healing problems due to poor perfusion.

After checking all wounds for hemostasis, a closed drainage system is placed for both the donor and recipient sites. A chest tube is placed in the pleural space and brought out through a separate stab incision. The flap is inset using a two-layered closure and the donor site closed in the usual manner.

POSTOPERATIVE CARE

The patient is usually kept in the intensive care unit (ICU) for 24–48 hours. Patients usually do not require assisted ventilation unless a large chest wall defect was reconstructed with soft tissue alone. The chest tube is placed to underwater seal with −20 cm of water suction and a portable upright chest x-ray film is obtained to evaluate chest tube placement and lung inflation. Baseline blood gas levels should be determined on arriving in the ICU and as often as needed thereafter. Wounds are cleaned every shift, and hydrogen peroxide and bacitracin ointment are applied.

In most cases, the patient is positioned in bed either semi-supine or in a lateral decubitus position on the contralateral side of the reconstruction. This avoids inadvertent compression of the pedicle of the flap by the weight of the arm if the patient is in a lateral decubitus position or compression of the back skin by the weight of the body against the bed.

The chest tube is usually removed within the first 24–48 hours if there is no air leak or pneumothorax; a follow-up chest x-ray film should be obtained after tube removal. After transfer to the surgical floor, the patient receives routine wound care; catheters are removed when the drainage decreases to 30 mL or less in a 24-hour period.

If external sutures or staples were used, they are usually removed on the eighth postoperative day; if absorbable buried dermal sutures were placed. Alternatively, using an absorbable mono-filament suture, such as Monocryl, placed in a subcuticular fashion, makes suture removal unnecessary.

The most common problems associated with the use of the latissimus dorsi flap are the prolonged serous drainage and seroma formation at the donor site. Drains are usually left in place for 2–3 weeks before the drainage decreases enough to remove them. Small seromas (50 mL or less) that form after drain removal are usually observed; larger seromas usually require one or more aspirations under sterile technique in the clinic.

REHABILITATION

In most cases, rehabilitation is minimal. Some patients may have a decreased range of motion in the ipsilateral shoulder if they do not begin range of motion exercises at the end of the third postoperative week. Patients may have a brachial plexus stretch injury if the arm is hyperabducted and the neck flexed toward the opposite shoulder during flap dissection. This can be avoided by limiting the amount of abduction of the arm and by proper positioning of the head.

CAVEATS

Although the latissimus dorsi myocutaneous flap is very reliable, there are certain caveats that should be remembered to avoid complications. These include:

1. Avoid placing skin islands over the distal end of the muscle because the blood supply to the distal end (origin) of the latissimus dorsi muscle arises from paraspinal perforators, which are usually beyond the watershed area of the thoracodorsal vessels.

2. Avoid postoperative hematomas by ligating all large posterior branches of the intercostal and paraspinous perforating vessels that enter the latissimus dorsi muscle.

3. Avoid elevating the serratus anterior muscle by dissecting the latissimus dorsi muscle from a lateral to medial direction over the serratus anterior muscle.

4. Avoid excessive tension on the vascular pedicle by suturing the insertion of the muscle to a secure location on the chest wall, if the insertion was divided. In such

cases, also consider dividing the thoracodorsal nerve to prevent excessive muscle contraction and subsequent traction injury of the pedicle which can lead to flap loss.

5. For an extended latissimus dorsi flap, leave the back skin at least 1 cm thick and limit the inferior dissection of the skin island to not more than 10 cm below the inferior border of the skin island to avoid poor perfusion of the skin and subsequent wound-healing problems.

OMENTAL FLAP

ASSESSMENT OF THE DEFECT

There are several factors about the defect that must be considered before selecting an omental flap for chest wall repair. These factors include the size, location, and depth of the chest wall resection; the radiation therapy history; the presence of infection; and the need for a chest wall implant. Because the omentum is thin and very pliable in most patients, it is ideally suited for repair of small- to medium-sized anterior chest wall defects. The most common location for these defects is in the lower anterior chest wall and lower two-thirds of the sternum. In most cases, the defect is closed by folding the omentum on itself one or more times to increase the thickness of the soft tissue cover over the wound before it is covered with a split-thickness skin graft.

For large chest wall defects, especially those located in the upper chest area, there is usually insufficient omentum to fold on itself and only a thin layer of vascularized tissue is available for skin grafting. This is not a problem if the defect is superficial, as occurs with removal of shallow radiation-induced chest wall ulcers; the skin graft heals well to the omentum and the flap protects the chest wall. In contrast, full-thickness chest wall defects usually require an implant covered with a relatively thick layer of soft tissue or, if an infection is present, a thick, bulky flap to repair the chest wall. The omentum does not usually provide enough soft tissue to accomplish either of these goals, and another flap option should be considered.

To reach defects in the upper chest region, the omentum must be cut to lengthen its pedicle, which decreases the amount of omentum available to cover anything but a small chest wound. If the patient has not received radiation therapy, the soft tissues around a large chest wall defect can sometimes be undermined and advanced to decrease the size of the defect, which may allow the rest of the wound to be closed with an omental flap and skin graft. This maneuver is usually not reliable if the patient has had a significant dose of radiation to the chest wall.

Only after considering these potential problems and the contraindications listed later can the reconstructive surgeon successfully use the omental flap for chest wall coverage.

INDICATIONS

The omental flap is most commonly used for repair of sternal defects, especially of the lower two thirds of the sternum. However, this flap can be extended to cover small chest wall defects almost anywhere on the anterior chest wall.

CONTRAINDICATIONS

Harvesting the omentum requires a laparotomy; thus, patients who have had multiple laparotomies are not good candidates for this flap. Absolute contraindications for an omental flap include a patient history of abdominal adhesions; ascites resulting from cardiac or malignant causes, or from protein malnutrition; and liver cirrhosis. Previous surgical staging laparotomy for ovarian cancer is also an absolute contraindication. Relative contraindications for the omental flap are (1) previous gastric surgery in which the gastroepiploic vessels may have been ligated and (2) morbid obesity. The omentum of obese patients tends to be much thicker and less pliable than desired because of significant quantities of adipose tissue; mobilization and rotation of the flap are much more difficult than in nonobese patients.

ROOM SETUP

The patient is placed in a supine position on the operating table such that the reconstructive surgeon and an assistant can work on either side of the table. The chest and abdomen are sterilely prepared and draped.

PATIENT MARKINGS

The omental flap is harvested through an upper midline abdominal incision. No other markings are required unless other flaps are to be used to repair the chest wall defect.

SURGICAL TECHNIQUE

With the patient's abdomen and chest sterilely prepared and draped, an upper midline abdominal incision is made and a Balfour retractor is placed to provide exposure. The greater omentum and transverse colon are mobilized and delivered through the incision. The omentum is a continuation of the parietal peritoneum of the stomach and the first part of the duodenum that extends caudally over the small bowel toward the pelvis for a variable distance and then turns upward to invest the transverse colon. The descending and ascending layers of the omentum are fused and inseparable. The left and right gastroepiploic vessels are the primary blood supply to the omentum. These vessels course along the greater curvature of the stomach to anastomose with each other and form the gastroepiploic arterial arch. The short gastric arteries branch off of the arterial arcade along the gastric side of the arch. The right, middle, and left omental arteries branch off of the omental side of the gastroepiploic arch to form the vascular network of the omentum and anastomose with each other along the caudal end of the omentum. The right side of the omentum is also supplied by an accessory omental artery that is not part of the main omental vascular network (Figure 69.4).

If the chest wall defect is located in the lowest third of the sternum and the patient has a long omentum, the flap will occasionally reach the defect without tension. If it does not reach or the defect is located higher on the chest wall, the following procedures may be performed to progressively lengthen the pedicle to reach the defect.

The first maneuver is to separate the omentum from the transverse colon. This procedure is relatively quick and without significant blood loss if dissection is confined to the avascular plane located between these structures. If a longer pedicle is still required, the left and right gastroepiploic vessels are identified and the short gastric vessels between the greater curvature of the stomach and the gastroepiploic vascular arch are ligated and divided (Figure 69.5). If the chest wall defect is located in the lowest third of the sternum, the defect can usually be covered without any further dissection of the omentum. The pedicle may be lengthened further by ligating and dividing the left gastroepiploic artery and vein so that the right gastroepiploic vessels become the vascular pedicle of the flap (Figure 69.5). Rarely, the omentum is used to cover distant defects that require an extended vascular pedicle. In these circumstances, the omental pedicle can be lengthened by ligating and dividing the gastroepiploic vascular arch between the middle omental branches, extending out toward the free end of the omentum. Because these vessels form a vascular arcade along the free end of the omentum, the pedicle can be lengthened further by dividing the gastroepiploic arcade between the take off of the right and middle omental vessels and dividing the middle omental vessels just before the communication with the terminal vascular arcade. Although this last maneuver will lengthen the vascular pedicle so that it can reach the neck, the flap size is decreased.

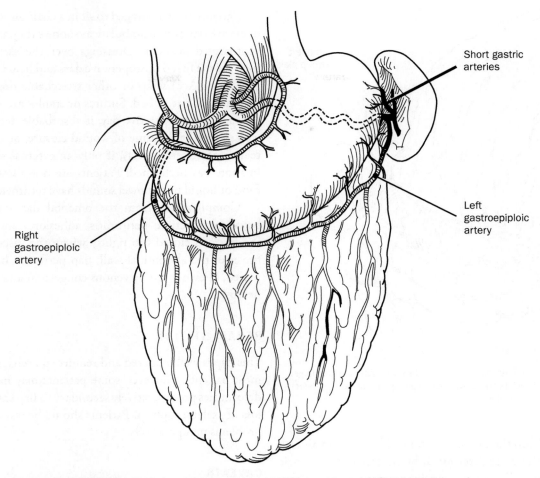

Figure 69.4. Blood supply to omentum arises from left and right gastroepiploic arteries and from short gastric arteries.

Short gastric arteries

Left gastroepiploic artery

Right gastroepiploic artery

A generous subcutaneous tunnel is created between the abdominal cavity and the sternal or chest wall defect. The omentum is passed through the tunnel and inset into the chest wall or sternal defect with absorbable suture. If there is any suspicion that the tunnel is too restrictive or may become restrictive later secondary to edema, the tunnel should be opened for its entire length and skin grafted with the omentum over the defect. Alternatively, the omentum may be passed through the diaphragmatic defect, if the patient has had a portion of the anterior diaphragm resected with the sternum. The diaphragmatic defect should be repaired so that the omental pedicle may pass through the diaphragm without restriction but a diaphragmatic hernia is prevented.

Before insetting the flap, chest tubes may be placed through stab incisions located on either side of the abdominal incision, if required. The abdominal incision is then closed with a strong permanent suture. To avoid compression of the vascular pedicle as it exits the abdomen, the fascia must not be closed too tightly around the vascular

pedicle, but it must be closed tightly enough to prevent a hernia. The abdominal skin is closed in the usual fashion. The omentum is then inset into the defect with absorbable suture, and a split-thickness skin graft is fixed over the omentum, using either staples or chromic gut suture (Figure 69.6).

Because of the delicate nature of the omental flap, we do not routinely place a bolster dressing to apply pressure to the skin graft. In most cases, a petroleum jelly gauze is applied over the graft followed by wet-to-wet dressings. The weight of these dressings applies sufficient pressure to the graft to ensure skin graft "take" without obstructing blood flow through the flap.

POSTOPERATIVE CARE

If the patient has significant medical problems or requires postoperative ventilation, the patient is taken to ICU until stable. Otherwise, most patients are returned to their hospital room after recovery from anesthesia. Chest tubes are

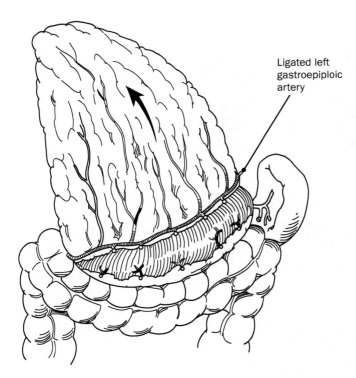

Figure 69.5. Ligation of left gastroepiploic artery and vein results in larger arc of rotation, which is sufficient to close almost any chest wall defect located below sternal manubrium.

Ligated left gastroepiploic artery

removed within the first 24–48 hours if there is no air leak or pneumothorax as determined by clinical and radiologic examination. All patients receive aggressive pulmonary care, consisting of incentive spirometry and deep breathing exercises.

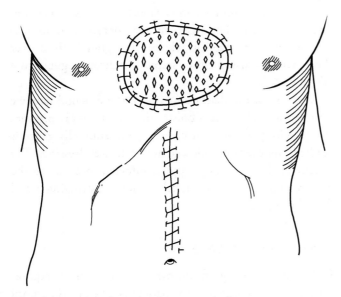

Figure 69.6. Omental flap is inset into defect and covered with skin graft. Chest tubes are placed, if indicated, and donor site incision is closed primarily.

Patients are encouraged to sit in a chair on the first postoperative day and to ambulate as soon as they are no longer ventilator-dependent. Dressings over the skin grafts are used for the first 5 postoperative days and held in place with an elastic (Ace) wrap or other stretchable dressing when patients get out of bed. Sutures or staples are removed on the eighth postoperative day, if absorbable dermal sutures were placed at the time of wound closure, or on the fourteenth postoperative day, if only an external skin approximation was performed. Patients are not allowed to have food or liquid until bowel sounds have returned.

Complications from the omental flap include ileus, bowel obstruction, peritonitis, adhesions, and hernia. If the fascia is closed too tightly where the vascular pedicle traverses the abdominal wall, flap perfusion becomes impaired, as evidenced by venous congestion and subsequent necrosis.

REHABILITATION

This flap is well tolerated and requires no rehabilitation for most patients. However, some patients may have contour deformities postoperatively secondary to flap shrinkage and loss of skeletal support. Patients should be warned of these problems preoperatively.

CAVEATS

The omental flap is very reliable as long as the surgeon carefully assesses the defect and thoroughly understands the flap's limitations. Also, the surgeon must make sure that the subcutaneous tunnel and fascial or diaphragmatic openings around the pedicle are not excessively tight and that there is sufficient room to allow for postoperative swelling, which can occlude blood flow.

RECTUS ABDOMINIS FLAP

ASSESSMENT OF THE DEFECT

The rectus abdominis muscle and its myocutaneous flaps have wide application in the reconstruction of anterior chest wall defects. Sternal wound infection after median sternotomy, radiation-induced chest wall necrosis, and tumors of the thorax make up most of the clinical scenarios requiring reconstruction of the anterior chest. As in other chest wall defects, chest wall stability and coverage of vital structures top the list of priorities. Consideration to chest wall stabilization before soft tissue coverage should be given to patients with more than four ribs resected and those patients undergoing total sternectomy. The depth of the wound and the thickness of the defect should be evaluated. The subcutaneous tissue of the anterior abdominal wall is thicker than that of the chest wall, and the advantages of harvesting the rectus muscle with or without its overlying subcutaneous layer and skin should be weighed.

Repair of the soft tissue defect in the chest is first determined by assessing the dimensions of the wound. The skin paddle of the myocutaneous flap should be planned well in advance of raising the flap by measuring and transposing the dimensions of the chest defect to the abdominal site. Selection of any flap must be based on the provision of an adequate amount of tissue in reasonable proximity to the wound. A superiorly based rectus abdominis flap rotates about a point just caudal to the costochondral arch and a few centimeters lateral to the midline. The length of the rectus muscle, especially if designed with a cutaneous component, can reach the entire anterior chest wall.

INDICATIONS

The rectus abdominis flap has first-line applicability for the reconstruction of lower sternal and parasternal defects and full-thickness anterolateral chest wall defects. The flap is useful in covering the heart and other lower mediastinal structures in those sternotomy patients with a long thoracic cage where coverage with pectoralis flaps is insufficient. The rectus abdominis is a thick and durable muscle and can be expected to provide adequate protection to vital mediastinal structures. In these and other cases where skin coverage is not an issue, transfer of the rectus muscle alone can provide vascularized bulk for dead space obliteration and the treatment of chronic or infected wounds.

When skin coverage or the repair of a deep defect is required, the vertical rectus abdominis myocutaneous (VRAM) or transverse rectus abdominis myocutaneous (TRAM) flaps are considered (Figure 69.7). The rectus muscle with a vertically oriented skin paddle is an extremely reliable flap with a straightforward dissection. It is the first choice for defects of lower sternal and parasternal regions that may require additional volume and skin replacement. Provided that the ipsilateral internal mammary vessels have not been disrupted or damaged during tumor resection, the blood supply to the flap is excellent. When this vessel has been divided, it is possible to raise the flap on the seventh and eighth intercostal arteries. The muscle can be expected to live on this secondary superior blood supply, but blood flow to overlying skin and subcutaneous tissues may be tenuous, and a skin paddle should be considered unreliable

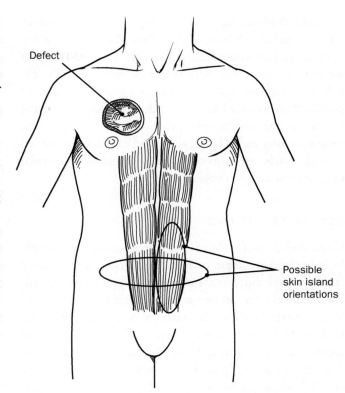

Figure 69.7. For moderate- to large-sized chest wall defects located on one side or other of sternum, vertical or transverse rectus abdominis myocutaneous (VRAM or TRAM, respectively) flap is good reconstructive option. To ensure flap viability, blood supply of flap should be based on contralateral muscle.

in this setting. With intact internal mammary vessels, a myocutaneous flap with a very large skin component can be raised, making this flap a workhorse in the reconstruction of large anterior chest wall defects. With sufficient planning, the donor site can be closed primarily even in very thin patients. Ipsilateral shift of the umbilicus will occur and should be discussed with the patient preoperatively.

The TRAM flap has become the flap of choice for postmastectomy breast reconstruction. This flap can transfer a very large amount of tissue to the chest wall in a relatively reliable manner with less of a donor site deformity than the VRAM flap. The skin portion of the TRAM flap, however, enjoys a less vigorous blood supply than that of the VRAM flap. The portion of the skin paddle located across the midline may be vascularly compromised, especially in patients with a history of smoking or obesity. A double-pedicled transverse rectus flap proves much more reliable in the transfer of a large, bilateral abdominal skin paddle to the chest. Because of the width of the skin paddle, the transverse rectus flap has a wider arc of rotation and the spectrum of reconstructible defects is larger than in the vertically designed flap.

The free rectus flap, based on the inferior epigastric artery and vein, has been well described. The use of this flap in chest wall reconstruction is, however, limited. The great majority of chest wall defects can be repaired with reliable pedicled flaps. Still, there are cases where the standard pedicle flap options have been exhausted and use of the free rectus flap may be appropriate. The inferior epigastric vessels are long and of large caliber and can be anastomosed to neck vessels, remnants of the internal mammary vasculature, or even the great vessels.

CONTRAINDICATIONS

Contraindications to the use of the rectus abdominis muscle include the destruction or high transection of the muscle from previous abdominal surgery or the presence of an ipsilateral intestinal or urinary ostomy. A relative, but compelling, contraindication is the removal or obliteration of the ipsilateral internal mammary artery and vein. As discussed earlier, the transfer of a rectus abdominis myocutaneous flap with an absent ipsilateral mammary artery should be avoided, although the rotation of a muscle-only flap is usually safe. Transfer of a rectus abdominis myocutaneous flap is contraindicated in a patient who has previously undergone a significant abdominal wall undermining procedure, such as an abdominoplasty. Preoperative radiation to the chest, in which portals may have included internal mammary vessels, was previously thought to be a contraindication to harvesting of the rectus muscle based on its superior blood supply. Recent work has shown that the rectus muscle can be reliably elevated on an intact internal mammary–superior epigastric axis even with a history of direct radiation to the vessel.

Use of a transversely oriented skin paddle on the rectus muscle (TRAM flap) is relatively contraindicated in obese patients and smokers. All skin and subcutaneous tissue on the opposite side of the midline is at risk of necrosis. Even the lateral projection of skin and soft tissue on the ipsilateral side can be at risk in patients with significant small vessel disease.

ROOM SETUP

The rectus muscle is best harvested with the patient placed in the supine position. Chest wall defects that extend laterally around the thorax may require the patient to be placed in a one-quarter lateral decubitus position. This can provide access to the chest wall defect and also leave the abdominal wall adequately exposed for muscle harvest. When this type of positioning is used, the arm ipsilateral to the defect can

be prepared into the field or can be abducted and flexed and fixed to a sterile-covered Mayo stand. If the surgery is to be performed with the patient in a supine position, arms should be fully abducted and fixed to armboards.

The chest and abdomen should be shaved, and the preparation should encompass the entire chest (including shoulders and axillary region), abdomen, and groin.

PATIENT MARKINGS

Harvesting the rectus muscle only for chest wall reconstruction should be performed through a right paramedian incision. This incision, designed approximately 3 cm lateral to the midline, provides adequate access to the anterior surface of the muscle as well as adequate medial and lateral access in raising the flap. At its superior aspect, the incision may be connected directly with the thoracic defect or the muscle may be passed through a comfortably sized subcutaneous tunnel in the xiphoid region.

If a cutaneous component to the flap is required, the dimensions of the defect on the chest wall should be measured and a template should be made and transposed to the appropriate location on the abdominal wall. Relatively long, thin defects (especially those oriented in a cephalocaudal direction) are best repaired with the VRAM flap (Figure 69.8). Horizontally oriented skin defects, unless immediately adjacent to the upper abdomen, are often best reconstructed with the TRAM flap. Since most of the musculocutaneous perforating vessels are centered around the umbilicus, the design of any skin paddle should include this region to maximize the number of perforating vessels captured. Some reconciliation between an oddly shaped defect and the creation of a donor wound that can be sufficiently closed must be made. Often the cutaneous portion of the TRAM flap is designed in the standard elliptical fashion, the size of which accommodates a pattern for a particular chest wall defect, and the excess can be trimmed away. The donor site in this case can be closed in a simple and reliable fashion.

SURGICAL TECHNIQUE: RECTUS MUSCLE FLAP

A paramedian incision is made and dissection is carried down to the level of the anterior rectus fascia, which is incised vertically approximately 2–3 cm lateral to the linea alba, exposing the muscle underneath. The anterior rectus sheath with skin and subcutaneous tissue intact is lifted off the muscle. The medial border of the rectus muscle is identified and dissected in a cephalic and caudal direction. The tendinous inscriptions are sharply divided closely to lateral neurovascular contributions to the muscle should be identified and divided, taking care not to inadvertently damage the superior epigastric vessels. Previous obliteration of the internal mammary vessels, however, mandates identification and careful preservation of these uppermost intercostal vascular contributions. Division of the muscle from the costochondral arch is the final step. Since the blood supply to the muscle emerges *posterior* to the thoracic cage, division of the muscle should take place on the *anterior* surface of the lowest rib. Careful downward traction of the muscle and transection of muscle fibers over the anterior surface of the lowermost aspect of the thoracic cage will prevent inadvertent damage to the vascular pedicle. The superior epigastric vasculature can now be identified. Any remaining attachments can be divided, and the muscle is now free to rotate into the chest. As noted, the donor and recipient sites can be connected by a skin incision, or a generous subcutaneous tunnel can be created through which the muscle may be passed.

SURGICAL TECHNIQUE: VERTICAL RECTUS ABDOMINIS (VRAM) FLAP

If a cutaneous component is planned with the rectus flap, a vertically oriented skin paddle is first designed over the surface of the muscle (Figure 69.8). Even in thin patients, a skin paddle with a width of 9 cm will permit adequate donor site closure. After skin incisions are made, dissection toward the center of the flap (in a medial direction for the lateral incision and a lateral direction for the medial incision) should be undertaken at the level just above the fascia. The medial and lateral rows of perforators are approximately 4 cm apart and the width of anterior rectus fascia that must be sacrificed is equal to or more than this. Time taken to identify the medial and lateral rows will, however, allow the surgeon to decide whether the blood supply of the skin island can be based on a single row of perforators and thus save sufficient fascia for a tension-free primary closure. If both rows of perforators are required for the blood supply, the surgeon should be prepared to repair the missing anterior rectus sheath with an inlay or onlay of acellular dermal bioprosthetic implant. Care should be taken to design the skin incision around the umbilicus. The umbilicus itself, plus a small amount of subcutaneous tissue at its base, should be maintained.

When a muscle-only flap is harvested and there is minimal subcutaneous undermining, the anterior rectus sheath can be closed directly and the wound need not be drained. If there is significant subcutaneous undermining (as is usually the case in the harvest of a myocutaneous flap), the

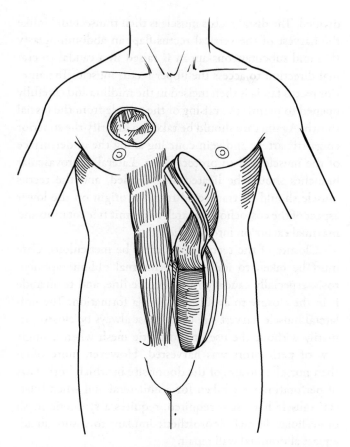

Figure 69.8. The skin island is elevated with muscle and passed through a subcutaneous tunnel dissected between donor site and chest wall defect. One or more closed suction drains are placed to drain both surgical sites before closure.

the muscle surface. Care must be taken not to disrupt vasculature, which can be quite superficial at the level of the inscriptions. The anterior rectus sheath is then raised laterally. Care should be taken to identify, ligate, and divide the neurovascular bundles, which enter the muscle along its posterolateral surface. The muscle may then be raised entirely to the pubic ramus or may be divided at the level of the arcuate line. If this is done, suturing of the cut upper edge of the inferior rectus muscle to the arcuate line is suggested to help prevent abdominal wall herniation below this level. If the entire muscle is harvested, the inferior epigastric artery and vein are ligated and transected. Leaving an adequate length of the epigastric artery and vein on the muscle flap provides the opportunity for microsurgically "supercharging" the flap in the chest, although this is more applicable to the TRAM flap with its precarious skin paddle. The flap is then carefully raised in a caudad to cephalad direction, taking care to identify the epigastric vessels, which run on the undersurface of the muscle. If the internal mammary artery is intact, the upper anterior rectus sheath should be repaired and the potential space above it should be drained postoperatively. Mesh closure in this situation is rarely indicated.

SURGICAL TECHNIQUE: TRANSVERSE RECTUS ABDOMINIS (TRAM) FLAP

In designing the cutaneous portion of the TRAM flap, care must be taken to maximize the number of musculocutaneous perforators included in the flap. The vascular pattern of these perforators is well understood. Since there is a predominance of perforating vessels in the periumbilical region, the skin paddle must include this area. Whether a mid-abdominal skin ellipse or a lower abdominal skin ellipse is planned is not so important, as long as an adequate number of periumbilical perforators are included. The upper line of the ellipse should pass above the umbilicus. The apices at the lateral extents of the design of the ellipse are oriented at the level of the anterior-superior iliac spines. The lower incisional component of the TRAM flap ellipse can vary in its positioning. The best way to estimate this placement is by slightly flexing the table and gripping the lower abdominal skin and subcutaneous tissue with both hands to assess the amount of flap tissue to be harvested. Corresponding points on the abdominal wall skin should be marked, which will help plan the proper positioning of the inferior curve of the ellipse. Conservative estimation of the placement of this line rarely leaves the surgeon in a situation in which donor site closure is difficult.

After the flap is outlined on the abdominal wall, the incisions for the TRAM flap are made and dissection is carried out on both sides of the flap in a lateral to medial direction. The umbilicus is circumcised and a plug of fat is left at the base of the umbilicus to ensure its viability. The contralateral aspect of the flap is elevated first. Dissection is carried above the abdominal fascia medially to the linea alba, ligating all perforators from the contralateral rectus muscle. Dissection is then carried across the linea alba for approximately 1 cm until the medial row of perforators from the donor rectus muscle is identified. The rectus sheath is then incised vertically, just medial to this row of perforators. Once the red muscle of the rectus abdominis is identified through a small fascial window, a hemostat and cautery or fine scissors can be used to open the fascia vertically. A similar lateral to medial dissection of the skin paddle lateral to the muscle is also performed until the lateral perforator row is identified. Similarly, only that fascia required to maintain the musculocutaneous perforators should be sacrificed. The inferior epigastric artery and vein should be dissected free to the level of the iliac vessels and

divided. The distal rectus muscle is then transected. Unlike the harvest of the vertical rectus flap, an abdominoplasty skin and subcutaneous apron is raised in a caudal to cranial direction to access the upper rectus muscle. The anterior rectus fascia is then incised in the midline and carefully opened to permit the raising of the muscle from the fascial sheath. Again, care should be taken to identify the superior epigastric artery and vein coursing along the undersurface of the muscle and to protect them. Lateral neurovascular branches should be ligated and divided, and the rectus muscle should be transected from its origin on the lower aspect of the costochondral arch to permit free rotation and maximal excursion into the chest.

Closure of the rectus fascia must be meticulous. Care must be taken to identify the internal oblique aponeurosis, especially caudal to the arcuate line, and to include it in the closure to avoid later hernia formation. The unilateral muscle harvest site can almost always be closed primarily without the use of prosthetic mesh when a single row of perforators was harvested. However, more often than not, the closure of the donor site in which both rows of perforators were taken for a unilateral and when bilateral muscle harvest is required, requires a synthetic mesh or acellular dermal bioprosthetic implant to ensure an adequate abdominal wall repair.

POSTOPERATIVE CARE

Rectus flaps that are used for chest wall reconstruction should be monitored as any muscle or musculocutaneous flap. Obviously, those flaps that are buried cannot be visually inspected to check their status. Buried flap monitoring systems, which may be useful in monitoring free tissue transfers, are of limited value in monitoring buried pedicle flaps. These flaps are most often subject to partial flap loss, which may not be detected through any internal monitoring system. Those flaps transferred for surface coverage should be evaluated regularly for warmth, edema, color, and capillary refill. Hematoma formation around the vascular pedicle or edema within a subcutaneous tunnel may contribute to flap compromise. Regular observation and quick and deliberate response predicts the salvage of most of these flaps. Drains in the deeper subcutaneous tissues should be removed when total daily drainage does not exceed 35 mL per drain.

REHABILITATION

Patients who undergo the harvest of one or both rectus muscles should be cautioned to avoid unnecessary exertion for 6 weeks. Patients may walk about and go up and down stairs with care, but any lifting or straining is prohibited. Adequate fascial healing can be expected at 6 weeks, and the patient may begin a therapy-guided program to return to normal daily and athletic activities. It is recommended that patients in whom the rectus abdominis muscle has been harvested undergo a graduated program of abdominal strengthening after the initial 6-week period. Nearly all patients return to their normal preoperative levels of abdominal strength and power after the harvest of this muscle.

CAVEATS

The rectus abdominis muscle and myocutaneous flaps are highly dependable and versatile for use in chest wall repair. Such flaps are almost always available for use as a pedicled flap and can be transferred in a variety of configurations to suitably reconstruct many lower and lateral thoracic defects. A few points must be reemphasized:

1. Obliteration of the ipsilateral internal mammary vessels may preclude use of the flap with a cutaneous paddle.

2. Skin defect dimensions of the chest wound should be transferred to the abdomen, taking care to include the perforator-dense region near the umbilicus.

3. Only anterior rectus fascia, including essential perforating vessels, should be sacrificed.

4. Meticulous abdominal fascial closure (inclusive of the internal oblique layer) is imperative.

PECTORALIS MAJOR MUSCLE FLAP

ASSESSMENT OF THE DEFECT

The pectoralis major muscle is most useful for the reconstruction of the lower neck, the upper anterior chest (specifically the upper two thirds of the sternal area), and the shoulder and axillary areas. Because of its relatively long length as an island muscle flap (30 cm after mobilization), the muscle is also useful for intrathoracic use.

ANATOMY

The pectoralis major muscle is a thick, broad, fan-shaped muscle with both clavicular and sternal components. The clavicular portion of the muscle originates in the medial one-half to two-thirds of the clavicle, traveling laterally, forming the anterior lamina of the muscle that inserts on the bicipital humeral groove. The sternal portion of the muscle originates from the anterior surface of the sternum from ribs two through six. As one follows it superolaterally, it forms the middle and posterior laminae, which also insert on the bicipital groove. The muscle's vascular anatomy is similar to that of the latissimus dorsi muscle, in which the thick superior lateral aspect of the muscle is fed by a single dominant vascular pedicle and the broad, flat medial region is fed by a series of segmental perforators. When raised, the entire muscle can be expected to live on either of these vascular systems. This vascular anatomy makes the muscle particularly useful and gives the operator significant flexibility with flap design, rotation, and transfer.

INDICATIONS

Because of the large number of median sternotomies for open heart surgery, the pectoralis major muscle is most commonly used for the closure of sternal dehiscences. Tumor resection or trauma that leaves a significant soft tissue or bony defect in the upper two-thirds of the chest can also be repaired with the pectoralis muscle. Because it is thick, broad, and well-vascularized and has an excellent arc of rotation in the upper chest, it can be used to cover mesh or rib grafts used in chest wall reconstruction, or it can be passed into the thorax to cover bronchopleural fistulae, obliterate dead space, and separate or protect vital structures.

The muscle can also be harvested as a myocutaneous flap by including overlying skin. The donor site of small skin paddles can often be concealed in the inframammary or former subpectoral fold, but the harvesting of a large segment of skin requires skin grafting. Such grafting is likely to be placed directly onto the thoracic wall, however, which is often undesirable. Caution must also be taken in women in whom breast tissue will be interposed between the muscle and skin of a myocutaneous flap, compromising the dependability of the overlying skin. Vascularized clavicle and vascularized rib can also be included in the elevation of the pectoralis muscle. Often used for soft and hard tissue reconstruction in the head and neck, such myo-osseous flaps have limited use in the chest. However, if the transfer of muscle with one or two relatively short segments of bone is required, this flap may be so designed.

Upper central chest defects with a large dead space may require the use of both pectoralis muscles. Each muscle may be raised on the thoraco-acromial vessels superolaterally and advanced into an upper sternal wound defect as a so-called *sliding pectoralis flap*. One or both of the pectoralis muscles (depending on the status of the internal mammary artery) may be raised on the medial segmental vasculature and "rolled over" into the defect. Many surgeons use a combination of these techniques for the obliteration of a large upper midline chest defect, where one pectoralis flap is raised on an intact internal mammary system and rolled into the defect, while the contralateral muscle is elevated on its thoraco-acromial artery and slid over the first pectoralis muscle to augment bulk and provide further coverage.

CONTRAINDICATIONS

Absolute contraindications to the use of the pectoralis muscle flap in chest wall reconstruction are (1) congenital or acquired absence of the muscle, (2) a chest wound substantially outside the arc of rotation of the muscle, and (3) the absence or obliteration of both vascular pedicles. Relative contraindications include a surgical or traumatic scar dividing or crossing a substantial portion of the muscle belly, loss of function of the other major muscles of the shoulder girdle, the obliteration of one set of vascular pedicles (mandating raising of the flap on its remaining vasculature), and the requirement for a large myocutaneous flap, which would leave a donor site requiring skin grafting.

ROOM SETUP

Patients who are to have one or both pectoralis muscles harvested should be placed in the supine position with arms abducted and firmly fixed to armboards. The entire anterior thorax, axillae, and shoulder regions should be prepared and draped into the operative field. If the muscle is to be harvested from a midsternal incision, long instruments, including a set of lighted retractors, are mandatory. The operator may also choose to wear a surgical headlight to provide adequate visualization into what will be a deep and dark surgical cavity.

PATIENT MARKINGS

When one or both pectoralis muscles are harvested to repair sternal defects, each of the muscles can be accessed from the edge of the wound itself, and often no surface markings are required. Many operators prefer to release the insertion of the pectoralis muscle at the anterior axillary fold through a separate counterincision. This incision may be designed by grasping the pectoralis muscle between the thumb and forefinger where it forms the anterior axillary fold at the level of the apex of the axilla. A vertical incision 6–8 cm in length should be marked on the skin over the muscle at this region. The inferior aspect of this incision should curve down over the caudal aspect of the muscle toward the axillary fossa. The upper pole of the incision is extended to the deltopectoral groove, which may be digitally palpated.

If the pectoralis muscle is not to be harvested via a preexisting sternal wound, it may be (1) approached from the margin by another thoracic wound to be repaired or (2) harvested through a separate incision. Depending on the choice of vascular supply, the location of the thoracic defect and the plan for inclusion of a cutaneous paddle, incisions may be varied. A most useful incision is often placed along the lateral border of the pectoralis muscle. This can be curved medially under the breast in the subpectoral groove on a male or in the inframammary fold on a female. Through this incision, adequate access to the entire surface of the muscle can be gained, and the muscle can then be raised on either set of vascular pedicles.

In a male, the design of a cutaneous paddle should be centered on a line drawn from the tip of the acromion to the xiphoid process. This line represents the course of the pectoral branch of the thoracoacromial artery. The donor site for a skin paddle of 8 cm in width can be expected to be closed in most individuals (Figure 69.9).

SURGICAL TECHNIQUE

In those patients with sternal wounds, the muscle is best raised in a medial to lateral fashion. Dissection should begin at the sternal wound edge by identifying the plane between the subcutaneous tissue of the chest wall and the anterior surface of the pectoralis fascia. Dissection over the surface of the pectoralis fascia continues in a superolateral direction toward the axilla. The entire anterior surface of the muscle should be exposed. Dissection near the insertion of the muscle can be difficult from the medial approach. In most patients, the placement of a counterincision over the anterior axillary fold is recommended. From this vantage, the anterior surface of the muscle in this region can be exposed by elevating the subcutaneous tissue, and this zone of dissection can then be connected to the primary zone. The muscle is now raised from the chest wall. Because the muscle inserts on the anterior surface of the sternum and on the upper portion of the external oblique aponeurosis, establishing the correct submuscular plane of dissection can initially be difficult, working in the medial to lateral direction. Inspection of the lateral aspect of the pectoralis muscle, however, reveals an easily identifiable subpectoral plane, which can be entered by the surgeon's fingers. It is suggested that the raising of the muscle itself be initiated

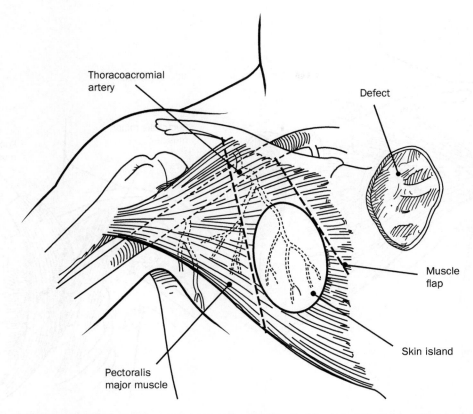

Thoracoacromial
artery

Defect

Muscle
flap

Skin island

Pectoralis
major muscle

Figure 69.9. To ensure viability of skin island of pectoralis major myocutaneous flap, the skin island should be designed just medial to nipple and must be large enough to capture as many cutaneous perforating blood vessels as possible. Even if skin defect is small, a large skin island is designed; unneeded portion of skin island is de-epithelialized and buried under intact skin.

by retracting the skin of the chest wall and raising the lower portion of the pectoralis muscle in a lateral to medial direction, where this initial plane of dissection is readily identifiable. As the dissection progresses superolaterally, the muscle becomes easier to raise. Care must be taken to identify the pectoralis minor muscle and leave it in situ. Dissection along the anterior surface of the pectoralis minor muscle leads the operator to the pectoralis minor branch of the thoraco-acromial artery. This is a reliable way to locate this pedicle. This vessel must be divided close to the surface of the pectoralis minor muscle to avoid damaging the artery's main trunk. The medial portion of the clavicular head of the muscle is then dissected off the clavicle, again working in a medial to lateral fashion. Care must be taken when approaching the junction of the medial and lateral thirds of the clavicle, where not only do the thoracoacromial artery and vein emerge, but the subclavian vein can be found just deep to this landmark. The safest dissection in this region may therefore proceed in a lateral to medial direction. If used, the counterincision is accessed to divide the muscle's insertion. Care is taken to identify and spare the cephalic vein. After division, the thick head of the muscle can be grasped with an Allis or Babcock forceps and rolled

into the medial wound. Careful dissection of the upper portion of the muscle then proceeds. The thoracoacromial artery should be identified as it exits the subclavicular space and enters the underside of the pectoralis major muscle. All muscle fibers lateral to this vessel are expendable and should in fact be divided to maximize excursion of the muscle flap. Careful inspection of the pedicle reveals that its initial course as it emerges from deep in the subclavicular space is in an inferolateral direction before it turns back medially to course downward in the direction of the pectoralis fibers. Careful dissection of connective tissues lateral to the "elbow" of this vessel will permit the surgeon to straighten the pedicle and maximize its length. All of the tough, muscular attachments to the clavicle should be divided to fully mobilize the pectoralis muscle flap.

The first phase in raising the pectoralis muscle that is to be based medially is identical to that described earlier (Figure 69.10). The entire anterior surface should be dissected free of overlying subcutaneous tissue. The muscle must, of course, be left attached to the chest wall at its medial aspect. Raising of the muscle, therefore, should begin with division of the insertion at the anterior axillary fold. Again, a small counterincision in this region is highly useful. Once

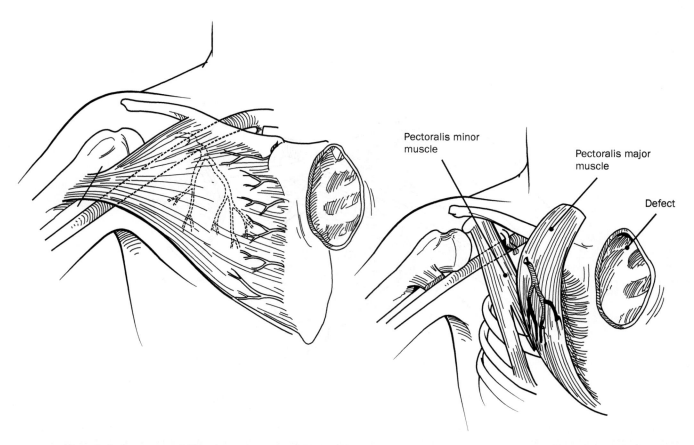

Pectoralis minor muscle

Pectoralis major muscle

Defect

Figure 69.10. Alternatively, thoracoacromial blood vessels may be divided, and insertion and clavicular attachments of pectoralis major muscle may be dissected so that muscle can be reflected into sternal defect immediately adjacent to sternum. Because blood supply to this design of pectoralis major flap depends on integrity of intercostal perforating blood vessels coming up from internal mammary blood vessels, and because undersurface of muscle will be exposed, skin island is not possible and muscle must be skin-grafted. This type of repair is contraindicated if internal mammary vessels were previously used for coronary bypass procedure or ligated during tumor resection.

the muscle has been divided, it is carefully dissected off the chest wall in a lateral to medial direction. This is a well-defined plane and dissection proceeds smoothly. When the thoraco-acromial artery and vein are encountered entering the underside of the pectoralis muscle, they are ligated and divided. The muscle is then further retracted medially while the fibrous attachments to the clavicle are carefully divided. The filmy attachments to the chest wall from the lower aspect of the muscle are likewise divided. As the muscle is rolled medially, perforating vessels from the internal mammary artery projecting from the intercostal spaces come into view. Care should be taken to identify and protect these vessels. No attachments medial to these perforators need be divided since these vessels themselves limit the medial transposition of the muscle (Figure 69.10).

If a myocutaneous flap is planned, the skin paddle should be designed either (1) as described earlier (Figure 69.9) or (2) in the inframammary region, centered over the inframammary fold. If the ellipse is centered over a line connecting the acromion to the xiphoid process, an

inferomedial and superolateral extension from the central skin paddle is used for access to the muscle. The skin is incised down to muscle, circumscribing the ellipse and extending the incision to the anterior axillary fold. Skin flaps are elevated and the muscle is exposed (Figure 69.9). Submuscular dissection is then initiated from lateral to medial, dividing the inferior attachments first and working up the lateral aspect of the sternum, dividing muscular fibers and ligating perforating vessels. Maximal mobilization is again achieved by dividing the insertion of the pectoralis muscle and freeing all clavicular attachments. Again, the thoraco-acromial artery should be identified emerging from the subclavicular fossa and entering the pectoralis muscle on its posterior surface (Figure 69.11).

All major areas of dissection should be drained with closed suction drains. Since the patient will be supine for a period of time, drainage of dependent spaces, such as mediastinal depressions, certain intrathoracic locations, and axillary regions, should be included. Sternal dead space obliterations should be well drained above and below

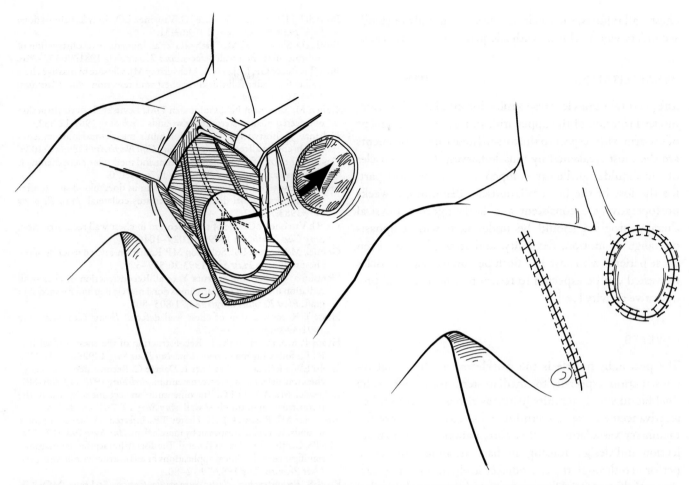

Figure 69.11. Portion of pectoralis major muscle that contains skin island is carefully dissected to include branch of thoracoacromial blood vessels supplying flap. Subcutaneous tunnel is dissected from pectoralis major donor site to defect, and flap is transposed and inset in defect. One or more closed suction drains are placed to drain both surgical sites before closure.

the muscle flap. All wounds should be closed in layers. Those sternotomy wounds that have been opened for a prolonged period of time may have scarred and retracted edges, making skin closure tighter than is desirable. In such cases, it is recommended that large-gauge monofilament, nonabsorbable sutures be placed as "stay sutures" to reinforce the closure and support the suture line during healing. These can be left in place, if needed, for 4–6 weeks while the tensile strength of the wound improves.

POSTOPERATIVE CARE

Postoperative dressings may be removed on the second day and suture lines cleansed with half-strength hydrogen peroxide solution. Some surgeons support the discontinuation of intravenous antibiotic therapy soon after surgery if there has been adequate debridement of the sternum. Others promote a prolonged course of intravenous antibiotic therapy to treat those patients with a diagnosis

of sternal osteomyelitis. If the osteomyelitis is not long-standing and if aggressive debridement of nonviable bone and cartilage from the chest wound has been undertaken, it is reasonable to discontinue antibiotics after a brief perioperative course.

Drains should undergo regular care and output measurements. They can be removed when daily output falls below 35 mL per day. Extra care must be taken with drains that communicate with intrathoracic spaces since these drains need to be maintained on constant low suction to discourage the development of pneumothorax until they are removed.

Any areas of superficial wound separation should be treated by the removal of skin sutures in the affected area, frequent wound irrigations, and light gauze packing. Correctly performed, muscle flap chest wall reconstruction provides adequate coverage of all deep vital structures. A significant wound separation would therefore, at worst, expose healthy skeletal muscle. Even in radiation-induced chest wall injuries, such a clinical scenario usually portends secondary wound closure with adequate conservative care.

REHABILITATION

The pectoralis muscle is responsible for shoulder adduction, internal rotation of the upper arm, and anterior movement of the arm with respect to the torso. These three movements are the most weakened by muscle harvest. Other muscles of the shoulder girdle can compensate, for the most part, for the loss of the pectoralis muscle. Beginning 6 weeks postoperatively, a consistent and fairly rigorous physical therapy program should be undertaken with emphasis on range of motion, flexibility, and strengthening. Even those patients who have had both pectoralis major muscles harvested can be expected to return to a near-normal preoperative activity level.

CAVEATS

The pectoralis muscle is the workhorse of chest wall reconstruction, especially for median sternotomy defects. Its dual blood supply permits its use as either a "turnover" or an advancement flap. Determining the status of the internal mammary vasculature is, therefore, paramount in flap selection and design. Raising the flap can almost always be performed through the chest defect itself, minimizing scarring and the potential for poor wound healing and skin flap necrosis. Division of the muscle's insertion medial to the humerus is recommended in virtually all cases to maximize mobility of the flap.

SELECTED READINGS

Al-Captain KM, Breach NM, Kaplan DO, Goldstraw P. Soft tissue reconstruction in thoracic surgery. *Ann Thoracic Surg* 1995;60: 1372–1375.

Alday ES, Goldsmith HS. Surgical technique for omental lengthening based on arterial anatomy. *Surg Gynecol Obstet* 1972;135:103.

Arnold PG, Lovich SF, Pairolero PC. Muscle flaps in irradiated wounds: an account of 100 consecutive cases. *Plast Reconstr Surg* 1994;93:324–327.

Arnold PG, Pairolero PC. Intrathoracic muscle flaps in the surgical management of life-threatening hemorrhage from the heart and great vessels. *Plast Reconstr Surg* 1988;81:831.

Arnold PG, Pairolero PC. Reconstruction of the radiation-damaged chest wall. *Surg Clin North Am* 1989;69:1081–1089.

Arnold PG, Pairolero PC. Surgical management of the radiated chest wall. *Plast Reconstr Surg* 1986;77:605–612.

Arnold PG, Pairolero PC. Use of pectoralis major muscle flaps to repair defects of anterior chest wall. *Plast Reconstr Surg* 1979;63:205.

Bobin JY, Crozet B, Ranchere JY. Using the costal muscle flap with latissimus dorsi muscle to repair full-thickness anterior chest wall defects. *Ann Plast Surg* 1988;20:471–476.

Bostwick J III, Nahai F, Wallace JG, Vasconez LO. Sixty latissimus dorsi flaps. *Plast Reconstr Surg* 1979;63:31.

Boyd AD, Shaw WW, McCarthy JG, et al. Immediate reconstruction of full-thickness chest wall defects. *Ann Thorac Surg* 1981;32:337–346.

Bury TF, Reece GP, Janjan NA, McMurtrey MJ. Closure of massive chest wall defects after full-thickness chest wall resection. *Ann Plast Surg* 1995;34:409–414.

Cohen M, Silverman NA, Goldfaden DM, Levitsky S. Reconstruction of infected median sternotomy wounds. *Arch Surg* 1987;122:323.

Coleman JJ, Bostwick J. Rectus abdominis muscle-musculocutaneous flaps in chest wall reconstruction. *Surg Clin North Am* 1989;667:1029.

Das SK. The size of the human omentum and methods of lengthening it for transplantation. *Br J Plast Surg* 1976;29:170.

Fisher J, Bostwick J III, Powell RW. Latissimus dorsi blood supply after thoracodorsal vessel division: the serratus collateral. *Plast Reconstr Surg* 1983;72;502.

Fix RJ, Vasconez LO. Use of the omentum in chest-wall reconstruction. *Surg Clin North Am* 1989;69:1029–1046.

Granick MS, Larson DL, Solomon MP. Radiation-related wounds of the chest wall. *Clin Plast Surg* 1993;20:559–571.

Harashina T, Takayama S, Ikuta Y, et al. Reconstruction of chest-wall radiation ulcer with free latissimus dorsi muscle flap and meshed skin graft. *Plast Reconstr Surg* 1983;71:805–808.

Hasse J. Reconstruction of chest wall defects. *Thorac Cardiovas Surg* 1991;39(suppl 3):241–247.

Hyans P, Moore JH, Sinha L. Reconstruction of the chest wall with e-PTFE following major resection. *Ann Plast Surg* 1992;29:321–327.

Jacobs EW, Hoffman S, Kirschner P, Danese C. Reconstruction of a large chest wall defect using greater omentum. *Arch Surg* 1978;113:886–887.

Jurkiewicz MJ, Arnold PG. The omentum: an account of its use in the reconstruction of the chest wall. *Ann Surg* 1977;185:548–554.

Jurkiewicz MJ, Bostwick J III, Hester TR. Infected median sternotomy wounds: successful treatment by muscle flaps. *Ann Surg* 1980;191:738.

Kim PS, Gottlieb JR, Harris GD, et al. The dorsal thoracic fascia: anatomic significance with clinical applications in reconstructive microsurgery. *Plast Reconstr Surg* 1987;79:72–80.

Kroll S. *Reconstructive Plastic Surgery for Cancer.* St Louis, MO: CV Mosby, 1996.

Kroll SS, Schusterman MA, Larson DL, et al. Long-term survival after chest-wall reconstruction with musculocutaneous flaps. *Plast Reconstr Surg* 1990;86:697–701.

Kroll SS, Walsh G, Ryan B, et al. Risks and benefits of using Marlex mesh in chest wall reconstruction. *Ann Plast Surg* 1993;31:303–306.

Larson DL, McMurtrey MJ. Chest wall reconstruction. *Adv Plast Reconstr Surg* 1987;2:217–244.

Larson DL, McMurtrey MJ. Musculocutaneous flap reconstruction of chest wall defects: an experience with 50 patients. *Plast Reconstr Surg* 1984;73:734–740.

Larson DL, McMurtrey MJ, Howe HJ, Irish CE. Major chest wall reconstruction after chest wall irradiation. *Cancer* 1982;49:1286–1293.

Magee WP, McCraw JB, Horton CE, et al. Pectoralis "paddle" myocutaneous flaps, the workhorse of head and neck reconstruction. *Am J Surg* 1980;140:507.

Maxwell GP, McGibbon BM, Hoopes JE. Vascular considerations in the use of a latissimus dorsi myocutaneous flap after a mastectomy with an axillary dissection. *Plast Reconstr Surg* 1979;64:771.

McCormack PM. Use of prosthetic materials in chest-wall reconstruction. *Surg Clin North Am* 1989;69:965–973.

McCraw JB, Arnold PG. *Atlas of Muscle and Musculocutaneous Flaps.* Norfolk, VA: Hampton Press, 1986:265.

McCraw JB, Penix JO, Baker JW. Repair of major defects of the chest wall and spine with the latissimus dorsi myocutaneous flap. *Plast Reconstr Surg* 1978;62:197.

Miller LB, Bostwick J III, Hartrampf CR, et al. The superiorly based rectus abdominis flap: predicting and enhancing its blood supply based on an anatomic and clinical study. *Plast Reconstr Surg* 1988;81:713.

Miyamoto Y, Hattori T, Niimoto M, Toge T. Reconstruction of full-thickness chest wall defects using rectus abdominis musculocutaneous flap. *Ann Plast Surg* 1986;16:90–97.

Nahai F, Morales L, Bone DK, Bostwick J III. Pectoralis major muscle turnover flaps for closure of the infected sternotomy wound with preservation of form and function. *Plast Reconstr Surg* 1982;70:471.

Neal HW, Kreilein JG, Schreiber JT, Gregory RO. Complete sternectomy for chronic osteomyelitis with reconstruction using a rectus abdominis myocutaneous island flap. *Ann Plast Reconstr Surg* 1981;6:305.

Pairolero PC, Arnold PG. Bronchopleural fistula: treatment by transposition of pectoralis major muscle. *J Thorac Cardiovasc Surg* 1980;79:142.

Pairolero PC, Arnold PG. Thoracic wall defects: surgical management of 205 consecutive patients. *Mayo Clin Proc* 1986;61:557.

Pierce WS, Tyers GFO, Waldhausen JA. Effective isolation of a tracheostomy from a median sternotomy wound. *J Thorac Cardiovasc Surg* 1973;66:841.

Press BHJ. Reconstruction of a large chest wall defect with a musculocutaneous free flap using anterolateral thigh musculature. *Ann Plast Surg* 1988;20:238–241.

Roswell AR, Davies DM, Eisenberg N, Taylor GI. The anatomy of the subscapular-thoracodorsal arterial system: study of 100 cadaver dissections. *Br J Plast Surg* 1984;37:574.

Roswell AR, Eisenberg N, Davies DM, Taylor GI. The anatomy of the thoracodorsal artery within the latissimus dorsi muscle. *Br J Plast Surg* 1986;39:206.

Rouanet P, Fabre JM, Tica V, et al. Chest wall reconstruction for radionecrosis after breast carcinoma therapy. *Ann Plast Surg* 1995;34:465–470.

Samuels L, Granick MS, Ramasastry S, et al. Reconstruction of radiation-induced chest wall lesions. *Ann Plast Surg* 1993;31:399–405.

Spear SL, Oldham RJ. A lengthened omental pedicle in facial reconstruction. *Plast Reconstr Surg* 1986;77:828.

Tobin GR. Pectoralis major muscle-musculocutaneous flaps for chest wall reconstruction. *Surg Clin North Am* 1989;69:991.

Tobin GR, Bland KI, Adcock R. Surgical anatomy of the pectoralis major muscle and neurovascular supply. *Surg Forum* 1981;32:573.

Weinzweig N, Yetman R. Transposition of the greater omentum for recalcitrant median sternotomy wound infections. *Ann Plast Surg* 1995;34:471–477.

70.

GLUTEAL FLAP FOR PRESSURE SORES

Sanam Zahedi, Jillian M. McLaughlin, and Linda G. Phillips

ASSESSMENT OF THE DEFECT

Pressure sores can occur anywhere along the body where there is compression of the overlying soft tissue causing ischemia, which eventually leads to necrosis and ulceration. Based on deep tissue pressure recordings, the necrosis visualized on the skin surface is the "tip of the iceberg" with exam findings out of proportion to the degree of necrosis underlying the skin defect. Pressure sores usually occur over bony prominences. Based on the distribution of pressure, sacral pressure sores are more common in supine patients, and ischial pressure sores are more common in sitting patients. Patients in acute care settings, in nursing homes, or with spinal cord injuries are among the most commonly affected populations.

Pressure sores are a recurrent problem with multiple risk factors including direct pressure, friction, shearing forces, immobility, and moisture. Malnutrition, anemia, and chronic illness can also contribute to their formation by the impairment of blood supply and delayed wound healing. As such, patients must be medically optimized preoperatively. Laboratory studies include a complete blood cell count, assays for total protein and albumin, coagulation profiles, urinalysis, cultures, and radiographs of the bones. Any abnormalities must be corrected prior to surgery. Particularly in diabetic patients, medications should be adjusted to improve glucose and hemoglobin A1C levels. Patients should be placed on a high-protein, low-residue diet.

All pressure sores are considered colonized, and granulation tissue is an immunologic reaction against these microorganisms. Wound biopsy is obtained and an organism count of greater than 10^5 is diagnostic of invasive infection and predictive of failure of surgical closure. If wound infection is present, wound closure should be deferred until the bacterial counts diminish with the use of topical or systemic antibiotics. Pulmonary and urinary sources of infection cause seeding and subsequent infection of pressure sores and should be treated prior to surgical intervention. If infection of the bone is suspected, bone biopsy is required to rule out osteomyelitis. Hip joint osteomyelitis necessitates treatment of the infected bone with ostectomy as well as wound closure.

Pressure sores must be examined manually to assess size, depth, bursa, underlying bony prominences, and proximity to the rectum. Care must be taken to evaluate the patient for previous surgical scars and flap surgery. Frequently, previous surgery may preclude the use of a flap because of compromised vascular supply. Spasticity must also be assessed. The placement of a flap in a spastic patient is doomed to failure because of the constant battle of muscle contracture on suture line closure. Treatment options for spasticity include baclofen, diazepam, dantrolene, and botulinum toxin injections. Due to frequent rates of recurrence, patients often require multiple surgeries during their life spans. Therefore, our goal in the treatment of pressure sore must be to provide the least invasive and most durable coverage at the first operation while preserving future sites for flap coverage for recurrent disease.

INDICATIONS

Myocutaneous flaps were previously the first-line treatment for pressure sores. The theoretical advantages include rich vascular supply and thick muscular bulkiness, which eliminates dead space and provides cushion over pressure-bearing areas. The gluteus muscle flap can be used for coverage of sacral and ischial defects. Trochanteric defects can also be addressed; however, mobilization of the muscle with minimal tension may be difficult in this area. The flap is frequently rotated on the superior gluteal vessels for

747

sacral defects and on the inferior gluteal vessels for ischial coverage.

Over the past decade, fasciocutaneous flaps have emerged as a treatment option for pressure sores because they preserve muscle for later surgeries. It cannot be emphasized enough that pressure sores are a recurrent problem, and the surgeon must consider this fact during operative planning. In addition, studies have demonstrated no difference in the rates of ulcer recurrence, infection, hematoma, seroma, and dehiscence between these two types of flaps. The major advantage of fasciocutaneous flaps is their ability to preserve the gluteus maximus muscle, which is critical for ambulatory patients. Additionally, the flap offers greater arc of rotation, decreased donor site morbidity, decreased postoperative pain, shorter hospital stay, and reduced cost. Typically, pressure sores develop in areas without much underlying muscle, and a theoretical advantage of fasciocutaneous flaps is the ability to mirror normal anatomy by only covering the defect with fascia, subcutaneous tissue, and skin.

CONTRAINDICATIONS

Because of the potential functional loss with the rotation of the muscle, the use of the gluteus maximus muscle in ambulatory patients is not advised. Strong hip stabilization is necessary for climbing, and sacrifice of the gluteal muscle can lead to a significant deformity. Dissection of the inferior or superior portion of the muscle separately may allow use of the muscle and preserve ambulation. Use of the muscle for lateral and anterior defects is not practical due to the limited arc of rotation. Unlike myocutaneous flaps, fasciocutaneous flaps are not bulky and therefore are not good candidates for large and deep defects.

PATIENT MARKINGS AND ROOM SETUP

Bowel preparation can be performed. In spinal cord injury patients, the creation of a diverting colostomy should be considered in select patients to prevent fecal soiling of the wound. A new indwelling urinary catheter should be placed before surgery.

Local anesthesia or sedation can be used in paraplegic patients; however, general anesthesia is preferred to reduce patient anxiety. Paraplegic patients have wide fluctuations in blood pressure and pulse rate, and the lack of a physiologic compensatory sympathetic response requires careful management and correction of hypovolemia. In addition, the use of succinylcholine as a depolarizing paralytic in this patient population can lead to life threatening hyperkalemia. After undergoing general anesthesia, the patient is then placed in the prone position on the operating table. Due to the length of the procedure, padding to protect all bony prominences must be utilized.

OPERATIVE TECHNIQUE

DEBRIDEMENT

All pressure sore wound edges are lined with pale, shiny, unhealthy granulation tissue. In many patients, a variable degree of undermining may be present around the periphery of the ulcer. After excision of the overlying skin, the depth of the decubitus ulcer can be determined by applying slight upward pressure to a clamp placed within the wound. The entire bursa must be excised. Injection of methylene blue into the ulcer cavity identifies granulation tissue and the bursa. The surgeon should remove all blue-stained tissue for complete debridement. Failure to adequately debride the wound can lead to recurrent disease and poor healing. After bursa excision, the wound defect should be measured and documented.

Since underlying bony prominences play a major role in both the formation and recurrence of pressure sores, partial excision is required. All osteomyelitis must be excised. If a total resection of the sacrum is required, the presacral venous plexus must be avoided to prevent bleeding.

If the wound is infected, debridement and flap closure are completed as staged operations. First, all necrotic and contaminated material must be debrided and packed with Kerlix gauze soaked in antibiotic solution or povidone iodine. The patient recovers with frequent wet-to-dry dressing changes and assessment of the wound. Pharmacologic or enzymatic debridement is generally not effective in these cases. Once the infection is cleared, flap closure is performed as the second stage.

ANATOMY AND PREOPERATIVE MARKINGS

The gluteus maximus is a broad, thick, superficial, quadrilateral muscle that forms the prominence of the buttocks. The muscle insertion and origin are determined by marking the lateral edge of the sacrum and greater trochanter of the femur. The posterior superior iliac spine (PSIS) and the ischial tuberosity are marked to determine the medial limit.

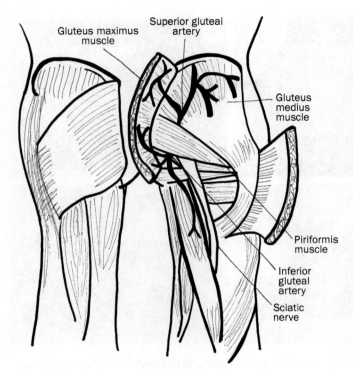

Figure 70.1. Anatomy of gluteus maximus.

The anterior superior iliac spine (ASIS) and greater trochanter mark the lateral limit of the muscle. The crista iliac determines the superior limit, while the inferior buttock fold sets the inferior limit (Figure 70.1).

The gluteus maximus is a type III muscle with two dominant pedicles, the inferior and superior gluteal arteries, which are direct branches of the internal iliac artery. These vessels arise separately from the internal iliac artery and exit the pelvis together with the superior and inferior gluteal nerves and their vena comitantes through the lateral border of the sacrum.

The skin territory of the gluteus maximus muscle can extend from T12 to the popliteal fossa and laterally from the ASIS to the lateral thigh overlapping the territory of the tensor fascia lata (TFL). The inferior gluteal artery supplies the lower two thirds of the gluteus muscle and the skin through perforators. Consequently, the entire gluteus maximus muscle with overlying skin may be advanced vertically based only on the inferior gluteal artery. Cadaveric studies demonstrate that about 20–25 perforators supply the entire gluteal region.

Motor innervation of the whole gluteus maximus muscle is from the inferior gluteal nerve (L5 to S2). The fibers of the gluteus maximus have sufficient laxity to allow advancement in different directions. After detachment of the origin of the fibers, up to 10 cm of medial advancement bilaterally can be obtained without disrupting the insertion and vascular pedicle. Similarly, detaching the inserting fibers allows significant lateral advancement. The gluteus maximus muscle is a strong extensor and lateral rotator of the thigh.

OPERATIVE TECHNIQUE FOR ROTATIONAL FLAP

Following debridement, elevating a larger flap than anticipated (at least 2–3 cm) allows for a tension-free closure. Flap preoperative markings can be made (Figure 70.2).

For elevation of a myocutaneous gluteal rotational flap (Figure 70.3), an incision is performed through the skin, subcutaneous tissues, and muscle insertion. The gluteus maximus muscle is divided at the inferior and lateral borders without undermining the subcutaneous tissues. The muscle is then elevated in a bloodless plane over the gluteus medius in a superomedial direction. The piriformis muscle is key in pedicle and sciatic nerve identification and protection. The superior gluteal artery and vein are identified and protected.

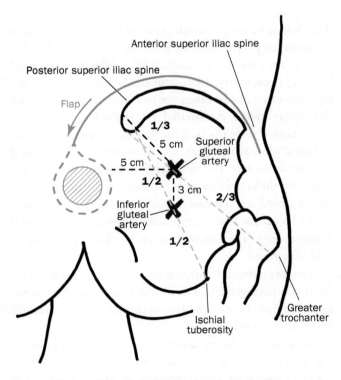

Figure 70.2. Gluteal rotation flap markings. Superior: Iliac crest. Inferior: Gluteal fold. Medial: Posterior superior iliac spine (PSIS) and ischial tuberosity (IT). Lateral: Anterior superior iliac spine (ASIS) and greater trochanter (GT). Superior gluteal artery (SGA) lies 5 cm inferior to the PSIS and 5 cm lateral to the midline or a point lying one-third of the way between the PSIS to the GT. The inferior gluteal artery (IGA) lies 3 cm inferior to the SGA. The IGA may be marked by a point halfway along a line drawn from the PSIS to the IT. Gluteal rotational skin flap skin incision marked just superior to the iliac crest and descends inferiorly, staying posterior to the GT. Advanced over defect.

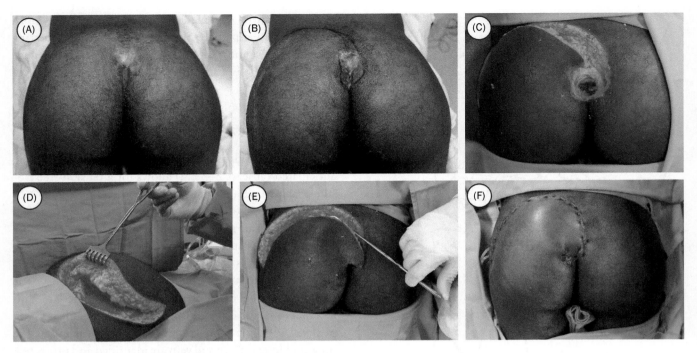

Figure 70.3. Sacral ulcer with gluteal rotation flap. (A) Preoperative photo. (B) Preoperative markings. (C) Incision. (D) Flap elevation. (E) Rotation. (F) Inset.

The gluteus maximus muscle is detached from its origin to allow for the proper rotation of the myocutaneous flap. For ambulatory patients, the inferior half of the muscle should be kept in continuity. A back-cut can be done for easy rotation, but care must be taken not to injure the pedicle. Once the flap is elevated, it is rotated over the sacral defect. After hemostasis, muscle fibers of the flap are sutured to the contralateral gluteus maximus muscle without tension, using absorbable sutures. The subcutaneous portion of the flap is inset into the sacral defect and sutured to the margins. The skin is closed using nonabsorbable suture. Drains (usually no. 15 French, or larger) are placed within the recipient and donor defects. The donor sites can be closed primarily or with skin grafts.

Fasciocutaneous rotation flaps are constructed in a similar fashion as myocutaneous rotation flaps. However, as the name implies, the incision stops at the fascia and the muscle insertion is never incised.

In addition, after rotation, the flap is then sutured to the contralateral fascia without tension. If needed, bilateral fasciocutaneous or musculocutaneous rotation flaps can be made.

OPERATIVE TECHNIQUE FOR V-Y ADVANCEMENT FLAP ("SLIDING" GLUTEAL FLAP)

In the ambulatory patient, the division of both the muscle origin and insertion can lead to hip instability and significant deformity. V-Y advancement of the flap or extending the skin to the posterior thigh can allow rotation of large amounts of skin without sacrifice of the muscle. If the sliding myocutaneous gluteal flap is used, it is designed to maintain integrity of the muscle, its insertion, and three main arterial systems (superior and inferior gluteal arteries plus cruciate anastomoses). Preoperative markings are made (Figure 70.4).

The V-Y advancement flap (Figure 70.5) is dissected down to the muscle after a skin paddle is designed. Wide subcutaneous dissection is then performed away from the skin island. Elevation of the gluteus muscle is performed along with its periosteal origin on the sacrum and coccyx. Dissection is continued inferiorly until the sacrotuberous ligament is identified and the branches of the pudendal artery are ligated.

The gluteus muscle is divided off the ligament, but the ligament itself should not be divided to avoid losing the dissection and potentially injuring the pedicle. The inferior and superior neurovascular pedicles are identified. The remaining fibers of the muscular origin are detached. If the size of the defect is large, the gluteus maximus muscle can be separated from the gluteus medius to increase the degree of advancement of the flap. The flap and the muscle are advanced into the defect and closed with absorbable suture. The skin edges are approximated with nonabsorbable sutures after the placement of large drains. The donor site is closed in a V-Y fashion. Patients are able to ambulate if

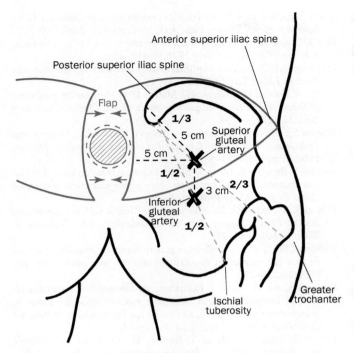

Figure 70.4. Gluteal V-Y flap markings. Superior: Iliac crest. Inferior: Gluteal fold. Medial: Posterior superior iliac spine (PSIS) and ischial tuberosity (IT). Lateral: Anterior superior iliac spine (ASIS) and greater trochanter (GT). Superior gluteal artery (SGA) lies 5 cm inferior to the PSIS and 5 cm lateral to the midline or a point lying one-third of the way between PSIS to the GT. The inferior gluteal artery (IGA) lies 3 cm inferior to the SGA. The IGA may be marked by a point halfway along a line drawn from the PSIS to the IT. V-shaped flap designed. Advanced, and donor site closed in V-Y fashion.

insertion and the neurovascular pedicle are preserved. In a nonambulatory patient, more advancement can be obtained by dividing the muscles' insertion.

The fasciocutaneous V-Y advancement flap is constructed in a similar fashion to its myocutaneous counterpart; both the superior and inferior arms of the flap are elevated, advanced, and closed in layers. Once again, the muscular origin is remains intact, and no incision is made in the muscular layer for fasciocutaneous flaps.

POSTOPERATIVE CARE

Patients are routinely discharged to a skilled nursing facility or a long-term acute care facility for 2–4 weeks to evaluate wound healing and improve physical rehabilitation. Rehabilitation is vital in the treatment protocol of these patients. In many patients, lifestyle changes are necessary to prevent recurrence. Direct pressure on the flap must be avoided, and the general nutritional condition of the patient must be optimized. The patient can remain prone or more preferably placed in an air-fluidized bed. Drains are generally kept in place for several weeks to avoid the potential for recurrent dead space. Pharmacologic agents may be required to prevent contamination of the wound with feces and to provide protection from hip spasticity.

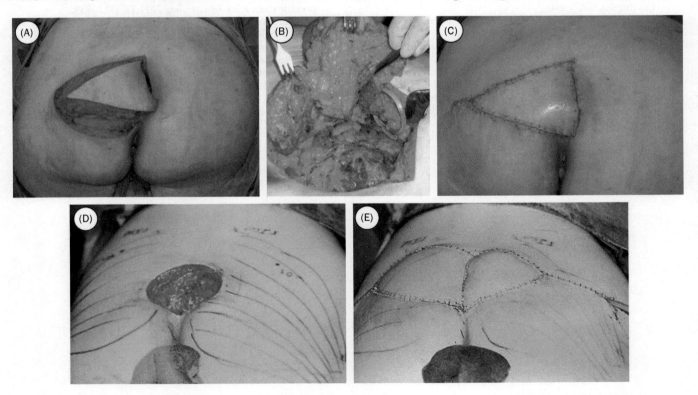

Figure 70.5. Sacral ulcer with V-Y advancement flap. (A) Incision. (B) Flap elevation and advancement. (C) Inset. (D) Preoperative bilateral V-Y advancement flap. (E) Postoperative bilateral V-Y advancement flap.

Stitches are removed at the end of the second or third week postoperatively. By the end of the second or third postoperative week, the patient is placed in physical therapy and mobilized. Avoiding pressure to the surgical site is essential for a successful result.

CAVEATS

Hematoma, partial or total flap loss, skin graft loss, wound dehiscence; recurrence, seroma, and infection are the leading complications. Suction drains are routinely left in place 10–14 days postoperatively to obliterate the dead space. Spasticity can lead to both seroma and hematoma formation; therefore, control of muscle spasms via methods mentioned previously is important. When diagnosed, infections should be aggressively treated with drainage and appropriate antibiotics. Rehabilitation and patient and family education are key to the prevention of recurrence.

SELECTED READINGS

Barth P, Le K, Madsen B, et al. Pressure profiles in deep tissue. *Proceedings of the 37th Annual Conference in Engineering in Medicine and Biology.* Los Angeles, CA, 1984.

Bauer J, Phillips LG. MOC-PSSM CME article: pressure sores. *Plast Reconstr Surg.* 2008;121:1–10.

Buhanan DL, Agris J. Gluteal plication closure of sacral pressure ulcers. *Plast Reconstr Surg* 1983;72:49–54.

Cormack GC, Lamberty BG. *The Arterial Anatomy of Skin Flaps.* 2nd ed. Edinburgh: Churchill Livingstone, 1994: 218–224, 234–238.

Diaz S, Li X, Rodriguez L, Salgado CJ. Update in the surgical management of decubitus ulcers. *Anaplastology* 2:3. Available at: http://dx/doi.org/10.4172/2161-1173.1000113.

Evans GRD, Gurlek A. Gluteal flap for pressure sores. In: Evans GRD, ed. *Operative Plastic Surgery.* New York: McGraw-Hill; 2000:719–729.

Ger R, Levine SA. The management of decubitus ulcers by muscle transposition. *Plast Reconstr Surg* 1976;58:419–428.

Heywood AJ, Quaba AA. Modified gluteus maximus V-Y advancement flaps. *Br J Plast Surg* 1989;42:263–265.

Keys KA, Daniali LN, Warner KJ, Mathes DW. Multivariate predictors of failure after flap coverage of pressure ulcers. *Plast Reconstr Surg* 2010;125:1725–1734.

Mathes SJ, Nahai F. *Reconstructive Surgery: Principles, Anatomy and Technique.* New York: Churchill Livingstone/Quality Medical Publishing, 1997:500–535.

Parkash S, Banerjee S. The total gluteus maximus rotation and other gluteus maximus musculocutaneous flaps in the treatment of pressure ulcers. *Br J Plast Surg* 1986;39:66–71.

Powers K, Phillips LG. Pressure sores. In: Thorne CH, ed. *Grabb and Smith's Plastic Surgery.* 7th ed. Philadelphia, PA: Williams & Wilkins; 2014:989–997.

Ramirez OM. The sliding plication gluteus maximus musculocutaneous flap for reconstruction of sacrococcygeal wounds. *Ann Plast Surg* 1990;24:223–230.

Sameem A, Au M, Wood T, Farrokhyar F, Mahoney J. A systematic review of complication and recurrence rates of musculocutaneous, fasciocutaneous, and perforator-based aps for treatment of pressure sores. *Plast Reconstr Surg* 2012;130: 67e–77e.

Seyhan T, Ertas NM, Bahar T, Borman H. Simplified and versatile use of gluteal perforator flaps for pressure sores. *Ann Plast Surg* 2008;60:673–678.

Stevenson TR, Pollock RA, Rohrich RJ, VanderKolk CA. The gluteus maximus musculocutaneous island flap: refinements in design and application. *Plast Reconstr Surg* 1987;79:761–768.

Stratton RJ, Ek AC, Engfer M, et al. Enteral nutritional support in prevention and treatment of pressure ulcers: a systematic review and meta-analysis. *Ageing Res Rev* 2005;4:422–450.

Tchanque-Fossuo CN, Kuzon WM Jr. An evidence-based approach to pressure sores. *Plast Reconstr Surg* 2011;127:932–939.

Thiessen FE, Andrades P, Blondeel PN, et al. Flap surgery for pressure sores: should the underlying muscle be transferred or not? *J Plast Reconstr Aesthet Surg* 2011;64:84–90.

Wilk A, Rodier C, Beau C, et al. Gluteus maximus muscular flap in the treatment of sacral pressure sores: a 10-year review. *Ann Chir Plast Esthet* 1991;36:132–137.

Yamamoto Y, Ohura T, Shintomi Y, et al. Superiority of the fasciocutaneous flap in reconstruction of sacral pressure sores. *Ann Plast Surg* 1993;30:116–121.

71.

POSTERIOR THIGH FLAP FOR PRESSURE SORES

Christopher L. Ellstrom and Gregory R. D. Evans

INTRODUCTION

The management of pressure sores is a challenging medical and surgical problem that requires a multifaceted approach for both prevention and treatment. Decubitus ulcers occur in a wide variety of patients and place an enormous economic burden on the healthcare system. Education of healthcare providers and at-risk patient populations about the importance of pressure offloading is an integral component of prevention. Despite best practices, pressure sores still occur with regular frequency. In managing these wounds, the plastic surgeon must initially focus on addressing the risk factors that led to the original wound to prevent further progression as well as the development of wounds at other sites. The wound itself should then be addressed to minimize the potential for complications, particularly infection. Surgical closure of the wound should only be considered after optimization of all risk factors and of the wound bed. One must keep in mind that, even under the best circumstances, ischial ulcers have a reported recurrence rate of up to 30% after surgical wound closure with the posterior thigh flap.[1]

ASSESSMENT OF THE DEFECT

Decubitus ulcers are primarily the result of prolonged, unrelieved pressure in a given area that that exceeds capillary perfusion pressure (32 mm Hg) and results in tissue ischemia and breakdown. Irreversible tissue damage occurs in as little as 2 hours. Wounds are most likely to occur over bony prominences, with the ischium the most commonly affected, followed, in descending frequency, by the trochanter, sacrum, heels, occiput, scapula, and elbows. Certain injuries or positioning tendencies may increase the likelihood of wound development in a given area. Hip injuries or fractures can predispose patients to development of trochanteric wounds. Bedbound patients have a higher probability of sacral wounds, while patients who spend more time in wheelchairs have an increased probability of ischial ulcer formation. Proper methods for pressure reduction and offloading should be incorporated for both prevention and treatment of pressure wounds and these include the use of turning and repositioning every 2 hours, low air loss or fluidized air mattresses, and proper padding on wheelchairs and other assistive devices.

In addition to pressure, friction, shear, and moisture work in combination to contribute to wound development. Excess friction may lead to blistering, abrasions, or skin tears, while shear forces can lead to deeper injury of the underlying subcutaneous tissue and its vascular supply. Care must be utilized in the handling and transfer of at-risk patients to avoid skin injury. Excess moisture from uncontrolled wounds or urinary or fecal incontinence can lead to irritation, dermatitis, and skin breakdown. Additionally, fecal incontinence can significantly increase the bacterial burden, which increases the probability of wound formation and impairs healing in already formed wounds. To avoid fecal soilage, particularly in the case of incontinent patients, consideration should be given for placement of a temporary or permanent colostomy.

Given the propensity for recurrence, surgical intervention for pressure sores should only be considered after a thorough evaluation and optimization of all medical comorbidities. Malnutrition is often present in the chronically ill patients who present with pressure wounds. Albumin and prealbumin levels should be checked to determine nutritional status. If appropriate, a high-protein diet along with appropriate supplementation should be started in an attempt to improve wound healing; however, there is only limited evidence to support improved outcomes with diet supplementation.[2]

Spinal cord injury patients are at increased risk due to prolonged immobility, muscle wasting, and loss of protective sensation. Muscle spasticity is present in a large percentage of the spinal cord injury population, and it must be controlled with anti-spasmodic agents due to the risk of flap failure from wound dehiscence. Additionally, this population suffers from a high rate of flexion contractures that must be addressed, surgically in some cases, to avoid pressure on a future flap from positioning limitations.

WOUND ASSESSMENT

Pressure sores should be thoroughly examined to determine the wound size and depth, as well as the presence of undermining, underlying or exposed bony prominences, necrotic tissue, slough, and infection. All necrotic or grossly infected tissue should be debrided. If there is concern for osteomyelitis a bone scan or magnetic resonance imaging (MRI) scan can be obtained; however, a bone biopsy should be obtained for definitive diagnosis and for determining the most appropriate antibiotic regimen. A variety of wound care regimens have been evaluated, but none has been shown to be definitively superior.[3] An appropriate wound care regimen should be instituted to keep the wound clean and to minimize bacterial burden. For chronically nonhealing wounds, consideration should be given to performing a wound biopsy to rule out malignant transformation.

INDICATIONS

The posterior thigh flap is a useful option for reconstruction of defects in the ischium or trochanter. It is particular well suited for ambulatory individuals because it avoids any muscle sacrifice and has the potential for protective sensation if the posterior femoral cutaneous branch is included. Prior to surgical intervention, preventative measures and local wound care should be fully explored to avoid an unnecessary operation. The patients must be highly motivated and compliant with care regimens to ensure a successful outcome. A well-functioning support care network should be in place to ensure optimal outcomes and recovery.

CONTRAINDICATIONS

Caution should be exercised when dealing with patients who have had multiple surgical procedures in the posterior thigh and buttock as the underlying blood supply may be compromised. Poor self-care and a history of recurrent ulcerations are also relative contraindications. Since the risks factors that predispose patients to the development of pressure ulcers are the same as those that lead to postoperative complications and recurrence, surgery should not be considered until the patient's medical and social issues are addressed.

OPERATIVE TECHNIQUE

ANATOMY OF THE POSTERIOR THIGH

The posterior thigh is an ill-defined region that extends from the inferior gluteal crease superiorly to the popliteal fossa inferiorly and is bordered by the iliotibial band laterally and abductor musculature medially. The hamstring muscles of the posterior thigh are made up of the biceps femoris, semimembranosus, and semitendinosus. The posterior thigh vascular supply is primarily via profunda artery perforators with secondary contribution via the inferior gluteal artery. Typically four to five profunda artery perforators can be found in a diagonal line from the ischium to the lateral femoral condyle. The most proximal perforators are at the level of the inferior gluteal fold, and the most distal are found approximately 10 cm proximal to the lateral femoral condyle.[4] The first and second perforators are generally the largest at 1.0–2.0 mm diameter and supply the majority of the cutaneous territory.[5] The inferior gluteal artery is located at the midpoint between the greater trochanter and ischial tuberosity, exiting the sciatic foramen between the piriformis and coccygeus muscles. A descending branch may accompany the posterior femoral cutaneous nerve of the thigh in some patients.[4,6] Vascular dye studies have shown the cutaneous territory of the inferior gluteal artery to be limited to the inferior gluteal region.[5]

POSITIONING

To provide optimal exposure the patient is positioned in a prone or semiprone position with a rolled towel or soft support under the chest and iliac spine to provide a 20-degree rotation of the pelvis to the recipient side. This not only allows the surgeon to expose and debride the trochanteric lesion, but it also aids flexibility in flap harvest. Appropriate protective padding must be in place on all potential pressure points. The surgeon is positioned at the same side as the ulcer and the assistant on the opposite side (Figures 71.1 and 71.2).

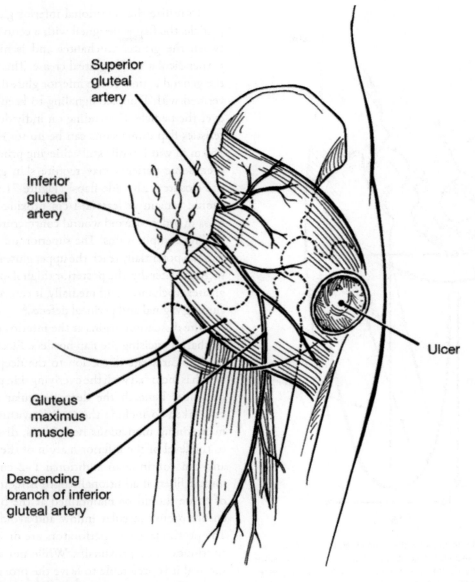

Superior
gluteal
artery

Inferior
gluteal
artery

Gluteus
maximus
muscle

Descending
branch of inferior
gluteal artery

Ulcer

Figure 71.1. Anatomy of gluteal and posterior thigh area with an example trochanteric defect.

DEBRIDEMENT

Most pressure ulcers are heavily colonized with bacteria in addition to significant eschar and debris in the wound bed. The wounds are often surrounded by poorly vascularized scar tissue and may tunnel for significant length. The initially step of pressure sore reconstructions should be a careful debridement of all nonviable structures and excision of prior scar to allow for healthy wound edges in order to minimize the chance for wound breakdown and recurrence. Grossly infected wounds should have staged debridements to optimize reconstructive success. It is helpful to place a methylene blue or brilliant green solution into the wound bed to aid in visualization and allow

for a complete excision of the bursa. Bony prominences should be osteomized or rasped to obtain smooth edges and prevent focal pressure points. If there is suspicion for potential osteomyelitis, then a bone biopsy should be obtained and the nonviable infected bone should be excised. Appropriate antibiotics should then be tailored to culture results. Care should be taken to avoid overresection of the bone because it may increase the chance for a contralateral pressure wound or for urethral damage. If there is suspicion for malignancy in the wound bed, then a biopsy should be sent to the pathology and consideration given to delaying the reconstructive portion of the case until a tissue diagnosis can be obtained.

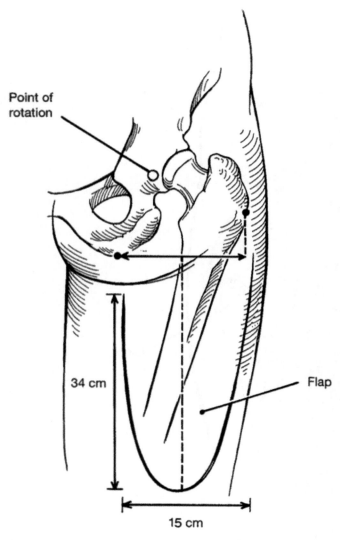

Point of rotation

34 cm

Flap

15 cm

Figure 71.2. The posterior thigh flap is designed on an extrapelvic course of the inferior gluteal vessel. The point of rotation of flap is 5 cm above ischial tuberosity with a central axis of the flap midway between greater trochanter and ischial tuberosity and perpendicular to gluteal crease.

FLAP DESIGN AND HARVEST

The posterior thigh flap was first described by Hurwitz as a superiorly based myocutaneous flap centered on the inferior gluteal artery.[6] It has since been described with an assortment of different names and in a variety of different configurations including rotational, advancement, island, and free flaps in both myocutaneous and fasciocutaneous forms. Flap design will ultimately depend on the nature of the defect and any potential limitations from prior wounds or surgeries. The flap can be based on either the profunda perforators or the inferior gluteal artery or both (Figure 71.3).

To utilize the traditional inferior gluteal artery–based pedicle, the flap is designed with a central axis halfway between the greater trochanter and ischial tuberosity and perpendicular to the gluteal crease. This trajectory follows the general course of the inferior gluteal artery and can be verified with Doppler signaling to keep the flap centered over the pedicle. Depending on individual patient characteristics flap dimensions can be up to 34 cm in length by 15 cm in width while still achieving primary closure; however, some patients may require skin grafting for donor site closure with wide flaps[7] (Figure 71.4), The dissection should remain at least a 4 cm proximal to the popliteal fossa in order to avoid wound contractures or other wound healing complications. The superior arc of rotation of the flap can potentially reach the upper gluteal region and lower sacrum. Laterally, the posterior thigh flap can extend to the greater trochanter, and medially, it can cover the pubis, including vaginal and perineal defects.[6]

The dissection begins at the inferior margin of the flap by sharply incising the flap borders. Electrocautery is then used to carry the dissection to the deep muscular fascia, which is included with the overlying skin paddle. Dissection continues beneath the deep muscular fascia with great care taken to include the pedicle within the flap. While maintaining meticulous hemostasis, dissection continues to the level of the inferior margin of the gluteus maximus and can continue an additional 1–2 cm by dividing the muscle fibers if additional length is required. A small cuff of tissue should be maintained at the base of the flap to ensure robust vascular inflow and avoid pedicle kinking. The profunda artery perforators are divided as dissection continues more proximally. While not necessary for flap survival it is preferable to leave the proximal profunda artery perforators intact for more collateral blood flow if the design permits. During transposition of the flap, the skin bridge separating the flap from the defect can be divided or a subcutaneous tunnel can be created above the level of the fascia. Tunneled flaps must be carefully evaluated for signs of pedicle compression, in which case the overlying skin bridge should be divided. The buried portion of the flap should be de-epithelized prior to final inset. Care also should be taken not to injure the branches of the inferior gluteal artery or sciatic nerve. The donor defect is closed primarily in the majority of cases; however, split-thickness skin grafts can be used for wider flaps. Alternatively, the posterior thigh flap can be elevated as an island flap. In this circumstance, the island is incised and the neurovascular pedicle is carefully dissected subfascially to reach the

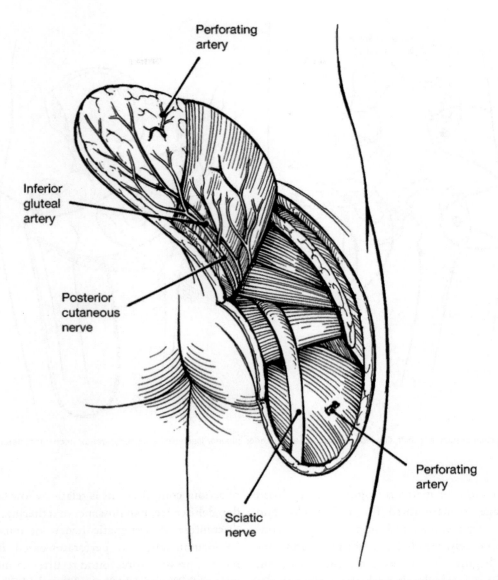

Figure 71.3. Vascular anatomy of inferior gluteal artery may vary. Larger perforators are usually encountered at level of inferior margin of gluteus maximus and can be divided if more length is required. The gluteus maximus can be partially divided and included with the flap.

appropriate length. Fully islandizing the flap on the inferior gluteal artery may lead to increased rates of complication. Subcutaneous drains should be placed in both the donor and recipient sites.

To develop a flap based primarily on the profunda artery perforators, a line is drawn between the ischial tuberosity and lateral femoral condyle. Using a hand-held Doppler, perforators are then identified beginning at the inferior gluteal crease and extending to 10 cm proximal to the lateral femoral condyle. Usually four to six perforators can be found, with the most proximal two generally being the most robust. A flap is then centered over the identified perforators and designed to appropriately fill the nearby defect. The skin is

sharply incised and the deep muscular fascia is included as a part of the flap with the remaining dissection continued in the typical fashion for a perforator flap. The distal perforators are divided as necessary in order to provide sufficient mobility to translate the flap into the defect. The donor site is then closed primarily or with a skin graft. Subcutaneous drains are placed in both the donor and recipient sites.

POSTOPERATIVE CARE

Patients are kept completely flat and supine in an air fluidized mattress for at least 5–7 days, then may be

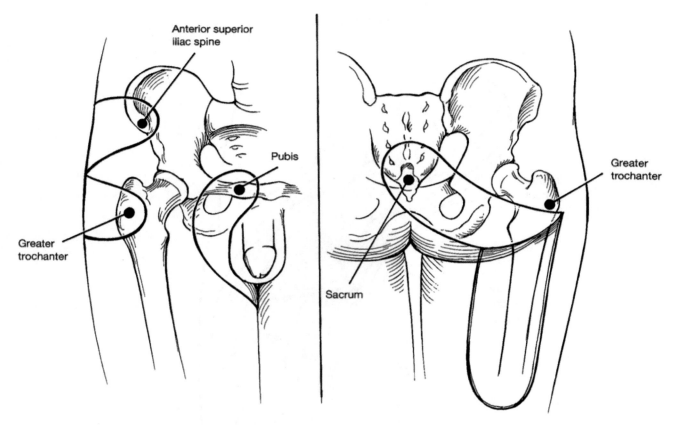

Figure 71.4. Arc of rotation of posterior thigh flap includes sacrum and anterior superior iliac spine superiorly, greater trochanter laterally, and pubis medially.

transitioned to a low air mattress (Figure 71.5). Closed suction drainage is maintained for 1–2 weeks, and culture-specific intravenous antibiotic coverage is continued postoperatively. Graded rehabilitation and mobilization are begun 2–3 weeks after the operation. Physical therapists work closely with the patient to develop an appropriate schedule for returning to daily activity, wheelchair use, and transfers to and from the chair. Education for prevention of recurrence continues after discharge, with follow-up care by all involved specialists. Home care, if necessary, can be coordinated by a visiting nurse.

CAVEATS

The technique for posterior thigh flap harvest is relatively easy to perform and provides reliable coverage of trochanteric and ischial wounds with low donor site morbidity. When done under optimized conditions, the rate of serious complications is relatively low but may include flap dehiscence, flap floss, nerve tethering, and donor site discomfort. A systematic review of musculocutaneous, fasciocutaneous, and perforator-based flaps for treatment of pressure sores found recurrence and complication rates of 8.9% and 18.6%, 11.2% and 11.7%, and 5.6% and 19.6%, respectively.[8] A series of posterior thigh flaps based on the inferior gluteal artery reported a wound healing complication rate of 54%, but only one flap loss out of 27 patients.[7] Early wound dehiscence should be treated with debridement and readvancement of the flap with primary closure.

The treatment of pressure sores involves a comprehensive approach of patient education, rehabilitation, and preoperative and postoperative intervention. The posterior thigh flap alone is not enough to permanently treat trochanteric and ischial ulcers; these complex wounds demand a team of specialists to facilitate all aspects of care and address the emotional, physical, and financial burdens on patients.

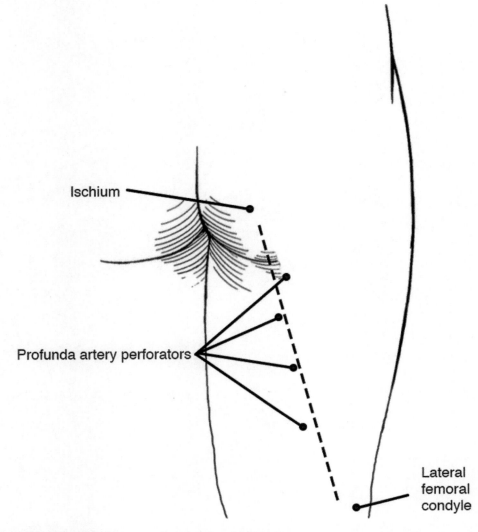

Ischium

Profunda artery perforators

Lateral
femoral
condyle

Figure 71.5. Profunda artery perforators can generally be found in a line between the ischium and lateral femoral condyle. A perforator-based flap is usually designed over the more robust proximal perforators to fill a given defect.

REFERENCES

1. Homma K, Murakami G, Fujioka H, Fujita T, Imai A, Ezoe K. Treatment of ischial pressure ulcers with a posteromedial thigh fasciocutaneous flap. *Plast Reconstr Surg* 2001;108:1990–1996; discussion 1997.
2. Langer G, Fink A. Nutritional interventions for preventing and treating pressure ulcers. *Cochrane Database Syst Rev* 2014: CD003216.
3. Norman G, Dumville JC, Moore ZE, Tanner J, Christie J, Goto S. Antibiotics and antiseptics for pressure ulcers. *Cochrane Database Syst Rev* 2016;4:CD011586.
4. Ahmadzadeh R, Bergeron L, Tang M, Geddes CR, Morris SF. The posterior thigh perforator flap or profunda femoris artery perforator flap. *Plast Reconstr Surg* 2007;119:194–200; discussion 201–202.
5. Rubin JA, Whetzel TP, Stevenson TR. The posterior thigh fasciocutaneous flap: vascular anatomy and clinical application. *Plast Reconstr Surg* 1995;95:1228–1239.
6. Hurwitz DJ, Swartz WM, Mathes SJ. The gluteal thigh flap: a reliable, sensate flap for the closure of buttock and perineal wounds. *Plast Reconstr Surg* 1981;68:521–532.
7. Friedman JD, Reece GR, Eldor L. The utility of the posterior thigh flap for complex pelvic and perineal reconstruction. *Plast Reconstr Surg* 2010;126:146–155.
8. Sameem M, Au M, Wood T, Farrokhyar F, Mahoney J. A systematic review of complication and recurrence rates of musculocutaneous, fasciocutaneous, and perforator-based flaps for treatment of pressure sores. *Plast Reconstr Surg* 2012;130:67e–77e.

72

SURGICAL TREATMENT OF POSTMASTECTOMY LYMPHEDEMA

Chad M. Teven and David W. Chang

Secondary lymphedema is a common complication of cancer treatment, particularly in breast cancer patients. Its prevalence has been reported at up to 28% of patients after lumpectomy and up to 49% of patients who have undergone mastectomy.[1] Postsurgical lymphedema is a significant source of morbidity and is often progressive in this setting. Factors that predispose to this condition include extensive of axillary dissection, trauma, infection, obesity, postoperative seroma, and radiotherapy.[2] In an effort to minimize the morbidity associated with axillary lymph node dissection (ALND) without compromising survival, sentinel lymph node biopsy (SLNB)—which consists of considerably less axillary surgery than ALND—has been offered to breast cancer patients who meet criteria for its use. The rate of upper extremity lymphedema in these patients is still significant, however, at 4–10%.[3]

Postsurgical lymphedema can arise in the immediate postoperative setting but more commonly develops after a latent period. Despite the identification of major risk factors (e.g., extensive axillary surgery, radiotherapy), the cause of lymphedema remains elusive.[4] Symptoms of lymphedema include increased volume and weight of the affected limb, increased skin tension, and a subjective feeling that the affected limb is heavy relative to the normal limb. Patients may report difficulty wearing their normal clothing or performing activities that involve the use of the affected extremity. Lymphedema may also affect psychological and emotional well-being, often because of the embarrassment associated with the enlarged limb and need for compression garments.

There is no cure for secondary lymphedema. However, several treatment options exist that attempt to attenuate this condition. The mainstay of conservative lymphedema management includes compression garments and complex decongestive therapy (CDT). These treatments aim to provide symptomatic relief and prevent disease progression and are generally considered to be palliative. Several factors are responsible for high rates of patient dissatisfaction and noncompliance associated with conservative approaches.[5] In response, surgical treatments have gained popularity over the past half-century. Many surgical procedures have been offered for the treatment of extremity lymphedema. Currently, the most widely used procedures consist of variations of a lymphatic shunt operation using microsurgical technique.[3] This chapter will highlight surgical treatment options for postmastectomy lymphedema, with a focus on vascularized lymph node transfer and lymphovenous bypass.

ASSESSMENT OF THE DEFECT

Patients with postmastectomy lymphedema commonly present with swelling of the affected upper extremity, which may be soft and pitting, or indurated and fibrotic as the condition progresses. Skin changes, including acanthosis and warty overgrowths, may develop with longstanding disease. Recurrent cellulitis and/or lymphangitis may cause severe discomfort. The International Society of Lymphology has developed a clinical classification system for lymphedematous swelling (Table 72.1).[6]

The diagnosis of lymphedema is generally made by history, physical examination, and overall clinical assessment. Advanced-stage disease is often straightforward to identify, but early lymphedema can be difficult to distinguish from other common causes of limb swelling (Box 72.1).[7,8] Characteristically unique to lymphedema on examination are a positive Stemmer sign (a thickened skin fold at the base of the second finger) and peau d'orange of the skin (indicative of subcutaneous and cutaneous fibrosis).[7] Also, the affected arm will usually have a larger circumference than the contralateral, unaffected arm. Serial circumferential

TABLE 72.1 CLINICAL CLASSIFICATION OF LYMPHEDEMATOUS SWELLING

Stage 0	Latent or subclinical condition where swelling is not evident despite impaired lymph transport. May exist for months or years before overt edema occurs.
Stage 1	Early accumulation of fluid relatively high in protein content (when compared with venous edema), and which subsides with limb elevation. Pitting may occur.
Stage 2	Pitting may or may not occur with the development of tissue fibrosis. Limb elevation rarely reduces tissue swelling.
Stage 3	Lymphostatic elephantiasis with absence of pitting. Trophic skin changes may occur (e.g., acanthosis, fat deposits, warty overgrowths).

measurements are used to follow disease progression. Additional information that should be documented on a regular basis includes severity of symptoms, degree of functional impairment, episodes of cellulitis, skin breakdown, and response to treatment.

Radiographic methods for diagnosis are rarely necessary but can be helpful in selected patients. Examples include computed tomography, magnetic resonance

BOX 72.1 DIFFERENTIAL DIAGNOSIS FOR LYMPHEDEMA AS THE CAUSE OF LIMB EDEMA

Local etiologies

Acute deep venous thrombosis

Postthrombotic syndrome

Chronic venous insufficiency

Myxedema

Lipedema

Limb hypertrophy

Tumor

Psoriatic arthritis

Idiopathic edema

Systemic causes of edema

Cardiac failure

Renal failure

Protein-losing conditions

imaging, venous Doppler studies, and lymphoscintigraphy. Lymphoscintigraphy provides information regarding lymphatic anatomy and function and is considered the gold standard for diagnosing lymphedma.[9] Nevertheless, it is rarely required to diagnose acquired lymphedema after cancer treatment.

ANATOMY AND PATHOPHYSIOLOGY

The lymphatic system parallels the cardiovascular system anatomically but is unique in that it flows unidirectionally to return lymph to the cardiovascular system. Lymph fluid is derived from blood plasma as hydrostatic and oncotic forces push it through capillary walls into the interstitial space. It is a complex mixture of proteins, nutrients, oxygen, bacteria, toxic byproducts, and metabolic waste that is returned to the cardiovascular system for eventual elimination by end-organs. Lymphatic vessels are endothelial-lined, thin-walled vessels that originate in the extremities and resorb lymph from the interstitial space. Pressure gradients that arise from skeletal muscle action, smooth muscle contraction, and respiratory movement transport lymph proximally. When lymphatic channels are subject to obstruction or destruction (e.g., by surgery and/or radiation), there is a disruption of normal lymph transport.

Under physiologic conditions, the amount of lymph flowing into the interstitium equals the amount removed. When this balance is disrupted, lymph accumulates and swelling results. Perpetuating the build-up of fluid is the aggregation of proteins and other macromolecules typically transported from the interstitium by lymphatic channels. An increased protein concentration causes elevated oncotic pressures within the interstitium, further driving fluid into the interstitum.[7] Moreover, a result of disrupted lymph transport is elevated compartment pressures within the subcutaneous and intramuscular spaces, which further compounds this condition by obstructing low-pressure lymphatic channels.[10]

Although the underlying mechanisms causing lymphedema are unknown, several studies have shed light on key pathologic factors. Inflammation and fibrosis, for example, are critical to its development and progression.[11] Over time, chronic lymphedema results in tense, fibrotic tissue, prone to injury and breakdown. Recurrent infections, due to impaired bacterial clearance, result in further lymphatic destruction. A feared complication of long-standing lymphedema is the development of lymphangiosarcoma and other cutaneous malignant tumors.[7] Therefore, early and effective treatment is necessary to prevent progression and potential malignant degeneration of lymphedema.

INDICATIONS AND CONTRAINDICATIONS FOR SURGERY

Surgical therapy for postmastectomy lymphedema is palliative, not curative. Generally, conservative efforts are attempted first. Surgical management is offered to selected patients who are refractory to medical management. Indications include localized primary lesions (e.g., microcystic and macroscopic lymphatic malformations), recurrent cellulitis, deformity or disfigurement, pain, limitation of function, and diminished quality of life.[12] It should be noted that, regardless of the therapy undertaken, meticulous hygiene is mandatory. Also of great importance is avoidance of injury to the affected limb. Injury to or breach of the skin barrier can cause a rapid cellulitis or deeper soft tissue infection. Recurrent infection or inflammation may cause obliteration of more lymph collaterals, thus worsening the condition.

MEDICAL MANAGEMENT

Medical therapies are offered initially for postmastectomy lymphedema. Indeed, the majority of patients will respond favorably to conservative measures, thereby avoiding the need for surgery. Integral to medical management is the finding that compression reduces the pitting edema associated with lymphedema. Multilayer inelastic lymphedema bandaging has been shown to reduce edema volume by 31%,[13] and controlled compression therapy by 46%.[14] Additional noninvasive methods, including limb elevation and weight reduction in obese patients, may also help. A widely offered treatment for secondary lymphedema is CDT or decongestive lymphatic therapy (DLT). These techniques rely on manual massage of the trunk adjacent to the affected limb and have changed little since their introduction by Vodder nearly a half-century ago.[15] He hypothesized that these methods stimulate lymphatic flow through cutaneous lymphatics, thereby reducing lymphatic fluid from the extremity. Results with these techniques have been fairly positive. Randomized controlled studies have reported a mean decrease in excess volume from 40% to 60% in selected patients.[7] However, not all patients respond favorably to DLT.[16] This may be due an increased level of fibrosis but has not been definitively proved.

CDT, which primarily consists of manual lymphatic drainage (MLD) by experienced therapists to guide lymph fluid toward lymph collaterals, is generally offered as part of a treatment regimen. The regimen often includes meticulous skin care, active participation in physical therapy, and compression garments. There are several challenges associated with CDT, including the need for multiple highly trained healthcare providers, an intensive time and labor commitment, and compliance issues. Patients may become disappointed that their hard work only reduces symptoms and does not lead to a cure.

In cases of severe swelling, sequential pneumatic compression may be offered as part of the overall treatment strategy. Although this has proved successful in both the short-term[17] and with longer follow-up,[18] there are reports suggesting that there is limited benefit in postmastectomy lymphedema.[19]

Many pharmacologic agents have also been attempted to reduce the symptoms of lymphedema. Among the commonest drugs offered are benzopyrones, which facilitate protein breakdown by increasing macrophage proteolysis.[20] The theory underlying the beneficial effect of this class of drugs is that protein breakdown will reduce the volume of high-protein lymphedema fluid. Studies are mixed as to how effective these drugs are, although a well-designed randomized control trial comparing the benzopyrone Coumarin to placebo demonstrated that the drug significantly reduced extremity edema and uncomfortable symptoms and increased limb mobility.[21] These drugs are not without limiting side effects, however, such as hepatoxicity. Diuretics are also occasionally offered, but must be used with caution. While they may provide some benefit in cases of severe systemic hypervolemia, long-term use has been associated with worsening of protein accumulation and increased fibrosis.

Additional noninvasive therapies have also been reported. Nutritional supplements, such as sodium selenite and vitamin E in combination with pentoxifylline, have shown modest albeit nonsignificant benefit. Other methods include extremity heating and intraarterial autologous lymphocyte infusion. Further research is warranted to identify a beneficial role for these and other novel therapies.

SURGICAL MANAGEMENT

Surgical techniques have been developed in an effort to treat patients with lymphedema that is refractory to conservative measures. Because the indications for surgical treatment remain controversial, the responsibility falls to physicians to educate patients about the available options and timing for surgical intervention. The two main approaches are excisional procedures and physiologic procedures.

In 1912, Charles published the first report of a surgical procedure to treat severe lymphedema of the scrotum and of the lower limb (elephantiasis).[22] The procedure consisted of circumferential resection of all skin and soft tissue above the deep fascia in the affected area followed by grafting of the raw surface with skin harvested from the resected specimen or opposite leg. Fifteen years later, Sistrunk reported the first procedure specifically for breast cancer–related upper extremity lymphedema.[23] In this procedure, an elliptical incision is made on the ulnar side of the limb in order to remove excess skin, soft tissue, and deep fascia. This and later refinements by Thompson attempted to facilitate the creation of new lymphatic drainage pathways so that retained lymphatic fluid in the superficial lymphatic system would drain into the deep lymphatic system.[24] However, objective data that these techniques induce new pathway creation are lacking. Although relatively simple to perform, these excisional procedures are associated with significant morbidity, including gross aesthetic deformity, keloid or unstable scar formation, destruction of remnant lymphatics, and return of swelling. Therefore, they are used in extreme cases only.

A recently developed excisional technique for lymphedema management that has gained favor due to its less invasive nature is suction-assisted lipectomy or liposuction. Liposuction, which was originally developed for cosmetic body contouring, employs cannulas connected to a vacuum suction machine to aspirate subcutaneous fatty tissue in the affected limb. In addition to reducing the volume of subcutaneous tissue, liposuction may replace compliant soft tissue with scar that is less dispensable. The largest series of liposuction in breast cancer patients with upper extremity lymphedema reported a 106% mean edema volume reduction at 4 years[25] and 10 years postoperatively.[7] However, patients undergoing liposuction must wear compression garments continuously to avoid recurrence of limb edema.[14] Liposuction is also associated with the potential risks of exacerbating the lymphedema and damaging residual lymphatic vessels.[26]

Physiologic operations include techniques in which new lymph channels are created to increase the capacity to transport lymph fluid. Many procedures have been attempted in an effort to drain lymph trapped within a lymphedematous limb into the venous system or functional lymphatic basins. Early reports utilized tissues containing lymphatics, such as greater omentum, local skin, and pedicled fasciocutaneous or musculocutaneous flaps, to drain lymph from surrounding affected areas.[3] However, many of these approaches lack objective evidence supporting their efficacy, are associated with high morbidity, and therefore have become unfavorable. The use of microsurgical techniques has been more successful and is now among the most effective treatments offered for lymphedema.

Two commonly offered microsurgical procedures for lymphedema are vascularized lymph node transfer (VLNT) and lymphovenous bypass (LVB). VLNT was first described in 1979, by Shesol and colleagues[27] in a rat model and applied clinically by Clodius and colleagues[28] in 1982. In this procedure, vascularized tissue and healthy lymph nodes from one region are transferred to the affected area by microsurgically repairing the arterial and venous (but not lymphatic) blood supply. Healthy lymph nodes are most commonly harvested from the groin or contralateral supraclavicular region. Becker et al. microsurgically transferred vascularized lymph nodes from the groin to the axilla in 24 female patients with postmastectomy lymphedema and found that upper limb perimeter returned to normal in 10 cases and was significantly decreased in 12.[29] Other authors have similarly found promising results with VLNT for secondary lymphema.[10,30–32] Potential theories to explain these findings are that transplanted lymph nodes produce growth factors that facilitate lymphangiogenesis and also that transferred lymph nodes act as a lymphatic pump.[33] The release of scar tissue at the recipient site is also significant in reducing lymphatic obstruction. In addition to the usual risks associated with a long surgical procedure, one potential devastating complication of VLNT is lymphedema development at the donor site.

LVB is form of lymphovenous shunting aimed at bypassing obstructed lymphatics. It consists of the direct anastomosis of obstructed lymphatics to a regional vein by microsurgical techniques. Most authors report modest improvements in limb volumes (30–50%) with lymphatic bypass procedures. In patients with upper extremity lymphedema, Chang and colleagues reported symptom improvement in 96% of patients, quantitative improvement in 74% of patients, and a mean volume differential reduction of 42% at 12 months postoperatively.[34] A recent advancement in LVB surgery is the use of fluorescence lymphangiography for intraoperative mapping of lymphatic vessels.

Both VLNT and LVB are effective surgical techniques in reducing lymphedema, particularly in the early stages of disease. However, patient selection is key. Patients must be evaluated for their ability to withstand long bouts under anesthesia and must demonstrate willingness to participate in postoperative rehabilitation. Also, patients must be counseled that these treatments may provide symptom relief and reduce swelling but are not a cure for lymphedema. Other microsurgical procedures that have been described for lymphedema management but that are rarely offered include lympho-lymphatic bypass (i.e., connection of obstructed lymphatic channels to nonobstructed channels) and lymphatic vessel transfer. Finally, surgeons have recently begun performing simultaneous VLNT with microvascular breast reconstruction in select patients with promising results.[35] Patients for whom this may be appropriate are those who have developed postmastectomy lymphedema and are also interested in delayed breast reconstruction. Performing the procedures simultaneously requires that patients undergo only one major surgery.

ROOM SETUP

The room is organized as for a standard autologous breast reconstruction using microsurgical techniques. Patients undergoing VLNT only (with or without concomitant breast reconstruction) are placed in the supine position with their extremities tucked. For patients undergoing LNB, the arms are abducted and access is provided to the affected limb. An operating microscope is available in the room to be sterilely brought into the field when needed. General anesthesia and a Foley catheter are routinely used. Preoperative antibiotics and thromboembolic prophylaxis (mechanical and chemical) are administered.

PATIENT MARKINGS

Patients undergoing LVB receive intradermal injections of indocyanine green into each finger web of the affected limb. An infrared camera is used to visualize fluorescent images of lymphatic vessels (Figure 72.1). Fluorescent stains are identified proximal to injection sites. The visible lymphatic pathways and sites for LVB incisions are marked with a pen.

In VLNT, the donor and recipient sites should be marked. Donor sites are usually the groin or contralateral supraclavicular region. For patients undergoing lymph node transfer from the groin, preoperative injection of Tm99 is given to the lower extremity to identify sentinel nodes during the surgery using a "reverse mapping" technique to avoid secondary donor site lymphedema. Patients undergoing simultaneous autologous breast reconstruction are marked appropriately.

OPERATIVE TECHNIQUE

As in any microsurgical procedure, sterile prepping, draping, and technique are used throughout the operation. For LVB surgery, local anesthetic with epinephrine is injected at the incision sites for its hemostatic effect. A 30-gauge needle is used to inject isosulfan blue dye (0.1–0.2 mL) intradermally into each finger web space and/or 1–2 cm distal to each incision to aid in visually identifying lymphatic vessels. The procedure is performed entirely using a surgical microscope. At the predetermined sites, 3 cm incisions are made with a no. 15 blade. The subdermal region is dissected in order to identify lymphatic vessels, which are either blue with isosulfan dye or clear if no dye has been taken up (Figure 72.2). Lymphatics also can be seen with the fluorescent mode of the microscope if that is available. (Figure 72.3) Once identified, lymphatic

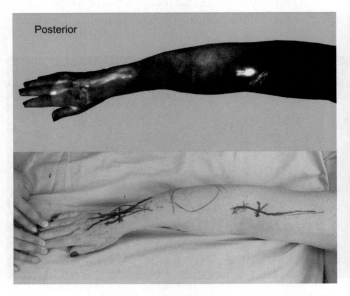

Figure 72.1. Fluorescent images of lymphatic vessels are visualized with an infrared camera.

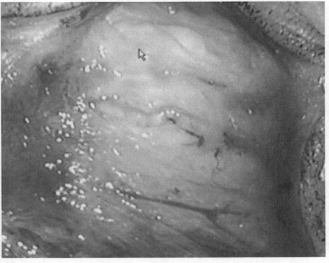

Figure 72.2. The subdermal region is dissected in order to identify lymphatic vessels, which are either blue with isosulfan dye or clear if no dye has been taken up.

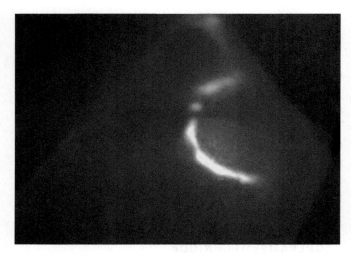

Figure 72.3. Lymphatics also can be seen with the fluorescent mode of the microscope if that is available.

avoid violating the deep inguinal lymphatic system. In addition, technetium-99m is injected intradermally into the leg to identify the sentinel lymph nodes. Once lymph nodes are identified, a gamma probe is used to ensure that the sentinel nodes are not included in the flap. These techniques will reduce the risk of postoperative lymphedema at the donor site. Dissection of the pedicle to the abdominal flap should be performed to maximize pedicle length.

At the recipient site, adequate axillary scar removal and release will enhance outcomes and is often necessary to identify recipient vessels for the VLNT. Generally, the thoracodorsal vessels or branches (e.g., serratus branch) or lateral thoracic vessels are used. The primary pedicle to the abdominal flap is generally anastomosed to the internal mammary vessels. Taking into account the recipient vessels, an algorithmic approach to simultaneous VLNT with microvascular breast reconstruction has been published.[36]

vessels are anastomosed to similarly sized venules that are adjacent in an end-to-end or end-to-side fashion. End-to-side anastomoses are especially useful if there is a substantial size mismatch between the lymphatic vessel and venule. Superfine microsurgical instruments are used and anastomoses are created with 11-0 or 12-0 nylon sutures with 50 μm needles. Patency of the bypass is confirmed by observing isosulfan blue dye or ICGN travel from the lymphatic vessel through the anastomosis into the venule (Figure 72.4).

For simultaneous VLNT and microvascular breast reconstruction, abdominal free flaps are based off of the deep inferior epigastric or superficial inferior epigastric pedicle. Lymph nodes are harvested en bloc with the abdominal flap along the superficial circumflex iliac vessels (Figure 72.5). It is important to not go below the inguinal ligament and to

POSTOPERATIVE CARE

Patients undergoing free tissue transfer (i.e., VLNT) generally remain in the hospital for 3 days postoperatively for monitoring while patients undergoing LVB only may be discharged as early as postoperative day 1 if standard criteria for discharge are met. Following surgery, patients are given 24 hours of intravenous antibiotics, and the affected limb is wrapped with short-stretch bandaging by a lymphedema therapist. Patients are seen in clinic for follow-up within the first week after surgery.

It is important to note that the approach to lymphedema treatment is multidisciplinary. Patients should be instructed

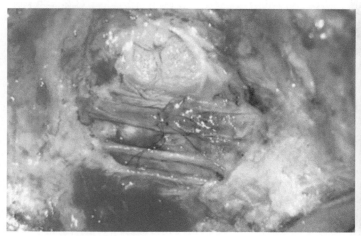
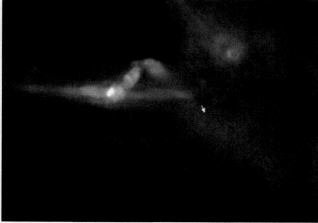

Figure 72.4. Patency of the bypass is confirmed by observing isosulfan blue dye or ICGN travel from the lymphatic vessel through the anastomosis into the venule.

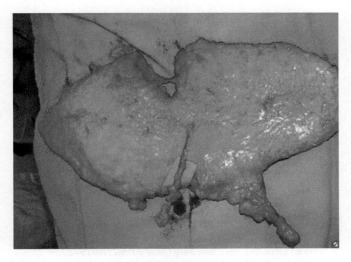

Figure 72.5. Lymph nodes are harvested en bloc with the abdominal flap.

to follow-up with a skilled lymphedema therapist at a time deemed safe by the surgeon (usually 4 weeks after surgery). The degree of residual swelling will guide the need for further therapy, which often includes compression garments and massage.

CAVEATS

In most cases, microsurgical techniques do not cure lymphedema. However, they do improve severity, reduce the number of complications associated with lymphedema, and improve quality of life. With respect to patient selection, LVB is best for clinical stages 1 or 2. In patients who are poor candidates for LVB (i.e., no functional lymphatic channels can be identified) or for those who are also interested in combined breast reconstruction, VLNT may be offered. Combined LVB and VLNT is often reserved for patients with advanced-stage (stage 3 or 4) lymphedema. Patients with less severe disease and those treated in a multidisciplinary center tend to respond more favorably. Nevertheless, there is no optimal solution. Further research is necessary for a better understanding of lymphatic anatomy and physiology and lymphedema pathophysiology.

REFERENCES

1. Becker C, Vasile JV, Levine JL, et al. Microlymphatic surgery for the treatment of iatrogenic lymphedema. *Clin Plast Surg* 2012;39: 385–398

2. Cormier JN, Rourke L, Crosby M, et al. The surgical treatment of lymphedema: a systematic review of the contemporary literature (2004–2010). *Ann Surg Oncol* 2012;19:642–651
3. Suami H, Chang DW. Overview of surgical treatments for breast cancer-related lymphedema. *Plast Reconstr Surg* 2010;126:1853–1863
4. Sakorafas GH, Peros G, Cataliotti L, et al. Lymphedema following axillary lymph node dissection for breast cancer. *Surg Oncol* 2006;15:153–165
5. Shih YC, Xu Y, Cormier JN, et al. Incidence, treatment costs, and complications of lymphedema after breast cancer among women of working age: a 2-year follow-up study. *J Clin Oncol* 2009;27:2007–2014
6. The diagnosis and treatment of peripheral lymphedema: 2013 Consensus Document of the International Society of Lymphology. *Lymphology* 2013;46:1–11
7. Warren AG, Brorson H, Borud LJ, et al. Lymphedema: a comprehensive review. *Ann Plast Surg* 2007;59:464–472
8. Mohler ER. Clinical features and diagnosis of peripheral lymphedema. *UpToDate* [serial online]. 2015;2015.
9. Weissleder H, Weissleder R. Lymphedema: evaluation of qualitative and quantitative lymphoscintigraphy in 238 patients. *Radiology* 1988;167:729–735
10. Lin CH, Ali R, Chen SC, et al. Vascularized groin lymph node transfer using the wrist as a recipient site for management of postmastectomy upper extremity lymphedema. *Plast Reconstr Surg* 2009;123:1265–1275
11. Torrisi JS, Joseph WJ, Ghanta S, et al. Lymphaticovenous bypass decreases pathologic skin changes in upper extremity breast cancer-related lymphedema. *Lymphat Res Biol* 2015;13:46–53
12. Mehrara BJ, Zampell JC, Suami H, Chang DW. Surgical management of lymphedema: past, present, and future. *Lymphat Res Biol.* 2011; 9(3):159–67. doi: 10.1089/lrb.2011.0011. Review. PMID: 22066746
13. Mortimer PS. Swollen lower limb-2: lymphoedema. *BMJ* 2000;320: 1527–1529
14. Brorson H, Svensson H. Liposuction combined with controlled compression therapy reduces arm lymphedema more effectively than controlled compression therapy alone. *Plast Reconstr Surg* 1998;102:1058–1067; discussion 1068
15. Vodder E. Lymohdrainage ad modem Vodder. *Aesthet Med* 1965;14:190
16. Williams AF, Vadgama A, Franks PJ, et al. A randomized controlled crossover study of manual lymphatic drainage therapy in women with breast cancer-related lymphoedema. *Eur J Cancer Care (Engl)* 2002;11:254–261
17. Miranda F, Jr., Perez MC, Castiglioni ML, et al. Effect of sequential intermittent pneumatic compression on both leg lymphedema volume and on lymph transport as semi-quantitatively evaluated by lymphoscintigraphy. *Lymphology* 2001;34:135–141
18. Szuba A, Achalu R, Rockson SG. Decongestive lymphatic therapy for patients with breast carcinoma-associated lymphedema. A randomized, prospective study of a role for adjunctive intermittent pneumatic compression. *Cancer* 2002;95:2260–2267
19. Dini D, Del Mastro L, Gozza A, et al. The role of pneumatic compression in the treatment of postmastectomy lymphedema. A randomized phase III study. *Ann Oncol* 1998;9:187–190
20. Brennan MJ, Miller LT. Overview of treatment options and review of the current role and use of compression garments, intermittent pumps, and exercise in the management of lymphedema. *Cancer* 1998;83:2821–2827
21. Casley-Smith JR, Morgan RG, Piller NB. Treatment of lymphedema of the arms and legs with 5,6-benzo-[alpha]-pyrone. *N Engl J Med* 1993;329:1158–1163
22. Charles RH. *Elephantiasis Scroti.* London: Churchill; 1912.
23. Sistrunk WE. Contribution to plastic surgery: removal of scars by stages; an open operation for extensive laceration of the anal sphincter; the kondoleon operation for elephantiasis. *Ann Surg* 1927;85:185–193

24. Thompson N. Buried dermal flap operation for chronic lymphedema of the extremities. Ten-year survey of results in 79 cases. *Plast Reconstr Surg* 1970;45:541–548
25. Brorson H. Liposuction in arm lymphedema treatment. *Scand J Surg* 2003;92:287–295
26. Frick A, Hoffmann JN, Baumeister RG, et al. Liposuction technique and lymphatic lesions in lower legs: anatomic study to reduce risks. *Plast Reconstr Surg* 1999;103:1868–1873; discussion: 1874–1865
27. Shesol BF, Nakashima R, Alavi A, et al. Successful lymph node transplantation in rats, with restoration of lymphatic function. *Plast Reconstr Surg* 1979;63:817–823
28. Clodius L, Smith PJ, Bruna J, et al. The lymphatics of the groin flap. *Ann Plast Surg* 1982;9:447–458
29. Becker C, Assouad J, Riquet M, et al. Postmastectomy lymphedema: long-term results following microsurgical lymph node transplantation. *Ann Surg* 2006;243:313–315
30. Gharb BB, Rampazzo A, Spanio di Spilimbergo S, et al. Vascularized lymph node transfer based on the hilar perforators improves the outcome in upper limb lymphedema. *Ann Plast Surg* 2011;67:589–593
31. Althubaiti GA, Crosby MA, Chang DW. Vascularized supraclavicular lymph node transfer for lower extremity lymphedema treatment. *Plast Reconstr Surg* 2013;131:133e–135e
32. Cheng MH, Huang JJ, Nguyen DH, et al. A novel approach to the treatment of lower extremity lymphedema by transferring a vascularized submental lymph node flap to the ankle. *Gynecol Oncol* 2012;126:93–98
33. Raju A, Chang DW. Vascularized lymph node transfer for treatment of lymphedema: a comprehensive literature review. *Ann Surg* 2015;261:1013–1023
34. Chang DW, Suami H, Skoracki R. A prospective analysis of 100 consecutive lymphovenous bypass cases for treatment of extremity lymphedema. *Plast Reconstr Surg* 2013;132:1305–1314
35. Saaristo AM, Niemi TS, Viitanen TP, et al. Microvascular breast reconstruction and lymph node transfer for postmastectomy lymphedema patients. *Ann Surg* 2012;255:468–473
36. Nguyen AT, Chang EI, Suami H, et al. An algorithmic approach to simultaneous vascularized lymph node transfer with microvascular breast reconstruction. *Ann Surg Oncol* 2015;22:2919–2924

73.

SENTINEL LYMPH NODE DISSECTION

Shadi Lalezari, Vivian V. Le-Tran, and Karen T. Lane

ASSESSMENT OF THE DEFECT

Regional lymph node status is an important prognostic factor in breast cancer and melanoma.[1,2] To determine the appropriateness of sentinel lymph node dissection (SLND) in the setting of these tumors, assessment should include a complete history and physical examination of the patient. Any history of radiation therapy or surgery in the region(s) under consideration for SLND should be noted by the surgeon as these factors may alter the anatomy of the surgical site. Physical examination should include palpation of lymph nodes to determine the presence of any clinically enlarged nodes. Pathology results and imaging, such as mammography, computed tomography (CT) scans, and/or magnetic resonance imaging (MRI), should be reviewed to determine important characteristics of the tumor, including its pathological type, its size, and the presence of any nodal or distant metastasis.

INDICATIONS FOR SURGERY

SLND is indicated in the surgical staging of the clinically negative axilla in patients with clinical stage I, stage IIA, stage IIB, or stage IIIA T3, N1, M0 breast cancer.[1] SLND is recommended in patients with melanoma with Breslow depth of greater than 1 mm and should also be discussed with and offered to patients with melanomas that are 0.76–1.0 mm thick in the appropriate clinical context.[2] High-risk features for positive sentinel lymph nodes include ulceration, high mitotic rate, and lymphovascular invasion.[2]

Tumors drain through the lymphatic system in an orderly manner, and the sentinel lymph node is the first to be affected if a tumor has spread.[3,4] Due to this drainage pattern, a tumor-free ("negative") sentinel node indicates that it is unlikely that other nodes are affected.[4] While the concept of the sentinel node had been introduced previously, Morton et al. first described SLNB for patients with melanoma in 1992.[3,5] Giuliano et al. later developed a modified technique to detect axillary lymph node metastases in patients with breast cancer.[3,6] This technique has eliminated the need for axillary lymph node dissection (ALND) or complete lymph node dissection (CLND) for the determination of tumor metastasis to regional lymph nodes in many patients. SLND is now a widely used, minimally invasive technique that allows accurate staging of regional lymph nodes with decreased morbidity and better quality of life for cancer patients.[7,8]

CONTRAINDICATIONS FOR SURGERY

SLND should not be performed in patients with a history of allergic reaction to blue tracer dyes or radioactive colloids, or in those with inflammatory breast cancer.

A history of allergic reaction to blue dyes or radioactive colloids is an absolute contraindication to SLND. Commonly used agents for sentinel lymph node detection in the United States are isosulfan blue dye (sold under the trade name Lymphazurin) and Technetium 99m (^{99m}Tc) labeled sulfur colloid. The reported incidence of allergic reactions, including anaphylaxis, to blue dyes used in lymphatic mapping has been reported as high as 2.7%.[9] Methylene blue is a less expensive and effective alternative to isosulfan blue with a lower risk of anaphylaxis and other allergic reactions.[10] However, intradermal injection of methylene blue dye can cause skin necrosis and other skin lesions.[11] Avoidance of intradermal injection can prevent skin necrosis.[12]

Inflammatory breast cancer typically presents with diffuse infiltration of the breast, dermis, and lymphatics. Involvement of the lymphatic channels in the breast may cause a blockage in these channels, making it difficult to identify the sentinel nodes.[13] Therefore, SLND should not be performed in patients with this type of breast cancer.[14] Patients with inflammatory breast cancer should undergo mastectomy and level I/II ALND.[1]

PREOPERATIVE PREPARATION AND ROOM SETUP

Special equipment is necessary in the operating room based on the technique used for lymphatic mapping. The combined use of radioactive colloid and blue dye has consistently been shown to have a better sentinel lymph node identification rate than blue dye alone.[15–18] In our practice, radiocolloid is often used alone to avoid the chance of an allergic reaction to the blue dye. In addition, the blue dye can temporarily tattoo the skin, which may make skin flap monitoring difficult in the immediate postreconstruction period. The use of radiocolloid alone is an accepted technique.

If radioactive colloid is to be used for sentinel node identification, the patient must be injected with the radionuclide prior to surgery. The radionuclide can be injected the morning of, or day prior to, surgery. For breast cancer, radiocolloid can be injected deep, at a peritumoral or intratumoral site, or superficial, at intradermal, subdermal, periareolar, or subareolar sites.[4] In the setting of melanoma, radiocolloid should be injected intradermally around the primary tumor (Figure 73.1) or in four parts

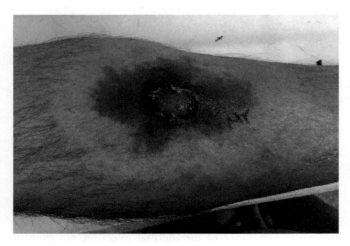

Figure 73.1. Intradermal injection of isosulfan blue dye at the site of the primary tumor. Photo courtesy of Dr. Maki Yamamoto.

around a biopsy scar.[19,20] Preoperative lymphoscintigraphy can be performed for improved accuracy.[4] This imaging modality is beneficial in identifying sentinel nodes that drain cancers in areas of the body with ambiguous and varied lymph node drainage such as tumors of the trunk, shoulder, and head and neck.[19,21,22] Melanomas of the trunk for example, can drain to one or more lymph node sites, including axillary, groin, cervical, supraclavicular, and others.[22] Similarly head and neck melanomas may drain to parotid, cervical, supraclavicular, occipital, or axillary lymph nodes.[22] Melanomas of the trunk and head and neck may also have sentinel nodes in contralateral basins, as drainage of the tumor may cross midline for these primary tumor sites.[22,23] Lymphoscintigraphy can also improve detection of malignant melanomas with aberrant sentinel lymph node drainage—such as upper extremity melanomas that drain to supraclavicular or epitrochlear nodes instead of the expected axillary nodes, or lower extremity melanomas that drain to popliteal nodes instead of nodes in the groin.[22,24]

Further imaging may include single-photon emission computed tomography/computed tomography (SPECT/CT), a technique that combines radioactivity detected by SPECT with CT images.[25] This imaging modality can be beneficial when lymphoscintigraphy shows an unusual drainage pattern, is difficult to interpret, or fails to show a sentinel node as SPECT/CT has better contrast and resolution than lymphoscintigraphy and allows for detection of nodes that may not be visualized on conventional imaging.[26,27] The improved detection of sentinel lymph nodes with SPECT/CT allows for improved operative planning and easier excision of the sentinel nodes; however, the use of these images is associated with increased costs and time.[25–27]

The operating room should be equipped for general anesthesia. Two instruments setups are required if immediate reconstruction is planned—one for the oncologic portion of the procedure and one for the reconstructive portion. Five milliliters of blue dye of the surgeon's choice and/or a gamma probe should be available in the operating room in preparation for lymphatic mapping. Preoperative prophylaxis using a glucocorticoid, diphenhydramine, and famotidine can be given intravenously just before or at the induction of general anesthesia to reduce the severity, but not incidence, of adverse reactions caused by isosulfan blue.[28] The patient is placed supine on the operating table. For axillary SLND, both arms are placed on padded arm boards, with the arm on the affected side abducted to 90 degrees. The surgical site (e.g., the axilla, groin, or neck) should be clipped prior to skin preparation and draping in a standard sterile fashion.

PATIENT MARKINGS

Three to five milliliters of blue dye can be injected in the same manner as radiocolloid, although methylene blue should not be injected intradermally due to the risk of skin necrosis described earlier.[11] The area of injection should be massaged for at least 5 minutes in order to allow the dye to reach the sentinel node through the lymphatic channels. A hand-held gamma probe is used to identify the area of greatest radioactivity. A 3–5 cm line is drawn to mark the appropriate skin incision. In the axilla, this is typically made transversely at the level of the distal hair-bearing area.

OPERATIVE TECHNIQUE

A 3–5 cm incision is made in the skin. The gamma probe and/or visualization of blue lymphatic channels are used to help guide dissection and identification of the sentinel nodes (Figure 73.2). The sentinel nodes will be blue and radioactive, or "hot." All blue nodes and nodes with significant radioactivity should be removed.[29] An ex-vivo radioactivity count should be determined for each excised node.[29] The node should be inspected with the gamma probe from multiple angles, and the highest radioactivity count is recorded. Removal of all blue nodes and all nodes with 10% or more

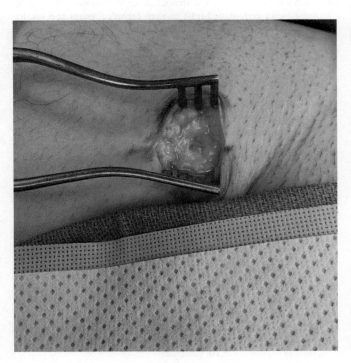

Figure 73.2. Identification of lymphatic channel in inguinal nodal basin by uptake of isosulfan blue dye. Photo courtesy of Dr. Maki Yamamoto.

of the ex-vivo radioactivity count of the hottest node allows for optimal detection of nodal metastases.[29–31] Prior to closure of the wound, the surgical area should be visually inspected and assessed with the gamma probe to ensure removal of all appropriate nodes. The nodal basin should be palpated, and any suspicious nodes should be considered for excision as the sentinel lymph node. Hemostasis is obtained and the wound is irrigated. The wound is closed in layers, with 3-0 absorbable sutures used to close the subcutaneous tissue and deep dermis. The skin is closed with a 4-0 absorbable monofilament suture in a running subcuticular fashion. A frozen section can be sent to pathology if an intraoperative result is needed. For breast cancer, a positive sentinel lymph node(s) may necessitate an ALND during the same procedure. Patients are always consented for both procedures. Excised nodes not sent for frozen section are sent for permanent pathology. In cases where the sentinel lymph node cannot be identified intraoperatively, ALND should be performed.[32]

POSTOPERATIVE CARE

Prior to discharge, patients should be given instructions regarding routine wound care and follow-up with their surgeon. They can typically be discharged on the day of surgery. The patient should be informed about the pathology results of their sentinel nodes once they are available. Patients with positive sentinel nodes will often require further workup and surgery.[1,2] The results of the American College of Surgeons Oncology Group Z0011 trial indicate that a subset of breast cancer patients may not need to undergo ALND despite having positive sentinel nodes. The study found "that women with a positive SLN and clinical T1-T2 tumors undergoing lumpectomy with radiation therapy followed by systemic therapy do not benefit from the addition of ALND in terms of local control, disease-free survival, or overall survival."[33]

CAVEATS

There are several areas of continuing research focusing on SLND. These include the appropriate use of this procedure for breast cancer patients in the setting of pregnancy, clinically positive lymph nodes, prior axillary surgery, ductal carcinoma in situ (DCIS), and neoadjuvant chemotherapy.[4]

The American Society of Clinical Oncology continues to recommend that clinicians should not perform SLND on patients with early-stage breast cancer who are pregnant.[14] There are various concerns regarding SLND in pregnancy, including fetal harm from radiation exposure due to radiocolloid use and possible teratogenicity of blue dyes.[34] However, available data indicate that this procedure can be safely performed during pregnancy.[34] Based on these findings, pregnant patients with breast cancer should be offered SLND when it is indicated.[35] Radiocolloid should be injected on the day of surgery to minimize radiation exposure, and blue dye should not be used.[35]

There are areas of continued investigation with respect to SLND for melanoma patients as well. Although thin melanomas (≤1 mm) represent the majority of melanomas diagnosed in most developed countries, including the United States, the role of SLND in these patients remains unclear.[2,36,37] Despite some controversy regarding the value of SLND for patients with thick melanomas (>4 mm), the procedure is recommended in these patients as it provides important staging information and facilitates regional disease control.[36,37]

There is ongoing research regarding the use of SLND for tumors other than breast cancer and melanoma. These include colon, gastric, and esophageal cancers.[3] The expansion of this minimally invasive technique to other types of cancer may decrease the challenging side effects of more invasive procedures, as it has for breast cancer and melanoma patients.

For breast cancer and melanoma patients in need of surgical staging of regional lymph nodes, SLND has significantly lowered the rates of surgical complications and morbidity compared to the more invasive lymph node dissection. Studies have shown that CLND, or SLND with CLND, results in higher rates of seromas, nerve injury, and lymphedema compared to SLND alone.[8,38,39] It is important to counsel patients preoperatively that the risk of lymphedema from SLND is 0–3%.

New techniques for SLND, such as the use of a magnetic tracer or indocyanine green fluorescence imaging, are being actively investigated and may play a more significant role in this procedure in the future.[40–42]

REFERENCES

1. NCCN Clinical Practice Guidelines in Oncology (NCCN Guidelines) Breast Cancer. Version 2.2016
2. NCCN Clinical Practice Guidelines in Oncology (NCCN Guidelines) Melanoma. Version 1.2016.
3. Chen SL, Iddings DM, Scheri RP, Bilchik AJ. Lymphatic mapping and sentinel node analysis: current concepts and applications. *CA: Cancer J Clinicians* 2006;56(5):292–309.
4. Manca G, Rubello D, Tardelli E, et al. Sentinel lymph node biopsy in breast cancer: indications, contraindications, and controversies. *Clin Nucl Med* 2016;2(41):126–133.
5. Morton DL, Duan-Ren Wen D-R, Wong JH, et al. Technical details of intraoperative lymphatic mapping for early stage melanoma. *Arch Surg* 1992;127(4):392–399.
6. Giuliano AE, Kirgan DM, Guenther JM, Morton DL. Lymphatic mapping and sentinel lymphadenectomy for breast cancer. *Ann Surg* 1994;220(3):391.
7. Mansel RE, Fallowfield L, Kissin M, et al. Randomized multicenter trial of sentinel node biopsy versus standard axillary treatment in operable breast cancer: the ALMANAC Trial. *J Natl Cancer Inst* 2006;98(9):599–609.
8. Kretschmer L, Thoms K-M, Peeters S, Haenssle H, Bertsch HP, Emmert S. Postoperative morbidity of lymph node excision for cutaneous melanoma-sentinel lymphonodectomy versus complete regional lymph node dissection. *Melanoma Res* 2008;18(1):16–21.
9. Bézu C, Coutant C, Salengro A, Daraï E, Rouzier R, Uzan S. Anaphylactic response to blue dye during sentinel lymph node biopsy. *Surg Oncol* 2011;20(1): e55–e59.
10. Simmons R, Thevarajah S, Brennan MB, Christos P, Osborne M. Methylene blue dye as an alternative to isosulfan blue dye for sentinel lymph node localization. *Ann Surg Oncol* 2003;10(3):242–247.
11. Stradling B, Aranha G, Gabram S. Adverse skin lesions after methylene blue injections for sentinel lymph node localization. *Am J Surg* 2002;184(4):350–352.
12. Varghese P, Abdel-Rahman AT, Akberali S, Mostafa A, Gattuso JM, Carpenter R. Methylene blue dye—a safe and effective alternative for sentinel lymph node localization. *Breast J* 2008;14(1):61–67.
13. Stearns V, Ewing CA, Slack R, Penannen MF, Hayes DF, Tsangaris TN. Sentinel lymphadenectomy after neoadjuvant chemotherapy for breast cancer may reliably represent the axilla except for inflammatory breast cancer. *Ann Surg Oncol* 2002;9(3):235–242.
14. Lyman GH, Temin S, Edge SB, et al. Sentinel lymph node biopsy for patients with early-stage breast cancer: American Society of Clinical Oncology clinical practice guideline update. *J Clin Oncol* 2014;32(13):1365–1383.
15. Canavese G, Gipponi M, Catturich A, et al. Sentinel lymph node mapping in early-stage breast cancer: Technical issues and results with vital blue dye mapping and radioguided surgery. *J Surg Oncol* 2000;74(1):61–68.
16. Gershenwald JE, Tseng C-h, Thompson W, et al. Improved sentinel lymph node localization in patients with primary melanoma with the use of radiolabeled colloid. *Surgery* 1998;124(2):203–210.
17. Kapteijn B, Acca E, Omgo E, et al. Localizing the sentinel node in cutaneous melanoma: gamma probe detection versus blue dye. *Ann Surg Oncol* 1997;4(2):156–160.
18. Wong SL, Edwards MJ, Chao C, et al. Sentinel lymph node biopsy for breast cancer: impact of the number of sentinel nodes removed on the false-negative rate. *J Am Coll Surg* 2001;192(6):684–689.
19. Norman JC, Cruse W, Espinosa C, et al. Redefinition of cutaneous lymphatic drainage with the use of lymphoscintigraphy for malignant melanoma. *Am J Surg* 1991;162(5):432–437.
20. Albertini JJ, Cruse CW, Rapaport D, et al. Intraoperative radio-lympho-scintigraphy improves sentinel lymph node identification for patients with melanoma. *Ann Surg* 1996;223(2):217.
21. Even-Sapir E, Lerman H, Lievshitz G, et al. Lymphoscintigraphy for sentinel node mapping using a hybrid SPECT/CT system. *J Nucl Med* 2003;44(9):1413–1420.
22. Uren RF, Howman-Giles R, Thompson JF. Patterns of lymphatic drainage from the skin in patients with melanoma. *J Nucl Med* 2003;44(4):570–582.
23. Chao C, Wong SL, Edwards MJ, et al., and Sunbelt Melanoma Trial Group. Sentinel lymph node biopsy for head and neck melanomas. *Ann Surg Oncol* 2003;10(1):21–26.

24. Lieber KA, Standiford SB, Kuvshinoff BW, Ota DM. Surgical management of aberrant sentinel lymph node drainage in cutaneous melanoma. *Surgery* 1998;124(4):757–762.
25. Doepker MP, Zager JS. Sentinel lymph node mapping in melanoma in the twenty-first century. *Surg Oncol Clin N Am* 2015;24(2):249–260.
26. van der Ploeg IMC, Valdés Olmos RA, Kroon BBR, et al. The yield of SPECT/CT for anatomical lymphatic mapping in patients with melanoma. *Ann Surg Oncol* 2009;16(6):1537–1542.
27. van der Ploeg IMC, Nieweg OE, Kroon BBR, et al. The yield of SPECT/CT for anatomical lymphatic mapping in patients with breast cancer. *Eur J Nucl Med Mol Imag* 2009;36(6):903–909.
28. Raut CP, Hunt KK, Akins JS, et al. Incidence of anaphylactoid reactions to isosulfan blue dye during breast carcinoma lymphatic mapping in patients treated with preoperative prophylaxis. *Cancer* 2005;104(4):692–699.
29. Martin RCG, Edwards MJ, Wong SL, et al. Practical guidelines for optimal gamma probe detection of sentinel lymph nodes in breast cancer: results of a multi-institutional study. *Surgery* 2000;128(2):139–144.
30. Carlson GW, Murray DR, Thourani V, Hestley A, Cohen C. The definition of the sentinel lymph node in melanoma based on radioactive counts. *Ann Surg Oncol* 2002;9(9):929–933.
31. McMasters KM, Reintgen DS, Ross MI, et al. Sentinel lymph node biopsy for melanoma: how many radioactive nodes should be removed? *Ann Surg Oncol* 2001;8(3):192–197.
32. Abdollahi A, Jangjoo A, Dabbagh Kakhki VR, et al. Factors affecting sentinel lymph node detection failure in breast cancer patients using intradermal injection of the tracer. *Revista española de medicina nuclear* 2010;29(2):73–77.
33. Giuliano AE, Hunt KK, Ballman KV, et al. Axillary dissection vs no axillary dissection in women with invasive breast cancer and sentinel node metastasis: a randomized clinical trial. *JAMA* 2011;305(6):569–575.
34. Gropper AB, Zabicki Calvillo K, Dominici L, et al. Sentinel lymph node biopsy in pregnant women with breast cancer. *Ann Surg Oncol* 2014;21(8):2506–2511.
35. Loibl S, Schmidt A, Gentilini O, et al. Breast cancer diagnosed during pregnancy: adapting recent advances in breast cancer care for pregnant patients. *JAMA Oncol* 2015;1(8):1145–1153.
36. Wong SL, Balch CM, Hurley P, et al. Sentinel lymph node biopsy for melanoma: American Society of Clinical Oncology and Society of Surgical Oncology joint clinical practice guideline. *J Clin Oncol* 2012;30(23):2912–2918.
37. Thompson JF, Shaw HM. Sentinel node mapping for melanoma: results of trials and current applications. *Surg Oncol Clin N Am* 2007;16(1):35–54.
38. Purushotham AD, Upponi S, Klevesath MB, Bobrow L, Millar K, Myles JP, Duffy SW. Morbidity after sentinel lymph node biopsy in primary breast cancer: results from a randomized controlled trial. *J Clin Oncol* 2005;23(19):4312–4321.
39. Langer I, Guller U, Berclaz G, et al. Morbidity of sentinel lymph node biopsy (SLN) alone versus SLN and completion axillary lymph node dissection after breast cancer surgery: a prospective Swiss multicenter study on 659 patients. *Ann Surg* 2007;245(3):452.
40. Douek M, Klaase J, Monypenny I, et al. Sentinel node biopsy using a magnetic tracer versus standard technique: the SentiMAG multicentre trial. *Ann Surg Oncol* 2014;21(4):1237–1245.
41. Kitai T, Inomoto T, Miwa M, Shikayama T. Fluorescence navigation with indocyanine green for detecting sentinel lymph nodes in breast cancer. *Breast Cancer* 2005;12(3):211–215.
42. Fujiwara M, Mizukami T, Suzuki A, Fukamizu H. Sentinel lymph node detection in skin cancer patients using real-time fluorescence navigation with indocyanine green: preliminary experience. *J Plast Reconstr Aesthet Surg* 2009;62(10): e373–e378.

74

NIPPLE-SPARING SURGERY

Karen T. Lane and David A. Daar

Techniques for the surgical management of breast cancer have significantly transformed in recent years. While the primary goal is to effectively remove the cancerous lesion or provide risk-reducing prophylaxis in high-risk patients, recent years have focused on minimizing the morbidity of the procedure and improving the aesthetic outcome. Nipple-sparing mastectomy (NSM) has gained increasing popularity as an option for treatment over the typical skin-sparing mastectomy (SSM).[1] As such, the proper identification of eligible patients for treatment with NSM is the most crucial aspect of caring for breast cancer patients and has been the subject of much scrutiny. Moreover, while there is no standard operative technique, various incision locations have proven advantageous depending on patient and oncologic characteristics. NSM has benefited from advances in technology (e.g., intraoperative laser angiography, acellular dermal matrices [ADM], and the lighted retractor). Consideration of the appropriate reconstructive method must be included, and the possibility of nipple-areolar complex (NAC) necrosis and locoregional recurrence require diligent postoperative assessment. To ensure successful treatment and recovery, the surgeon must encourage enhanced coordination among all members of the breast cancer treatment team along with shared decision-making with each individual patient.

ASSESSMENT OF THE DEFECT

Assessment ultimately involves similar preoperative measures for any breast cancer patient, including consultations with each member of the multidisciplinary treatment team. Key measures focus on determining whether or not it is safe—based on oncologic and patient factors—to preserve the NAC as well as the prospect of a superior aesthetic outcome. Physical exam of the breast and axilla must be performed, paying particular attention to evidence of tumor involvement of the nipple and adjacent area. Skin changes suggestive of Paget's disease or inflammatory breast cancer must be identified, and, if present, any nipple discharge should be examined for blood or other contents.

Dimensions of the breast should be measured, including breast size and size of footprint, degree of ptosis, nipple characteristics, sternal notch-to-nipple distance, nipple-to-inframammary crease distance, and nipple-to-nipple distance. Breast asymmetry should be noted to aid in determining proper reconstructive options as well as to counsel the patient later regarding managing expectations of her outcome.

The use of preoperative magnetic resonance imaging (MRI) has been examined in the literature; while some consider it routine, others prefer a patient-specific approach and even use a shared decision model/tool.[1] The proposed benefits of preoperative MRI are twofold: (1) to identify possible NAC involvement and (2) to evaluate the patient's vascularity to determine the risk of necrosis. Several studies have shown the utility of MRI in identifying tumor-to-NAC distance (TND), a key predictor for occult NAC involvement, with a high specificity and negative predictive value ranging from 87.5% to 100% and 82% and 94.9%, respectively.[2–6] There is still question regarding its superiority to thorough clinical evaluation. Preoperative MRI can also be used to identify breast vascular patterns; presence of a dual vascular supply seen on MRI has been associated with a decreased risk of NAC and skin flap necrosis.[7]

Intraoperative evaluation of the NAC margin should be assessed to determine appropriateness of NSM (see "Operative Technique" section for further discussion).

INDICATIONS FOR SURGERY

Proper patient selection is the key to performing NSM safely and effectively. While there is no concrete set of indications for the procedure, National Comprehensive Cancer Network (NCCN) practice guidelines for 2016 propose that NSM eligibility be "selected by experienced, multidisciplinary teams."[8] Partially as a result of this lack of consensus, indications for NSM have been rapidly expanding in recent years and vary among institutions.[1,9,10]

NSM may be indicated in prophylactic or risk-reducing surgeries, as well as in therapeutic surgeries for oncologic resection. Patients with germline mutations in BRCA1 and BRCA2 are proven candidates for NSM, with recurrence rates comparable to SSM.[10,11] Also, as patients increasingly opt for contralateral prophylactic mastectomy, the superior aesthetic outcome of NSM favors its use in this setting.

Several other trends may be related to increasing eligibility for NSM. The advent of new technologies for both oncologic resection and reconstruction, including preoperative MRI and intraoperative laser-assisted indocyanine green angiography, has helped with patient selection.[12] Improvements in genetic testing have identified a greater number of high-risk patients.[1] Advances in systemic treatment have decreased locoregional recurrence rates and offer more effective neoadjuvant and adjuvant therapy for patients undergoing NSM. The growing rate of breast cancer patients being treated with NSM has allowed for heightened technical expertise among surgeons.

CONTRAINDICATIONS FOR SURGERY

The contraindications for NSM vary widely in the literature and have continued to evolve in recent years. The various considerations can be categorized into (1) clinical or oncologic considerations and (2) patient and anatomic factors.

CLINICAL OR ONCOLOGIC FACTORS

The only proven absolute contraindication for NSM is overt evidence of NAC involvement or Paget's disease on preoperative imaging or clinical examination.[9] Other widely accepted contraindications include inflammatory breast cancer, bloody nipple discharge, evidence of multifocal disease, and axillary lymph node involvement.[13,14]

The TND has been intensely studied, with institutional guidelines recommending against NSM for tumors less than 2–2.5 cm from the NAC and, more recently, as close as 1 cm.[2,13,15] Recent evidence has shown this contraindication

may be considered relative rather than absolute as long as intraoperative pathology of the NAC margin is proven negative.[9,16]

Tumor size has been considered a traditional contraindication to NSM due to its implication in nipple involvement. Debate over maximum cutoff for exclusion from NSM continues, ranging between 3 and 5 cm as a predictive factor for NAC involvement.[17,18] Nonetheless, other institutional experience suggests NSM can be safely performed for any tumor size if both clinical and radiologic evidence excludes NAC or skin involvement.[9]

History of prior breast irradiation or the prospect of postmastectomy radiation therapy previously deemed patients ineligible for NSM due to various concerns affecting aesthetic outcomes (e.g., skin tightening as well as risk of fat, skin, or NAC necrosis, incision breakdown, and nipple malposition).[10] A study of patients from the Surveillance, Epidemiology, and End Results (SEER) database found that patients treated with therapeutic NSM were more likely to undergo postmastectomy radiation therapy compared with SSM patients, possibly due to concern for NAC involvement.[19] Recent studies have demonstrated successful outcomes with NSM in irradiated patients, although level of evidence is limited to case series.[10,20,21] Proponents for NSM in this setting argue that patients undergoing SSM with implant-based reconstruction typically experience unsuccessful nipple reconstruction, and the increased skin envelope in NSM enhances the ability for single-stage reconstruction.[20]

PATIENT AND ANATOMIC FACTORS

Patient comorbidities that increase the risk of NAC necrosis or impaired wound healing are relative contraindications for NSM, including smoking, obesity, and the like.[22]

The utility of NSM in excessively large or ptotic breasts continues to be debated. Concerns regarding an unacceptable aesthetic outcome include poor skin quality leading to increased risk of skin flap or NAC necrosis as well as the challenge of proper NAC positioning.[23] Yet surgeons are continuing to push the boundary as to what degree of ptosis or breast size is unacceptable. Recent individual surgeon experiences show that this decision requires input from both the breast surgeon and plastic surgeon as well as a long discussion with the patient. In many cases, the patient and plastic surgeon have agreed on a smaller breast size, which would result in the need for the nipple to be placed in a more superior position to optimize the cosmetic result. This factor may ultimately be informed by clinical judgment and the surgeon's assessment of his or her own technical expertise because large, ptotic breasts can prove a more challenging dissection.

Prior breast surgery or augmentation is a relative contraindication, with recent evidence demonstrating conflicted outcomes regarding risk for complications after NSM.[24,25] One study identified an increased rate of hematoma and mastectomy flap ischemia in prior cosmetic breast surgery patients.[24] Thus, if chosen to proceed with NSM, it may be crucial to preserve the periprosthetic capsule in these patients.

Surgeon experience may also play a role in deciding to perform NSM. Studies have shown a decreasing rate of complications as well as lower rates of positive NAC margins over time among surgeons performing NSM at their respective institutions.[1,21] This may correlate with increased volume of procedures leading to enhanced surgical expertise and improved coordination among treatment teams. Therefore, inexperienced surgeons may be better suited to attempt NSM in patients who are early-stage cancer patients with low risk for complications and lack of relative contraindications.

Many more breast cancer patients are receiving neoadjuvant chemotherapy even in the setting of early-stage breast cancer, with treatment based on tumor markers. It is important to make a decision regarding the patient's suitability for NSM prior to initiating neoadjuvant chemotherapy. While many patients have an excellent response to treatment, it seems prudent to base decisions regarding the role for NSM on their initial tumor size and position. This will more than likely change as more patients undergo NSM after neoadjuvant chemotherapy and data become available regarding nipple recurrence.

ROOM SETUP

The patient is placed in the supine position with arms out to 90 degrees in supination. The patient's arms are wrapped from shoulder to the elbows to prevent sliding, leaving adequate exposure of the axilla as a sentinel lymph node dissection may also be indicated. The patient is prepped in sterile fashion from the chin to the navel on both sides. Draping is performed first with surgical towels to square off areas of the breast footprint, and two split drapes are then laid down. Other materials/supplies to consider include:

- Lighted fiberoptic retractor
- (Insulated) retractors (Army/Navy, small Rich, small Deaver)

- Electrocautery
- Skin hooks
- Surgical clips
- Aliss clamps
- (Insulated) DeBakey forceps
- Freeman rake retractors
- Tonsil, right-angle

PATIENT MARKINGS

Preoperative markings should be discussed and agreed upon by both the oncologic and reconstructive surgeons involved, and the specific incision choice (see "Operative Technique" further discussion) should be reconfirmed on day of operation.

Mark the sternal notch, midline from sternal notch to inframammary fold (IMF), anterior axillary line, and proposed incision (varies). Identifying the breast outline preoperatively ensures the surgeon adequately removes all breast tissue while avoiding unnecessary excision.

OPERATIVE TECHNIQUE

The patient is placed under general anesthesia, and prophylactic intravenous antibiotics are administered. Some surgeons advocate for the use of local anesthetic (e.g., 1% lidocaine with epinephrine or a more dilute concentration). Proponents of this cite its utility in hydrodissection of the mastectomy flap as well as hemostasis during dissection, while others may consider its masking effect on easier recognition of poorly perfused skin flaps. It is debated whether the NAC is to be infiltrated, but, if performed, it is done so in a subareolar plane. In some cases, a thoracic paravertebral block may be performed to assist with pain control as well as potentially reduce postoperative opioid use and nausea/vomiting.

There is no proven superior incision location for NSM, and techniques vary considerably. The transareolar approach has fallen out of favor due to disruption of blood supply to the NAC and subsequently high necrosis rates.[26] Similarly, it is imperative to avoid making an incision greater than 180 degrees around the NAC.

The periareolar incision has been used to provide adequate access to the axilla for sentinel lymph node and axillary dissections, when necessary, and may be better suited for larger breasts or those with higher grade ptosis.[17] Other benefits included enhanced scar camouflage due to areolar texture and color and easier bleeding control.[27] Despite these advantages, its use has decreased due to its consistently proven significance as a risk factor for NAC necrosis and complications.[27,28] Caution must be taken when performing a periareolar incision to prevent disrupting the blood supply to the NAC, and patients may experience decreased NAC sensitivity compared to other incisions.[29]

In cases where autologous reconstruction is planned, the radial incision may be appropriate in that it provides substantial access to the internal mammary vessels.[30] Most commonly placed in a lateral radial approach, it offers ease in reaching the axillary tail and upper breast pole and can allow for sentinel node biopsy without a necessary counterincision. However, scarring is more obvious with radial incisions, and contraction can result in nipple malposition—particularly lateral displacement.[31,32] Retraction must be handled carefully to avoid causing ischemia to mastectomy skin flaps.

The IMF incision has increased in popularity due to its superior cosmetic outcome.[27,33,34] The mastectomy scar can be well-hidden in the IMF, and its inferior placement prevents compromise of blood supply to the NAC. Some authors report its superiority in implant-based reconstruction as well as in small-breasted patients due to easy of resection and dissection for implant or expander placement. However, it may prove a more challenging dissection with regard to accessing the upper breast pole and performing an axillary node dissection, often requiring a counterincision.[17,31] Lateralizing the IMF incision can offer improved access and cosmesis, assuaging some of the technical difficulty.[27,33] The inferolateral IMF incision is placed along the curvilinear skin crease and may range in extension from the 6 o'clock position to the 3 o'clock position laterally (for the left breast). Moreover, the use of the lighted retractor has enhanced visualization of the upper breast pole and may increase utility of the IMF incision in patients with larger breast footprints.

For larger breasts with moderate to severe ptosis, a mastopexy incision can provide better access to breast tissue as well as offer superior nipple aesthetics and positioning.[35] Reducing the skin envelope and dead space offers enhanced shaping during reconstruction. Nevertheless, risks include compromise to lateral and medial skin flaps; some authors suggest it may be better as a secondary mastopexy procedure.[23]

In cases requiring a sentinel lymph node dissection, this may be carried out first through a separate axillary incision at the inferior aspect of the axillary hairline. After this is complete, the breast incision is made and dissection of the glandular breast tissue off the mastectomy skin flap is performed. This can be done sharply with scissors or using electrocautery. Sharp dissection may offer less risk to the mastectomy skin flap but will result in increased bleeding to be controlled before immediate reconstruction is performed. The use of a lighted retractor (e.g., Invuity, Invuity, Inc., San Francisco, CA) is used to increase visualization and exposure of tissue planes. Care must be taken to retract gently on the skin flaps as excessive tugging may cause tissue damage and potential necrosis, particularly at the skin edges. In an inframammary incision, the skin edges may be trimmed judiciously to reduce risk of wound breakdown.

Once the breast tissue is fully dissected off the mastectomy flap, the flap should comprise skin and subcutaneous tissue 2–3 mm in approximate thickness. Optimal NAC thickness to ensure viability and adequate oncologic resection has not been proven, although most studies suggest no greater than 3 mm behind the NAC.[17]

Intraoperative pathologic evaluation of the NAC margin is performed next. While various techniques exist for harvesting the subareolar margin, at our institution we shave a small margin from under the NAC using a no. 15 blade and send the specimen to pathology for frozen section. Taking a frozen section provides rapid feedback for the surgeon and therefore the ability to convert to SSM if margins prove positive. Prophylactic NSM does not preclude taking an intraoperative nipple margin. While the risk is quite low, several studies have found ductal carcinoma in situ within the NAC margin, ranging from 0.4% to 0.8%.[17,21,36]

Petit et al. have used electron intraoperative radiation (ELIOT) to reduce the risk of locoregional recurrence after NSM.[37] While results have been positive, the technology is not widely available.

The dissection proceeds with removal of the breast tissue from the chest wall. The pectoralis major fascia should be removed with the breast tissue while maintaining the integrity of the underlying muscle as it may be a necessary aspect of the breast reconstruction. Once the mastectomy has been completed and breast tissue has been removed completely, NAC margins have returned, and no further oncologic resection is warranted, care should be taken to ensure adequate hemostasis. If not achieved, even minor extravasation can lead to hematoma and compromise reconstruction. However, beware of causing thermal injury to the NAC and mastectomy flaps; grasping bleeding vessels on the skin flaps with an insulated DeBakey forceps to achieve hemostasis can reduce this risk.

At this point, the plastic surgery team proceeds with the reconstruction portion of the operation.

POSTOPERATIVE CARE

Postoperative course after NSM is primarily dictated by the reconstructive method. Generally, patients undergoing prosthetic reconstruction remain hospitalized for 1–2 nights postoperatively, while autologous reconstruction often requires 3–5 days depending on plastic surgeon protocol (see chapters 65–66 on Autologous Breast Reconstruction for further details). Patients are given intravenous fluids until adequate oral intake is established, and they are encouraged to ambulate immediately afterward. Pain control with acetaminophen, opioids, and +/− diazepam for muscle spasm are used.

Drain management is generally guided by the plastic surgeon. Typically, dressings include surgical adhesive strips along incisions, nonadhesive gauze, and an occlusive dressing. Surgeon preference dictates when dressings are removed as well as whether the NAC is to be covered. Some surgeons may prefer to monitor the nipple and allow patients to see that their nipple has been preserved, while others prefer to cover it to prevent patients from fixating on it.

Final pathology is returned typically within 1 week when the patient returns for first follow-up appointment. With this information, further discussion is had with the patient regarding need for adjuvant therapy (i.e., chemotherapy and/or radiation). In particular, postmastectomy radiation is recommended in high-risk breast cancer patients undergoing NSM, including those with positive margins, axillary lymph node involvement, and large tumors (>5 cm).[38]

It is important both pre- and postoperatively to have an in-depth, frank discussion with the patient regarding nipple preservation. Patients should be counseled that while there is a likelihood of maintaining nipple erection, studies have shown NAC sensitivity is often overrated and does not necessarily correlate with erection.[29] Despite its lack of function, nipple preservation can provide patients with a more natural feel to their breast, nevertheless.

CAVEATS

Consider whether NSM makes sense from a cosmetic standpoint. If there is concern for postoperative nipple malposition (e.g., due to severe ptosis), NSM may not be the appropriate operation. Active discussions are essential with the patient and breast surgeon regarding data available and limited or no long-term data.

A breast/plastic surgeon should be able to utilize more than one incision.

In patients who present with unilateral breast cancer requiring skin-sparing mastectomy, it may not achieve optimal cosmesis, in our experience, to perform NSM on the contralateral (prophylactic side). Be cautious in counseling your patients, as there may be difficulty in matching the shape and position of the nipples upon completion of reconstruction.

Patients may hold unrealistic expectations about postoperative nipple sensation and function. These expectations must be addressed preoperatively.

REFERENCES

1. Krajewski AC, Boughey JC, Degnim AC, et al. Expanded indications and improved outcomes for nipple-sparing mastectomy over time. *Ann Surg Oncol* 2015;22(10):3317–3323. doi:10.1245/s10434-015-4737-3.
2. Steen ST, Chung AP, Han S-H, Vinstein AL, Yoon JL, Giuliano AE. Predicting nipple–areolar involvement using preoperative breast MRI and primary tumor characteristics. *Ann Surg Oncol* 2013;20(2):633–639. doi:10.1245/s10434-012-2641-7.
3. Byon W, Kim E, Kwon J, Park YL, Park C. Magnetic resonance imaging and clinicopathological factors for the detection of occult nipple involvement in breast cancer patients. *J Breast Cancer* 2014;17(4):386. doi:10.4048/jbc.2014.17.4.386.
4. Ponzone R, Maggiorotto F, Carabalona S, et al. MRI and intraoperative pathology to predict nipple–areola complex (NAC) involvement in patients undergoing NAC-sparing mastectomy. *Eur J Cancer* 2015;51(14):1882–1889. doi:10.1016/j.ejca.2015.07.001.
5. Cho J, Chung J, Cha E-S, Lee JE, Kim JH. Can preoperative 3-T MRI predict nipple–areolar complex involvement in patients with breast cancer? *Clin Imaging* 2016;40(1):119–124. doi:10.1016/j.clinimag.2015.08.002.
6. Piato JRM, Jales Alves de Andrade RD, Chala LF, et al. MRI to predict nipple involvement in breast cancer patients. *Am J Roentgenol* 2016;206(5):1124–1130. doi:10.2214/AJR.15.15187.
7. Bahl M, Pien IJ, Buretta KJ, et al. Can vascular patterns on preoperative magnetic resonance imaging help predict skin necrosis after nipple-sparing mastectomy? *J Am Coll Surg* 2016;223(2):279–285. doi:10.1016/j.jamcollsurg.2016.04.045.
8. NCCN Clinical Practice Guidelines in Oncology. https://www.nccn.org/professionals/physician_gls/#site. Accessed December 28, 2017.
9. Coopey SB, Tang R, Lei L, et al. Increasing eligibility for nipple-sparing mastectomy. *Ann Surg Oncol* 2013;20(10):3218–3222. doi:10.1245/s10434-013-3152-x.

10. Peled AW, Wang F, Foster RD, et al. Expanding the indications for total skin-sparing mastectomy: is it safe for patients with locally advanced disease? *Ann Surg Oncol* 2016;23(1):87–91. doi:10.1245/s10434-015-4734-6.

11. Yao K, Liederbach E, Tang R, et al. Nipple-sparing mastectomy in BRCA1/2 mutation carriers: an interim analysis and review of the literature. *Ann Surg Oncol* 2015;22(2):370–376. doi:10.1245/s10434-014-3883-3.

12. Dua MM, Bertoni DM, Nguyen D, Meyer S, Gurtner GC, Wapnir IL. Using intraoperative laser angiography to safeguard nipple perfusion in nipple-sparing mastectomies. *Gland Surg* 2015;4(6):497.

13. Spear SL, Hannan CM, Willey SC, Cocilovo C. Nipple-sparing mastectomy. *Plast Reconstr Surg* 2009;123(6):1665–1673. doi:10.1097/PRS.0b013e3181a64d94.

14. Cyr AE. Safely expanding the use of nipple-sparing mastectomy in BRCA mutation carriers. *Ann Surg Oncol* 2015;22(2):353–354. doi:10.1245/s10434-014-4007-9.

15. Dent BL, Miller JA, Eden DJ, Swistel A, Talmor M. Tumor-to-nipple distance as a predictor of nipple involvement: expanding the inclusion criteria for nipple-sparing mastectomy. *Plast Reconstr Surg* 2017;140(1):1e–8e. doi:10.1097/PRS.0000000000003414.

16. Ryu JM, Nam SJ, Kim SW, et al. Feasibility of nipple-sparing mastectomy with immediate breast reconstruction in breast cancer patients with tumor-nipple distance less than 2.0 cm. *World J Surg* 2016;40(8):2028–2035. doi:10.1007/s00268-016-3487-0.

17. Manning AT, Sacchini VS. Conservative mastectomies for breast cancer and risk-reducing surgery: the Memorial Sloan Kettering Cancer Center experience. *Gland Surg* 2016;5(1):55.

18. Zhang H, Li Y, Moran MS, Haffty BG, Yang Q. Predictive factors of nipple involvement in breast cancer: a systematic review and meta-analysis. *Breast Cancer Res Treat* 2015;151(2):239–249. doi:10.1007/s10549-015-3385-4.

19. Agarwal S, Agarwal J. Radiation delivery in patients undergoing therapeutic nipple-sparing mastectomy. *Ann Surg Oncol* 2015;22(1):46–51. doi:10.1245/s10434-014-3932-y.

20. Reish RG, Lin A, Phillips NA, et al. Breast reconstruction outcomes after nipple-sparing mastectomy and radiation therapy. *Plast Reconstr Surg* 2015;135(4):959–966. doi:10.1097/PRS.0000000000001129.

21. Tang R, Coopey SB, Merrill AL, et al. Positive nipple margins in nipple-sparing mastectomies: rates, management, and oncologic safety. *J Am Coll Surg* 2016;222(6):1149–1155. doi:10.1016/j.jamcollsurg.2016.02.016.

22. Lohsiriwat V, Rotmensz N, Botteri E, et al. Do clinicopathological features of the cancer patient relate with nipple areolar complex necrosis in nipple-sparing mastectomy? *Ann Surg Oncol* 2013;20(3):990–996. doi:10.1245/s10434-012-2677-8.

23. DellaCroce FJ, Blum CA, Sullivan SK, et al. Nipple-sparing mastectomy and ptosis: perforator flap breast reconstruction allows full secondary mastopexy with complete nipple areolar repositioning. *Plast Reconstr Surg* 2015;136(1):1e–9e. doi:10.1097/PRS.0000000000001325.

24. Dent BL, Cordeiro CN, Small K, et al. Nipple-sparing mastectomy via an inframammary fold incision with implant-based reconstruction in patients with prior cosmetic breast surgery. *Aesthet Surg J* 2015;35(5):548–557. doi:10.1093/asj/sju158.

25. Frederick MJ, Lin AM, Neuman R, Smith BL, Austen WG, Colwell AS. Nipple-sparing mastectomy in patients with previous breast surgery: comparative analysis of 775 immediate breast reconstructions. *Plast Reconstr Surg* 2015;135(6):954e–962e. doi:10.1097/PRS.0000000000001283.

26. Endara M, Chen D, Verma K, Nahabedian MY, Spear SL. Breast reconstruction following nipple-sparing mastectomy: a systematic review of the literature with pooled analysis. *Plast Reconstr Surg* 2013;132(5):1043–1054. doi:10.1097/PRS.0b013e3182a48b8a.

27. Colwell AS, Tessler O, Lin AM, et al. Breast reconstruction following nipple-sparing mastectomy: predictors of complications, reconstruction outcomes, and 5-year trends. *Plast Reconstr Surg* 2014;133(3):496–506. doi:10.1097/01.prs.0000438056.67375.75.

28. Algaithy ZK, Petit JY, Lohsiriwat V, et al. Nipple-sparing mastectomy: can we predict the factors predisposing to necrosis? *Eur J Surg Oncol EJSO* 2012;38(2):125–129. doi:10.1016/j.ejso.2011.10.007.

29. van Verschuer VMT, Mureau MAM, Gopie JP, et al. Patient satisfaction and nipple-areola sensitivity after bilateral prophylactic mastectomy and immediate implant breast reconstruction in a high breast cancer risk population: nipple-sparing mastectomy versus skin-sparing mastectomy. *Ann Plast Surg* 2016;77(2):145–152. doi:10.1097/SAP.0000000000000366.

30. Stolier AJ, Sullivan SK, Dellacroce FJ. Technical considerations in nipple-sparing mastectomy: 82 consecutive cases without necrosis. *Ann Surg Oncol* 2008;15(5):1341–1347. doi:10.1245/s10434-007-9753-5.

31. Sisco M, Yao KA. Nipple-sparing mastectomy: a contemporary perspective: Nipple-Sparing Mastectomy. *J Surg Oncol* 2016;113(8):883–890. doi:10.1002/jso.24209.

32. Small K, Kelly KM, Swistel A, Dent BL, Taylor EM, Talmor M. Surgical treatment of nipple malposition in nipple-sparing mastectomy device-based reconstruction. *Plast Reconstr Surg* 2014;133(5):1053–1062. doi:10.1097/PRS.0000000000000094.

33. Blechman KM, Karp NS, Levovitz C, et al. The lateral inframammary fold incision for nipple-sparing mastectomy: outcomes from over 50 immediate implant-based breast reconstructions. *Breast J* 2013;19(1):31–40. doi:10.1111/tbj.12043.

34. Salibian AH, Harness JK, Mowlds DS. Inframammary approach to nipple-areola–sparing mastectomy. *Plast Reconstr Surg* 2013;132(5):700e–708e. doi:10.1097/PRS.0b013e3182a4d64f.

35. Munhoz AM, Aldrighi C, Montag E, et al. Optimizing the nipple-areola sparing mastectomy with double concentric periareolar incision and biodimensional expander-implant reconstruction: aesthetic and technical refinements. *Breast* 2009;18(6):356–367. doi:10.1016/j.breast.2009.09.008.

36. Camp MS, Coopey SB, Tang R, et al. Management of positive subareolar/nipple duct margins in nipple-sparing mastectomies. *Breast J* 2014;20(4):402–407. doi:10.1111/tbj.12279.

37. Petit JY, Veronesi U, Orecchia R, et al. Nipple-sparing mastectomy in association with intra operative radiotherapy (ELIOT): a new type of mastectomy for breast cancer treatment. *Breast Cancer Res Treat* 2006;96(1):47–51. doi:10.1007/s10549-005-9033-7.

38. Orecchia R. The use of postoperative radiation after nipple-sparing mastectomy. *Gland Surg* 2016;5(1):63.

75.

DIEP AND MUSCLE SPARING BREAST FREE FLAP

Maurice Y. Nahabedian

Breast reconstructions using the deep inferior epigastric perforator (DIEP) or the muscle-sparing (MS) free transverse rectus abdominis musculocutaneous (TRAM) flaps have become routine procedures following mastectomy. Indications for these flaps are primarily based on the availability of sufficient abdominal skin and fat, the patient's desire to use her own tissues rather than implants, and the plastic surgeon's recommendation. Many women with moderate to excessive volume are interested abdominal free flaps because of the abdominoplasty appearance that is usually achieved. Other indications for the free TRAM and DIEP flaps include women with increased body mass index (BMI), a history of tobacco use, prior radiation therapy, and failed prosthetic reconstruction. The main benefit of the DIEP and the muscle-sparing free TRAM is that the patient will have an autologous reconstruction that lasts forever, improves over time, and that retains abdominal function and contour. The principal advantage of the DIEP over the MS free TRAM is that no portion of the rectus abdominis muscle is removed (Figure 75.1). This chapter will review the preoperative, intraoperative, and postoperative factors that make these two autologous options the most desired and commonly performed.

In general, the abdomen is the preferred donor site for the majority of microvascular reconstruction procedures. The normal blood supply to the intact anterior abdominal wall is derived from the deep inferior epigastric as well as the superficial inferior epigastric systems (Figure 75.2). The deep system is usually more dominant and is therefore preferred in the majority of cases. The adipocutaneous component of the free TRAM and DIEP flaps is perfused via the perforating branches of the inferior epigastric artery and vein.

Classification of muscle-sparing is based on the amount of rectus abdominis preserved. The rectus abdominis muscle can be separated into three longitudinal segments: medial, lateral, and central. MS-0 (muscle sparing—none) includes the full width of the muscle; MS-1 includes preservation of the medial or lateral segment of the muscle (Figure 75.3); MS-2 includes the medial and lateral segment of the muscle (Figure 75.4); and MS-3 includes preservation of all three segments (Figure 75.5).

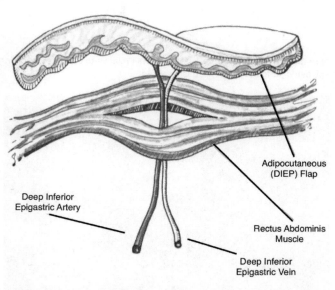

Adipocutaneous
(DIEP) Flap

Rectus Abdominis
Muscle

Deep Inferior
Epigastric Vein

Deep Inferior
Epigastric Artery

Figure 75.1. A schematic illustration of the deep inferior epigastric perforator (DIEP) flap with the primary source vessel perforating the rectus abdominis muscle.

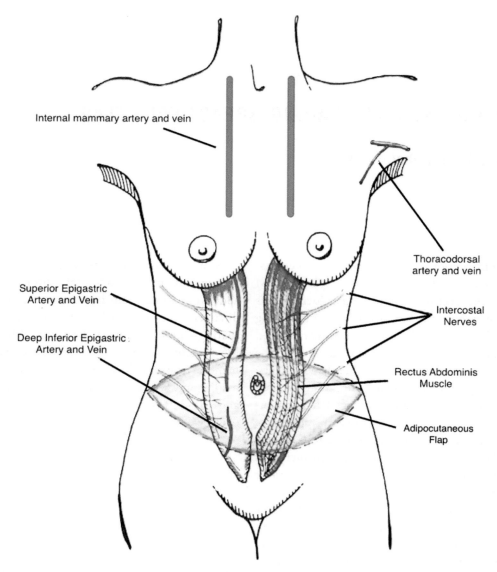

Figure 75.2. The anatomy of the abdominal wall relative to the muscle-sparing free transverse rectus abdominis myocutaneous (TRAM) and deep inferior epigastric perforator (DIEP) flap is depicted.

Internal mammary artery and vein

Thoracodorsal artery and vein

Superior Epigastric Artery and Vein

Intercostal Nerves

Deep Inferior Epigastric Artery and Vein

Rectus Abdominis Muscle

Adipocutaneous Flap

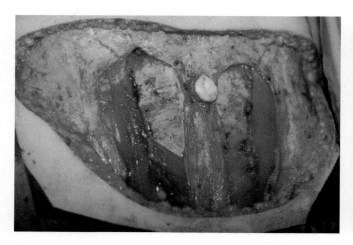

Figure 75.3. The appearance of the rectus abdominis muscle following harvest of a muscle sparing flap (1). The central and medial segments were harvested preserving the innervated lateral segment.

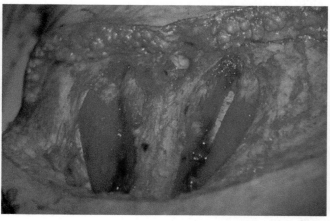

Figure 75.4. A bilateral muscle-sparing (2) free transverse rectus abdominis myocutaneous (TRAM) flap is depicted. The central segment of the rectus abdominis muscle has been harvested.

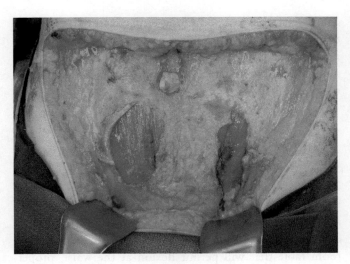

Figure 75.5. A bilateral muscle-sparing (3) deep inferior epigastric perforator (DIEP) flap is depicted. A myotomy without muscle removal has been performed.

TABLE 75.1 ALGORITHM FOR SELECTING THE FREE TRANSVERSE RECTUS ABDOMINIS MUSCULOCUTANEOUS (TRAM) OR DEEP INFERIOR EPIGASTRIC PERFORATOR (DIEP) FLAP BASED ON QUANTITY OF ABDOMINAL TISSUE, BREAST VOLUME REQUIREMENTS, AND QUALITY OF PERFORATORS

Factor	Free TRAM	DIEP
Breast volume requirements		
<800 grams	+	+ +
>800 grams	+ +	+
Abdominal fat		
Mild to moderate	+	+ +
Severe	+ +	+
Perforators >1.5 mm		
0	+	no
> 1	+	+ +
Bilateral	+	+ +

ASSESSMENT OF THE DEFECT

There are several decision points to be considered when determining candidacy for a free TRAM or DIEP flap. In general, women considered candidates for a DIEP or MS free TRAM flap are in good to excellent general health and will be able to tolerate an operation that may range in duration from 3 to 10 hours. Ideally, women should have a mild to moderate excess of skin and fat in the abdominal area. A slender woman with a paucity of abdominal fat may still be a candidate for an abdominal flap if the reconstructive requirements are low. Women who are obese or morbidly obese may not be ideal candidates for pedicled abdominal flaps but may be candidates for a free TRAM or DIEP flap because of the improved vascularity and perfusion provided by the deep inferior epigastric artery and vein. The flap, however, must be tailored appropriately to sustain adequate perfusion to minimize fat necrosis.

Traditional indications for autologous tissue include patients who are not interested in prosthetic reconstruction, patients who have had prior radiation therapy, and patients who have had multiple revisions or failures with prosthetic reconstruction. The authors' indications for a MS free TRAM include women who will require a breast volume exceeding 800 g, an abdominal pannus with a thickness greater than 6 cm, and in situations where there is no dominant perforator. The authors' indications for a DIEP flap include a reconstruction volume that is less than 800 g, presence of a dominant perforator, and all bilateral reconstructions (Table 75.1)

Many patients are choosing to have bilateral mastectomy and reconstruction in the setting of unilateral breast cancer or following bilateral prophylactic mastectomy. The quantity of abdominal skin and fat should be of sufficient volume to reconstruct two breasts. In some cases of bilateral free flap reconstruction, a hemi-abdominal flap may not provide adequate volume and adjunct procedures such as implants or autologous fat grafting are considered.

CONTRAINDICATIONS

In assessing the indications, relative contraindications, and contraindications for the DIEP or MS free TRAM, a thorough history and physical examination are necessary. These should include patient age, assessment of comorbidities, tobacco use, BMI, breast size and volume, prior surgical history, prior radiation therapy history, and stage of the breast cancer. Patient age, in and of itself, is not an indication or contraindication for these operations. Advanced patient age (>65 years) may be a relative contraindication for microvascular breast reconstruction, but personal experience and the existing literature demonstrate that these techniques are safe and effective in properly selected patients. Women of advanced age are required to obtain medical clearance from their primary physicians. Women with multiple medical comorbidities such as poorly controlled diabetes mellitus, chronic obstructive pulmonary disease, hypertension, connective tissue disorders, and cardiac disease are usually discouraged from pursuing complex microvascular procedures and directed toward simpler methods such as mastectomy alone or implant reconstruction. Patients who use tobacco products are at increased risk for adverse events such as delayed healing, fat necrosis, and flap failure. These patients are instructed to refrain from using tobacco products for 1 month prior to and 2 weeks following breast reconstruction. Obesity is not a contraindication for women considering autologous reconstruction with an abdominal flap; however, studies have demonstrated that complication rates are increased and include delayed healing, infection, seroma, and flap failure. In women with a BMI ranging from 30 to 40, decisions regarding microvascular breast reconstruction are individualized based on body fat distribution. In women with a BMI of greater than 40, immediate reconstruction following mastectomy is usually not recommended, and weight loss measures are encouraged. Delayed reconstruction is sometimes recommended. Prior operations, such as open cholecystectomy, abdominoplasty, or coronary artery bypass grafting (with use of internal mammary vessels), may preclude the use of the abdomen as a donor site as well as limit the options regarding recipient vessels. The use of computerized tomographic angiography (CTA) or magnetic resonance angiography (MRA) is sometimes considered in women who have had prior abdominal surgery or have an elevated BMI to assess the patency and location of the deep inferior epigastric artery and vein and perforators (Table 75.2).

Performing a DIEP or free TRAM also depends on the timing of reconstruction. Immediate reconstruction may be considered a contraindication in patients with inflammatory breast cancer or locally advanced breast cancer because of the risk of local recurrence as well as the need for postoperative radiation therapy. Whether to radiate a flap is

controversial because of the long-term effects that radiation therapy may cause, which include flap shrinkage, distortion, fibrosis, and skin contracture. Delayed autologous reconstruction following radiation therapy is often preferred in these patients.

ROOM SETUP

The successful execution of a DIEP or free TRAM flap requires a thorough knowledge of the equipment needed and the staff/personnel that will be assisting with the operation. Proper equipment includes a functional operating room table that will permit flexion at the waist, proper overhead lighting, instruments that are specific for microsurgery, and an operating microscope. The other important aspect is making sure that the operating room team is well-versed in microsurgical procedures. It is a well-known fact that a group will function optimally when working in a milieu of camaraderie, teamwork, competence, and consistency. When a surgeon enters the operating room, it is expected that the operating crew will be constant, knowledgeable, and competent. There are fewer mishaps, patient safety is optimized, and the operations tend to progress more smoothly.

PATIENT MARKINGS

The patient is marked in the upright position (Figure 75.6). The anterior superior iliac spine (ASIS) is palpated and marked bilaterally. The upper extent of the abdominal flap is delineated connecting the two ASIS marks across the abdomen and staying approximately 1 cm above the umbilicus. The lower abdominal marking is an estimation that extends from the two ASIS markings in a curvilinear fashion. The inferior limit of this line is the pubic

TABLE 75.2 INDICATION AND BENEFITS OF THE VARIOUS PREOPERATIVE IMAGING MODALITIES FOR ASSESSING THE VASCULARITY OF THE ABDOMINAL DONOR SITE

Test	XR	Contrast	Caliber	Location	Flow	Course	Accuracy
Doppler	No	No	No	Yes	No	No	Low
Color Duplex	No	No	No	Yes	Yes	No	Moderate
Computed tomography angiography (CTA)	Yes	Yes	Yes	Yes	No	Yes	High
Magnetic resonance angiography (MRA)	No	Yes	Yes	Yes	No	Yes	High

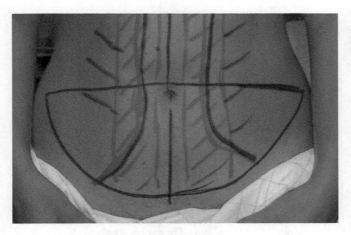

Figure 75.6. The preoperative patient markings for a free transverse rectus abdominis myocutaneous (TRAM) or deep inferior epigastric perforator (DIEP) are identical. The lateral apices are at the anterior superior iliac crest.

symphysis. The final inferior incision is determined in the operating room after the upper skin flap is redraped. The markings for a free TRAM flap and a DIEP flap are identical.

OPERATIVE TECHNIQUE

RECIPIENT VESSEL DISSECTION

Recipient vessels for the microvascular anastomosis include the internal mammary and thoracodorsal artery and vein. The most commonly used recipient vessels are the internal mammary system. The internal mammary vessels run paramedian to the sternum directly beneath the costal cartilage. The thoracodorsal vessels are posterior in the axillary space and traverse along the anterior surface of the latissimus dorsi muscle. The exposure technique described will be for the internal mammary system.

Exposure of the internal mammary artery, vein, and perforators is usually at the level of the third or fourth interspace. In some patients, a very large perforating artery and vein can be seen and considered; however, in most patients, the deep source vessels are preferred and exposed. The pectoralis major muscle overlying the desired rib is divided along the direction of the fibers using electrocautery. An adequate window is made allowing for safe rib and vessel dissection. The perichondrium overlying the costal portion of the rib is removed, and the dissection proceeds in a subperichondrial fashion. Doyen clamps are used to release the posterior perichondrium from the

cartilaginous rib. Inadvertent passage through the posterior perichondrium can result in IMA/V vessel injury or entry into the pleural space. A rib cutter is used to remove the lateral segment of costal cartilage. The medial cartilage is excised with a bone rongeur and proceeds from lateral to medial. Following complete removal of the costal cartilage segment extending to the sternal meniscus, the posterior perichondrium is divided, elevated, and excised. The internal mammary artery and vein are visualized. In some cases, a venae comitans is present that may be used for a second venous anastomosis. The recipient vessels are further dissected to clear the perivascular tissue using loupe magnification.

FLAP HARVEST: COMMON PATHWAY

Flap elevation begins with the upper abdominal incision. The dissection extends to the anterior rectus sheath using electrocautery. The upper abdominal adipocutaneous flap is usually undermined to the midpoint between the umbilicus and the xiphoid process, although, in some cases, the undermining may extend to the xiphoid process and costal margin. The patient is flexed 10–30 degrees and the lower abdominal ellipse is definitively delineated and incised. The umbilicus is incised and preserved on its stalk. Flap elevation begins from a lateral to medial direction at the level of the anterior rectus sheath. The "safe zone" of flap elevation extends to the lateral edge of the linea semilunaris. Medial to the linea semilunaris, precautions are taken to preserve and avoid injury to perforating vessels from the deep inferior epigastric system. A decision at this stage must be made to determine if an MS free TRAM flap or a DIEP flap will be performed. In either case, the lateral innervation to the rectus abdominis muscle is preserved.

DIEP FLAP

The DIEP flap is characterized as an adipocutaneous flap without muscle (Figure 75.7). The dissection proceeds between the adipocutaneous flap and the anterior rectus sheath, with identification and preservation of the deep inferior epigastric perforators. The number of perforators included with the flap ranges from 1 to 3. The anterior rectus sheath is divided inferior to the presumed course of the perforators. The fibers of the rectus abdominis muscle are divided using bipolar or monopolar cautery. The authors preferred technique is to use monopolar cautery and fine-tip Jacobsen clamps when dividing through the

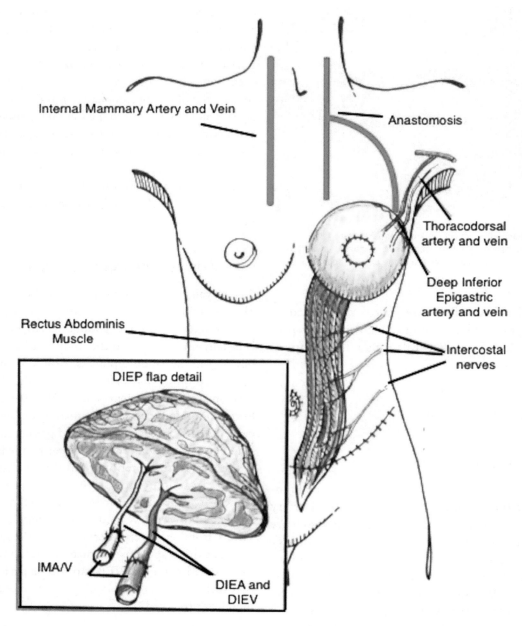

Internal Mammary Artery and Vein

Anastomosis

Thoracodorsal
artery and vein

Deep Inferior
Epigastric
artery and vein

Intercostal
nerves

Rectus Abdominis
Muscle

DIEP flap detail

IMA/V

DIEA and
DIEV

Figure 75.7. A schematic illustration of a unilateral deep inferior epigastric perforator (DIEP) flap. The anastomosis can be performed to the internal mammary or the thoracodorsal vessels. A myotomy is performed but no muscle is harvested.

rectus abdominis muscle. When the perforator joins the deep inferior epigastric vessels, a submuscular dissection is initiated (Figure 75.8). The desired length of the vascular pedicle is variable and based on surgeon preference. Some surgeons prefer a short 6–8 cm pedicle whereas others prefer a longer 11–14 cm pedicle (Figure 75.9). The advantage of the longer pedicle is that vessel diameter increases as the dissection approaches the external iliac vessels. There are multiple side branches along the course of the deep

inferior epigastric artery and vein that must be identified, clipped, and divided.

MS FREE TRAM

The MS free TRAM flap is characterized as a musculocutaneous flap that includes variable amounts of muscle but not the full width (Figure 75.10). A MS free TRAM flap is usually considered when the quality of the

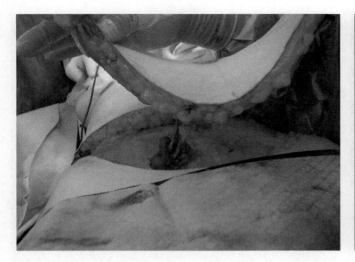

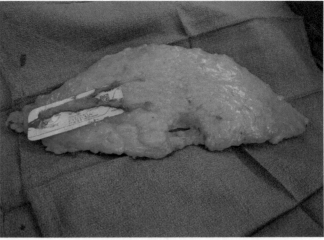

Figure 75.8. A two-perforator deep inferior epigastric perforator (DIEP) flap is harvested in-situ.

Figure 75.9. A two-perforator deep inferior epigastric perforator (DIEP) flap is detached with a pedicle length of approximately 10 cm.

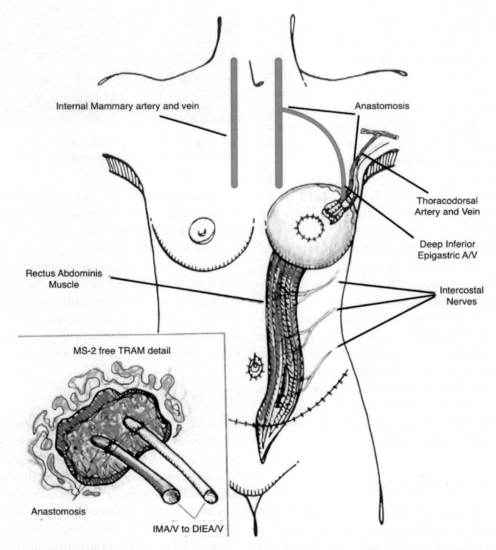

Figure 75.10. A schematic illustration of a unilateral muscle-sparing free transverse rectus abdominis myocutaneous (TRAM) flap. A small segment of the rectus abdominis muscle is harvested with the flap. The microvascular anastomosis is performed to the internal mammary or the thoracodorsal artery and vein.

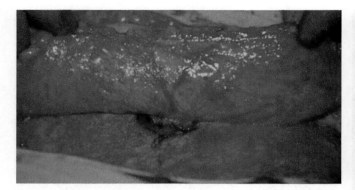

Figure 75.11. The island of perforators is incised at the perimeter.

perforating vessels are deemed inadequate, the patient is morbidly obese, flap volume requirements exceed 800 g, or when the thickness of the flap exceeds 6 cm. With the MS free TRAM technique, an island of perforators is defined, and the anterior rectus sheath surrounding the island of perforators is incised (Figure 75.11). The medial and lateral aspects of the anterior rectus sheath are elevated off the muscle and the retrorectus space is defined. The central segment of muscle is divided using monopolar or bipolar cautery. The superior portion of the rectus muscle is cauterized, and the superior epigastric artery and vein cephalad to the flap is identified, clipped, and divided. Palpation beneath the muscle will help identify the pulse and location of the pedicle to ensure that the pedicle is within the muscle segment. Following division of the superior epigastric artery and vein, the perfusion to the flap is solely based on the deep inferior epigastric system. Cautery dissection proceeds at low current. The distal portion of the flap pedicle can be visualized traveling toward the lateral edge of the rectus muscle. All side branches are clipped or ligated. Care must be taken to avoid injury to the vessels and intercostal nerves at this stage as diathermic injury may result in vessel thrombosis or neural injury. Pedicle dissection is continued distal to the flap as deemed necessary for adequate pedicle length (Figure 75.12). Slightly increased caliber of the DIEA/DIEV is seen with more proximal dissection. Approximately 10–12 centimeters may be obtained if dissection is continued to the external iliac vessels. Muscle sparing free TRAM flaps and DIEP are frequently performed bilaterally (Figure 75.13).

MICROSURGICAL ANASTOMOSIS

Intravenous heparin is usually administered prior to division of the inferior epigastric vessels. The harvested flap is positioned over the chest wall such that the inferior epigastric artery and vein are aligned with the internal

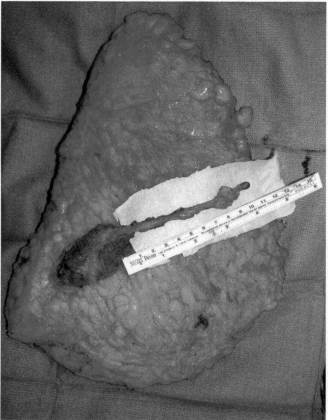

Figure 75.12. The muscle-sparing (2) free transverse rectus abdominis myocutaneous (TRAM) flap is harvested with a pedicle length of 11 cm.

mammary artery and vein. The medial anastomosis is usually performed first, which is typically the venous anastomosis. This is followed by the lateral or arterial anastomosis. The decision to use the vascular coupler or to perform a hand-sewn anastomosis is based on surgeon preference. If a coupler is chosen, a 2.0–3.0 mm ring is usually recommended. If a hand-sewn venous anastomosis is chosen, 8-0 or 9-0 sutures are used in an interrupted or continuous fashion. Avoidance of back wall sutures is critical. Usually 8–10 sutures are needed to complete the artery.

FLAP INSETTING

Following completion of the arterial and venous anastomoses, the vascular pedicle must be appropriately positioned on the chest wall to prevent twisting and kinking in order to minimize pedicle-related complications such as thrombosis. Positioning of the flap on the chest wall is an important step to recreate the breast contour and shape. Fortunately, with free flaps, there are no points that tether the flap, and mobility of the flaps is maintained for optimal shaping. When insetting the flap following a unilateral or

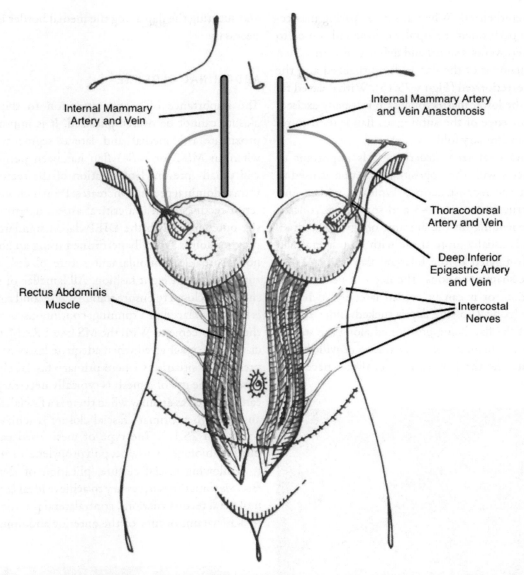

Figure 75.13. A schematic illustration of a bilateral muscle-sparing free transverse rectus abdominis myocutaneous (TRAM) flap. The flap is divided along the midline into two halves.

Internal Mammary Artery and Vein

Internal Mammary Artery and Vein Anastomosis

Thoracodorsal Artery and Vein

Deep Inferior Epigastric Artery and Vein

Intercostal Nerves

Rectus Abdominis Muscle

bilateral reconstruction, it is recommended to sit the patient upright to approximately 45 degrees to assess the position, symmetry, contour, and projection of the breast. The medial edge of the flap is usually positioned along the sternal border, and the lateral aspect of the flap is positioned on the lateral chest wall. (Figure 75.14) Suturing of the flap to the chest wall is sometimes necessary with immediate reconstruction, especially when the footprint of the old breast is larger than the footprint of the flap. These sutures can be placed superomedially, inferomedially, and laterally. With delayed reconstruction, the dimensions of the created subcutaneous pocket are made to match that of the flap.

In cases of a skin-sparing mastectomy, the skin territory to be exteriorized is delineated, and the remainder of

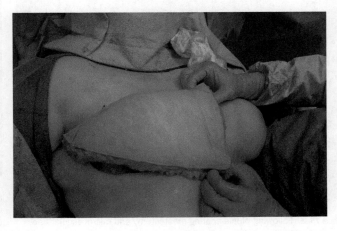

Figure 75.14. The medial border of the flap is positioned along the sternal border during the initial stage of flap insetting.

the flap is de-epithelized. When a nipple-sparing mastectomy has been performed, a Doppler ultrasound is used to identify an arteriovenous signal and delineated with a 2 cm circle. The remainder of the flap is de-epithelized and the skin paddle is exteriorized (Figure 75.15). With delayed reconstruction, the lower mastectomy skin is usually excised, and the inferior edge of the autologous flap is used to recreate the inframammary fold.

With a unilateral reconstruction, it is important to achieve symmetry with the opposite breast that is used as a template for the reconstruction. Typically, with a unilateral reconstruction, zones 1–3 and sometimes zones 4 are utilized depending on the amount of tissue required. Because there is usually more tissue with a unilateral flap (zones 1–3) compared to the bilateral flap (zones 1–2), there are more shaping options. The flap can be folded in a conical fashion, or it can be folded laterally such that apical portion (zone 2) of the flap is tucked under zone 1 with zone 3 of the flap being positioned along the sternal border. With both maneuvers, the goal is to provide better projection. Suturing the flap laterally is always necessary,

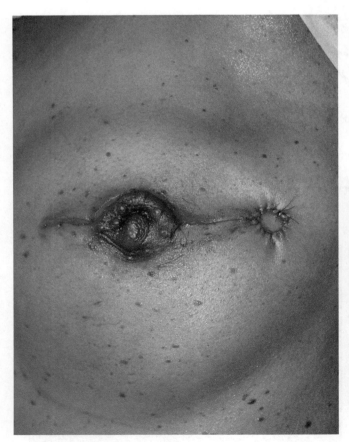

Figure 75.15. Following nipple-sparing mastectomy and microvascular flap reconstruction, a small island of skin overlying the Doppler signal is retained for monitoring.

and suturing the flap along the medial border is sometimes necessary.

ABDOMINAL CLOSURE

The importance of proper attention to the abdominal closure cannot be overemphasized. It is important to approximate the medial and lateral segments of muscle when an MS-2 or MS-3 flap has been performed. This will usually prevent lateralization of the rectus muscle as intraabdominal pressure increases. Proper closure of the anterior rectus sheath is a critical aspect determining donor site outcomes. With the DIEP flap, a standard fascial approximation is typically performed using an absorbable or nonabsorbable monofilament suture placed in an interrupted figure-of-eight fashion. All lamellae of the anterior sheath are closed to ensure stability. A second row of sutures is typically placed in a running, continuous fashion for further reinforcement. With the MS free TRAM, primary fascial closure is achieved when adequate laxity of the fascia is present. In situations where primary fascial closure is not possible, the use of a mesh is typically necessary. The mesh can be placed as an inlay when there is a fascial deficit and as an onlay when primary fascial closure is achieved (Figures 75.16 and 75.17). The type of mesh used can vary and includes biologic synthetic, polypropylene, or resorbable.

Following fascial closure, plication of the remaining fascia is sometimes necessary to achieve ideal contour. With unilateral reconstructions, contralateral plication will serve to achieve uniformity of the anterior abdominal wall and

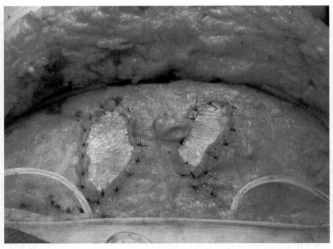

Figure 75.16. Following a bilateral muscle-sparing free transverse rectus abdominis myocutaneous (TRAM) flap, a biologic (or synthetic) mesh is often used to replace the excised anterior rectus sheath. This will retain or improve the contour of the anterior abdominal wall and minimize the incidence of bulge or hernia.

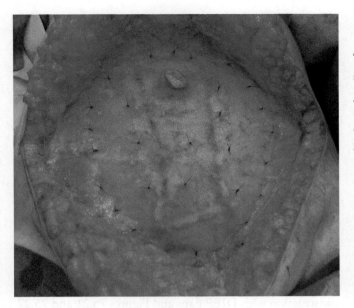

Figure 75.17. A synthetic mesh is sometimes placed over the anterior abdominal wall to further reinforce the fascial repair following bilateral flap reconstruction to reduce the incidence of a bulge or hernia.

to centralize the umbilicus. With bilateral reconstructions, the supraumbilical fascia is often plicated along the midline to prevent an upper abdominal bulge. These sutures are usually monofilament and placed in a figure-of-eight fashion. Infraumbilical midline sutures are also sometimes useful to achieve ideal contour.

In obese women, the Scarpa's fascial layer is sometimes in excess along the pubic area as well as the upper abdomen. This fat is often less vascularized than the fat above the Scarpa's layer and is sometimes excised. The thickness of the upper and lower adipocutaneous layers of the abdominal wall should be similar to prevent any step-off deformity. The slight depression of the midline anterior abdominal wall can be recreated by excision a few millimeters of fat along the midline of the adipose layer. This maneuver will also tend to provide a more natural abdominal contour.

Skin closure is the final stage of abdominal closure and includes the umbilicus and the incisions. The insetting of the umbilicus is another important step to achieve ideal abdominal aesthetics. Various skin incision patterns are possible that include circular, oval, and "U" designs all of which are capable delivering good results. Skin closure is performed in three layers that include Scarpa's fascia, dermis, and epidermis. Monofilament sutures are used for the dermis and subcuticular layers. Lateral dog-ears should be identified at time of closure and addressed. This will lead to lengthening of the abdominal incision but an improvement in abdominal contour. Two closed suction drains are always used to minimize the occurrence of a fluid collection.

POSTOPERATIVE CARE

The postoperative care of the patient following free TRAM and DIEP flap breast reconstruction is identical. In the postanesthesia care unit (PACU), adequate resuscitation and ensuring flap perfusion is prioritized. Factors that can result in anastomotic failure include hypotension, hypothermia, pressure, patient position, infection, and medications. A fresh microvascular anastomosis is prone to clot formation when the flow is sluggish. Fluid bolus may be necessary if hypotension is present. Anticoagulation in the form of intravenous heparin or dextran is usually not necessary following free flap reconstruction. Subcutaneous heparin is usually considered, especially in women with a BMI of greater than 30 and may provide benefit in minimizing venous outflow issues. Aspirin is usually started on postoperative day 1 because of its antiplatelet properties.

Patient positioning following free abdominal flap reconstruction is another important consideration. Patients are positioned with the head of the bed at 30 degrees to minimize the stress placed on the abdominal closure. They are also instructed to ambulate slightly flexed at the waist for a few days until the skin elasticity improves. When the thoracodorsal artery and vein have been used as recipient vessels, patients should avoid lying on their side to avoid compression of the anastomosis that is located in the axillary region. External compression of the reconstructed breast is avoided as this may occlude the anastomosis. Internal compression from a fluid collection such as a hematoma can occlude the anastomosis. Following any of the abdominal flaps, an abdominal binder or fitted garment may be applied postoperatively for support and comfort.

Pain management strategies include patient-controlled analgesics and enhanced recovery after surgery (ERAS) protocols. Patients are typically instructed to ambulate on postoperative day 1 and encouraged to sit in a chair. The dressings are typically removed on postoperative day 2. Patients are encouraged to shower on postoperative day 3. Most patients are discharged home on postoperative day 3 except when an adverse event such as an operative takeback has occurred.

POSTOPERATIVE FLAP MONITORING

One of the most important aspects of free flap breast reconstruction is proper monitoring of the flap during the acute postoperative period. The critical period for flap monitoring is usually the first 24 hours as most anastomotic issues occur during this time, although they can still occur after that time frame. Compromised perfusion is more common with the venous system because it is a low-pressure system that is vulnerable to compression and kinking.

Techniques of flap monitoring include physical examination as well as external monitoring devices. Physical examination includes the assessment of color, capillary refill, turgor, and temperature. External flap monitoring can be performed with various devices that include a hand-held pencil Doppler, implantable Doppler, or a transcutaneous oxygen sensor. The hand-held Doppler is used by most nurses and physicians to assess the vascular perfusion of a free flap. Implantable Doppler devices can be considered with buried flaps following nipple-sparing mastectomy. Near-infrared spectroscopy for monitoring permits continuous real-time assessment of oxygen saturation within the cutaneous layer of the flap

THE COMPROMISED FLAP

When alterations in perfusion occur, the patient is prepared for operative exploration. With the MS free TRAM, there is approximately a 2-hour window of ischemia before irreversible damage occurs to muscle fibers. With a DIEP flap, there is a 3- to 6-hour window because there is no muscle. The majority of reoperations are due to venous obstruction (Figure 75.18). Chang et al. (2014) have demonstrated that

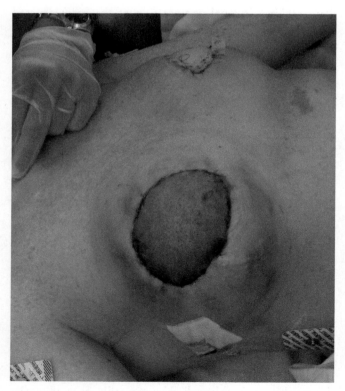

Figure 75.18. The typical appearance of a congested flap due to venous outflow obstruction.

the likelihood of flap salvage is highest when compromised flow is identified within the first 24 hours of the anastomosis (83.7%) and identified early. Successful salvage is less between days 1 and 3 (38.6%; $P < 0.0001$) and beyond 4 days (29.4%; $P < 0.0001$).

OUTCOMES

The benefit of the MS free TRAM and the DIEP flap is that the reconstructed breast will usually achieve excellent outcomes and result in high patient satisfaction. Figures 75.14 and 75.15 illustrate a patient following immediate bilateral breast reconstruction with DIEP flaps and Figures 75.16 and 75.17 illustrate a patient following a delayed unilateral MS free TRAM flap. Figures 75.19 and 75.20 illustrate a patient following immediate bilateral breast reconstruction with DIEP flaps and Figures 75.21 and 75.22 illustrate a patient following a delayed unilateral MS free TRAM flap.

CONCLUSION

The DIEP and MS free TRAM flaps are excellent options for women considering autologous reconstruction following mastectomy. Both flaps can provide excellent aesthetic outcomes, achieve high patient satisfaction, and maintain a low incidence of adverse events.

CAVEATS

Ensure a thorough preoperative consultation and explain to the patient the need to perform either a DIEP or a MS free TRAM. Consider preoperative imaging studies using CTA or MRA to map the perforators.

Consider a MS free TRAM flap when the patient has a large reconstructive requirement exceeding 800 g, the patient has a moderate to large abdominal pannus, and the perforator diameter is small and less than 1.5 mm. Consider a DIEP flap when perforator diameter is sufficient to perfuse the desired flap volume and in bilateral reconstructions,

Appropriate fascial closure is important to minimize the risk of a bulge or contour abnormality. Mesh materials are sometimes necessary.

Postoperative monitoring is an essential component with any free flap and can be adequately performed via clinical examination, hand-held Doppler probe, internal Doppler probe, or near-infrared spectroscopy.

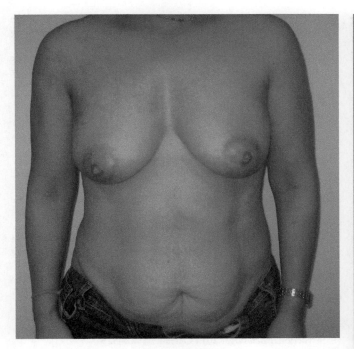

Figure 75.19. Preoperative image of a woman with right breast cancer scheduled for bilateral skin-sparing mastectomy and immediate reconstruction with deep inferior epigastric perforator (DIEP) flaps.

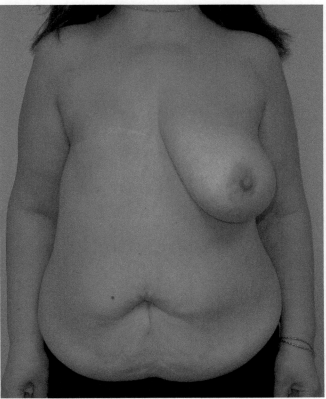

Figure 75.21. Preoperative image of a woman following right mastectomy presenting for delayed breast reconstruction.

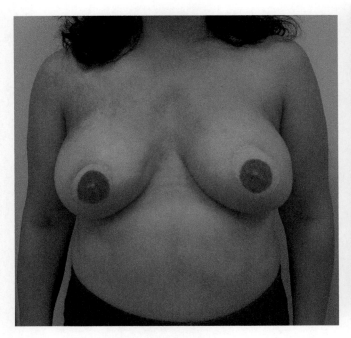

Figure 75.20. Two-year postoperative photograph following bilateral breast reconstruction with deep inferior epigastric perforator (DIEP) flaps.

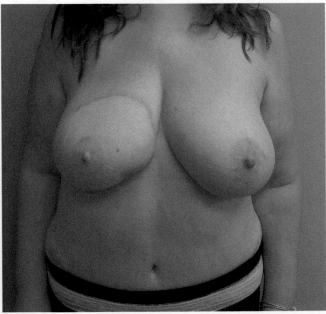

Figure 75.22. Postoperative image following unilateral muscle-sparing free transverse rectus abdominis myocutaneous (TRAM) flap and contralateral reduction mammaplasty for symmetry.

It is important to promptly return to the operating room in the event of flap compromise. Maneuvers include redo anastomosis, Fogerty embolectomy, thrombolytic agents, and postoperative leech therapy.

SELECTED READINGS

Allen RJ, Treece P. Deep inferior epigastric perforator flap for breast reconstruction. *Ann Plast Surg* 1994 Jan;32(1):32–8.

Baldorf NJ, Lemaine V, Lovely JK, et al. Enhanced recovery after surgery in microvascular breast reconstruction. *J Plast Reconstr Aesthet Surg* 2015 Mar;68(3):395–402.

Bonde CT, Khorasani H, Elberg J, Kehlet H. Perioperative optimization of autologous breast reconstruction. *Plast Reconstr Surg* 2016 Feb;137(2):411–414.

Chang E, Chang E, Soto-Miranda MA, et al. Comprehensive evaluation of risk factors and management of impending flap loss in 2138 breast free flaps. *Ann Plast Surg* 2014 Jul 4 [Epub ahead of print].

Chen Y, Shen Z, Shao Z, Yu P, Wu J. Free flap monitoring using near-infrared spectroscopy: a systemic review. *Ann Plast Surg* 2015 Feb 7 [Epub ahead of print].

Grotting JC, Urist MM, Maddox WA, Vasconez LO. Conventional TRAM flap versus free microsurgical TRAM flap for immediate breast reconstruction *Plast Reconstr Surg* 1989 May; 83(5):828–841.

Henderson PW, Fernandez JG, Cemal Y, et al. Successful salvage of late anastomotic thrombosis after free tissue transfer. *J Reconstr Microsurg* 2016 Feb 12 [Epub ahead of print].

Lee KT, Mun GH. The efficacy of postoperative antithrombotics in free flap surgery: a systematic review and meta-analysis. *Plast Reconstr Surg* 2015 Apr;135(4):1124–1139.

Nahabedian MY. Overview of perforator imaging and flap perfusion technologies. *Clin Plast Surg* 2011;38(2):165–174.

Nahabedian MY, Momen B, Galdino G, Manson PN. Breast reconstruction with the free tram or diep flap: patient selection, choice of flap, and outcome. *Plast Reconstr Surg* 2002;110:466–475.

Nahabedian MY, Momen B, Manson PN. Factors associated with anastomotic failure following microvascular reconstruction of the breast. *Plast Reconstr Surg* 2004;114:74–82.

Nahabedian MY, Momen B, Tsangaris T. Breast reconstruction with the MS (MS-2) free TRAM and the DIEP flap: Is there a difference? *Plast Reconstr Surg* 2005;115:436–444.

Nahabedian MY, Patel K. Maximizing the use of the handheld Doppler in autologous breast reconstruction. *Clin Plast Surg* 2011;38(2):213–218.

Nahabedian MY, Schwartz J. Autologous breast reconstruction following mastectomy. *Handchirurgie, Mikrochirurgie, Plastische, Chirurgie.* 2008;40(4):248–254.

Pannucci CJ, Nelson JA, Chung CU, et al. Medicinal leeches for surgically uncorrectable venous congestion after free flap breast reconstruction. *Microsurger* 2014 Oct;34(7):522–526.

Rao SS, Stolle EC, Sher S, Wang LC, Momen B, Nahabedian MY. A multiple logistic regression analysis of complications following microsurgical breast reconstruction. *Gland Surg* 2014;3(4): 226–231.

76.

BREAST RECONSTRUCTION WITH NON-ABDOMINAL–BASED FREE TISSUE FLAPS

Erica Bartlett and Aldona J. Spiegel

Abdominal-based free tissue transfer accounts for the majority of autologous breast reconstruction. However, other sources need to be considered in situations where the abdomen is not a suitable donor site, such as in the face of previous abdominal operations, inadequate tissue, or patient preference. Alternative donor sites include the buttocks and thighs, which can provide expendable soft tissue without leaving a conspicuous scar or significant deformity. Like abdominal-based free tissue transfer, many alternative tissue sources consist of perforator flaps, which can maximize tissue gain while minimizing donor site morbidity. Non-abdominal–based tissue sources for breast reconstruction are gaining in popularity as reliable second-line flap options when abdominal tissue is not available. Discussed in this chapter are the most common non-abdominal–based free flaps used in breast reconstruction by location.

GLUTEAL-BASED OVERVIEW

Gluteal-based flaps were first introduced in 1975 as the first myocutaneous free tissue transfer for breast reconstruction. However, they were not commonly utilized until perforator flaps were popularized in the early 1990s. Two types of gluteal artery perforator (GAP) flaps have been described by their vascular pedicle: the superior gluteal artery perforator (SGAP) and inferior gluteal artery perforator (IGAP) flap. These flaps have also been utilized for sacral and lumbar defect coverage as well as for breast reconstruction.

Gluteal-based flaps offer the advantage of providing a large volume of fat relative to skin. Various orientations and dimensions have been designed ultimately providing a projected breast mound. Volumes of tissue exceeding mastectomy weights have been described and can exceed 600

g in the appropriately selected patient. Ideal candidates are those with a pear-shaped body habitus to reconstruct a B or C cup breast. No absolute contraindications exist, but liposuction to the buttocks represents a relative contraindication as perforator viability may be compromised.

The dissection of a GAP flap can be tedious and carries with it a steep learning curve. Preoperative imaging with the use of computed tomography angiography (CTA) is invaluable for identification of perforator anatomy and can expedite dissection.

ANATOMY

The gluteal region or "buttocks" is bound superiorly by the iliac crest, inferiorly by the inferior border of the gluteus maximus, medially by the sacral cleft, and laterally by the greater trochanter. Gluteal muscles function in hip extension, although the deeper gluteus medius and minimus act to laterally rotate the hip. The superior and inferior gluteal arteries are terminal branches of the internal iliac system and exit the pelvis through the greater sciatic foramen.

The superior gluteal artery passes above the piriformis muscle, where it splits into deep and superficial branches. It enters the buttocks at the junction of the proximal and middle third of a line from the posterior superior iliac spine (PSIS) to the greater trochanter of the femur. The superficial branch proceeds through the upper portion of the gluteus maximus, where it gives off perforators to the overlying fat and skin. On average, five perforators emanate from the superior gluteal artery, predominately musculocutaneous although septocutaneous perforators are present to a lesser degree. Perforators are found consistently around the intersection of a line drawn from the PSIS to the greater trochanter and a line extending halfway from the PSIS to the coccyx to the greater trochanter.

The inferior gluteal artery passes below the piriformis, adjacent to the sciatic nerve as well as to the internal pudendal vessels and the posterior femoral cutaneous nerve. It proceeds through the lower third of the gluteus maximus, where it gives off musculocutaneous and septocutaneous perforators. On average, eight perforators emanate from the inferior gluteal artery and are more obliquely oriented compared to the more vertical superior gluteal artery perforators. The inferior gluteal artery perforators are focused around the middle third of a line drawn from the posterior superior iliac spine and the medial gluteal fold.

SURGICAL TECHNIQUE

SGAP

The patient is marked in the preoperative holding area in the same position that the patient will lie on the operating table. A pencil Doppler is used to locate the dominant perforators in correlation with preoperative imaging. A skin island is then drawn as an ellipse in a superolateral position, centered around the dominant perforators. The more lateral the skin paddle, the longer the pedicle. Careful pinch test approximation should be performed when planning flap incisions. Skin islands with a height of 7–10 cm and length of 18–22 cm can safely be closed but ultimately depend on available laxity. Care should be taken to keep the upper border of the incision below the underwear line in order to conceal the postsurgical scar.

The patient is placed in the lateral decubitus position for unilateral procedures or prone for bilateral. After incisions made, the flap is raised from lateral to medial in the suprafascial plane. Contour deformities can be created if aggressive beveling is performed superiorly. To prevent this, the flap can be beveled inferiorly to recruit additional bulk, knowing that the flap will be rotated 180 degrees for inset. One must consider overall flap shape during dissection in order to maximize breast contour while minimizing donor site deformity.

The gluteus maximus fascia is then encountered and the subfascial plane is entered to identify the main perforator. Once an adequate perforator has been identified, it is dissected through the gluteus maximus muscle with the fibers split longitudinally to minimize injury. Care should be given during intramuscular dissection as small thin side branches can cause considerable bleeding. These must be carefully ligated with microclips as it is very important to keep a dry surgical field with deeper dissection. Dissection proceeds deep to the gluteus maximus into the subgluteal plane where another fascial plane is entered. This fascia needs to be incised to access the main pedicle. One must carefully orient one's self toward the main pedicle as many venous branches exist in this plane which can be inadvertently transected at the main pedicle or cause bleeding. The pedicle is transected as proximally as needed to accommodate microanastomosis. Pedicle length averages between 5 and 7 cm. The remainder of the subcutaneous tissue can then be elevated in the suprafascial plane to minimize risk of seroma.

If a sensate flap is desired, segmental lumbar sensory nerves from L2 or L3 can be chosen and included into the flap design. These are located above the deep muscular fascia at the upper edge of the flap for most designs. Sensory nerves run with small vessels, but there is considerable variability in their course.

If the flap is to be based on a purely septocutaneous perforator (septocutaneous gluteal artery perforator [scGAP] flap), as described by Tuinder, the skin island is centered appropriately. This tends to be more cephalad and lateral than the standard SGAP flap. Generally, these perforators are located 13 cm from the midline and 5 cm inferior to the iliac crest. The pedicle tends to be slightly longer than a standard SGAP flap, averaging 8 cm with equivalent volumes.

After the flap is dissected free, the buttock is then closed in layers over a closed suction drain. The patient is then turned supine and anastomosis typically performed to the internal mammary artery and vein. Since the pedicle length is relatively short, the recipient vessels are dissected with removal of the rib, and not in the rib sparing manner, in order to increase vessel length and facilitate inset. The flap is rotated 180 degrees for inset, which maximizes upper medial pole fullness and correlates with the caudal extend of gluteal beveling.

IGAP

Similarly to the SGAP flap, preoperative markings are of paramount importance. The gluteal fold is noted in the standing position and the inferior limit of the flap marked 1 cm above this line. If performing an in-the-crease IGAP flap, the inferior limit is marked at the gluteal fold. A pencil Doppler is used to identify the major perforators within the inferior gluteal artery limits. A skin ellipse is marked incorporating these perforators, paralleling the gluteal fold or including it for an in-the-crease IGAP flap. Markings should be shifted laterally for saddlebag correction as indicated. Average flap dimensions are 7 cm in height and 18 cm in length but again are patient dependent. One should be considerate of the location of the ischial tuberosity as this fat pad should not be disturbed or an undue pressure point can be created postoperatively.

The procedure is carried out in the lateral decubitus position for unilateral flaps or prone for bilateral. After the skin incision is made, the subcutaneous tissue is beveled as needed for volume. Additional soft tissue can be recruited from the saddlebag area, laterally. Once down to the gluteus maximus, dissection proceeds in the subfascial plane until a dominant perforator is identified. Muscle is spread in the direction of its fibers and dissection is carried through the lower third of the gluteus maximus until the pedicle is identified. The lighter colored fat over the ischium should be avoided. The pedicle is followed to its origin; however, care should be given not to over retract on surrounding tissue as the sciatic nerve is in the vicinity. The pedicle is transected as desired for length and can reach 7–10 cm. The buttock is then closed in layers over a closed suction drain and microanastomosis performed after the patient is turned supine.

COMPARISON BETWEEN FLAPS

At our institution, gluteal-based flaps, primarily the SGAP flap, are the second most common free tissue transfer used for breast reconstruction if abdominal tissue is not available. The donor site morbidity for both SGAP and IGAP flaps can be minimal as there is no sacrifice of muscle. Additionally, the skin paddle can be flexible in terms of its location and dimensions. Volume of subcutaneous tissue can also be tailored to individual needs but is limited based on patient habitus. Perfusion studies show a larger cutaneous territory with the IGAP flap compared to the SGAP flap. The quality of the fat is different and more dense when compared to the abdomen, which can allow for a more projecting breast mound.

Scar placement can be confined under a woman's bathing suit or undergarment with the SGAP flap, but dissection can cause flattening up the upper buttock. The IGAP flap places the scar roughly at the gluteal crease which can be visible to many patients and may leave a contour deformity. It can, however, potentially improve the saddlebag area. Additionally, the gluteal crease incision can be accompanied by discomfort while sitting for several weeks during the postoperative period or more permanently if the fat pad over the ischial tuberosity has been disturbed.

Pedicle length of the IGAP flap is longer than that of the SGAP flap, which allows a more flexible inset or sparing of the costal cartilage for microanastomosis. There is potential for sciatic nerve injury with the IGAP flap harvest, although this is uncommon. However, patients may develop temporary weakness from sciatic nerve traction close to the pedicle origin during dissection. Ultimately, the decision to use the SGAP or the IGAP flap comes from surgical experience and preference.

TECHNICAL PEARLS

- Ensure paralysis during intramuscular dissection to minimize injury to the perforator.

- Preferable artery and vein diameters for microanastomosis are 2.0–2.5 mm and 3.0-4.0 mm, respectively.

- Only one main perforator is needed to maintain the flap. If two perforators are used, care should be taken so they are not tethered when insetting the flap.

- Keep in mind final breast shape when sculpting the flap while minimizing donor site contour deformity.

THIGH-BASED OVERVIEW

The female thigh makes a suitable donor site for breast reconstruction as it is typically a site of soft tissue abundance. Numerous thigh-based flaps have been designed for breast reconstruction but only a few are used in standard practice. In this section, relevant thigh-based flaps are discussed and include the transverse upper gracilis (TUG) flap, profunda artery perforator (PAP) flap, and the lateral thigh perforator (LTP) flap. Other less common, historical thigh-based flaps have been utilized for breast reconstruction, but these will not be discussed.

TUG

The transverse upper gracilis (TUG) flap allows the transfer of a horizontal ellipse of skin and soft tissue from the upper medial thigh with a resultant scar confined to the anterior and medial groin crease. It is best utilized by women with small to medium-sized breasts and larger hips who could benefit from a cosmetic thigh lift. Dissection is straightforward with minimal anatomical variance. It also allows a two-team approach which can significantly shorten operative time.

Originally described in 1992 by Yousif, this flap remains a viable alternative in breast reconstruction for the appropriately selected individual. The TUG flap is not without its drawbacks. Numbness of the leg (temporary or permanent), seroma, chronic lymphedema, scar widening, and contour deformities are known complications that need to be considered when evaluating potential candidates.

Preoperative imaging is not mandatory as the vascular anatomy is consistent.

Anatomy

The gracilis is a type II muscle, fed by the ascending branch of the medial femoral circumflex artery. This long, thin muscle takes its origin from the ischiopubic ramus and inserts on the pes anserinus of the medial tibia. The axis of the muscle is defined by drawing a line from the ischium to the medial femoral condyle. Its location is superficial in the medial compartment of the thigh and sits lateral to the adductor longus. It functions as a thigh adductor, medial rotator, and weak hip flexor. The musculocutaneous TUG flap relies on a transversely oriented upper thigh skin paddle which is only limited in size by the ability to close the donor site. Cutaneous perforators are located 8–12 cm distal to the symphysis along a line connecting the pubis to the medial tibial condyle. The pedicle enters the proximal third of the gracilis muscle, approximately 10 cm distal to the pubic tubercle. The obturator nerve travels obliquely from the obturator foramen to innervate the muscle; however, this nerve is transected when used for breast reconstruction. The anterior cutaneous nerve of the thigh, a branch from the anterior division of the femoral nerve, provides sensation to the anterior and medial thigh through medial and intermediate branches.

Surgical Technique

The patient is marked in the preoperative holding area. The ipsilateral side is typically chosen based on pedicle orientation. Major anatomical landmarks are marked and include the pubic tubercle and medial tibial condyle. Dominant cutaneous perforators are marked with the assistance of a hand-held Doppler. A crescent-shaped skin paddle is marked at the upper medial thigh, centered over these perforators. The upper limit of the flap extends from a line parallel and 1–2 cm inferior the inguinal ligament to the gluteal crease at the midpoint of the gluteal fold. The width of the flap depends on donor soft tissue and volume requirements for breast reconstruction, although it averages 10–12 cm.

Dissection proceeds in the frog-leg position after the leg is circumferentially prepped. Incisions are made and the anterior wing of the flap is elevated. The subcutaneous tissue is elevated in the suprafascial plane to minimize disruption of lymphatics. The posterior branch of the saphenous vein travels within the substance of the

flap and is divided. The anterior branch should be spared if amenable. The muscular fascia is incised at the posterior limit of the adductor longus muscle and retracted medially. The dominant pedicle is then found deep to the adductor longus as it courses into the medial and deep surface of the gracilis. The pedicle is subsequently dissected back to the origin of the profunda artery with care to clip the small muscular branches to the adductor longus and magnus. The anterior branch of the obturator nerve is then ligated. Care is taken not to undermine over the gracilis muscle, otherwise skin paddle perforators will be disrupted. The posterior wing of the flap can then be elevated in the suprafascial plane over the semimembranous and semitendinosus muscles. The bulk of soft tissue is harvested with posterior dissection as the fat is thicker and contour deformities are better tolerated. Additionally, there is less potential lymphatic disruption. The muscle is then transected at its proximal and distal ends and the pedicle divided. Pedicle length is short, ranging from 6 to 8 cm with a small-caliber artery ranging from 1 to 2 mm.

The flap is inset onto the chest with both wings folded onto themselves to increase projection. The donor site must be closed cautiously as it is prone to wound separation and dehiscence. The superficial thigh fascia should be secured to the perineal Colles fascia to prevent labial separation and scar migration. Final closure is in a layered fashion over closed suction drains as would be done in a cosmetic thigh lift.

Technical Pearls

- Extension of the anterior limit of the flap beyond the femoral neurovascular bundle can result in flap tip necrosis.

- The gracilis can be identified approximately three finger breadths posterior to the adductor longus muscle.

- The saphenous vein should be preserved in order to prevent prolonged leg swelling.

- Bipedicled flaps can be utilized to increase the volume of reconstruction.

- The gracilis muscle should be transected at its insertion to prevent contour deformities in thin patients.

- Care must be taken to preserve the anterior cutaneous nerve of the thigh in order to maintain sensation to its anterior medial aspect.

PAP

The PAP flap was introduced in 2010 by Allen as an alternative to the TUG flap. It is indicated in women with a pear-shaped body habitus with reconstruction of small to medium-sized breasts. A horizontal ellipse of tissue is removed from the posterior thigh over the "banana roll." Tissue volumes can be variable but average 200–400 g. Incisions are more posterior than the TUG flap, and the scar is relatively well hidden in the gluteal crease. The procedure results in a posterior thigh lift which also improves gluteal contour. Additionally, lymphatic injury is minimized as medial dissection is not required. Pitfalls include difficult positioning and inconsistent dominant perforator location. Preoperative imaging with CTA or magnetic resonance angiography (MRA) is highly recommended for determining the intramuscular course of perforators to help guide dissection.

Anatomy

The posterior thigh derives its dominant blood supply from medial perforators of the profunda femoris system. Landmarks of the posterior thigh include the gluteal fold superiorly, iliotibial tract laterally, thigh adductors medially, and popliteal fossa inferiorly. The medial femoral circumflex pedicle enters the thigh posterior and deep to the gracilis, where it travels through the adductor magnus to supply the skin. Two to five perforators are present in each thigh and are clustered 3–6 cm inferior to the gluteal fold. Perforators are described as being medial or lateral. Medial perforators exit the fascia at the level of the adductor magnus; lateral perforators exit in the vicinity of the biceps femoris and vastus lateralis. Roughly half of the perforators follow a musculocutaneous path, the others septocutaneous. The posterior femoral cutaneous nerve lies in the subfascial plane at the midline, approximately over the long head of the biceps femoris, and provides sensation to the posterior thigh.

Surgical Technique

The patient is marked in the preoperative holding room. The course of the cutaneous perforators is marked with a hand-held Doppler which should correlate with preoperative CTA or MRA. The superior marking is made 1 cm inferior and parallel to the gluteal fold with extension medially to the gracilis muscle. The inferior marking is drawn roughly 7 cm below the superior, but is limited by available laxity. The flap is designed as an ellipse, averaging 27 cm transversely, with care not to extend past the lateral gluteal fold or medial thigh. The flap can be harvested in the prone position or lithotomy. The latter allows less position changes and can decrease operative time. The prone position affords the ability to convert to a TUG flap if adequate perforators are not identified.

Incisions are made and dissection is carried from medial to lateral. Medially, elevation is at the subfascial level in order to identify the dominant perforator. Medial perforators are more commonly dominant and found on average 3.8 cm from midline and 5 cm below the gluteal fold. Lateral perforators are found, on average, 1.2 cm from midline and 5 cm below the gluteal fold. Perforator dissection follows an intramuscular course through the adductor magnus or a septal course between the adductor magnus and thigh flexors in a loose areolar plane. Pedicle dissection then proceeds in order to gain sufficient length and vessel diameter. Care is given to ligate small intramuscular branches to prevent bleeding. The average pedicle length is 10 cm and, when taken down to the profunda takeoff, can have a diameter of greater than 2 mm. Vena comitantes accompany the artery with a diameter greater than 2.5 mm. A longer pedicle can be achieved if a lateral perforator is chosen. Lateral flap elevation is then performed at the level of Scarpa's fascia in order to preserve the posterior femoral cutaneous nerve of the thigh, beveling as needed to recruit additional soft tissue bulk.

The donor site is closed in a layered fashion over a closed suction drain. The superior donor flap should be tacked down to the underlying fascia to reinforce the gluteal fold and prevent scar migration into the thigh. The flap can be coned on the chest to create a projected breast mound, similar to the TUG flap. Microanastomosis can be performed on the ipsilateral or contralateral side and can even afford thoracodorsal microanastomosis given sufficient pedicle length.

Technical Pearls

- Limit beveling superiorly to avoid distorting the gluteal fold and buttock.

- The posterior femoral cutaneous nerve is found in the subfascial plane in the posterior midline and can be used for a sensitized flap.

- Lateral perforators are larger, but a longer intramuscular dissection is required.

- More than 98% of patients have appropriate perforators on imaging to proceed with flap harvest.

LTP

The LTP flap, also known as the septocutaneous tensor fasciae lata (sc-TFL) flap, was devised through a suggestion by a patient who wanted excess thigh tissue used for her breast reconstruction after mastectomy. The original musculocutaneous flap was performed in the 1980s, although was associated with instability of the knee joint. It was later described as a perforator-based flap by Hubner in 2009, which avoided instability associated with iliotibial band transection. The flap was later popularized by Tuinder and with Allen, who have the largest patient series. The flap, like many of the other thigh-based flaps, utilizes excess tissue from the saddlebag region. A transverse island of skin and soft tissue is resected from the upper outer thigh. The resultant scar, ideally, is hidden within the underwear line. Flap dimensions can be variable but depend on laxity. Flap volumes average 500 g in one report but can be variable based on patient size. Preoperative imaging with either CTA or MRA is necessary to identify perforator anatomy. Drawbacks include a change in hip shape from convex to concave, seroma, wound healing complications, and visible scar.

Anatomy

The TFL is a hip stabilizer that aids in hip flexion. It also acts in synergy with the gluteus medius and minimus muscles. It originates from the iliac crest and inserts into the iliotibial tract. The TFL is bordered by the vastus lateralis anteriorly and the gluteus maximus and medius posteriorly. It is innervated by the superior gluteal nerve. It is a type I muscle supplied by the ascending branch of the lateral femoral circumflex artery, a branch of the profunda system. Musculocutaneous and septocutaneous perforators from this system supply the skin and soft tissue of the lateral midthigh directly over the TFL. Limits of this perfusion zone are the anterior superior iliac spine (ASIS) anteriorly, lateral half of the inferior buttocks posteriorly, within 5 cm of the iliac crest superiorly, and lower thigh inferiorly. Septocutaneous perforators that supply this area enter at two locations: ventral or posterior septum. The ventral septum is found between the rectus femoris, vastus lateralis, and TFL. The posterior septum is found between the TFL and gluteus medius. One to three septocutaneous perforators are found in each thigh. More than 50% of patients have only one septocutaneous perforator, 40% have two, and 4% have three. The distance the perforator enters the fascia from the ASIS is variable, but it averages around 8–9 cm in the vertical plane. The lateral femoral cutaneous nerve enters the thigh at the level of the ASIS below the inguinal ligament to provide sensation to the lateral thigh.

Surgical Technique

The patient is marked in the preoperative holding area. Septocutaneous perforators are located with a hand-held Doppler at the posterior thigh over the posterior septum. An S-shaped skin island is drawn around the marked perforator. The medial extent should not exceed the ventral edge of the TFL. The lateral extent should include as much gluteal fat as possible. The pinch test is used to determine the maximum width but averages 7 cm. A pillow is placed under the lumbar spine to maximize exposure to the lateral thigh.

After incisions are made, the flap is elevated from superior to inferior and medially to laterally. Limit beveling medially to minimize contour deformities. Dissection is performed in the suprafascial plane until the posterior septum is encountered between the TFL and gluteus medius. Once the septocutaneous perforators are identified, the septum is opened and the perforator traced to the ascending branch of the lateral femoral circumflex pedicle using blunt dissection. A small cuff of fascia is taken to avoid damage to the vessel. Musculocutaneous branches are ligated. Dissection stops when adequate pedicle length is achieved or at the origin of the ascending branch. The average length of the pedicle is around 8 cm but ranges from 6 to 10 cm. Perforator size range from 1.5 to 2.0 mm.

Once the flap is freed, the donor site is closed in layers over a closed suction drain. The use of progressive tension sutures has been shown to minimize seroma and wound dehiscence. The flap can be inset much like a TUG, with wings sutured to themselves to increase projection. Microanastomosis is performed in the usual fashion.

Technical Pearls

- The flap may not be ideal if the perforator exits too far distal from the ASIS as the resultant scar will be more visible on the thigh.

- If more than one perforator is present, the one closest to the ASIS should be chosen to shift the scar higher on the thigh.

- A thin layer of fat should be left laterally on the gluteus maximus to improve overall postoperative shape.

- The leg can be manipulated during dissection to change tension on the TFL fascia.

- A lighted retractor can be helpful to retract the vastus lateralis during pedicle dissection.

- A ventral septal perforator can be used, but the pedicle is shorter and there is less available fat volume.

CONCLUSION

Abdominal-based free tissue transfer remains the first-line reconstructive choice for autologous breast reconstruction. Due to improved surgical techniques, comparable results can also be achieved by using non-abdominal–based tissue. Each type of flap presents its own unique surgical advantages as well as certain disadvantages. Ultimately, the decision of which non-abdominal–based flap to utilize depends on the surgeon's experience as well as patient habitus and expectations. As microsurgical techniques continue to advance, gluteal- and thigh-based flaps will become part of the plastic surgeons armamentarium for breast reconstruction as comparable alternatives to abdominal-based free tissue transfer.

SELECTED READINGS

Ahmadzadeh R, Bergeron L, Tang M, Morris SF. The superior and inferior Gluteal artery Perforator flaps. *Plast Reconstr Surg* 2007;120(6):1551–1556.

Allen RJ, Haddock NT, Ahn CY, Sadeghi A. Breast reconstruction with the Profunda artery Perforator flap. *Plast Reconstr Surg* 2012;129(1):16e–23e.

Arnež ZM, Pogorelec D, Planinšek F, Ahčan U. Breast reconstruction by the free transverse gracilis (TUG) flap, *Br J Plast Surg* 2004;57(1):20–26.

Buchel EW, Dalke KR, Hayakawa TE. The transverse upper gracilis flap: Efficiencies and design tips. *Can J Plast Surg* 2013;21(3):162–166.

Chen CM, LoTempio M and Allen RJ. *Profunda Artery Perforator (PAP) Flap for Breast Reconstruction, Breast Reconstruction*. Aldona J. Spiegel, IntechOpen. DOI: 10.5772/56332. https://www.intechopen.com/books/breast-reconstruction-current-perspectives-and-state-of-the-art-techniques/profunda-artery-perforator-pap-flap-for-breast-reconstruction

DeLong MR, Hughes DB, Bond JE, Thomas SM, Boll DT, Zenn MR. A detailed evaluation of the anatomical variations of the profunda artery perforator flap using computed tomographic angiograms. *Plast Reconstr Surg* 2014;134(2):186e–192e.

Elliott LF, Beegle PH, Hartrampf CR. The lateral transverse thigh free flap. *Plast Reconstr Surg* 1990;85(2):169–178.

Gagnon AR, Blondeel PN. Superior gluteal artery perforator flap. *Semin Plast Surg* 2006;20(2):79–88.

Georgantopoulou A, Papadodima S, Vlachodimitropoulos D, Goutas N, Spiliopoulou C, Papadopoulos O. The microvascular anatomy of superior and inferior gluteal artery perforator (SGAP and IGAP) flaps: a fresh cadaveric study and clinical implications. *Aesthet Plast Surg* 2014;38(6):1156–1163.

Haddock NT, Greaney P, Otterburn D, Levine S, Allen RJ. Predicting perforator location on preoperative imaging for the profunda artery perforator flap, *Microsurgery* 2012; 32(7):507–511.

Hubmer MG, Justich I, Haas FM, Koch H, Parvizi D, Feigl G, Prandl E. Clinical experience with a tensor fasciae latae perforator flap based on septocutaneous perforators. *J Plast Reconstr Aesthet Surg* 2011;64(6):782–789.

Hubmer MG, Schwaiger N, Windisch G, et al. The vascular anatomy of the tensor fasciae latae perforator flap. *Plast Reconstr Surg* 2009;124(1):181–189.

Hunter C, Moody L, Luan A, Nazerali R, Lee GK. Superior gluteal artery perforator flap. *Ann Plast Surg* 2016;76: S191–S195.

Hunter JE, Lardi AM, Dower DR, Farhadi J. Evolution from the TUG to PAP flap for breast reconstruction: comparison and refinements of technique. *J Plast Reconstr Aesthet Surg* 2015;68(7):960–965.

Hur K, Ohkuma R, Bellamy JL, et al. Patient-reported assessment of functional gait outcomes following superior gluteal artery perforator reconstruction. *Plast Reconstr Surg Global Open* 2013;1(5):e31.

Lakhiani C, DeFazio M, Han K, Falola R, Evans K. Donor-site morbidity following free tissue harvest from the thigh: a systematic review and pooled analysis of complications. *J Reconstr Microsurg* 2015;32(05):342–357.

LoTempio MM, Allen RJ. Breast reconstruction with SGAP and IGAP flaps. *Plast Reconstr Surg* 2010;126(2):393–401.

Pan W-R, Taylor GI. The angiosomes of the thigh and buttock. *Plast Reconstr Surg* 2009;123(1):236–249.

Saadeh FA, Haikal FA, Abdel-Hamid Fathiyya AM. Blood supply of the tensor fasciae latae muscle. *Clin Anat* 1998;11(4):236–238.

Satake T, Muto M, Ogawa M, et al. Unilateral breast reconstruction using bilateral inferior gluteal artery perforator flaps. *Plast Reconstr Surg Global Open* 2015;3(3): e314.

Tuinder S, Baetens T, De Haan MW, Piatkowski de Grzymala A, Booi AD, Van Der Hulst R, Lataster A. Septocutaneous tensor fasciae latae perforator flap for breast reconstruction: radiological considerations and clinical cases. *J Plast Reconstr Aesthet Surg* 2014;67(9):1248–1256.

Tuinder S, Chen CM, Massey MF, Allen RJ, Van Der Huist R. Introducing the septocutaneous gluteal artery perforator flap: a simplified approach to microsurgical breast reconstruction. *Plast Reconstr Surg* 2011;127(2):489–495.

Wong C, Nagarkar P, Teotia S, Haddock NT. The profunda artery perforator flap. *Plast Reconstr Surg* 2015;136(5):915–919.

Yaghoubian A, Boyd JB. The SGAP flap in breast reconstruction: backup or first choice? *Plast Reconstr Surg* 2011;128(1):29e–31e.

Yousif NJ, Matloub HS, Kolachalam R, Grunert BK, Sanger JR. The transverse gracilis musculocutaneous flap. *Ann Plast Surg* 1992;29(6):482–490.

PART XI.

GROIN AND PENILE RECONSTRUCTION

77

GROIN DISSECTION AND REGIONAL LYMPHADENECTOMY

Darlene M. Sparkman and W. John Kitzmiller

ASSESSMENT OF THE DEFECT

Groin dissection with regional lymphadenectomy is indicated as a diagnostic or therapeutic procedure in patients who have a primary malignant neoplasm that has known or suspected lymphatic drainage to the superficial or deep inguinal lymph nodes. These pathologic entities can include anal, vaginal, urethral, vulvar, uterine, penile, ovarian, rectal, and cutaneous cancers. The most common of these neoplasms plastic surgeons must manage is melanoma.

INDICATIONS

The recommended method for lymph node analysis continues to evolve. All patients should undergo basic clinical evaluation for the presence of palpable nodes. Sentinel node biopsies are suggested for any stage I melanoma with a thickness of greater than 0.75 mm and recommended for thickness of greater than 1 mm and stage II melanoma so long as patient comorbidities do not prevent it.[1] Regional lymphadenectomy in patients with nonpalpable nodes and negative sentinel lymph node biopsies has failed to demonstrate survival benefits and is thus not indicated. Although the impact of completion lymph node dissection on regional control and survival has not been clearly delineated, additional positive nodes beyond positive sentinel nodes can be found in 18% of patients following node dissection.[2,3] Thus, consistent clinical agreement exists that if the patient's general condition is good, groin dissection should be performed in the presence of palpable nodes and strongly considered with positive sentinel lymph node biopsies.[1] Fine-needle aspiration may confirm histologic metastatic involvement of clinically positive nodes or nodes suspicious of recurrence before lymphadenectomy with no significant increase in morbidity. Isolated limb perfusion has been performed at the time of regional lymphadenectomy with no appreciable increase in morbidity.[4]

Although a complete lymphadenectomy of the involved nodal basin should be performed, separate and specific indications for deep iliac or obturator node dissections exist. Even with no clinical or radiologic evidence of pelvic nodal involvement, patients with clinically positive superficial node involvement, three or more superficial nodes histologically involved, or a positive Cloquet node are candidates for elective iliac and obturator lymph node dissection.[5,6] In addition, iliac and obturator lymph node dissection is indicated if a pelvic positron emission tomography (PET)/computed tomography (CT) or stand-alone CT scan is positive.

Regional lymphadenectomy is contraindicated if there is evidence of widespread visceral metastases.

PATIENT PREPARATION, ROOM SETUP, AND PATIENT POSITIONING

Groin dissection with regional lymphadenectomy is usually performed under general anesthesia, although it may be performed under epidural anesthesia in selected patients. Perioperative antibiotics are recommended. We prefer a first-generation cephalosporin, but in the presence of a local chronic open wound that is drained by the involved lymph nodes, perioperative antibiotic choice may be guided by preoperative cultures. Prophylaxis against deep venous thrombosis is recommended. We routinely use sequential compression devices and reserve anticoagulant therapy for high-risk patients based on their risk assessment score. Patients should take special care to thoroughly wash the operative field with antibacterial soap the evening before surgery. We routinely provide patients with chlorhexidine

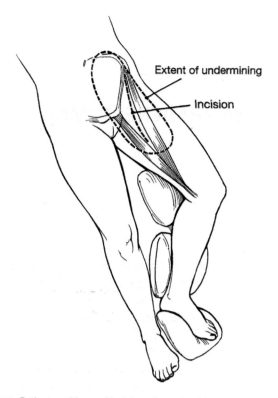

Figure 77.1. Patient position and incisions for regional lymphadenectomy.

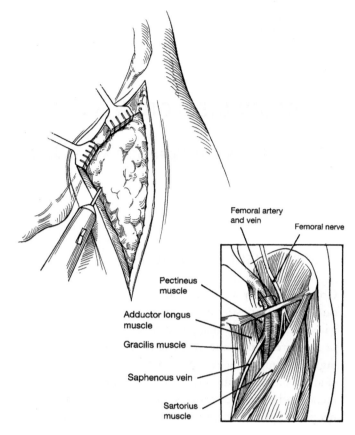

Figure 77.2. Elevation of skin flaps at proper plane is critical to minimize complications.

soap. Hair is clipped from the operative field the morning of surgery by a member of the surgical team.

The patient is positioned on the operating room table in the supine position with the hip flexed, abducted and externally rotated (so-called frog-leg position). The leg and ankle are supported by a pillow or sandbags (Figure 77.1). A Foley catheter is inserted into the bladder. In males, the scrotum is secured to the contralateral thigh. The surgical field is prepared from the level of the knee superiorly to the costal margins, medially to the contralateral pubic tubercle, and laterally to the greater trochanter.

OPERATIVE TECHNIQUE

The incision is made along an oblique line from 3 cm medial to the anterior superior iliac spine to the apex of the femoral triangle, defined by the sartorius muscle laterally and the adductor longus muscle medially. The floor of the femoral triangle is the abductor longus and iliopsoas muscles.[7] If there has been a previous biopsy site, this should be included in the incision. T-incisions and parallel incisions are not recommended because of a higher risk of skin slough. A vertical incision over the femoral vessels is not recommended because of an increased risk

of wound-healing problems over the most critical area for coverage. The level of undermining begins just superficial to Scarpa's fascia, maintaining 2–3 mm of subcutaneous fat on the skin flaps (Figure 77.2). As the dissection continues laterally and medially, the flaps are made gradually thicker. If there is bulky disease in the groin, skin is excised along with the lymph nodes, rather than maintaining skin flaps of questionable viability and possibly compromising the oncologic resection. Undermining is completed laterally to the anterior superior iliac spine, medially to the pubic tubercle, superiorly to just below the umbilicus, and inferiorly to the apex of the femoral triangle.

Superficial lymphadenectomy is initiated laterally by incision of the fascia overlying the sartorius muscle (Figure 77.3). The dissection is carried medially. The lateral cutaneous nerve of the thigh is identified and preserved unless it is grossly invaded by tumor. It courses under the inguinal ligament and over the sartorius muscle into the thigh before dividing into anterior and posterior branches. It can generally be found about 10–15 cm medial to the anterior superior iliac spine. At the inferior margin of dissection, the saphenous vein is identified and

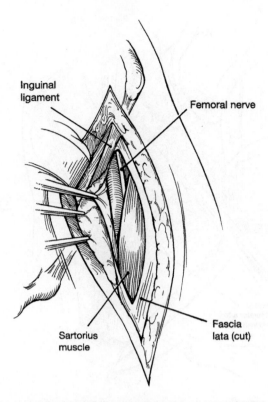

Figure 77.3. Superficial lymphadenectomy progressing lateral to medial, with incision of fascia of sartorius muscle proceeding medially superficial to femoral nerve.

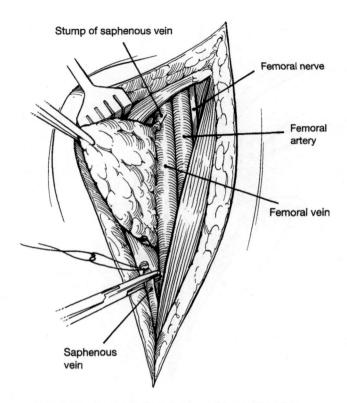

Figure 77.4. Saphenous vein is ligated at apex of femoral triangle.

ligated—although some recent studies have suggested sparing the vein (Figure 77.4).[8] Beginning inferiorly, the fibrolymphatic contents of the femoral triangle are reflected superiorly and the anterior femoral sheath is incised and included in the specimen. Branches of the femoral artery and vein are suture ligated and divided as they are encountered. The dissection continues superiorly to the level of the inguinal ligament. The specimen is maintained in continuity with the fatty areolar tissue medial to the femoral vein. The superficial dissection is completed by sweeping the fatty tissue from above the inguinal ligament inferiorly and medially off the anterior abdominal wall musculature, maintaining continuity with the lower part of the specimen (Figure 77.5).

When deep iliac and obturator node dissection is indicated, the inguinal ligament can be divided 2 cm medial to its attachment to the anterior superior iliac spine. The external oblique, internal oblique, and transversus abdominis muscles are split longitudinally and the retroperitoneal plane is developed. The inguinal ligament is retracted, and the inferior epigastric artery and vein are ligated and divided, allowing medial retraction of the anterior abdominal wall musculature and the peritoneum (Figure 77.6). The ureter is identified and

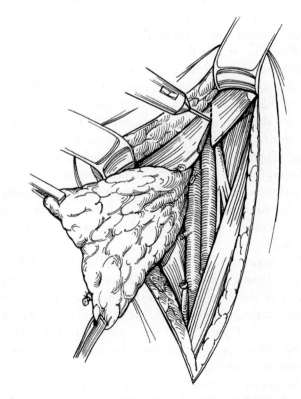

Figure 77.5. After completion of superficial inguinal dissection, lateral abdominal wall muscles are incised along with inguinal ligament.

GROIN DISSECTION AND REGIONAL LYMPHADENECTOMY

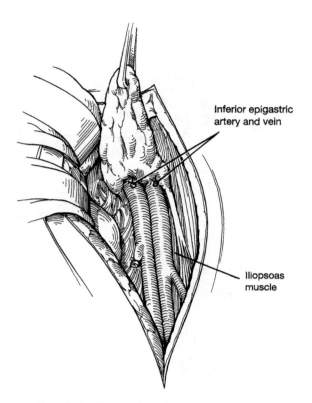

Figure 77.6. Abdominal wall and peritoneal contents are reflected medially, allowing exposure of retroperitoneal space.

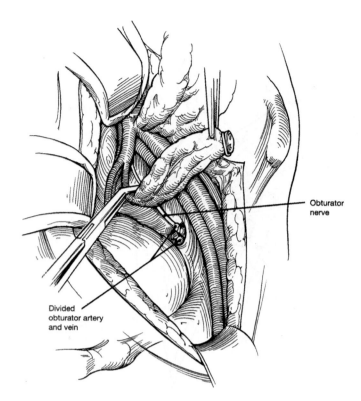

Figure 77.7. Obturator node dissection is completed as final step of dissection.

reflected medially. With this exposure, the dissection is carried along en bloc superiorly to the bifurcation of the external and internal iliac arteries. The floor of the dissection at this level is the iliopsoas muscle. The genitofemoral nerve is the lateral boundary of dissection. Medially, dissection is completed to the medial aspect of the external iliac vein. Posterior to the external iliac vein the obturator nodes are identified and resected. The obturator nerve is identified posteriorly and preserved (Figure 77.7). The specimen is left attached and in continuity with the superficial specimen medial to the femoral vein. If necessary, the dissection may be easily extended to the level of the aortic bifurcation. The specimen is removed en bloc, labeled, and oriented for the pathologist.

The inguinal ligament is repaired and sutured to Cooper's ligament medial to the femoral vein. A relaxing incision in the anterior rectus sheath facilitates closure without excessive tension, as performed in a McVey hernia repair (Figure 77.8). The transversus abdominis, internal oblique, and external oblique muscles are closed in layers with absorbable suture. The sartorius muscle may be elevated, incised proximally, and turned over the femoral vessels for added protection (Figure 77.9). Skin is closed in two layers over two closed suction drains.

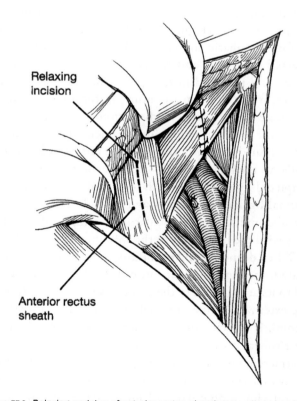

Figure 77.8. Relaxing excision of anterior rectus sheath may relieve tension on abdominal wall closure.

GROIN AND PENILE RECONSTRUCTION

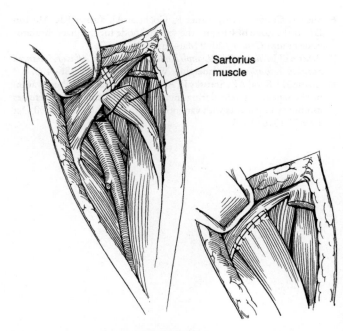

Figure 77.9. Sartorius muscle is commonly used as turn-over for flap coverage of femoral vessels.

If there is any question of viability of skin flaps, fluorescein may be administered intravenously and flaps inspected with a Wood's light. If there is any question of viability, skin flaps should be debrided intraoperatively. Once skin closure is accomplished, the drains are connected to suction. Primary closure is possible in the majority of cases.

POSTOPERATIVE CARE

Compression dressings are avoided by the use of closed suction drains. Light gauze dressings are taped in place, and the patient is transferred to the hospital bed from the operating room table. For the first 12–24 hours, the patient is maintained at bed rest. The use of a footboard and an overhead trapeze helps facilitate recovery. Sequential compression devices are continued until the patient is ambulatory. Patients are allowed to ambulate on a limited basis the day after surgery. The involved lower extremity is wrapped with elastic (Ace) bandages from the toes to the groin, and prolonged sitting or standing is avoided. While the patient is resting in bed, the semi-Fowler's position is recommended. Parenteral antibiotics are maintained until drains are removed. The drains are removed after the patient is ambulating and the drainage is less than 30 mL in 24 hours. If seromas occur after drainage, they are intermittently and sterilely

aspirated. Sutures are removed 10 days to 2 weeks after surgery.

Graduated compression stockings are recommended to minimize risk of edema. If edema is noted despite these measures, a serial compression pump is prescribed.

Common postoperative complications are skin slough, wound infection, wound seroma, and postoperative edema of the lower extremity. Skin slough is minimized by avoiding wound closure under tension with flaps of questionable viability. Flap viability is maintained by careful skin flap elevation and resection of skin that is of questionable viability or involved by tumor. Rather than close wounds under tension, the use of myocutaneous flaps readily allows obliteration of dead space and provides for tension-free wound closure. Wound infection may be minimized by the use of prophylactic antibiotics. Seroma may be minimized by careful ligation of the areolar tissue around the femoral and iliac vessels. The use of closed suction drains kept in place until after the patient is ambulatory also helps minimize this complication. Postoperative edema may be minimized by keeping the patient at bed rest for the day and allowing minimal ambulation with meticulous use of compression stockings.

CAVEATS

Groin dissection with regional lymphadenectomy using this technique is based on sound surgical principles: en bloc removal of the involved lymphatic chain and tension-free wound closure with well-vascularized tissue. If there is any question of skin involvement over the involved nodes, the skin should be resected with the specimen. Skin flap viability is judged by the presence of dermal bleeding. Skin edges should be debrided back to clearly viable tissue. If the edges cannot be approximated without excessive tension, a regional myocutaneous flap is recommended to allow proper closure. This approach allows an aggressive resection of the involved lymphatics and the best chance of uncomplicated wound healing.

SELECTED READINGS

1. National Comprehensive Cancer Network, Inc. Melanoma. NCCN Guidelines Version 2.2016.
2. Cascinelli N, Bombardieri E, Bufalino R, et al. Sentinel and nonsentinel node status in stage IB and II melanoma patients: two-step prognostic indicators of survival. *J Clin Oncol* 2006 Sep 20;24(27):4464–4471.
3. Lee JH, Essner R, Torisu-Itakura H, Wanek L, Wang H, Morton DL. Factors predictive of tumor-positive nonsentinel lymph nodes after

tumor-positive sentinel lymph node dissection for melanoma. *J Clin Oncol* 2004 Sep 15;22(18):3677–3684.

4. Lens MB, Dawes M. Isolated limb perfusion with melphalan in the treatment of malignant melanoma of the extremities: a systematic review of randomised controlled trials. *Lancet Oncol* 2003 Jun;4(6):359–364.

5. Coit DG, Brennan MF. Extent of lymph node dissection in melanoma of the trunk or lower extremity. *Arch Surg* 1989 Feb;124(2):162–166.

6. Shen P, Conforti AM, Essner R, Cochran AJ, Turner RR, Morton DL. Is the node of Cloquet the sentinel node for the iliac/obturator node group? *Cancer J* 2000 Mar–Apr;6(2):93–97.

7. Beattie EJ Jr. *Ilioinguinal Lymph Node Dissection: An Atlas of Advanced Surgical Techniques*. Philadelphia: WB Saunders, 1968:386–403.

8. Zhang SH, Sood AK, Sorosky JI, Anderson B, Buller RE. Preservation of the saphenous vein during inguinal lymphadenectomy decreases morbidity in patients with carcinoma of the vulva. *Cancer* 2000 Oct 1;89(7):1520–1525.

78.

TENSOR FASCIAE LATA FOR GROIN RECONSTRUCTION

Peter C. Neligan

Patients with large groin wounds pose a particular reconstructive problem. The groin is a unique area, combining elements of myofascial strength, which influences the integrity of the abdominal cavity, with the role of being a conduit for neurovascular structures to the lower limb. Groin reconstruction thus demands that the repair be strong as well as provide adequate soft tissue to protect these structures.

ASSESSMENT OF THE DEFECT

The defect must be carefully examined and the reconstructive requirements assessed based on this examination. The cause of the defect is important as is its current status: the presence of infection, the status of the surrounding tissue, or the requirement for further debridement are all important issues to be determined. For groin wounds, it is important to ascertain whether the defect includes all the layers of the abdominal musculature, whether vascular structures are exposed, whether or not skin cover is required, and what the demands on reconstruction are going to be (e.g., whether the patient is likely to undergo postoperative irradiation, the patient's level of physical activity, etc.). These factors determine not only the type of reconstruction that is most appropriate but also, as in the case of exposed vascular structures, the urgency of the closure.

The tensor fasciae lata (TFL) and rectus femoris flaps are both ideally suited to groin reconstruction. However, in recent years, the anterolateral thigh flap (ALT) has become more popular for these reconstructions.[1] The choice of which flap to use is as often determined by the choice of the surgeon as by the particular requirements of the repair. The amount of tissue transferred with these flaps can be enlarged by incorporating a fascial extension. Indeed, for large defects, a combination of these flaps may be used.

INDICATIONS

The major indications for use of the TFL flap are in reconstruction of the trochanteric area as well as reconstruction of the lower abdomen. Because of the abundance of fascia that can be transferred with this flap, it is particularly suited to situations where closure of a defect involving the muscular integrity of the abdominal wall is concerned. As a myofascial flap, it is particularly useful for reconstructing defects where skin cover is not an issue. It has an arc of rotation which includes the lower abdomen, groin, the anterior perineum, the trochanter, and the hip[2] (Figure 78.1). Only the rectus femoris, TFL, and ALT

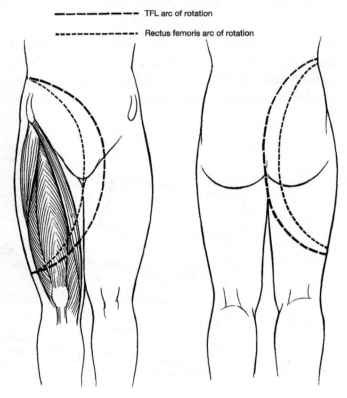

----------- TFL arc of rotation

------------ Rectus femoris arc of rotation

Figure 78.1. Arc of rotation of tensor fascia lata and rectus femoris.

replace infected mesh. Its use in reconstructing abdominal defects in patients who have previously been irradiated is recognized.[2] The flap can be raised as a myofascial flap or as a myofasciocutaneous flap with either an isolated skin island or, more commonly, with a skin bridge (Figure 78.2).

CONTRAINDICATIONS

The use of a large skin paddle may preclude direct closure of the donor defect that consequently requires grafting with an undesirable cosmetic defect. The skin paddle may be unreliable distally so that the flap should not extend beyond 8 cm from the knee. If the defect to be reconstructed includes extensive soft tissue loss, a bulkier flap such as the rectus femoris may be preferred. One can also argue that such a muscular flap may be preferable in a contaminated bed. Use of the TFL flap in an athletic individual may lead to some lateral instability of the knee. With extensive wounds of the groin resulting from trauma, tumor ablation, and vascular reconstruction involving the femoral vessels the TFL flap cannot be used.[3]

ROOM SETUP

The patient is placed supine on the operating table. The flap can also be elevated quite easily with the patient in the lateral decubitus position. The choice of position will be determined by the defect to be closed. For groin reconstruction, the supine position is preferred. Placing the hip and knee in flexion with the hip internally rotated facilitates flap elevation (Figure 78.3). The leg is

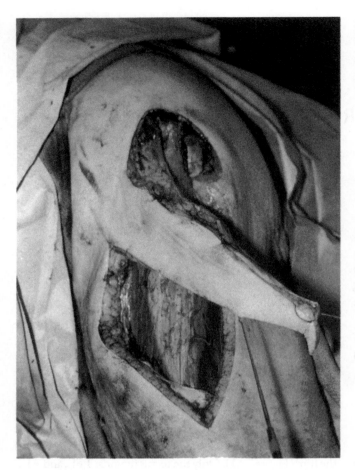

Figure 78.2. Tensor fascia lata being raised with intact skin bridge.

can compete for lower abdominal reconstruction in terms of the quality of strong fascia, which they provide. As with the rectus femoris, the TFL can be used for reconstructing fascial defects in which the use of mesh is contraindicated or to

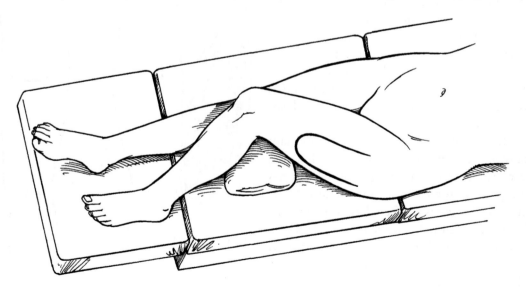

Figure 78.3. Patient in position for flap harvest.

free-draped so that its position can be changed during the procedure to maximize exposure of the defect and to facilitate insetting of the flap. This is not a two-team procedure, so there are no specific recommendations for room setup.

PATIENT MARKINGS

The origin of the TFL is from the lateral aspect of the anterior superior iliac spine and the anterior aspect of the adjacent iliac crest, as well as from the deep surface of the

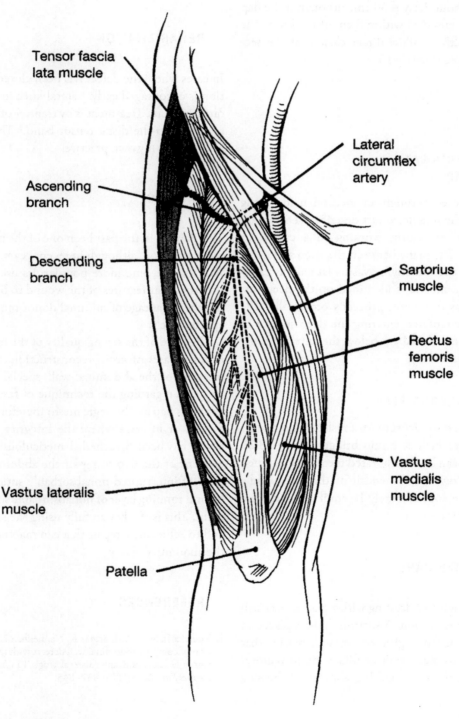

Figure 78.4. Anatomy of tensor fascia lata.

fascia lata.[4] The insertion is into the lateral aspect of the knee, and it functions as a lateral stabilizer of the knee. The TFL muscle lies between the biceps femoris posteriorly and rectus femoris anteriorly. The vastus lateralis muscle is attached to the deep surface of the fascia lata but does not contribute to the vascular supply of the fascia lata.[5] The distal end of the cutaneous portion of the flap is somewhat unreliable. The maximum length of the skin flap that can be safely raised without delay is 30 cm, although if the flap is delayed it can be raised to within 8 cm of the knee. The maximum skin width to allow direct closure of the secondary defect is approximately 10 cm.

TECHNIQUE

THE TENSOR FASCIA LATA MYOFASCIAL FLAP

The muscle is exposed through an incision made along the central axis of the muscle, as just described. Dissection begins distally and anteriorly, working in a caudal to cephalad direction. The plane between the deep surface of the fascia lata and the underlying vastus lateralis is easily identified. The TFL muscle is identified on the deep surface of the fascia as dissection proceeds proximally. The main pedicle is encountered entering the deep surface of the muscle approximately 10 cm below the anterior superior iliac spine (Figure 78.4).

MYOFASCIOCUTANEOUS FLAP

The flap can be raised to incorporate an island skin paddle or, more usually, can include a skin bridge (Figure 78.2). A large skin paddle can be incorporated measuring as much as 20 × 30 cm. However, the width of the skin paddle should be limited to approximately 10 cm if direct closure of the donor defect is desired.

POSTOPERATIVE CARE

The leg is placed in a bulky dressing with a plaster backslab holding the knee in extension. A suction drain is placed in the leg and brought out through a separate stab incision that I prefer to place proximally as it facilitates drain removal without disturbing the dressing. The abdominal dressing depends on whether or not a skin graft has been used, in which case a tie-over dressing is used to secure the graft to the underlying muscle. Again, a suction drain placed in the abdominal wound is brought out through separate stab incision as described for the rectus femoris flap. Drains are removed when drainage has become minimal, which is usually in about 3 or 4 days. Management of the abdominal wound is as described for the rectus femoris flap.

REHABILITATION

In cases where the defect has been closed directly, ambulation is encouraged early. Lateral knee instability can infrequently occur. Treatment is by transfer of the rectus femoris tendon into the distal tensor band.[5] This has never been necessary in my own practice.

CAVEATS

This flap has in the past been one of the mainstays for groin reconstruction, although in recent years, as mentioned, the ALT has become more popular. Its use is determined by the particular features of the wound to be reconstructed. It has the advantage of minimal donor morbidity when used appropriately.

Because of the strong quality of the fascia and the need, in most cases of groin reconstruction, to reconstruct the integrity of the abdominal wall, special mention needs to be made regarding the technique of fascial insetting. I regard this flap as a biologic mesh; therefore, in full-thickness defects or in cases where the integrity of the abdominal cavity has been breached, I meticulously inset the fascial element of the flap to repair the abdominal defect with a layer of interrupted nonabsorbable sutures, followed by a second running layer of nonabsorbable suture for reinforcement. This is the key to fully using the strength of the flap and to achieving a repair that can maintain the integrity of the abdominal cavity

REFERENCES

1. Vranckx JJ, Stoel AM, Segers K, Nanhekhan L. Dynamic reconstruction of complex abdominal wall defects with the pedicled innervated vastus lateralis and anterolateral thigh PIVA flap. *J Plast Reconstr Aesthet Surg* 2015;68(6):837–845.

GROIN AND PENILE RECONSTRUCTION

2. Bostwick J, 3rd, Hill HL, Nahai F. Repairs in the lower abdomen, groin, or perineum with myocutaneous or omental flaps. *Plast Reconstr Surg* 1979;63(2):186–194.

3. Ger R, Duboys E. The prevention and repair of large abdominal-wall defects by muscle transposition: a preliminary communication. *Plast Reconstr Surg* 1983;72(2):170–178.

4. McCraw J. Tensor fascia lata. In: Phillip G. Arnold, John B. McCraw, eds. *McCraw and Arnolkd's Atlas of Musclke and Musculocutaneous Flaps.* Norfolk, VA: Hampton Press, 1986: 423.

5. Nahai F, Hill L, Hester TR. Experiences with the tensor fascia lata flap. *Plast Reconstr Surg* 1979;63(6):788–799.

79.

THE RECTUS FEMORIS FLAP FOR GROIN RECONSTRUCTION

Peter C. Neligan

The rectus femoris muscle is an important but expendable knee extensor. It is a bipennate muscle with a dense and strong fascia on its undersurface. This feature makes it extremely attractive for the repair of defects of the lower abdominal wall and groin as a pedicled flap (Figure 79.1). It can also be transferred as a free flap, and this expands its reconstructive potential. The muscle can be transferred alone as a muscle flap or with a skin paddle as a myocutaneous flap.

ASSESSMENT OF THE DEFECT

The defect must be carefully examined and the reconstructive requirements assessed based on this examination. The history and origin of the defect is important, as is its current status: Is the wound infected, is the surrounding tissue healthy, or will further debridement be necessary? For groin wounds, it is important to determine whether the defect includes all the layers of the abdominal musculature, whether vascular structures are exposed, whether or not skin cover is required, and what the demands on reconstruction are going to be (e.g., is the patient likely to undergo postoperative irradiation? How physically active is the patient?).

INDICATIONS

The major indication for use of the rectus femoris flap is in reconstruction of the lower abdomen and groin, particularly where closure of a full-thickness defect or a defect involving the muscular integrity of the abdominal wall is concerned.[1], which is ideally suited for reconstruction of these defects (Figure 79.2). It has been used for lower abdominal and groin reconstruction since the early 1970s and appeared early in the evolution of musculocutaneous flaps.[2] It has an arc of rotation that includes the groin, the anterior perineum, the trochanter, and the hip.

The umbilicus is the upper limit of the flap's reach. This reach can be increased when the muscle is flipped over rather than rotated. While there are several regional flaps that can reach these areas, only the rectus femoris and the tensor fascia lata can compete for lower abdominal reconstruction in terms of the quality of strong fascia that they provide. This is especially useful in reconstructing fascial defects in which the use of mesh is contraindicated or, as is frequently the case, to replace infected mesh. Its arc of rotation allows it to reach comfortably to the umbilicus, and it can reach across the midline in the groin (Figure 79.1). The flap can be raised as a muscle flap or as a myocutaneous flap with either an isolated skin island or with a skin bridge (Figure 79.3).

CONTRAINDICATIONS

With appropriate care, the donor defect is acceptable,[3]. The use of a large skin paddle may preclude direct closure of the donor defect, which consequently requires grafting with an undesirable cosmetic defect. Because of the issues with potential damage to knee extension, this flap has been largely superseded by the anterolateral thigh flap (ALT).[4] However it is still a useful flap to have available.

ROOM SETUP

The patient is placed supine on the operating table. Depending on the configuration of the defect to be

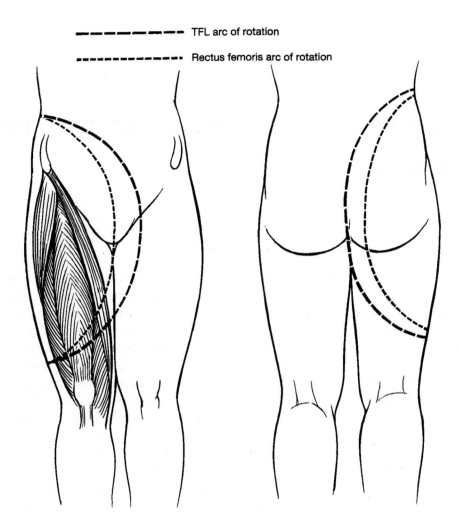

Figure 79.1. Arc of rotation of tensor fascia lata and rectus femoris.

reconstructed, it is often easiest to free-drape the leg so that its position can be changed during the procedure to maximize exposure of the defect and to facilitate insetting of the flap. This is not a two-team procedure so there are no specific recommendations for room setup.

PATIENT MARKINGS

The origin of the rectus femoris muscle is from the anterior inferior iliac spine and the adjacent acetabular rim. Its insertion is into the upper pole of the patella, running down the anterior thigh between vastus lateralis and medialis[5] (Figure 79.4). The tendon of insertion is separated from the femur by the suprapatellar bursa and becomes confluent with the quadriceps tendon that also incorporates the vastus group of muscles. A line drawn between the anterior superior iliac spine and the patella represents the central

axis of the muscle. The skin paddle of the flap is drawn relative to this central axis (Figure 79.3). The distal end of the flap is a minimum of 6 cm above the upper pole of the patella. The maximum dimensions of the skin paddle are 20 × 30 cm but the maximum width to allow direct closure of the secondary defect is approximately 10 cm.

TECHNIQUE

ANATOMY

The rectus femoris has a single dominant vascular pedicle that arises from the descending branch of the lateral circumflex femoral artery. Descriptions of the vascular anatomy in the literature vary.[5,6] There may be a number of nondominant secondary pedicles; superiorly, they form the ascending branch of the lateral circumflex femoral artery,

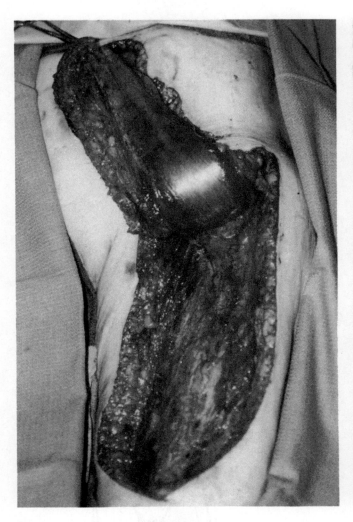

Figure 79.2. Dense fascia on undersurface of rectus femoris muscle.

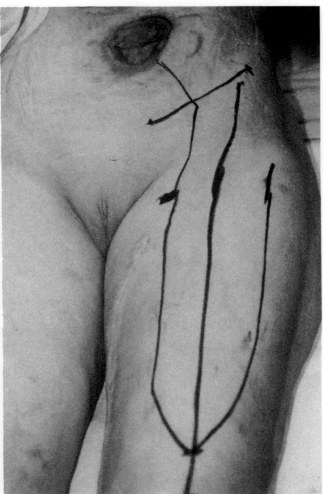

Figure 79.3. Surface markings for rectus femoris flap. Flap is being used with intact skin bridge.

and, inferiorly, they form both the descending branch of the lateral circumflex femoral artery and the femoral artery (Figure 79.4).

THE RECTUS FEMORIS MUSCLE FLAP

The muscle is exposed through an incision made along the central axis of the muscle, as described earlier. Dissection begins distally by identifying the tendinous insertion of the muscle (Figure 79.4). Division of the muscle should be carried out at least 6 cm above the patella in order to preserve the integrity of the tendon and of the suprapatellar bursa. The vastus muscles must be separated from the rectus at this level. Dissection then proceeds from distal to proximal and from lateral to medial. The secondary pedicle from the descending branch of the lateral circumflex femoral artery will be encountered and can be ligated. The main pedicle is encountered entering the deep surface of the muscle approximately 10 cm below the anterior superior iliac spine

(Figure 79.4). At this level, the sartorius muscle crosses the medial border of the muscle.

MYOCUTANEOUS FLAP

The flap can be raised to incorporate an island skin paddle or can include a skin bridge (Figure 79.3). A large skin paddle can be incorporated measuring as much as 20 × 30 cm. However, the width of the skin paddle should be limited to approximately 10 cm if direct closure of the donor defect is desired. The skin paddle should be centered over the proximal two-thirds of the muscle. Proximally, the sartorius muscle crosses over the origin of the rectus femoris, and this must be borne in mind in designing the skin paddle.

Of vital importance is centralization of the quadriceps mechanism prior to closure. Using strong, nonabsorbable interrupted sutures, the vastus medialis and lateralis muscles are plicated in the midline for approximately 15 cm above

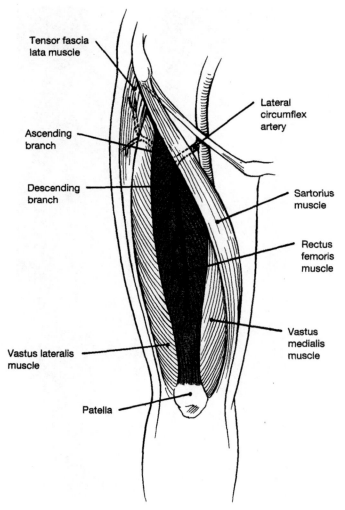

Figure 79.4. Anatomy of rectus femoris muscle.

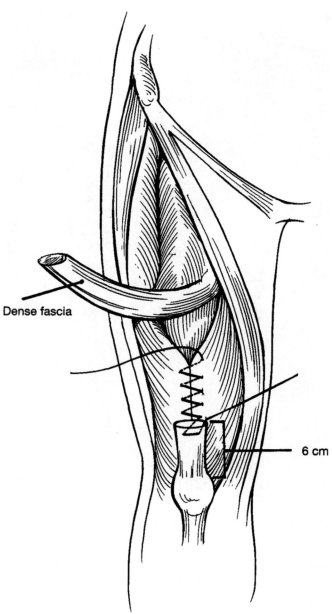

Figure 79.5. Centralization of extensor mechanism.

the point of distal muscle harvest. By having the leg free-draped, one can satisfy oneself that this plication, which is designed to maximize knee extension, is not so tight as to limit knee flexion (Figure 79.5).

A suction drain is placed in the leg and brought out through a separate stab incision that I prefer to place proximally as it facilitates drain removal without disturbing the dressing.

POSTOPERATIVE CARE

The leg is placed in a bulky dressing with a plaster backslab holding the knee in extension. The abdominal dressing depends on whether or not a skin graft has been used, in which case a tie-over or VAC dressing is used to secure the graft to the underlying muscle. Again, a suction drain

placed in the abdominal wound is brought out through separate stab incision.

Drains are removed when drainage has become minimal, which is usually in about 3–4 days. If a tie-over dressing or VAC has been used over a grafted muscle, it is left in place for a minimum of 5 days unless factors such as surrounding cellulitis or odor demand that the site be inspected sooner. An abdominal binder is used to provide support during healing, and this is worn for 3 weeks postoperatively. Care must be taken that this does not cause undue pressure on the pedicle.

REHABILITATION

It is very important to ensure that knee extension is preserved with minimal deficit.[3] To this end, the patient is splinted for 2 weeks. Following this, range of motion is increased actively and passively in all joints with particular attention being paid to the knee. Quadriceps strengthening exercises are initiated. Patients frequently have difficulty climbing stairs initially, and these exercises are helpful for this activity.

CAVEATS

The rectus femoris flap has been one of the mainstays of groin reconstruction in the past, although, as mentioned above, the ALT flap has largely replaced it in recent years. Its use is determined by the particular features of the wound to be reconstructed. It has the advantage of minimal donor morbidity when used appropriately. Because of the strong quality of the fascia and the need, in most cases, of groin reconstruction to reconstruct the integrity of the abdominal wall, special mention needs to be made of the technique of fascial insetting. I regard this flap as a biologic

mesh, therefore, in full-thickness defects or in cases where the integrity of the abdominal cavity has been breached, I meticulously inset the fascial element of the flap to repair the abdominal wall defect with a layer of interrupted nonabsorbable sutures, followed by a second layer of running nonabsorbable suture for reinforcement. This is the key to fully using the strength of the flap and to achieving a repair that can maintain the integrity of the abdominal cavity.

REFERENCES

1. Ramasastry SS, Liang MD, Hurwitz DJ. Surgical management of difficult wounds of the groin. *Surg Gynecol Obstet* 1989;169(5):418–422.
2. Bhagwat BM, Pearl RM, Laub DR. Uses of the rectus femoris myocutaneous flap. *Plast Reconstr Surg.* 1978;62(5):699–701.
3. Caulfield WH, Curtsinger L, Powell G, Pederson WC. Donor leg morbidity after pedicled rectus femoris muscle flap transfer for abdominal wall and pelvic reconstruction. *Ann Plast Surg* 1994;32(4):377–382.
4. Vranckx JJ, Stoel AM, Segers K, Nanhekhan L. Dynamic reconstruction of complex abdominal wall defects with the pedicled innervated vastus lateralis and anterolateral thigh PIVA flap. *J Plast Reconstr Aesthet Surg* 2015;68(6):837–845.
5. McCraw J. Tensor fascia lata. In: *McCraw and Arnolkd's Atlas of Muscle and Musculocutaneous Flaps*, John B. McCraw and Phillip G. Arnold, eds. 1986, Norfolk, VA: Hampton Press, 1986:423.
6. Arai T, Ikuta Y, Ikeda A. A study of the arterial supply in the human rectus femoris muscle. *Plast Reconstr Surg* 1993;92(1):43–48.

80.

PENILE (RE)CONSTRUCTION WITH THE RADIAL FOREARM FREE FLAP

Lawrence J. Gottlieb and Deana S. Shenaq

INTRODUCTION

The goals of total penile (re)construction are to provide a semblance of a penis which is cosmetically acceptable and psychologically satisfying. Ideally, it should incorporate a neourethra that allows for micturition while standing through a meatus at the end of the neophallus, provide erogenous and protective sensation, include an autologous stiffener or be able to accommodate a mechanical prosthesis, and have adequate length and girth to allow for sexual intercourse.

The history of total penile reconstruction has paralleled that of flap development in plastic and reconstructive surgery. The multistage tube pedicle flap reconstruction has given way to axial pattern skin and muscle flaps. These procedures have subsequently yielded to the tube-within-a-tube design of the neurosensory radial forearm free flap phalloplasty, which has achieved the idealized goals just listed. Since its initial description, several modifications of the radial forearm free flap technique for penile construction have been described. The main disadvantage of the radial forearm procedure is the unsightly donor site. Alternative donor sites have emerged to avoid the forearm scars and perceived stigmata by some patients. However, the radial forearm free flap continues to be our preferred method for neophallus (re)construction and will be the subject of this chapter.

ASSESSMENT OF THE DEFECT

Careful preoperative assessment of the anatomy is essential. In patients with gender dysphoria, verification of normal anatomy is necessary, especially if any preliminary procedures such as metoidioplasty have been performed. In the genetic male who has a deformity or loss from surgery or trauma, the key is to not only determine what has been lost, but also to evaluate what is present and if it is normal. It is imperative to determine the level of injury and whether it was limited to the shaft or more proximal. The components that are most important to focus on include the quality of the surrounding skin and soft tissue, recipient vascular anatomy, pudendal nerves, urethra, bladder, sphincter, ejaculatory system and the corpora cavernosae. A careful sensory examination will help determine the level of nerve injury and a urodynamics study, as well as a radiologic genitourinary examination may be necessary. In patients with ambiguous genitalia, it is important to assess whether any Wolffian or Müllerian structures are present. In addition to any anatomical defect that may be present, most patients with concerns related to their genitalia have psychological stress and are best served with a multidisciplinary team that includes mental health providers, reconstructive plastic surgeons, and urologists, as well as endocrinologists and gynecologists as needed.

INDICATIONS

Patients with severe penile deformities or loss, either congenital or acquired secondary to trauma, infection, or malignant neoplasm, are potential candidates for penile reconstruction. Gender dysphoric patients may become candidates for penile construction if they meet guidelines established by the World Professional Associate for Transgender Health, a nonprofit, interdisciplinary professional and educational organization devoted to transgender health.

CONTRAINDICATIONS

Elective complex microneurovascular penile construction is inappropriate in patients with major cardiac, vascular, or metabolic diseases as well as in those with major psychiatric or psychological problems that would not improve with this procedure. Consideration must also be given to the patient's level of expectation and ability to deal with potential complications and significant donor site deformity. Previous injury to both forearms or to the upper extremity vasculature would obviously preclude the use of the radial forearm free flap. In addition, morbidly obese patients with a significant amount of subcutaneous fat are poor candidate for radial forearm flaps because it is very difficult, if not impossible, to create a tube-within-a-tube because of excess tissue bulk.

ROOM SETUP

The patient is placed supine on the operating table with the donor (usually nondominant) arm extended on an arm table. Transsexuals and men with perineal urethrostomies are placed in the lithotomy position during the "recipient site preparation" portion of the case (Figure 80.1.) Other patients may be positioned supine or in a frog-leg position. Sequential pneumatic lower extremity compression boots should be used to decrease the risk of deep venous thrombosis. While in lithotomy, the lateral leg should be appropriately padded to prevent pressure on the common peroneal nerve. The thighs should be prepped into the sterile field to

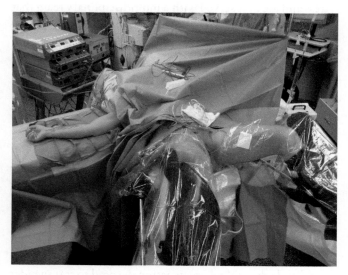

Figure 80.1. Room setup to accommodate two teams working simultaneously on forearm and perineum.

allow for harvesting of saphenous vein grafts as well as skin graft harvest for donor site closure.

PATIENT MARKINGS

The nondominant arm is generally chosen as the donor site. A preoperative Allen's test should be performed on all patients for whom a radial forearm flap is being considered. Arteriograms are usually unnecessary. Patients with an equivocal Allen's test may undergo duplex Doppler imaging to delineate the vascular anatomy of the palmar arch of the hand.

Many patients elect to undergo preoperative laser hair removal; in those patients who do not, the arm should not be shaved, as this allows for neourethral markings to be planned reliably in an area with the least amount of hair. It is also helpful to mark the course of the radial artery and any visible veins during this time.

The flap is designed on the volar aspect of the forearm. The neourethra is planned in a central location in continuity with a neoglans. This design avoids a circumferential meatal suture line without sacrificing length and leads to an improved aesthetic result. The dimensions of the flap depend on the patient's needs and desires, as well as the size of the forearm and the amount of subcutaneous tissue present. The width of the flap should vary directly with the amount of subcutaneous tissue present; the more subcutaneous tissue, the wider the flap needs to be to allow for constructing the tube-within-a-tube design. In most cases, our flap dimensions are a minimum of 15 × 17 cm. The circumference of the wrist may limit flap width distally, where it must be tapered to 13–14 cm. Generally, the decreased amount of subcutaneous tissue in this area allows for tubing and folding despite the narrow width (Figure 80.2).

SURGICAL TECHNIQUE

The extremity is elevated and a sterile tourniquet is inflated to 250 mm Hg. Two strips of skin, each 1 cm wide, on either side of the planned centrally positioned neourethra are de-epithelialized from the proximal edge of the flap to within 3–5 cm of the distal portion. The de-epithelialization should be extended around the proximal end of the planned neourethra (Figure 80.3).

The distal portion of the flap is then incised, and the radial artery is identified at the wrist and isolated with vessel loops. The distal venae comitantes and other small veins are

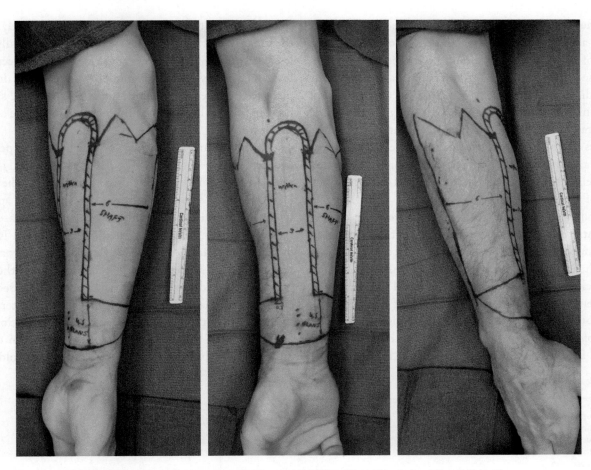

Figure 80.2. Flap design marked on nondominant forearm. Note that increase in width requires almost circumferential elevation.

clipped and divided. The distal cephalic vein is dissected for an additional centimeter or two and then clipped and divided. An incision is then made along the radial border of the flap and carried down to the deep fascia. Care must be taken

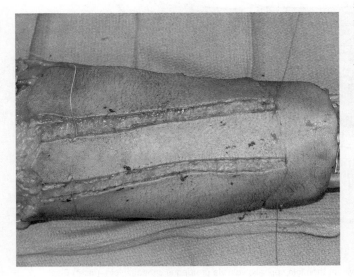

Figure 80.3. Area around the planned neo-urethra is de-epithelialized.

to include the cephalic vein and the lateral antebrachial cutaneous nerve with the flap elevation and to identify and preserve the superficial branch of the radial sensory nerve beneath the flap as it courses close to the cephalic vein at the wrist. Suprafacial dissection then continues until the ulnar side of the brachioradialis, where the fascia is incised and the brachioradialis muscle is retracted radially, exposing the radial artery and its venae comitantes. Muscular and periosteal branches coming off the radial side of the radial artery and venae comitantes are clipped and divided. The septocutaneous perforators are usually concentrated at the distal and proximal portion of the flap with a paucity of perforators in the center.

The proximal incision is then made to help facilitate the elevation of the proximal part of the flap, taking care to identify and preserve the superficial venous system as well as the sensory nerves. The lateral antebrachial cutaneous nerve is located adjacent to the cephalic vein, and the medial antebrachial cutaneous nerve is adjacent to the basilic vein. These sensory nerves should be dissected an additional 4 cm proximal to the skin paddle, tagged with 7-0 Prolene, and divided.

Next, the ulnar border of the flap is incised and elevated radially above the deep fascia. The cutaneous perforating vessels of the ulnar artery should be ligated and divided. The dissection is continued to the radial side of the flexor carpi radialis, where the fascia is incised and the flexor carpi radialis muscle is retracted ulnarly, exposing the ulnar side of the radial artery and its venae comitantes. Muscular branches coming off the ulnar side are ligated and divided, and the radial artery and its venae comitantes are elevated from their bed, beginning distal to proximal until the bifurcation of the brachial artery is identified.

The dissection of the proximal venae comitantes proceeds until the two veins coalesce into one. If this dissection is continued more proximally, the venae comitantes join the cephalic vein via the profundus cubitalis vein, which is a valveless vein connecting the superficial (cephalic) and deep (venae comitantes) venous systems of the radial side of the forearm (Figure 80.4). This added dissection makes it possible for one large-caliber vein to drain both venous systems. Due to the large width of the flap, it is imperative to include veins from the basilic system to adequately drain the ulnar side of the flap. These veins will occasionally coalesce with the cephalic system at the level of the antecubital fossa, as demonstrated in Figure 80.4, but, if they do not, plans to drain veins from both the ulnar and radial side of the flap need to be made to minimize the incidence of partial necrosis.

The tourniquet is released, allowing the flap to perfuse, and hemostasis is obtained. The flap is attached only by its radial vascular bundle proximally and distally and the proximal superficial veins. Microvascular clamps are applied to the distal radial artery, and hand perfusion is observed. Only after adequate ulnar circulation to the hand is confirmed is the distal radial artery divided 1–2 cm beyond the skin paddle. If, in the unusual circumstance that the perfusion of the radial side of the hand is compromised, the microvascular clamp is removed from the radial artery and a vein graft is harvested for radial artery reconstruction.

The neophallus is then fashioned while still in continuity with its proximal vascular supply. A neoglans fold-over

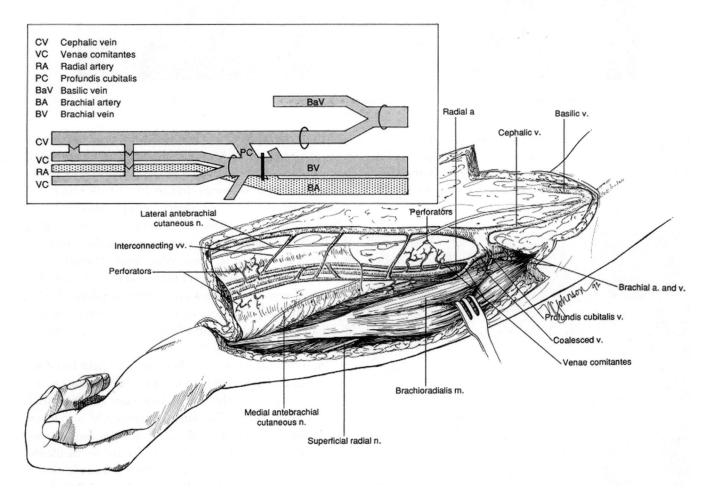

Figure 80.4. Venous anatomy of flap. Note coalescence of venae comitantes, which then join cephalic vein via profundus cubitalis vein. (Inset) Black vertical bar depicts site of transection; circles depict possible venous anastomotic sites.

GROIN AND PENILE RECONSTRUCTION

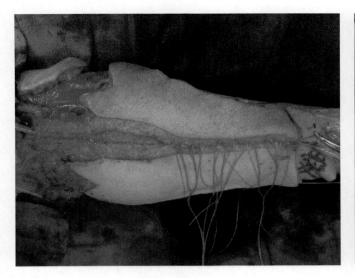

Figure 80.5. Multiple layer closure of neo-urethral tube.

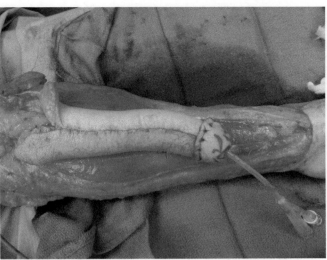

Figure 80.7. Distal portion of flap folded back and wings of neo-glans trimmed. Neo-glans secured with 3-0 Maxon mattress sutures.

flap is created by making full-thickness transverse incisions that connect the distal portion of the centrally placed neourethral skin with the radial and ulnar edges of the flap. The central portion of the flap forming the neourethra is then "tubed" over a no. 10 French silastic urinary catheter and closed in multiple layers (Figure 80.5).

The flap is then turned over and the dorsal skin is closed creating a tube-within-a-tube. To augment venous flow, the distal radial artery is anastomosed to the cephalic vein at the wrist creating an arterial-venous fistula (Figure 80.6).

The wings of the neoglans are rolled-back on the shaft and trimmed to the appropriate shape. The neoglans is then secured in its rolled-back position with full-thickness

Maxon mattress sutures leaving the edge raw to heal by secondary intention (Figure 80.7).

Of note, if the patient has a relatively small forearm with a significant amount of subcutaneous fat, then the shaft suture lines may not close without tension. In this situation, the outer layer of the volar suture line may be opened and a full-thickness graft placed. Placement of the graft on the ventral surface allows with dorsal suture line to be closed primarily for a better aesthetic result (Figure 80.8). The constructed neophallus is left on the arm, attached to its proximal vascular pedicle, until the recipient site has been prepared.

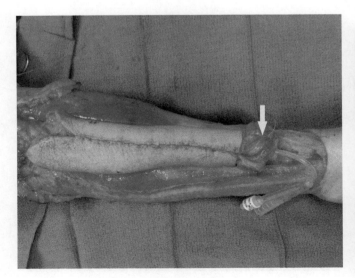

Figure 80.6. Flap turned over and dorsum closed. A-V anastomosis (*arrow*) between distal radial artery and cephalic vein to augment venous flow.

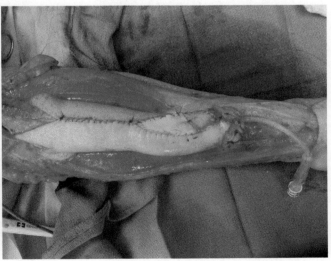

Figure 80.8. Tension relieved with full thickness skin graft.

PENILE (RE)CONSTRUCTION WITH THE RADIAL FOREARM FREE FLAP

RECIPIENT SITE PREPARATION

At the beginning of the case, the urological team places a suprapubic catheter into the bladder and a sterile Foley catheter through the native urethra, if present. During flap elevation, a second surgical team prepares the recipient site, vessels and nerves. In the genetic male, if a portion of the native phallus exists, a degloving procedure is performed. The dorsal penile branches of the pudendal nerve are isolated. If the nerves are not apparent, dissection is continued toward the perineum and the pudendal nerves are identified as they emerge from Alcock's canal and travel along the inferior ramus of the pubis.

In female-to-male transgender patients, inverted V-incisions are made in the superior portion of the labia majora (Figure 80.9). Neoscrotum are created by performing V-Y retrodisplacement flaps of the bilateral labia majora. If the vagina is still present, then a vaginectomy is performed, preserving a small area of distal anterior vaginal wall for possible use in native urethral extension as necessary. The vaginal cavity is then collapsed by re-approximating its walls with absorbable sutures and placing closed suction drains. The medial aspects of the labia majora are secured together, creating a neoscrotal median raphe.

The skin over the shaft of the clitoris is then incised and the dorsal clitoral nerves are identified and surrounded with vessel loops (Figure 80.10). A urethral extension is then created by tubularization of the vestibular mucosal plate between the native urethra and the clitoral glans. This is occasionally supplemented with an anterior vaginal flap and the medial aspect of the labia minora. The dorsal clitoral skin and skin of the glans is removed.

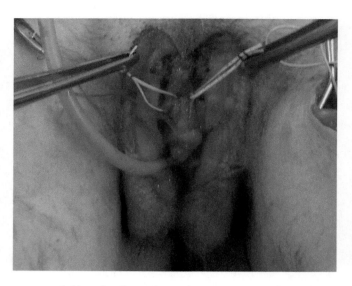

Figure 80.10. Labia majora flaps inferiorly displaced to create site for phallic attachment and start of neo-scrotal construction. Vessel loops around clitoral nerves.

An incision is then made in the thigh in the region of the femoral artery and vein. Along with the saphenous vein, these vessels are identified and surrounded with vessel loops. Approximately 20 cm of the greater saphenous vein is harvested from the thigh and left attached to the femoral vein at the fossa ovalis. In addition, large proximal branches of the saphenous vein are preserved for additional venous anastomoses as needed. Typically, a 10 cm segment of the vein of Giacomini, which is the posterior branch of the saphenous vein, is harvested, leaving it attached proximally to the greater saphenous vein (Figure 80.11).

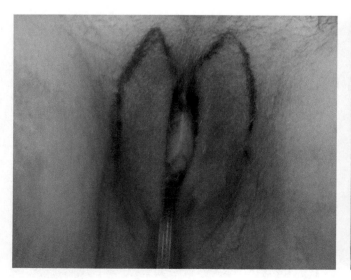

Figure 80.9. Skin markings for recipient site in female-to-male transgender patients.

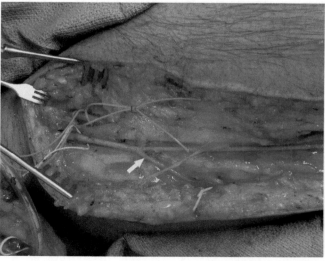

Figure 80.11. Incision in left thigh. Arrow points to the posterior branch of greater saphenous vein (vein of Giacomini.)

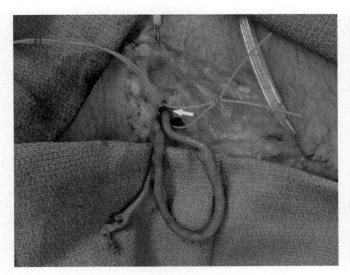

Figure 80.12. Temporary A-V loop. Connecting distal end of greater saphenous vein (*arrow*) to femoral artery.

The divided end of this saphenous vein is then anastomosed to the superficial femoral artery to create a temporary arteriovenous (AV) loop fistula (Figure 80.12). This is allowed to flow for at least 20 minutes, until the flap is ready for transfer.

The incision used for the recipient vessel harvest is connected to the flap recipient bed incision to prevent compression, torqueing, or kinking of the vein grafts or flap pedicle (Figure 80.13).

When both the neophallic construct and recipient site preparation are complete, the proximal radial artery and any proximal veins still connected are ligated or clipped and divided. The neophallus is then detached from the arm, moved to the recipient site and secured with tacking sutures. The previously placed Foley catheter through the native urethra is removed, and the 10-French Foley catheter, now inside the reconstructed neophallus is placed into the bladder through the urethral extension and balloon inflated. An end-to-end spatulated urethral anastomosis with 4-0 absorbable sutures is performed. This suture line is reinforced by tacking the de-epithelialized edge over the repair.

Attention is then directed to the nerve repair. Epineural neurorrhaphies are performed between the antebrachial cutaneous nerves and the dorsal clitoral nerves with 8-0 monofilament polypropylene sutures. The clitoral nerves are not transected totally but approximately 80% so that some of the nerve fibers continue through the clitoris.

An end-to-end microvascular anastomosis is performed between the basilic vein and the vein of Giacomini. One thousand units of heparin is given intravenously before the temporary AV loop is clamped and divided to avoid clotting of the stagnant blood in the loop while it is clamped. An end-to-end microvascular anastomosis is then performed between the radial artery and the arterial limb of the saphenous loop. Upon releasing the microvascular clamps, good flow into and out of the flap should be observed. An end-to-end microvascular anastomosis between the cephalic vein and the venous limb of the saphenous loop is then performed.

The remaining wounds about the proximal shaft of the neophallus and femoral vessels are closed over closed suction drains (Figure 80.14).

The percutaneous suprapubic catheter remains in place to divert urinary flow from the healing neourethra. The 10 French Foley catheter is left in place but capped.

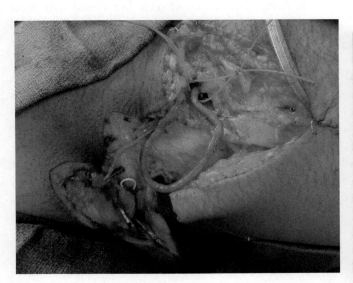

Figure 80.13. The thigh and perineal incisions are connected to prevent compression, torquing, or kinking of the vein grafts or flap pedicle.

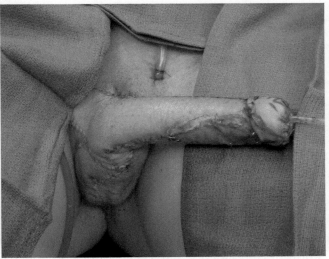

Figure 80.14. Neo-phallus at completion of operation.

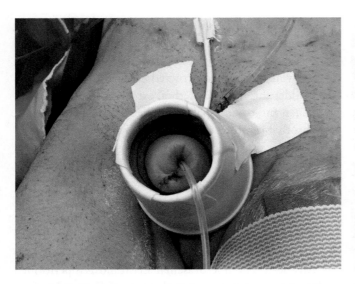

Figure 80.15. Postoperative dressing includes a cup to keep construct from bending and kinking while allowing for monitoring of the neo-glans. Note the noncircumferential meatal suture line.

The forearm muscles in the bed of the donor site are approximated and placed over any exposed tendons with absorbable suture to minimize contour irregularities. A thick split-thickness skin graft is then harvested from the hip or thigh and applied to the forearm. It is covered with negative pressure wound therapy and a volar resting splint is fashioned.

The postoperative dressing incorporates an upside down large Styrofoam cup with the bottom cut off, secured with foam tape to lower abdomen, to keep the neophallus supported in the erect position during the early postoperative period (Figure 80.15).

POSTOPERATIVE CARE

Flap viability is assessed by clinical signs including: skin color, turgor, and capillary refill of the neoglans, which emerges out of the cut-off Styrofoam cup dressing. In addition to hourly pulse checks and bedside Doppler examinations, flap perfusion is monitored using ViOptix Tissue Oximeter (ViOptix, Incorporated Fremont, CA).

Perioperative antibiotics, subcutaneous heparin, and low-dose aspirin are employed in all cases. Intravenous antibiotics are discontinued on the second postoperative day, and suppressive oral antibiotics are administered until the urethral and suprapubic catheters are removed.

Physical therapy for the donor upper extremity begins once the initial dressings are removed on the fifth postoperative day. A compression garment is fashioned and worn for 3–6 months, and a removable wrist splint is worn for 2 weeks.

Urine is drained via the suprapubic catheter, allowing the urethral catheter to be capped. This reduces tension on the neophallus and meatus. In the third to fourth postoperative week, a retrograde urethrogram is performed by inserting a small catheter alongside the indwelling urethral catheter. The urethral catheter may be removed if there is no evidence of extravasation or fistula. The suprapubic catheter is then removed 1–2 days after normal micturition is established.

The neophallus is insensate postoperatively and care must be taken not to inadvertently injure the flap through trauma or by pressure from elastic garments until protective sensation returns. Most patients recover gross tactile sensation at 4–6 months. A penile prosthesis is inserted only after protective sensation is present to decrease the incidence of prosthetic erosion and extrusion. At 6–9 months, patients are usually able to stimulate the shaft of the neophallus to orgasm.

Typically, at 3 months postoperatively, neoscrotal tissue expander(s) are place in the previously retro-displaced labia majora. At the time of penile implant insertion, the expander(s) are removed, one testicular implant is placed on one side of the neoscrotal sac, and the pump of the inflatable penile prosthesis is placed on the other side.

CAVEATS

The most common complications are related to the proximal urethral anastomosis, including sinuses, fistulae, strictures, and hairy urethras, which have been reported to be as high as 80%. Reporting on their series of radial forearm phalloplasties, Monstrey et al. had a urological complication rate of 41% but found that most early fistulae closed spontaneously. Proximal urethral anastomotic suture line strictures may be treated with internal urethrotomy, followed by a short period of self-catheterization. Recurrent proximal urethral suture line complications require surgical correction with local flaps or buccal mucosal grafts; unfortunately, recurrent stricture is common.

Meatal stenosis has not been problematic in these patients since a circumferential meatal suture line is avoided. Likewise, urethral stone formation has not been observed in these patients, despite the hair present on the forearm. It is presumed that the fine hair on forearm skin does not have the same propensity to form stones that the thick coarse hair of scrotal skin has.

Erosion and extrusion of penile prostheses has been described. The key to success here is to delay insertion of penile prosthesis until protective sensation returns.

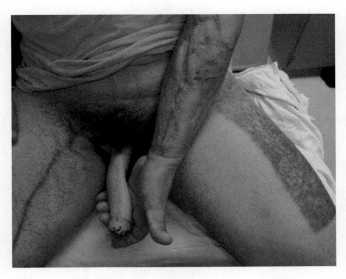

Figure 80.16. Donor sites at 3 months postop. Skin graft on left forearm, left thigh skin graft donor site, right thigh greater saphenous incision.

Maintaining a good coronal ridge is difficult. Secondary procedures are frequently required to obtain the best results.

The greatest drawback of the radial forearm flap is the unsightly donor site scar (Figure 80.16).

Suprafascial dissection and thicker skin grafts improve aesthetics. Functional disability of the donor extremity is rare.

Some patients may not be candidates for radial forearm flap penile reconstruction or refuse to have the forearm donor site. In this situation, although perhaps less optimal in sensation, girth, and quality of urethra, alternative methods of penile reconstruction should be considered.

SELECTED READINGS

Biemer E. Penile construction by the radial arm flap. *Clin Plast Surg* 1988;15:425.

Chang T-S, Hwang WY. Forearm flap in one-stage reconstruction of the penis. *Plast Reconstr Surg* 1984;74:251.

Cherup LL, Gottlieb LJ, Zachary LS, Levine LA. The sensate functional total phallic reconstruction. *Plast Surg Forum* 1989;25.

Gilbert DA, Horton CE, Terzis JK, et al. New concepts in phallic reconstruction. *Ann Plast Surg* 1987;18:128.

Gilbert DA, Williams MW, Horton CE, et al. Phallic innervation via the pudendal nerve. *J Urol* 1988;41:160.

Gottlieb LJ, Levine LA. A new design for the radial forearm free flap phallic construction. *J Plast Reconstr Surg* 1993;92:276.

Gottlieb LJ, Tachmes L, Pielet RW. Improved venous drainage of the radial artery forearm free flap: use of the profundus cubitalis vein. *J Reconstr Microsurg* 1993;9:281.

Khouri RK, Young VL, Casoli VM. Long-term results of total penile reconstruction with a prefabricated lateral arm free flap. *J Urol* 1998;160(2):383–388.

Koshima I, Tai T, Yamasaki M. One-stage reconstruction of the penis using an innervated radial forearm osteocutaneous flap. *J Reconstr Microsurg* 1986;3:19.

Levine LA, Zachary LS, Gottlieb LJ. Prosthesis placement after total phallic reconstruction. *J Urol* 1993;149:593.

Lumen N, Monstrey S, Goessaert A-S, et al. Urethroplasty for strictures after phallic reconstruction: a single-institution experience. *Eur Urol* 2011;60:150–158.

Meyer R, Daverio PJ, Dequesne J. One-stage phalloplasty in transsexuals. *Ann Plast Surg* 1986;16:472.

Monstrey S, Hoebeke P, Selvaggi G, et al. Penile reconstruction is the radial forearm flap really the standard technique? *Plast Reconstr Surg* 2009;124:510–518.

Morrison SD, Shakir A, Vyas KS, et al. Phalloplasty: a review of techniques and outcomes. *Plast Reconstr Surg* 2016 138(3):594–615.

Pariser JJ, Cohn JA, Gottlieb LJ, Bales GT. Buccal mucosal graft urethroplasty for the treatment of urethral stricture in the neophallus. *Urology* 2015; 85: 927–931

Sadove RC, Sengezer M, McRoberts JW, et al. One-stage total penile reconstruction with a free sensate osteocutaneous fibula flap. *J Plast Reconstr Surg* 1993;92:1314.

Selvaggi G, Monstrey S, Hoebeke P, et al. Donor-site morbidity of the radial forearm free flap after 125 phalloplasties in gender identity disorder. *Plast Reconstr Surg* 2006;118(5):1171–1177.

Sengezer M, Oztürk S, Deveci M, Odabaşi Z. Long-term follow-up of total penile reconstruction with sensate osteocutaneous free fibula flap in 18 biological male patients. *Plast Reconstr Surg* 2004;114(2):439–450–discussion451–452.

Shenaq SM, Dinh TA. Total penile and urethral reconstruction with an expanded sensate lateral arm flap. Case report. *J Reconstr Microsurg* 1989;5:245.

Van Caenegem E, Verhaeghe E, Taes Y, et al. Long-term evaluation of donor-site morbidity after radial forearm flap phalloplasty for transsexual men *J Sexual Med* 2013;10(6):1644–1651.

PART XII.

VAGINAL AND PERINEAL RECONSTRUCTION

81.

RECTUS ABDOMINIS FLAP FOR PERINEAL AND VAGINAL RECONSTRUCTION

Brogan G. A. Evans and Gregory R. D. Evans

Reconstruction of the vagina is usually performed in patients undergoing abdominal-perineal resection or pelvic exenteration for carcinoma of the cervix, vagina, or rectum. Vaginal reconstruction is indicated for both psychological rehabilitation and perineal wound healing. Immediate reconstruction after partial or total vaginal resection facilitates primary healing of the perineal defect, decreases fluid loss from the pelvis, reduces infection rate, prevents herniation of abdominal contents into the perineum, and decreases nutritional demands. Additionally, flap closure provides neovascularization of the remaining pelvic tissue, which is particularly important in successful wound healing for patients who have either had radiation to the area or who are having postoperative radiation therapy. Moreover, even in the sexually inactive patient, this surgery provides patients with faster healing and overall enhanced self-esteem.

ASSESSMENT OF THE DEFECT

Reconstruction of the vagina with the rectus abdominis myocutaneous flap technique after abdominal-perineal resection or pelvic exenteration is most easily performed at the time of resection.[1-13] Delayed reconstruction requires repeat laparotomy and redissection of the pelvis. Communication with the resecting surgeon before, as well as during, the operative procedure ensures accurate assessment of the vaginal defect. Depending on the extent of the disease, a simple vertical ellipse of the rectus myocutaneous flap can be used to repair a partial vaginal loss, such as only the anterior or posterior wall. Loss of the vaginal introitus as well as part of the vault requires careful planning to provide a flap design with adequate length and width to prevent stenosis of

the vaginal entrance. Defects of the perineal floor sometimes require additional reconstruction with Marlex mesh, acelluarlized dermis, an omental flap, or a second rectus abdominis flap to remove the dead space and seal the abdominal cavity. Additionally, total vaginal reconstruction usually necessitates reconstruction with a large skin component of the rectus abdominis myocutaneous flap.

INDICATIONS

The rectus abdominis myocutaneous flap is appropriate for both larger partial and complete vaginal vault reconstructions (Figure 81.1), as small or medium-sized defects can usually be repaired using local flaps from the thigh or buttocks. This flap is particularly useful in reconstruction after supralevator exenteration, in which the retained distal vagina makes use of gracilis flaps difficult. Although this procedure can also be used for reconstruction in vaginal agenesis, usually simpler methods of skin grafts or dilation are used.

The rectus flap can be designed in the area of a planned colostomy or ileostomy. In this situation, the reconstruction flap is harvested and the fascial donor defect closed before placement of the conduit. Hernia, or compromise of the conduit, has not been a problem. Furthermore, the colostomy or ileostomy can be placed more lateral for increased stability.

Preoperative discussions include the potential complications and expected results of the reconstructed vagina. The patient is counseled that the rectus flap will lack normal sensation and to anticipate the effects of this change on sexual intercourse. Patients can experience chronic pain after surgery, especially if there is pain preoperatively and the patient has undergone radiation therapy. Surgical reconstruction cannot be expected to relieve chronic pain.

CONTRAINDICATIONS

The rectus abdominis myocutaneous flap cannot be used for reconstruction if designed on the side of the abdomen where surgical scars interrupt the blood supply of the skin paddle (i.e., paramedian scars) or of the inferior epigastric blood supply (i.e., appendectomy scars). If the blood supply of the inferior epigastric vessels is divided during the pelvic resection, the contralateral flap can be used. Use of the flap on the side of a prior colostomy is contraindicated because of probable disruption of major umbilical perforators at the time of conduit placement. Vaginal reconstruction in the obese patient requires careful consideration of the smaller volume of the pelvis and vaginal vault, as well as assessment of the thickness of the skin paddle. Excessive bulk may result in collapse of the vaginal canal or vascular compromise of the cutaneous paddle.

ROOM SETUP

The patient is placed in the dorsal lithotomy position for the resection and subsequent reconstruction (Figure 81.2). The abdomen and perineum are prepared and draped. Placement of two or more grounding pads for electrocautery

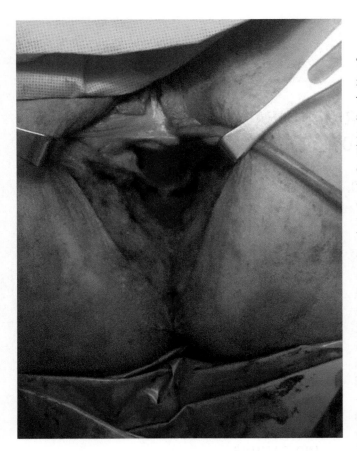

Figure 81.1. Patient with rectal and posterior vaginal wall resection following extirpation for squamous cell carcinoma.

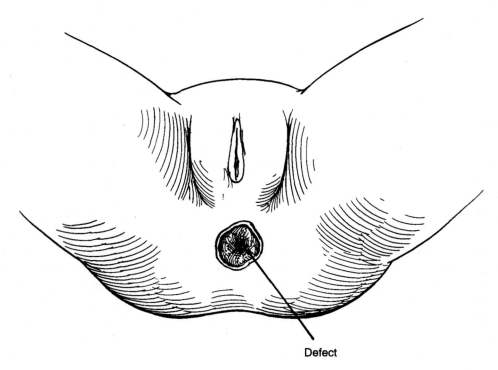

Defect

Figure 81.2. Patient on operating room table in dorsal lithotomy position for simultaneous resection and elevation of rectus abdominis myocutaneous flap.

VAGINAL AND PERINEAL RECONSTRUCTION

allows both the resecting and reconstructive surgeons to operate simultaneously.

PATIENT MARKINGS

After the extent of the defect is defined, the skin paddle is marked as a vertical ellipse centered over the upper half of the rectus muscle, being sure to include the periumbilical perforators; this provides the longest pedicle length. Adequate skin at the costal end of the skin paddle is maintained to prevent the potential problem of stenosis because this area will reconstruct the vaginal entrance. It is helpful to temporarily staple the midline incision together, after the resection and before marking the patient, in order to stabilize the flap. The medial border of the skin paddle should be the midline laparotomy incision, allowing for a single midline abdominal closure. The dimensions of the skin paddle depend on the width and length of the vaginal defect. For a total vaginal reconstruction a skin paddle of 12–14 cm in width provides a neovaginal diameter of 4 cm when tubed. The flap spans from the costal margin to just below the umbilicus (Figure 81.3).

In addition to flap design, sites for the colostomy and ileal conduit should be marked preoperatively and agreed upon by both the plastic and oncologic surgeons as well as the enterostomal nurse to ensure that the conduits do not transverse the rectus abdominis muscle that will be used for the reconstruction. If conduits are required on both sides, the markings for placement are made preoperatively, but the flap is harvested before placement of the colostomy or ileal conduit.

SURGICAL TECHNIQUE

After the oncologic surgeons have completed the abdominal part of the resection and defined the extent of the vaginal defect, the markings for the rectus abdominis myocutaneous flap are made. Alternately, if the resecting surgeons can accurately describe the planned defect before resection, the flap can be raised before the laparotomy incision. The perimeter of the skin island is incised to the anterior rectus fascia, and the cutaneous paddle is undermined at the level just above the fascia medially and laterally until both rows of perforators are identified (Figure 81.4). The epigastric skin is supplied by the perforators of the inferior epigastric vessels of the rectus abdominis muscle that exit through the anterior rectus fascia. The inferior and superior epigastric vessels join by an anastomotic network just above the umbilicus, providing the blood supply to the entire rectus muscle and the overlying skin paddle. The anterior rectus fascia is incised, including the perforators, usually leaving 1 cm of fascia medially, adjacent to the linea alba, and 3 cm laterally, adjacent to the external oblique aponeurosis.

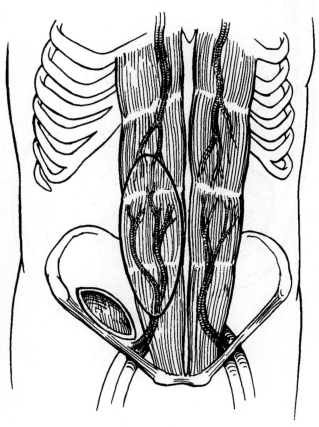

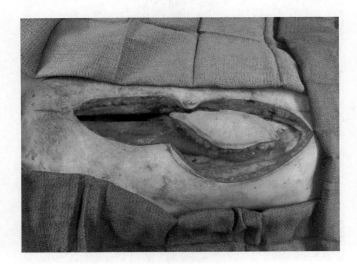

Figure 81.3. Skin paddle is marked as vertical ellipse to include periumbilical perforators and to provide adequate length and width for total vaginal reconstruction.

Figure 81.4. Blood supply for cutaneous paddle is the myocutaneous perforators of inferior epigastric vessels of the rectus abdominis muscle.

The muscle is transected at the costal margin near the apex of the skin paddle, which divides the superior epigastric vessels. The rectus muscle with the skin paddle is dissected off the posterior rectus sheath in a retrograde manner, dividing the lateral neurovascular bundles sequentially until the pedicle is long enough to reach the vaginal defect without tension.

The flap is then inset into the vaginal defect after positioning the skin paddle, wherein partial defects (anterior or posterior) can be sutured at the apex from the abdominal exposure and completed from the lithotomy position (Figure 81.5). This allows completion of a colostomy while the remainder of the flap is being inset. Usually the most distal aspect (toward the costal margin) of the skin paddle is placed at the introitus of the vagina, with the apex being formed from the proximal part of the skin flap. Ultimately, inset will depend on the least tension on the vascular pedicle and the rectus abdominis muscle. Adequate skin from the costal end of the flap is inset at the vaginal introitus to prevent stenosis. The flap is rotated 180 degrees into the pelvic defect, with the insertion of the rectus abdominis

to the pubis usually remaining attached to prevent tension on the inferior epigastric pedicle. The flap enters the pelvis through the posterior rectus fascia and peritoneum. This fascial plane is reapproximated loosely around the rectus pedicle, allowing for flap edema without strangulation of the blood supply. Continued inspection of the inferior epigastric vessels during inset allows for modification of the reconstruction to prevent tension on the vascular pedicle. Interrupted absorbable sutures, such as 2-0 or 3-0 polyglactin monofilament, are used to approximate the flap skin edge to the vaginal mucosa. Frequently 4-0 chromic is used to approximate the skin edges. This prevents the necessity of removing the stitches in an area in which it may be difficult to obtain visualization (Figure 81.6).

If a total neovagina is reconstructed, the flap is transposed to the groin area to form the vaginal pouch, while the second surgical team constructs the colostomy. The vaginal pouch is formed by folding the flap longitudinally into a tube by approximating the medial and lateral edges of the skin paddle along a single suture line to recreate a vaginal tube. The skin surface is sutured with simple or mattress interrupted absorbable sutures. The

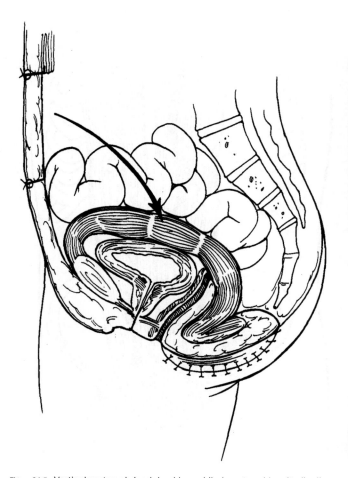

Figure 81.5. Vertical rectus abdominis skin paddle is sutured longitudinally, and apex is formed with infolding before delivery into pelvis.

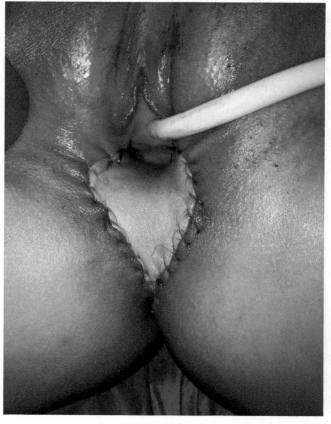

Figure 81.6. Reconstruction of a posterior vaginal and rectal defect with the rectus abdominis myocutaneous flap.

VAGINAL AND PERINEAL RECONSTRUCTION

apex of the neovagina is fashioned by turning the terminal inverted "V" shape of skin at the pubic end of the skin ellipse back into the suture line of the tube to form a blind pouch (Figure 81.5). The flap is passed into the pelvis through the midline peritoneal incision, and the open end is sutured into the perineal defect (Figure 81.7).

The anterior rectus fascial defect is usually closed primarily with a nonabsorbable suture such 0-Ethibond with a second layer of 1 or 0 Prolene. Alternatively a barbed suture may be utilized. We generally tend to interrupt the 0-Ethibond suture and "run" the Prolene or barbed suture over the top. Usually the midline fascial incision is closed, but if this closure prevents the midline laparotomy incision closure because of tension, a Marlex mesh or acellularized dermis is interposed to recreate the anterior rectus fascia. The cutaneous skin paddle defect is closed directly in continuity with the laparotomy incision. Additionally, closed suction drains are used at the donor and recipient sites. If the muscle is only required for pelvic exclusion along with bolstering the vaginal closure, then the rectus muscle alone can be turned down into the pelvis. We have harvested the muscle alone by incising the fascia investing the rectus muscle along the

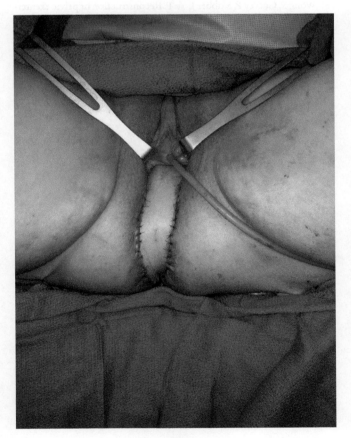

Figure 81.7. Orientation of myocutaneous flap through posterior rectus fascial defect into peritoneum.

midline. This allows the fascia to be elevated anteriorly off the rectus muscle, and the rectus muscle can then be elevated off the posterior fascia without any fascial defects.

Postoperatively, the vascularity of the flap is followed by inspection of the skin paddle at the vaginal introitus. Examination of the proximal flap is adequate to ensure viability of the entire skin paddle since this is the most distal segment of the cutaneous pedicled flap.

POSTOPERATIVE CARE

Postoperative monitoring of the flap includes examination by visual inspection of the proximal flap at the bedside for 48–72 hours to assess the circulation. Capillary refill of 2–3 seconds and a pink color are expected. A light source (flashlight or penlight) is required to adequately see the skin paddle, and, if the flap appears congested, the patient should have a more complete examination and possibly return to the operating room. After 7–10 days, the postoperative edema has resolved enough to perform a more thorough examination using the speculum.

No special dressings are required, and bacitracin or a dry absorbent dressing should be applied to the abdominal incision. Colostomy or ileal conduit bags are secured to prevent contamination of the wound. Because the neovagina is reconstructed with well-vascularized tissue from the myocutaneous flap, no vaginal stents are used. Dressings are not used on the perineum, allowing the skin to air dry. Drains are removed when drainage is less than 30 mL in 24 hours.

The patient should remain at bed rest for 48–72 hours before beginning ambulation, and sitting is restricted until 1 week after surgery. We frequently utilize an abduction pillow between the legs that permits less compression on the flap. A physical therapist is helpful in assisting the patient in getting out of bed without sitting on the perineal area. The patient is advised to refrain from lifting heavy objects for 4–6 weeks to decrease the chances of abdominal hernia formation. Patients may begin a vaginal douche beginning the third postoperative week, provided that the vaginal wounds are healed appropriately. Sexual intercourse can be resumed 5–6 weeks after surgery, if the patient has resolution of her postoperative pain.

CAVEATS

Successful vaginal reconstruction using the rectus abdominis myocutaneous flap is facilitated by good communication with the resecting surgeons regarding the size of the defect and the potential placement of a colostomy. This is important for the correct planning of the skin paddle and to facilitate the possibility of the two surgical teams working simultaneously. The rectus abdominis skin flap is designed to both include the periumbilical perforators for the blood supply and to provide adequate length and width to reconstruct the vaginal vault and introitus, if needed. During surgery, the surgeon continually monitors the position of the flap vascular pedicle, as well as the perfusion and capillary refill of the flap, as it is inset into the vaginal defect to prevent tension on the pedicle or shear of the cutaneous perforators. Efforts to prepare the patient for the necessary postoperative monitoring by medical personnel should be taken. Additionally, the patient should be advised on a gradual, supervised return to her activities of daily life after a dictated period of strict bed rest due to the reconstruction of this difficult area.

REFERENCES

1. Carlson JW, Soisson AP, Fowler JM, et al. Rectus abdominis myocutaneous flap for primary vaginal reconstruction. *Gynecol Oncol* 1993;51:323.
2. Tobin GO, Parcel SH, Day TG Jr. Refinements in vaginal reconstruction using rectus abdominis flaps. *Clin Plast Surg* 1990;17:705.
3. Tobin GR, Day TG. Vaginal and pelvic reconstruction with distally based rectus abdominis myocutaneous flaps. *Plast Reconstr Surg* 1988;81:62.
4. McCraw J, Kemp G, Given F, Horton CE. Correction of high pelvic defects with the inferiorly based rectus abdominis myocutaneous flap. *Clin Plast Surg* 1988;15:449.
5. Xiong S, Zhan W, Cheng X, et al. Vaginal reconstruction with an island flap of the inferior epigastric vascular pedicle. *Plast Reconstr Surg* 1993;92:271.
6. Evans GRD. Rectus abdominis flap for vaginal reconstruction. In: Evans GRD, ed. *Operative Plastic Surgery*. New York: McGraw Hill, 2000: chapter 68, 781–787.
7. Mericli AF, Martin JP, Campbell CA. An algorithmic anatomical subunit approach to pelvic wound reconstruction. *Plast Reconst Surg* 2016;137:1004–1017.
8. Frasson M, Flor-Lorente B, Carreno O. Reconstruction techniques after extralevator abdominoperineal rectal excision or pelvic exenteration: meshes, plasties and flaps. *Cir Esp* 2014;92:48–57.
9. Horch RE, Hohenberger W, Eweida A, et al. A hundred patients with vertical rectus abdominis myocutaneous (VRAM) flap for pelvic reconstruction after total pelvic exenteration. *Int J Colorectal Dis* 2014;29:813–823.
10. Holman FA, Martijnse IS, Traa MJ, Boll D, Nieuwenhuijzen GA, de Hingh IH, Rutten HJ. Dynamic article: vaginal and perineal reconstruction using rectus abdominis myocutaneous flap in surgery for locally advanced rectum carcinoma and locally recurrent rectum carcinoma. *Dis Colon Rectum* 2013;56:175–185.
11. Crosby MA, Hanasono MM, Feng L, Butler CD. Outcomes of partial vaginal reconstruction with pedicled flaps following oncologic resection. *Plast Reconstr Surg* 2011;127:663–669.
12. Shukla HS, Tewari M. An evolution of clinical application of inferior pedicle based rectus abdominis myocutaneous flap for repair of perineal defects after radical surgery for cancer. *J Surg Oncol* 2010;102:287–294.
13. Wong S, Garvey P, Skibber J, Yu P. Reconstruction of pelvic exenteration defects with anteriolateral thigh-vastuc lateralis muscle flaps. *Plast Reconstr Surg* 2009;124:1177–1185.

82

GRACILIS FLAP FOR VAGINAL RECONSTRUCTION

Natalie Barton and Gregory R. D. Evans

Reconstruction of the vagina is performed for patients undergoing abdominoperineal resection or pelvic exenteration for carcinoma of the cervix, vagina, or rectum.[1-8] Other causes of acquired pelvic defects include locally advanced cancers of the genitalia or perineal skin, lichen sclerosis, or necrotizing soft tissue infections. Nevertheless, acquired pelvic defects present complex reconstructive challenges secondary to the combination of significant pelvic dead space, the need for perineal soft tissue resurfacing, and the shear forces associated with the dependent pelvis. Vaginal reconstruction is unique in that the creation of a neovagina is also important for the psychological well-being of many women, especially those who wish to remain sexually active and who thus require a functional reconstruction.

Immediate reconstruction after partial or total vaginal resection facilitates primary healing of the perineal defect, decreases fluid loss from the pelvis, reduces infection rate, and decreases nutritional demands. Additionally, flap closure provides neovascularization of the remaining pelvic tissue, an important consideration for successful wound healing. Of note, the majority of these patients have attempted and failed chemotherapy and radiation therapy preoperatively, which may influence postoperative wound healing. All of these factors, both alone and in combination, explain the frequent failure of primary perineal wound closure and emphasize the importance of durable and reliable soft tissue reconstruction.

The gracilis flap is one of the most commonly used flaps for reconstruction of perineal/vaginal defects as it is versatile, has minimal donor site morbidity, and often lies outside the field of radiation.

ASSESSMENT OF THE DEFECT

In total pelvic exenteration, the pelvic contents including the rectum, bladder, vagina, uterus, and adnexa are removed en bloc. The operation results in two permanent ostomies or, in some cases, a urinary diversion and a low rectal anastomosis.

To achieve primary wound healing and restore urogenital and anorectal function, the location of the defect and the presence of pelvic dead space should dictate the flap(s) selected.[7] When assessing the defect, one must also consider several other factors including whether the reconstruction will be performed in an immediate or delayed setting; whether the vaginectomy will result in a partial or total defect; whether the defect will be located in the posterior, anterior, or distal vaginal wall; whether a concomitant cystectomy or abdominoperineal resection will be performed; and the size of the "dead space" created by the tumor resection.[1-8] The location of the ileal conduit or colostomy on the abdominal wall with respect to the rectus abdominis muscle, the orientation of abdominal scars from previous surgeries, and the total dosage of previous radiation therapy and portals used for delivery must also be considered.

INDICATIONS

The gracilis myocutaneous flap is indicated for vaginal reconstruction as a means of wound closure after tumor resection, to fill an anatomic "dead space," to improve wound healing in irradiated tissue, and to improve the psychological well-being of the patient by restoring her anatomy to a functional state.[1-8]

CONTRAINDICATIONS

In general, the gracilis myocutaneous flap is not an acceptable option for vaginal or perineal reconstruction if the patient has had previous surgery that violated the blood supply to the gracilis muscle or its skin island, the patient is morbidly obese, or the patient has a significant history of tobacco use.

Because the medial femoral circumflex system provides the vascular supply to the gracilis flap, previous surgery that required ligation of these vessels should be considered an absolute contraindication to using this flap for reconstruction. Similarly, procedures, such as previous surgery or high-dose irradiation to the area of the skin island, and conditions that make the skin island unreliable, such as morbid obesity and tobacco use, are relative contraindications.

ROOM SETUP

The patient should be positioned in a dorsal lithotomy position, allowing access to the both the abdomen and the perineum so the oncologic and reconstructive surgeons may work simultaneously. In this position, the medial thighs may be prepared and draped such that the gracilis flaps may be raised from their beds and transposed into the vaginal area without repositioning the patient. To prevent a peroneal nerve compression injury, the lateral side of the knee and upper calf must be carefully padded when positioning the patient's legs in the operating stirrups.

PATIENT MARKINGS

The skin island of the gracilis myocutaneous flap may be designed preoperatively with the patient standing or intraoperatively, with the patient's thighs abducted and knee flexed at 45 degrees (dorsal lithotomy position) (Figure 82.1).

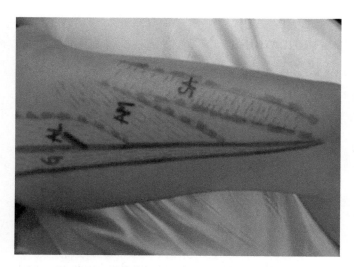

Figure 82.1. Preoperative markings of the gracilis flap may be performed with the patient either standing or in dorsal lithotomy position.

The standing position allows the patient to assist in marking the flap by contracting the muscle, which allows the surgeon to accurately design the skin island to include the perforators. The gluteal crease is marked as the upper border of the cutaneous part of the flap, and the distal end of the flap is located between the middle and lateral thirds of the posterior thigh.

Marking the flap during surgery allows the skin island to be designed according to the actual defect. Of note, when the skin island is marked with the patient in a supine position, care must be taken to allow for the gravitational shift of the true skin island inferior (posterior) to the muscle. Failure to account for this shift can result in poor tissue perfusion and subsequent necrosis of the skin island.

The gracilis muscle originates from the pubic symphysis and inserts on the medial tibial condyle. The gracilis origin is located behind the origin of the adductor longus. The distal gracilis tendon passes behind the medial femoral condyle and inserts at the upper medial tibia below the medial tibial condyle.

The gracilis is a type II muscle with the dominant nutrient vessels to the flap arising from the medial femoral circumflex system. These vessels are the dominant blood supply to the muscle and enter the muscle approximately 8–10 cm below its origin. The average length of the dominant pedicle is reported to be 6–7 cm with an average diameter of 1.5 mm. Additional branches of the femoral vessels enter the muscle in its distal third. Perforators off the superficial femoral artery supply the blood to the skin overlying the muscle; however, only the skin of the proximal two-thirds of the overlying skin of the flap are reliably perfused when the flap is based on its dominant blood vessels.

The flap is designed by drawing a line along the anterior border of the gracilis muscle, locating the posterior border of the adductor longus at the pubic tubercle and drawing the line from this point to the distal end of the gracilis tendon at its insertion on the medial tibial condyle (Figure 82.2). The anterior limits of the flap can extend 2–3 cm anterior to the initial design and 6–8 cm posterior (Figure 82.2). Although a skin island as large as 11 × 27 cm can be designed, the skin island is usually no wider than 8–9 cm, permitting primary closure of the donor site in most cases.

The vertical height of the skin island needed for vaginal reconstruction is typically around 6–7 cm, providing a vaginal circumference of 12–14 cm when bilateral flaps are used.[4]

Because a rectus muscle flap may be required, the reconstructive surgeon should always be aware that many surgeons and enterostomal nurses prefer to have the colostomy

VAGINAL AND PERINEAL RECONSTRUCTION

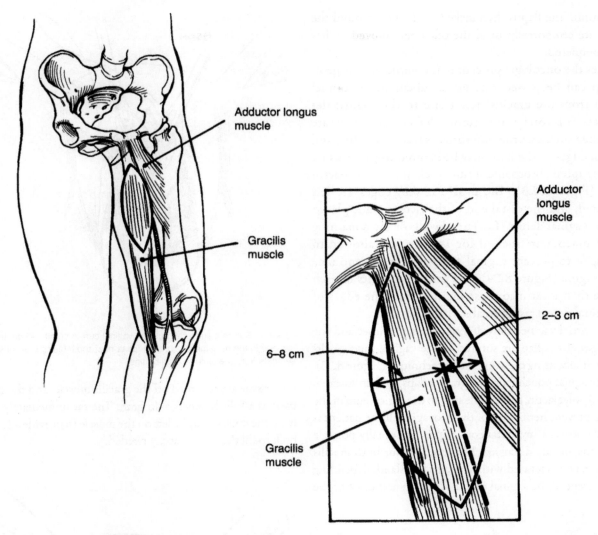

Figure 82.2. The skin island is designed over the proximal two-thirds of the muscle; the skin island over the distal third of the gracilis has very few perforator blood vessels and is unreliable. The line drawn from the pubic tubercle to the medial tibial condyle just posterior to the easily palpable adductor longs muscle. The line delineates the anterior border of the gracilis muscle.

and ileal conduit traverse the rectus abdominis muscle. Thus, in addition to flap design, sites for the colostomy and ileal conduit must be marked with the patient in the standing position and agreed upon by the plastic surgeon, surgical oncologist, and enterostomal nurse.

OPERATIVE TECHNIQUE

With the patient in the dorsal lithotomy position, the gracilis myocutaneous flaps are raised while the surgical oncologist is performing the abdominal portion of the oncologic procedure. If only a partial vaginectomy is planned, only the gracilis flap on the same side as the vaginal procedure is harvested; otherwise, both flaps are harvested. The anterior skin incision is first made down to the fascia of the adductor

longus muscle, beveling away from the flap for 1 or 2 cm, until the fascia of the adductor muscle is exposed. The fascia over the adductor longus is then incised longitudinally over the middle portion of the muscle and elevated posteriorly. The adductor longus muscle is retracted.

The main vascular pedicle and anterior motor branch of the obturator nerve to the gracilis muscle are visualized. The septum is always included with the flap as it contains septocutaneous perforators that supply the overlying skin. The posterior incision is then performed down through the subcutaneous tissue to the gracilis muscle, and a thin skin flap is harvested carefully without including much of the subcutaneous tissue.

The proximal gracilis musculocutaneous flap is then elevated. It is important to separate the skin paddle from the muscle in a posterior to anterior direction until reaching the septum. The flap is then tacked to the skin around the donor site temporarily, until the oncologic procedure has been completed.

After the oncologic procedure is completed, the gracilis flap can be passed through a subcutaneous tunnel created from the gracilis donor site to the vaginal defect site. For total vaginectomy defects, the flaps are positioned such that the skin surfaces face each other, and the skin edges of the flaps may be sutured together using an interrupted absorbable suture, such as 3-0 polyglactin suture (Figure 82.3). The proximal skin edges are left unsutured, and the distal end of the neovagina is placed into the vaginal defect. The lateral walls of the remaining vaginal mucosa are incised for 1–2 cm and allowed to splay open to prevent vaginal stenosis near the entrance of the vagina (Figure 82.4). The proximal points of each flap are then inset into these incisions and the edges of the vaginal defect using an absorbable suture.

For partial vaginectomy defects, the flap is inset and the skin edges of the flap are sutured to the vaginal mucosa circumferentially, using the same suture technique (Figure 82.5). The neovaginal pouch (sutured gracilis flaps) is then sutured, using 3-0 polyglactin, at multiple sites to the periosteum of the pubis to prevent herniation of the neovagina. If the patient is morbidly obese, a myocutaneous flap is not usually possible for reasons already discussed. However, one or both gracilis muscles may be elevated with a small skin island, depending on the extent of the vaginal defect. The skin and most of the

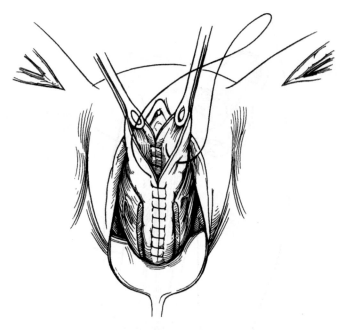

Figure 82.4. Before placing the sutured vaginal cuff, a small 1–2 cm incision is made in the remaining vaginal mucosa near the labia to prevent vaginal stenosis from the circular incision line.

fatty tissue are trimmed off the gracilis muscle, and the skin is used as a full-thickness skin graft. The fat immediately overlying the muscle may be left on the muscle to provide adequate bulk to fill the dead space, if needed.

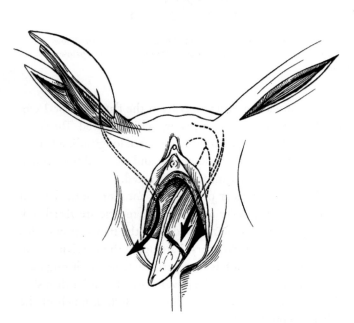

Figure 82.3. If total vaginal reconstruction is being performed, skin islands are sutured together using absorbable suture. This maneuver is more easily performed with flaps exteriorized before inserting neo-vaginal cuff into the vaginal defect.

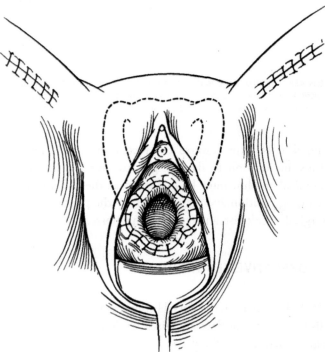

Figure 82.5. Flap is inset into the defect using interrupted polyglactin suture to approximate the skin of the gracilis flap to the remaining vaginal mucosa or labial skin. Tabs of gracilis skin island are inset into small incisions placed in the labial skin laterally on each side.

VAGINAL AND PERINEAL RECONSTRUCTION

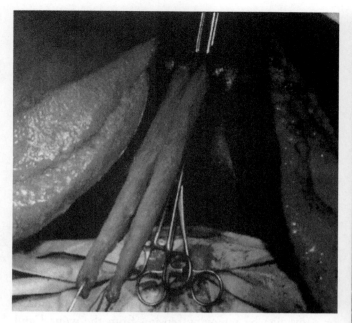

Figure 82.6. In obese patients, gracilis muscles, with or without overlying subcutaneous tissue, are sutured together with polyglactin suture in continuous fashion from proximal to distal (distal end held by Allis clamps) on each side of the two muscles, forming a muscular cuff for inserting the soft vaginal stent covered with the skin graft. The flap containing the stent and graft is inserted into the vaginal defect.

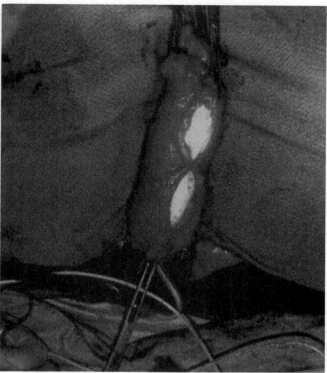

Figure 82.7. The soft vaginal stent is covered with split-thickness skin graft (dermis side out) and is placed in the muscular cuff, which is closed. The proximal end of the muscular cuff is left open for removal of the stent after the skin graft has taken, approximately 1 week postoperatively.

For total vaginectomy defects, the gracilis muscles are passed into the perineal aspect of the vaginal defect and sutured together along their longitudinal perimeter to create a muscular pouch (Figure 82.6). If fat was left on the muscle, the side without the fat is used to form the inner aspect of the muscular pouch. The subdermal fat is sharply removed from the undersurface of the skin grafts, and both skin grafts are sutured together (dermal side out) around a large, soft vaginal stent (Figure 82.7). The stent is inserted into the muscular defect with the skin grafts. The skin-grafted vaginal stent is placed into the muscular pouch, and the pouch and stent are placed into the vaginal defect. The labia majora are sutured together temporarily for approximately 7 days to allow the skin graft to take and to prevent the stent from inadvertently being extruded out of the neovagina. This same procedure is used for partial vaginal defects except that only one gracilis flap and skin graft is required. Although the skin can be used off the cutaneous portion of the flap as a full-thickness graft, sometimes a split-thickness graft may take more easily. It is important to remember that graft contracture will be more prominent with a split-thickness graft.

Drain catheters are placed on each side through the subcutaneous perineal tunnel and along the side of each flap. These drains can exit the skin in the upper posterior thigh through a small stab incision. The skin of the gracilis donor site is closed in a two-layered fashion; the dermis is closed using interrupted polyglactin suture and the epidermal layer with a subcuticular approximation with a polyglactin monofilament suture.

DRESSINGS

Absorbent dry dressings may be applied to the gracilis donor site incisions. Because the neovagina is lined by healthy, nonirradiated vascularized skin, a vaginal stent is typically not necessary. Vaginal stents are used only when the neovagina is skin grafted.

POSTOPERATIVE CARE

Routine postoperative care involves checking the microcirculation of the myocutaneous flaps during the first 24–48 hours postoperatively and keeping the perineal wounds and drain catheter sites clean. Flap monitoring is best performed by visual inspection to check for a pink color and a 2- to 3-second capillary refill. This can be done by gently retracting the labia to see the proximal edges of the flap under good lighting. Because the vulvar area may be markedly edematous and somewhat painful, inspection of the distal end of the flaps is usually reserved until some of the edema and postoperative pain have resolved. This usually occurs by postoperative day 7. Although this approach to flap monitoring does not permit examination of the entire neovagina immediately after surgery, we have found that if the proximal end of the gracilis flap appears to be well-perfused, the distal end is usually adequately perfused as well. If there is any question about flap perfusion, the patient should undergo complete inspection of the neovagina and be returned to the operating room, if required.

Postoperative activity modification is very important for the success of pelvic soft tissue reconstruction. The patient is restricted to the supine and lateral recumbent positions, changing positions every 2 hours in a low-pressure bed when not ambulating. Often an abduction pillow is placed between the legs to prevent further pressure on the flaps. As a general rule, ambulation is permitted on postoperative day 1. A physical therapist is consulted to teach the patient how to safely transition from the supine to the standing position. Moreover, sitting is typically not allowed for the first 3–5 postoperative days as this position may result in significant flap congestion and edema.

Drains are removed when the drainage is less than 30 mL over a 24-hour period.

The patient is not permitted to sit upright greater than 30 degrees for 3 weeks, after which a graduated sitting protocol is initiated until full activity is permitted at 6 weeks after surgery. If there are areas of delayed wound healing, the restriction from sitting may be increased until it is certain that the wound is not increasing in size. Complete pelvic rest is required for a minimum of 6 weeks. Patients may begin sexual intercourse after the wounds are healed, typically at the 6-week mark. Patients who have had a skin-grafted vaginal reconstruction require more time for the skin grafts to heal. The skin graft postoperative protocol is typically started approximately 2–3 weeks later than that for a myocutaneous flap.

REHABILITATION

For most patients, vaginal reconstruction results in an excellent rehabilitation. After reconstruction, the patient usually will not have sensation in the neovagina. This can be distressing to some patients, and they should be counseled preoperatively. Paradoxically, some patients have chronic pain postoperatively; this is more prevalent in patients who have had chronic pain often related to preoperative radiation therapy. Patients who are well-healed but have unexplained pain should be referred to a chronic pain or rehabilitation specialist. Patients who have vaginal stenosis require splinting or twice-daily dilations.

Patients with recalcitrant stenosis that does not respond to repeated dilations may require partial excision of the stenosis and labia minora skin flaps or a split-thickness skin graft. Of note, incising the mucosa of the lateral vaginal walls near the vulva and insetting the proximal portion of the flap at the time of vaginal reconstruction may help prevent vaginal stenosis.

As studied by computed axial tomography, the natural course for the gracilis muscle is to atrophy. Despite this fact, the gracilis flap does help prevent fistulas from forming between the rectum and vagina (partial reconstruction) or neovagina by removing tension from the wound and filling the pelvic "dead space" with well-vascularized, nonirradiated tissue. Removal of the gracilis myocutaneous flap seldom causes a significant problem at the donor site. Although abduction strength of the hip joint was decreased by 11% in one study of 42 patients who underwent elevation of their gracilis muscles, the patients do not typically notice the relative decrease in strength. However, 41% of the patients in this study did complain of some hypoesthesia corresponding to the cutaneous territory of the obturator nerve. Nevertheless, reconstruction with this flap in appropriately selected patients restores normalcy to most patients and is worth the minor problems associated with this flap.

CAVEATS

The gracilis myocutaneous flap is a reliable flap in carefully selected patients; however, the following caveats should be remembered: (1) the skin overlying the distal one-third of the flap is unreliable, especially in patients who are morbidly obese or use tobacco products; and (2) the surgeon must account for the inferior shift of the true skin island of the gracilis flap when marking the patient in a supine position or a poorly perfused skin island will be harvested. Wound healing in this region has historically been poor, with dehiscence rates reported up to 66%.[7]

Vaginectomy defects may communicate with the intrapelvic and intraabdominal space; therefore, flap reconstruction serves a dual purpose: to obliterate dead space and prevent herniation and to provide the patient with a functional neovagina.[4-7] Bulky flaps offer the appropriate soft tissue fullness and skin to reconstruct the vagina and perineal raphe. In addition, the pedicled omental flap may be useful to close the pelvic inlet to prevent inferior displacement of the intraabdominal viscera.[7] With the advent of acelluarized dermis, many of these procedures can utilize these new biomaterials for similar prevention of displacement of the intraabdominal viscera. The omental flap can be combined with an additional regional flap to provide muscle for further dead space obliteration and a skin paddle for either external or vaginal canal reconstruction, depending on the defect type.

REFERENCES

1. Deutinger M, Kuzbari R, Paternostro-Sluga T, et al. Donor-site morbidity of the gracilis flap. *Plast Reconstr Surg* 1995;95: 1240–1244.
2. Epstein DM, Arger PH, LaRossa D, et al. CT evaluation of gracilis myocutaneous vaginal reconstruction after pelvic exenteration. *Am J Roentgenol* 1987;148:1143–1146.
3. Freshwater MF, McCraw JB. Intraoperative identification of the gracilis muscle for vaginal reconstruction. *Plast Reconstr Surg* 1980;65:358–395.
4. Kaartinen IS, Vuento MH, Hyöty MK, et al. Reconstruction of the pelvic floor and the vagina after total pelvic exenteration using the transverse musculocutaneous gracilis flap. *J Plast Reconstr Aesthet Surg* 2015 Jan;68(1):93–97.
5. McCraw JB, Horton CE, Horton CE Jr. Basic techniques in genital reconstructive surgery. In: McCarthy JG, ed. *Plastic Surgery*. Vol. 6. The Trunk and Lower Extremity. Philadelphia: WB Saunders, 1990:4128–4137.
6. McCraw JB, Massey FM, Shanklin KD, Horton CE. Vaginal reconstruction with gracilis myocutaneous flaps. *Plast Reconstr Surg* 1976;58:176.
7. Mericli AF, Martin JP, Campbell CA. An algorithmic anatomical subunit approach to pelvic wound reconstruction. *Plast Reconstr Surg* 2016 Mar;137(3):1004–1017.
8. Sezeur A, Hautefeuille P, Trevidic P. Immediate vaginal reconstruction with a musculocutaneous flap from the gracilis muscle after extended abdomino-perineal resection. *Ann Chir* 1995;49:534–538.

83.

GRACILIS FLAP FOR PERINEAL RECONSTRUCTION AND FUNCTIONAL RESTORATION FOR THE TREATMENT OF FECAL INCONTINENCE

Ryan M. Moore and Gregory R. D. Evans

The plastic surgeon is confronted by several challenges when tasked with the reconstruction of complex perineal wounds. Previous surgery, radiation, or trauma; large size and surface area following resection or debridement; and loss of structural integrity are factors common to these defects. The proximity of the gracilis muscle affords an opportunity to utilize local, well-vascularized tissue for perineal reconstruction. In addition, the transposition of functional gracilis muscle has served a historic role in anal sphincter reconstruction for the treatment of fecal incontinence.

ASSESSMENT OF THE DEFECT

A variety of factors must be considered in perineal reconstruction.[1] The local burden of enteric organisms demands secure, watertight closure with well-vascularized tissue. Failure to meet these demands predisposes any reconstructive efforts to a greater likelihood of infection or dehiscence. Urinary and fecal diversion may be necessary to further mitigate the risk of wound contamination.

Frequently, the area has been irradiated prior to tumor extirpation.[2] Local flaps should be avoided in such circumstances, and the rotation of the gracilis with its excellent blood supply may avoid the combined deleterious effects of irradiated and contaminated tissue beds.[3,4] Wound healing may be further augmented by sharp debridement of irradiated tissue at the time of reconstruction.

In assessing the defect following surgical excision, the type and quantity of deficient soft tissue, including specialized structures such as the pelvic floor or anal sphincter, or bone must be considered.[1] When designed as a pedicled

flap, the gracilis muscle or myocutaneous flap can be used to selectively reconstruct the perineum according to the nature of the defect. It is possible to import skin, subcutaneous tissue, and muscle using the gracilis flap.[3,4] For defects not requiring skin replacement, the muscle, subcutaneous fat, and de-epithelialized skin from the flap can be used to obliterate dead space (Figure 83.1).

Further assessment of perineal defects requires a tissue capable of preventing pelvic organ prolapse. The de-epithelialized dermal layer of the gracilis flap is ideal for this purpose. If the flap is not sufficient for structural

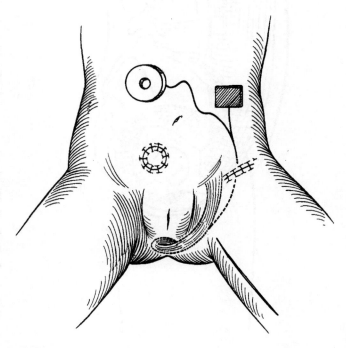

Figure 83.1. New perineal defect.

849

support, the placement of synthetic grafts (e.g., polypropylene mesh) may allow added stability (Figure 83.2). Of note, there is little role for the use of biologic materials (e.g., porcine dermis or cadaveric fascia lata) over synthetic mesh or native tissue in urogynecologic reconstructive surgery.[5] In these instances, the gracilis myocutaneous flap serves as a vascularized barrier, preventing possible contamination and erosion. Contraindications to synthetic grafts include local infection and conditions associated with impaired wound healing (e.g., diabetes mellitus).

All patients being considered for anal sphincter reconstruction undergo preoperative assessment that assess the nature, severity, and impact of fecal incontinence on quality of life using validated scoring instruments (e.g., Cleveland Clinic Fecal Incontinence Score and Fecal Incontinence Quality of Life scale).[6] Following a complete disease history and detailed physical examination, anorectal physiology evaluation is recommended to direct management. This may include anal manometry, endoanal ultrasound, pudendal nerve terminal motor latency testing, defecogram, or magnetic resonance imaging (MRI).[7]

INDICATIONS

The thin, pliable gracilis muscle or myocutaneous flap is ideally suited for moderately sized perineal defects involving skin, soft tissue, and bone following tumor extirpation, pressure injury, pelvic exenteration, abdominoperineal resection, radical prostatectomy, and osteoradionecrotic bony pelvis resection (Figure 83.3A,B). Small bony defects following partial pubic symphyseal resection, for example, can be bridged using a de-epithelialized skin paddle.

Due to the relatively small size of the muscle, occasionally the gracilis myocutaneous flap is of insufficient bulk to fill larger defects. Additionally, the size of the skin paddle is constrained by the unreliable blood supply to the skin overlying the distal third of the muscle, thus the myocutaneous flap should be used with caution.[4] Accordingly, rectus abdominis, tensor fascia lata, or rectus femoris flaps may be more suitable.

This versatile flap may also be used for wound coverage of the groin, ischium, and lower abdomen, or even in reconstruction of male and female external genitalia.[8] Finally, the gracilis muscle flap may be indicated in anal sphincter reconstruction in selected patients with severe fecal incontinence resulting from significant neurologic, traumatic, or iatrogenic injury, as well as congenital abnormalities.[9–15]

CONTRAINDICATIONS

Patients with multiple comorbidities (e.g., smoking, diabetes, obesity, malnutrition) should be identified because they are greatest risk for flap failure. Patients should be advised to abstain from smoking for 4 weeks preoperatively and postoperatively so as to decrease risk of overall complications, including dehiscence and wound infection. Nicotine replacement therapy cessation is also imperative as nicotine is a potent vasoconstrictor capable of inducing local ischemia, although its overall effects on wound healing remain to be seen. A delay procedure to enhance the blood supply of the flap and increase the surviving length of the

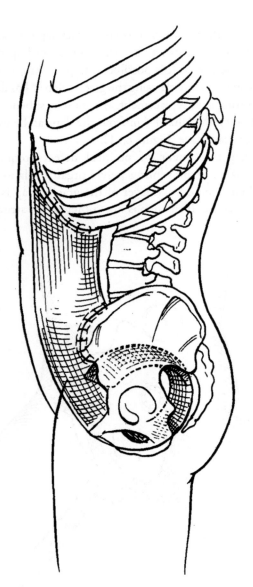

Figure 83.2. Example of synthetic mesh lining pelvic floor for structural support.

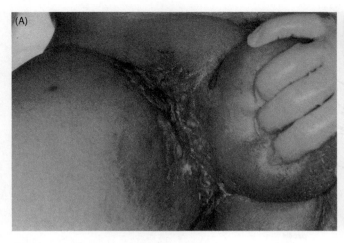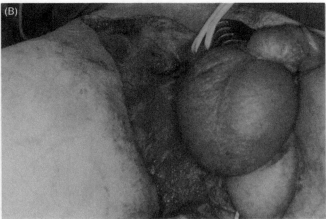

Figure 83.3. (A) Squamous cell carcinoma that has metastasized to right groin in 43-year-old male. (B) Defect in groin and perineum following surgical excision of squamous cell carcinoma.

flap should be considered in these case. (Flap division is often safe between 10 days and 3 weeks following surgical delay.) Preoperative intervention to tighten glucose control and optimize nutrition is also imperative.[16]

In a rare anatomic variant, the dominant blood supply originates from a proximal minor pedicle branching from the profunda femoris artery––not the typically dominant pedicle arising from the terminal branch of the medial circumflex femoral artery. Alternatively, the dominant pedicle may enter the muscle belly too far distal, thus restricting the arc of rotation of the flap and precluding its use in perineal reconstruction. Although flap harvest is often performed without vascular mapping, magnetic resonance angiography may be useful.[17]

The reliability of the skin paddle of the gracilis myocutaneous flap may not be adequate in obese patients. Frequently, the dissection in these patients is difficult and septocutaneous perforators are variable; thus, harvesting the gracilis muscle without a skin paddle may be more prudent. Furthermore, direct closure of the donor site may not be possible in obese patients.

Previous surgery that required ligation of the medial circumflex femoral or profunda femoris arteries should be viewed as an absolute contraindication to using this flap. Finally, consideration should be given to an alternative flap if a proposed gracilis flap is within a previously irradiated field.

ROOM SETUP

The flap can be harvested with the patient in lithotomy position with the thighs prepared circumferentially. This allows the reconstructive surgeon to work while surgical extirpation proceeds. To prevent peroneal nerve compression, the lateral side of the knee and the upper calf muscle must be carefully padded when positioning the patient's legs. Alternatively, the patient can be placed in the supine position with the hips partially flexed and abducted.

PATIENT MARKINGS

The flap can be elevated as either a muscle or myocutaneous flap. The patient should be standing when marked; however, markings can also be made intraoperatively with the patient's thighs abducted. The advantage of marking the patient standing is the ability of the patient to contract the muscle and thus allow the surgeon to design the skin island with more precision. Frequently, marking the skin island with the patient in the supine position places the skin paddle too anterior. This must be kept in mind when designing the flap (Figure 83.4).

A line is drawn from the pubic tubercle to the medial tibial condyle, and a second line is drawn 2–3 cm posterior to this original marking. This second, more posterior line represents the surface marking of the longitudinal axis of the muscle. The terminal branch of the medial circumflex femoral artery (dominant pedicle) courses deep to the adductor longus muscle before entering the posteromedial surface of the muscle approximately 6–12 cm inferior the pubic tubercle. If a muscle flap alone is desired, an incision is made along the surface marking of the longitudinal axis of the muscle. For a myocutaneous flap, the skin paddle can be oriented in a transverse or vertical direction. If a vertical skin paddle is desired, it can be designed up to

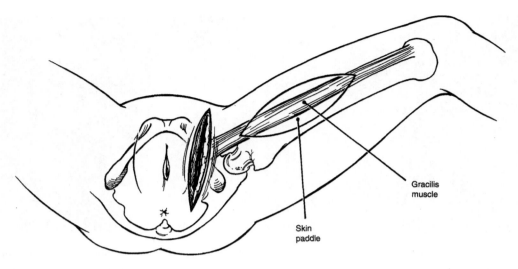

Figure 83.4. Design of skin paddle for myocutaneous gracilis flap.

15 × 8 cm centered over the proximal third of the inner thigh. The reliability of this skin paddle, however, must be viewed with caution. If a transverse skin paddle is needed, it can measure up to 20 × 6 cm centered over the dominant pedicle of the gracilis muscle bounded by the superficial femoral artery anteriorly and posterior midline of the thigh posteriorly.

OPERATIVE TECHNIQUE

A muscle flap can be elevated by making a skin incision along the surface marking of the longitudinal axis of the muscle. The muscle is easily identified posterior to the taut adductor longus muscle, which can be palpated with the medial thigh abducted. If a skin paddle is desired, it is essential to center the skin paddle over the proximal two-thirds of the gracilis muscle, which measures about two-thirds of the medial thigh. Dissection is begun by an incision made distal to the skin paddle, and the myotendinous insertion of the muscle is identified. The gracilis muscle belly can then be confirmed by applying traction to the distal gracilis muscle while distinguishing the straight muscle fiber orientation of the gracilis from the oblique orientation of sartorius muscle fibers. At this point, if a skin paddle is desired, the anterior portion of the skin paddle is incised. While applying tension, with the muscle identified, the posterior portion of a skin paddle can then be incised (Figure 83.5).

Defects in the anterior and posterior fascia are created and carried down to the edge of the gracilis muscle. Care is taken to include the septum between the gracilis and adductor longus muscle as this preserves septocutaneous perforators that supply the overlying skin paddle. In fact, wide inclusion of perigracilis fascia to include septae between the gracilis and sartorius and adductor magnus muscles permits harvest of a longer, full-size skin paddle, if desired. The skin island is then anchored to the underlying muscle to minimize shear forces on the perforators. The muscle is raised from a distal to proximal direction. The minor pedicle from the superficial femoral vessels should be ligated after the more proximal dominant primary pedicle is identified. The vascular pedicle is easily located by retracting the adductor longus medially at a point approximately 10 cm below the pubic tubercle. The flap can be rotated by dividing the skin paddle proximally or by creating an island flap and rotating the flap on the vascular pedicle (Figure 83.6).

Care must be taken to avoid twisting of the vascular pedicle. The flap is inset into the wound using absorbable

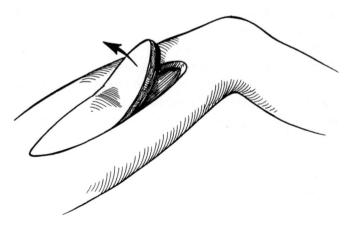

Figure 83.5. Initial elevation of flap. Skin island is secured to underlying muscle. Flap is elevated from caudal to cranial direction.

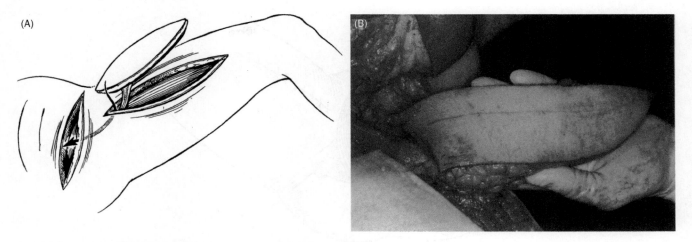

Figure 83.6. (A) Flap can be rotated by directing skin paddle proximally or by creating island flap by rotating on vascular pedicle. (B) Photograph demonstrates rotation of ipsilateral gracilis myocutaneous flap for closure of right groin and perineal defect after surgical excision.

sutures. While insetting the flap, the skin paddle should be tailored to fit the perineal skin defect (Figure 83.7).

Any excess skin can be de-epithelialized to obliterate dead space and restore the integrity of the pelvic floor as needed. This will prevent pelvic organ prolapse into the perineum. If a synthetic mesh is used for pelvic stability, the gracilis muscle flap should adequately prevent exposure.

The distal skin paddle must be assessed for viability before flap inset. If further length on the flap is required (especially for lower abdominal defects), the pedicle can be lengthened by dissection to its take-off at the profunda femoris vessels.[8]

ANAL SPHINCTER RECONSTRUCTION

Gracilis muscle transposition for anal sphincter reconstruction for the treatment of severe fecal incontinence was originally described by Pickrell et al. in 1952.[9] As the procedure proved incapable of producing sustained and forceful contraction due to the fatigue-prone nature characteristic of striated skeletal muscle (e.g., gracilis), Williams et al. and Baeten et al. later independently developed dynamic graciloplasty in 1991.[11,12] By delivering continuous electrical stimulation through a subcutaneous neurostimulator connected to implanted intramuscular electrodes, they transformed the once fatigue-prone gracilis

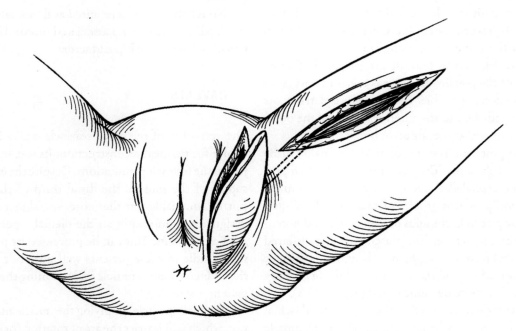

Figure 83.7. Insetting of flap. Excess skin can be de-epithelialized to fill dead space and reconstruct pelvic floor.

GRACILIS FLAP FOR PERINEAL RECONSTRUCTION AND FUNCTIONAL RESTORATION

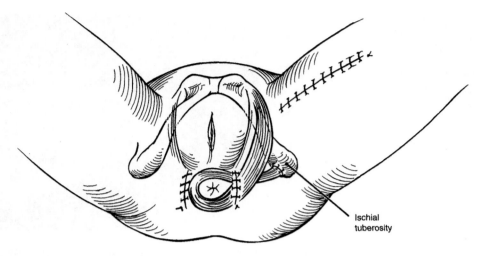

Figure 83.8. Placement of gracilis muscle in sling around anus for restoration of fecal continence.

Ischial tuberosity

muscle into a fatigue-resistant functional neosphincter. Though dynamic graciloplasty achieved significant improvement in fecal incontinence in 55–78% of patients, due to significant morbidity (e.g., infection, device erosion, and obstructed defecation) and procedural complexity, the neurostimulator and leads are not currently approved for use in North America.[18,19] (Dynamic graciloplasty is still frequently used for the management of severe fecal incontinence in Europe.) Recently, modified dynamic graciloplasty via external electrical stimulation and biofeedback has been shown to restore and maintain continence.[20]

Gracilis muscle transposition is historically performed in three stages.[9] The first stage involves creation of a diverting stoma and gracilis flap delay. The distal two to three blood vessels to the gracilis muscle are divided. The second stage is performed 4–6 weeks later. The innervated gracilis flap is elevated in the standard fashion. The abdomen, chest, perineum, and leg to the midcalf are prepared. During the elevation of the gracilis flap, care is taken to harvest as much distal tendon as possible. The gracilis is isolated on its neurovascular pedicle, and the anterior branch of the obturator nerve is exposed at the adductor brevis.

Two anteroposterior 3–4 cm counterincisions are made on either side of the anus. The dissection should then proceed lateral and cephalad. A clamp is then used to connect the anterior and posterior aspects of each lateral incision. A finger can be placed in the anus or vagina to avoid potential injury to these structures. The muscle is then transferred through a tunnel from the thigh, and the muscle (without tendon) is wrapped around the anus in an alpha (α) configuration to confer a more dynamic repair (Figure 83.8).

The muscle is then anchored to the contralateral ischial tuberosity with nonabsorbable sutures. The final muscle wrap is then placed in a deep subcutaneous plane. The third—and final stage—is closure of the stoma.

POSTOPERATIVE CARE

A dressing of Kerlix and Ace bandages can be used to reduce donor site swelling. The dressing should not be applied proximally as it may cause pedicle compression and flap vascular compromise of the flap. Drains (no. 15 French) are placed in the thigh to prevent seroma. Patients are kept immobile for 3–5 days, depending on the inset location of the gracilis flap. Ambulation is begun after this period.

No rehabilitation is required as donor site morbidity is minimal, and there is no associated motor deficit given the gracilis is one of five hip adductors.

CAVEATS

The versatility of the gracilis muscle makes it an excellent choice for perineal reconstruction. Its use, however, is subject to the following limitations. Despite the excellent blood supply of the muscle, the distal third of the skin paddle can be unreliable. Furthermore, the skin paddle is often designed too anteriorly on the medial aspect of the thigh in obese patients. This can be prevented by positioning the skin paddle in these patients well posterior to the axis of the adductor longus muscle and outlining the flap while the patient is standing.

The main pedicle supplying the muscle may be too inferior, which will restrict the arc of rotation for defect closure.

Finally, in cases of anal sphincter reconstruction, care must be taken to place the muscle in a deep subcutaneous pocket. Placement of the muscle in too superficial a plane predisposes to overlying skin necrosis, exposure of the flap, and failure.

REFERENCES

1. Labandter HP. The gracilis muscle flap and musculocutaneous flap in the repair of perineal and ischial defects. *Br J Plast Surg* 1980;33:95.
2. Granick MS, Solomon MP, Larson DL. Management of radiation associated pelvic wounds. *Clin Plast Surg* 1993;20:581.
3. Giordano PA, Abbes M, Pequignot JP. Gracilis blood supply: anatomical and clinical re-evaluation. *Br J Plast Surg* 1990;43:266.
4. Whetzel TP, Lechtman AN. The gracilis myofasciocutaneous flap: vascular anatomy and clinical application. *Plast Reconstr Surg* 1997;99:1642.
5. Yurteri-Kaplan LA, Gutman RE. The use of biological materials in urogynecologic reconstruction: a systematic review. *Plast Reconstr Surg* 2012;130 (Suppl. 2):242S
6. Rockwood TH, Church JM, Fleshman JW, et al. Fecal incontinence quality of life scale: quality of life instrument for patients with fecal incontinence. *Dis Colon Rectum* 2000;43:9–16.
7. Paquette IM, Varma MG, Kaiser AM, Steele SR, Rafferty JF. The American society of colon and rectal surgeons' clinic practice guideline for the treatment of fecal incontinence Fecal Incontinence Quality of life scale: quality of life instrument for patients with fecal incontinence. *Dis Colon Rectum* 2015;58(7):623–636.
8. Ducic I, Dayan JH, Attinger CE, Curry P. Complex perineal and groin wound reconstruction using the extended dissection technique of the gracilis flap. *Plast Reconstr Surg* 2008;122: 472.
9. Pickrell KL, Broadbent TR, Masters FW, Metzger JT. Construction of a rectal sphincter and restoration of anal continence by transplanting the gracilis muscle: a report of four cases in children. *Ann Surg* 1952;135:853–862.
10. Caviina E, Seccia M, Evangelista G, et al. Construction of a continent perineal colostomy by using electrostimulated gracilis muscles after abdominoperineal resection: personal technique and experience with 32 cases. *Ital J Surg Sci* 1987;17: 305–314.
11. Williams NS, Patel J, George BD, Hallan RI, Watkins ES. Development of an electrically stimulated neoanal sphincter. *Lancet* 1991;338:1166–1169.
12. Baeten CGMI, Konsten J, Spaans F, et al. Dynamic graciloplasty for treatment of faecal incontinence. *Lancet* 1991;338:1163–1165.
13. Baeten CG, Geerdes BP, Adang EM, Heineman E, et al. Anal dynamic graciloplasty in the treatment of intractable fecal incontinence. *N Engl J Med* 1995;332:1600–1605.
14. da Silva GM, Jorge JM, Belin B, et al. New surgical options for fecal incontinence in patients with imperforate anus. *Dis Colon Rectum* 2004;47:204–209.
15. Wexner SD, Gonzalez-Padron A, Teoh TA, Moon HK. The stimulated gracilis neosphincter for fecal incontinence: a new use for an old concept. *Plast Reconst Surg* 1996;98:693
16. Harrison B, Khansa I, Janis JE. Evidence-based strategies to reduce postoperative complications in plastic surgery. *Plast Reconstr Surg.* 2016;137: 351.
17. Schwartz JA, Smith M, Dayan JH, et al. Utility of pre-operative MRA in assessing gracilis flap vascular anatomy. *Plastic Surgery Research Council* 2013;131(5)(Abstract Supplement).
18. Van Koughnett JA, Wexner SD. Current management of fecal incontinence: choosing amongst treatment options to optimize outcomes. *World J Gastroenterol* 2013;19(48):9216–9230.
19. Wexner SD, Baeten C, Bailey R, et al. Long-term efficacy of dynamic graciloplasty for fecal incontinence. *Dis Colon Rectum* 2002;45(6):809–818.
20. Hassan MZ, Rathnayaka MM, Deen KI. Modified dynamic gracilis neosphincter for fecal incontinence: An analysis of functional outcome at a single institution. *World J Surg* 2010;34:1641–1647.

84.

PUDENDAL ARTERY FLAP (SINGAPORE) FOR PERINEAL RECONSTRUCTION

Gregory R. D. Evans

INTRODUCTION

Perineal reconstruction can be challenging. Fraught with bacterial contamination, limitation of tissue advancement, and often tissues subjected to previous adjuvant therapy, perineal reconstruction is frequently accompanied by complications. Knowledge of the appropriate anatomy has, however, reduced morbidity.[1] There are a variety of options for reconstruction depending on the extent of perineal involvement. Extensive myocutaneous flaps or perforator flaps are probably the two most common forms of repair. If laparotomy is required, the rectus abdominis flaps seem the most reasonable for reconstruction as the abdominal wall tissue is already available. This will be covered in another chapter and the techniques for reconstruction are appropriately outlined therein. If, however, the abdominal contents are not exposed, options for perforator flaps are available. This chapter will focus on the pudendal (Singapore) artery flap for reconstruction.

ASSESSMENT OF THE DEFECT

Resection of the perineal area is challenging. Not only is there a component of loss of skin and muscle, but one must also consider reconstruction in an immediate or delayed fashion, whether a vaginal resection will result in partial or a total defect, and, if partial, whether the vaginal loss will be on the anterior, posterior, or distal vaginal wall. The pudendal flap may not be the best option for some of these defects. Loss of the vaginal introitus as well as part of the vault requires careful planning to provide a flap design with adequate length and width to prevent stenosis.

INDICATIONS FOR SURGERY

This flap is ideal for perineal and vaginal reconstruction. Large vaginal defects, however, may be more amenable to alternative myocutaneous flap options. Vaginal stenosis in the Western world is often due to trauma, overzealous repair, and radiation therapy. Alternatively, in developing countries, tropical diseases and circumcision may create issues of vaginal stenosis (Figures 84.1 and 84.2). Several authors have reported using the axial patterned flaps in a bilateral component for vaginal reconstruction and atresia.[1–17] The technique is simple, safe, and reliable. Bilateral reconstruction can be utilized for vaginal reconstruction, whereas unilateral flap design can be used for rectovaginal fistulas. Nature has provided a rich blood supply to the area fed by the femoral and iliac arteries. Branches from these vessels offer a unique

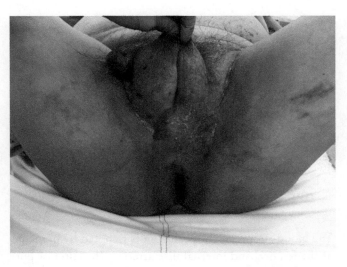

Figure 84.1. A 69-year-old man with Paget's disease of the perineum.

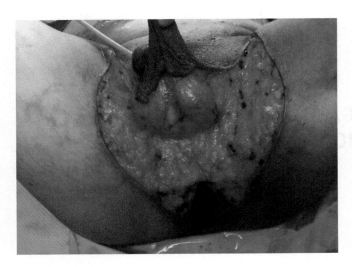

Figure 84.2. Following surgical resection.

opportunity, enabling surgeons to base reconstruction on these vessels.[2]

The ideal flap for any perineal defect should be of like tissue, not bulky but reliable and robust. Protective sensation should be available to provide normal function and cosmesis.[9] For defects in the upper quadrant, the donor flaps can come from the groin and/or mons area; for the lower quadrant, the donor can be from the gluteal fold and/or the gluteal area. The midthigh can also provide a flap for these defects.

CONTRAINDICATIONS FOR SURGERY

Extensive radiation, previous surgery, or other factors that might interfere with the blood supply of the flap should be considered. Lack of rotation or deep vaginal reconstruction may lend itself to alternative flap design.

ROOM SETUP

The patient is placed in the lithotomy or prone position. This allows excellent access to the flap as well as the defect. These flaps depend on the integrity of the vascular territories of the internal pudendal artery.[3] The location and extent of the resection usually determine the requirements for reconstruction.

OPERATIVE TECHNIQUE

The blood supply of the perineum is rich, fed by branches of the femoral and internal iliac arteries. The anterior portion of the perineum is supplied by the superficial and deep external pudendal arteries.[2] The internal pudendal artery and branches of the inferior gluteal artery supply the posterior half. The internal pudendal artery terminates into two branches—the perineal or clitoral branch and the perineal artery. The perineal artery supplies the labia/scrotal part of the perineum by the terminal branches that anastomose with their counterparts from the opposite side.[2] Other branches of the perineal artery are the medial and lateral branches. All of these provide the rich vascular network of the perineum and provide the basis of the development of perforator flaps.

The pudendal thigh fasciocutaneous flap is an axial patterned and potentially sensate flap based on the groin crease.[1–9] It frequently is used for perineal reconstruction. Although some advocate it for vaginal reconstruction, alternative options may be more appropriate, such as the gracilis and rectus abdominis myocutaneous flaps.[4] The well-tolerated scar located in the inguinal crease is characterized by its thin adaptable options for reconstruction.

The arterial supply of the flap is through (1) a direct cutaneous branch of the deep external pudendal artery, which is a branch of the femoral artery lying deep to the fascia lata, which it pierces on the medial side of the thigh[5]; (2) the anterior branch of the obturator artery, which curves down along the anterior margin of the obturator foramen and supplies the gracilis and the adductor muscles of the overlying skin; and (3) the medial femoral circumflex artery, which supplies muscular branches to the gracilis and adductor muscles and is a musculocutaneous artery from the femoral or profunda femoral artery.[6–17]

Once the dimensions of the defect are available, the required flap is planned over the donor area. The success of perforator flap reconstruction depends mainly on the selection of the perforator vessel at or around the base of the selected flap.[2] Perforators can be identified before surgery with a handheld Doppler. Once the perforator is identified within an axial flap, the cutaneous vessels should be identified.

The advantage of the use of the superomedial thigh flap is that it ensures normal sensation since both the genital branch of the genitofemoral nerve and the ilioinguinal nerve are likely to be retained with these flaps.

With the patient in a lithotomy position, the flap is outlined adjacent to the defect. The base of the flap overlies the adductor longus muscle while distally the flap reaches lateral to the perineum. The width of the flap roughly corresponds to the width of the defect although some mobility of the tissues at the defect should make flap design smaller. The flap is raised off the underlying fat distally and more proximally off the fascia lata covering the origins of the adductor longus and gracilis muscles. Care is taken not

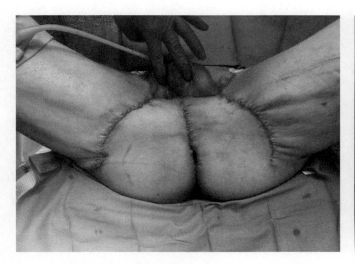

Figure 84.3. Reconstruction followed with bilateral pudendal artery flaps.

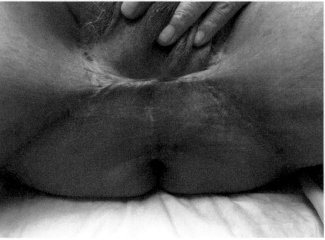

Figure 84.4. Six months postoperatively.

to destroy any perforating vessels. The more inferior portion of the flap can be rotated to close the defect in the suprapubic area. Flaps may be sutured together after developing them from each side, closing the defect. Primary closure is often possible. If closure is not possible, skin grafting is required (Figure 84.3).

POSTOPERATIVE CARE

The patient remains in bed rest for 2–3 days on some form of pressure-reducing mattress or bed. Often an abduction pillow is used to prevent potential compromise of the vascular flow. Thighs are kept abducted and the knees slightly flexed. Patient-controlled analgesia is often required for the first 3 days. Most patients can be mobilized after 24–48 hours. The requirement for bed rest is to ensure that the movement of the patient does not tear the flap from its inset. Once several days have passed, assistance by physical therapy is key in getting the patient out of bed. Care must be taken not to pull or drag the patient across the mattress. While the patient is sitting, continued pressure-relieving measures should be instituted in a chair. This can be done by placing donuts or other alternative forms of cushioned support.

Ambulation occurs when the patient is ready. Again, slow progress is important to avoid loss of the continuity of the flap. Drains are maintained until the drainage is less than 30 mL in 24 hours. If skin grafts have been used in conjunction with the pudendal flap, continued bolstering of the grafts through the use of negative-pressure dressings or other alterative support is critical.

Once the patient is discharged home, vascularity is less of an issue; however, we recommend continued pressure

relief options for several weeks. Losses of small areas of the flap usually heal by secondary intention (Figure 84.4).

CAVEATS

Plastic surgeons today are involved in reconstructive surgery as part of a multidisciplinary team. Reconstruction is challenging because one has to maintain both important functional and aesthetic options. Anatomically, there are multiple perforators and subcutaneous vessels arising from the superficial external pudendal artery, deep external pudendal artery, and internal pudendal arteries with accompanying veins.

REFERENCES

1. Sinna R, Qassemyar Q, Benhaim T, Lauzanne P, Sabbach C, Regimbeau JM, Mauvais F. Perforator flaps: a new option in perineal reconstruction. *J Plast Reconstr Aesthet Surg* 2010;63:e766–e774.
2. Niranjan NS. Perforator flaps for perineal reconstructions. *Semin Plast Surg* 2006;20(2):133–144.
3. Wong DS. Reconstruction of the perineum. *Ann Plast Surg* 2014;73:S74–S81.
4. Benito P, De Juan A, Cano M. The pudendal thigh flap as YV advancement flap for the release of perineum burns contractures. *J Plast Reconstr Aesthet Surg* 2012;65:681–683.
5. Hashimoto I, Goishi K, Abe Y, Takaku M, Seike T, Harada H, Nakanishi H. The internal pudendal artery perforator thigh flap: a new freestyle pedicle flap for the ischial region. *Plast Reconstr Surg Glob Open* 2014;2:e142.
6. Mopuri N, O'Connor EF, Iwuagwu FC. Scrotal reconstruction with modified pundendal thigh flaps. *J Plast Reconstr Aesthet Surg* 2016;69:278–283.
7. Zhang W, Zeng A, Yang J, et al. Outcome of vulvar reconstruction in patients with advanced and recurrent vulvar malignancies. *BMC Cancer* 2015;15(5):851.

8. Huang JJ, Chang NJ, Chou HH, Wu CW, Abdelrahman M, Chen HY, Cheng MH. Pedicle perforator flaps for vulvar reconstruction—new generation of less invasive vulvar reconstruction with favorable results. *Gynecol Oncol* 2015;137:66–72.

9. Coltro PS, Ferreira MC, Busnardo FF, et al. Evaluation of cutaneous sensibility of the internal pudendal artery perforator (IPAP) flap after perineal reconstruction. *J Plast Reconstr Aesthet Surg* 2015;68:252–261.

10. Selcuk CT, Evsen MS, Ozalp B, Durgun M. Reconstruction of vaginal agenesis with pudendal thigh flaps thinned with liposuction. *J Plast Reconstr Aesthet Surg* 2013;66:e246–e250.

11. Lee SH, Rah DK, Lee WJ. Penoscrotal reconstruction with gracilis muscle flap and internal pudendal artery perforator flap transposition. *Urology* 2012;79:1390–1394.

12. Ugburo AO, Mofikoya BO, Oluwole AA, Fedeyibi IO, Abidoye G. Pudendal thigh flap in the treatment of acquired gynatresia from caustic pessaries. *Int J Gynaecol Obstet* 2011;115:44–48.

13. Scott JR, Liu D, Mathes DW. Patient-reported outcomes and sexual function in vaginal reconstruction: a 17-year review, survey, and review of the literature. *Ann Plast Surg* 2010;64:311–314.

14. Pakiam AI. Medial thigh skin flaps for repair of vaginal stenosis. In: Strauch B, Vasconez L, Hall-Findlay E, eds. *Encyclopedia of Flaps*. Boston: Little, Brown and Company, 1990:1431–1433.

15. Hirshowitz B. Bilateral superomedial thigh flaps for primary reconstruction of the vulva. In: Strauch B, Vasconez L, Hall-Findlay E, eds. *Encyclopedia of Flaps*. Boston: Little, Brown and Company, 1990:1434–1436.

16. Monstrey SM, Blondeel P, Van Landuyt K, Verpaele A, Tonnard P, Matton G. The versatility of the pundendal thigh fasciocutaneous flap used as an island flap. *Plast Reconstr Surg* 2001;107:719–725.

17. Joseph VT. Pundendal-thigh flap vaginoplasty in the reconstruction of genital anomalies. *J Pediatr Surg* 1997;32;62–65.

PART XIII.

EXTREMITY RECONSTRUCTION

85.

GASTROCNEMIUS FLAP FOR PROXIMAL LEG RECONSTRUCTION

Howard N. Langstein, Elaina Y. Chen, and Nicholas A. Wingate

A quantum improvement in technique over the cross-leg flap for lower extremity reconstruction was advanced by McCraw, Ger, and others, in which a "myoplasty" of the gastrocnemius muscle was used to cover exposed defects.[11,26,34] This strategy was popularized by the landmark work of Mathes, Nahai, Arnold, McCraw, and Vasconez, which established the safety and applicability of muscle and musculocutaneous transfers.[1,26,36] Muscle flaps were shown to enhance antibiotic delivery to infected locations, and it became standard to treat osteomyelitis and open wounds of the proximal tibia with gastrocnemius flaps.[11,20,31] The use of the gastrocnemius flap has also been described to salvage exposed knee prostheses and also to provide coverage for hardware used in limb-sparing surgery for bone sarcomas around the knee.[19,27,32] The cutaneous territories overlying the gastrocnemius muscle flap were defined by McCraw who, along with Arnold, later published refinements of the myocutaneous flap harvest and use.[1,25] Most surgeons, however, now agree with Nahai, who has advocated the use of a muscle flap without a skin paddle and a skin graft to avoid donor site deformities.[28] Because of its dependability and ease of transfer, the gastrocnemius muscle remains the workhorse tissue transfer for defects in the upper third of the lower extremity.

ASSESSMENT OF THE DEFECT

Assessing the defect begins with an inventory of which elements of the leg are missing. If subcutaneous tissue of reasonable quality remains in the bed of the wound, then a skin graft might suffice for coverage. In the case of an irradiated wound, skin grafts and fasciocutaneous flaps are often unreliable. In the case of exposed bone, tendons, or neurovascular structures, more stable and substantial resurfacing is needed. It is important to anticipate if the debrided defect will be significantly larger than the existing defect; this will represent the actual tissue requirement. In many cases, a single aggressive debridement followed by wet-to-dry dressings or a negative-pressure wound therapy (NPWT) device is adequate to prepare the wound for closure. Of course, this depends on the degree of contamination. If bone viability is in question, more than one debridement may be required to remove all potentially nonviable bone. After final debridement, simple measurement of the cutaneous deficit and wound depth will supply the reconstructive surgeon with the necessary information to choose or reject the gastrocnemius flap.

Rarely will a radiographic study be required, with the exception of assessment of bony abnormality. The neurovascular bundles are usually preserved in most cases of peripheral vascular disease, and an angiogram is typically unnecessary. An angiogram should be considered if femoral pulses are absent, chiefly to evaluate whether an inflow procedure, surgical bypass, or angioplasty can be done. When resecting a tumor of the proximal third of the leg, an angiogram may be required to plan the resection and can be used to determine if inflow exists to the gastrocnemius muscles. Most of the time, the only reliable method of vascular assessment of the flap is to actually raise the flap and evaluate bleeding at the distal cut edge.

INDICATIONS

The gastrocnemius muscle flap or one of its variants should be thought of as the first-option tissue transfer for reconstruction of defects located from the lower thigh to the junction of the upper and middle thirds of the lower extremity.[7] As seen in Figure 85.1A,B, the reach of the heads

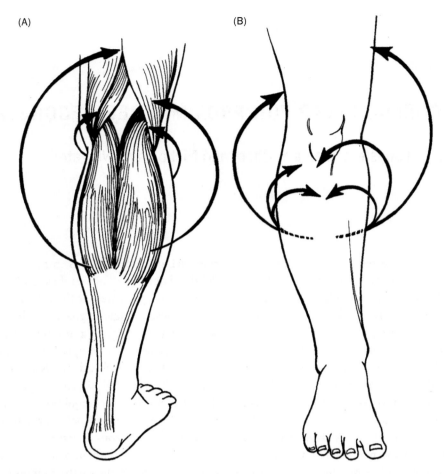

Figure 85.1. (A,B) Limits of gastrocnemius muscle flaps. Reach of gastrocnemius muscles is from distal thigh to around patella, generally reconstructing upper third of lower leg. Arc of rotation and size of available muscle dictate reach, which is longer for medial head.[17]

of the gastrocnemius muscles comfortably extends from the lower thigh to most of the upper third of the leg. When the defect is closer to the middle third of the leg, the soleus flap is customarily chosen. Bear in mind that both heads of the gastrocnemius may be transposed anteriorly to meet each other to cover the entire patellar region.[8] For anterior defects, the width of the heads of the gastrocnemius muscles dictates the available tissue in the superior-inferior dimension because of the geometry of a 90-degree rotation. For this reason, the senior author has found that medial defects up to approximately 9 cm and lateral defects of nearly 5–7 cm can be closed by applying the typical widths of these structures. To extend these dimensions, it is possible to use maneuvers such as stretching the muscle or orienting it obliquely. When larger defects are encountered, the soleus can be used in addition to the medial head of the gastrocnemius. Long, narrow defects of the upper tibia can be closed by bringing both heads together over the bone, through a posterior incision.

CONTRAINDICATIONS

Rarely will the gastrocnemius muscle be contraindicated. However, if the patient has sustained recent trauma to the calf, it is possible that the muscle is in the zone of injury and would not tolerate transposition. Typically, the rich anastomotic network around the knee allows use of the gastrocnemius flap even in the setting of peripheral vascular disease (PVD). Hence, PVD is not specifically a contraindication, and use of the gastrocnemius, even in the setting of arterial reconstruction, has been described. Essentially, the only contraindication is too large a defect to be covered by a gastrocnemius flap or one of its variants.

ALTERNATIVES

Fasciocutaneous flaps may be used for upper-third lower extremity defects instead of muscle or musculocutaneous flaps.

However, these flaps often require a skin-grafted donor site and may not be preferable in many clinical situations.

Pedicled perforator or "propeller" flaps are gaining popularity for select soft tissue defects where a gastrocnemius might have previously been utilized or where a gastrocnemius flap alone is unable to cover the entire defect.[16] Function preservation is their major advantage, as no muscle need be included. However, partial flap necrosis has been reported to be 7–11%, and complete flap loss is reported at 1–5%,[4,5,13,30] with some evidence that complication rates are higher in diabetics, the elderly (>60 years old), and arteriopaths.[4] Additionally, Bekara recently found that although the overall complication rate of propeller flaps is comparable to free flaps, partial necrosis is significantly more likely in propeller flaps compared to free flaps (6.88% vs. 2.70%, $p = 0.001$).[5] Hence, these flaps should be used with careful patient selection.

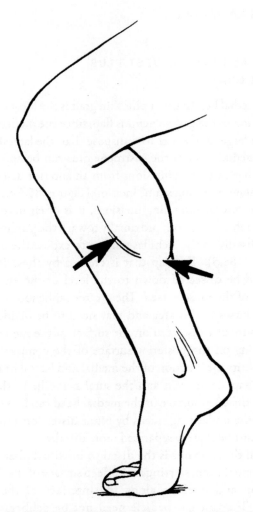

Figure 85.2. Surface markings of gastrocnemius muscles. With plantar flexion, limits of gastrocnemius muscles are evident on surface and are easily marked.

As a final alternative, a wide variety of free tissue transfer options can be considered if the gastrocnemius flap cannot be utilized.

PATIENT MARKINGS AND POSITIONING

The surface landmarks of the gastrocnemius muscles are quite obvious with the foot in plantarflexion and serve as a rough guide for incision placement (Figure 85.2). Depending on the location of the defect, the approach can be anterior or posterior. The medial head can be comfortably harvested via an anteromedial incision with the leg abducted in the unilateral "frog-leg" position. An anterolateral incision may be used to retrieve the lateral head. Both heads can also be approached through a posterior "stocking seam" incision; this requires prone positioning.

PREPARING THE WOUND

In the case of traumatic injuries to the upper tibial area, coverage should not be undertaken until debridement of all devitalized tissue is accomplished. This is especially difficult when deciding how much bone to remove since significant removal may require a subsequent bone graft for stability. However, this is an invaluable step and, if not done, can leave an inoculum of bacteria sufficient to ruin the most meticulously prepared flap. The success or failure of the gastrocnemius flap in preventing or treating osteomyelitis rests on the appropriateness of the debridement.

OPERATIVE TECHNIQUE

SURGICAL ANATOMY

The landmarks of the gastrocnemius complex can be seen on the surface of the posterior calf, especially on plantarflexion (Figure 85.2). Each head originates from its respective femoral condyle and joins the other in the midline before coalescing with the underlying soleus muscle to insert into the calcaneal tendon (Figure 85.3). Upon flexion, the heads of the gastrocnemius muscles serve to plantarflex the ankle and, to a lesser degree, flex the knee. In all but athletic patients, adequate plantarflexion can be preserved with maintenance of one of these muscles—the soleus or one of the heads of the gastrocnemius. The medial head is

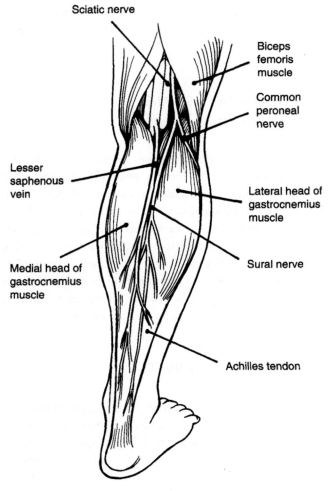

Figure 85.3. Superficial posterior leg anatomy. View of posterior calf with skin and subcutaneous tissue removed demonstrates position of heads of gastrocnemius muscle bellies, their attachment to Achilles tendon, and course of lesser saphenous vein and sural, common peroneal, and sciatic nerves.

The course of the common peroneal nerve is also relevant to the harvest of the lateral head of the gastrocnemius muscle. This nerve splits off from the sciatic nerve in the popliteal fossa to travel over the head of the fibula, between the proximal portion of the lateral head of the gastrocnemius and the tendon of the biceps femoris muscle (Figure 85.4). Division of this nerve denervates the lateral and anterior compartments, chiefly resulting in foot drop and sensory loss to the dorsum of the foot.

Deep to the gastrocnemius is the soleus muscle, which fuses with the distal gastrocnemius muscle itself and also inserts along the Achilles tendon. In the upper leg, there is a plane between the gastrocnemius and the soleus, but more distally these muscles must be sharply separated. The tendon of the plantaris muscle lies between the soleus and the medial head of the gastrocnemius and helps to confirm this anatomic plane.

FLAP VARIANTS

MEDIAL HEAD HARVEST PLUS SKIN GRAFT

The medial head harvest plus skin graft is the most common variation of the gastrocnemius flap, since the medial head is much larger and easier to transpose than the lateral head.[28] The medial head of the gastrocnemius can be approached by either extending incisions from an anterior defect or by a separate "stocking seam" incision (Figures 85.5 and 85.6). In the case of extending incisions, it is often necessary to obliquely extend both proximally toward the popliteal fossa and distally to the Achilles tendon to expose the insertion (Figure 85.5). The flap that is created by these incisions should be dissected down to the level of the enveloping fascia of the muscle itself. The greater saphenous vein usually courses in this area and may need to be divided. This flap is further dissected on the surface of the medial head, stopping on the posterior surface of the complex, which represents the junction of the medial and lateral heads. The lesser saphenous vein and the sural nerve lie in this cleft. Next, the deep surface of the medial head can be separated from the underlying soleus by blunt dissection proximally but must be sharply separated more distally.

All that remains is the distal to proximal liberation of the medial head, starting at the deep surface of the Achilles tendon and working along the interface of the lateral head. The vascular pedicle need not be deliberately uncovered because separation of the heads usually provides

the larger of the two components. The neurovascular pedicle, varying from 2 to 5 cm in length, consists of a sural artery and veins along with branches from the tibial nerves. The pedicles enter the muscle bellies proximally, from their tibial surfaces, just a few centimeters distal to the condylar origins (Figure 85.4). The gastrocnemius muscle is thus considered a Mathes and Nahai type 1 muscle and can survive completely as an island flap based on this proximal pedicle.[9]

An important anatomic landmark is the course of the lesser saphenous vein and the sural nerve, which travel together from the lateral malleolar region to ascend up the leg in the cleft between both heads of the gastrocnemius muscle along the posterior surface. If possible, the sural nerve should be spared since its sacrifice can result in a troubling anesthesia along the lateral aspect of the foot.

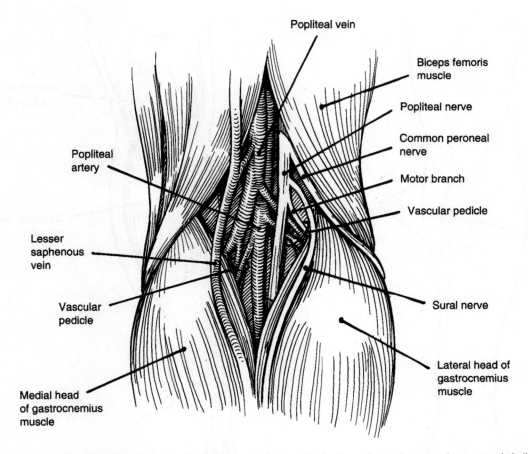

Figure 85.4. Deeper anatomy of popliteal region. Neurovascular bundles arise from popliteal artery, veins, and nerve and enter muscle bellies from their proximal undersurface.

enough length for transposition into most defects. In young ambulatory patients, it may be advisable to dissect out the nerve from the pedicle and divide it to prevent an unwanted anterior muscle contraction of the transposed calf muscle.

The next maneuver to increase the reach of the muscle, even before dividing the origin, is to score or even completely remove the fascia on either the deep or superficial surfaces, or both. Not only does this increase the length of the muscle by as much as 4 cm, but it allows for a better bed for the "take" of a skin graft and permits muscle to come into contact with raw bony surfaces to help deliver antibiotics to tissue at risk.

When even more length is desired, the origin of the muscle can be taken off the femur by a proximal extension of the incision into the popliteal fossa to create an island flap (Figure 85.7). It is advisable to locate the sural pedicle and protect it when dividing the muscular origin. The flap that was elevated to uncover the gastrocnemius muscle is then draped back into position and invariably needs to be trimmed to allow pressure-free passage of the muscle to the

defect. Thus, the defect is made larger, with the flesh of the muscle being exposed where a constricting tunnel would be.

If one chooses to harvest the muscle through a posterior "stocking seam" incision, then this line is placed over a palpable cleft in the calf and drawn from the distal third of the leg to a "lazy S" extension into the popliteal fossa (Figure 85.6). The incision is quickly taken down to the muscle complex, locating and preserving the sural nerve and lesser saphenous vein while the heads are sharply separated. Then the plane superficial to the muscle is opened. Next, dissection is directed over the medial head to the deep surface. This plane is readily separated bluntly more superiorly, but this must be done sharply at the distal-most aspect. The distal muscle is divided off the Achilles tendon and liberated proximally. The subcutaneous tunnel, which must not be excessively constricting and is required to deliver the muscle, is then created. Inset of the flap proceeds.

If the distal end of the defect is still not adequately filled with the medial head, harvest of the soleus muscle should be considered. Alternatively, the medial head can be advanced

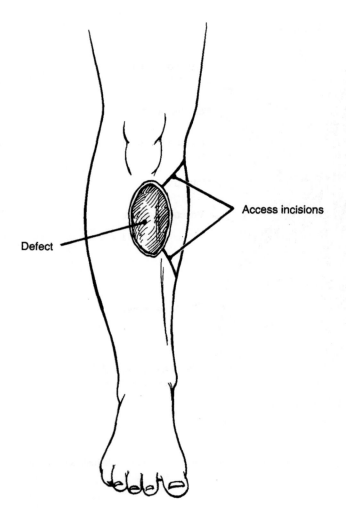

Figure 85.5. Typical medial approach for harvest of gastrocnemius medial head. Proximal and distal oblique incisions are made from typical anterior defect revealing medial head of gastrocnemius.

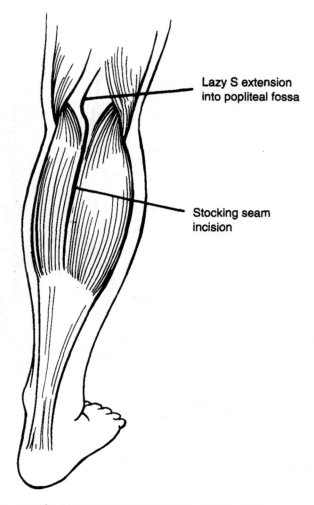

Figure 85.6. "Stocking seam" incision with extension into popliteal fossa. Both heads of gastrocnemius muscle can be approached through incision. It is easier to use this approach, but it requires prone positioning and perhaps additional change of position for flap inset.

more distally by dividing the vascular pedicle and inserting vein grafts as a "local" free flap.[17]

The inset of the muscle is facilitated by leaving a rim of fascia on the perimeter of the muscle to allow for better purchase of sutures. A simple way to secure the muscle flap to the margins of the defect is to use nonabsorbable heavy monofilament sutures tied over a Xeroform bolster, fashioning the bites to hold the muscle to the undersurface of the defect, the skin edges of which must be undermined slightly. These bolster sutures should be left in place for at least 2 weeks and preferably longer to help ensure strong union of the muscles to the defect. The exposed muscle is skin-grafted with a meshed split-thickness piece of skin from the thigh. Closed suction drains are used to drain the region under the muscle flap as it overlays the defect and also the posterior location from where the medial head was harvested.

LATERAL HEAD OF GASTROCNEMIUS MUSCLE HARVEST

Because the lateral head of the gastrocnemius muscle is substantially smaller than the medial head, its use will be limited to smaller defects and to those on the lateral aspect of the upper third of the leg.[8,32] The posterior stocking-seam incision is preferred, through which the lateral head is separated from the medial head. The key to the lateral harvest is to continue the incision more proximally into the popliteal fossa to visualize the neurovascular bundle and the common peroneal nerve. This nerve courses between the biceps femoris and the lateral head before wrapping around the head of the fibula. The remainder of the procedure is the same as for the medial head.

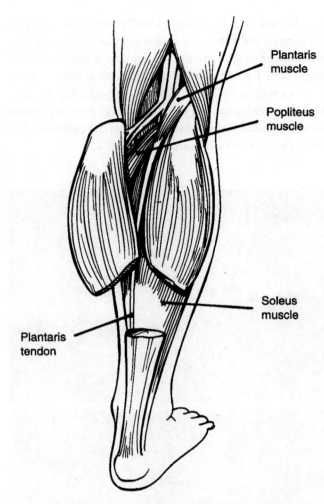

Figure 85.7. Island muscle flap of medial head of gastrocnemius muscle. If scoring of fascia of muscle does not achieve desired length, muscle can be made into pure island flap. It is advisable to locate and protect the pedicle when dividing the origin off the femur. Courtesy of Ramon Llull, MD, PhD.

GASTROCNEMIUS MYOCUTANEOUS FLAP HARVEST

Recognizing that keeping the skin and subcutaneous tissue attached to the gastrocnemius muscle generally necessitates a skin graft for closure of the donor site, there may be situations where this is preferred.[7,10,14,26,33] Remember that the cosmetic outcome, especially of the donor defect, can be inferior to that accomplished with a muscle flap and a skin graft. The skin paddle is centered on the head to be transferred and, if reasonably small, may be primarily closed. Usually, a large paddle is chosen, which is harvested similarly to the methods described earlier. While not related to proximal third reconstruction, the entire calf tissue can be advanced distally to cover distal-third posterior defects by simply dividing both muscular attachments and freeing the complex from the underlying soleus. In this case, the donor site is closed with a V-Y advancement.[1]

FLAP CONTOURING

The gastrocnemius muscle, especially the medial head, can be excessively bulky for many defects. Fortunately, much muscle bulk subsides with time, and the need for revision is rare. However, if the muscle exceeds the level of the defect by more than 2–3 cm, it is reasonable to sharply plane excess bulk at the initial reconstruction. This could be bloody, and hematomas may jeopardize the "take" of the skin graft. Fortunately, the initially bulky muscle atrophies considerably and contours well in time.

DRESSINGS

Dressing this inset flap is quite simple. A tight tie-over bolster dressing is to be avoided since this could choke the flap; rather, a piece of bacitracin-impregnated gauze can be placed directly on the graft and covered with layers of gauze or a negative-pressure wound dressing. Following this, a well-padded posterior plaster splint, from above the knee to the toes, is placed and not removed until the fifth postoperative day, at which time the gauze is removed and appropriate rehabilitation instituted. Until the interstices of the skin graft have epithelialized, the patient needs nonadherent gauze dressings and a moisturizing agent. An elastic (Ace) bandage is routinely wrapped from the toes to above the flap site to limit edema of the leg, which notoriously accompanies such a reconstruction.

FLAP MONITORING

Since the gastrocnemius is a very robust flap, it is usually unnecessary to monitor the flap closely for viability. Occasionally, if the insetting is too aggressive, flap viability may be challenged, but this is usually evident in the operating room. It is necessary to evaluate the flap for an underlying hematoma, which could jeopardize the flap and also result in an infected collection beneath the flap. Therefore, a small opening should be made in the nonstick gauze through which the muscle and skin graft can be periodically observed. Naturally, a significant hematoma should prompt a return visit to the operating room for evacuation.

REHABILITATION

Depending on the underlying bony status, which could preclude weight-bearing for a considerable amount of time, the gastrocnemius flap does not require a complicated rehabilitation regimen. If the flap and skin graft are viable when the dressings and splint are removed on the fifth postoperative day, it is reasonable to begin gradual limited weight-bearing in a few days with crutches or a walker. The sutures are still in place at this point and afford some mechanical strength to the wound. Of course, if the patient has any risk factors for poor wound healing, then a corresponding period of immobilization is warranted. Usually, the condition that precipitated the need for a gastrocnemius flap dictates the avoidance of weight-bearing activity on the affected leg for longer than 1 week, so early mobilization is often a moot point. Certainly, by 3 weeks after surgery, the flap is secure enough to withstand full weight-bearing. Another month or two is typically reserved for strengthening exercises, after which the leg may be maximally stressed.

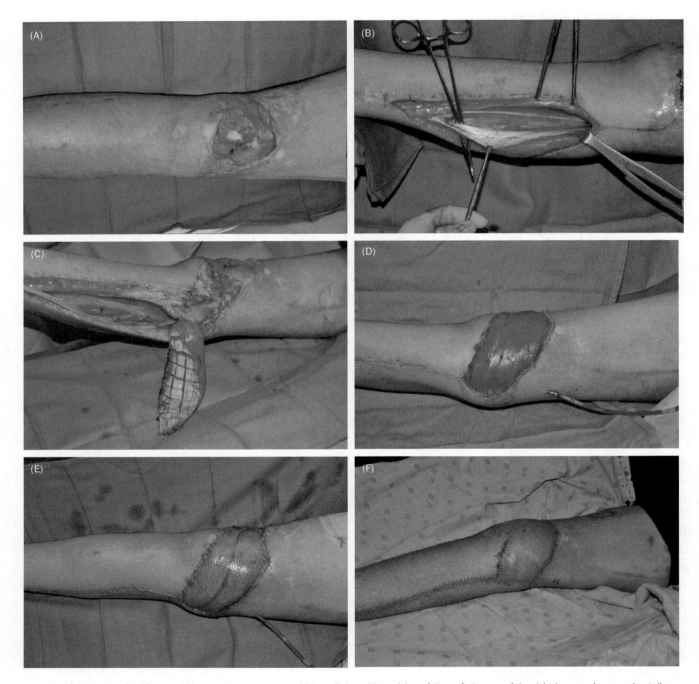

Figure 85.8. Case study of a 15 year old boy status post motor vehicle collision with avulsion of the soft tissues of the right knee and exposed patellar fracture as well as hardware (A). The medial gastrocnemius is exposed (B). After division of the distal tendon, the fascia of the gastrocnemius is scored to allow expansion of its length and width (C). Inset of the flap with closure of the donor site (D), followed by the placement of a skin graft (E). Appearance at 3 weeks postoperatively (F). Courtesy of Clinton Morrison, MD.

EXTREMITY RECONSTRUCTION

CAVEATS

This flap transfer is routinely easy and reliable, but there are a few potential areas where minor complications may arise. Complete flap loss is rare but will occur with excessive kinking of the pedicle or with overaggressive insetting. More commonly, partial flap necrosis results from a constricting tunnel and frank pressure on the muscle itself. This can be prevented by the judicious opening of any tight tunnel that might cause ischemia. Fortunately, the vascular pedicle arborizes shortly after it enters the proximal muscle, and this arrangement allows aggressive trimming. Rarely, this can be overdone and the distal muscle rendered nonviable.

The common peroneal and sural nerves are vulnerable during muscle harvest and should be carefully avoided. Also, the tibial nerve is potentially at risk during distal dissection, although more commonly when the soleus needs to be harvested. The Achilles tendon can be injured but will be left intact if one removes only muscle fibers from the distalmost junction with the tendon. Of course, dissection in the correct anatomic plane is critical to properly harvest either head; if too deep, the soleus can be uncovered by mistake.

CONCLUSION

The gastrocnemius flap is a versatile and reliable flap that has been the workhorse for reconstructing proximal-third leg defects for decades. With the advent of pedicled perforator (propeller) flaps and the availability of free vascularized tissue transfer, plastic surgeons have a wide armamentarium of options to reconstruct any defect in the leg.

Case Study

This 15-year-old boy was status post motor vehicle collision with avulsion of the soft tissues of the right knee and exposed patellar fracture. This was reduced and fixated with patellar screws, but, despite several rounds of negative-pressure wound vac therapy, there remained a persistently exposed patellar screw. A medial gastrocnemius muscle flap and skin graft was chosen for reconstruction (Figure 85.8A–F). The medial gastrocnemius flap was found to be deficient in length to reliably cover the most superolateral portion of the wound, as well as deficient in width to span the entire height of the wound. As such, the decision was made to score the fascia in a checkerboard pattern. This allowed an additional 1–2 centimeters of length and width to be obtained, therefore resulting in a tension-free and reliable

inset of the flap. A split-thickness meshed skin graft was then placed upon the muscle and the surgical site was dressed with negative-pressure wound therapy. The donor site was closed primarily. The patient recovered uneventfully, and the postoperative appearance at 3 weeks is shown. The patient is now ambulatory and has a very satisfactory quality of life.

SELECTED READINGS

Barfod B, Pers M. Gastrocnemius-plasty for primary closure of compound injuries of the knee. *J Bone Joint Surg* 1970;52B: 124–127.

Barfred T, Reumert T. Myoplasty for covering exposed bone or joint on the lower leg. *Acta Orthop Scand* 1973;44:532–538.

Byrd H, Cierny G, Tebbets JB. The management of open tibial fractures with associated soft-tissue loss: external pin fixation with early flap coverage. *Plast Reconstr Surg* 1981;68:73–79.

Ger R. Surgical management of ulcerative lesions of the leg. *Curr Probl Surg* 1972:1–52.

Hallock G. Local knee random fasciocutaneous flaps. *Ann Plast Surg* 1989;23:289–296.

Lentz M, Noyes FR, Neale HW. Muscle flap transposition for traumatic soft tissue defects of the lower extremity. *Clin Orthop Related Res* 1979;143:200–210.

Mathes S, McCraw JB, Vasconez LO. Muscle transposition flaps for coverage of lower extremity defects. *Surg Clin North Am* 1974;54:1337–1354.

Mathes SJ, Nahai F. Classification of the vascular anatomy of muscles: experimental and clinical correlation. *Plast Reconstr Surg* 1981;67:177.

Mathes S, Vasconez LO, Jurkiewicz MJ. Extensions and further applications of muscle transposition. *Plast Reconstr Surg* 1977;60:6–13.

McCraw J, Arnold PG. *McCraw and Arnold's Atlas of Muscle and Musculocutaneous Flaps.* Norfolk: Hampton Press, 1986:733.

Neale H, Stern PJ, Kreilein JG, et al. Complications of muscle flap transposition for traumatic defects of the leg. *Plast Reconstr Surg* 1983;72:512–515.

Strauch B, Yu HL. *Atlas of Microvascular Surgery.* New York: Thieme Medical, 1993:560.

REFERENCES

1. Arnold P, Mixter RC. Making the most of the gastrocnemius muscles. *Plast Reconstr Surg* 1983;72:38–48.
2. Bekara F, Herlin C, Mojallal A, et al. A systematic review and meta-analysis of perforator-pedicled propeller flaps in lower extremity defects: identification of risk factors for complications. *Plast Reconstr Surg.* 2016 Jan;137(1):314–331.
3. Bekara F, Herlin C, Somda S, de Runz A, Grolleau JL, Chaput B. Free versus perforator-pedicled propeller flaps in lower extremity reconstruction: what is the safest coverage? A meta-analysis. *Microsurgery.* 2016 Mar 28.
4. Dibbell D, Edstrom LE. The gastrocnemius myocutaneous flap. *Clin Plast Surg* 1980;7:45–50.
5. Elsahy N. Cover of the exposed knee joint by the lateral head of the gastrocnemius. *Br J Plast Surg* 1978;31:136–137.
6. Ersek R, Abell JM, Calhoon JH. The island pedicle rotation advancement gastrocnemius musculocutaneous flap for complete coverage of the popliteal fossa. *Ann Plast Surg* 1984;12:533–536.
7. Feldman J, Cohen BE, May JW. The medial gastrocnemius myocutaneous flap. *Plast Reconstr Surg* 1978;61:531–539.

8. Ger R. Muscle transposition for treatment and prevention of chronic post-traumatic osteomyelitis of the tibia. *J Bone Joint Surg* 1977;59A:784–791.

9. Gir P, Cheng A, Oni G, Mojallal A, Saint-Cyr M. Pedicled-perforator (propeller) flaps in lower extremity defects: a systematic review. *J Reconstr Microsurg.* 2012 Nov;28(9):595–601.

10. Gryskiewicz J, Edstrom LE, Dibbell DG. The gastrocnemius myocutaneous flap in lower extremity injuries. *J Trauma* 1984;24:539–543.

11. Hallock GG. A paradigm shift in flap selection protocols for zones of the lower extremity using perforator flaps. *J Reconstr Microsurg.* 2013 May;29(4):233–240.

12. Keller A, Shaw W. The medial gastrocnemius muscle flap: a local free flap. *Plast Reconstr Surg* 1984;73:974–976.

13. Malawer M, Price WM. Gastrocnemius transposition flap in conjunction with limb-sparing surgery for primary bone sarcomas around the knee. *Plast Reconstr Surg* 1984;73:741–750.

14. Mathes S, Alpert BS, Chang N. Use of the muscle flap in chronic osteomyelitis: experimental and clinical correlation. *Plast Reconstr Surg* 1982;69:815–828.

15. McCraw J, Dibbell DG, Carraway JH. Clinical definition of independent myocutaneous vascular territories. *Plast Reconstr Surg* 1977;60:341–352.

16. McCraw J, Fishman JH, Sharzer LA. The versatile gastrocnemius myocutaneous flap. *Plast Reconstr Surg* 1978;62:15–23.

17. Meller I, Ariche A, Sagi A. The role of the gastrocnemius muscle flap in limb-sparing surgery for bone sarcomas of the distal femur: a proposed classification of muscle transfers. *Plast Reconstr Surg* 1997;99:751–756.

18. Nahai F, Mathes SJ. Musculocutaneous flap or muscle flap and skin graft? *Ann Plast Surg* 1984;12:199–203.

19. Nelson JA, Fischer JP, Brazio PS, Kovach SJ, Rosson GD, Rad AN. A review of propeller flaps for distal lower extremity soft tissue reconstruction: is flap loss too high? *Microsurgery.* 2013 Oct;33(7):578–586.

20. Russell R, Graham DR, Feller AM, et al. Experimental evaluation of the antibiotic carrying capacity of a muscle into a fibrotic cavity. *Plast Reconstr Surg* 1988;81:162–170.

21. Saliban A, Anzel SH. Salvage of an infected total knee prosthesis with medial and lateral gastrocnemius muscle flaps. *J Bone Joint Surg* 1983;65:681–684.

22. Saunders R, O'Neill T. The gastrocnemius myocutaneous flap used as a cover for the exposed knee prosthesis. *J Bone Joint Surg* 1981;62B:383–386.

23. Stark R. The cross-leg flap procedure. *Plast Reconstr Surg* 1952;9:173–204.

24. Vasconez L, Bostwick J, McCraw J. Coverage of exposed bone by muscle transposition and skin grafting. *Plast Reconstr Surg* 1974;53:526–533.

86.

SOLEUS FLAP FOR LOWER LEG RECONSTRUCTION

Jeffrey D. Friedman and Eric S. Ruff

ASSESSMENT OF THE DEFECT

Physical examination of the involved extremity remains the cornerstone for evaluation and future treatment of the wound. Gross inspection of the leg is first carried out and usually provides a significant amount of useful information. Signs of residual soft tissue infection, chronic or acute ischemia, and persistent edema should be identified. In these circumstances, such changes should be corrected before attempting permanent wound coverage. Strict bedrest for 48–72 hours improves and often resolves significant soft tissue swelling in the leg, which makes mobilization and transfer of the involved tissues much easier. Preoperative arteriography is not routinely performed or recommended. In most cases, clinical evaluation of the dorsalis pedis and posterior tibial pulses gives an accurate assessment of distal perfusion to the extremity. Simple palpation of the pulses, however, does not suffice. Alternate compression of the posterior tibial and dorsalis pedis arteries must be performed to assure prograde, not retrograde, flow in these vessels. Absence of prograde, pulsatile flow in the posterior tibial vessel should, however, raise suspicion as to the adequacy of the soleus flap for reliable soft tissue coverage of extremity defects.

As is true of most infected wounds, control of the local wound environment is of paramount importance. This translates into the need for operative debridement should any necrotic tissue or localized infection exist. Should the soleus reside in the zone of injury, one must be prepared to explore the posterior compartment to evaluate the viability of the muscle. This is particularly true when there has been significant trauma in the region of the proximal vascular pedicle. However, given the segmental nature of the blood supply, one cannot accurately assess the presence or absence of sufficient inflow at this level. Similarly,

previous radiation therapy to this area affects decision-making with regard to coverage options. Severely scarred and ischemic radiated tissues often take grafts poorly, and, in this situation, more reliable soft tissue coverage with muscle flaps may be necessary. As a general rule, previous radiation to the area of the soleus muscle and pedicle does not limit its use as a rotation flap. However, consideration of the dosages and types of radiation as well as the gross appearance of the muscle may alter the decision whether to use this flap.

Evaluation of the underlying or exposed bone is particularly needed in cases of osteomyelitis. Optimal treatment would dictate that all nonviable tibia or fibula be removed before the wound is covered. This may result in the creation of large gaps between the proximal and distal tibia; however, this can be effectively managed with future distraction or with nonvascularized bone grafts. In cases of osteomyelitis, the bone is debrided until a negative residual bone culture is identified; however, it may require repeated debridements to achieve this.[1] Segmental defects in the fibula are of little consequence, particularly when localized away from the ankle or knee articulation.

Once the wound is prepared for coverage, a careful evaluation of the underlying tissues and the dimensions of the particular defect is carried out. Assessment of the longitudinal dimension of the wound is critical as the soleus muscle has a narrow arc of rotation, thereby limiting the use of this muscle for long defects. Splitting the muscle in the midline may improve this arc of rotation, but this reduces the volume of muscle available to close any specific open wound. Although there are no specific surface area dimensions that prohibit use of the soleus flap, wounds measuring more than 10 cm in length must be approached with caution.

INDICATIONS

The soleus muscle is generally used for soft tissue reconstruction in the lower extremity. In most circumstances, this involves coverage of exposed tibial segments. Although these defects are typically located in the middle third of the tibia, at times this flap can be used for coverage of wounds located in the distal third of the leg and around the medial and lateral malleoli. Most of these middle-third defects are located in the anterior pretibial region since the posterior aspect of the leg has ample soft tissue for coverage with either a skin graft or various local fasciocutaneous flaps. These defects usually result from open fractures, chronic osteomyelitis, tumor resection, burns, and, in some cases, soft tissue loss about the ankle with exposure of the underlying joint space and Achilles tendon. Clearly, the nature and cause of the wound influence the treatment options with regard to timing and specific flap options.

As the dominant blood supply is located proximally in the leg, the soleus flap is ideal for coverage of middle-third defects.[2] The arc of rotation is usually made at the transition zone between the proximal and middle thirds of the leg where the vascular pedicle is located.[1] This necessarily creates a flap with a broad base, subsequently producing a narrow arc of rotation, which limits the movement of the flap. Short and relatively narrow defects can be easily closed; however, wide defects in this area may not be amenable to this form of coverage. Should the soleus muscle extend to the level of the ankle, this will allow for coverage of defects in the distal third of the leg and ankle. In these cases, it has been helpful to explore the distal muscle first, before resorting to alternative techniques.

Hemi-soleus flaps, which are often mentioned in the literature, obviously provide even less bulk than more standard techniques. Although this can be a reliable transfer, this author finds this dissection to be quite tedious, and it is not frequently used in clinical practice. From an anatomic standpoint, there are clear advantages to the use of hemi-soleus flaps.[3] As mentioned, dividing the muscle along the intermuscular septum clearly improves the arc of rotation and reach of the flap. Distally based flaps, specifically medially based hemi-soleus flaps, can be raised on the distal medial perforators arising from the posterior tibial artery. Reversed transfer of the lateral hemi-soleus muscle is questionable as there are no major distal segmental peroneal perforators to the lateral segment, and there are few vascular connections from the posterior tibial vessels that cross the distal midline. The entire soleus muscle can be transferred in a reverse fashion using a technique in which the posterior tibial vessels are divided at their popliteal origin and the posterior tibial vessels and soleus muscle are reversed together. However, this technique involves sacrifice of a major vessel to the lower extremity and, as such, is rarely utilized. Distally based flaps can be raised on the distal medial perforators arising from the posterior tibial artery. Care must be taken to ensure the adequacy of these perforators before transfer. The proximal musculature of the soleus is relatively unreliable in these transfers and must not be relied on for soft tissue coverage of the specific wound. As such, use of these flaps is limited to the area of the ankle and particularly the medial malleolus. Preoperative Doppler examination of this pedicle is quite helpful in planning this distally based flap.

CONTRAINDICATIONS

There are relatively few absolute contraindications to the use of the soleus flap. As previously mentioned, the dimensions of the wound may obviate the use of this flap for lower extremity coverage. Exploration and evaluation of the muscle may give the surgeon an insight into the relative size of this muscle and the appropriateness of the transfer. Should this result in an inadequate amount of soft tissue needed for coverage, consideration for the use of additional regional tissue or a free tissue transfer must be considered.

Clearly, lack of adequate inflow contraindicates the use of this flap. This may occur in the setting of both chronic and acute ischemia of the lower extremity. Patients with claudication and rest pain must be evaluated preoperatively to determine the degree of impaired perfusion. Noninvasive Doppler studies can delineate areas of segmental obstruction and regional areas of hypoperfusion. Should multiple levels of proximal occlusion be identified, caution must be used before considering this flap as an option. In many cases, revascularization with bypass grafts or angioplasty may provide the inflow necessary to achieve a successful transfer. Acute ischemia, generally following trauma, is usually corrected at the time of the initial injury. Vascular repairs performed above the knee should not affect the use of this flap. The more troublesome situation occurs when the vascular insult involves the segment of the leg below the knee. In this situation, there is usually direct injury to the soleus muscle itself and the possibility for interruption of the major segmental perforators. Severe muscular contusion and areas of discontinuity of the muscle may also occur and significantly limit its potential use. A history of a previous compartment syndrome also in effect denotes a significant injury to this region. In most such cases, prompt compartment release without further evidence of muscle necrosis allows for the use of this flap. When these situations occur, the prudent course of action typically involves exploration of the muscle before transfer, which can often be performed at the time of wound debridement. Should any doubt exist regarding the integrity of the flap, other options for soft tissue coverage, such as free tissue transfer, should be considered.

ROOM SETUP

Since the majority of these procedures are performed for anterior defects, the patient is best positioned supine. Prone positioning can be used; however, this makes inset of the flap quite difficult. An extension placed at the foot of the operating table is essential. This simple maneuver allows the surgeon ample room to sit comfortably near the operating field without being restricted by the joints of the table. A tourniquet is always used, which allows for operation in a bloodless field. Patients who have undergone proximal vascular bypass grafts, particularly those that have been recently performed, may be an exception to this standard practice. The use of a sterile tourniquet facilitates using the ipsilateral extremity for harvest of a split-thickness skin graft when needed. Placing a hip roll under the contralateral hip allows easy access to the medial aspect of the involved limb. This simple maneuver makes dissection of the proximal half of the soleus much simpler.

PATIENT MARKINGS

A medial approach to the soleus muscle remains the simplest and safest method for harvesting this flap. Although a posterior approach can be used, this makes dissection from the overlying gastrocnemius quite tedious. As previously mentioned, inset of the flap into an anterior defect, given this positioning, would be quite cumbersome for the surgeon as well as the assistant. A lateral dissection is limited by the presence of the fibula, not to mention the close proximity of the peroneal nerve, and is generally not recommended.

Given that the soleus is densely attached to the posterolateral aspect of the tibia, the incision is marked in a vertical direction along the posterior lip of the tibia. This extends from the origin of the Achilles tendon to an area approximately 6 cm below the knee. Should additional length

be needed, the incision can be extended in both a proximal and distal direction. A lateral approach can be used, and a linear incision just posterior to the fibula is recommended.

OPERATIVE TECHNIQUE

PERTINENT ANATOMY

The soleus muscle is a long, broad, flat muscle located within the posterior compartment of the leg. The muscle is situated between the two heads of the gastrocnemius posteriorly and the intermuscular septum of the deep posterior compartment anteriorly. The plantaris tendon, when present, lies between the soleus and gastrocnemius muscles and serves to roughly identify the median raphe between the medial and lateral heads of the soleus. The soleus takes its origin from the proximal posterior surface of the fibula and from the posterior and medial surface of the tibia. Distally, the soleus joins the fascial extensions of the gastrocnemius to form the Achilles tendon. The muscular portion of the soleus extends well beyond the fascial zone of the gastrocnemius and, in many cases, may be found at the level of the ankle.

The blood supply to the soleus is segmental, with what is considered a dominant proximal vascular blood supply. This muscle is therefore classified as a type II muscle. The segmental vessels arise from the popliteal, posterior tibial, and peroneal vessels. Proximally, all three vessels contribute to the blood supply and remain the dominant source of nutrient flow. These axial vessels provide sufficient flow to allow successful harvesting of the muscle along its entire anatomic course. In the distal aspect of the leg, the posterior tibial artery supplies the distal medial head of the soleus, with the peroneal artery supplying the lateral segment. This distal perfusion serves as the basis for the reverse soleus flap. Similarly, the innervation to the two heads of the muscle is independent; the medial popliteal and tibial nerves provide this innervation. Myocutaneous flaps can also be raised, based on the accompanying cutaneous vessels, particularly in the distal-most portions of the leg.

TECHNIQUE

Gaining access to the soleus in the posterior compartment is rather straightforward. With the leg exsanguinated and the tourniquet inflated, the anterior wound is usually extended proximally and distally at a level just posterior to the tibia along the medial aspect of the leg (Figure 86.1).

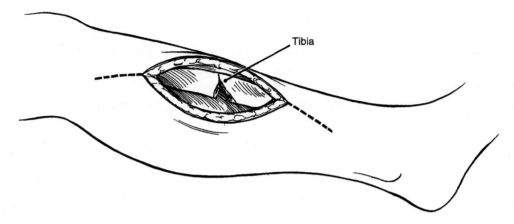

Figure 86.1. Large open fracture and soft tissue deformity in middle third of leg. Debridement has been completed and tourniquet inflated. Incisions are extended proximally and distally below posterior edge of tibia to gain access to underlying posterior compartment.

Using cautery dissection, the subcutaneous tissue is opened down to the level of the fascia of the posterior compartment. Often the greater saphenous vein can be spared by simply retracting the vein posteriorly. Proximally, the medial head of the gastrocnemius muscle is identified and the plane between the gastrocnemius and soleus is opened (Figure 86.2). Multiple perforating branches between these two muscles are controlled with surgical clips or with cautery, being careful to avoid injuring the plantaris tendon (Figure 86.3). Again, the plantaris tendon identifies the median raphe of the soleus muscle, which is helpful when

performing a hemi-soleus rotation flap. Anteriorly, the soleus is dissected from the tibial origin. Care must be taken to avoid entering the deep posterior compartment, located just anterior to the soleus muscle, where injury to the posterior tibial and peroneal neurovascular bundles can occur.

Elevation of the soleus is most easily begun at the distal extent of the muscle at its junction with the Achilles tendon. Self-retaining retractors are placed between the tibia anteriorly and the gastrocnemius and Achilles tendon posteriorly to enhance exposure. A scalpel is used to gently dissect the soleus fibers from the anterior aspect of the

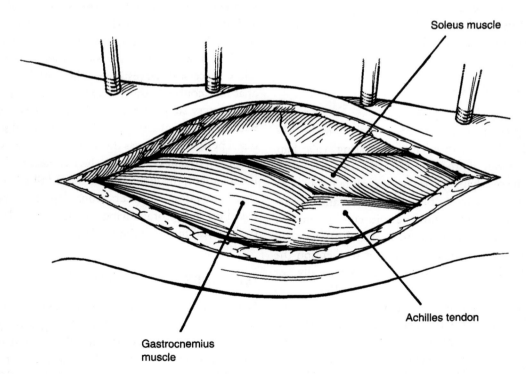

Figure 86.2. Plane between gastrocnemius and soleus muscle is identified and opened. This is best accomplished in middle third of leg, proximal to Achilles tendon.

EXTREMITY RECONSTRUCTION

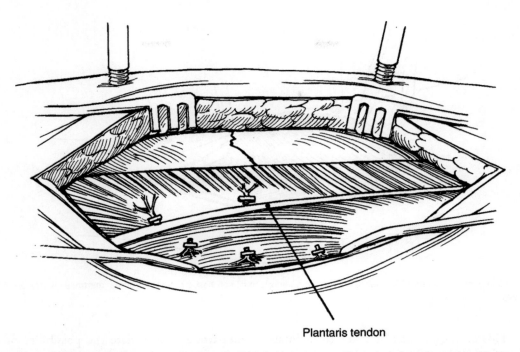

Plantaris tendon

Figure 86.3. Perforating vessels between gastrocnemius and soleus are divided with cautery or with surgical clips, allowing identification of plantaris tendon in midline.

tendon. This dissection can be facilitated by using a gentle stroking motion with the bevel of the scalpel directed at a 45-degree angle to the Achilles tendon. As the dissection proceeds proximally, small vessels are controlled with the bipolar or simple cautery, which makes obtaining hemostasis easier when the tourniquet is deflated. An Allis clamp is placed at the distal aspect of the muscle to provide traction, which also facilitates this sharp dissection. If a hemi-soleus flap is chosen, the median raphe is divided as the dissection proceeds proximally. Larger perforators from the posterior tibial and peroneal vessels are controlled, as they are encountered, with surgical clips. This dissection must be carried proximally, far enough to allow sufficient anterior rotation into the adjacent defect

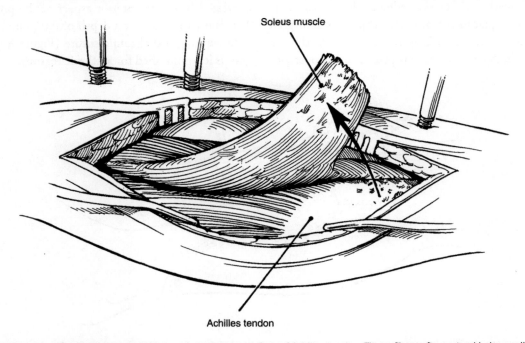

Soleus muscle

Achilles tendon

Figure 86.4. Terminal fibers of soleus are sharply dissected from anterior surface of Achilles tendon. These fibers often extend below malleolus in children and some adults. Dissection proceeds proximally until appropriate arc of rotation is achieved.

SOLEUS FLAP FOR LOWER LEG RECONSTRUCTION

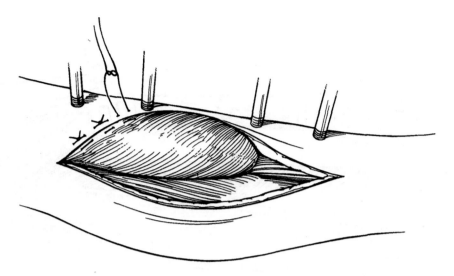

Figure 86.5. Following complete dissection of flap, soleus is rotated anteriorly to fill soft tissue defect. Horizontal mattress sutures are placed to bring muscle beneath adjacent skin margin.

(Figure 86.4). However, care must be taken to maintain the proximal perforating branches to avoid devascularizing the flap. Lateral release of the soleus from the tibia can improve this arc of rotation without the potential for injuring the blood supply. If this is performed quite proximal in the leg, care must be taken to avoid injuring the peroneal nerve as it enters the lateral compartment. When sufficient rotation is achieved, the muscle can be inset into the defect. Horizontal mattress sutures of 3-0 nylon are used for this purpose (Figure 86.5).

By suturing behind the free muscle border, the flap is brought beneath the free skin edge as these sutures are tied. This makes placement of a split-thickness skin graft much simpler and easier to keep in contact with the underlying muscle. A suction drain is placed in the posterior

compartment to obviate the possibility of postoperative hematoma. An additional drain can be placed beneath the flap if significant drainage is expected. Access incisions are closed in two layers without reapproximation of the posterior compartment fascia.

Once the flap is secured into position, the tourniquet is released and an assessment of perfusion to the muscle is made. Excess tension on the muscle may prevent sufficient blood flow; therefore, additional proximal release may be needed. If the flap is well-perfused, a split-thickness skin graft is then placed. As previously noted, this can be harvested from the anterior aspect of the proximal thigh. This is usually taken at a depth of 0.016 inch and secured with running 5-0 chromic suture (Figure 86.6). The skin graft is left unmeshed for aesthetic reasons.

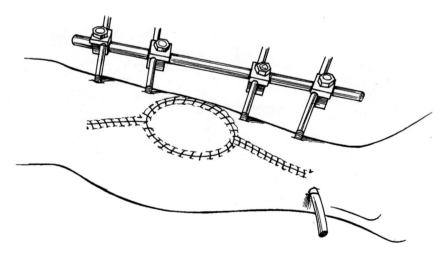

Figure 86.6. Split-thickness skin graft is placed and secured with running 5-0 chromic sutures. Sheet grafts are preferable. Closed suction drain is routinely used.

EXTREMITY RECONSTRUCTION

DRESSINGS AND SPLINTS

At the completion of the operative procedure, placement of adequate dressings is essential to a successful outcome. The skin graft is covered with a nonadherent dressing impregnated with antibiotic ointment. This nonadherent gauze is also used to cover the remaining suture lines and to surround each drain site. Circumferential coverage with gauze rolls and cast padding are placed extending from the midthigh to the level of the metatarsal heads. The heel must be further padded with soft foam to prevent pressure ulceration in this area. The dressing is completed by placing a long-leg plaster splint, which is held in place with Ace wraps. It is essential that the ankle be placed in a neutral position to maintain the remaining gastrocnemius musculature out to length and to avoid the potential for an equinus deformity. A slight amount of knee flexion also avoids the tendency to develop localized pressure effects in the popliteal fossa.

POSTOPERATIVE CARE

The primary component of the postoperative treatment involves the strict elevation of the involved extremity. This maneuver avoids significant edema within the flap and the potential for wound separation and hematoma formation. The splint and original dressing are left in place for 5 days, at which time the dressing is changed and the drains removed. Careful removal of the dressing allows for observation of the flap and assessment of the viability of the skin graft. Nonadherent dressings are replaced and are maintained for 10–14 days. The continued use of a splint beyond the first week is based on the underlying orthopedic status of the involved tibia and fibula. The remaining sutures are removed 2–3 weeks postoperatively, during which time continued elevation of the involved extremity is recommended. At this point, progressive dangling for periods of 5–10 minutes is started. If no significant flap edema results, these time periods of leg dependency can be rapidly increased over the next 1–2 weeks. At this point, full weight-bearing can be started should the orthopedic status of the extremity permit. During this time, it is often helpful to keep the leg wrapped in an Ace bandage to avoid unnecessary edema in the lower extremity. Physical therapy may commence at any point in the patient's recovery, as long as the preceding guidelines are followed.

CAVEATS

The soleus muscle flap is a reliable method for soft tissue coverage in the middle third of the leg and, in some cases, the distal third. Careful analysis of the wound's dimensions can greatly influence the suitability of this flap for the specific defect. Flap elevation is best performed under tourniquet control, using sharp dissection to elevate the distal muscle from the Achilles tendon. Horizontal mattress sutures allow secure inset of the muscle behind the skin margin, and unmeshed skin grafts provide an improved cosmetic appearance of these transfers in the long term. The efficacy of postoperative anticoagulants in the postoperative period to prevent thromboembolic events is generally favored by this author.

REFERENCES

1. Patzakis MJ, Abdollahi K, Sherman R, et al. Treatment of chronic osteomyelitis with muscle flaps. *Orthop Clin North Am* 1993;24:505–509.
2. McCraw JB, Arnold G. *McCraw and Arnold's Atlas of Muscle and Musculocutaneous Flaps.* Norfolk, VA: Hampton Press, 1986:545–547.
3. Tobin GR. Hemi-soleus and reversed hemi-soleus flaps. *Plast Reconst Surg* 1985;76:87–96.

87.

LATISSIMUS DORSI FLAP FOR LEG RECONSTRUCTION

Marek K. Dobke and Gina A. Mackert

The latissimus dorsi (LD) myocutaneous flap is one of the most popular and reliable anatomical units used for reconstruction of extensive tissue defects. The advantages are its consistent anatomy, its long and versatile vascular pedicle (with vascular side branches), its large size, and its ease in the obliteration of three-dimensional defects. Additionally, the LD flap can be raised as a chimeric flap or as multiple small "subflaps" from a single donor site, with all constituent parts originating from the single vascular pedicle. This then can be utilized for a simultaneous repair of lining, the obliteration of dead space, and for coverage, which presents an alternative to raising multiple free flaps resulting in multiple donor sites.

The LD flap is classified as a type V flap, displaying a dominant pedicle consisting of the thoracodorsal vessels and secondary segmental perforating vessels consisting of branches of the posterior intercostal vessels. The LD flap can be transferred either as a pedicled or a microvascular anastomosis requiring a free flap. Its composition can be solely muscle tissue, but it can be also dissected as a musculocutaneous or even an osteomyocutaneous flap, including a scapular or rib bone segment. With a size of up to 20 × 35 cm and the possibility of combining it with other components nourished by the subscapular system such as the serratus anterior muscle, it is one of the most versatile flap options available.

ASSESSMENT OF THE DEFECT AND WOUND PARAMETERS

There are many criteria that need to be taken into account when considering reconstruction of a complex defect. Location, size, structure(s) damaged or missing, trauma or other etiology, and postoperative functional requirements all need to be considered and the reconstructive options carefully weighed out in terms of benefits and drawbacks. The essential parameters to understanding a particular wound in the lower extremity include the size and location of the defect, the specific tissues lost, and the type of tissues or implants exposed. Large composite defects of the lower extremity, regardless of whether they are in and around the knee or closer to the ankle, will, more often than not, require a microsurgical reconstruction, while small, contained defects (i.e., sinus tracts) with little or no actual tissue loss may be amenable to local rotational flaps.

Additionally, comorbidities and rehabilitation potential, as well as the social and cultural considerations of the patient, need to be incorporated into the equation to develop a comprehensive and optimally tailored strategy for defect reconstruction. Assessment of any particular defect before deciding on reconstructive alternatives should begin with taking a thorough history and performing a thorough physical examination. The assessment of a patient and his or her lower extremity problem and wound should not just be about the "flap surgery" but must be undertaken in the context of strategy for leg salvation. Previous operative procedures and any previous history of trauma, compartment syndrome type of problems, irradiation, smoking, or long-term drug therapy must be taken into account. The patient's occupational, family, and social history are crucial for the development of a long-term strategy for lower extremity reconstruction because all reconstructive efforts must have as their ultimate goal not only the closure of the wound, but also the return to a productive, premorbid lifestyle, and this must be carefully measured against the standard of early amputation with functional prosthetic fitting.

Reconstruction utilizing the LD flap for leg reconstruction implies microsurgical tissue transfer for the repair of extensive or composite tissue defects.

The most common causes of soft tissue and bone loss requiring the LD flap for microsurgical reconstruction are injuries with open fractures and concomitant soft tissue loss. The discussion of multiple classifications for detailed stratification of soft tissue and bone injuries is beyond the scope of this chapter. However, for operative planning, one must take into account not only the size of the wound and the nature of the exposed structures, but also the extent of the zone of injury resulting from the strength and velocity of the injuring force. A progressive increase in the extent of the tissue loss and a concomitant perfusion decrease is common for high-impact wounds. Whenever possible, microvascular anastomoses should be performed away from the zone of injury (or tissue damaged by infection, radiation, etc.). The extent of the true zone of injury, including vascular injury, can be judged best by a tissue assessment during serial debridements.

Intraoperative laser angiography using the SPY System (LifeCell Corporation, Branchburg, NJ) is useful for the assessment of tissue perfusion and frequently for the determination of the extent of wound debridement. The SPY System uses the contrast agent indocyanine green, which has an excellent safety profile and pharmacokinetic characteristics that allow for repeated evaluations during the same surgical procedure. The SPY System has demonstrated high sensitivity and specificity for the detection of tissues at risk for ischemia and necrosis during reconstructive surgery, which could have otherwise complicated definitive microsurgical repairs.

Other defects, such as those resulting from chronic osteomyelitis, unstable soft tissue coverage of skeletal structures, postablative defects after tumor resection, and exposed or infected total joint prostheses, frequently require microvascular repairs. Infrequently, microsurgical reconstruction might play a role after severe thermal or radiation injury to the extremity and, in rare cases, for corrective surgery of congenital abnormalities.

Neurovascular status assessment is of paramount significance while planning leg reconstruction. The quality of arterial inflow or venous outflow, as well as any insufficiency, should be analyzed. Peripheral pulses should be documented and quantitated. Vascular examination can be further documented noninvasively with duplex Doppler imaging. Angiography remains a definitive radiologic test for the examination of the arterial tree, especially at the infrapopliteal level.

Sensory examination is mandatory and should focus on weight-bearing surfaces. Range of motion of each joint should be assessed in comparison to the opposite, normal side. Any additional limb-length discrepancy must be noted. Supplemental evaluations beyond the physical examination are limited to plain x-ray films in the traumatic setting and can be supplemented by computed tomographic scans, magnetic resonance imaging, or specialized bone scanning (whichever is most appropriate regarding the oncologic situation).

Even large but "skin-level" wounds, such as abrasions, burns, and degloving injuries, after adequate debridement(s), can result in a wound that is eminently closed using split-thickness skin grafts. However, composite tissue losses resulting in exposure or defects of osseous or neurovascular structures, joint spaces, and denuded tendons are all candidates for microsurgical tissue transfer for defect repair. Most commonly, type III open fractures of the tibia with bony comminution and overlying soft tissue loss demand free tissue transfer for adequate wound healing and minimization of subsequent chronic osteomyelitis. In acute circumstances, an accurate tabulation of each structure that is damaged or lost helps the reconstructive surgeons focus their decision-making toward reconstructive alternatives. In chronic wounds, it is imperative to assess the defect only after complete and thorough debridement has been undertaken. Choosing a reconstructive option before completing debridement inevitably leads to underappreciation of the size and complexity of the wound requirements. When evaluating wounds in and around the foot and ankle, ambulation dynamics must be taken into account: (1) Is the defect on a weight-bearing surface, and (2) how will this affect the choice of tissue transfer options?

INDICATIONS AND PLANNING TIPS

The LD muscle has become one of the main workhorses on the free tissue transfer market for good reasons (Figure 87.1).

Its large size, thickness, and tissue robustness, and its overall flat configuration allows its conformation to leg defects of virtually any size and shape. It is thin and quickly broadens from its insertional fibers to provide a large rhomboid muscle that can be transferred almost entirely on its proximal pedicle. The thoracodorsal artery, usually 2–4 mm in diameter, is joined by two venae comitantes to form a single large thoracodorsal vein, 3–5 mm in diameter, prior to entering the subscapular vein. The neurovascular hilum is approximately 9 cm from the axillary vessels and enters the deep LD muscle surface 2–3 cm from its anterior

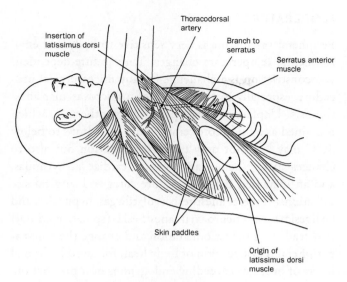

Figure 87.1. The latissimus dorsi flap can be harvested as muscle or myocutaneous flap. It may be accompanied by serratus muscle and a scapular/parascapular flap (with or without bone), all of which are perfused by the subscapular system. Typically, the latissimus dorsi free flap is raised and transferred on the thoracodorsal vascular pedicle. Perforating branches to the skin are clustered over intramuscular branches of the thoracodorsal vessels: these branches parallel the anterior and the superior border of the muscle. Nevertheless, when designing the skin paddle, hand-held Doppler examination should be performed to verify the location of perforating branches.

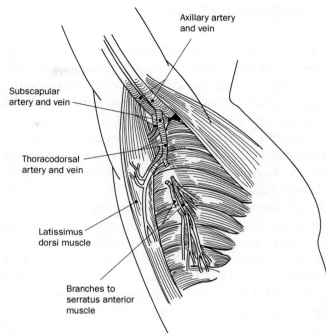

Figure 87.2. When harvesting the latissimus dorsi flap, the muscle is extensively mobilized before the pedicle is visualized. For even better visualization of the pedicle, it can be detached distally and lifted cranially. The serratus branch should be taken near its origin to maximize pedicle length.

border. Components of the subscapular system, which can be included in the pedicle dissection, allow the creation of flow-through flaps and the restoration of vascular defects. The flap can also be dissected as part of the large monobloc (fasciocutaneous parascapular flap, together with an ipsilateral latissimus dorsi muscle flap harvested on a common neurovascular pedicle). In large defects (e.g., after posterior compartment resection for sarcoma), the vessels of the monobloc transfer serve as a segmental interposition to restore arterial continuity: proximally, the subscapular artery, and, distally, the thoracodorsal artery are used to bridge the tibial artery defect. To achieve Achilles tendon motor function, the LD muscle flap can be reinnervated by anastomosing the tibial nerve stump to the thoracodorsal nerve.

The thoracodorsal vessels and the nerve usually bifurcate within the muscle with one main descending branch usually located parallel and just behind the anterior border of the muscle and the upper, transverse branch directed medially below the superomedial border of the muscle. This typical topography provides the anatomic basis for the partial muscle-sparing LD flap or the split-flap dissection variants. Thoracodorsal vessel perforator flaps are based on the capillary perforators arising from the descending

vascular branches; the diameter of these perforators passing through the anterior border of the LD muscle is usually 0.3–0.5 mm.

The LD muscle can be elevated solely as a muscle flap or with an overlying cutaneous paddle. The latter option is rarely used in reconstruction of lower extremity defects because of its bulk. A skin paddle can restrict muscle folding if a three-dimensional defect is being reconstructed. It is easier to complete the surgery with subsequent skin grafting of the muscle surface. The serratus anterior branch coming off the thoracodorsal vessels allows for companion harvest of the inferior portion of the serratus anterior muscle in circumstances in which an extremely large surface area must be covered (Figure 87.2).

If needed (because of the surface requirement), coverage of leg amputation stumps using a free LD flap (optionally with a serratus anterior muscle) provides durable coverage allowing the preservation of functional joints and bony stump length. Another prime indication for the latissimus dorsi flap involves the acute coverage of an endoprosthesis placed after musculoskeletal tumor ablation. Coverage of the prosthesis requires a surprisingly large amount of tissue, which, when deep defect repair and resurfacing are added into the equation, leaves few options other than the LD.

CONTRAINDICATIONS

Contraindications for the LD flap are based on donor site tissue suitability. Donor site contraindications for LD muscle flaps are rare. It would be relatively contraindicated to harvest the LD from a patient who is entirely dependent on the shoulder girdle musculature for locomotion (i.e., paraplegics). Previous thoracic surgery in the form of a posterolateral thoracotomy for lung resection usually divides the latissimus in its mid-substance. The presence of a scar consistent with a previous thoracotomy incision should steer the reconstructive microsurgeon away from this donor site. Previous axillary dissection or irradiation for breast cancer should signal a possible transection of the thoracodorsal pedicle or loss of proximal blood flow secondary to obliterative fibrosis, respectively. In either case, if the LD is to be considered as a reconstructive option, patency of the thoracodorsal artery must be assured preoperatively and back-up options should be well planned in case of an intraoperative circulatory problem. In circumstances like these, the most practical methods are physical and Doppler ultrasound examinations. During the examination, the patient may be asked to contract the muscle, which—if its vascularity and, by default, robustness is unimpaired—should form a solid posterior axillary fold. If there is still doubt, the Doppler blood flow evaluation should be done. Overall, removal of the muscle is associated with surprisingly minimal functional deficit, however, individuals active in skiing, tennis, and sports requiring throwing may notice a decrease in their strength and velocity.

ROOM SETUP

Throughout these often very lengthy and complex operations, it is crucial that the surgeon retains his or her ability to concentrate optimally on each part of the procedure. While many technical factors are under limited control, it is imperative that all possible controllable variables regarding the physical and situational configuration of the operating room are adjusted to favor the comfort and functionality of the surgical team. These elements include room temperature, lighting, surgeon comfort, and tool quality. Briefing the surgical team about the case and checking on microscope and instruments well before the surgery itself helps to minimize the potential for downtime during the procedure.

TEMPERATURE

Peripheral vasculature is very sensitive to body and environmental temperature changes. Temperature-dependent vasoconstriction is a challenge for any microsurgical procedure, especially in the middle of a microvascular anastomosis. Unplanned intraoperative hypothermia, which is defined as a body core temperature that drops to below 36°C may lead not only to vasoconstriction but also to changes in the hemostatic system, cardiac arrhythmias, and an increased risk for pressure sores and surgical site infections. General anesthesia (volatile gas, hypnotics, and analgesics) and neuroaxial anesthesia (spinal, epidural) may lead to initial vasodilatation and change the core-to-peripheral redistribution of body heat, followed by several hours of heat loss exceeding endogenous heat production. This can lead to a reduction in core body temperature and ultimately to hypothermia and peripheral vasoconstriction which is difficult to reverse. Prewarming of the operating room and the body prior to anesthesia induction reduces the core-to-peripheral temperature gradient, increases total body heat, and thus is essential to the prevention of intraoperative hypothermia. Circulating warm water, resistive heating circuits, heated local air (e.g., "Bear Hugger"), and forced warm air into the operating room are effective warming techniques applicable to microsurgery. It is important to remember that by the time the patient's body temperature has dropped, a simple rise in room temperature will not yield sufficiently fast results, while the surgeon, already sweating from physical strain, shining operative lights, and layers of surgical garments, will find himself in an uncomfortable, subjectively overheated situation possibly impacting the technical stamina of himself and the surgical team.

LIGHTING

Optimal visualization of the surgical site is the most crucial aspect regarding the operating environment. If the lighting is suboptimal, even the most delicate instruments and most high-tech microscopes are of little value, and the surgeon's work, regardless of his degree of skill, may be compromised. Thus, preoperatively, the overhead lights should be inspected for functionality and level of brightness and placed in a favorable position for the illumination of the anticipated area of the defect to be addressed. The microscope should be set up to allow the surgeon(s) to see the target without quitting the eyepiece of the microscope (e.g., to adjust the field of vision). New models of surgical loupes with such technical features as prismatic design, are lightweight, small, and provide maximum peripheral vision, adjustable neutral white light, increased contrast and depth of field, and blue cable technology for surgeon's protection from burns are particularly useful for assisting surgeons.

SURGEON COMFORT

With the stereotype of the surgeon seen as an indestructible human being working tirelessly without sentiments of hunger, stiffness, pain, or fatigue, the basic and ergonomic needs of the surgeon are often last on the list of priorities. Microsurgical procedures are demanding both mentally and physically. They often require the surgeon to work for hours and pose a strain on the entire body due to unusual and often uncomfortable positions, with various attached gadgets. This can lead to premature physical and mental fatigue and loss of concentration when needed most (during the microsurgery part).

One of the variables that can be optimized to enhance ergonomics is patient positioning. Time spent on optimal patient positioning always pays off. The surgeon must be able to access freely all operative sites on the patient without restrictions. This can be aided by a flexible and height-adjustable operating table, with enough room underneath to accommodate the surgeon's lower extremities, especially during the microsurgical part. There should be enough room provided for the instrumentation stands and Mayo tables, and the instrumenting nurse should be placed in such a fashion that she or he can hand out and receive instruments in an ergonomically favorable manner. Similarly, it should be ensured that other equipment is up to satisfactory standards. For example, the surgeon should request a comfortable chair, ergonomically cushioned, that is adjustable in height and, depending on the surgeon's preference, is equipped with an arm or backrest. Options should be considered for optimal arm, elbow, and wrist supports to allow the surgeon to comfortably focus on the delicate manipulation involved in the microsurgical part of the procedure and prevent muscular fatigue and possible subsequent muscular tremors.

Even though all of these aspects can be established in a work-flow protocol, it is advisable for the surgeon to personally involve himself in the preoperative check and setup. It is the surgeon's responsibility to brief the team, and convey requests for unusual equipment, and enforce an operating room setup that will foster efficiency.

INSTRUMENTATION

Every microsurgeon has come to prefer different types of instrumentarium for grasping, cutting, and suturing under the microscope. There are many aspects that can be customized; for example, the length of the shaft, the weight (for balance), and the shape of the handle of the instrument chosen can play an important role and all are subject of individual preference. The surgeon, wielding the most delicate instruments, may still feel extremely awkward if the length of the instrument is not adjusted correctly and is not ergonomic considering the size of her or his hands. Generally, mid-length shaft instruments (13 cm) work well for anastomosis in the distal lower extremity. Some helpful features seem to be more universal: nonmagnetic or demagnetized instruments with matte or nonreflective surfaces make work more enjoyable and less tiring for the eyes under a high-intensity microscope. Certain accessories such as colored background sheets, microsurgical flexible suction mats, and colored vessel loops can facilitate the operation. Bipolar forceps with gold tips (e.g., Aesculap, Center Valley, PA) to reduce tissue and coagulated tissue adherence to the forceps surface seem luxurious but are a useful tool to avoid microstructural damage secondary to adherence and inadvertent pull.

Instruments must be functioning flawlessly. A cutting tool that does not cut with ease has a tendency to rip tissue apart, which is a serious problem especially in microsurgery, potentially doing an uncontrollable amount of damage detrimental to the whole surgical outcome. The same holds true for suture quality, Doppler probe, and other equipment and supplies used during the surgery.

LATISSIMUS DORSI FLAP

PATIENT MARKINGS AND POSITIONING

The LD muscle flap is almost always harvested with the patient in the lateral decubitus position, although LD flap harvest is also possible in supine and prone positions. Preoperative patient markings of the unit—outline, perforators, and skin paddle—should reflect understanding of the anatomy of the flap and the surgical plan objectives. The ipsilateral extremity should be placed on a well-padded stand (e.g., Mayo stand) and included into the operative field to allow maneuvering. The insertion of the muscle into the bicipital groove of the humerus, the trapezius muscle, and the LD anterior border extending from the posterior aspect of the posterior axillary fold to the iliac crest should be identified and marked. The trapezius muscle should be marked superiorly and medially, tracing it inferiorly where it overlaps the superomedial origin of the latissimus. The inferior tip and edges of the scapula should be marked as the next landmark. These markings help to identify the insertion of the rhomboid muscles and their subsequent separation from the LD. If a skin portion is to be used, its design and position over the muscle will determine the cutaneous incision and the resultant donor site scar. Elliptical (providing ease of direct closure) skin paddles can be designed over the subtending latissimus, usually centered on the rich perfusion through perforators along the anterior or superior borders of the muscle.

TECHNIQUE

In the lateral approach, the patient's body should be supported by an inflatable bean bag, with padding over the bony prominences, kidney rests, or total arthroplasty supports and axillary soft rolls. In the lateral position approach, the patient should be shifted close to the edge of the operating table and close to the flap-dissecting surgeon. The entire hemithorax should be prepared and draped out with the arm prepared into the field and preferably covered with a tube stockinette. Manipulation of the extremity allows for optimal visualization during pedicle dissection. The assistant and the primary surgeon must avoid excess abduction or extension of the shoulder to prevent excessive stretching of the brachial plexus. A heating blanket or mattress and a warmed-up operating room prevent problems resulting from peripheral vasoconstriction.

Typically, the initial incision line for muscle elevation can be placed obliquely, parallel to and approximately 3–4 cm behind to its anterior border for a direct LD exposure. By palpation, the exact location of the axillary artery can be appreciated. The hilum of the thoracodorsal artery as it enters the muscle is approximately 10 cm distal to this point with the arm in the abducted position and should be remarked. The skin and subcutaneous tissue should be elevated off the muscle fascia. If the skin paddle is part of the LD flap, it should be dissected as an island over the muscle. Any shearing of both structures against each other, which will potentially disrupt perforator integrity, should be avoided. For this same reason, an outward beveling of the blade from the skin edge to the muscle helps to ensure maximum capture of the musculocutaneous perforators.

After the skin and subcutaneous tissue incision, as well as the exposure of the muscle edge, a plane between the lateral chest and LD should be developed, preferably

distal to the presumed entry of thoracodorsal vessels into the muscle and proximal to the fusion of the LD muscle and the serratus anterior muscle. At this point, the decision has to be made whether the serratus anterior muscle and the LD flap will be harvested together. If not, then the arterial and venous branches to the serratus anterior muscle should be identified and divided. The LD tissue should be separated from its attachments to the serratus anterior and the lower ribs. Prior to the commitment to the level of distal and medial LD muscle division, the LD muscle flap length should be reassessed and some extra tissue taken to avoid a situation where the flap is too small because the muscle will retract upon division of its distal and medial borders. Actually, the LD flap should be harvested in an oversized fashion. The flap can be lifted toward the posterior neck to allow access for dissection of the areolar tissue and the neurovascular thoracodorsal bundle within, toward the axilla and providing adequate exposure of the neurovascular pedicle components. Medially, identification of the rhomboid muscle fibers, oriented in different directions than those of the LD, will allow for the separation of both structures. Once the desired extent of the vascular pedicle is exposed, vessel loops should be placed around the artery, vein, and nerve (if not divided at this point) separately, as well as soaks with vasodilating agent (e.g., papaverine or plain lidocaine solution or other agents).

The humeral attachment of the LD muscle should be divided above the neurovascular pedicle: vessel loops help to retract and protect the vessels while the manipulation of the upper extremity orientation helps to identify the LD tendon and its differentiation from the teres major and minor muscles. It is worth mentioning that with the muscle freed along its lateral, distal, and medial borders, many recommend folding the muscle upward and outward to begin the pedicle dissection. The completion of the LD muscle release superiorly along the lateral edge of the scapula, paying attention to the identification of the rhomboid muscles and leaving these important for scapula positioning muscles intact, ultimately allows muscle cranial lift for much greater ease in exposing the entire length of the thoracodorsal and proximal subscapular pedicles (and their inclusion into the vascular pedicle if needed).

With the LD flap as an island, it should be left in situ without any tension on the vascular pedicle, and the flap unit should be observed for any signs of perfusion problems (Figure 87.3). If no perfusion problems are encountered, the flap is ready for transfer.

Although it is possible to raise and transfer the LD muscle flap on the serratus branch alone when the

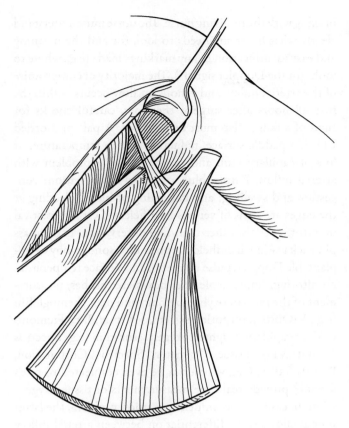

Figure 87.3. The flap muscle can be completely islandized, which maximizes the arc of rotation if used as a pedicled flap and allows for maximum length of pedicle harvest if used as microvascular transfer. Muscle or myocutaneous flap variants are the most common.

proximal thoracodorsal artery and vein are not patent, it is not a commonly held practice and should be reserved for exceptional circumstances (e.g., for breast reconstruction). It would be very impractical and probably unsafe to utilize such an anatomical LD flap variant for leg reconstruction.

FLAP VARIATIONS

Split Latissimus Dorsi

The consistent proximal branching of the LD neurovascular anatomy with the bifurcation of the thoracodorsal vessels (>90%) forming two intramuscular branches permits the surgical splitting of the myocutaneous unit into two flaps. Either or both branches of the split flap can be independently transferred. There are advantages and applications of this relatively consistent anatomy, and they include split-muscle branches, preservation of motor function in the flap donor site with one split muscle branch, and microvascular free tissue transfer of the branched flap or of individual branches.

Pedicled Descending Branch Muscle-Sparing Latissimus Dorsi Flap

The pedicled muscle-sparing LD flap can be a useful adjunct to the reconstructive armamentarium when a relatively small unit with a long vascular leash is needed (e.g., for leg, foot, or partial breast reconstruction). Typically, the skin paddle is centered over the axis of the descending branch of the thoracodorsal vessels. The lateral edge of the skin paddle should be 1–2 cm anterior to the muscle edge to capture lateral perforators. The course of the descending branch should be marked using a handheld Doppler. The skin paddle is raised off the muscle in the subfascial plane with the necessary strip of the muscle, with the thoracodorsal vessels coursing on its undersurface (in a similar fashion to a pedicled muscle-sparing transverse rectus abdominis flap dissection). With well-marked perforators, the pedicled muscle-sparing flap even with the transversely oriented skin paddle may be designed.

Perforator and Perforator-Chimeric Latissimus Dorsi Flap

With the increased popularity of perforator flaps, the chimeric flap's design has benefited from the "perforator flap" concept. In the chimeric flap subset, each component of the unit can be separately placed because each is supplied by a distinct branch off a common source vessel. The LD flap elevation from the lateral thoracic area and composed of a skin LD perforator flap and a minuscule muscular portion harboring vessels is a similar dissection to that of the source vessels of a muscle-sparing flap but more demanding technically when perforating vessels have to be isolated.

Actually, the size of the muscle segment is determined by the size and configuration of the dead space to be obliterated at the recipient site, while the skin portion is determined by the size that needs to be covered. The LD chimeric flap is an example of a classical chimeric flap including source vessels and one perforator flap. If one begins dissection from a source vessel or branch vessels (as opposed to from perforators toward the feeding vessels), then the LD chimeric flap is a classic example of this type of unit. Doppler ultrasound or, even better, color Doppler ultrasonographic preoperative mapping of the capillary perforators from the descending branch of thoracodorsal artery facilitates a safe flap dissection.

Flow-Through Flap

Flow-through flaps are useful when the continuity of distal circulation must be maintained or restored and the steal phenomenon (caused by the flap) minimized. Interposing a "Y" configured vascular network into the leg circulatory system (e.g., with the subscapular artery ensuring inflow and the circumflex scapular artery ensuring distal runoff, and with the thoracodorsal artery also ensuring inflow to the flap), arterial circulation to both distal leg and the flap can be secured. The subscapular vessels (SSV), angular branch, circumflex scapular artery and vein (CSV), and the serratus anterior branch can be all available for combinations of flow-through conduits (Figure 87.4). Interposed arteries may allow bridging of a vascular defect or replacement of an atherosclerotic segment of an artery at the time of free tissue transfer.

MONITORING AND DRESSINGS

After the microvascular tissue transfer surgery has been completed, the critical postoperative period begins. Complications leading to surgical exploration and anastomoses revision have the best chance to succeed if done within the first hour after their occurrence. Postoperative care and monitoring starts with the patient's careful transportation to the recovery room and hospital unit and a

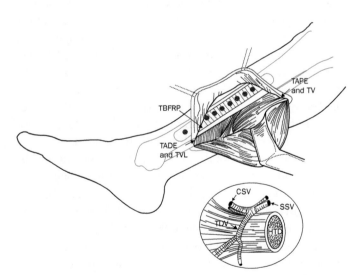

Figure 87.4. Schematic of latissimus dorsi (LD) arterial flow-through flap and its inset in a lower leg. A relatively long vessel defect is depicted. Distal tibial vein end (TVL) is ligated. The tibial artery proximal end (TAPE) and tibial vein (TV) proximally and the tibial artery distal end (TADE) present three recipient sites for microvascular anastomoses to one of the LD flap vessels (two arterial anastomoses and one venous). This enables the conduction of the flap inset and vascular defect bridging by anastomosing the subscapular artery and vein (SSV) to the TAPE and TV, respectively, and the circumflex scapular artery to the TADE. The circumflex scapular vein can be used for supercharging the venous outflow. Other anatomic components shown are the tibial fracture site which is plated (TBFRP), circumflex scapular vessels (CSV), subscapular vessels (SSV), and thoracodorsal vessels (TDV). and humeral tendon divided (HTD).

briefing with the receiving nurse. The nurse must understand clearly what he or she needs to look for and the meaning and easy identification of any markings made (e.g., where to look "for the Doppler signal"). The majority of compromise of the arterial inflow and venous outflow occurs within the first 48 hours after surgery, therefore, careful checks for signs of a failing flap must be followed. A pale or mottled LD skin paddle surface, reduction in flap temperature, or loss of capillary refill and turgor signify a problem with arterial inflow. Purple, blue, or dusky discoloration; congestion and swelling; and darkening of blood bleeding at the edges are signs of venous insufficiency. Other practical monitoring tools, other than flap observation, encompass pinprick testing, handheld Doppler ultrasonography or implantable Doppler, pulse oximetry, and surface temperature monitoring. Implantable laser flowmeter probes, measurement of the ratio of oxyhemoglobin and deoxyhemoglobin (e.g., ViOptix monitoring system, ViOptix, Inc., Fremont, CA), or capillary-weighted oxygen saturation (e.g., Spectros T Stat VLS Tissue Oximeter, Spectros Corporation, Portola Valley, CA, which can be even connected to one's iPhone) provide real-time measurements of tissue oxygenation. In case of an imminent perfusion problem, the latter system allows early differentiation between arterial inflow versus venous outflow compromise. Overall, it is important that the flap is monitored on a regular basis and that the dressing (if any) be nonconcealing and easy to lift or change to expose the flap (e.g., sheet of Xeroform or translucent Biobrane or equivalent material). If the leg is splinted, then "surveillance windows" in the dressing and/or splint are necessary. It is preferred to dress the flap in a manner adherent to "as much as needed, but as little as possible." Circumferential dressings should be avoided whenever possible. Dressing-induced "compartment problems" may lead to the disastrous cessation of blood flow into, from, or through the LD flap.

EXTERNAL FIXATORS AND DRAINS

Many microsurgical cases are complex, so it is not uncommon that defects are not limited to soft tissues only. Bone defects may require temporary stabilization, restoration, or definitive reconstruction. Technical options may include spacers, antibiotic beads, grafts, prostheses, plates, and, in many trauma cases, an external fixator. It is vital to understand that the external fixator serves not only as a tool for fracture reduction and alignment, but also provides a means for wound management.

Understanding the full potential of the usage of an external fixator and the appropriate indications makes it a very powerful tool. The reconstructive microsurgeon should be part of the fixator selection, its spatial configuration, and placement design, all to allow dissection and microsurgical reconstruction, including wound management and the anatomical as well as functional aspects of the postoperative course. The reconstructive surgeon should be aware of the different kinds of external fixation available, such as additional half-frame extensions which will allow elevation of the leg to facilitate wound and flap monitoring as well as dressing changes. External ring fixators may allow dynamic axial loading and bone distraction and may be useful in the absence of longer bone segments in the lower extremity (e.g., extensive tibial bone defect). External fixation devices may be, dependent on the situation, removed and replaced with casts or splints or internal fixation once wound parameters permit this.

Drains may be placed intraoperatively to prevent hematoma formation and the subsequent risk of infection and impaired wound healing. Each institution and even each reconstructive microsurgeon may have a specific protocol regarding drains and drain removal. However, if a closed drain system is used, a common guideline is to remove it once the daily output is 30 mL or less.

DANGLING PROTOCOLS, PHYSICAL THERAPY, AND REHABILITATION

The postoperative course following free tissue transfer to the lower extremity is often dictated by concomitant fracture healing and sometimes other problems (e.g., nerve injury and restoration). However, such measures as dependency training do not necessarily include weight-bearing and ambulation and can therefore be initiated much earlier. To train a flap's circulation toward maturity and resilience, compression by wrapping and simultaneous dangling is utilized. Dangling the extremity (e.g., from the edge of the bed) for a certain amount of time utilizes gravity to increase the intravenous pressure and acquaint the new tissue to the hydrostatic pressures it will be faced with once vertical posture, standing, or weight-bearing are possible again. This is indeed a challenge for the tissue, and it should be implemented and advanced gradually. Most surgeons initiate dangling 7–14 days after surgery and begin with 1–2 minutes per session every few hours. The frequency of dangling is variable, and concomitant injuries (e.g., pelvic fractures) may preclude aggressive rehabilitation. When dangling is initiated, flaps have to be carefully monitored.

Immediately after unwrapping, the LD skin paddle should be assessed for color, capillary refill speed, turgor, signs of venous congestion, and sometimes surface temperature (the comparison with the contralateral extremity is helpful) and a Doppler (conventional or laser) assessment of blood flow within the pedicle. If the flap surface is skin grafted, the dependency protocol should start 10–12 days after surgery. By then, the skin grafts should tolerate wrapping. The length of dangling is increased to 10 minutes every hour for a few days and ends with the leg held dependent for 15 minutes out of every hour. Then, if not contraindicated by other reasons, the patient begins a program of weight-bearing, ambulation, and indicated physical therapy (e.g., range of motion of knee joints, ankles, etc.).

CAVEATS

It is essential to provide a large operating room, good access to the patient from all sides and by more than one team, and ergonomic surgeon positioning to ensure comfort and avoid premature fatigue and drop in focus during these long and meticulous procedures.

For the LD flap dissection, inclusion of the entire upper extremity helps to maximize visualization of the pedicle during pedicle dissection by moving the patient's arm. However, excessive and prolonged arm abduction (and brachial plexus stretching) should be avoided.

Complete LD muscle release prior to the completion of neurovascular pedicle dissection allows maximal exposure of the thoracodorsal, proximal subscapular, and distal circumflex scapular vessels (if needed).

SELECTED READINGS

Bullocks J, Naik B, Lee E, Hollier L. Flow-through flaps: a review of current knowledge and a novel classification system. *Microsurgery* 2006;26(6):439–449.

Buncke HJ. Latissimus dorsi muscle transplantation. In: Buncke HJ, ed. *Microsurgery: Transplantation-Replantation*. Philadelphia, PA: Lea & Febiger, 1991:394–433.

Godina M. *A Thesis on the Management of Injuries to the Lower Extremity*. Prezernova Druzba, Ljubljana, Slovenia, 1991.

Kim JT, Kim YH, Ghanem AM. Perforator chimerism for the reconstruction of complex defects: a new chimeric free flap classification system. *J Plast Reconstr Aesth Surg* 2015;68(11):1556–1567.

Manktelow R. *Microvascular Reconstruction*. Berlin: Springer-Verlag, 1986.

Serafin D. *Atlas of Microsurgical Composite Tissue Transplantation*. Philadelphia, PA: W. B. Saunders, 1996:205–216.

Watanabe K, Kiyokawa K, Rikimaru H, Koga N, Yamaki K, Saga T. Anatomical study of latissimus dorsi musculocutaneous flap vascular distribution. *J Plast Reconstr Aesth Surg* 2010;63(7):1091–1098.

Yaremchuk M, Manson P. Local and free flap donor sites for lower extremity reconstruction. In: Yaremchuk M, Burgess A, Brumback R, eds. *Lower Extremity Salvage and Reconstruction*. New York: Elsevier, 1989:117–157.

88

PLANTAR FLAP FOR FOOT RECONSTRUCTION

Benjamin T. Lemelman and David W. Chang

The medial plantar flap is an axial pattern flap from the non–weight-bearing area of the sole of the foot between the heel and the metatarsal heads. It has also been called the "instep flap," but this name is misleading since the "instep" is actually located on the dorsal aspect of the arch of the foot. Thus, the flap is more appropriately termed "the midsole," "midplantar," or "medial plantar flap."

The flap can be raised as a pedicle or a free flap, based on either the medial or lateral plantar arteries, or both. It was initially designed to provide protective sensation for reconstruction of the heel, but it has also been used as a musculocutaneous free flap for thenar muscle reconstruction of the hand. Sensory or motor function is provided by including branches of the medial plantar nerve.

In 1979, Shanahan and Gingrass first reported transposing a medial plantar sensory flap based on the medial plantar artery and nerve for coverage of heel defects. In 1981, Harrison and Morgan subsequently described the use of an island medial plantar flap for the coverage of plantar defects. The free transfer of the medial plantar flap was first described by Morrison in 1983. Ibraraki and Kanayi described its use for thenar reconstruction for hand defects in 1995.

INDICATIONS

The main indication for the medial plantar flap is the need for a sensate coverage of the weight-bearing portion of the heel. Its special anatomic features make it ideal for the coverage of the weight-bearing area: the keratinized skin is fixed by many fibrous septa to a thick fibrofatty subcutaneous tissue and strong plantar fascia, providing durable tissue for weight-bearing (Figure 88.1); and, based on the medial plantar neurovascular pedicle, the flap can be used as a sensate flap.

POSSIBLE USES OF THE MEDIAL PLANTAR FLAP

Fasciocutaneous Island Flap

This fasciocutaneous flap based on the medial plantar neurovascular bundle provides a sensate and similar local

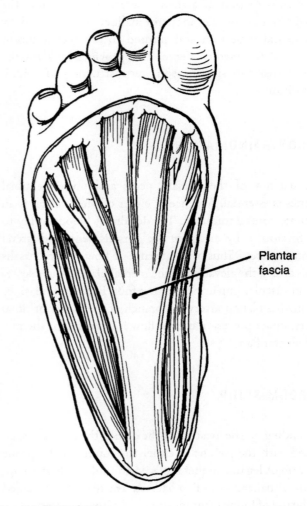

Plantar fascia

Figure 88.1. Plantar fascia.

tissue for the ipsilateral foot. Uses include the plantar heel, tendocalcaneus, and lower leg; and on the plantar forefoot, as a reverse island flap.

Free Fasciocutaneous Flap

The free fasciocutaneous flap provides coverage of the opposite foot when a local flap is not available; for example, when both the instep and the heel have been lost or when inadequate circulation from the posterior tibial or dorsalis pedis artery preclude the use of an island flap. It can also be used to repair palmar or volar digital defects on the foot or hand or to cover amputation stumps on the foot or hand.

Musculofasciocutaneous Flap

The flexor digitorum brevis muscle or abductor hallucis muscle can be included in the flap. The abductor hallucis muscle can be included as a musculofasciocutaneous flap for reconstruction of a thenar defect on the hand. The motor branch of the abductor hallucis is preserved by intraneural dissection and sutured to the thenar motor branch of the median nerve. This provides bulk for the thenar area and simultaneous reconstruction of thumb opposition.

CONTRAINDICATIONS

The patency of the dorsalis pedis and posterior tibial arteries is essential. Absence of either of these vessels is an absolute contraindication. The dominant blood supply to the forefoot is by means of the dorsalis pedis and lateral plantar arteries. Thus, with absence of flow in the dorsalis pedis artery, the elevation of the medial plantar flap may result in vascular impairment of the foot. Furthermore, since the medial plantar artery is a branch of the posterior tibial artery, intact posterior arterial flow is essential for the medial plantar flap.

ROOM SETUP

Depending on the location of the defect, the flap can be elevated with the patient in either the supine or the prone position. A leg tourniquet is placed around the thigh to optimize visualization of flap harvest. The dissection is aided by the use of loupe magnification and bipolar cautery.

PATIENT MARKINGS

The flap is designed on the non–weight-bearing area of the sole between the heel and the metatarsal heads. The lateral border of the sole overlying the fifth metatarsal is weight-bearing, and this area should be avoided. Although the medial plantar flap is usually based on the medial plantar artery, it can also be raised on the lateral plantar artery (Figure 88.2).

OPERATIVE TECHNIQUE

RELEVANT ANATOMY

The posterior tibial artery passes beneath the flexor retinaculum and divides into the medial and lateral plantar arteries under the origin of the abductor hallucis. The medial plantar artery, the smaller of the two branches, runs between the abductor hallucis and flexor digitorum brevis. It sends nutrient branches to the abductor hallucis, and its cutaneous branches perforate the plantar fascia and supply the skin overlying the medial plantar surface. At the base of the first metatarsal bone, it passes along the medial side of the big toe and ultimately terminates in branches to the first and second toes. The lateral plantar artery, the larger branch, travels obliquely under the proximal third of the flexor digitorum brevis, supplying this muscle. It then continues distally between the flexor digitorum brevis and abductor digiti minimi to join the deep plantar arch. Venous drainage is maintained by means of venae comitantes accompanying these arteries.

The medial plantar nerve originates from the tibial nerve 1–3 cm inferior to the medial malleolus and accompanies the medial plantar artery. The nerve courses distally to the tarsal tunnel, where motor branches to the flexor digitorum brevis and the abductor hallucis muscle arise. The nerve then divides into two branches. The medial division of the nerve is medial to the plantar fascia and thus does not actually lie in a "subfascial" location. It gives rise to subcutaneous sensory branches that curve around the plantar fascia to innervate the skin over its medial half. The lateral division of the nerve courses below the plantar fascia and terminates as branches to web spaces and toes. The lateral plantar nerve passes obliquely forward, accompanying the lateral plantar artery. Its cutaneous branches supply the lateral one third of the sole.

PREOPERATIVE EVALUATION

The presence of dorsalis pedis and posterior tibial artery pulses is essential. Both arteries should be palpated for

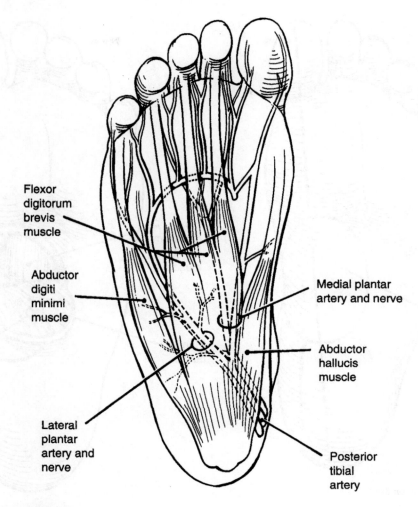

Flexor
digitorum
brevis
muscle

Abductor
digiti
minimi
muscle

Medial plantar
artery and nerve

Abductor
hallucis
muscle

Lateral
plantar
artery and
nerve

Posterior
tibial
artery

Figure 88.2. Relevant anatomy of plantar foot.

pulses. Calculation of arterial indices is helpful: an ankle-to-arm blood pressure ratio of more than 0.8 is acceptable. In doubtful cases, preoperative Doppler examination and angiography should be performed to assess the functional patency of these arteries.

TECHNIQUE

The dissection is aided by a leg tourniquet and loupe magnification. A skin island is designed based on the medial plantar artery. The region of the sole between the heel and the metatarsal heads, except for the lateral border overlying the fifth metatarsal, can provide a maximum area of about 10 × 10 cm. Before raising the flap, locate the medial edge of the plantar aponeurosis. It can be marked by drawing a line between the center of the heel posteriorly and the medial sesamoid of the big toe. This line indicates the area where the perforators emerge from the medial plantar artery (Figure 88.3).

The distal edge of the flap is incised and the plantar fascia is transversely divided. The medial plantar neurovascular bundle is identified in the cleft between the abductor hallucis and flexor digitorum brevis. The cutaneous nerve branches to the flap skin are identified as they arise from the medial plantar nerve. The vascular bundle is separated from the medial plantar nerve and divided. The flap is raised at the level between the plantar fascia and the flexor digitorum brevis muscle, keeping the medial plantar vascular bundle and the cutaneous nerve branches intact with the flap. The flap is raised in a distal-to-proximal and dorsal-to-plantar direction (Figure 88.4). Attention should be paid to the cutaneous branches from the nerve to the flap. As the flap is raised proximally, these cutaneous nerve fascicles are retained with the plantar flap by a meticulous interfascicular dissection, leaving the nerve trunk in the foot. Tracing the medial plantar neurovascular bundle proximally, dissection proceeds to expose its bifurcation with the lateral plantar neurovascular bundle. The abductor

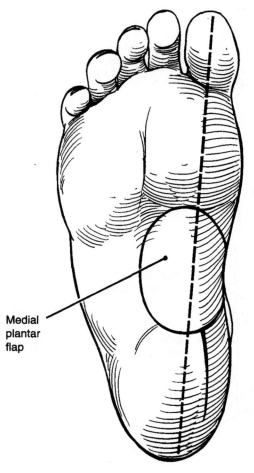

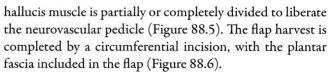

Figure 88.3. Design of medial plantar flap.

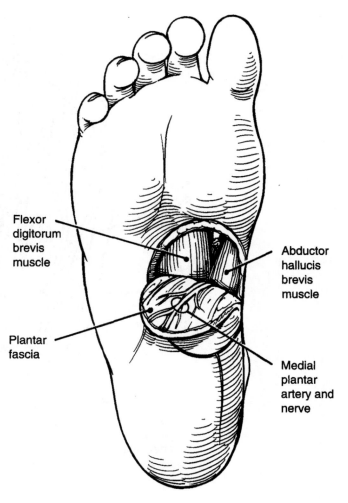

Flexor digitorum brevis muscle

Abductor hallucis brevis muscle

Plantar fascia

Medial plantar artery and nerve

Figure 88.4. Flap is raised distal to proximal.

hallucis muscle is partially or completely divided to liberate the neurovascular pedicle (Figure 88.5). The flap harvest is completed by a circumferential incision, with the plantar fascia included in the flap (Figure 88.6).

Once the flap harvest is completed, the divided muscle is reattached, and the donor defect of the foot is covered with a split-thickness skin graft. The skin graft is secured with a bolster dressing. A closed suction drain is placed beneath the flap. The foot and ankle are immobilized in a posterior splint.

Alternatively, a V-Y islanded medial plantar flap has been described for heel reconstruction, eliminating the need to skin graft the donor site.

Free Flap

For free flap transfer, the pedicle is divided at its origin, just distal to the division into medial and lateral plantar arteries.

If a longer and larger vascular pedicle is required, the patency of the dorsalis pedis artery should be confirmed

before ligation of the lateral plantar artery and division of the posterior tibial artery. If needed, the posterior tibial artery can be reconstructed with a vein graft.

Tendocalcaneus and Distal Tibia

The dissection follows the same format as outlined earlier, with some variations. No attempt is made to preserve the cutaneous branches of the medial plantar nerve to the flap. An interfascicular dissection is not usually possible for this distance. To move the flap further and retain these cutaneous fascicles would require sacrificing the common digital branches of the medial plantar nerve at the metatarsal side of the flap.

The abductor hallucis muscle is divided near the calcaneus to gain an increased degree of pedicle freedom. The lateral plantar artery is divided just after it branches from the posterior tibial artery. The flap, now based on the posterior tibial artery, has a long enough vascular pedicle length

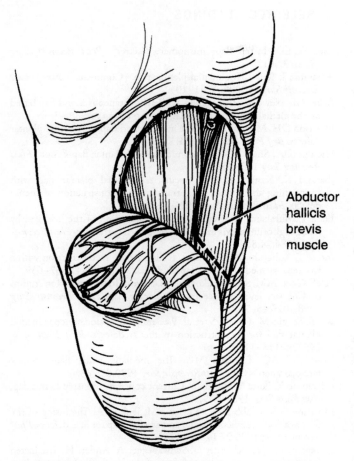

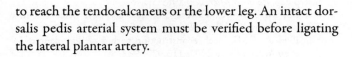

Abductor
hallicis
brevis
muscle

Figure 88.5. Abductor hallucis muscle is divided to expose underlying pedicle.

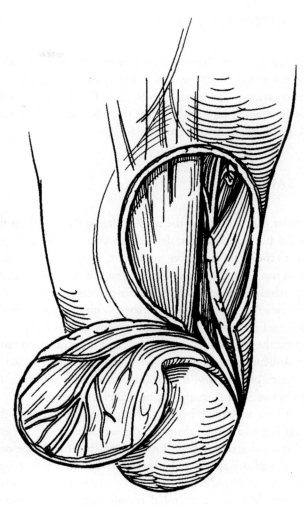

Figure 88.6. Flap is completed by circumferential incision.

to reach the tendocalcaneus or the lower leg. An intact dorsalis pedis arterial system must be verified before ligating the lateral plantar artery.

Plantar Forefoot: A Reverse Island Flap

In this application, the flap is raised from proximal to distal. Following flap design, an incision is made first on the proximal margin of the flap. After identification of the medial plantar artery, this vessel is temporarily interrupted with a vascular clamp. Viability of the flap can thus be evaluated by means of retrograde flow into the distal portion of the medial plantar artery. The dorsalis pedis artery, by means of the first dorsal metatarsal communicating vessel, and the lateral plantar artery, by means of the distal plantar arch, provide the retrograde flow. The division of the proximal medial plantar vascular pedicle allows the medial plantar flap to be rotated distally. This distal rotation provides satisfactory soft tissue cover for the weight-bearing forefoot. The medial plantar nerve and its digital components are preserved intact.

Lateral Plantar System

The lateral plantar neurovascular bundle is identified and divided at the distal part of the flap in the cleft between the flexor digitorum brevis medially and the abductor digiti minimi laterally. Proximally, the flexor digitorum brevis is divided and the vascular branches to the muscle are ligated to allow the release of the vessels and nerves.

Musculofasciocutaneous Flap

The abductor hallucis muscle can be included with the medial plantar artery system, or the flexor digitorum brevis can be included with the lateral plantar artery system, as either pedicled or free flaps. Motor branches to these muscles can be preserved for potential functional musculofasciocutaneous free tissue transfer.

POSTOPERATIVE CARE

The leg is strictly elevated and immobilized in a posterior splint for 7–10 days. If a skin graft is used, the bolster dressing is removed in 5–7 days. The drain is usually removed when its output is less than 30 mL in 24 hours. Weight-bearing is not permitted for 4 weeks.

CAVEATS

In most patients, raising the medial plantar flap based on the medial plantar neurovascular pedicle does not significantly disturb the blood and nerve supply of the foot. The dominant blood supply to the forefoot is by means of the dorsalis pedis and lateral plantar arteries. The medial plantar artery plays only a minor role in circulation to the toes. With the intact dorsalis pedis and posterior tibial arterial systems, the medial plantar flap can be raised on its pedicle without subsequent vascular impairment of the forefoot. Likewise, innervation provided by the lateral plantar nerve is more important for sensibility of the weight-bearing area than is the medial plantar nerve.

When extended beyond the plantar surface to the distal leg and ankle, many of the advantages of the medial plantar artery flap are lost. Innervation cannot be preserved without forefoot denervation, and the thick, tough tissues are not specifically required on non–weight-bearing surfaces. Moreover, extended transfer of this flap on the posterior tibial vascular pedicle leaves the foot dependent on the dorsalis pedis artery.

The donor site defect in the foot has caused no difficulty except for occasional marginal hyperkeratosis. Hyperkeratosis seems more likely if the suture line is at the weight-bearing area or is under tension.

The sensate flap often seems fairly insensitive in the early postoperative period. This, however, improves over the succeeding few weeks to provide protective sensation.

SELECTED READINGS

Altchek ED. Instep flap: misnomer? [Letter]. *Plast Reconstr Surg* 1984;73:501.

Amarante J, Reis J. The medial plantar flap. [Comment. Letter.] *Plast Reconstr Surg* 1990;86:1041–1042.

Baker GL, Newton ED, Franklin JD. Fasciocutaneous island flap based on the medial plantar artery. *Plas Reconstr Surg* 1996;85:47.

Harrison DH, Morgan BDG. The instep island flap to resurface plantar defects. *Br J Plast Surg* 1981;34:315.

Hidalgo DA, Shaw WW. Anatomic basis of plantar flap design. *Plast Reconstr Surg* 1986;78:627.

Ibararki K, Kanaya F. Free vascularized medial plantar flap with functioning abductor hallucis transfer for reconstruction of thenar defects. *Plast Reconstr Surg* 1995;95:108.

Ikata Y, Murakami T, Yoshioda K. Reconstruction of the heel pad by flexar digitorum brevis musculocutaneous flap transfer. *Plast Reconstr Surg* 1984;74:86.

Inoue T, Kobayahi M, Harashina T. Finger pulp reconstruction with a free sensory medial plantar flap. *Br J Plast Surg* 1988;41:657–659.

Isik S, Gular MM, Selmanpakoglu N. Salvage of foot amputation stumps of Chopart level by free medial plantar flap. *Plast Reconstr Surg* 1998;101:745–750.

Isik S, Sezgin M, Ozturk S, et al. Free musculofasciocutaneous medial plantar flap for reconstruction of thenar defects. *Br J Plast Surg.* 1997;50:116–1120.

Masquelet AC, Romana MC. The medialis pedis flap: a new fasciocutaneous flap. *Plast Reconstr Surg* 1990;85:765.

Miyamoto Y, Ikuta Y, Shigeki S. Current concepts of instep island flap. *Ann Plast Surg.* 1987;19:97.

Morrison WA, Crabb DM, O'Brien BM, Jenkins A. The instep of the foot as a fasciocutaneous island and as a free flap for heel defects. *Plast Reconstr Surg* 1996;97:1489–1493.

Ninkovic M, Wechselberger G, Schwabegger A, Anderl H. The instep free flap to resurface palmar defects of the hand. *Plast Reconstr Surg* 1996;97:1489–1493.

Nohira K, Shintomi Y, Sugihara T, Ohura T. Replacing losses in kind: improved sensation following heel reconstruction using the free instep flap. *Reconstr Microsurg* 1989;5:1–6.

Reiffel RS, McCathy JG. Coverage of heel and sole defects: a new subfascial arterialized flap. *Plast Reconstr Surg* 1980;66:250.

Roblin P, Healy CMJ. Heel reconstruction with a medial plantar V-Y flap. *Plast Reconstr Surg* 2007; 113:927–932.

Shanahan RE, Gingrass RP. Medial plantar sensory flap for coverage of heel defects. *Plast Reconstr Surg* 1979;64:295.

Shaw WW, Hidalgo DA. Anatomic basis of plantar flap design: clinical applications. *Plast Reconstr Surg* 1986;78:637.

Strauch B, Yu HL. Medial plantar flap. In: *Atlas of Microvascular Surgery. Anatomy and Operative Approaches.* New York: Thieme Medical, 1993:341.

89

GRACILIS AND RECTUS ABDOMINIS FLAPS FOR LEG AND FOOT RECONSTRUCTION

Alessandro G. Cusano, Lee L. Q. Pu, and Michael S. Wong

INTRODUCTION

Wounds of the lower extremity are some of the most challenging to reconstruct, particularly those in the distal leg, ankle, and foot. Vital structures are frequently exposed, vascularity is often compromised, and local options are seldom available due to a paucity of adequate local tissue. As such, free tissue transfer is regarded as the reconstructive gold standard for defects of the distal leg, ankle, and foot, with the gracilis and rectus abdominis being two flaps that have proved reliable in such circumstances.

This chapter focuses on reconstruction of distal lower extremity defects utilizing the gracilis and rectus abdominis muscle flaps. To better appreciate the utility of these flaps, an understanding of the generalized approach to lower extremity reconstruction is warranted. A comprehensive review of the subject is beyond the scope of this chapter; a brief overview is presented herein.

GENERAL APPROACH TO THE LOWER EXTREMITY

Ideally, the goal of any reconstructive effort should be to restore form and function. Nowhere is this more apparent than in the lower extremity, where restoration of an intact but otherwise nonfunctional limb is considered a reconstructive failure. This raises the issue of limb salvage, a topic that continues to spark much debate. With advances in surgical technique, extremities that would have previously been amputated are now routinely salvaged. But, it should be asked, at what cost?

In Francel's review of 72 patients with Gustillo grade IIIB open tibial fractures, despite a 93% limb salvage rate, only 28% returned to work at a mean follow-up of 42 months. This is in contrast to the 68% of patients who returned to work following below-knee amputation. Georgiadis et al. compared 27 patients who had attempted limb salvage with 18 patients who had primary below-knee amputation. The patients with limb salvage took longer to achieve full weight-bearing status, were less willing to return to work, and had higher hospital charges than those with primary amputation. In Khouri and Shaw's 10-year experience with microvascular free flaps for lower extremity reconstruction, they report a more promising return to work rate of more than 60%. Only 66 of 128 patients, however, were available for long-term follow-up, and the time to return to work, for some, was as great as 10 years. What is interesting to note is that, despite the lengthy and often incomplete recovery, only 3 patients were dissatisfied with their reconstruction, and none was willing to convert to an amputation.

Despite the reluctance to amputate, it must be stressed that the goal of lower extremity salvage is to preserve a limb that is more functional than if it is amputated. While in some cases the decision is obvious, in others it is equivocal. Attempts to objectively predict, through risk assessment scores, which limbs should be salvaged and which should be amputated have, unfortunately, been largely unsuccessful. In the absence of such a concrete measure to direct management, lower extremity salvage is typically approached algorithmically with multidisciplinary collaboration advocated.

The remainder of the chapter will highlight the gracilis and rectus abdominis muscle and musculocutaneous flaps and their roles in reconstruction of the distal lower extremity.

THE GRACILIS FLAP

INTRODUCTION

The gracilis flap is perhaps best appreciated for its versatility, and its numerous and varied applications. While it can be used locally, it is more often applied distantly as a free flap. It has a long neurovascular pedicle, making it a first-line choice for functional free muscle transfer. The inconspicuous donor site scar and lack of functional deficit further contribute to the popularity of this flap.

INDICATIONS

In lower extremity reconstruction, the gracilis is most commonly used as a free flap for wound coverage of the distal leg, ankle, and foot. It has added utility as an adjunct in the management of osteomyelitis. The ability to provide a neurotized reconstruction makes restoration of extensor function of the foot and ankle another attractive application.

CONTRAINDICATIONS

As a dependable flap with a constant and reliable blood supply, contraindications to gracilis transfer are rather infrequent. Flap–defect mismatch or a concern for a compromised vascular pedicle (e.g., from previous surgery or vascular disease) may preclude its use.

ANATOMY

Muscle

The gracilis is a long, flat, thin, unipennate muscle that runs superficially down the length of the medial thigh. It has its origin at the pubic tubercle and inferior ramus of the pubis and its insertion into the pes anserinus at the medial knee. In the proximal thigh, the gracilis can be found medially and posterior to the adductor longus muscle, while distally it lies immediately posterior to the sartorius. At its insertion just inferior to the tibial condyle, the gracilis occupies a position between the sartorius anteriorly and the semitendinosus posteriorly.

The gracilis functions as an accessory adductor of the thigh and an accessory flexor of the knee. With four other thigh adductors (pectineus, adductor longus, adductor brevis, adductor magnus) and seven other knee flexors (biceps femoris, semitendinosus, semimembranosus, sartorius, gastrocnemius, plantaris, popliteus), the entire gracilis

muscle can be harvested with little deficit in thigh or knee function.

In the adult patient, the width of the gracilis is approximately 5–8 cm proximally at the level of the vascular hilum. The muscle then tapers distally to 2–3 cm near its tendinous insertion. The length of the muscle belly is typically 20–30 cm, with an additional 15 cm or more of distal tendon. The thickness of the muscle is 2–3 cm.

Vascular Supply

The gracilis flap is a type II Mathes and Nahai muscle flap, having both dominant and minor vascular pedicles. The dominant pedicle is typically the terminal branch of the medial femoral circumflex artery, but it may also arise directly from the profunda femoris. The pedicle can be seen to enter the muscle anywhere from 10–15 cm below the inguinal ligament. Pedicle length averages 6–8 cm and diameter 1–1.5 mm, giving it sufficient length and caliber for microvascular anastomosis.

Minor pedicles are typically two in number, one proximal and one distal to the main pedicle. The proximal of the two is a branch off of the profunda femoris and is quite variable in its relation to the main pedicle. The distal minor pedicle is a branch of the superficial femoral artery. It is more constant and can be found entering the muscle 10–15 cm distal to the dominant pedicle.

The vast majority of cutaneous perforating vessels are confined to the proximal third of the muscle, making a proximal skin paddle the most reliable. The length of the skin territory does not exceed two-thirds of the muscle length, limiting the size and distal extent of skin harvest. One or two distinct perforators can be found exiting medial and/or lateral to the proximal portion of the muscle, allowing design of transversely oriented skin paddle and harvest of a musculocutaneous perforator flap if so desired.

Venous Drainage

Venous drainage is via the paired venae comitantes that accompany the main arterial pedicle. They have a diameter of 1.5–2.5 mm. In some circumstances, additional outflow may be gained by inclusion of the greater saphenous vein, although this is not typically required.

Innervation

The gracilis muscle is innervated by the anterior branch of the obturator nerve. The nerve runs between the adductor longus and brevis muscles and enters the gracilis 1–2 cm proximal to the dominant vascular pedicle. If additional nerve length is required, retrograde dissection to the level of the bifurcation of the obturator nerve, or further to the obturator foramen, will yield an additional 2–4 cm of nerve length for a total of 12 cm of harvestable nerve.

Sensibility to the skin of the proximal, medial thigh is supplied by the medial cutaneous nerve of the thigh, also a branch of the obturator nerve.

PREOPERATIVE PREPARATION

Routine preoperative imaging, angiography, or other vascular studies are not typically indicated when harvesting the gracilis muscle or musculocutaneous flap. A handheld unidirectional Doppler is helpful, however, for perforator identification and subsequent skin paddle design if the medial circumflex femoral artery perforator flap is to be used.

ROOM SETUP

The gracilis flap is harvested with the patient in the supine position with the ipsilateral hip flexed, abducted, and externally rotated in the "frog-leg" position. Not only does this provide exposure, but it accentuates the prominence of the adductor longus, which serves as a key anatomical landmark for gracilis harvest.

FLAP DESIGN

The gracilis may be harvested as a "muscle-only" or musculocutaneous flap. In distal leg and foot reconstruction, where contour is often more important than bulk, the muscle-only flap with split-thickness skin graft is typically the preferred approach.

With the patient supine and in the frog-leg position, the tight band that can be appreciated in the proximal medial thigh is the adductor longus. The gracilis is found just posterior to the adductor longus. Its origin at the pubic tubercle can be marked.

The distal gracilis tendon inserts onto the proximal medial tibia just inferior to the medial tibial condyle. Before doing so, however, it passes posterior to the medial femoral condyle in the distal medial thigh. The path of the gracilis can be marked, therefore, as a straight line from its origin at the pubic tubercle to the medial condyle of the femur. If one requires additional exposure for an extended gracilis harvest, one may continue the marking inferiorly, in a curvilinear fashion, to the medial condyle of the tibia.

With the course of the gracilis identified, the transition point between its muscle belly and distal tendon is now marked; a point two-thirds the way down the medial thigh marks the transition. If a muscle-only flap is to be used, a single, 10 cm straight-line incision is drawn proximally over the course of the muscle. In the event that an extended gracilis flap is required, a second straight-line incision may be placed distally to facilitate harvest of the entire muscle and tendon.

When a skin paddle is to be included with the flap, it should be centered over the proximal portion of the muscle or, just anterior to it, over the intermuscular septum. The intermuscular septum can be appreciated as a palpable cleft between the gracilis and the adductor longus muscles. The septocutaneous perforators that nourish the skin paddle travel within the intermuscular septum, and are more numerous proximally. The skin paddle is, thus, preferentially designed proximally; a longitudinal or transverse orientation may be used. It should be noted, however, that the skin paddle for the gracilis musculocutaneous flap is occasionally unreliable. Perforator identification with a handheld unidirectional Doppler may be helpful, therefore, in confirming skin paddle design.

Finally, the position of the dominant vascular pedicle, where it enters the muscle, is marked 8–10 cm below the pubic tubercle.

FLAP HARVEST

Muscle Flap

Under general anesthesia, a straight-line incision is made in the proximal medial thigh, overlying and paralleling the gracilis muscle. The incision continues to the overlying fascia, preserving the greater saphenous vein as it is encountered. The junction of the gracilis and the adductor longus is now identified, and, with a longitudinal fascial incision, the interspace between the two muscles is exposed. This allows anterior retraction of the adductor longus, exposing the main vascular pedicle and the anterior branch of the obturator nerve. It should be noted that the main pedicle to the gracilis muscle is occasionally absent. This underscores the importance of early pedicle identification prior to flap elevation.

If required for whole muscle/tendon harvest, or to facilitate identification of the gracilis muscle belly, a second distal incision can be used. At this point, the distal musculotendinous portion of the gracilis will lie between the sartorius anteriorly and the semimembranosus posteriorly. Inferior traction on the gracilis' distal tendon will confirm the position of its proximal muscle belly, providing reassurance as to the proper plane of dissection.

With the vascular pedicle identified and the gracilis confirmed, the muscle is freed of its proximal fascial attachments. This requires release from the adductor longus anteriorly, the adductor magnus posteriorly, and the adductor brevis on its deep surface. The distal tendon is now divided, and, with proximal dissection, it can be delivered into the proximal incision, facilitating completion of the dissection.

The proximal gracilis is now divided, and the dominant vascular pedicle is dissected to its origin at the takeoff of the medial femoral circumflex vessels. Proximally, the pedicle gives off a branch to the vastus medialis, which should be ligated. If a neurotized flap is to be harvested, the anterior branch of the obturator nerve may be included in the flap; it can be found 2 cm proximal to the vascular hilum. The flap is now isolated on its vascular pedicle and is ready for transfer.

Musculocutaneous Flap

The skin paddle is typically designed in a lenticular fashion and is centered over the proximal portion of the gracilis muscle. Depending on reconstructive needs, it may be designed longitudinally or transversely. With a longitudinal design, the anterior and posterior borders of the skin flap may extend 2–3 cm anterior to and 6–9 cm posterior to the anterior border of the muscle. Craniocaudally, to ensure adequate perfusion, the skin island is confined to the proximal two-thirds of the muscle belly. While a larger skin paddle may be supported, the preferred design is one that has its center at the level of the vascular hilum and its width determined by the ability to achieve primary closure of the donor site defect.

For a transversely designed skin paddle, the long axis is placed perpendicular to the orientation of the gracilis muscle. It is similarly designed over the proximal portion of the muscle belly with its center at the level of the vascular hilum. The anterior extent is the superficial femoral artery; the posterior extent is the posterior midline of the thigh. Primary closure of the donor site again limits the short-axis of the paddle, with a "pinch test" used to define the width in the craniocaudal dimension.

Flap harvest begins with a skin incision at the anterior margin of the skin paddle down to the fascia of the adductor longus muscle. The fascia is incised longitudinally in the mid-axis of the muscle, and the anterior aspect of the skin paddle is dissected subfascially towards the intermuscular septum. The intermuscular septum, which is to be included with the flap, is then freed from the posterior surface of the adductor longus, allowing the muscle be retracted anteriorly and exposing the vascular pedicle.

If required, the distal incision is now made in the same fashion as described previously for harvest of the "muscle-only" flap. Distal traction on the gracilis tendon confirms the identification of the gracilis muscle belly, providing reassurance for accurate skin paddle design. The posterior margin of the skin island is now safely incised down to and through the gracilis fascia. Flap harvest now proceeds as it would for the gracilis muscle flap outlined in the preceding section.

If increased mobility of the skin paddle is desired, it may be freed from the underlying muscle. The posterior aspect, as it was done for the anterior portion, can be dissected subfascially toward the intermuscular septum. Musculocutaneous perforators will be encountered during the dissection and should be coagulated and divided as necessary. Once the intermuscular septum is reached, the row of septocutaneous perforators supplying the skin paddle will be seen coursing through the septum.

DONOR SITE MANAGEMENT

For the gracilis muscle flap, the donor site is closed primarily. For the musculocutaneous flap, if the width of the skin paddle is limited to 6–8 cm, the wound can usually be closed primarily. Undermining of the skin flaps is typically required. A three-layer closure is performed over a suction drain, and a mild compressive dressing is applied.

THE RECTUS ABDOMINIS FLAP

INTRODUCTION

The abdominal region has a rich blood supply and an abundance of expendable soft tissue, making it a preferred donor site for soft tissue transfer. The rectus abdominis flap is the workhorse of the region and has relevance in numerous applications. In breast reconstruction, as a musculocutaneous, muscle-sparing, or perforator flap, it provides supple tissue for the reconstructed breast while offering the advantage of an "abdominoplasty-like" closure at the donor site. In distal lower extremity reconstruction, however, where contour is favored over bulk, the "muscle-only" option is typically preferred. While it is true that muscle harvest adds to the morbidity profile of the flap, it is still a valuable tool for complicated lower extremity wounds, particularly those of the distal leg and foot.

INDICATIONS

Like the gracilis, the rectus abdominis, in lower extremity reconstruction is used as a free flap for defects of the distal third, ankle, and foot. Because of its dimensions, the "muscle-only" flap is well suited for wounds that are long and narrow and, with a split-thickness skin graft, can provide a reasonably well-contoured reconstruction. When additional bulk is desired, a musculocutaneous rectus flap may be used. This is particularly relevant in large cavitary defects with significant soft tissue deficit. In such cases, having a muscular component for bony coverage and dead space obliteration, and a cutaneous component to restore the soft tissue envelope, single-flap reconstruction of even the most complicated lower extremity defects is possible.

CONTRAINDICATIONS

An absolute contraindication to the free rectus abdominis flap is previous abdominal surgery that has compromised the vascular pedicle. In elderly patients or in those with chronic obstructive pulmonary disease, postoperative abdominal discomfort may increase the risk of atelectasis and pneumonia. Use of an alternative flap in these patients may be prudent. Finally, donor site morbidity is not negligible. This has led some surgeons to abandon the rectus abdominis flap for lower leg reconstruction in favor of other flaps with improved donor site profiles.

ANATOMY

Muscle

The paired rectus abdominis muscles are the major longitudinal muscles of the anterior abdominal wall. They originate at the symphysis pubis and the pubic crest and insert onto the anterior aspect of the fifth, sixth, and seventh costal cartilages and the xiphoid process. The muscles are approximately 25 cm in length with a thickness of approximately 0.6 cm. The width is 6 cm at its origin, 8 cm at its midpoint, and tapers to 3 cm at its insertion.

The rectus muscles are enclosed within an investing fascia, the rectus sheath. The sheath comprises the aponeuroses of the external oblique, internal oblique, and transversus abdominis muscles and the transversalis fascia. This creates a multilayered, myofascial construct giving the abdominal wall its support. The rectus muscle has three inscriptions: one at the xiphoid, one at the umbilicus, and one in between. The arcuate line is of interest and is found at the level of the anterior superior iliac spines. It marks a transition in the integrity of the posterior rectus sheath. While the posterior sheath above the arcuate line has contributions from the internal oblique, transversus abdominis, and transversalis fascia, below it is composed of only the transversalis fascia. This has particular relevance as this area is more prone to postoperative hernia or bulge.

Vascular Supply

The rectus abdominis is a type III Mathes and Nahai muscle, having two dominant vascular pedicles: the deep superior epigastric artery (DSEA) and the deep inferior epigastric artery (DIEA). The DSEA is a branch of the internal mammary artery. It is the smaller of the two pedicles and enters the rectus on its deep surface between the xiphoid and the eighth rib. The DIEA is the more dominant vascular pedicle, and the pedicle is better suited for microvascular anastomosis.

The DIEA arises from the external iliac artery immediately above the inguinal ligament. It travels superomedially, deep to the posterior rectus sheath, piercing the transversalis fascia just above the arcuate line. It then enters the lateral undersurface of the rectus muscle, where it ramifies and travels cephalad to communicate with the DSEA, contributing to the watershed in the periumbilical region. Retrograde dissection of the DIEA to its origin will yield a pedicle length of approximately 8–10 cm. The diameter of the pedicle at its origin is approximately 3–3.5 mm.

Venous Drainage

Venous drainage is typically via the deep system. Two venae comitantes accompany the DIEA, each of which has a diameter of approximately 3 mm at its origin. If a musculocutaneous rectus flap is to be used, supplementary drainage of the skin paddle may be desired. If this is the case, the superficial inferior epigastric vein may be included with the flap.

Innervation

The rectus abdominis is supplied by the ventral rami of the seventh through twelfth segmental thoracic spinal nerves. The intercostal nerves enter the muscle at various points and divide into motor and sensory branches. The sensory branches join the vascular perforators to supply the skin. Segmental motor innervation of the rectus precludes its use in functional free muscle transfer.

PREOPERATIVE PREPARATION

Used as a free flap for reconstruction of the distal lower extremity, the rectus abdominis flap, like the gracilis, does not routinely require preoperative vascular imaging. In situations where a deep inferior epigastric perforator (DIEP) flap is preferred, precise knowledge of perforator location can expedite flap harvest. Preoperative vascular studies in these cases, while not mandatory, may be desired.

ROOM SETUP

Like the gracilis, the rectus abdominis flap is harvested with the patient in the supine position, offering the advantage of a simultaneous, two-team approach for flap harvest and recipient site preparation.

FLAP DESIGN

Depending on the application, the blood supply to the rectus abdominis can be the source of numerous flap designs with various flap components. For distal leg and foot reconstruction, the inferiorly based free rectus flap is, by far, the most applicable. It is typically harvested as a "muscle-only" flap, used in conjunction with a split-thickness skin graft. In rare cases, however, where substantial bulk is desired, a skin paddle may be included. Depending on reconstructive needs, vertical, transverse, or obliquely designed skin islands may be used.

FLAP HARVEST

MUSCLE FLAP

The rectus abdominis muscle flap can be harvested through a median, paramedian, or low transverse incision. While the median and paramedian incisions offer the benefit of a direct approach, the low transverse incision is preferred for its inconspicuous scar placement.

An incision is made through skin and subcutaneous tissue down to the rectus fascia. In an abdominoplasty-type fashion, the superior skin flap is dissected and reflected cephalad, exposing the anterior rectus sheath. The anterior rectus sheath is longitudinally incised, 2 cm lateral to the linea alba, thereby exposing the rectus muscle. Caudally, the medial border of the rectus is elevated to identify the vascular pedicle.

Once the pedicle is located, the rectus muscle can be completely freed of its fascial attachments. Anteriorly,

the rectus sheath is quite adherent, particularly in the region of the tendinous inscriptions. Perforating vessels are often present at the inscription sites, and their release is facilitated with bipolar electrocautery. On the deep surface of the rectus, the sheath is less adherent. An avascular plane is entered between the posterior sheath and the muscle, permitting a more rapid dissection.

With the muscle now isolated, it is divided at its proximal insertion and progressively reflected distally toward the pubis. Segmental branches entering the rectus on its lateral aspect will be encountered; they should be ligated and divided. At the distal extent of the muscle, the deep inferior epigastric vessels will be visible coursing along the deep surface of muscle before they enter at the vascular hilum.

Harvest continues with dissection of the pedicle. The pedicle is dissected inferiorly to the inguinal ligament where it has its origin at the external iliac artery. Once pedicle dissection is complete, the rectus is transected distally at the symphysis pubis and pubic crest. The flap is now isolated on its vascular pedicle and is ready for harvest.

MUSCULOCUTANEOUS FLAP

The vertical rectus abdominis (VRAM) flap, with its vertically oriented skin paddle designed longitudinally over the rectus muscle, is harvested in much the same manner as previously described for the "muscle-only" rectus flap. Harvest of a transverse rectus abdominis (TRAM) flap, in which the skin paddle is designed at right angles to the long axis of the muscle, has some minor differences. It is described later.

The skin paddle for the TRAM flap is designed transversely in the lower abdomen, similar to the skin resection of an abdominoplasty. The inferior incision is placed in the pubic hairline and the superior incision just above or below the umbilicus. Supraumbilical placement incorporates the paraumbilical perforators, while an infraumbilical incision may permit a lower and more concealed scar. Craniocaudally, the width is defined by a "pinch test": the lateral borders of the skin island extend just shy of the anterior superior iliac spines.

The skin paddle is circumferentially incised down to the rectus fascia, and the superior "abdominoplasty" flap is reflected superiorly. Dissection of the skin paddle commences at its lateral poles, reflecting them subfascially to the medial and lateral borders of the carrier rectus muscle. The portion of the anterior rectus sheath that overlies the carrier rectus and that is immediately below the skin paddle will be included in the flap; it is incised accordingly. The portion of the rectus inferior to the skin island is then dissected, facilitating exposure of the vascular pedicle. Flap harvest then proceeds as previously described.

DONOR SITE MANAGEMENT

To prevent postoperative herniation and bulge, particular attention should be paid to closure of the anterior rectus sheath. The incision is closed over a closed suction drain, which should exit through a separate incision in the mons pubis. With a "muscle-only" rectus flap, the anterior rectus sheath is incised but spared. In this fashion, the standard technique of nonresorbable, interrupted figure-of-eight stitches, reinforced with a running, nonresorbable stitch will suffice. A monofilament 2-0 polypropylene is commonly used. The remainder of the incision is closed in the typical three-layered fashion.

In the musculocutaneous rectus flap, a portion of the anterior rectus sheath is harvested with the flap, leaving a fascial defect. If possible, this is closed in the same fashion as just described. This will, however, displace the umbilicus to the ipsilateral side. Fascial plication along the length of the contralateral rectus will correct the asymmetry. In fascial defects that are too large for primary closure, inlay mesh reinforcement is required. In circumstances where primary fascial closure is accomplished but there is concern for the possibility of postoperative bulge, an "onlay" configuration can be used, tacking the mesh into position with interrupted sutures and securing it with a running circumferential stitch.

FLAP INSET AND ANASTOMOSIS

Flap inset is at least partially performed prior to microvascular anastomosis to prevent undue tension on the pedicle during inset. Whenever possible, the anastomosis is performed outside the zone of injury. An end-to-side anastomosis is preferred, having the advantage of negating vessel size mismatch and minimizing distal vascular compromise

With respect to recipient site preparation, wound edges are freshened and undermined to ensure a smooth transition between flap and native skin. The flap is then inset with a resorbable suture in a half-buried, horizontal mattress fashion. A closed suction drain is placed, and a split-thickness skin graft applied. A bolster dressing or negative pressure wound therapy device is used over the graft to facilitate graft take.

POSTOPERATIVE CARE

An appropriate postoperative care regimen is critical to the outcome of any reconstructive effort, particularly those involving free-tissue transfer, but nowhere is this more apparent than in the distal lower extremity.

Dressings can be problematic if particular attention is not paid to their application. If the dressing is too constricting, it may compromise vascular inflow or venous drainage. With movement, an ill-fitting dressing or splint has the potential to cause shearing of the underlying graft or flap. And by concealing the surgical site, clinical assessment of the reconstruction is limited. As these issues are all particularly troublesome, especially in the setting of an acute free-tissue transfer, when it comes to dressings, a "less is more" approach is often favored.

Skeletal traction is ideally suited for these cases. Not only does it provide elevation and immobilization of the extremity, but it also permits continuous, unobstructed, 360-degree access to the leg and flap. If a musculocutaneous flap is used, no other dressings are required, and the flap is freely accessible for clinical assessment. If a skin-grafted muscle flap is used, a petrolatum gauze and cotton fluff dressing is used to "bolster" the graft to facilitate graft take. Alternatively, negative-pressure wound therapy may be used, provided that a low continuous setting (75 mm Hg) is applied.

In the case of skin-grafted muscle flaps, the negative-pressure wound therapy device or bolster dressing (whichever used) is discontinued on postoperative day 5. Topical antibiotic ointment with petrolatum gauze may then be applied until complete epithelialization of the grafted muscle has occurred. Strict leg elevation and immobilization is continued for 10–14 days postoperatively, after which a dangling protocol is initiated to gently introduce the reconstructed extremity to a position of dependency.

To initiate the dangling protocol, the foot and leg of the reconstructed extremity are wrapped circumferentially (in a distal to proximal fashion) with an elastic (Ace) bandage. Care must be taken to monitor the tension with which the bandage is applied to avoid overcompression of the flap and/or pedicle. The extremity is then dangled for a period of 10–15 minutes each day for the first 2 days. After each dangling episode, the extremity is immediately returned to the suspended position and monitored for signs of venous congestion. Depending on how this is tolerated, progressive periods of protected dependency are allowed, increasing by 5 minute increments every 1–2 days, until a total of 30 minutes of protected dependency is reached. The patient is then allowed to begin non–weight-bearing ambulation (with crutches or a walker) provided that sufficient strength has been gained to do so. Periods of non–weight-bearing ambulation should not exceed 30 minutes in a given session, and the foot and leg should remain in a circumferential

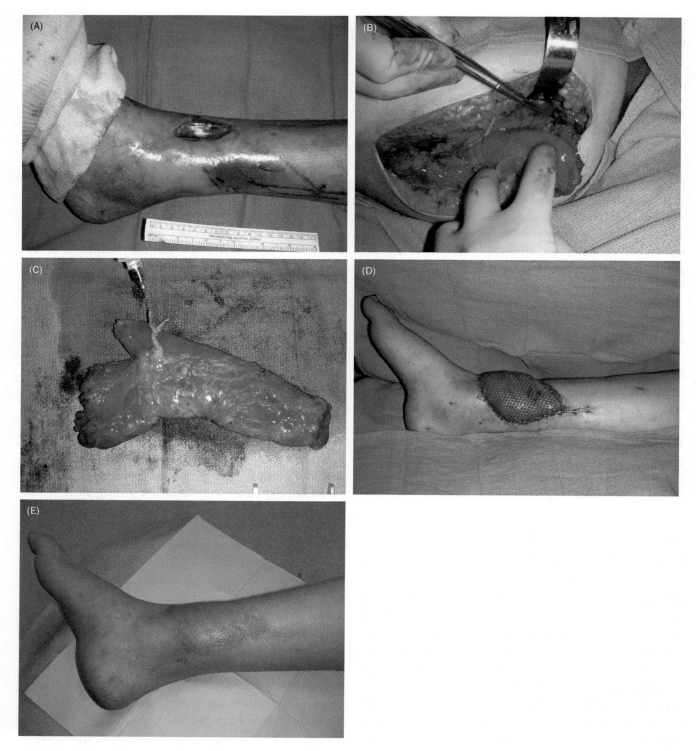

Figure 89.1. A 34-year-old woman after fall from height with delayed presentation of comminuted pilon fracture. The patient sustained bilateral pilon fractures with comminution on the right side. The left-sided fracture was repaired at an outside hospital at the time of initial admission. The patient was subsequently transferred to the authors' institution for higher level of care and management of the comminuted right-sided pilon fracture. A staged approach was used, requiring temporary external fixation, followed by open-reduction internal fixation and definitive soft tissue reconstruction with a free tissue transfer using a gracilis muscle flap. (A) Distal third defect with bone and hardware exposure. Area of compromised skin can be seen superomedial to the defect (darkened area). This was excised. (B) Flap harvest: The right gracilis muscle flap has been raised and remains attached via its vascular pedicle (shown). The flap is ready for division and transfer. (C) Right free gracilis muscle flap after harvest. The vascular pedicle is clearly seen. (D) Final inset: Microvascular anastomosis is complete, and the flap is inset and covered with a split-thickness skin graft. (E) The final healed wound.

elastic wrap during this time. This routine is continued for 3 weeks, after which unrestricted ambulation is allowed. Elastic support, in the form of either Ace bandages or compression stockings, is continued for 3 months or longer as indicated.

Flaps placed on the weight-bearing areas of the foot or pressure-bearing areas of the ankle warrant special consideration as these areas are particularly prone to pressure and shear injury. Patient participation in the form of understanding and compliance, and flap protection with a well-fitting shoe and orthotic, are of paramount importance in maintaining the longevity of the reconstruction. Consultation with a podiatric specialist is extremely helpful in this regard. Strict foot hygiene and daily inspections are also essential, with areas of redness, blistering and/or ecchymosis mandating a change in shoe, orthotic, or ambulatory activity.

CASE EXAMPLES

CASE 1: A 34-year-old woman after fall from height with delayed presentation of comminuted right pilon fracture. The patient was treated with a free gracilis muscle flap with split-thickness skin graft (Figure 89.1).

CASE 2: A 14-year-old girl struck by motor vehicle with open left tibial fracture complicated by extensive soft

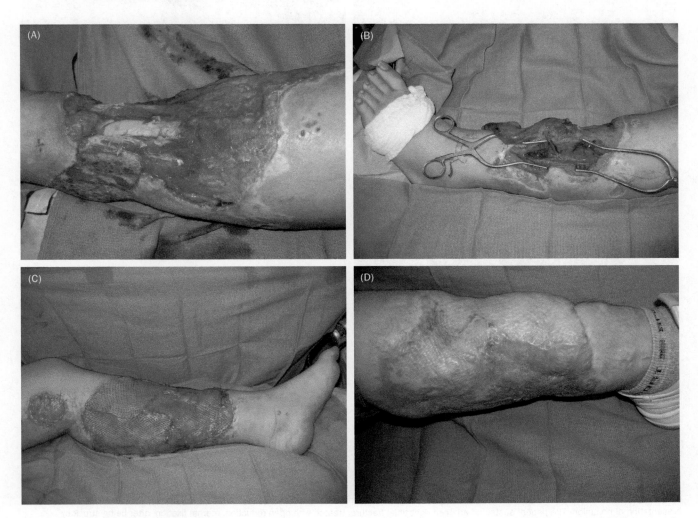

Figure 89.2. A 14-year-old girl struck by vehicle with open left tibial fracture complicated by extensive soft tissue loss. The fracture was initially managed with external fixation and an antibiotic spacer, followed by definitive repair with open reduction internal fixation via intramedullary nail. This was complicated by extensive soft tissue loss requiring serial debridement, negative pressure wound therapy, and, ultimately, free tissue transfer. (A) Defect at time of free tissue transfer after serial debridement and negative-pressure wound therapy. Significant soft tissue deficit can be appreciated involving proximal, middle, and distal thirds. Area of bone exposure is clearly seen and is confined to the distal third of the leg. (B) An ipsilateral free gracilis muscle flap has been harvested and microvascular anastomosis has been performed. (C) Final flap inset with split-thickness skin grafting of the flap and all exposed native muscle. (D) The final healed wound.

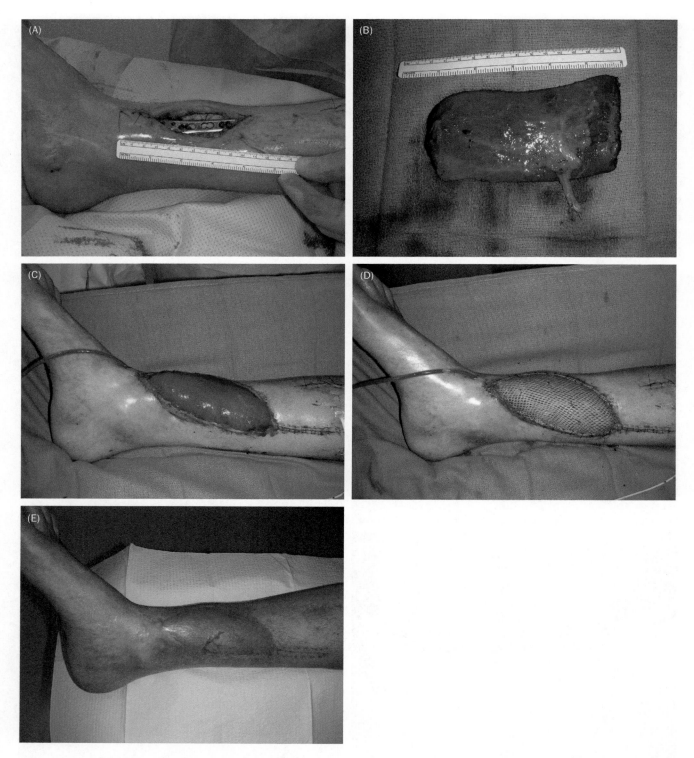

Figure 89.3. A 54-year-old man with history of old open right tibial fracture treated with open reduction internal fixation, complicated by a delayed presentation of nonunion. The patient sustained an open right tibial fracture, treated with open reduction internal fixation, after being struck by a motor vehicle more than 20 years prior. Decades later, he presented with a draining wound of the right leg, with radiographic confirmation of nonunion at the fracture site. This was managed with hardware removal, tibial ostectomy, and placement of antibiotic spacer with a bridging plate for fixation. A significant soft tissue deficit ensued requiring free tissue transfer for definitive reconstruction. (A) Distal third defect with bridging plate and underlying antibiotic spacer clearly seen. (B) Free rectus abdominis muscle flap after harvest. The vascular pedicle is clearly seen. (C) Final inset: Microvascular anastomosis is complete and the flap inset over a closed suction drain. (D) A split-thickness skin graft is applied to the transplanted muscle. (E) The final healed wound.

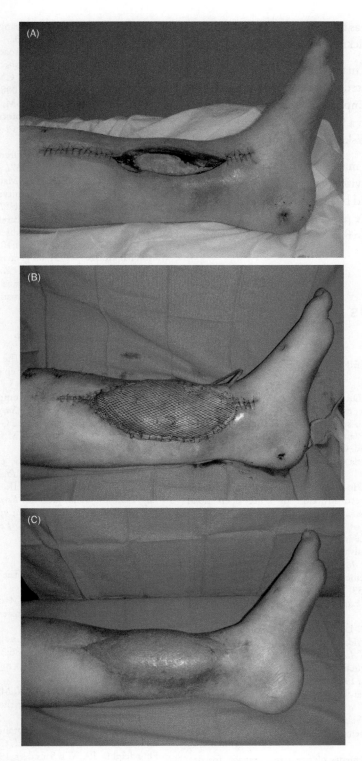

Figure 89.4. A 70-year-old man with history of old left tib-fib fracture after open reduction internal fixation complicated by nonunion, osteomyelitis, and failed hardware. This was treated with hardware removal, bony sequestrectomy, and placement of antibiotic spacer. Definitive soft tissue reconstruction required free tissue transfer with a free rectus abdominis muscle flap. (A) Distal third defect measuring 15 × 6 cm with exposed bone and antibiotic spacer. (B) Final inset of free rectus abdominis flap. Microvascular anastomosis is complete, and the flap is inset and skin-grafted over a closed suction drain. (C) The final healed wound.

tissue loss. The patient was treated with a free gracilis muscle flap with split-thickness skin graft (Figure 89.2).

CASE 3: A 54-year-old man with history of old open right tibial fracture treated with open reduction internal fixation and complicated by nonunion. The patient was treated with a free rectus abdominis muscle flap with split-thickness skin graft (Figure 89.3).

CASE 4: A 70-year-old man with history of an old left tib-fib fracture treated with open reduction internal fixation and complicated by nonunion, osteomyelitis, and failed hardware. The patient was treated with a free rectus abdominis muscle flap with split-thickness skin graft (Figure 89.4).

SELECTED READINGS

LIMB SALVAGE AND LOWER EXTREMITY RECONSTRUCTION

Cordiero PG, Neves RI, Hidalgo DA. The role of free tissue transfer after oncologic resection in the lower extremity. *Ann Plast Surg* 1994;33:9.

Drake D. Reconstruction for limb-sparing procedures in soft-tissue sarcoma of the extremities. *Clin Plast Surg* 1995;22:123.

Fallico N, Somma F, Cigna E, et al. Coverage of exposed hardware after lower leg fractures with free flaps or pedicled flaps. *Eur Rev Med Pharmacol Sci* 2015;19:4715.

Francel TJ, Vander Kolk CA, Hoopes JE, et al. Microvascular soft tissue transplantations for reconstruction of acute open tibial fractures: timing of coverage and long-term functional results. *Plast Reconstr Surg* 1992;89:478.

Giorgiadis GM, Behrens FF, Joyce MJ, et al. Open tibial fractures with severe soft tissue loss. Limb salvage compared with below-the-knee amputations. *J Bone Joint Surg Ann* 1993;75:1431.

Hallock GG. Evidence-based medicine: lower extremity trauma. *Plast Reconstr Surg* 2013;132(6):1733.

Heller L, Kronowitz SJ. Lower extremity reconstruction. *J Surg Onc* 2006;94:479.

Higgins TF, Klatt JB, Beals TC. Lower extremity assessment project (LEAP)—The best available evidence on limb-threatening lower extremity trauma. *Orthop Clin N Am* 2010;41:233.

Khouri RK, Shaw WW. Reconstruction of the lower extremity with microvascular free flaps. *J Trauma* 1989;29:1086.

Klebuc M, Menn Z. Muscle flaps and their role in limb salvage. *MDCVJ* 2013;9(2):95.

Korompilias AV, Lykissas MG, Vekris MD, Beris AE, Soucacos PN. Microsurgery for lower extremity injuries. *Int J Care Injured* 2008;395: S103.

Marek CA and Pu LLQ. Refinements of free tissue transfer for optimal outcome in lower extremity reconstruction. *Ann Plast Surg* 2004;52:270.

Momoh AO, Chung KC. Measuring outcomes in lower limb surgery. *Clin Plast Surg* 2013;40(2):323.

Pu LLQ. A comprehensive approach to lower extremity free tissue transfer. *Plast Reconstr Surg Global Open* 2017: In press.

Reddy V, Stevenson T. MOC-PS CME article: lower extremity reconstruction. *Plast Reconstr Surg* 2008;121(4):1.

Rhode C, Howell BW, Buncke GM, Gurtner GC, Levin LS, Pu LLQ, Levine JP. A recommended protocol for the immediate postoperative care of lower extremity free flap reconstruction. *J Reconstr Microsurg* 2009;25:15.

Sagerbien CA, Rodriguez ED, Turen CH. The soft tissue frame. *Plast Reconstr Surg* 2007;119(7):2137.

Schiro GR, Sessa S, Piccioli A, Maccauro G. Primary amputation vs limb salvage in mangled extremity: a systematic review of the current scoring system. *BMC Musculoskel Dis* 2015;16:372.

Swaminathan A, Vemulapalli S, Patel MR, et al. Lower extremity amputation in peripheral artery disease: improving patient outcomes. *Vascul Health Risk Manag* 2014;10:417.

Walton RL, Rothkopf DM. Judgement and approach for management of severe lower extremity injuries. *Clin Plast Surg* 1991;18:525.

Yazar S, Lin CH, Wei FC. One-stage reconstruction of composite bone and soft tissue defects in traumatic lower extremities. *Plast Recontr Surg* 2004;114(6):1457.

RECTUS ABDOMINIS FLAP

Boyd JB, Taylor GI, Corlett RJ. The vascular territories of the superficial epigastric and deep inferior epigastric systems. *Plast Reconstr Surg* 1984;73:1.

Hartrampf CR. Abdominal wall competence in transverse abdominal island flap operations. *Ann Plast Surg* 1984;12:139.

Kroll SS, Schusterman MA, Reece GP, et al. Abdominal wall strength, bulging and hernia after TRAM flap reconstruction. *Plast Reconstr Surg* 1995;96:616.

Meland NB, Fisher J, Irons GB, et al. Experience with 80 rectus abdominis free-tissue transfers. *Plast Reconstr Surg* 1989;84:108.

Taylor GI, Corlett RJ, Boyd JB. The extended deep inferior epigastric flap: a clinical technique. *Plast Reconstr Surg* 1983;72:751.

Taylor GI, Corlett RJ, Boyd JB. The versatile deep inferior epigastric (inferior rectus abdominis) flap. *Br J Plast Surg* 1984;37:330.

GRACILIS FLAP

Harii K, Ohmari K, Sekiguchi J. The free musculocutaneous flap. *Plast Reconstr Surg* 1976;57:294.

O'Brien BC, Morrison WA, Macleod AM, Weiglein OV. Free microneurovascular muscle transfer in limbs to provide motor power. *Ann Plast Surg* 1982;9:381.

Manktelow RT. *Gracilis in Microvascular Reconstruction.* New York: Springer-Verlag, 1986:37–44.

Mathes SJ, Albert BS. Advances in muscle and musculocutaneous flaps. *Clin Plast Surg* 1980;7:15.

May JW, Gallico GG, Lukash FN. Microvascular transfer of free tissue for closure of bone wounds of the distal lower extremity. *N Engl J Med* 1982;306:253.

Serafin D. The gracilis musculocutaneous flap. Chapter 24. In: Serafin D, ed. *Atlas of Microsurgical Composite Tissue Transplantation.* Philadelphia, PA: WB Saunders, 1996:293–302.

PART XIV.

HAND SURGERY

90

NAIL BED INJURY

Gennaya L. Mattison and Amber R. Leis

INTRODUCTION

Fingertip injuries, which are often associated with nail bed damage, are one of the most common injuries to the upper extremity. Successful treatment of such injuries requires an understanding of the anatomy, function, injury extent, and mechanism, as well as of the techniques available for reconstruction. Surgical judgment also comes into play, incorporating factors such as medical history, occupation, age, hand dominance, and expected outcome for the degree of damage.

Nail bed injuries occur most commonly in males 4–30 years old. They most frequently affect the middle finger and occur with equal frequency to both the dominant and nondominant hand. Most presentations are secondary to crush injuries and lacerations. Other causes of nail bed deformity can include infection, congenital anomaly, systemic disease, tumor, and iatrogenic causes.

FUNCTIONAL IMPORTANCE

Fingernails serve an important role in both mechanical and sensory function. They provide an edge against which to pick up small objects. They supply a counterforce to the fingertip pad that improves sensation. Without a fingernail in place, two-point discrimination is decreased. They also contribute to peripheral circulatory regulation and function in cosmetic adornment and defensive or protective mechanisms.

KEY ANATOMY

The nail matrix, also known as the nail bed, is the thin and critical layer of tissue deep to the nail plate. It is subdivided into the germinal and sterile matrix. The germinal matrix begins proximally and deep to the nail fold and is adherent to the distal phalanx. It extends to the distal end of the lunula and produces more than 90% of the nail. The

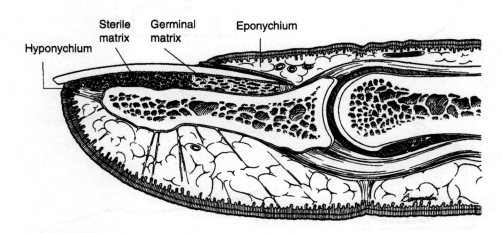

Figure 90.1. Cross-section of nail anatomy. Reproduced with permission, from The Christine M. Kleinert Institute for Hand and Microsurgery, Inc.

remaining 10% of the nail is contributed by the sterile matrix laying distal to the lunula and compensates for dorsal wear. The nail fold adds to the shine of the nail while the ventral floor produces the cells that push upward and flow distally. Nail growth occurs at approximately 3–4 mm per month (Figure 90.1).

ASSESSMENT

Nail bed injuries may range in severity from subungual hematomas and simple lacerations to more complex stellate lacerations, severe crush injuries, and complete nail bed avulsion. The mechanism contributes significantly

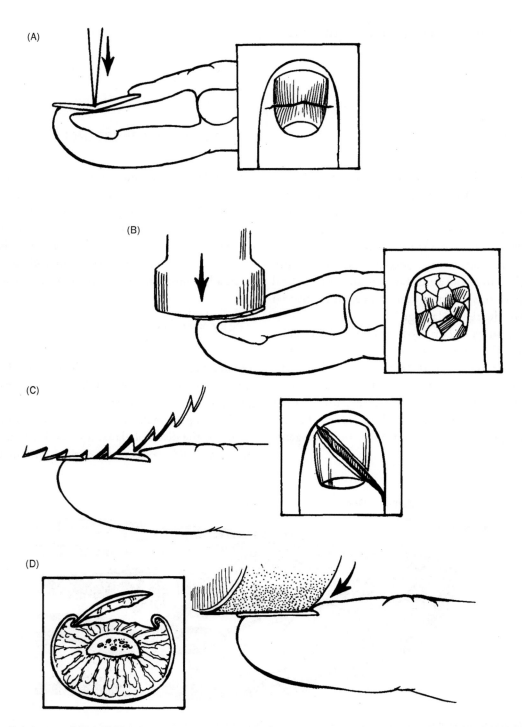

Figure 90.2. Types of injuries to nail bed. (A) Linear or crush laceration caused by narrowly applied forces. (B) Explosion of nail bed caused by more broadly applied forces. (C) Nail bed and perionychial crush and multiple lacerations caused by fast-moving, irregular tools such as saws or drills. (D) Avulsion injury caused by belts and sanders.

HAND SURGERY

to the injury pattern. Disruption of the nail bed beneath an intact nail plate may result in a subungual hematoma. Narrowly applied forces cause a linear crush with laceration, whereas more broadly applied forces produce an explosion of the nail bed. Fast-moving, irregular tools, such as saws and drills, produce a nail bed and perionychial crush injury with multiple lacerations (Figure 90.1A–D). When force is applied to the distal end of the phalanx, the germinal and sterile matrix may be dislocated with the nail plate. This type of injury can be deceptive, as the nail plate may otherwise be intact (Figure 90.2). Although a multitude of classification schemes for nail bed injury exist, they are not tied to outcome or management and are not included in this discussion.

Assessment of all injuries should begin with a thorough history and physical. Be sure to obtain details regarding the mechanism of injury. It is important to note the injury timeline, patient's age, handedness, medical comorbidities, smoking status, and occupation. Patient evaluation should include vaccination status. For patients with unclear or outdated vaccinations, a tetanus vaccination should be provided. A careful examination following adequate cleaning of the injured site should follow. Due to the position of the nail bed between two protective structures—the distal phalanx and the nail plate—generally, the force to damage the nail bed is great enough to cause a fracture of the distal phalanx. As such, up to 50% of nail bed injuries are associated with distal phalanx fractures, and radiographic evaluation of the involved finger is required. If necessary, a digital block may be utilized to assist in obtaining a thorough evaluation. Prior to any type of digit block, sensation should be tested to evaluate for nerve damage. During the exam, tendon function should also be noted to ensure that the extensor and flexor insertions on the distal phalanx have not been disrupted.

INDICATIONS, CONTRAINDICATIONS, AND INJURY MANAGEMENT

PREOPERATIVE CONSIDERATIONS

Indications for nail bed repair include any crush or avulsion of the nail bed, injury to the nail fold, distal phalangeal fractures associated with nail bed injury, complete or partial avulsion of the nail plate, and associated soft tissue injury with exposed bone. Contraindications to nail bed repair include soft tissue or bone infections that necessitate a more significant intervention and medical instability to tolerate the appropriate procedure (Table 90.1).

PREOPERATIVE PREPARATION

Assessment of the patient and injury assists in determination of anesthesia needs for repair. In a noncomplicated, single-digit injury, repair in the emergency department (ED) under digital nerve block is sufficient. In children, anxious adults, uncooperative patients, complex injuries, multidigit involvement, or severely contaminated injuries, the repair may be performed in the operating room or under sedation in the ED. Anesthetic options in these cases include wrist blocks, regional anesthesia, intravenous sedation, or general anesthesia.

Additional preoperative considerations include antibiotic prophylaxis. There is limited data regarding antibiotic utilization in these injuries. A short course of oral antibiotics is usually recommend if there is an associated underlying

TABLE 90.1 MANAGEMENT OF SECONDARY DEFORMITY AFTER NAIL BED INJURY

Complication	Cause	Treatment
Nail ridges	Scar under nail bed	None if asymptomatic
Dull nail	Damage to dorsal roof	None
Nonadherence	Scar in sterile matrix	None if asymptomatic
Split nail	Scar (longitudinal) or ridge in germinal or sterile matrix	Scar excision and nail bed repair or replacement
Short nail	Shortening of sterile matrix	Osteoonychocutaneous free graft from toe
Hook-nail deformity	Loss of bony support	Excision of scarred tissue and replacement with a local flap, bone grafting with local flap, or full thickness skin graft
Nail spurring	Residual nail matrix	Ablation

phalanx fracture. Additionally, they can be considered in settings of severe contamination or in patients with medical complications such as uncontrolled diabetes.

GENERAL APPROACH TO NAIL BED REPAIR AND FINGERTIP INJURY

PREOPERATIVE PREPARATION IN THE EMERGENCY DEPARTMENT

The required supplies for nail bed repair in the ED are as follows:

- Trash bin, Mayo stand, sitting stool, proper lighting
- Additional towels for the floor and bed
- Two packs of sterile fluffs
- Two 1-liter bottles of saline
- Povidone-iodine (Betadine) prep solution
- Freer elevator, iris scissors, needle driver, pickups, fine rongeur if bone shortening needed, bandage scissors
- 18-gauge and 27-gauge needle, 10 cc syringe, Lidocaine, Marcaine, and bicarbonate
- Fingercot or other type of finger tourniquet (Note: Be sure that, whatever type of tourniquet is utilized, it is easily visualized to ensure removal at the end of the procedure)
- Loupe magnification
- 4-0 chromic suture for skin repair
- 6-0 or 7-0 fast suture for nail bed repair
- Two pairs of sterile gloves
- Sterile drapes/towels
- Xeroform, bacitracin, 2-inch cling, 2 × 2 gauze, plastic tape

Prior to setting up, have the patient sign an informed consent. Be sure to discuss the possible risks of any procedures as well as the risks of long-term complications such as nail deformities, numbness, hypersensitivity, long-term cold sensitivity, loss of graft if a graft is to be utilized for repair, osteomyelitis, malunion, and need for revision. If the nail plate has been or will be removed, educate the patient that it will take several months for the nail plate to grow out again.

After obtaining informed consent, perform the digit block. Use a half-and-half mixture of Lidocaine and Marcaine with or without epinephrine. Traditional teaching was to avoid epinephrine in digit injury, but subsequent studies have confirmed its safety. For every 10 cc of this mixture, buffer the solution with 1 cc of 8.4% bicarbonate solution. 10 cc will be more than adequate for a single-digit block. Prep the skin with an alcohol pad prior to performing the block. If the dorsum of the hand is grossly contaminated, wash it gently with Betadine and rinse with normal saline prior to prepping. Our preferred approach is to perform the block on the dorsum of the hand, first with a distracting skin pinch before introducing the needle to the skin (Figure 90.1A–D). The radial skin is blocked first by slowly infusing a few cc's of the mixture. After an adequate wheal has been created, the needle may be gradually advanced into the volar digital neurovascular bundles.

After the block, allow for onset of analgesia while you prepare the Mayo stand with the required supplies: fill one pack of fluffs with Betadine and the second one with saline. Apply the ointment to an edge of the table and prepare a few pieces of tape, which you can place on the edge of the Mayo stand for easy access (Figures 90.2 and 90.3). Having

(A)

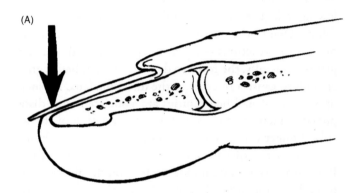

(B)

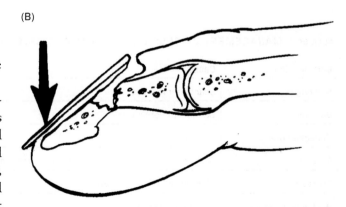

Figure 90.3. Injuries from force applied to distal end of intact nail. (A) Distal phalanx is bent without fracture, but dislocation of germinal and sterile matrix occurs. (B) Distal phalanx is fractured and dislocation of germinal and sterile matrix, linear tears, or stellate lacerations may occur.

everything in place prior to the start of the procedure will maximize efficiency.

Once prepared, have the patient extend the arm over the trash bin. With the first pair of sterile gloves, prep the patient's entire hand with povidone-iodine (Betadine), allowing the runoff to be caught in the waste bin (Figure 90.4). Keeping one hand sterile, use the other hand to open the bottles of saline. Use your still-sterile hand to rub and clean the patient's hand while pouring saline over the wound with your unsterile hand, again allowing the rinse to collect in the waste bin (Figure 90.5). Ask the patient to keep the hand elevated over the waste bin while changing into the second pair of sterile gloves. Next, lay out the drapes and prepare your procedure field. (Figure 90.6).

Depending on the anesthesia/repair technique and injury extent, the tourniquet may only be at the level of the injured digit, or it may be placed on the forearm tor upper arm. Upper extremity tourniquet pressure is determined by adding 100–150 mm Hg to the patient's systolic blood pressure. A tourniquet may not be left inflated for more than 2 hours. An unanaesthetized patient will generally only tolerate about 20 minutes of a forearm or brachial tourniquet. If only utilizing a finger tourniquet, the hand can be prepped and draped prior to tourniquet application (Figure 90.7). If a larger area is to be under tourniquet, the exsanguination and application of a tourniquet occurs prior to prepping and draping the involved extremity. If a finger tourniquet is utilized, be certain to remove it at the end of the case as the combination of an anesthetized finger with a forgotten tourniquet will result in digit loss.

Nail bed repair should always be performed under loupe magnification.

NAIL REMOVAL

After anesthetizing, prepping, and draping the finger, the nail plate is removed by inserting a Freer elevator beneath the free distal edge of the nail at the hyponychium. Using a gentle, fanning motion work proximally to remove the nail (Figure 90.8). Perform this maneuver carefully to avoid further disruption of the nail matrix. In most cases, removal of the entire nail is required to allow for adequate

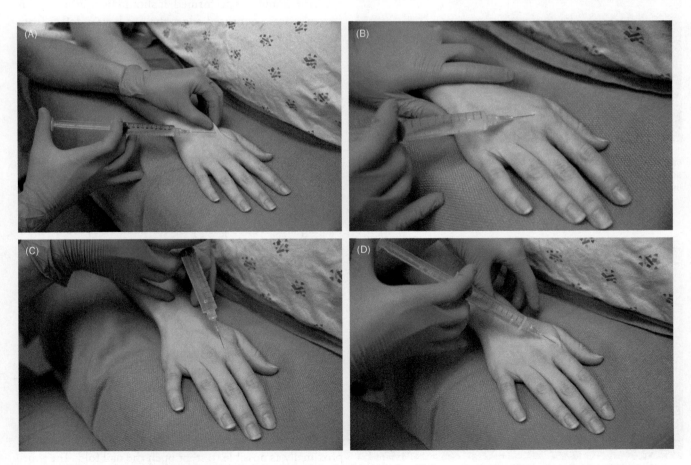

Figure 90.4. Demonstration of the digital nerve block performed for repair of nail bed injuries. (A) Demonstrates the "distracting pinch" performed prior to radial nerve block. (B) Blockade of the radial sensory branches. (C) Slow advancement through the same puncture hole to perform the ulnar digital nerve branch block. (D) Shows the radial digital nerve branch block.

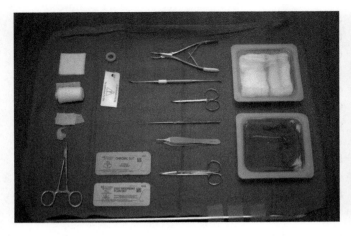

Figure 90.5. Typical mayo stand setup. Setup includes essential instruments, saline moistened gauze, betadine moisened gauze, dressing supplies, sutures, finger tourniquet, and tape.

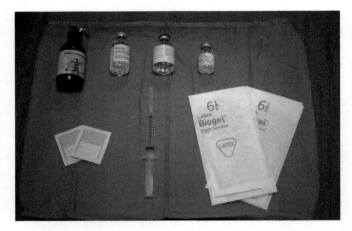

Figure 90.6. Typical non-sterile supply setup. Non-sterile supplies needed: 2 sets of sterile gloves, local anesthesia, alcohol preps, and skin refrigerant useful for patient comfort.

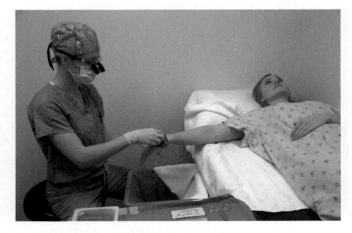

Figure 90.7. Technique for preparing the patient's hand. The patient's hand is prepared with Betadine over waste bin to catch runoff.

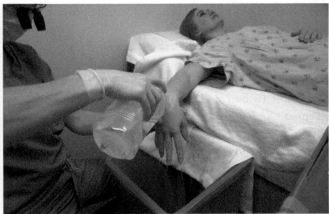

Figure 90.8. Irrigation of wounds with normal saline.

assessment and repair of the nail bed. Once removed, the nail plate should be trimmed of any ragged edges and then the undersurface scraped with the Freer elevator to remove any excess soft tissue or debris. The nail plate should then be placed in povidone-iodine (Betadine) solution during the nail bed repair. The nail bed is then examined. If debridement must be performed, it should be minimal—it is better to leave contused edges than to have a defect from debridement.

DRESSING

Once the repair is complete, an eponychial fold splint should be applied to preserve the nail fold and prevent synechial adherence of the germinal matrix dorsal roof to the ventral floor that would block nail regrowth. The splint can be created by reapplying the nail plate, which is the best option if available. The nail plate is a perfect mold of the nail bed and serves as a biologic dressing that can promote healing and reduce postoperative pain. A figure-of-eight suture is our preferred technique for holding the nail in place (Figure 90.9). Alternatively, the nail can be secured with 4-0 chromic suture through the edge of the nail and the hyponychium or with a mattress suture through the nail and nail fold. This technique risks further scarring and damage to the nail matrix and as such is not our preferred method. If the nail plate is too badly injured to replace, or is missing, a substitute should be fabricated (Figures 90.11, 90.13, and 90.16). This can be created from nonadherent gauze (Xeroform, Adaptic), metal foil from the suture package, or a sterile 0.020-inch silicon sheet. In either case, care must be taken to ensure that the splint is placed as proximally as possible to stent open the nail fold. The tourniquet is then removed and fingertip vascularity noted. Both the duration of time of tourniquet application and the

HAND SURGERY

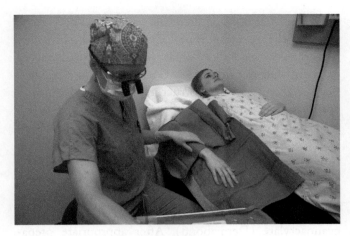

Figure 90.9. Application of sterile drapes.

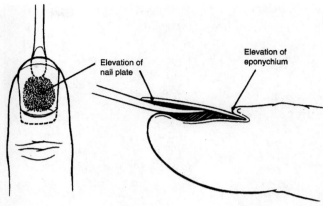

Elevation of nail plate

Elevation of eponychium

Figure 90.11. Elevation of the nail plate for exposure of the nail bed.

return of appropriate capillary refill should be documented in the procedure note. The finger is then wrapped in a loose dressing of nonadherent gauze, antibiotic ointment, and sterile gauze (FIGURE 9a–e). A protective aluminum foam cap may be applied for protection and comfort but should not immobilize any joint. If a fracture is present, a splint should be applied and kept in place for 2–3 weeks.

MANAGEMENT OF SPECIFIC NAIL BED INJURIES

SUBUNGUAL HEMATOMA

Subungual hematomas occur when injury of the nail bed causes bleeding beneath the nail plate. Inciting injuries are frequently minor crush injuries, but the confined space created by an intact nail can lead to severe pain. If the nail

plate is at all disrupted, it should be removed to allow for inspection of the injury with repair if needed. Additionally, if a widely displaced tuft fracture is concomitant or the nail matrix appears to be trapped in the fracture, the nail plate should be removed to allow for reduction and repair. Large hematomas are indicative of more substantial injury and are generally considered an indication for nail plate removal to inspect for possible nail bed injury. If the hematoma is small and there is no significant underlying fracture, trephination alone can be performed to alleviate the pressure and pain. Trephination should be performed under sterile conditions in order to avoid inoculation of the hematoma. If the patient is in severe pain and unable to tolerate the procedure, a digit block can be performed. After the finger is prepped and draped in sterile fashion, evacuation of the hematoma can be performed by creation of a hole in the nail plate by

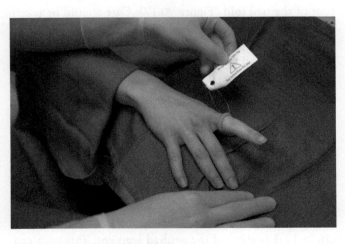

Figure 90.10. Finger tourniquet applied.

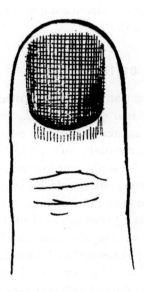

Figure 90.12. Figure of eight suture to hold nail fold stent in place.

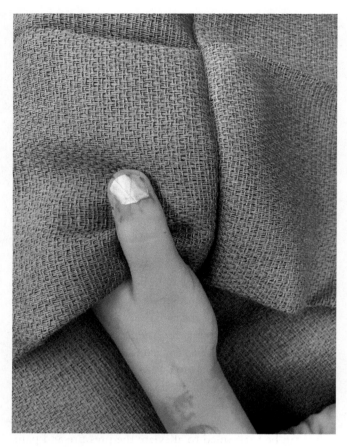

Figure 90.13. Splint creation to maintain nail fold. The splint should maintain the nail fold open once in place.

carefully twisting a no. 11 blade or applying gentle pressure with a battery-powered microcautery unit, taking care to avoid further injuring the underlying nail bed with the instrument of choice. The hole should be large enough to allow for drainage in order to avoid recurrence of the hematoma (Figure 90.15).

LACERATIONS OF THE NAIL BED

The goal of laceration repair is to provide a smooth nail bed surface for nail plate regrowth. Precise alignment and repair of all injured structures is essential to maintain nail integrity. Undermining of the edges of the laceration by 1 mm allows for slight eversion with repair. Any protruding bone fragments should be leveled or removed, and exposed and contaminated bone is curetted prior to repair. Nondisplaced fractures of the tuft and distal phalanx are treated with repair of the nail bed and replacement of the nail plate as a splint. Displaced fractures of the distal phalanx should be anatomically reduced, and this is almost always achieved with adequate soft tissue repair.

If K-wire fixation is required, the patient will need to be taken to the operating room. Closure of the nail bed is performed with a 6-0 or 7-0 fast suture on a small tapered or spatulated needle (e.g., a GS-9 ophthalmic needle). Care is taken to repair all structures anatomically. Sutures are placed in a simple interrupted fashion (Figure 90.16). If the injury is more severe, devascularized areas of the nail bed should be replaced as free grafts. The nail fold skin should be repaired with fine chromic suture and the pulp skin may be repaired with a larger 4-0 chromic suture. An alternate option for nail bed repair, which has been described as equivalent to suture repair, is with 2-octyl-cyanoacrylate (Dermabond). After appropriate preparation, the nail bed fragments should be opposed gently using fine forceps or by gently cupping the digit pulp with the surgeon's fingers. The 2-octyl-cyanoacrylate should then be applied over the entire sterile matrix and reapplied three times with 30 second intervals between the layers. Care must be taken during application to not disrupt or displace the edges of the nail bed fragments with excessive pressure or movement to avoid adhesive entering the wound and compromising healing.

AVULSION INJURIES OF THE NAIL BED

Avulsion injuries of the nail bed are typically more severe and carry a worse prognosis for subsequent nail deformity. When force is applied to the nail plate dorsally and distally, an avulsion of the proximal nail bed from underneath the nail fold may occur. This results in a distally based nail bed flap (Figure 90.17). Repair should be performed using fine chromic horizontal mattress sutures to bring the avulsed germinal matrix back under the nail fold. The suture is passed through the proximal portion of the fold into the free margin of the nail bed and back out through the dorsal roof of the nail fold (Figure 90.17). Care should be taken when evaluating children with this type of injury because the nail matrix may become interposed between the growth plate of the distal phalanx. This injury, known as a Seymour fracture, requires operative intervention. When the nail plate is completely avulsed, it may take with it a portion of the nail bed adherent to the ventral surface. If possible, retrieve the nail plate and any amputated tissues to attempt repair. Replacing the nail and nail bed as a whole will allow for the best alignment and inosculation as well as compression on the graft. If the nail plate is overly damaged, carefully remove the avulsed nail bed from the plate and suture it in place (Figure 90.17). It is important to maintain the original orientation of the avulsed segment. This graft can

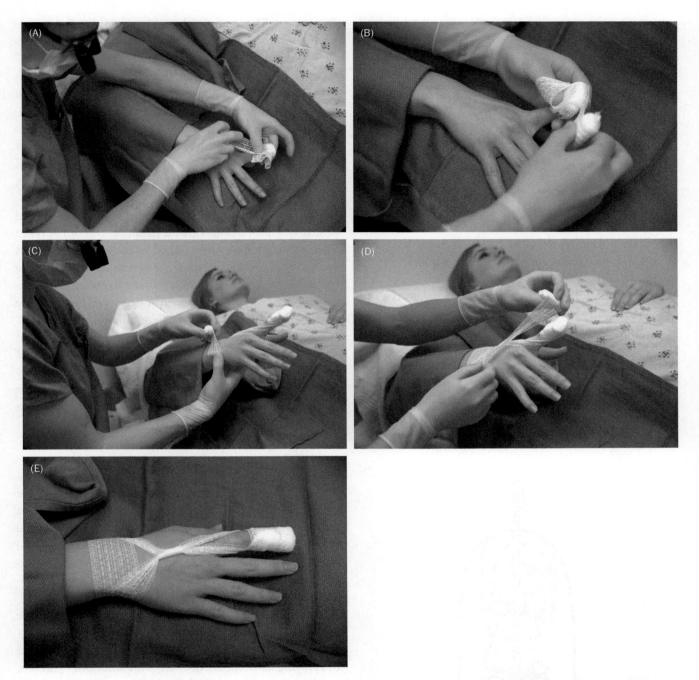

Figure 90.14. Application of gauze dressing. (A) The bulky wrap over the digit end. (B) Contouring of the wrap around the finger. (C-D) Extension of the wrap to the patient's wrist to prevent the dressing from becoming dislodged. (E) The final wrap, taped. This dressing allows for patient's to maintain full range of motion without risk of dislodging their dressing.

be held in place using a carefully applied dressing or a tie-over bolster.

INJURIES WITH NAIL BED DEFICITS

If the nail bed defect is split-thickness, it will regenerate and does not need closure. If a small area of full-thickness nail bed loss occurs, lateral release of the paronychial folds will allow for advancement of the germinal matrix toward the center of the nail and primary repair. This technique can be useful with a defect of less than 3–5 mm or in a patient for whom grafting isn't an option due to medical contraindications or patient preference.

For larger areas of nail bed loss, the cortical bone in the distal phalanx will accept a matrix graft. Results are inconsistent, and a careful discussion with the patient

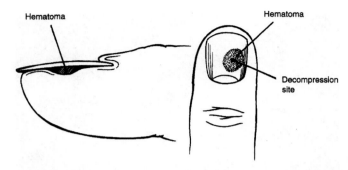

Figure 90.15. Evacuation by nail perforation is performed for a subungual hematoma.

regarding additional deformity at the donor site is required. For reconstruction of small defects of the sterile matrix, an adjacent uninvolved finger or the great toe can be used as a donor sites. The graft must be taken as a thin split-thickness sterile matrix graft because it will not take successfully and injury can occur to the donor site if the graft is too thick. Graft harvest is performed under loupe magnification in the operating room. The donor digit is anesthetized and prepared in the standard fashion. Only as much of the nail plate as necessary is removed to harvest the graft. Leave the proximal nail intact within the nail fold. A template of the defect is transposed to the

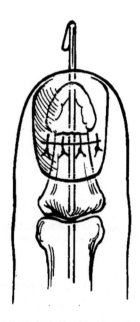

Figure 90.16. Treatment for nail bed injuries with distal phalanx fractures. The nail plate is removed to examine nail bed injury. Displaced fractures of distal phalanx can be anatomically reduced and percutaneously fixed with K-wire. Repair is closed with interrupted 7-0 chromic sutures using a small, tapered or spatulated needle. The nail plate is reapplied. If the nail plate cannot be reapplied, nonadherent gauze, metal foil from suture package, or nail fabricated from a sterile 0.020-in. silicone sheet can be used in its place as a splint.

donor site. The graft is then harvested using a gentle sawing motion with a surgical blade with the scalpel parallel to the nail bed. The graft should be between 0.007 and 0.011 inches in depth, thin enough that the knife edge is visible through the graft (Figure 90.1). It should be 1–2 mm larger than the defect (Figure 90.18). The orientation of the graft should be maintained to avoid the appearance of a ridge where the recipient tissue and graft meet. The donor site is dressed by reapplication of the nail followed by nonadherent dressing and a protective cap, when applicable (Figure 90.18).

In germinal matrix defects greater than can be closed primarily, a full-thickness graft is required. This can be taken from an amputated, nonsalvaged finger or from the great toe nail bed. A longitudinal strip of germinal and sterile matrix along with a wedge of underlying tissue can be taken from the lateral aspect of a toenail bed with direct closure of the donor site, avoiding complete ablation of the toenail. If harvesting an entire toe nail bed, the donor site is closed with a split-thickness skin graft (Figure 90.18). A section of the donor nail plate or the original nail plate and a carefully applied nonadherent dressing are used to bolster the graft to the recipient fingertip. A small hole should be created in the nail plate to allow for adequate drainage.

INJURY OF THE NAIL BED AND FINGERTIP

The goals for reconstruction of any fingertip injury should be adequate sensory recovery, length preservation, joint function preservation, durable wound closure, and minimal donor site morbidity. Consideration of both the nature and function of the tissues lost and the patient's goals and expectations is vital in choosing the most appropriate reconstructive option (Figure 90.19).

Loss of palmar skin and pulp without exposed bone measuring less than 1 cm² may be allowed to heal by secondary intention with good results. Wound care consists of applying an occlusive dressing with antibiotic ointment and Xeroform gauze daily for several weeks. Larger wounds require coverage with a skin graft. Split-thickness grafts are preferred due to the additional secondary contraction resulting in a minimization of the insensate area. After graft inset, a conforming dressing or tie-over bolster is used for the recipient site. Though some sensory recovery may be possible, true tactile development likely never occurs, limiting the application of skin grafts in the hand to small, preferably nontactile areas.

Fingertip amputations involving only 2–3 mm of the distal phalanx can be treated by bone shortening and primary closure, also known as *revision amputation*. If fingertip

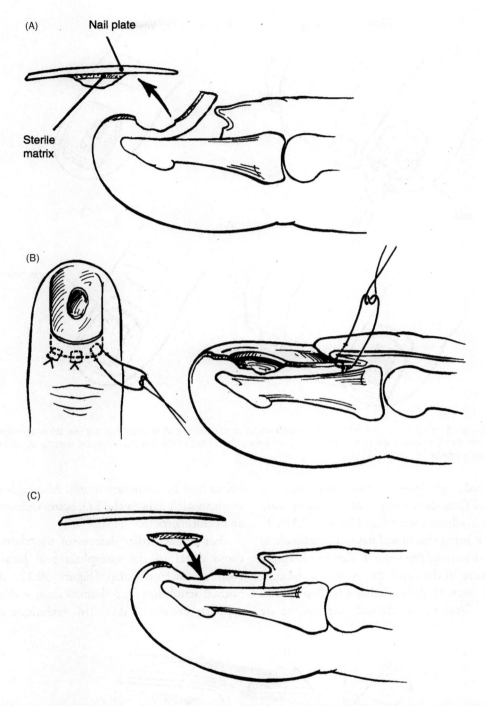

(A) Nail plate

Sterile matrix

(B)

(C)

Figure 90.17. Treatment for nail bed avulsion injuries. (A) Avulsion of proximal nail bed from nail fold, leaving distal nail bed flaps. (B) 7-0 chromic sutures are passed through proximal portion of fold into the free margin of the nail bed and back out through the dorsal roof of nail fold. (C) Avulsed section of the nail bed is removed from the plate and sutured into place.

pulp of more than one-third the length of the phalanx is lost, soft tissue replacement to support the distal nail is necessary to prevent a hook nail deformity. If the digit is to be shortened more significantly, care must be taken to completely ablate the germinal matrix and obliterate future nail growth.

For volarly angled amputations with large skin and pulp defects as well as exposed bone, primary closure would require an unreasonable amount of bone shortening. In such instances, extended Kutler flaps or regional flaps are often required for coverage (Figure 90.20). Dorsally angulated amputations are easier to repair than the palmarly angulated

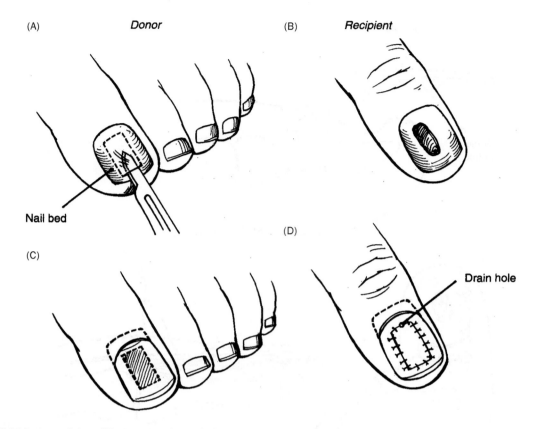

Figure 90.18. Split thickness graft for nail bed repair defects. (A) Split-thickness sterile matrix graft is taken form big toe. (B) Recipient site with defect. The graft should be so thin that the point of the knife can be visualized through it. (C) Reappliction of the nail at the donor site. (D) Graft sutured to the recipient site and the nail reapplied.

variety because dorsal fingertip amputation spares the more sensate palmar skin. These dorsal amputations may be managed with volar V-Y advancement flap (Figure 90.21). In practice, even when using these local flaps, it is difficult to achieve complete closure of the wound. Key to obtaining maximal advancement of the flap is full release of the connection of the soft tissue to the underlying tendon sheath. Often small areas at both the donor and recipient site are

left to heal by secondary intent. Although it is possible to perform such flaps in the ED, better outcomes are likely in an operating room.

For smaller volar defects of the thumb, particularly those distal to the interphalangeal joint, the Moberg volar advancement flap (Figure 90.22) maintains near normal sensibility. The thumb's unique dorsal circulation supports the dorsal skin. This technique often results in

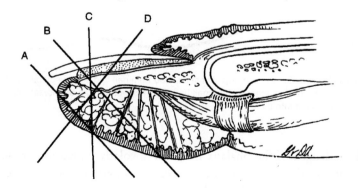

Figure 90.19. Levels and angles of amputation. (A) Volar skin and pulp loss without bone exposed. (B) Large amount of volar skin and pulp loss with distal phalanx exposed. (C) Guillotine fingertip amputation. (D) Dorsal fingertip amputation with little nail bed remaining. Reproduced, with permission, from The Christine M. Kleinert Institute for Hand and Microsurgery, Inc.

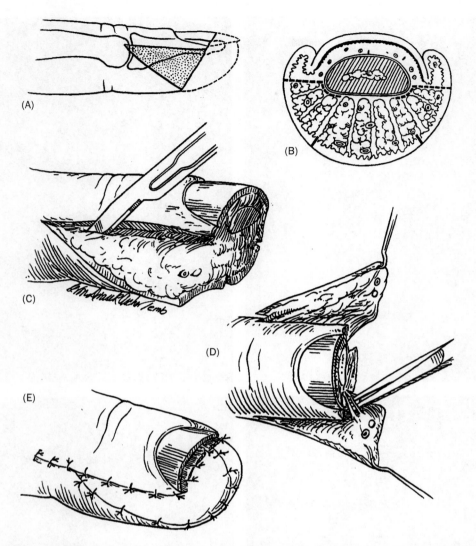

Figure 90.20. Extended Kutler flap. (A) Flap design. (B-C) Dorsal incision deepened to free flap from distal phalanx. (D) Septi divided while preserving nerves and vesels. (E) Flaps advanced and closed using V-Y technique. Reproduced, with permission, from The Christine M. Kleinert Institute for Hand and Microsurgery, Inc.

a mild flexion contracture of the thumb interphalangeal joint, which is generally well tolerated by patients and can be addressed with secondary splinting after the wound is healed. Larger volar thumb defects may be addressed with a sensate first dorsal metacarpal flap. The alternative sensate flap, the Littler flap, is infrequently used due to significant complications associated with the donor digit. Smaller volar defects of the fingers and thumb may be closed with a standard or modified cross-finger flap (Figure 90.23) or with a thenar flap. Dorsal roof and nail wall avulsion may be repaired by local dorsal rotation flaps or a reverse cross-finger flap, although results with the reverse cross-finger flap are often unsatisfactory. (Figure 90.24). These procedures require an operating room. For patients over the

age of 40, cross-finger flaps and thenar flaps are relatively contraindicated due to the frequent complication of joint flexion contracture and digit stiffness.

COMPLETE NAIL BED AMPUTATION

Replantation at or distal to the distal interphalangeal (DIP) joint has been reported to achieve 81% viability with adequate sensibility. This procedure, however, remains controversial as well as technically demanding. Replantation at the level of the lunula presents venous outflow problems, frequently requiring adjuncts such as medicinal leeches. Composite replacement of fingertip amputations in adults is much less successful than in children, with one study

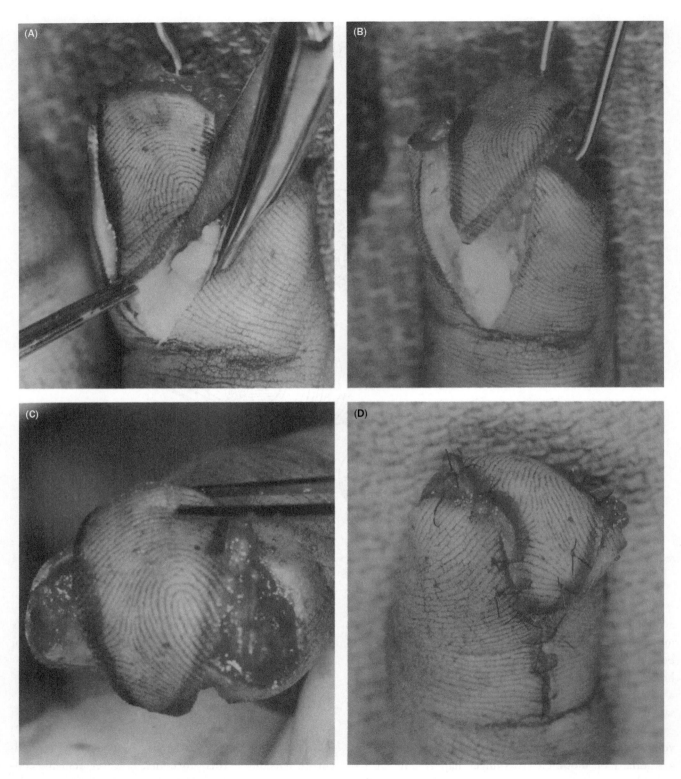

Figure 90.21. Volar V-Y advancement flap. (A) Skin incision. The apex of the flap is placed at the distal crease. The base is made as wide as the nail bed. (B-C) Flap mobilization. (D) The flap is advanced and the incision closed by converting the V to a Y. Reproduced, with permission, from The Christine M. Kleinert Institute for Hand and Microsurgery, Inc.

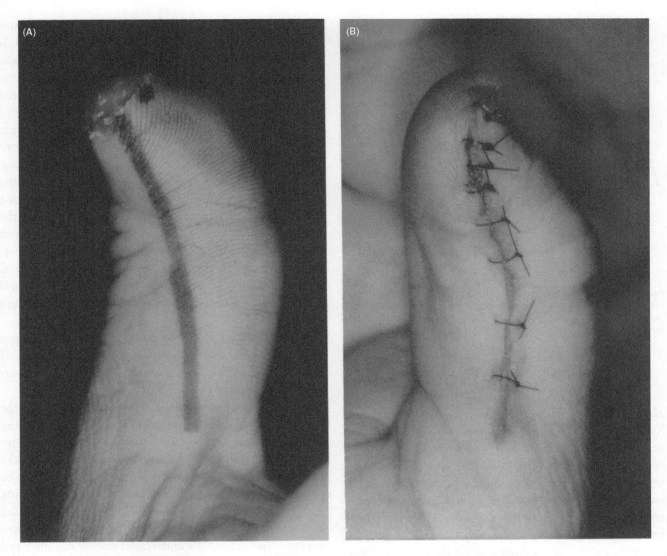

Figure 90.22. (A-B) Moberg volar advancement flap. Reproduced, with permission, from The Christine M. Kleinert Institute for Hand and Microsurgery, Inc.

showing only a 20% survival rate for amputations at the level of the lunula and a 25% incidence of at least partial necrosis distal to this level.

Rose proposed the "cap" technique, in which the amputated segment is filleted and reapplied as a cap over the distal phalanx bone peg (Figure 90.25). In this technique, approximately 6 mm of soft tissue was trimmed from the proximal stump of the distal phalanx, being careful to retain at least 2 mm of the germinal matrix. The concept is to increase the contact area between the composite and vascularized tissue. To avoid the sharp area of the volar aspect of the stump, the volar cortex can be trimmed, leaving

intact bone under the proximal nail. In the study by Rose, all six patients with lunula-level amputations had complete survival with an average two-point discrimination of 6.5 mm. However, composite grafting in the adult remains risky with a high chance of failure. Results are not evident until approximately 6 weeks after surgery. In the case of a patient who is unwilling to consent for revision amputation and not a candidate for replantation, it is a reasonable option.

Microsurgical toenail transfer has been reported to have high success rates and good cosmetic outcomes. However, the procedure is technically demanding and should be reserved for special situations.

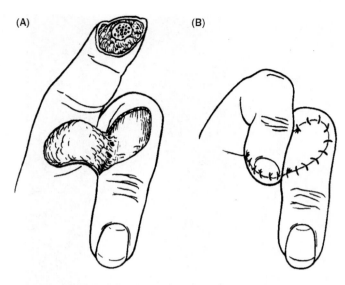

Figure 90.23. Cross-finger flap. (A) volar oblique amputation of the left index finger. Elevation of a cross-finger flap. (B) Flap sutured to edges of defect. Reproduced, with permission, from The Christine M. Kleinert Institute for Hand and Microsurgery, Inc.

NAIL BED INJURIES IN CHILDREN

Nail bed injuries comprise approximately two-thirds of hand injuries in children. These injuries should be addressed utilizing the same meticulous technique as in adults to avoid deformity. Extra care should be taken to avoid undue tension on soft tissue closure of the fingertip to prevent necrosis. Healing by secondary intention and composite grafts are more successful in children than adults, however. The repair should be protected with a long arm cast for any child under the age of 5 and a short arm cast for older children.

POSTOPERATIVE CARE

The patient should be instructed to keep the finger and dressing dry until follow-up and to elevate the hand when possible to reduce swelling. They are encouraged in range of motion exercises multiple times daily to prevent stiffness and contracture. Patients are seen in clinic 5–7 days following repair, at which time the dressing is carefully taken down. The dressing can be removed by soaking in normal saline. If a skin graft or nail matrix graft was performed, the dressing is left in place for 10 days unless there is a concern for infection. The suture holding the nail plate or splint in place under the nail fold should be removed at the first clinic visit, leaving the stent in place. The nail plate often adheres to the nail bed and the new nail growth will push the old nail off the nail bed, typically in 1–3 months. If nonadherent gauze or foil was used to stent the nail fold, it should be left in place for 2 weeks to prevent adhesion at the level of the nail fold. Approximately 1 year is required prior to reliable evaluation of final nail appearance.

Starting 1 week after injury, the patient should begin a standard desensitization and sensory reeducation program. This program is typically instituted with the assistance of a hand therapist and consists of fingertip tapping on firm surfaces in a progressively stronger fashion along with recognition of various objects in a bag using only the fingertips. Most patients respond well to these programs and do not have additional problems. For those with persistent complaints, the hand therapist may utilize several techniques, such as immersion, vibration, and electrical stimulation or transcutaneous electrical nerve stimulation (TENS).

Complications following repair include nail absence, split nail, ridges, short nail, dull nail, cold intolerance, or hook-nail deformity. These complications and their treatment are delineated in Table 90.1.

Nail ridges are caused by an uneven surface beneath the nail bed, leading to irregularity in growth and the formation of a ridge. These are typically a cosmetic complication unless symptomatic by causing elevation of the nail from the nail bed and nonadherence. If this occurs, correction can be performed by elevating the nail bed off the distal phalanx with surgical excision of the scar. Nonadherence is caused by a scar in the sterile matrix resulting in a lack of contribution of nail cells to the undersurface of the nail plate and subsequent lack of adhesion. The scared area of sterile matrix must be excised and either repaired or replaced with a split-thickness sterile matrix graft. A shortened nail and hook-nail deformity can be repaired with graft transfer from the toe. Nail spikes and spurs may be treated by revision nail matrix ablation.

CONCLUSION

Nail bed and fingertip injuries are extremely common and can be initially quite disabling. An understanding of the anatomy and physiology of the fingertip, the mechanism of injury, and the various techniques for repair is vital if deformity and long-term disability are to be avoided. When surgery is necessary, meticulous technique is essential for successful repair.

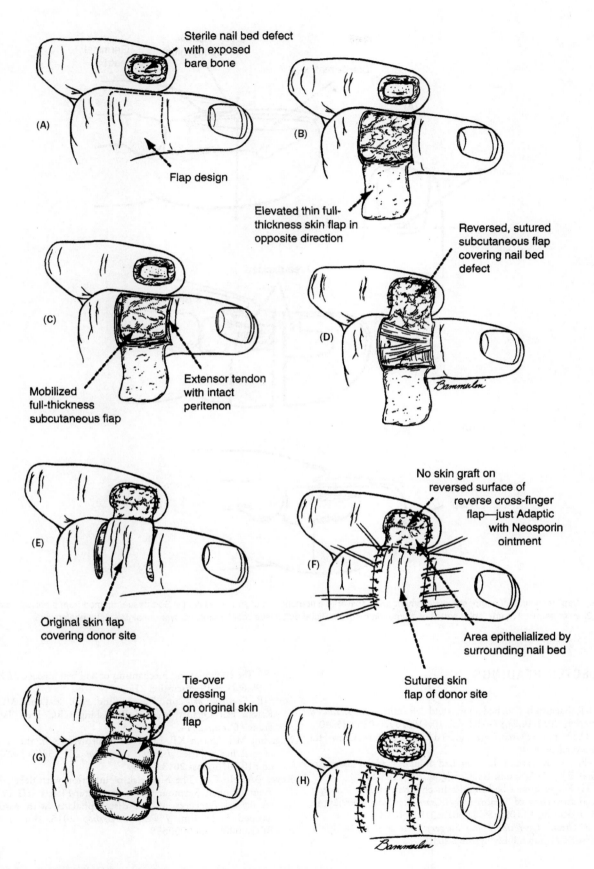

Figure 90.24. Reverse cross-finger flap. Reproduced, with permission, from The Christine M. Kleinert Institute for Hand and Microsurgery, Inc.

Labels within the figure:

(A) Sterile nail bed defect with exposed bare bone; Flap design

(B) Elevated thin full-thickness skin flap in opposite direction

(C) Mobilized full-thickness subcutaneous flap; Extensor tendon with intact peritenon

(D) Reversed, sutured subcutaneous flap covering nail bed defect

(E) Original skin flap covering donor site

(F) No skin graft on reversed surface of reverse cross-finger flap—just Adaptic with Neosporin ointment; Area epithelialized by surrounding nail bed; Sutured skin flap of donor site

(G) Tie-over dressing on original skin flap

(H)

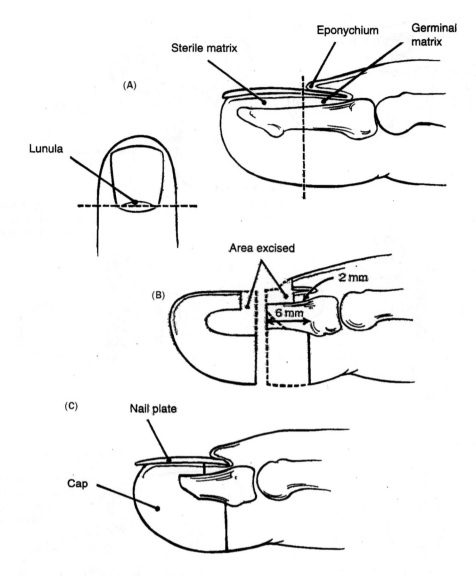

(A)

Sterile matrix

Eponychium

Germinal matrix

Lunula

(B)

Area excised

2 mm

6 mm

(C)

Nail plate

Cap

Figure 90.25. "Cap" technique of composite replacement. (A) Transverse amputation through the lunula. (B) Soft tissue trimmed from prodimal stump, retaining 2mm of germinal matrix. Volar cortex of stump trimmed. (C) Distal soft-tissue "cap" reapplied over remaining distal phalanx.

SELECTED READINGS

Bharathi RR, Bajantri B. Nail bed injuries and deformities of nail. *Indian J Plast Surg* 2011;44(2):97–202. doi: 10.4103/0970-0358.85340

Evans GRD. *Operative Plastic Surgery* (1st ed.). New York: McGraw-Hill Professional, 2000.

Fehrenbacher V, Blackburn E. Nail bed injury. *J Hand Surg Am* 2015;40(3):581–582. doi: 10.1016/j.jhsa.2014.10.024

Gellman H. Fingertip-nail bed injuries in children: current concepts and controversies of treatment. *J Craniofac Surg* 2009;20(4): 1033–1035. doi: 10.1097/SCS.0b013e3181abb1b5

Green DP. *Green's Operative Hand Surgery* (6th ed.). Philadelphia, PA: Elsevier/Churchill Livingstone, 2010.

Guy RJ. The etiologies and mechanisms of nail bed injuries. *Hand Clin* 1990;6(1):9–19; discussion 21.

Janis JE. *Essentials of Plastic Surgery* (2nd. ed.). St. Louis, MO/Boca Raton, FL: Quality Medical Publishing CRC Press/Taylor & Francis Group, 2014.

Mignemi ME, Unruh KP, Lee DH. Controversies in the treatment of nail bed injuries. *J Hand Surg Am* 2013;38(7):1427–1430. doi: 10.1016/j.jhsa.2013.04.009

Reyes BA, Ho CA. The high risk of infection with delayed treatment of open Seymour fractures: Salter-Harris I/II or juxta-epiphyseal fractures of the distal phalanx with associated nailbed laceration. *J Pediatr Orthop* 2015. doi: 10.1097/BPO.0000000000000638

Saito H, Suzuki Y, Fujino K, Tajima T. Free nail bed graft for treatment of nail bed injuries of the hand. *J Hand Surg Am* 1983;8(2): 171–178.

Van Beek AL, Kassan MA, Adson MH, Dale V. Management of acute fingernail injuries. *Hand Clin* 1990;6(1):23–35; discussion 37–28.

Yam A, Tan SH, Tan AB. A novel method of rapid nail bed repair using 2-octyl cyanoacrylate (Dermabond). *Plast Reconstr Surg* 2008;121(3): 148e–149e. doi: 10.1097/01.prs.0000300212.73022.9d

Zook EG. Anatomy and physiology of the perionychium. *Clin Anat* 2003;16(1):1–8. doi: 10.1002/ca.10078

Zook EG, Guy RJ, Russell RC. A study of nail bed injuries: causes, treatment, and prognosis. *J Hand Surg Am* 1984;9(2):247–252.

Zook EG, Van Beek AL, Russell RC, Beatty ME. Anatomy and physiology of the perionychium: a review of the literature and anatomic study. *J Hand Surg Am* 2980;5(6):528–536.

91.

EXTENSOR TENDON REPAIR

Scott D. Oates

The location of the extensor tendons on the dorsum of the hand and forearm make them especially vulnerable to injury. This is even more common over the interphalangeal and metacarpophalangeal joints, where the subcutaneous tissue is thinner. Because of the nature of their anatomy, extensor tendon repairs may be less technically challenging than flexor tendon repairs. However, careful surgical technique and postoperative care is still required to achieve excellent results.[1-7]

The repair and rehabilitation of severed extensor tendons is discussed relative to the zone of injury. The eight classic zones of extensor injury correspond to anatomic changes in the tendons and joint location. They can easily be recalled based on the odd numbers corresponding to the joints (zone I over distal interphalangeal [DIP], zone III over proximal interphalangeal [PIP], etc.).[2]

ZONES I AND II

ASSESSMENT OF THE DEFECT

Extensor tendon disruption in zones I and II is common. Injuries to the terminal tendon, triangular ligament, and conjoint tendons can be closed or open. Tearing or rupture of the terminal tendon usually results from a closed hyperflexion injury. The terminal tendon may be solely involved, or the injury may be concomitant with a chip fracture from the dorsum of the distal phalanx where the tendon inserts. An extensor lag develops with loss of active extension of the distal phalanx (known as a mallet finger) (Figure 91.1). Volar subluxation or dislocation of the distal phalanx may also be apparent if the collateral ligaments are disrupted. With bony mallet injuries, a fragment of the distal phalanx remains attached to

the terminal tendon. X-rays should be obtained to assess bony involvement. Open lacerations of the terminal tendon demonstrate a similar finger habitus as the closed injury. With open injuries, the DIP joint may be involved. Similarly, the germinal matrix of the nail bed may be injured, resulting from its close proximity to the terminal tendon's insertion. A thorough examination of these local structures is indicated if they are near the zone of injury. Partial tendon lacerations are common and can be diagnosed by eliciting pain on resisted extension. An extensor lag is not present because part of the tendon can still extend the distal phalanx. In all cases of isolated zone I and II injuries, there is normal range of motion and function of the PIP joint. Untreated, these injuries can lead to chronic, nonreducible mallet deformities. In addition, a secondary swan neck deformity (distal phalanx flexion and proximal interphalangeal joint hyperextension) may manifest itself as a result of laxity of the volar plate and overcompensation of the central slip at the PIP joint.

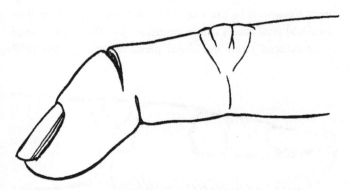

Figure 91.1. Mallet finger deformity. Extensor lag secondary to pull of profundus tendon.

OPERATIVE TECHNIQUE

The treatment of closed disruption of the terminal tendon should be nonoperative. A stack or figure-of-eight splint maintains extension of the distal phalanx (Figure 91.2). The phalanx is held in neutral or slight hyperextension for 6 weeks, at which time gentle active range-of-motion exercises can be initiated. The splint is then worn only at night or in protective situations. At 8 weeks, passive range-of-motion and blocking exercises are initiated. If an extensor lag is still present after the 6 weeks of initial splinting, then the splint should remain in place for another 2–4 weeks before initiating therapy.

The treatment of chip fracture avulsions with the terminal tendon depends on the stability of the interphalangeal joint and the size of the fragment. The bone fragment often achieves anatomic reduction by maintaining the distal phalanx in neutral or slight hyperextension. A single longitudinal 0.045-inch Kirschner wire from the distal phalanx through the DIP joint to the middle phalanx may be indicated if splinting is not feasible or felt to be inadequate alone to maintain proper position of the joint. Splinting is still used if possible in conjunction with percutaneous fixation for 6 weeks. The K-wire is removed and the therapy commences as just described. Larger bone fragments that involve more than 30% of the articular surface may be unstable and fail to maintain anatomic reduction if a closed technique is employed. Unstable volar subluxation of the distal phalanx with a chip fracture mandates open reduction. A curvilinear incision is made dorsally over the DIP joint. The flaps are dissected down to the paratenon and held in retraction with 5-0 nylon to visualize the fracture site. Anatomic reduction is obtained. A pull-through stainless steel wire (or 3-0 nylon) is passed through the terminal tendon, bone fragment, and distal phalanx to the volar aspect of the finger (Figure 91.3). The wire or suture is tied over a button (Figure 91.4). An alternative means of fragment fixation is to use a lag screw from the fragment into the distal phalanx. A single longitudinal 0.045-inch K-wire is introduced from the distal phalanx through the DIP

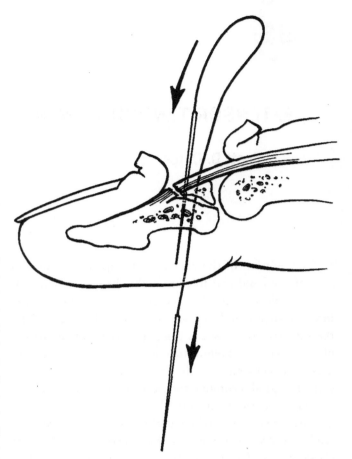

Figure 91.3. Pull-through wires pass through terminal tendon and dorsal bony fragment to volar distal finger.

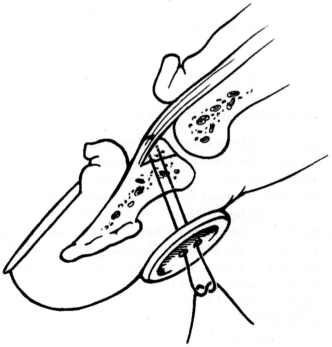

Figure 91.4. Terminal tendon and dorsal chip fracture maintained in anatomic position with pull-through wire over button.

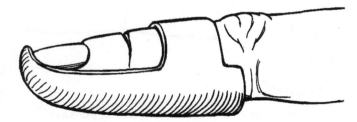

Figure 91.2. Stack splint. Distal phalanx is held in neutral or slight hyperextension. Proximal interphalangeal joint is fully mobile.

joint and into the middle phalanx. The wounds are closed with a 5-0 nylon suture, and antibiotic ointment is applied. A splint is fitted and worn for 6 weeks. The button and pull-through wires are removed at 4 weeks. The therapy regimen commences as described earlier, after the K-wire is removed at 6 weeks. Follow-up x-ray films confirm the appropriate integrity of the articular surface of the distal phalanx.

Open injuries should be addressed at the time of injury. Under local or general anesthesia, the hand is prepped and draped to allow for easy manipulation of the finger. Use of a hand table and turning the operating room table 45 degrees facilitates use of an assistant, and a tourniquet is used with gentle exsanguination. The wound is extended in a proximal and distal fashion. This is accomplished by incising proximally from one edge of the wound and distally from the other edge. The skin flaps are held in retraction with 5-0 nylon sutures. The flaps are mobilized at the level of the paratenon. Care should be taken not to injure the germinal matrix of the nail bed, which is immediately distal to the insertion of the terminal tendon. The joint is thoroughly irrigated with saline solution. The tendon is then repaired with 4-0 permanent suture in a figure-of-eight or horizontal mattress fashion (Figure 91.5). Two sutures may be required for appropriate coaptation. The tendon edge should not be bunched together. The skin is then redraped over

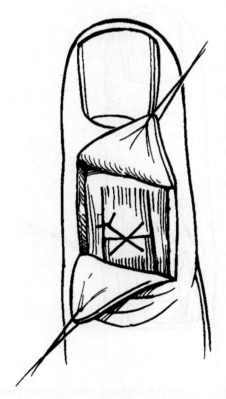

Figure 91.5. Exposed terminal tendon and repair with figure-of-eight 4-0 nylon suture.

the tendon and closed with a 5-0 nylon suture. The DIP is splinted in extension or held with a K-wire, while the PIP joint remains mobile.

POSTOPERATIVE CARE

At 4 weeks postoperatively, any K-wires are removed. At 6 weeks postoperatively, the splint is worn only at night or in protective situations. Additional continuous splinting for another 2–4 weeks is warranted should an extensor lag be present. Otherwise, gentle active range-of-motion therapy of the DIP joint is initiated at 6 weeks. Passive range of motion is started at 8 weeks, and blocking exercises may commence. It is important to continuously evaluate the splint to maintain correct finger posture.

ZONES III AND IV

ASSESSMENT OF THE DEFECT

Extensor injuries in Zone III can also be closed or open. The insertion of the central slip can be avulsed with or without a chip fracture of the proximal aspect of the middle phalanx. These closed injuries may be associated with a volar subluxation or dislocation of the middle phalanx. Central slip avulsions are often difficult to fully appreciate on initial examination but should be suspected with hyperflexion injuries at the PIP joint or in those patients with posttraumatic swelling of the PIP joints. There may or may not be an extensor lag at the PIP joint because, in an acute situation, the lateral bands still function to extend the PIP joint. A sign that the central slip is not functioning appropriately can be elicited by holding the PIP joint in full flexion and observing the passive flexion of the distal phalanx. The finger with a disrupted central slip shows an increased resistance to passive flexion of the DIP joint because of the relative increase in tension in the lateral bands pulling the terminal tendon—and thus the distal phalanx—into extension (Elson's test). Also, an extensor lag (15–20 degrees) may be noticeable if the metacarpophalangeal (MCP) joint and wrist are in flexion while attempting to extend the PIP joint.

Loss of the central slip creates an anatomic and physiologic imbalance of the flexor and extensor forces acting on the finger. The triangular ligament attenuates and the lateral bands soon migrate volarly. The transverse retinacular ligament foreshortens, as do the lateral bands and Landsmeer's ligament (oblique retinacular ligament). These ligaments now pull volar to the pivot axis of the PIP joint. This, in conjunction with the pull of the flexor digitorum sublimis tendon, acts to pull the PIP joint into flexion while the DIP is forced into extension. If left unattended, this boutonnière deformity may become irreducible as the volar plate contracts and bony articular changes occur. It is therefore important to recognize central slip injuries and the significance of repairing the central slip.

INDICATIONS AND CONTRAINDICATIONS

Contaminated wounds, such as human bites, require definitive treatment for the infection with irrigation, debridement, and appropriate antibiotics. Tendon repair in grossly infected wounds should be delayed until the infection resolves and any open areas are closed, usually by delayed secondary closure. Alternatively, the wounds are allowed to heal by secondary intent, and the tendons are repaired 4–6 weeks later. Stable soft tissue coverage in traumatic wounds with flaps or grafts should also be performed prior to definitive tendon repair.

OPERATIVE TECHNIQUE

Closed injuries can usually be managed by splinting the PIP joints in extension for 6 weeks. The DIP and MCP joints can remain mobile.

Open injuries to the extensor apparatus in zones III and IV should follow the same assessment as described previously. Tendon repair in these zones can usually be accomplished in an appropriately equipped emergency department under local anesthetic (digital block). Severely contaminated wounds or associated complex open fractures should be treated in an operative theater under regional or general anesthetic. For the isolated extensor injury, however, the digital block is instilled at the base of the finger and the hand is prepped and draped to allow for easy manipulation of the hand and finger. All nonviable tissue is debrided, and the wound is thoroughly irrigated with a saline solution. If the PIP joint has been entered, a thorough fluid irrigation is required to cleanse the joint. The tendon is repaired in a figure-of-eight, horizontal mattress, or modified Kessler fashion using 4-0 permanent buried sutures. Associated lateral band injury should be repaired similarly. The tendons are quite thin and relatively friable at this level, and therefore, adequate suture purchases are required to hold the repair. However, care should be taken not to telescope tendon edges. As little as 2 mm of extensor overlap or loss could lead to a marked decrease in PIP flexion. The skin is closed with a 5-0 nylon suture and the finger is splinted in extension. Again, if the lateral bands are not involved,

only the PIP joint should be kept in extension. If the lateral bands are involved, the DIP, PIP, and MCP joints should be included in the splint. The DIP and PIP joints are splinted in full extension, and the MCP joints are splinted in 70 degrees of flexion.

Avulsions of the central slip may not have sufficient tendinous substance distally to suture to the proximal segment. In these cases, a transverse hole is drilled in the dorsum of the proximal aspect of the middle phalanx. A suture is passed through the hole, and the central slip is advanced to the bone (Figure 91.6). Alternatively, a suture anchor can be placed in the middle phalanx to secure the tendon.

POSTOPERATIVE CARE

Isolated lacerations to the central slip require PIP splinting in full extension for 5–6 weeks. The DIP and MCP joints may remain mobile. Should the lateral bands also be lacerated, the DIP should be included in the splint. At 6 weeks, splinting continues only at nighttime, and active range-of-motion therapy is initiated. Passive flexion and blocking exercises start at 7–8 weeks at the PIP and DIP joints. After 8 weeks, resisted extension exercises are promoted.

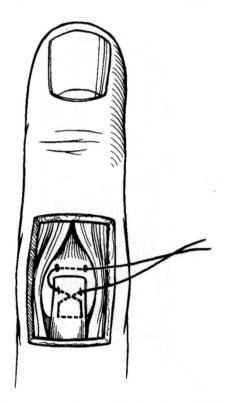

Figure 91.6. Transverse tunnel is created in dorsal aspect of base of middle phalanx. Horizontal suture (4-0 nylon) is passed through central slip and bone. Tightening suture reapproximates central slip tendon.

LACERATIONS OF THE EXTENSOR TENDON IN ZONES V AND VI

ASSESSMENT OF THE DEFECT

Lacerations of the extensor tendon over the MCP joint (zone V) or the dorsum of the hand (zone VI) are common injuries. Discontinuity of the extensor tendons in these zones is usually achieved by direct laceration, although ruptures of tendons have occurred. The patient usually presents with an open wound on the dorsum of the hand, usually over the tendon itself. There is often an inability to actively extend the proximal phalanx. Lacerations of the tendons in zone V are often concomitant with a joint capsule laceration, especially in cases of human bites from striking someone in the mouth with a closed fist. Irrigation of the MCP joint is mandatory, but the capsule can be left open to drain. Partial lacerations of the extensor tendon in these zones is not uncommon and can be ascertained by eliciting an increase in pain on resisted extension.

OPERATIVE TECHNIQUE

Complete or partial lacerations require exploration and irrigation of the wound. This is performed in a well-equipped emergency department with appropriate sterile technique. Alternatively, repair can be performed in the operating room, especially if multiple tendons are involved.

The wounds are irrigated and debrided of devitalized tissue. If necessary, the lacerations may be extended in a curvilinear fashion for increased exposure, but often the tendons can be repaired directly through the laceration since there is little retraction of the tendon ends at this level. The tendons generally are thick enough to use 3-0 core sutures, with either horizontal mattress or modified Kessler types utilized. Care is taken not to traumatize the extensor tendon by grasping the nonsevered areas to minimize postoperative adhesions.

POSTOPERATIVE CARE

For the first 4 weeks after surgery, the MCP joint is splinted in 10–20 degrees of flexion and the PIP joint is fully extended. The wrist is held in approximately 20–30 degrees of extension. Occupational therapy can be initiated after the first week, with limited passive range of motion of the MCP and PIP joints to prevent adhesions. At 4 weeks, day splints are discontinued and active flexion and extension is permitted in all joints. Night splints are continued

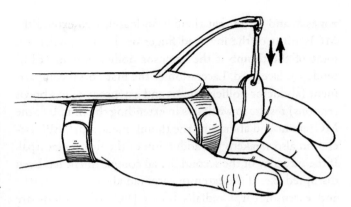

Figure 91.7. Dynamic split for immediate passive motion of fingers.

and passive extension is permitted, followed at 8 weeks by resisted extension exercises.

A more recent and alternate means of postoperative rehabilitation involves dynamic splinting. This is deemed by some to be more important in complex injuries with associated fractures and soft-tissue loss requiring secondary coverage. This form of rehabilitation, however, can also follow the more simple extensor tendon laceration in these zones. The dynamic splint should include all affected fingers in the outrigger apparatus, as well as adjacent fingers, to alleviate the pull of the adjacent junctura (Figure 91.7). A forearm-based, Orthoplast dynamic extension splint is applied within 3–5 days. The wrist is placed in 10–20 degrees of extension. The splint is fashioned to allow 30 degrees of active flexion at the MCP joint for the first 2 weeks and 45 degrees active flexion for the following 2 weeks. Extension is achieved passively with elastic bands. Several millimeters of extensor tendon excursion occurs in the dorsum of the hand with this protocol, helping to decrease the formation of adhesions and promote healing. Exercises are encouraged 10 times a day, with 25 repetitions per set. After 4 weeks, a rehabilitative regimen similar to static splinting is instituted.

EXTENSOR LACERATIONS IN ZONES VII AND VIII

ASSESSMENT OF THE DEFECT

Lacerations of the extensor tendons in zones VII and VIII are common. The close approximation of the dorsal compartments makes multiple tendon injuries common, as well as injury to other structures, such as the superficial radial nerve, the dorsal cutaneous branch of the ulnar nerve, and the antebrachial cutaneous nerves. The clinical findings of the extensor lacerations are similar to that of zones V and VI in that there is an inability to extend the MCP joints of the involved finger or the interphalangeal joint of the thumb if the extensor pollicis longus (EPL) tendon is lacerated. Laceration of the first dorsal compartment (abductor pollicis longus and extensor pollicis brevis tendons) results in weakness in extending the thumb at the MCP joint and abducting the thumb metacarpal. EPL laceration also weakens the adduction of the first metacarpal. If the integrity of the second dorsal compartment has been disrupted (i.e., if the extensor carpi radialis longus [ECRL] and extensor carpi radialis brevis [ECRB] tendons are severed), there is weakness in wrist extension. The index finger has two long extensors servicing the extension of the MCP joint (i.e., the extensor indicis proprius and the extensor digitorum communis). It is common for both of these tendons to be transected in zone VII. The extensor indicus proprius (EIP) tendon is volar and slightly ulnar to the index extensor digitorum communis (EDC) tendon in this area. Should only one tendon be transected, the patient would still be able to extend the MCP joint, although there may be a lag of approximately 10–15 degrees. Extension of the fifth finger MCP joint is also controlled by two extensor tendons, the extensor digiti quinti (EDQ) and the EDC. Should the EDQ tendon be transected, the MCP joint will still be extended by the EDC tendon, although there may again be a lag of approximately 10–15 degrees. Weakness on extension and radial deviation may ensue if the extensor carpi ulnaris tendon has been severed in the sixth dorsal compartment. For significant lacerations or injuries where extensor tendon injury is suspected a thorough exploration in the operating room should be done to help delineate the full extent of the extensor tendon and/or associated structure damage in zones VII and VIII.

OPERATIVE TECHNIQUE

Principles of tendon repair are similar to those for the other zones, with debridement of nonviable tissue and irrigation of wounds. These repairs should be performed in the operating room. A tourniquet is utilized. The wound is thoroughly irrigated and incisions are extended proximally and distally in a zigzag or curvilinear fashion, if necessary, to visualize the extent of any injured structures. If required, and for better access, the extensor retinaculum can be divided in a step-cut fashion so that the edges may transpose (in a modified Z-plasty fashion) after the repair. This maneuver makes tension-free closure of the retinaculum much easier. The severed tendons are identified, appropriately aligned, and the edges of the tendons debrided of frayed strands. Care should be taken not to remove more than 1 cm of the

total tendon length from the ends as this will interfere with the extension and flexion ability of the finger. Core sutures of 3-0 polypropylene or other permanent type in a buried horizontal mattress or modified Kessler pattern are used, utilizing atraumatic techniques. The retinaculum is then redraped over the repaired tendons and sutured in place with a nonabsorbable suture. In zone VIII, it may be difficult to find the proximal tendon ends because of retraction into the muscle bellies. In addition, the laceration may be at the musculotendinous junction, where suturing may be more difficult. The use of 2-0 or 3-0 braided polyester sutures, in a figure-of-eight fashion, rather than monofilament, will hold the muscle fibers more firmly without cutting through the muscle belly. The wounds are thoroughly irrigated with saline solution. Any concomitant injury to the nerves or vessels can be repaired at this time. The wounds are closed with a 4-0 nylon suture. A nonadherent gauze dressing and mupirocin are applied to the wounds, followed by an absorbent gauze dressing and splint.

POSTOPERATIVE CARE

The wrist is splinted in approximately 15–20 degrees of extension and the MCP joints are splinted in 50 degrees of flexion with the interphalangeal joints free. The patient is maintained in this splint for approximately 4 weeks, at which time the day splints are discontinued. Night splints are continued for another 2 weeks. Occupational therapy can be initiated after the first week, with limited passive range of motion of the MP joints and wrist to help prevent adhesions. Active flexion and extension can ensue at 4 weeks and resisted extension at 8 weeks.

CAVEATS

A high level of suspicion is required for tendon injury following any laceration of the back of the forearm, hand, or finger. The surgeon must obtain appropriate visualization by extending the lacerations so that each of the tendon ends can be carefully identified. Close attention to detail is required to restore anatomic alignment of the extensor mechanism. Several types of suture techniques and materials have been described, and the surgeon should use whatever method he or she is most comfortable with to regain proper alignment of the tendons with minimal additional trauma. One or two permanent core sutures, with or without additional running peritendinous sutures, depending on the size and character of the tendon, should be utilized. A close relationship with the hand therapist should be fostered to initiate and follow through with strict rehabilitation regimens. Splint modifications may be warranted depending on the patient's work status, motivation, and compliance with therapy. A good rapport with the patient is helpful to optimize results.

SELECTED READINGS

Anderson DJ. Extensor tendon repairs in zones 3-4. In: Blair WF, Steyers CM, eds. *Techniques in Hand Surgery*. Philadelphia: Lippincott, 1996:96–103.

Aulicino PL. Acute injuries of the extensor tendons proximal to the metacarpophalangeal joints. *Hand Clin* 1995;11:403–410.

Chang P. Extensor tendon repairs in zones 1-2. In: Blair WF, Steyers CM, eds. *Techniques in Hand Surgery*. Philadelphia: Lippincott, 1996:91–95.

Evans RB. An update on extensor tendon management. In: Hunter JM, Mackin EJ, Callahan AD, eds. *Rehabilitation of the Hand: Surgery and Therapy*. St. Louis: Mosby-Year Book, 1995:565–608.

Newport ML. Extensor tendon repair in zones 5-6. In: Blair WF, Steyers CM, eds. *Techniques in Hand Surgery*. Philadelphia: Lippincott, 1996:104–111.

Schneider LH. Extensor tendon injuries. *Hand Clin* 1995;11:3.

Strauch RJ. Extensor Tendon Injury. In: Wolfe SW, ed. *Green's Operative Hand Surgery*. 6th ed. Philadelphia: Churchill Livingstone, 2011: 159–188.

92

FLEXOR TENDON REPAIR

Michael W. Neumeister and Richard E. Brown

The disruption and subsequent repair of flexor tendons presents a formidable challenge to the hand surgeon. In an effort to regain excursion of the involved tendons, the definitive outcome depends on a number of variables, including the level of injury, the mechanism of injury, and associated trauma to the skin, pulleys, neurovascular bundles, and bone. The ultimate result, however, is directly proportional to scarring, fibrosis, adhesions, and gap formation that limit the return of normal tendon excursion and the final composite motion of the digit.

ZONE I INJURIES

ASSESSMENT OF THE DEFECT

The initial assessment of the injury should include an appropriate history. An awareness of the mechanism of injury allows the surgeon to be cognizant of injuries to local tissues, including skin, bone, nerve, and blood vessels. Injuries in zone I include avulsion and laceration injuries. Avulsion injuries of the flexor digitorum profundus (FDP) tendon typically result in forced extension during active flexion of the digit (i.e., football jersey injury), most commonly affecting the ring finger. Injury to the FDP tendon in this zone results in loss of flexion of the distal phalanx. An intact vinculum to the distal FDP tendon may prevent retraction and hold this tendon nearly out to length. Further proximal retraction can affect the movement at the proximal interphalangeal (PIP) joint. The FDP tendon may lodge near or at the PIP joint, restricting motion as a result of excess bulk within the fibro-osseous canal at this level. This excess bulk may be caused by a bone fragment or may occur secondary to edema. Should the tendon retract further proximally

into the palm, a palmar mass may be present. The flexor digitorum sublimis (FDS) tendon will then allow normal middle phalanx flexion at the PIP joint with loss of distal phalanx flexion only.

The independent action of the FDP should be assessed. The patient fails to actively flex the distal phalanx when maintaining the finger in extension at the PIP joint if the FDP tendon is severed at this level. In addition, the natural flexion cascade is lost in the involved finger because of the unopposed action of the terminal extensor tendon pulling the distal phalanx into extension (Figure 92.1). Flexion is lost at the distal interphalangeal (DIP) joint while testing the tenodesis effect when the wrist is extended (causing composite finger flexion). The neurovascular supply to the distal finger should also be assessed at this time.

OPERATIVE TECHNIQUE

The wounds are thoroughly irrigated in the emergency department, but the definitive repairs are performed in the operating room. The patient should receive a prophylactic antibiotic (e.g., cefazolin) preoperatively. The tetanus status should be ascertained while the patient is in the emergency department. Under general or regional (axillary or Bier block) anesthetic, the patient is prepared with a povidone iodine (Betadine) solution and draped in the appropriate fashion. The wounds are extended both proximally and distally in a Bruner fashion (in a zigzag fashion with the apices of each flap on the volar lateral edge of each skin crease) (Figure 92.2). Care must be taken not to injure the neurovascular bundles and the tips of the Bruner flaps. The subcutaneous tissue is freed from the overlying flexor sheath and the amount of distal tendon is ascertained. If 1 cm of distal tendon is available, primary suture repair can be performed. FDP tendons

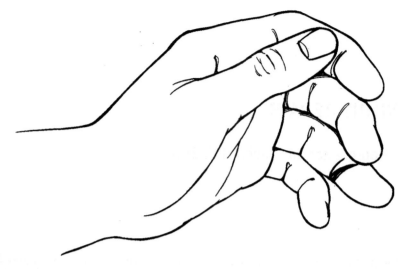

Figure 92.1. Ring finger has lost its normal posture in cascade of all digits. Distal phalanx remains extended because of unopposed action of terminal tendon.

held by intact vinculae may be easily retrieved through the flexor sheath with a hemostat or mosquito forceps. As the tendon is brought out distally, a Bunnell or 25-gauge needle is used proximally through the skin and flexor tendons to keep the FDP tendon out to length. The tendons are handled with care at their severed ends with Bishop-Harmon forceps

(Figure 92.3). Before repair, frayed ends are debrided. A 6-0 nylon or polyethylene suture is used to suture the posterior aspect of the coapted tendon ends, incorporating only the epitenon. The core suture of 4-0 polyethylene or nylon is used in a modified Kessler fashion: a single suture is passed through one of the lacerated ends extending out at a volar lateral edge, passed horizontally through the tendon to the other side, and then passed back through the cut edge of the tendon to continue through in a similar fashion at the proximal end of the tendon. The suture is tied to keep the knot buried within the substance of the repair. The tendon should not be bunched

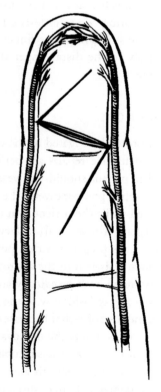

Figure 92.2. Bruner incision to gain appropriate access and visualization of flexor sheath. Neurovascular bundles lie quite volar and are situated near apices of Bruner flaps. Nerve is volar to artery in digits.

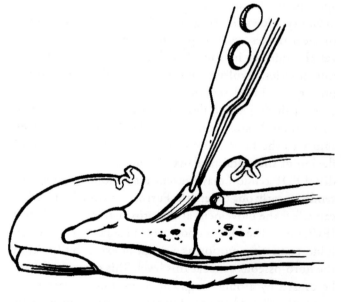

Figure 92.3. Careful handling of flexor tendon prevents further damage to epitenon. Severed edges are grasped with fine forceps.

HAND SURGERY

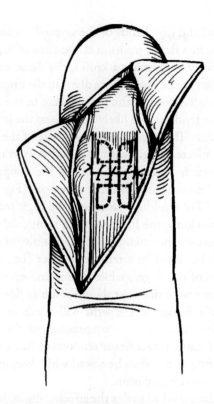

Figure 92.4. Core suture is tightened with care to prevent bunching of severed ends. Epitenon suture complements apposition. All knots are buried within repair site.

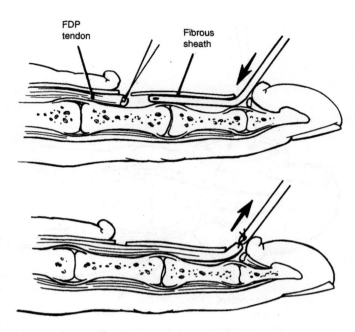

Figure 92.5. Pediatric feeding tube is introduced within fibro-osseous canal at distal end. Profundus tendon is sutured to tube, which is pulled out distally, pulling tendon along with it. Severed ends of the profundus tendon can now be coapted.

together when tightening the suture (Figure 92.4). The 6-0 epitenon suture can then be continued around the anterior surface of the tendon. The Bunnell needle is removed. The A4 pulley is repaired with a 6-0 nylon suture if it has been lacerated or incised to facilitate the tendon repair. The wounds are thoroughly irrigated with a saline solution. Any neurovascular injury can be repaired at this time under the microscope and the skin closed definitively with a 5-0 nylon suture.

A nonadherent dressing and bacitracin are applied and the hand is splinted with a dorsal blocking splint. The wrist is splinted in 10–20 degrees of flexion, the metacarpal phalangeal (MCP) joints are in 60–70 degrees of flexion, and the interphalangeal joints are extended. If the repair will not pass under the A4 pulley, motion may actually be improved by dividing and lengthening the A4 pulley, although some bowstringing may occur. Alternatively, one slip of the FDS may be flipped distally to enlarge or reconstruct an A4 pulley.

The FDP tendon can retract further in the finger and occasionally into the palm. Further Bruner incisions on the volar aspect of the finger are usually required to visualize the proximal tendon. It may be necessary to incise part of the pulley to allow the tendon to funnel into the

fibro-osseous canal and be pulled up to the distal wound. Often a pediatric feeding tube can be used for this purpose. It is passed from distal to proximal (Figure 92.5A). The tendon is sutured to the tube's proximal end and pulled up through the fibroosseous canal (Figure 92.5B). The repair is then done as described earlier.

Occasionally, the FDP is lacerated at its insertion or very close to it, necessitating a different means of coapting the tendon ends. A tendinous periosteal flap is elevated off the distal phalanx for a distance of approximately 5–6 mm. The cortex of the bone is roughened with a rongeur (Figure 92.6). The tendon is retrieved as described earlier and held at length with a Bunnell needle. The suture (braided polyethylene or 4-0 pull-out wire) is placed in the proximal tendon end in a Bunnell (crisscross) fashion. Two holes are drilled through the distal phalanx from the volar aspect to the dorsum of the finger. The suture is then passed through these drill holes and tied over a surgical button on the dorsum of the distal finger or through the nail plate. As the suture is pulled tightly, the FDP tendon must be pulled underneath the periosteal tendon flap and into the pocket made by roughening the phalangeal cortex. The wounds are irrigated and closed in a similar fashion as previously described.

The button is left in place for approximately 4–6 weeks. The patient follows the same rehabilitation protocol as described in the following section.

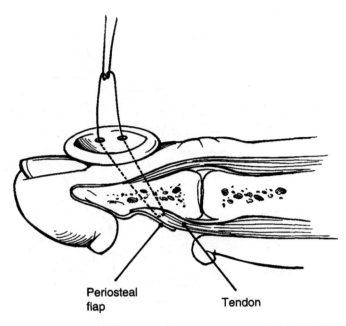

Figure 92.6. Tendinous periosteal remnant flap is elevated distally. Cortex is roughened with rongeur to allow appropriate seating of profundus tendon. Pull-through wires are tied over dorsal button after tendon is well-seated.

Closed FDP tendon avulsions follow similar surgical principles except in cases where a chip fracture has avulsed off the distal phalanx with the FDP tendon. Should the fragment be large enough, the tendon can be brought out to length as described earlier, and the fracture reduced and maintained in reduction with a small lag screw, 0.028-inch pins, or interosseous wire. Smaller fragments should be debrided and the FDP tendon attached to the distal phalanx with a pull-through suture as described earlier.

ZONE II INJURIES

The goal in tendon repairs in zone II is to obtain a functional gliding tendon within the fibro-osseous canal. This mandates not only minimizing adhesion formation, but also preserving the tendon pulleys. Flexor tendons severed in zone II should be primarily repaired. It is acceptable, however, to perform delayed primary repair without the need for tendon grafting. This delayed repair should be performed within the first 7–14 days for optimal results.

ASSESSMENT OF THE DEFECT

An appropriate history and physical examination in the emergency department can usually identify the extent of the injury. Identifying the position of the fingers at the time of injury will help the surgeon anticipate the location of

the proximal and distal ends of the severed tendons. If the fingers were in a flexed position at the time of injury (e.g., if the patient was grasping a knife), the distal end of the tendon is likely to be much more distal in the finger relative to the skin lacerations. If the fingers were in the extended position, the tendons will likely be close to the level of the skin laceration. The normal resting cascade of the fingers is lost in the affected finger with the tendon laceration. The finger will rest in extension because of the unopposed action of the extrinsic and intrinsic extensors (Figure 92.7). If only the FDP tendon is lacerated, the digit maintains a posture of flexion at the PIP and MCP joints, although the distal phalanx will be extended. The continuity of the flexor tendon can be tested by a tenodesis effect (i.e., observing the position of the fingers while flexing and extending the wrist). Extension of the wrist should result in flexion of the fingers, while flexion of the wrist will result in extension of the digits. Alternatively, compression of the proximal forearm will cause intact flexor tendons to flex the fingers. Individual fingers can then be tested while keeping the adjacent digits in full extension.

The patient is asked to flex the affected digits. If the FDS tendon is intact, the middle phalanx should flex at the PIP joint. The DIP joint is isolated by holding the PIP joint in extension with the examiner's index finger while the thumb presses on the middle phalanx. The patient is asked to flex the affected digit. An intact FDP tendon will flex the distal phalanx. A severed FDP tendon will result in the distal phalanx remaining in extension.

Occasionally, the proximal end of the tendon can be palpated at its limit of retraction. The extent of the retraction depends on a number of factors. If the vinculum is still intact, the tendon will remain at the level of the A2 pulley, and, rarely, a fullness may be present in the proximal finger. The tendons will retract into the palm if the vincula are not

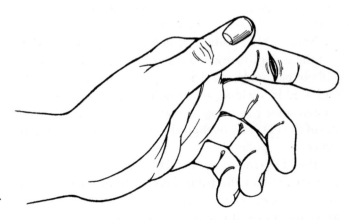

Figure 92.7. Loss of normal digital cascade resulting from unopposed pull of extensors.

preserved, and a fullness may occasionally be palpable in the palm. The tendon retraction may be greater if the fingers were in active flexion at the time of injury.

The sensory and vascular supply to the fingers should be carefully assessed. The neurovascular bundles are volar, yet slightly lateral to the tendons. The digital nerve is volar to the digital artery, and both structures (usually together) may be involved in the injury. Bilateral neurovascular bundle laceration will render the finger insensate and ischemic. It is possible, however, for the finger to remain viable in this circumstance, living off dorsal and collateral blood supply. Relative ischemia of the finger may compromise tendon or skin flap healing. One artery suffices to revascularize the finger, although the digit may be more susceptible to cold intolerance, flap and tendon healing may be compromised, and reinnervation may take longer.

Partial tendon lacerations may not be apparent unless a careful examination is performed. The postural cascade of the fingers may not be altered. The tenodesis effect and individual tendon examination may also be normal. Usually, there is tenderness and pain in attempting to flex the involved digit, especially against resistance. This is often difficult to assess because there is likely pain present from the skin laceration itself. Exploration of the wound can confirm the diagnosis of partial tendon laceration.

INDICATIONS AND CONTRAINDICATIONS

There are few contraindications to primary or delayed primary repair of the involved severed flexor tendons in zone II. The tendons should be repaired in conjunction with nerve or artery laceration repair. Phalangeal fractures also do not preclude repairing the flexor tendons. However, infection is a contraindication to primary repair, whereas severe contamination of wounds and volar skin and subcutaneous skin loss are *relative* contraindications to primary repair.

OPERATIVE TECHNIQUE

The wounds are extended both proximally and distally as needed. This is performed with a Bruner type of zigzag incision alone or in conjunction with a lateral longitudinal incision, depending on the location and direction of the lacerations. The wounds are deepened with sharp and blunt dissection to the flexor sheath. Care is taken not to breach the integrity of the neurovascular structures. The Bruner flaps must be kept thin over the neurovascular bundles to prevent injury to these structures. However, flaps that are

too thin may result in flap necrosis, especially in crush injuries. The skin is handled delicately with skin hooks and held in retraction with nylon sutures. The dissection should leave the flexor sheath free of subcutaneous tissue. The proximal and distal extent of the incisions depends on where the severed tendon ends are located. It is usually possible to retrieve the proximal end of the tendon with a fine mosquito forceps, hemostat, or tendon retriever. This must be done with care since grasping of the flexor sheath may promote adhesions. The tendons should be grasped at their severed edge only; otherwise, fraying of the tendons can occur, necessitating tendon shortening on repair. The tendons are pulled out to length and their position maintained by introducing a Keith or Bunnell needle or a 25-gauge needle through the skin and tendon proximally. Care must be taken to avoid injury to the neurovascular bundles while passing these needles. The distal tendon remnant is often quite distal within the fibro-osseous canal, and passage of the proximal tendon through this canal can be quite difficult. A pediatric feeding tube can be passed from distal to proximal within the sheath. The tendon is sutured to this end and pulled through. Alternatively, a fine mosquito hemostat may work for grasping the tendons and pulling them through. The A2 and A4 pulleys need to be preserved to minimize the axis moment arms and subsequent bowstringing, ultimately maintaining appropriate tendon excursion to finger flexion ratio. It may be necessary, however, to incise part of the pulleys to allow for the passage of the tendons. This can usually be accomplished with a L-shaped incision transversely over the proximal edge of the pulley and longitudinally up the lateral edge. This acts as a funnel opening of the sheath to aid in tendon passage. The pulley is repaired with a 6-0 polyethylene or nylon suture after the tendon repair. Z-plasties in the pulley can also be performed to allow greater space within the canal for unrestricted tendon excursion (Figure 92.8).

Should both the FDS and FDP tendons be lacerated, the FDS slips, which are flat, are repaired first with a 5-0 nylon suture in a figure-of-eight fashion. The FDP tendon is then repaired (Figure 92.9). Grasping the tendons anywhere other than the severed end breaches the integrity of the epitenon and may promote adhesions, ultimately restricting tendon excursion. Therefore, fine forceps, such as the Bishop-Harmon, should be used to grasp the tendon at the freshened severed ends. Alternatively, small incisions in the edges of the tendon can be made at the freshening site. The suture is then placed while grasping the end that will be debrided (Figure 92.10). A 4-0 polyethylene or nylon core suture is placed in a modified Kessler fashion, making certain the tendons are not accordioned. A running

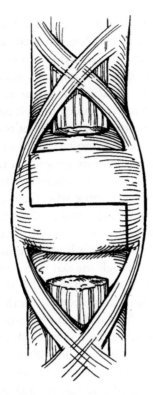

Figure 92.8. Z-plasty can be performed on pulley to increase volume of fibroosseous canal at this level.

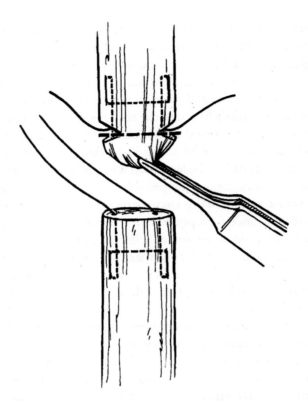

Figure 92.10. Fine forceps grasp only frayed severed end of tendon. Incisions are made in tendon near tendon ends; 4-0 nylon suture is passed through this near incision. Frayed end is completely excised after placement of core suture.

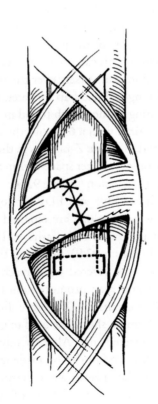

Figure 92.9. Transposition of pulley flaps after repair of sublimis and profundus tendons.

6-0 polyethylene or nylon suture circumvents the repair to minimize exposure of raw tendon edges.

As in zone I injuries, the epitenon repair on the back wall of the tendon can be performed initially with 6-0 polyethylene or nylon before core suture placement. The core sutures should be placed approximately 1 cm from the tendon ends in the volar two-thirds of the tendon, thereby preventing injury to the longitudinal vascularity of the tendon. Should the neurovascular structures require repair, this is performed under the microscope subsequent to the repair of the tendons.

POSTOPERATIVE CARE

The skin is closed with 5-0 nylon suture. The wounds are initially dressed with a nonadherent dressing and an antibiotic ointment. A gauze dressing is then applied, and all digits are splinted in the position of wrist flexion at 10–20 degrees and the MCP at 60–70 degrees, PIP joints in extension, and the DIP at 0–30 degrees of flexion. The fingers should be free to flex within the splint while awakening from anesthesia and while sleeping to prevent flexion against resistance. Patients are started on early range of motion therapy

48–72 hours after surgery. Most postoperative protocols for flexor tendon repairs call for early controlled motion programs. Traditionally, these early motion techniques are passive and have reportedly increased early tensile strength while preventing formation of restrictive adhesions. A Duran protocol can be initiated by the well-motivated and compliant patient. Otherwise, the Kleinert protocol is followed with elastic bands attached to hooks glued to the fingernails. The Duran technique requires the affected fingers to be immobilized with Velcro straps in the dorsally protected splint. During each waking hour, the patient passively flexes all joints and actively extends the digits. This is repeated 15–25 times per set. The Kleinert technique uses the same sequence of therapy, except the elastic bands attach to the fingernail hooks and then to the volar aspect of the splint, thus passively flexing the digits. The patient then extends against the minimal resistance of the elastic bands. Pulleys should be added at the level of the distal palm to obtain maximum DIP flexion. Elastic bands are removed at night. The patients are instructed to passively extend the PIP joint completely inside the splint to avoid flexion contractures.

The Mayo modifications of these techniques use an element of wrist extension. The Duran protocol is used but modified to allow 30 degrees of wrist extension in the splint. The digits are passively flexed, and the wrist is then extended. The patient actively holds this position of the fingers for 5 seconds, the wrist is flexed, and, by the tenodesis effect, the digits passively extend. This is repeated 25 times per hour. These techniques can be modified, or splints may be modified to regain full extension despite the initial splinting technique should flexion contractures develop.

These protocols are undertaken for 4 weeks after repair. During the fourth and sixth week, the base splint can be discontinued and worn only at night. The elastic traction can be discontinued completely. Gentle active range of motion at the PIP and DIP joints is initiated and passive flexion continued. Independent FDS and FDP excursion is exercised with blocking splints. From the sixth to the eighth week after repair, more vigorous exercises are begun, and night splinting is discontinued. Passive extension of the MCP, PIP, and DIP joints is initiated and blocking exercises are continued. At 8–10 weeks after repair, resisted flexion exercises are encouraged. Flexion contractures can be treated with dynamic extension splints while the patient is undertaking physical therapy. Finger compression and desensitization protocols are used to promote healing and facilitate composite range of motion. Digital nerves repaired at the initial surgery should not delay the postoperative therapy protocol. However, digital artery repair may delay therapy for 7–10 days, to lessen the chance of thrombosis.

Early active range of motion therapy may be of benefit in the healing and overall excursion of the flexor tendons. Volume studies of the flexor tendons have shown that during passive motion of the flexor tendon, there is little change in the diameter or circumference of the tendon. In fact, there may be a tendency to "bunch" at pulleys. During "active" excursion, the muscles powering the tendons pull them into a taut disposition, which decreases the overall tendon diameter, especially of the FDP tendon. The active range of motion must be controlled, of course, as too much tension will cause rupture of the tendons.

ZONES III, IV, AND V

ASSESSMENT OF THE DEFECT

Laceration of the flexor tendons in the palm, within the carpal tunnel, or in the distal forearm are often associated with other neurovascular injury. The median nerve is extremely vulnerable to injury within the palm and carpal tunnel. The radial artery, median nerve, and the ulnar nerve and artery are also vulnerable in the distal forearm. A complete evaluation is mandatory during the preoperative analysis. Typically, lacerations in zone III with severance of the flexor tendons will show the lack of normal digital cascade in the affected digits. The finger will be in the extended position if both FDS and FDP tendons are severed. Since the FDS tendon is superficial to the FDP tendon at this level, the normal cascade of the finger may be present if only the FDS tendon is severed. However, there will be tenderness on resisted flexion of the finger. The neurovascularity of the digits should be well documented because injury to the superficial palmar arch or the common digital vessels and nerves is common.

OPERATIVE TECHNIQUE

Primary repair of the structures in zones III, IV, and V is indicated. The wound is irrigated in the emergency department, but definitive repair should be performed in the operating room. Prophylactic antibiotics (generally, cefazolin) are administered. Under regional anesthesia (axillary or supraclavicular block) or general anesthesia, the upper limb is prepared with an antiseptic solution and a tourniquet is applied to the upper arm. The wound is then extended proximally in a zigzag fashion.

The transverse carpal ligament is released in zone IV injuries to identify the underlying pathologic condition. A thorough assessment of the median nerve is essential. The trifurcation of the median nerve is identified and the branches followed distally. The continuity of the superficial palmar arch and the common digital vessels is also inspected if they are within the zone of injury. The FDS and FDP tendons are repaired initially, followed by the vessels and nerves. On the ulnar side of the wrist, it is easier to repair the ulnar nerve and artery, followed by the flexor carpi ulnaris tendon. A modified Kessler or figure-of-eight suture is used to coapt the tendon ends. Care is taken to grasp only the severed edge of the tendon with Bishop-Harmon forceps, and a 4-0 polyethylene or monofilament suture is used for the suturing. The running 6-0 polyethylene or nylon epitenon suture is used to maintain the appropriate edge alignment of the tendon as well as to add strength. Any associated neurovascular injury is repaired using a microscope. The wounds are irrigated with a saline solution, hemostasis is secured, and the skin is closed definitively with 5-0 nylon suture. A nonadherent dressing and bacitracin are applied to the wound along with a bulky dressing and dorsal blocking splint. The splint is applied to maintain the wrist in approximately 10–20 degrees of flexion, the MCP joints in 60–70 degrees of flexion, and the interphalangeal joints in full extension.

Zone V injuries are treated in a similar fashion, although the tendinous edges are usually approximated with a figure-of-eight suture since the tendons are flatter. It is often difficult to initially locate these tendon ends at the muscular–tendinous junction because the tendons retract into the muscle belly. They can be grasped with a Halstead hemostat and the edges of the tendons freshened with a no. 15 blade; 4-0 polyethylene or nylon sutures are used. The postoperative course is similar to that of injuries in zones III and IV.

POSTOPERATIVE CARE

Patients are left in the initial dressing for approximately 3–5 days. An orthoplastic splint is then fitted to maintain the position of the digits and wrist. This position is maintained for approximately 4 weeks. A postoperative regime similar to the zone II rehabilitation protocol is followed from week 4 to week 10.

CAVEATS

The purpose of repairing flexor tendons in the hand is to restore and maintain function of the fingers and hand as a unit. One must maintain a high level of suspicion for tendon injury in all injuries to the hand while paying attention to detail in the physical examination. The normal cascade of the fingers will be lost when the flexor tendon has been lacerated. Appropriate visualization with adequate incisions is mandatory; it is never appropriate to work in a hole. Delicate handling of the tendons will help prevent further tendon injury and subsequent adhesions. It is prudent, therefore, to grasp only the lacerated ends of the tendon during manipulation. Careful placement of the core sutures and attention to detail will ensure strength and minimize trauma to the tendon. A running epitendinous suture not only adds to the strength, but improves the contour of the tendon repair. The A2 and A4 pulleys must be maintained or reconstructed so that bowstringing is prevented.

It is important to foster a close relationship with the hand therapist to initiate, maintain, and troubleshoot rehabilitation regimens. A good rapport is required with the patient to understand and respond to issues of compliance, motivation, and work status as well as potential complications. Therapy should be initiated immediately postoperatively to optimize the results.

SELECTED READINGS

Stewart KM, VanStrien G. Postoperative management of flexor tendon injuries. In: Hunter JM, Mackin EJ, Callahan AD, eds. *Rehabilitation of the Hand: Surgery and Therapy*. 4th ed. St. Louis: Mosby-Year Book, 1995:443–462.

Strickland JW. Flexor tendon injuries. In: Strickland JW, ed. *The Hand: Master Techniques in Orthopaedic Surgery*. Philadelphia: Lippincott-Raven, 1998:474–489.

Strickland JW. Flexor tendons—acute injuries. In: Green DP, ed. *Green's Operative Hand Surgery*. 4th ed. Philadelphia: Churchill Livingstone, 1999:1851–1897.

Taras J, Schneider LH. Flexor tendon repairs. *Atlas Hand Clin* 1996;1:1.

Wagner WF Jr, Carroll C, Strickland JW, et al. A biomechanical comparison of techniques of flexor tendon repair. *J Hand Surg (Am)* 1994;19:979–983.

Wang E. Tendon repair. *J Hand Ther* 1998;11:105–110.

93.

NERVE REPAIR

Amy M. Moore and Keith E. Brandt

The art of nerve repair goes beyond the simple mechanics of sewing two ends of a nerve together. In addition to a precise technical repair, a concentrated effort must be made to be outside the zone of injury, to avoid tension, and to consider the topography of the nerve—directing motor fibers to muscles and sensory fibers to sensory receptors. In this chapter, we review the key principles of nerve repair in order to maximize functional outcomes in patients with devastating nerve injuries.

ASSESSMENT OF THE INJURY

Managing nerve injuries requires careful patient evaluation and understanding of the degree, timing, and extent of nerve injury. Consideration of the mechanism of injury is also important. Was the injury open or closed? Was the trauma from a sharp injury, such as glass or knife, or was it from a gunshot wound blast? Blunt trauma can also cause significant nerve injuries. The mechanism and timing of the injury (acute or delayed presentation) will help determine the degree and zone of nerve injury and will ultimately influence the surgical versus nonsurgical management.

The degree of nerve injury was first described by Seddon, then later modified by Sunderland and then Mackinnon. In short, the nerve injury can range from a neurapraxia that will have complete spontaneous recovery to a complete transection that will require surgical intervention to restore function.[1,2] A description of each degree of nerve injury follows (Figure 93.1).

- *First-degree injury (neurapraxia)*. A first-degree injury produces a segment of demyelination, resulting in a localized conduction block. Since the axons themselves are not injured, regeneration is not required. After remyelination, usually within 12 weeks, recovery should be complete.

- *Second-degree injury (axonotmesis)*. In a second-degree injury, axonal injury occurs and the distal nerve segment undergoes Wallerian degeneration. By definition, the connective tissue layers of the endoneurium, perineurium, and epineurium are uninjured. Regeneration proceeds at the rate of a millimeter per day and 1 inch per month.[3] Nerve regeneration can be followed clinically by an advancing Tinel's sign. Recovery will be complete unless the distance between the injury and the end organ results in such prolonged denervation that motor recovery is adversely affected.

- *Third-degree injury*. In a third-degree injury, Wallerian degeneration is combined with fibrosis of the endoneurium. Recovery will be incomplete because scar within the endoneurium blocks or causes mismatching of regenerating fibers with the appropriate distal end organ. Often there is partial recovery with this injury, but incomplete restoration of function is expected.

- *Fourth-degree injury*. A complete scar block results after a fourth-degree injury to a nerve. Regeneration does not occur unless the block is excised and the nerve is reconstructed.

- *Fifth-degree injury (neurotmesis)*. The nerve is completely divided. Gapping occasionally occurs between the cut nerve ends—downgrading any recovery from the regenerating fibers attempting to cross the gap.

- *Sixth-degree injury*. This represents a combination of any of the previous five levels of injury. With the longitudinal nature of crush or blast injuries, different levels of nerve injury can be seen at various locations along the nerve.

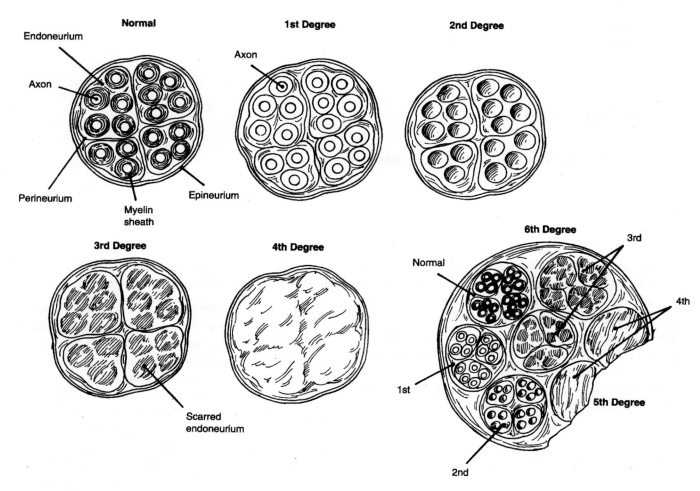

Figure 93.1. Schematic of degree of nerve injury.

It is often difficult to determine the degree of injury and zone of injury on physical exam. An open wound with a functional deficit should be considered a fifth-degree injury and explored. Blast injuries and closed injuries should be monitored for recovery over time. A thorough physical exam should be clearly documented at presentation and then repeated with serial exams. Key examination techniques include assessment of motor function (Medical Research Council muscle strength grading and pinch and grip strength testing with a dynamometer) and sensory function (two-point discrimination and Semmes-Weinstein filament testing). This documentation can then be correlated over time with electrodiagnostic studies to determine intervention.

INDICATIONS AND CONTRAINDICATIONS

Unrepaired nerve injuries can result in decreased function and pain from a neuroma of the proximal nerve stump.

Indications for surgical intervention are based on the timing of the injury, location of the injury, and zone of injury. In general, lack of motor recovery or sensation by 3 months from injury should trigger further workup and possible surgical intervention.[4]

Nerve regeneration progresses at a rate of 1–3 millimeters a day, or 1 inch per month, but, unfortunately, muscle atrophy begins immediately after denervation. There is a critical window of time for muscle reinnervation and recovery of function.[5,6] Depending on the distance the regenerating nerve must travel, there may be a considerable amount of time before the regenerating nerve reaches the muscle. Although the exact window is unknown, it is believed that muscle should receive nerve input by 18 months to avoid irreversible atrophy.[7] Therefore, recognizing a motor nerve injury early is important to maximize motor recovery. Sensation, in contrast, is not thought to be as time sensitive and one can allow more time for recovery before intervention.

Electrodiagnostic testing can be extremely helpful in determining which nerves are recovering or not. It should be used to complement the physical exam. Nerve conduction studies provide useful information about the degree of axonal loss and can identify concomitant nerve compression or diabetic neuropathy.[8,9] Electromyography (EMG) is another clinically useful tool that is used to understand the impact of the nerve injury on the distal muscle end organs. The EMG can detect subclinical recovery. We recommend obtaining neurodiagnostic testing at 10–12 weeks from injury when muscle reinnervation can be detected. If, at 12 weeks, there is no evidence of volitional motor unit potentials present—a fourth- or fifth-degree injury can be assumed and surgical intervention is indicated. We recommend developing a relationship with the electrodiagnostician for adequate interpretation of these tests.

The location and zone of the injury are also important in determining surgical indications. In the case of very proximal injuries or multiple nerve injuries, the surgeon needs to prioritize their reconstruction. For example, in a brachial plexus injury involving multiple roots, one would not expect recovery of the intrinsic muscles of the hand because they will have undergone irreversible atrophy by the time the nerve could regenerate down the length of the arm. Instead, the effort should focus on proximal muscle groups that the nerve can reach in a timely fashion. Furthermore, peripheral nerves commonly remain intact even after severe stretch or blast injuries. The nerve injury may extend for a considerable distance both proximally and distally from the site of injury. In these high proximal nerve injuries or in cases of large zones of injury, a direct repair may be prohibitive. Alternative reconstruction techniques such as nerve transfers should be considered.[4,10]

Contraindications for nerve repair include late presentation of a motor nerve injury where the muscle has already undergone irreversible atrophy. A relative contraindication is in high proximal nerve injuries where other reconstructive options exist that have demonstrated improved functional recovery.[11]

SURGICAL MANAGEMENT

PERIOPERATIVE CONSIDERATIONS

When preparing for the surgical case, it is important to have all diagnostic information available on the day of surgery (i.e., copies of the EMG, radiographs of the involved extremity, and previous operative reports if performed). Preoperatively, it is encouraged to discuss with the anesthesiologist about avoiding the use of muscle relaxants.

This is especially important in the reconstruction of motor nerves when electrical stimulation is desired. Dissection of the recipient and donor sites can be aided by proximal tourniquets, but it should be noted that a tourniquet palsy can also impede intraoperative stimulation of the motor nerves.

EQUIPMENT

The equipment needed for nerve repair includes microsurgical instruments and a microscope. Special nerve cutting devices are available, but use of these instruments should be left to surgeon preference. A fresh surgical scalpel or razor blade against a firm surface (wooden tongue blade) works nicely to freshen the nerve ends. A microsurgical bipolar cautery can be used to control small epineurial vessels, especially on larger nerves. Last, a colored background material is also helpful during the repair.

POSITIONING

The patient should be positioned to allow easy access to both the recipient and possible donor nerve graft sites. In nerve injuries involving the upper extremity, the patient is supine with the arm abducted on an arm board. The operating room microscope should be positioned to allow two surgeons to comfortably access the repair site. The microscope is usually brought into the field from a position at the end of the arm table.

OPERATIVE TECHNIQUE

Using careful dissection and operative technique, the injured nerve should be identified and exposed proximal and distal to the injury site. The exposure may need to be extended if the branching pattern of the nerve is needed to define the topography of the nerve. Once the nerve injury site is identified, the neuroma is excised sequentially or "bread loafed" back until a fresh uninjured fascicular pattern is identified (Figure 93.2). It is important to get outside of the zone of injury. A nerve repaired within the zone of injury will have a poor outcome.[12,13]

Knowledge of the internal topography of a nerve is helpful to direct functional or regional fascicles to their appropriate end target. For example, the ulnar nerve in the middle to distal forearm contains three distinct fascicles that maintain a predictable orientation (Figure 93.3). This knowledge can be used to correctly align the motor fascicle

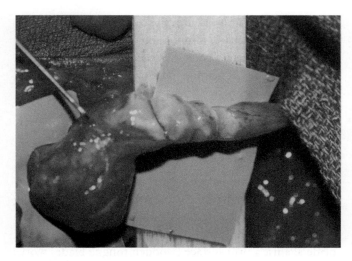

Figure 93.2. "Breadloafing" technique of excision of neuroma. A neuroma is identified in the ulnar nerve. In an effort to get outside of the zone of nerve injury, serial proximal excisions of nerve (i.e., like slicing bread) are performed along the length of the nerve until a clear, healthy fascicular pattern is visualized.

degeneration begins at approximately 72 hours after injury[4]), and distal dissection of the nerve branching pattern. The median, radial, peroneal, and sciatic nerves all have a predictable internal topography that can help correctly orient the fascicles during nerve repair.

Primary Nerve Repair

The nerve repair should be performed with the use of the operating microscope, and the coaptation should be tension-free.[14] The ability of microsuture to maintain the nerve ends in coaptation serves as a gauge to the appropriate tension.[15] If two 9-0 microsutures placed 180 degrees apart do not hold the nerve repair during full range of motion of the extremity then an interpositional nerve graft should be used. Postural positioning of the extremity, such as wrist or elbow flexion, to achieve a primary coaptation is discouraged. Increased tension or stretching of the nerve will result in significant ischemia and decreased regeneration.[16,17]

The nerve coaptation should be performed with either 8-0 or 9-0 epineurial sutures. If a fascicular repair is performed to align topography, 9-0 or 10-0 microsuture should be used. If fascicular matching is not needed to

in the proximal nerve stump to the correct fascicle distally and in the like manner to align the sensory fascicles. The distal nerve segment can be identified by topography, electrical stimulation (if performed before Wallerian

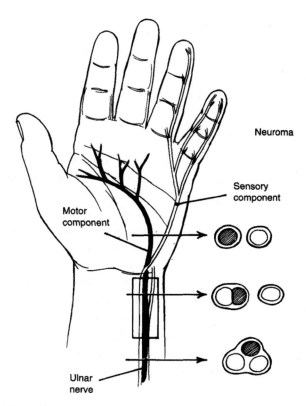

Figure 93.3. Schematic of the topography of the ulnar nerve in the forearm. The topographical arrangement of the sensory and motor fascicles of the ulnar nerve is consistent and reliably can be used for accurate nerve repair and/or grafting.

help direct regenerating fibers, there is no advantage of a fascicular repair over an epineurial repair.[13,18] In a freshly cut nerve, the fascicles protrude from the plane of the epineurium and perineurium because of normal endoneurial pressure. The protruding fascicles should be trimmed flush to the plane of the nerve in order to perform a clean epineurial repair and avoid misguidance of regenerating fibers (Figure 93.4).

Nerve Grafting

If a tensionless primary nerve repair cannot be achieved when the extremity is put through full range of motion, a nerve graft is indicated to bridge the nerve defect.[13] Traditionally, segmental nerve defects were repaired with autologous nerve grafts (i.e., autografts). However, with the development of off-the-shelf alternatives, use of nerve conduits and processed nerve allografts have become popular to treat nerve gaps.[19,20] The strengths and limitations of these nerve graft options are presented in Table 93.1.

Autografts

Autografts contain the nerve substrate to support regeneration including viable Schwann cells, endoneurial tubes, and extracellular matrix.[21] Donor autografts are chosen based on the size and length of the nerve defect as well as the donor site morbidity and ease of harvest. In general, the most common donor nerves include the sural nerve, the medial antebrachial cutaneous nerve, and the lateral antebrachial cutaneous nerve.[22]

"Spare part" nerve grafting can also be performed. For example, in a proximal radial nerve injury, restoration of

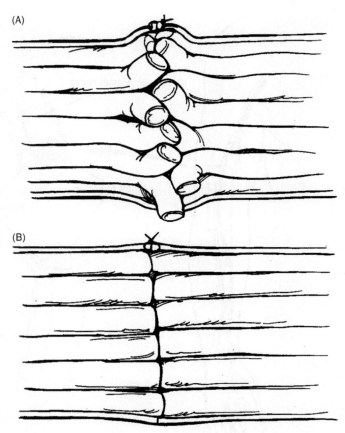

(A)

(B)

Figure 93.4. Direct end-to-end nerve repair. (A) Misdirection of nerve fibers can occur if there is lack of adequate excision of individual fascicles and/or if the epineurial sutures are tied too tightly. (B) Fascicular alignment is improved with trimming of the nerve fibers and gentle approximation of the epineurium.

extensor motor function is desirable and achievable, but restoration of radial sensory function is less important. If reconstruction requires nerve grafting, the donor morbidity could be limited by excluding the sensory fascicles

TABLE 93.1 OPTIONS FOR NERVE GAP RECONSTRUCTION

Material	Pros	Cons	Indication
Autograft	Gold standard Contains: Schwann cells Nerve vasculature Endoneurial structure	Donor site deficit Donor site scar Limited expendable supply	All nerve gaps lengths (Ideally <6 cm) Sensory, motor, mixed nerve injuries
Conduit	Available "off the shelf" Inexpensive	Lacks Schwann cells Lacks nerve architecture Lacks vasculature	Sensory nerves Short gap length (<3 cm) Small-diameter nerve (<3 mm)
Processed Nerve Allograft (i.e., Avance, AxoGen Nerve Graft)	Available "off the shelf" Retained nerve architecture (endoneurial tubes and extracellular matrix)	Expensive Lacks Schwann cells Lacks nerve vasculature	Short gap length (≤3 cm) Sensory nerves Alternative for motor or mixed nerve reconstruction when autograft not available and/or as studies demonstrate effectiveness

Source: Adapted from Reference 4.

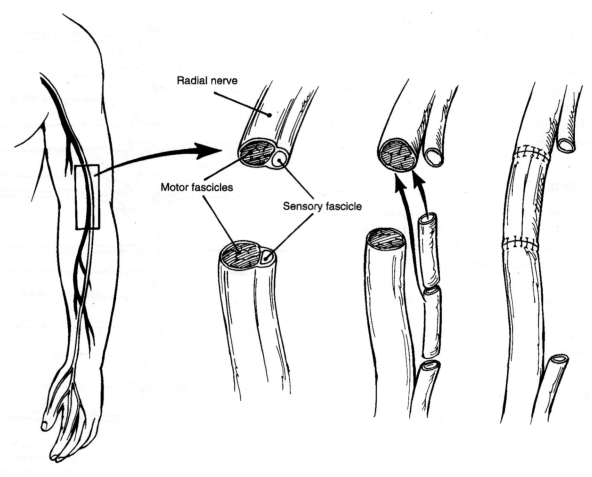

Figure 93.5. "Spare-part" nerve grafting. The topography of the radial nerve in the upper arm is depicted in the figure. The nerve has two major segments: the large multifascicular segment located medially contains almost all of the motor fascicles. The smaller lateral monofascicular segment contains the sensory fibers. This sensory nerve can be used as donor material to avoid a second surgical site.

Labels in figure: Radial nerve; Motor fascicles; Sensory fascicle

from the repair and harvesting these branches/fascicles to repair the motor fascicles (Figure 93.5).

Unless a branching nerve graft is specifically needed to repair a single proximal nerve to two or more nerve branches distally, donor autografts should be reversed. Reversing the grafts encourages all regenerating fibers to funnel to the distal nerve and to avoid loss at distal branch sites along the way. During autograft harvest, we paint the proximal nerve with a purple surgical marker and state "purple proximal" to remind ourselves of the orientation.

The surgical technique of autografting is similar to performing a coaptation as described earlier. There should be redundancy of the nerve graft to avoid tension across the repairs and allow for full range of motion of the extremity. In large nerves, such as the median nerve in the forearm, multiple grafts are needed to repair the defect. In these instances, cable grafting is performed. If fascicular topography is known, then each cable can be aligned and fascicular repairs performed to promote targeted regeneration. If the topography is questionable or unknown, then it is best to perform epineurial repairs allowing for preferential motor reinnervation to ensue.[23]

Autograft Alternatives

Synthetic conduits and processed nerve allografts are commercially available alternatives to autografting. They are appealing because they avoid the donor site morbidity of autografting, are easily available (i.e., can be taken "off the shelf"), and decrease operative times. They can be used to bridge nerve defects, and they can support regeneration across variable distances. Seven synthetic conduits and one processed nerve allograft are approved by the US Food and Drug Administration (FDA) and available for use (Figure 93.6).[24]

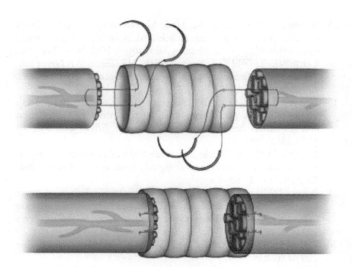

Figure 93.6. Schematic of a conduit assisted repair. Horizontal sutures are used to secure the conduit in place.

Research indicates that synthetic conduits should be limited to use in small-diameter nerves and for gaps of less than 3 cm.[25,26] The surgical technique for conduit use includes preparation of the nerve ends as described previously, and then choosing a proportionally sized (diameter) conduit. The nerve is secured 1–2 mm within the conduit with a horizontal mattress suture at each end. To improve nerve regeneration via the conduit, a small amount of proximal healthy nerve tissue can be mulched and placed within the tube to encourage axonal growth.[7]

Processed nerve allografts have gained significant appeal since the FDA approval of the Avance nerve graft in 2009.[19,27–29] These grafts preserve the three-dimensional scaffolding of the nerve, including endoneurial architecture, which supports nerve regeneration. They are also easy to use. Once defrosted, the nerve allograft has the similar consistency of autograft tissue and is coapted to the nerve ends as described earlier for nerve grafting.

Significant research is under way evaluating the efficacy of these products in comparison to autografts. Until further research demonstrates equivalent function as autografts in long nerve gaps (>3 cm) and for nerve defects in critical motor or mixed nerves, the authors advocate the use of autografts. In the authors' current practice, processed nerve allografts are used for small-diameter, small-gap nerve defects. More recently, as rodent data have demonstrated lack of regeneration across long processed nerve allografts (>4 cm), we have been using this product to successfully control aberrant nerve growth and neuroma formation.[30]

ADJUNCTIVE PROCEDURES

It is recommended to release all distal nerve entrapment points after a proximal nerve repair. For example, if the median nerve is repaired in the forearm, a carpal tunnel release should also be performed. This will improve functional recovery and decrease painful nerve compression when regeneration and associated edema of the nerve reaches the distal entrapment point.

POSTOPERATIVE CARE

Nerve repairs should be performed without tension, and thus immobilization of the extremity after an isolated nerve repair is often unnecessary. Splinting of the extremity can be performed to allow for tissue rest in the initial 2–3 days after surgery. Ideally, gentle range of motion exercises would begin within the first week of surgery to allow for nerve gliding and to avoid significant scarring of the nerve to the surrounding soft tissue. Range of motion, scar massage, and desensitization techniques should be initiated early in the postoperative course and under the guidance of a certified hand therapist.

If functional loss has resulted from a nerve injury, then protective splinting must be continued during the period of reinnervation to maintain ideal resting muscle length–tension ratio and to prevent joint contractures. Furthermore, if tendon repairs or bony procedures were also performed, then splinting and immobilization are implemented to protect these injuries.

Early referral to a hand therapist is recommended to maximize functional outcomes. Motor and sensory re-education can begin in the immediate postoperative period. Delays in this critical retraining can limit surgical outcomes. Furthermore, nerve injuries, even those after repair, are often associated with pain and hypersensitivity. Desensitization techniques, edema control, and scar massage can be initiated to assist with the discomforts of nerve injuries and neuropathic pain. Referral to a pain management specialist is also often helpful to treat patients with neuropathic pain after nerve injury.

CONCLUSION

Nerve injuries can be devastating and require an understanding of not only the mechanism and the degree of nerve injury, but also the key principles of repair techniques to enhance regeneration. A multidisciplinary team, including surgeons, neurologists, hand therapists, and pain specialists, is needed to adequately care for patients with nerve injuries. If nerve injuries are recognized early and safe surgical principles are applied, successful outcomes can be achieved.

REFERENCES

1. Fox IK, Mackinnon SE. Adult peripheral nerve disorders: nerve entrapment, repair, transfer, and brachial plexus disorders. *Plast Reconstr Surg* 2011;127(5):105e–118e.
2. Mackinnon SE. New directions in peripheral nerve surgery. *Ann Plast Surg* 1989;22(3):257–273.
3. Seddon HJ, Medawar PB, Smith H. Rate of regeneration of peripheral nerves in man. *J Physiol* 1943;102(2):191–215.
4. Moore AM, Wagner IJ, Fox IK. Principles of nerve repair in complex wounds of the upper extremity. *Semin Plast Surg* 2015;29(1):40–47.
5. Fu SY, Gordon T. Contributing factors to poor functional recovery after delayed nerve repair: prolonged denervation. *J Neurosci* 1995;15(5 Pt 2):3886–3895.
6. Fu SY, Gordon T. Contributing factors to poor functional recovery after delayed nerve repair: prolonged axotomy. *J Neurosci* 1995;15(5 Pt 2):3876–3885.
7. Boyd KU, Nimigan AS, Mackinnon SE. Nerve reconstruction in the hand and upper extremity. *Clin Plast Surg* 2011;38(4):643–660.
8. Campbell WW. Evaluation and management of peripheral nerve injury. *Clin Neurophysiol* 2008;119(9):1951–1965.
9. Willmott AD, White C, Dukelow SP. Fibrillation potential onset in peripheral nerve injury. *Muscle Nerve* 2012;46(3):332–340.
10. Mackinnon SE, Colbert SH. Nerve transfers in the hand and upper extremity surgery. *Tech Hand Up Extrem Surg* 2008;12(1):20–33.
11. Brown JM, Mackinnon SE. Nerve transfers in the forearm and hand. *Hand Clin* 2008;24(4):319–340, v.
12. Merle M, de Medinaceli L. Primary nerve repair in the upper limb. Our preferred methods: theory and practical applications. *Hand Clin* 1992;8(3):575–586.
13. Mackinnon SE. Surgical management of the peripheral nerve gap. *Clin Plast Surg* 1989;16(3):587–603.
14. Terzis J, Faibisoff B, Williams B. The nerve gap: suture under tension vs. graft. *Plast Reconstr Surg* 1975;56(2):166–170.
15. de Medinaceli L, Prayon M, Merle M. Percentage of nerve injuries in which primary repair can be achieved by end-to-end approximation: review of 2,181 nerve lesions. *Microsurgery* 1993;14(4):244–246.
16. Clark WL, Trumble TE, Swiontkowski MF, Tencer AF. Nerve tension and blood flow in a rat model of immediate and delayed repairs. *J Hand Surg Am* 1992;17(4):677–687.
17. Lundborg G, Rydevik B. Effects of stretching the tibial nerve of the rabbit. A preliminary study of the intraneural circulation and the barrier function of the perineurium. *J Bone Joint Surg Br* 1973;55(2):390–401.
18. Young L, Wray RC, Weeks PM. A randomized prospective comparison of fascicular and epineural digital nerve repairs. *Plast Reconstr Surg* 1981;68(1):89–93.
19. Brooks DN, et al. Processed nerve allografts for peripheral nerve reconstruction: a multicenter study of utilization and outcomes in sensory, mixed, and motor nerve reconstructions. *Microsurgery* 2012;32(1):1–14.
20. Taras JS, Nanavati V, Steelman P. Nerve conduits. *J Hand Ther* 2005;18(2):191–197.
21. Millesi H. Bridging defects: autologous nerve grafts. *Acta Neurochir Suppl* 2007;100:37–38.
22. Higgins JP, et al. Assessment of nerve graft donor sites used for reconstruction of traumatic digital nerve defects. *J Hand Surg Am* 2002;27(2):286–292.
23. Brushart TM, et al. Contributions of pathway and neuron to preferential motor reinnervation. *J Neurosci* 1998;18(21):8674–8681.
24. Kehoe S, Zhang XF, Boyd D. FDA approved guidance conduits and wraps for peripheral nerve injury: a review of materials and efficacy. *Injury* 2012;43(5):553–572.
25. Moore AM, et al. Limitations of conduits in peripheral nerve repairs. *Hand (N Y)* 2009;4(2):180–186.
26. Ray WZ, Mackinnon SE. Management of nerve gaps: autografts, allografts, nerve transfers, and end-to-side neurorrhaphy. *Exp Neurol* 2010;223(1):77–85.
27. Karabekmez FE, Duymaz A, Moran SL. Early clinical outcomes with the use of decellularized nerve allograft for repair of sensory defects within the hand. *Hand (N Y)* 2009;4(3):245–249.
28. Moran L, et al. Sonographic measurement of cross-sectional area of the median nerve in the diagnosis of carpal tunnel syndrome: correlation with nerve conduction studies. *J Clin Ultrasound* 2009;37(3):125–131.
29. Cho MS, et al. Functional outcome following nerve repair in the upper extremity using processed nerve allograft. *J Hand Surg Am* 2012;37(11):2340–2349.
30. Saheb-Al-Zamani M, et al. Limited regeneration in long acellular nerve allografts is associated with increased Schwann cell senescence. *Exp Neurol* 2013;247:165–177.

94.

REPLANTATION

Grant M. Kleiber and Keith E. Brandt

INTRODUCTION

Successful replantation depends on far more than the skill of the operating surgeon. A coordinated effort of emergency transport services, emergency room personnel, operating room staff, anesthesiologists and postoperative nursing is required for success. The need for this team approach has led to the development of several specialized replantation centers worldwide.

ASSESSMENT OF THE DEFECT

The first and most important step toward replantation is a thorough evaluation of the injury. Bleeding should be controlled with gentle pressure. Appropriate fluid resuscitation should be initiated. A thorough history and physical examination are performed to rule out associated injuries and medical comorbidities that may complicate replantation. Assessment of the mechanism of injury is crucial because outcomes vary between sharp, crush, and avulsion injuries. The time since injury and management of the amputated part are also important considerations that influence outcome. Proximal amputations containing muscle can tolerate up to 6 hours of warm ischemia. Digital amputations, which contain no muscle, can tolerate longer periods of ischemia. Successful digital amputation has been performed at as long as 42 hours of warm ischemia[1] and up to 94 hours of cold ischemia,[2] but the chance of success improves with shorter ischemia times. For proximal replantations of the hand or forearm, appropriate fasciotomies should be performed.

The amputated part should be placed in saline-soaked gauze and sealed in a plastic bag or specimen cup, which should then be placed in an ice slurry. The amputated part should never be placed directly on ice in order to avoid further cellular damage. If the injured part is devascularized but not completely amputated, it should be dressed with moistened gauze and surrounded with ice bags. Incomplete amputations should never be completed in the field.

A thorough history should be obtained from the patient at the time of evaluation. While many industrial and agricultural injuries may involve machines unfamiliar to the treating physician, these patients can often give a detailed description of the mechanism of the machine. The patient's hand dominance, occupation, and hobbies should be ascertained. Tobacco, drug, and alcohol use should also be documented. A detailed evaluation should be performed of the amputation site and the amputated part. In avulsion injuries, tendons and nerves are often seen dangling from the amputated part. Photographs and radiographs should be obtained of the amputated part as well as the affected hand, ideally on the same plate to allow simultaneous evaluation. Adjacent digits should also be thoroughly examined to rule out occult injury.

INDICATIONS

Replantation is indicated for any amputation of the thumb since the thumb is critical for hand function. Multidigit amputations are typically indicated for replantation because of the degree of function lost to these injuries. Amputations distal to the flexor digitorum sublimis (FDS) tendon insertion usually benefit from replantation as they can achieve excellent functional outcomes. Every effort should be made to replant any salvageable digit in a child as their outcomes far exceed adult replantations. For proximal amputations involving the hand or forearm, replantation should be attempted whenever possible.[3]

CONTRAINDICATIONS

STRONG CONTRAINDICATIONS

Replantation should not be attempted in patients with severe life-threatening injuries or with severe medical comorbidities who could be endangered by a prolonged surgical procedure. Additionally, replantation is rarely successful in multilevel amputations due to the decreased functional result. These injuries are often seen from rotary-blade mechanisms, such as industrial fans or lawnmowers.

RELATIVE CONTRAINDICATIONS

Mechanism of injury plays an important role in the eventual functional outcome. Crush injuries cause significant damage to bones and joints, as well as creating a wide zone of injury to nerves and vessels which may require extensive grafting. Avulsion injuries result in differential injuries to various structures: while skeletal injuries typically occur distally, tendinous avulsions are more likely to occur proximally at the musculotendinous junction, making meaningful functional recovery unlikely. Additionally, digital nerves are often avulsed out of the amputated part and vessels sustain extensive traction injury. This is often seen as a red streak along the digit, representing extravasated blood. Adequate assessment of the zone of injury cannot be overemphasized—the greater the zone of injury, the greater the likelihood of failure.

Replantation of a single border digit proximal to the PIP joint will likely result in a stiff replanted finger and may impair the overall function of the hand. It is important to recognize that single-digit replantation will require prolonged postoperative immobilization, potentially leading to stiffness of uninvolved digits and a decrease in overall function.

Certain patient factors must be considered prior to attempting replantation. Patients of advanced age have an overall poorer functional recovery. Peripheral vascular disease and atherosclerosis may preclude the possibility of replantation. Heavy smokers and cocaine users are more prone to vasospasm and should expect poorer outcomes.

ROOM SETUP AND MONITORING

A large room with adequate space for two operating teams is desirable. A back table with microsurgical instrumentation is necessary for preparation of the amputated part. The room should be warmed to prevent vasoconstriction.

Warming blankets and warmed intravenous fluids should be used as necessary. Tourniquets should be available for the injured extremity and any potential donor site. Donor sites for vascular, skin, and tendon grafts should be included in the sterile preparation and draping. Heparinized irrigation solution and topical vasodilators such as lidocaine or papaverine should be available. Kirschner wires, drills, and fluoroscopy should be available for bony fixation. An operating microscope and microsurgical instruments will be needed for vessel and nerve repair. Microsuture such as 9-0 and 10-0 nylon with small needles should be available. Bipolar electrocautery microforceps will aid in bloodless dissection and hemostasis.

A supraclavicular or axillary block may be performed preoperatively by the anesthesia team, and this will aid in vasodilation of the extremity. Placement of a continuous infusion catheter at the time of the block will allow for excellent postoperative pain control. The patient's temperature should be maintained above 36°C to prevent a sympathetic response. Systemic heparin administration can be considered in crush injuries but is not routinely necessary. Every effort should be taken by the anesthesia team to avoid vasoconstrictive agents, instead focusing on fluid resuscitation to maintain blood pressure. If vasopressors are required, this should be communicated with the surgical team.

OPERATIVE TECHNIQUE

OPERATIVE SEQUENCE

The usual sequence of repair begins with back-table preparation of the amputated part, followed by preparation of the injured extremity under tourniquet control. Bony fixation is performed first, followed by flexor tendon repair and extensor tendon repair. Within an acceptable timeframe, nerve repair may also be performed under tourniquet control. The tourniquet is then deflated and the arteries and veins are repaired under the operating microscope. If veins can be identified in the distal part, they may be repaired before the artery to minimize blood in the operating field. However, many surgeons prefer to perform arterial repair first to allow for easier venous identification.

Ideally, two teams of surgeons should be available to allow simultaneous preparation of the amputated part and the injured extremity. Preparation of the part may begin while the patient is being transported to the operating room and prepared for surgery. Amputated parts should be flushed with a heparinized saline solution. Debridement of all devitalized tissue should be performed. Nerves and vessels should be identified and tagged with microsuture to allow for later identification.

INCISIONS

Midlateral digital incisions allow for elevation of proximal and distal flaps, providing excellent exposure of all structures (Figure 94.1). The incisions should be placed dorsal to the neurovascular bundles to prevent exposure if the incisions cannot be completely closed. In ring avulsion amputations, a single midlateral incision at the level of the distal interphalangeal (DIP) joint allows for access to the joint for arthrodesis as well as vein grafting to the distal digital artery (Figure 94.2). In proximal amputations, incisions should be placed over muscle groups rather than directly over neurovascular structures as primary closure is often not possible. Fasciotomy incisions may be incorporated and used for exposure.

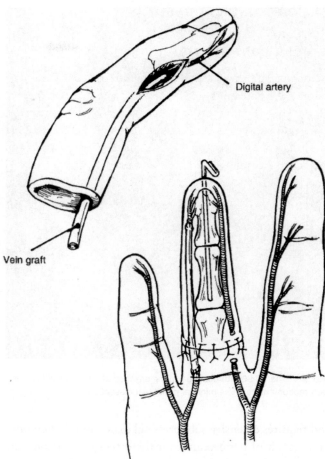

Figure 94.2. Single midlateral incision placed at the level of the distal interphalangeal (DIP) joint in ring avulsion allows for joint arthrodesis and vein grafting to distal artery.

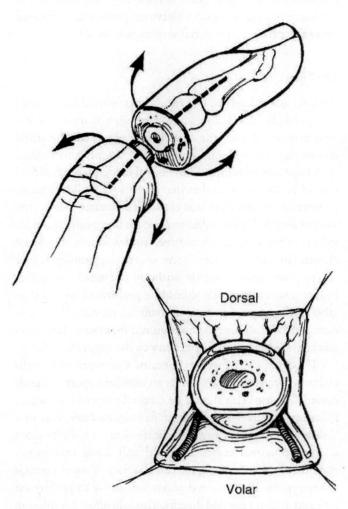

Figure 94.1. Midlateral incisions for exposure of volar and dorsal structures.

BONY FIXATION

In the case of amputations, unlike isolated fractures, anatomic alignment of bony fragments is not typically feasible. Prior to fixation, the fracture site should be debrided with a rongeur to remove any devitalized bone fragments and provide smooth bony edges for fixation. Osteosynthesis techniques depend on fracture geometry, surgeon preference, and availability of materials. Crossed K-wire fixation is typically the most efficient method of fixation, but it does not allow for early motion. Parallel longitudinal K-wires allow for the most rapid fixation but may lead to distraction at the fracture site. Use of 90-90 intraosseous wiring provides rigid enough fixation to allow for early movement. This technique is performed by passing two 24- or 26-gauge wires through parallel drill holes in the proximal and distal fragment at orthogonal angles to each other (Figure 94.3).[4] Internal fixation with plates and screws provides the most rigid fixation. However, this technique is time-consuming

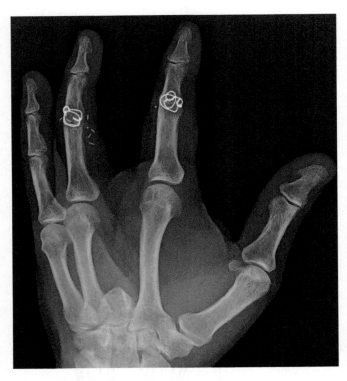

Figure 94.3. The 90-90 interosseous wiring provides stable fixation to allow early motion and requires minimal periosteal dissection.

and requires extensive subperiosteal dissection. When possible, repair of periosteum over the osteosynthesis site can improve union and prevent tendon adhesions. In periarticular amputations, arthrodesis of the involved joint should be strongly considered. Attempts at joint salvage rarely result in meaningful motion. Arthrodesis of DIP joints of the fingers or the metacarpophalangeal (MP) joint of the thumb typically does not result in significant loss of function.

TENDON REPAIR

Flexor tendon repair is a crucial portion of the replantation procedure as it has a direct influence on finger stiffness and motion; this part of the procedure should not be rushed through in anticipation of arterial revascularization. The proximal end of the tendons may be retrieved by flexing the wrist and milking the tendon distally or by using a tendon retriever. Once the tendon is pulled out to length, it may be transfixed using a small hypodermic needle. Every effort should be made to preserve the A2 and A4 pulleys. The FDP tendon should be repaired in all cases. In zone 2 amputations, many surgeons advocate repairing at least one slip of flexor digitorum sublimis (FDS) in addition to FDP. To prevent bunching of the tendons at the repair site, the epitendinous repair may be performed first followed by placement of core sutures. Popular core suture techniques include Kessler,

Tsuge, Bunnell, and cruciate. A four-strand repair should be performed whenever possible. Extensor tendon repair should be performed with mattress or figure-of-eight sutures.

NERVE REPAIR

If adequate tourniquet time remains, nerve repair should be performed under tourniquet to allow for a bloodless field. Nerve ends are trimmed distally and proximally until "pouting" fascicles are seen. In crush or avulsion injuries, there may be a significant zone of injury requiring debridement. Nerve gap should be assessed with the finger in extension. If a nerve gap exists, a nerve graft should be utilized. Potential donor sites for digital nerve grafts include the posterior interosseous nerve at the wrist level, which may be found in the floor of the fourth dorsal compartment and can provide 3–5 cm of nerve graft, or the lateral antebrachial cutaneous nerve, found in the proximal forearm adjacent to the cephalic vein, which may provide 8–12 cm of graft.[5] Acellular nerve allografts have also shown good results in digital nerve reconstruction.[6–8] Nerve coaptation is performed using three to four epineurial sutures, usually 9-0 or 10-0.

ARTERIAL REPAIR

Prior to arterial repair, the tourniquet should be released and pulsatile blood flow should be seen from the proximal arteries. If pulsatile flow is not observed, the distal end of the artery should be trimmed sharply and flushed with heparinized saline. If flow is still inadequate, the vessel should be treated with dilating agents such as lidocaine or papaverine. If this does not establish adequate inflow, the wound should be extended to look for a proximal vascular injury; otherwise, an alternative arterial source should be chosen. In sharp injuries, bone shortening usually allows for primary arterial repair without the need for grafts. End-to-end anastomosis should be performed with 9-0 or 10-0 microsuture. In crush or avulsion injuries, interposition grafts are almost always required for revascularization due to the extensive zone of injury to the digital vessels.

The distal volar forearm contains a network of superficial veins of varying sizes and is an excellent source of graft material. These veins should be marked prior to tourniquet inflation (Figure 94.4). Vein grafts may be harvested in a Y-shape to allow for revascularization of two digits from a single proximal vessel. Proximal and distal orientation should be marked during harvest to ensure proper reversal of vein grafts. The proximal anastomosis may be performed first and a clamp applied distally. This will allow for dilation and elongation of the vein graft, ensuring correct length

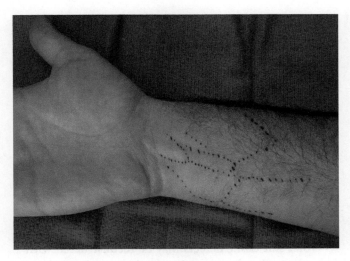
Figure 94.4. Volar wrist veins should be marked preoperatively. These veins are an excellent size match for digital artery reconstruction.

prior to distal anastomosis and preventing kinking due to excessively long grafts. If reconstruction of the palmar arch is necessary due to a mid-hand amputation, an arterial graft with branches may be harvested from the thoracodorsal or deep inferior epigastric systems. These branches may be directly anastomosed to common digital vessels.

Typically, the artery closest to the central ray of the hand will be the larger "dominant" digital artery, reducing technical difficulty of the anastomosis. Occasionally, in oblique amputations, there may be a proximal injury on one side of the digit and a distal injury on the other side. In this situation, cross-arterial repair is advised (Figure 94.5), which

may require vein grafting. If no suitable proximal inflow vessel can be identified, a digital artery may be harvested from an adjacent digit. However, this may lead to cold intolerance or stiffness in the uninvolved digit and is only recommended as a last resort. In thumb amputations at the metacarpal phalangeal (MCP) joint, the ulnar digital artery is significantly larger than the radial. However, this vessel can be very difficult to access once bony fixation is performed. In this case, it is recommended to use a vein graft, performing the distal anastomosis first on the back table, then the proximal anastomosis to the princeps pollicis artery or end-to-side to the radial artery at the anatomical snuffbox (Figure 94.6).[9]

Following arterial anastomosis and release of microvascular clamps, bleeding should be seen from the distal amputated part. This may occur immediately or it may take several minutes. If the digit does not appear perfused, apply topical vasodilating agents (lidocaine, papaverine) and warm gauze to the anastomosis. Digital arteries are highly prone to vasospasm when manipulated and therefore should be allowed to "rest" after anastomosis. If no flow is seen into the digit after dilating agents are allowed to take effect, the anastomosis should be checked for patency using the Acland test. Ensure that the vessel is not twisted, kinked,

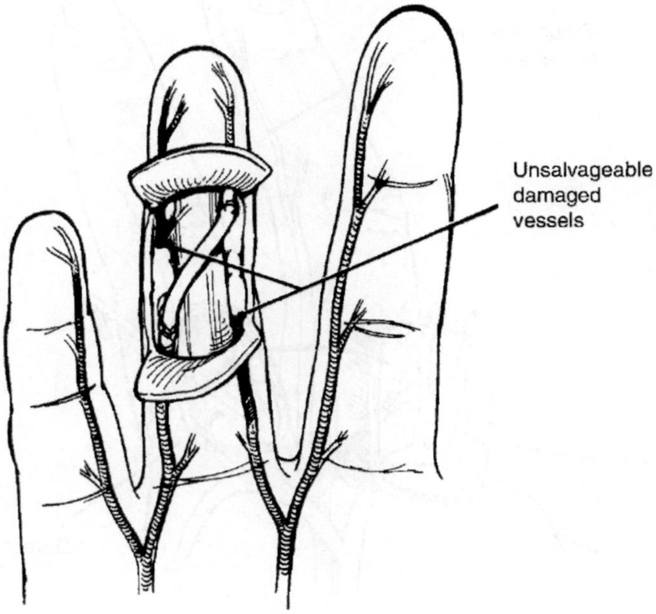

Unsalvageable damaged vessels

Figure 94.5. Certain injuries may require cross-arterial graft to provide inflow from undamaged contralateral artery.

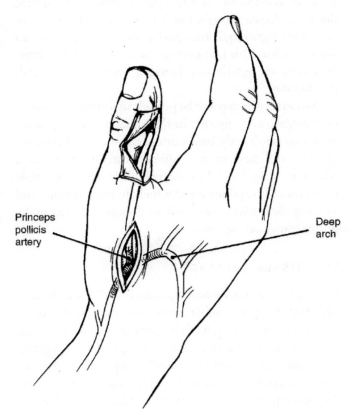

Princeps pollicis artery

Deep arch

Figure 94.6. Vein graft to ulnar digital artery of thumb, routed dorsally from princeps pollicis artery or radial artery end-to-side.

or under excess tension. If flow cannot be established the anastomosis may require revision. Systemic heparinization may be beneficial in cases of intraoperative anastomotic thrombosis but is not required in routine cases.

VENOUS REPAIR

If veins can be adequately identified and dissected proximally and distally prior to arterial anastomosis, the venous anastomoses may be performed first. This will allow for a clear, bloodless surgical field. However, distal veins will be collapsed and difficult to identify, particularly in more distal amputations. In these scenarios, the arterial anastomosis is performed first and bleeding distal veins are identified and prepared for anastomosis. Since venous insufficiency is a major factor in replantation failure, every effort should be made to repair at least two veins in each digit.

Dorsal digital veins suitable for anastomosis can be identified 4 mm proximal to the nail fold. Amputations distal to this point require anastomosis of volar veins, which form a superficial anastomotic network in the digital pulp.[10] Venous anastomosis typically requires 10-0 or 11-0 microsuture, high magnification, and fine-tip microsurgical instruments.

If an end-to-end venous repair cannot be performed due to inadequate length, a graft may be considered. An alternative to grafting is transposing an intact vein from an adjacent digit. This is also an excellent option when proximal veins are significantly damaged, such as in ring avulsion injuries.

Venous repair may not be possible in distal amputations or crush/avulsion injuries. In this situation, the replanted digit may be directly bled postoperatively to relieve congestion until new venous communications are formed, which may take 5–14 days and will likely require multiple transfusions.[11] Options for this include leech therapy and leeching alternatives, which will be discussed further in the postoperative care section.

SOFT TISSUE COVERAGE

Often amputations are accompanied by full-thickness skin defects with exposure of vital structures. In these situations, several options are available to provide wound coverage. Acellular wound matrices such as Integra dermal regeneration template provide a technically simple solution for select wounds without small exposed areas of tendon or bone. As the template becomes revascularized, it may bridge over these exposed areas, allowing for placement of a skin graft at 2–3 weeks.[12,13] However, these dermal regeneration

templates are expensive and require a second surgical procedure for definitive skin graft placement.

Dorsal soft tissue defects with accompanying venous defects may be reconstructed with a reverse cross-finger flap incorporating dorsal veins from the donor digit. These veins may be extended by 2–3 mm on either side of the flap to allow for anastomosis proximally and distally. The flap is then covered with a skin graft and must be divided 2–3 weeks later. Dorsal defects proximal to the proximal interphalangeal (PIP) joint may be reconstructed with a pedicled flag flap incorporating dorsal veins from an adjacent digit (Figure 94.7). Similarly, a vein-carrying kite flap may be used for defects of the dorsal thumb.

Volar soft tissue defects may be reconstructed with a cross-finger flap from an adjacent digit provided there is an available uninjured donor digit. Unlike with venous defects, vein-carrying cross-finger flaps are unsuitable for arterial reconstruction since the distal–proximal orientation cannot be reversed. In cases of volar soft tissue loss with an arterial defect, a small flow-through free flap may be harvested from the temporoparietal fascia, serratus fascia, or dorsal foot.[14] Vein-carrying free flaps may be harvested from the distal volar forearm. These may be used for either venous or arterial reconstruction. Excellent outcomes have been reported using arterialized venous free flaps for simultaneous revascularization and soft tissue coverage.[15]

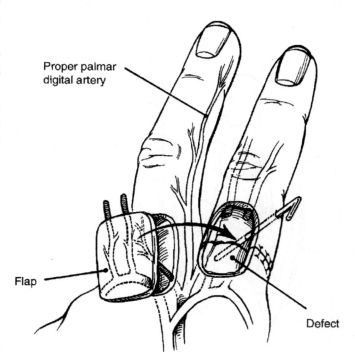

Figure 94.7. Pedicled flag flap can be used to provide soft tissue coverage and venous outflow.

POSTOPERATIVE CARE

Dressings or splints should be carefully applied to avoid circumferential compression proximal to the replanted part. Blood within the dressing may lead to constriction as it congeals, and dressings must be carefully changed. The patient's room should be kept warm to prevent vasoconstriction, and a warming blanket may be applied over the affected extremity. Continuous regional anesthesia catheters are useful for prevention of postoperative pain as well as a local sympathectomy effect leading to further vasodilatation.[16,17]

Replanted digits are carefully monitored with hourly vascular exams for the first 48 hours utilizing a Doppler probe to check vascular signals as well as monitoring for color, turgor, and capillary refill. Delayed capillary refill may be a sign of poor vascular inflow, whereas flash capillary refill signals venous congestion. Replantation patients are typically hospitalized for at least 5 days for monitoring. Continuous monitoring of replanted digits using pulse-oximetry or a temperature probe can provide real-time objective measures of perfusion.

Vascular inflow without outflow will lead to congestion, as is the case for artery-only replantation or postoperative venous insufficiency. Relief of congestion may be accomplished by causing temporary bleeding from the digit through several different methods. Medicinal leeches may be applied at regular intervals to suck blood from the replanted part. These leeches also secrete hirudin, a local anticoagulant. Leeches are colonized with *Aeromonas hydrophila*, and patients should be given antibiotic prophylaxis with a fluoroquinolone or third-generation cephalosporin. Alternatives to leeches include other methods of causing controlled bleeding from the digit, such as heparin scrubs to the exposed nailbed, fish-mouth incision at the fingertip, or local heparin injections. Controlled bleeding is required for 5–7 days until there is sufficient venous ingrowth into the digit support outflow. Although every effort should be made to repair veins during replantation, multiple studies have demonstrated successful protocols for artery-only distal replantation.[18,19]

Postoperative anticoagulation is often given based on institution-specific protocols. This may include aspirin, unfractionated or low-molecular-weight heparin, dextran, dipyridamole, or no anticoagulation. While single-institution studies report high levels of success with each of these methods,[18,20,21] there is no compelling data showing a superior method of anticoagulation.[22–24] Intravenous anticoagulation has been associated with a higher incidence of complications with no significant difference in success of replantation.[25]

As with all hand injuries, functional result depends on postoperative rehabilitation. This is complicated by concurrent injuries to flexor and extensor tendons as well as bony injuries with nonrigid fixation. Typically gentle active motion is initiated within the dressing after 2–3 days.[26] Formal hand therapy is initiated as allowed by the stability of bony fixation.

CAVEATS

Strict adherence to proper replantation indications has led to a high rate of success after digital replantation or revascularization. Nevertheless, replanted digits rarely attain a high level of function. Communication with patients about reasonable postoperative expectations is critical. The majority of lawsuits filed from replantation cases stem from the decision not to replant unsalvageable parts rather than failure of replantation, underscoring the importance of patient involvement in the decision to replant or amputate.[27]

REFERENCES

1. Baek SM, Kim SS. Successful digital replantation after 42 hours of warm ischemia. *J Reconstr Microsurg* 1992;8:455–458; discussion:459.
2. Wei FC, Chang YL, Chen HC, Chuang CC. Three successful digital replantations in a patient after 84, 86, and 94 hours of cold ischemia time. *Plast Reconstr Surg* 1988;82:346–350.
3. Pederson WC. Replantation. *Plast Reconstr Surg* 2001;107:823–841.
4. Zimmerman NB, Weiland AJ. Ninety-ninety intraosseous wiring for internal fixation of the digital skeleton. *Orthopedics* 1989;12:99–103; discussion:103–104.
5. Weber RV, Mackinnon SE. Bridging the neural gap. *Clin Plast Surg* 2005;32:605–616, viii.
6. Moore AM, et al. Acellular nerve allografts in peripheral nerve regeneration: a comparative study. *Muscle Nerve* 2011;44:221–234.
7. Lin MY, Manzano G, Gupta R. Nerve allografts and conduits in peripheral nerve repair. *Hand Clinics* 2013;29:331–348.
8. Cho MS, et al. Functional outcome following nerve repair in the upper extremity using processed nerve allograft. *YJHSU* 2012;37:2340–2349.
9. Chang J, Jones N. Twelve simple maneuvers to optimize digital replantation and revascularization. *Tech Hand Up Extrem Surg* 2004;8:161–166.
10. Jazayeri L, Klausner JQ, Chang J. Distal digital replantation. *Plast Reconstr Surg* 2013;132:1207–1217.
11. Chen Y-C, et al. Fingertip replantation without venous anastomosis. *Ann Plast Surg* 2012;1. doi:10.1097/SAP.0b013e3182321b81
12. Weigert R, Choughri H, Casoli V. Management of severe hand wounds with Integra® dermal regeneration template. *J Hand Surg (Eur Volume)* 2011;36:185–193.
13. Shores JT, Hiersche M, Gabriel A, Gupta S. Tendon coverage using an artificial skin substitute. *J Plast Reconstr Aesthet Surg* 2012;65:1544–1550.
14. Schwabegger AH, Hussl H, Rainer C, Anderl H, Ninković MM. Clinical experience and indications of the free serratus fascia flap: a report of 21 cases. *Plast Reconstr Surg* 1998;102:1939–1946.

15. Woo S-H, et al. A retrospective analysis of 154 arterialized venous flaps for hand reconstruction: an 11-year experience. *Plast Reconstr Surg* 2007;119:1823–1838.

16. Niazi AU, et al. Continuous infraclavicular brachial plexus blockade: effect on survival of replanted digits. *Hand Surg* 2013;18:325–330.

17. Kurt E, Ozturk S, Isik S, Zor F. Continuous brachial plexus blockade for digital replantations and toe-to-hand transfers. *Ann Plast Surg* 2005;54:24–27.

18. Buntic RF, Brooks D. Standardized protocol for artery-only fingertip replantation. *J Hand Surg Am* 2010;35:1491–1496.

19. Erken HY, Takka S, Akmaz I. Artery-only fingertip replantations using a controlled nailbed bleeding protocol. *J Hand Surg Am* 2013;38:2173–2179.

20. Veravuthipakorn L, Veravuthipakorn A. Microsurgical free flap and replantation without antithrombotic agents. *J Med Assoc Thai* 2004;87:665–669.

21. Ridha H, Jallali N, Butler PE. The use of dextran post free tissue transfer. *J Plast Reconstr Aesthet Surg* 2006;59:951–954.

22. Buckley T, Hammert WC. Anticoagulation following digital replantation. *J Hand Surg Am* 2011;36:1374–1376.

23. Khouri RK, et al. A prospective study of microvascular free-flap surgery and outcome. *Plast Reconstr Surg* 1998;102:711–721.

24. Chen Y-C, Chi C-C, Chan FC, Wen Y-W. Low molecular weight heparin for prevention of microvascular occlusion in digital replantation. *Cochrane Database Syst Rev* 2013;7:CD009894.

25. Nikolis A, et al. Intravenous heparin use in digital replantation and revascularization: the Quebec Provincial Replantation program experience. *Microsurgery* 2011;31:421–427.

26. Allen DM, Levin LS. Digital replantation including postoperative care. *Tech Hand Up Extrem Surg* 2002;6:171–177.

27. Bastidas N, Cassidy L, Hoffman L, Sharma S. A single-institution experience of hand surgery litigation in a major replantation center. *Plast Reconstr Surg* 2011;127:284–292.

95

TRIGGER FINGER

Rajiv Sood, Joshua M. Adkinson, and Brett C. Hartman

ASSESSMENT OF THE DEFECT

Stenosing flexor tenosynovitis of the digits, commonly known as "trigger finger," is one of the most common conditions affecting the hand. Trigger finger is characterized by painful locking or clicking of the finger during flexion or extension. Occasionally, the digit will lock in flexion and require a passive extension force to straighten the finger. If untreated, persistently locked digits may result in a secondary proximal interphalangeal (PIP) joint flexion contracture.

There are two types of trigger finger. The more common primary type occurs in middle-aged women and typically affects a single digit. The most frequently involved digit is the ring finger, followed by the thumb, long, small, and index fingers. The secondary form is associated with collagen vascular diseases, diabetes mellitus, gout, renal disease, rheumatoid arthritis, and mucopolysaccharidoses. Trigger digits in children most commonly affect the thumb and manifest as a fixed flexion deformity of the interphalangeal (IP) joint (Figure 95.1).

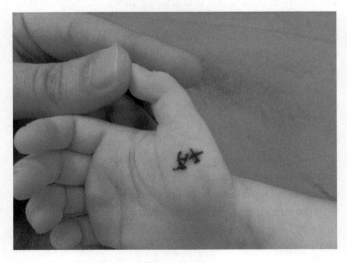

Figure 95.1. Congenital trigger thumb.

The flexor tendon sheath is comprised of five annular pulleys and three cruciate pulleys and contains the flexor digitorum superficialis (FDS) and flexor digitorum profundus (FDP) tendons (Figure 95.2). The most commonly accepted etiology of trigger finger is fibrocartilaginous metaplasia of the flexor tendons at the level of the first annular (A1) pulley in addition to pulley hypertrophy. These phenomena lead to increased friction and decreased tendon gliding. Congenital trigger thumb results from a nodular thickening of the flexor pollicis longus (FPL) tendon (i.e., Notta's node) catching on the A1 pulley, whereas congenital trigger digits result from abnormal thickening of the FDS and FDP tendons with possible anatomical variations of the FDS tendon decussation.

INDICATIONS

Patients with a trigger finger may have symptoms ranging from stiffness and pain at the A1 pulley to a fixed PIP joint flexion deformity. The most common presentation is mild pain with active flexion and intermittent triggering. The triggering is often worse in the morning or at night. On occasion, patients will describe symptoms localized to the PIP joint of the finger or interphalangeal joint of the thumb. A thorough history should be obtained to rule out other causes, such as trauma, Dupuytren's contracture, or rheumatoid arthritis.

Physical examination findings will vary depending on the severity. We ask the patient to actively flex the involved digit while we palpate over the level of the A1 pulley. This will commonly result in point tenderness over the A1 pulley. There is often a tender nodular mass that moves with FDS and FDP tendon excursion. In long-standing trigger finger, patients will limit PIP and DIP joint flexion to avoid pain associated with tendon gliding through the inflamed A1

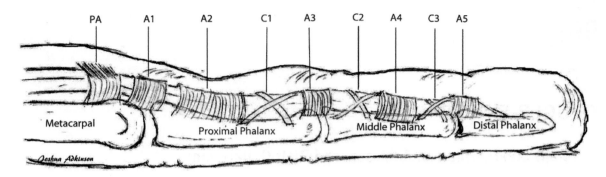

Figure 95.2. Anatomy of the flexor tendon sheath.

pulley. It is important to assess the other digits as they may have signs of early triggering masked by severe symptoms in one finger. A radiograph is only necessary in patients with long-standing flexion contractures to determine the extent of PIP joint involvement.

Treatment is based on the duration, severity, and etiology of triggering. Generally speaking, treatment may be either conservative (nonoperative) or operative (Table 95.1). Although there is no consensus treatment algorithm, most patients with the primary form of disease are initially offered conservative modalities. These consist of activity modification, splinting, nonsteroidal anti-inflammatory medication, iontophoresis, phonophoresis, and corticosteroid injection. The decision to pursue nonoperative treatment must be considered in light of the potential loss of time and income as a result of recurrent or persistent symptoms and the need for subsequent office visits.

The literature does not support the use of a specific orthosis for trigger finger. In patients who are candidates for an orthotic, we recommend a static metacarpophalangeal (MCP) joint extension splint for use at night, combined with activity modification and nonsteroidal anti-inflammatories. This combination theoretically alleviates the inflammatory response both pharmacologically and through minimizing

TABLE 95.1 OPTIONS FOR TREATMENT OF TRIGGER DIGITS

Conservative (nonsurgical)
Activity modification
Nonsteroidal anti-inflammatory drugs (NSAIDs)
Splinting
Corticosteroid injection
Surgical
Percutaneous release
Open release

tendon gliding. Our experience is consistent with the literature showing that, in patients with mild triggering and a short duration of symptoms, more than 50% of patients may have improvement.

Because noncompliance with a trigger finger orthosis is an unfortunate reality, many patients and surgeons instead opt for corticosteroid injection. Success after injection varies widely in the literature as a result of differences in corticosteroid type, solubility, and potency; duration and severity of symptoms; site of injection (proximal or distal to the A1 pulley, palmar vs. midaxial); intrasheath versus extrasheath delivery; and single versus multiple injections. There are also different rates of effectiveness in patients with a discrete nodular swelling as compared to those with diffuse swelling, and this distinction is rarely noted in the literature. The evidence is clear, however, that success rates after injection are lower (<40% success) in patients with insulin-dependent diabetes mellitus. Although some studies report success rates of up to 90% after injection, a recent systematic review of the best available evidence suggests an overall success rate of only 57%. A second injection may increase the success rate to well over 75%. Furthermore, Kerrigan and Stanwix concluded that management of trigger finger with two corticosteroid injections is the least costly treatment strategy. Based on these data, we will offer up to two injections for patients with a primary trigger finger before proceeding to surgery.

Once a patient has been deemed a surgical candidate, two options are available for A1 pulley release: percutaneous or open. Although the percutaneous technique was described nearly 60 years ago, it has gained recent popularity as a result of convenience, economics, a rapid recovery, and the office-based nature of the procedure. In general, the indications for percutaneous release are for patients with less than 4 months of symptoms and in triggering of the middle and ring fingers. The digital nerves to the thumb, index, and small fingers are at risk with percutaneous release, and we prefer an open release in these patients. The open technique has a long history of success and is technically straightforward. The success rates are nearly 100%, with a less than 1% risk for recurrence or persistent triggering.

Last, children with a flexible congenital trigger thumb should be treated with an orthosis that maintains the IP joint in full extension. Regardless of symptoms, we prefer observation in children younger than 2 years, given the evidence showing the possibility for spontaneous resolution in many cases. For children older than 2 years with persistent triggering or a fixed flexion deformity, A1 pulley release is offered. There is no role for a corticosteroid injection in children with a congenital trigger thumb.

CONTRAINDICATIONS

With the exception of a locked trigger digit, there are no contraindications to splinting. Obvious contraindications to corticosteroid injection include an allergy to the medication or an active infection. Diabetes mellitus is a relative contraindication, given the risk for corticosteroid-induced hyperglycemia. Systemic absorption of a corticosteroid injected into the palm is quite small, but diabetic patients can expect a hyperglycemic effect that lasts for at least 1–2 days. Patients with recent trauma to the hand should also be evaluated for other causes of "triggering," such as a partial flexor tendon laceration. Other mimickers of a trigger digit include a locked MCP joint, subluxation of the lateral bands or extensor tendon at the MCP joint, a tendon sheath mass (such as a giant cell tumor), and a rheumatoid nodule or synovitis. Although there is no consensus regarding the type of steroid, number of injections, or timing between injections, we prefer two or three injections with an interval of approximately 4 weeks. If there is no relief of symptoms, then percutaneous or open release is offered. Trigger digits in the rheumatoid patient should be approached with caution because an A1 pulley release may cause or exacerbate ulnar drift at the MCP joint. Triggering in this population may result from tenosynovitis, and is best treated by tenosynovectomy.

ROOM SETUP

Trigger finger or thumb release is performed as an outpatient procedure. Although some surgeons routinely use a forearm tourniquet, we prefer an upper arm tourniquet for trigger release. The benefit of decreased ischemic pain with the use of a forearm tourniquet is obviated by the extremely short duration of tourniquet use; usually only a few minutes for a single digit. The procedure can be performed under straight local anesthesia infiltrated around the surgical site, with or without the use of sedation. Percutaneous release can be performed in the office setting. An 18-gauge needle is all that is necessary for this procedure, although it requires experience to develop comfort with the technique. Ultrasound guidance may be helpful when performing a percutaneous release.

PATIENT MARKINGS

The proximal edge of the A1 pulley of the small and ring finger lie almost inline exactly with the distal palmar crease. The proximal edge of the A1 pulley of the index finger lies inline with the proximal palmar crease. The proximal portion of the A1 pulley of the middle finger lies between the distal and proximal palmar crease. For the thumb, the proximal portion of the A1 pulley is at the level of the MCP flexion crease (Figure 95.3). Another easy way of locating

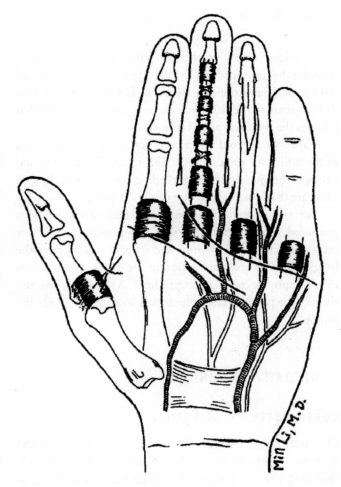

Figure 95.3. Location of A1 pulley.

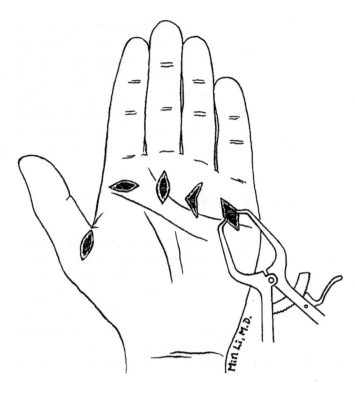

Figure 95.4. Incisions for open trigger digit release.

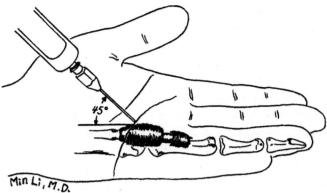

Figure 95.5. Percutaneous trigger finger injection sites.

the proximal extent of the A1 pulley of all digits is to measure the distance from the PIP crease to the palmar digital crease. That distance is then translated from the palmar digital crease to the palm over the metacarpal head and that point is the proximal aspect of each A1 pulley.

For corticosteroid injection, knowledge of the location of the pulley for each digit should suffice. For the percutaneous technique, I use the preceding measuring technique to locate the proximal portion of the A1 pulley.

For the open technique, many incisions have been proposed (Figure 95.4). Again, I preoperatively mark the pulley location and my proposed incisions. We prefer the longitudinal or oblique incision in the digits, which allows easier exposure to the longitudinal A1 pulley. For the thumb, we prefer a chevron-shaped incision to access the pulley.

OPERATIVE TECHNIQUE

CORTICOSTEROID INJECTION

Our technique involves the use of 1% lidocaine with/without epinephrine and Triamcinolone acetonide (Kenalog 10). A 1 mL mixture of 0.5 mL of lidocaine and 0.5 mL of Kenalog is placed in a 3 mL syringe. A 25- or

27-gauge needle is applied to the syringe. The hand to be injected is prepped with alcohol or chlorhexidine. The metacarpal head is palpated, and the needle is introduced directly into the flexor digitorum profundus and superficialis. Confirm the position by moving the digit and ensuring that the needle does not move with flexion or extension (Figure 95.5). Slowly withdraw the needle while exerting slight pressure on the syringe. You will feel some resistance at this level, and, upon withdrawing the needle from the tendons, you will feel a sudden decrease in resistance upon entry into the tendon sheath. It is important to aspirate to rule out rare intravascular placement. A total of 1 mL of the mixture is placed into each trigger digit. The needle is removed and pressure held for 1 minute. The injection can be repeated two or three times at 4–6 week intervals.

PERCUTANEOUS RELEASE

I strongly advise that surgeons unfamiliar with the percutaneous technique try it before the open releases (Figure 95.6). A skin incision can then be made to determine whether the technique has been successful. Once familiarity with the technique has been established, the percutaneous release can evolve into an office-based procedure. As mentioned earlier, we prefer not to percutaneously release the thumb pulley, although other authors do not hesitate to use the technique.

The technique for percutaneous release is as follows. Prepare and drape the patient as if performing a corticosteroid injection. The proximal edge of the A1 pulley and the path of the FDS and FDP tendons should be marked. Infiltrate the area of the A1 pulley with 1% lidocaine solution. Using an 18-gauge, 2.5 cm needle on a 3 mL syringe, locate the proximal end of the A1 pulley directly in the course of the flexor tendons. Some authors advocate making a small incision in the skin, but a needle can certainly be used

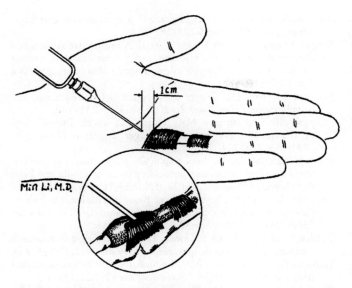

Figure 95.6. Percutaneous release techniques.

to avoid injury to the A2 pulley as greater than 25% release of the A2 pulley may result in bowstringing of the flexor tendons. Once adequate release is obtained, the tourniquet is released and hemostasis obtained. The skin is then closed with 4-0 nylon horizontal mattress sutures. We then apply Xeroform, a 4 × 4 gauze pad, 1-inch Kling wrap and Coban for our dressing.

POSTOPERATIVE CARE

After placement of the bulky dressing, the patient will leave that in place for 48 hours and then may remove the dressing and apply a smaller dressing at that time. The patient may then begin active range of motion. The patient is seen at the 2-week interval and the sutures removed.

CAVEATS

Despite the minimal surgical time and postoperative care, complications may occur in up to 7% of patients. Several authors have described complete sensory loss in the operated digit secondary to laceration of the digital nerve, particularly the radial digital nerve of the thumb. If identified, exploration and repair is warranted.

Bowstringing of the flexor tendons has also been reported secondary to inadvertent release of the A2 pulley. If this finding does not resolve, subsequent pulley reconstruction may be required.

A more common complication is pain at the operative site. We find this to be a relatively frequent complaint, but it resolves in a few weeks with reassurance and scar massage. Overall, we find the patients to be extremely satisfied with the management of trigger finger.

to make this stab wound. Move the needle either proximal to distal or distal to proximal depending on your position and locate the edge of the A1 pulley. Incise the A1 pulley with the tip of the needle. Continue the procedure until no clicking or locking is present with active motion. Patients who remain symptomatic after percutaneous release should undergo the open release technique.

OPEN TECHNIQUE

After marking the position of the A1 pulley as described earlier, we prefer either an oblique incision or a longitudinal incision over the A1 pulley for ease of access. For the thumb, we prefer a chevron-type incision with the apex at the MCP crease. We then place either a forearm or an upper arm tourniquet and local anesthesia. After chlorhexidine scrub and hand draping, the planned incision is then infiltrated with 1% lidocaine solution. The extremity is elevated and then exsanguinated with the tourniquet applied to a pressure of 250 mm Hg. A 1.0–1.5 cm incision is then completed with a no. 15 blade. Tenotomy scissors are then used to break apart the fibrous bands in a direction parallel to the neurovascular bundles until the flexor tendon sheath is encountered. Two Ragnell retractors are then used to expose the A1 pulley and flexor tendon sheath. The A1 pulley is 1.0–1.5 cm in length and is then incised with a no. 15 blade through the full thickness of the pulley. The FDS and FDP are now exposed. After release, the patient is then asked to flex and extend the digit to ensure adequate release and that no further triggering exists. If the patient is still actively triggering, ensure adequate release and examine the tendons for nodularity. Caution must be taken

SELECTED READINGS

Bauer AS, Bae DS. Pediatric trigger digits. *J Hand Surg Am* 2015 Nov;40(11):2304–2309.

Brito JL, Rozental TD. Corticosteroid injection for idiopathic trigger finger. *J Hand Surg Am* 2010 May 35(5):831–833.

Bruijnzeel H, Neuhaus V, Fostvedt S, et al. Adverse events of open A1 pulley release for idiopathic trigger finger. *J Hand Surg Am* 2012;37(8):1650–1656.

Colbourn J, Heath N, Manary S, et al. Effectiveness of splinting for the treatment of trigger finger. *J Hand Ther* 2008;21:336–343.

Evans RB, Hunter JM, Burkhalter W. Conservative management of the trigger finger: a new approach. *J Hand Ther* 1988;1:59–68.

Fahey JJ, Bollinger JA. Trigger-finger in adults and children. *J Bone Joint Surg Am* 1954 Dec;36-A(6):1200–1218.

Farnebo S, Chang J. Practical management of tendon disorders in the hand. *Plast Reconstr Surg* 2013 Nov;132(5):841e–853e.

Favre Y, Kinnen L. Resection of the flexor digitorum superficialis for trigger finger with proximal interphalangeal joint positional contracture. *J Hand Surg Am* 2012 Nov;37(11):2269–2272.

Ferlic DC, Clayton ML. Flexor tenosynovectomy in the rheumatoid finger. *J Hand Surg Am* 1978 Jul;3(4):364–367.

Fleisch SB, Spindler KP, Lee DH. Corticosteroid injections in the treatment of trigger finger: a level I and II systematic review. *J Am Acad Orthop Surg* 2007;15:166–171.

Freiberg A, Mulholland RS, Levine R. Nonoperative treatment of trigger fingers and thumbs. *J Hand Surg Am* 1989;14:553–558.

Kerrigan CL, Stanwix MG. Using evidence to minimize the cost of trigger finger care. *J Hand Surg Am* 2009 Jul-Aug;34(6):997–1005.

Lange-Riess D, Schuh R, Honle W, et al. Long-term results of surgical release of trigger finger and trigger thumb in adults. *Arch Orthop Trauma Surg* 2009;129(12):1617–1619.

Maury AC, Roy WS. A prospective, randomized, controlled trial of forearm versus upper arm tourniquet tolerance. *J Hand Surg Br* 2002 Aug;27(4):359–360.

Peters-Veluthamaningal C, Winters JC, Groenier KH, et al. Corticosteroid injections effective for trigger finger in adults in general practice: a double-blinded randomised placebo controlled trial. *Ann Rheum Dis* 2008 Sep;67(9):1262–1266.

Peters-Veluthamaningal C, van der Windt DA, Winters JC, et al. Corticosteroid injection for trigger finger in adults. *Cochrane Database Syst Rev* 2009 Jan 21;(1):CD005617.

Pope DF, Wolfe SW. Safety and efficacy of percutaneous trigger finger release. *J Hand Surg* 1995;20A:280–283.

Ring D, Lozano-Calderón S, Shin R, et al. A prospective randomized controlled trial of injection of dexamethasone versus triamcinolone for idiopathic trigger finger. *J Hand Surg Am* 2008 Apr;33(4):516–522.

Ryzewicz M, Wolf JM. Trigger digits: principles, management, and complications. *J Hand Surg Am* 2006 Jan;31(1):135–146.

Sampson SP, Badalamente MA, Hurst LC, et al. Pathobiology of the human A1 pulley in trigger finger. *J Hand Surg* 1991;16A:714–721.

Smith J, Rizzo M, Lai JK. Sonographically guided percutaneous first annular pulley release: cadaveric safety study of needle and knife techniques. *J Ultrasound Med* 2010 Nov;29(11):1531–1542.

Stepan JG, London DA, Boyer MI, et al. Blood glucose levels in diabetic patients following corticosteroid injections into the hand and wrist. *J Hand Surg Am* 2014 Apr;39(4):706–712.

Tarbhai K, Hannah S, von Schroeder HP. Trigger finger treatment: a comparison of 2 splint designs. *J Hand Surg Am* 2012;37:243–249.

Turowski GA, Zdankiewicz PD, Thomson JG. The results of surgical treatment of trigger finger. *J Hand Surg Am* 1997;22:145–149.

Wang AA, Hutchinson DT. The effect of corticosteroid injection for trigger finger on blood glucose level in diabetic patients. *J Hand Surg Am* 2006 Jul–Aug;31(6):979–981.

Wojahn RD, Foeger NC, Gelberman RH, et al. Long-term outcomes following a single corticosteroid injection for trigger finger. *J Bone Joint Surg Am* 2014 Nov 19;96(22):1849–1854.

96.

EXCISION OF GANGLION CYSTS

Shepard P. Johnson and Kevin C. Chung

INTRODUCTION

Ganglia are the most common soft-tissue masses of the hand and wrist.[1,2] They are not technically tumors but are benign, mucin-filled cysts associated with a tendon sheath or emanating from the wrist joint, which often communicate with a synovial compartment by a stalk.[2-4] These formations have fibrous walls that lack an epithelial lining and therefore are not considered true cysts, but rather *ganglia*.[3] Although many theories have been proposed, including articular stress and joint herniation, the pathophysiology remains unknown.[1-4]

Clinically, a ganglion presents as a visible and palpable rubbery subcutaneous mass that is mobile and tethered to an underlying structure. Although commonly asymptomatic, patients may present with pain on activity and palpation, decreased range of motion and grip strength, or paraesthesia from local nerve compression. Furthermore, patients may have aesthetic concerns or fears that the mass is malignant.[5-8]

Treatment algorithms of ganglia begin with patient education and nonsurgical management, owing to its low morbidity, high rate of spontaneous resolution, and risk of recurrence after intervention.[9,10] Surgical management is indicated in symptomatic patients when intervention outweighs risks and is generally accepted as a superior treatment over aspiration (with or without substance injections) for most ganglia.[9,10]

ASSESSMENT OF THE DEFECT

In order of frequency, ganglia occur at (1) the dorsal wrist, (2) the volar wrist, (3) the flexor tendon sheath at the area of the A1 pulley, and (4) the distal interphalangeal joint (DIP) (Figure 96.1).[1,11,12] Less common locations of ganglia are associated with carpometacarpal boss, ulnocarpal

joint (in conjunction with tears of the triangular fibrocartilage complex), first extensor compartment, proximal interphalangeal (PIP) joint, and inside the carpal tunnel or Guyon canal, causing nerve compression.

DORSAL WRIST GANGLION

Approximately 70% of ganglia are located on the dorsal radial aspect of the wrist between the third and fourth extensor compartment.[1-4] Clinically, they measure 1–2 cm and are best appreciated with flexion of the wrist. The lesion should transilluminate, and diagnosis is made by examination alone. Patients may complain of wrist discomfort at rest as a result of pressure on the posterior interosseous nerve in the fourth extensor compartment. Dorsal wrist ganglia occasionally are associated with scapholunate dissociation and may cause carpal instability by disrupting the scapholunate ligament after excision.

Occult dorsal ganglia refer to small ganglia (1–3 mm) that cannot be palpated but that may lead to chronic wrist pain.[11] Patients may report wrist aching exacerbated by activity, pain radiating proximally, or grip weakness. Patients often have palpable tenderness over the dorsal scapholunate ligament.[13] Ultrasound and magnetic resonance imaging (MRI) studies provide useful information for diagnosis of occult ganglia. Occult lesions are best treated nonsurgically with immobilization and corticosteroid injections into the dorsal wrist capsule.

VOLAR WRIST GANGLION

Twenty percent of ganglion cysts occur on the volar wrist and arise from the scaphoid articulations, the radiocarpal joint, or the scaphotrapezial joint.[14] They commonly appear proximal to the wrist flexion crease in the interval between the first extensor compartment and flexor carpi

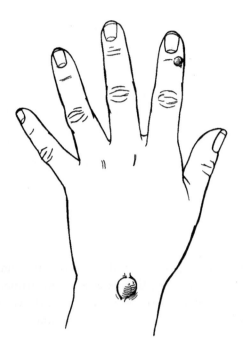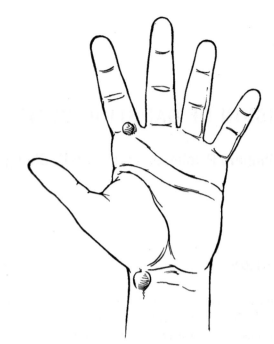

Figure 96.1. Common locations of ganglion cyst of the hand and wrist.

radialis (FCR) tendon sheath.[14–17] Volar wrist ganglia can be intimately related to the radial artery, and if a history of penetrating trauma is elucidated, auscultation and Doppler ultrasound should be used to distinguish a ganglion from a radial artery pseudoaneursym.[11] A third of volar wrist ganglia are associated with carpal arthritis. Furthermore, volar wrist ganglia have potential to cause median or ulnar nerve palsies, and ultrasound or MRI can help identify space-occupying lesions within the carpal or Guyon canal.[18]

DEGENERATIVE MUCOUS CYSTS

Mucous cysts arise from the DIP joint (typically the index and long fingers) and in association with osteoarthritis.[11] Characteristically, they present as a small, firm, rounded mass to the side of the extensor tendon and between the dorsal distal joint crease and eponychium. If they extend into the eponychial tissue, pressure on the nail matrix may result in nail plate deformity. They also have a propensity to rupture and drain clear fluid, placing the cyst at risk of infection. Removal of mucous cysts requires concomitant excision of adjacent osteophytes.[19] Radiographs are helpful to identify underlying degenerative arthritis in the DIP joint.[4]

VOLAR RETINACULAR CYSTS

Volar flexor sheath ganglia or retinacular cysts arise from the palmar digital sheath in the region of the A1 and A2 pulleys, and, therefore, patients present with a mass at the metacarpophalangeal flexion crease. As a result of this location, patients experience discomfort when gripping objects forcefully. They may arise secondary to repetitive digit flexion against resistance, tendon sheath injections, or in association with stenosing flexor tenosynovitis. Aspiration or injection with corticosteroids can be curative.[1,4]

INTRAOSSEOUS, INTRATENDINOUS, AND INTRANEURAL GANGLIA

Intraosseous ganglia may produce chronic pain. They are seen in carpal bones as well as in metacarpals and phalanges.[2] Diagnosis is of exclusion, but radiographs and computed tomographic (CT) scans may identify a sclerotic, well-defined lesion. If symptoms persist, curettage and bone grafting of intraosseous ganglia adequately treat the condition.[1,2] Intratendinous ganglia are diagnosed clinically by palpation of a distinct mass that moves with tendon excursion. Most are in extensor tendons.[11] When the diagnosis is made, excision is done with repair of tendon or tenosynovectomy (Figure 96.2). Intraneural ganglia are rare cysts that originate within the epineurium of peripheral nerves but are uncommon in the hands and wrist.[20] Effective treatment options include surgical excision, simple excision of the articular branch, and decompression of the cysts.

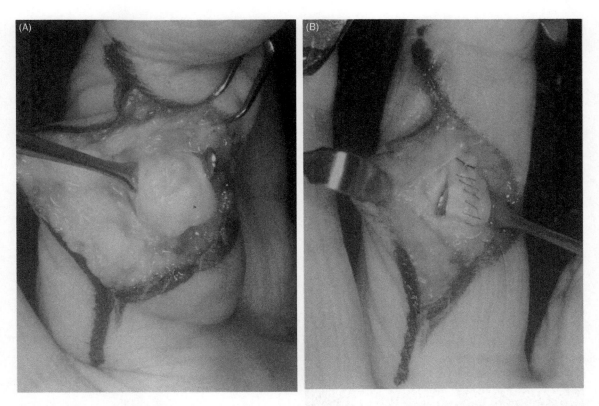

Figure 96.2. Intratendinous ganglion. (A) Ganglion is excised from within tendon through longitudinal splitting approach. Care is taken to avoid incising annular pulleys, especially A2 and A4. (B) A 6-0 nylon suture gently coapts tendon edges to produce smooth repair.

INDICATIONS

After diagnosis of a ganglion, patients should be reassured of their benign nature and that many resolve spontaneously. Following an initial period of observation, indications for treatment include persistent pain, enlargement, aesthetic concern, or symptoms suggestive of a concomitant nerve entrapment syndrome. Nonsurgical treatments include rupture by pressure, aspiration alone, or aspiration combined with injection of a substance (e.g., corticosteroid, ethanol, hyaluronidase), electrocautery, or multiple punctures.[21–24] Aspiration is done using a large needle, usually 16- or 18-gauge, to draw out the viscous fluid. Although there is wide variability in literature reports, recurrence rates after aspiration (with or without adjuncts) is approximately two-thirds. Excision of ganglia reduces recurrence rate by more than 50% in comparison with aspiration and therefore is recommended for definitive treatment.[9,25–27]

PREOPERATIVE EVALUATION

History-taking and physical examination are essential parts of patient evaluation. Examination should include thorough testing of the integrity of the musculoskeletal and neurovascular structures of the hand. This includes provocative maneuvers to identify carpal instability and an Allen's test to confirm the patency of the ulnar and radial arteries. A routine radiographic of the wrist and hand is not essential for diagnosis but may establish or confirm other diagnoses (e.g., intraosseous cysts, static wrist instability, and osteoarthritis). Transillumination or aspiration confirms the diagnosis.[12]

ROOM SETUP AND ANESTHESIA

Surgery is performed in an operating suite with loupe magnification. The patient is positioned supine with pneumatic tourniquet control and provided regional anesthesia.

OPERATIVE TECHNIQUE

DORSAL WRIST GANGLION

Dorsal wrist ganglia usually lie directly over the scapholunate ligament, but may occur anywhere on the

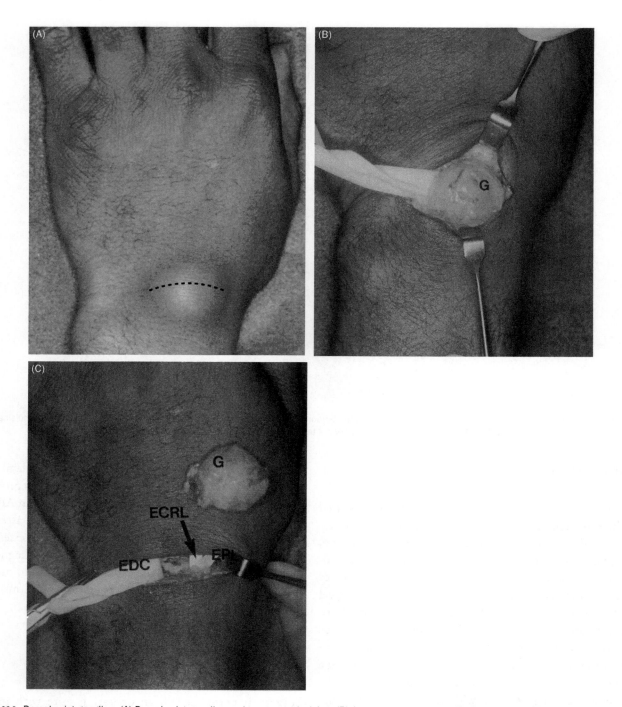

Figure 96.3. Dorsal wrist ganglion. (A) Dorsal wrist ganglion and transverse incision. (B) Appearance at surgery. (C) Ganglion usually appears between extensor pollicis longus and extensor carpi radialis longus radially and extensor digitorum communis ulnarly. ECRL, extensor carpi radialis; EDC, extensor digitorum communis (retracted with Penrose drain); EPL, extensor pollicis longus; G, ganglion.

dorsum of the hand (Figure 96.3A). Regardless, the stalk is presumed to be originating from the scapholunate joint.[1] The surgical approach is through a transverse incision centered over the cysts, which offers an excellent aesthetic result to expose the dorsal wrist capsule (Figure 96.3B). Dissection through subcutaneous tissues is delicately performed to avoid injury to the dorsal radial and ulnar sensory nerves. Typically, the ganglion appears in the interval of the third and fourth extensor compartments between the extensor pollicis longus and extensor digitorum communis tendons (Figure 96.3C). After the ganglion is identified, the extensor retinacular and a rim of dorsal joint capsular tissue around the cyst are excised (Figure 96.4).

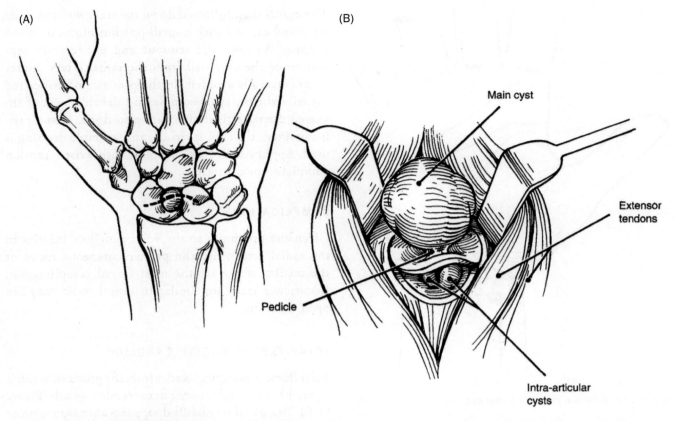

(A)   (B)

Main cyst

Extensor
tendons

Pedicle

Intra-articular
cysts

Figure 96.4. Surgical technique of dorsal wrist ganglion excision. (A) A transverse incision. (B) Extensor tendons are retracted to expose main cyst. Cyst and pedicle are mobilized to underlying joint and excised. All accessory cysts and portion of joint capsule are removed to minimize possibility of recurrence. Care is taken to preserve the scapholunate ligament. ECRL, extensor carpi radialis longus; EDC, extensor digitorum communis; EPL, extensor pollicis longus.

The ganglion is held with forceps while blunt dissection is used to mobilize the cyst from surrounding structures. The stalk is then identified arising from the scapholunate interosseous membrane proximal to the dorsal scapholunate ligament. The ganglion is elevated and transected at the stalk with a rim of the dorsal wrist capsule. The edges of the wrist capsule are cauterized thoroughly to avoid pesky bleeding that is difficult to identify when the tourniquet is let down. Smaller cysts, duct connections to the scapholunate ligament, intraarticular cysts, and excess capsular tissue may be identified and should be excised to minimize the possibility of recurrence. The joint capsule is not closed to avoid loss of wrist motion from tight capsular closure. The skin is closed and a dressing applied. A wrist splint in a neutral wrist position for 1 week is recommended for comfort and healing of the deep surgical wound.

COMPLICATIONS

Injury to the dorsal carpal arch can result in postoperative hematoma. Capsular closure may lead to wrist stiffness and therefore should not be performed. Other complications include persistent pain and hypertrophic scarring. Recurrence rates are widely reported, but estimated to be 10%.[9–12]

VOLAR WRIST GANGLION

Approximately two-thirds of volar wrist ganglia arise from the radiocarpal joint and one-third from the scaphotrapezial joint.[11] The varying locations make stalk identification critically important during surgery to avoid recurrence. The ganglion is approached through a Bruner curvilinear incision across the wrist (Figure 96.5), in the interval between the first extensor compartments and FCR tendon. This incision provides good visibility to extend into the carpal canal or base of the thenar muscles. If extension into the carpal canal is necessary, particular care must be taken to avoid cutting the palmar cutaneous nerves. After incision, the skin flaps are retracted and the underlying fascia is incised.

The ganglion is identified and mobilized with meticulous dissection to avoid injury to the radial artery and branches of the superficial radial nerve. (If the

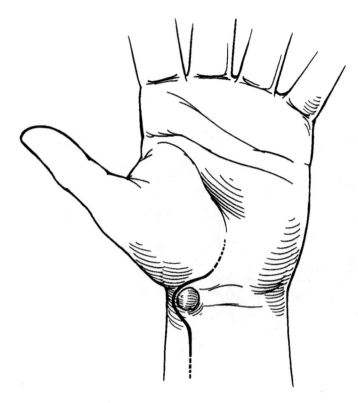

Figure 96.5. Usual incision to expose a volar ganglion.

radial artery is injured, it should be microscopically repaired.) All volar ganglia will be adherent to the radial artery and may share a common wall that makes injury to the radial artery common. We advocate for the ganglion to be opened, decompressed, and the wall between the ganglion and the artery kept intact.

The cyst is then followed down the stalk into the volar joint and excised with a small portion of the involved capsule. Without the tenuous and unnecessary separation of the cyst wall from the radial artery, injury to the artery is avoided. In the presence of associated carpal arthritis, synovectomy and debridement of involved carpal articulations are also done. Hemostasis is obtained, the skin is closed, and a simple dressing is used. Application of a volar splint with wrist extension completes the operation.

COMPLICATIONS

Given the proximity to the volar ganglion, injuries to the radial artery and the palmar cutaneous nerve of the median nerve are the most feared complications. Recurrence rates are similar to dorsal wrist ganglion open excisions.

VOLAR FLEXOR SHEATH GANGLION

Volar flexor sheath ganglia arise from the proximal annular ligament or A1 pulley of the flexor tendon sheath (Figure 96.6). This ganglion usually disappears after aspiration or injection. This can be done with a 20-gauge needle and 1% lidocaine (with or without methylprednisolone). The needle is introduced into the cyst, and local anesthetic is injected to induce cystic rupture. The remainder of local anesthetic can then be used to anesthetize the flexor sheath for pain control. If a volar flexor sheath ganglion recurs after aspiration, surgery is indicated. This is

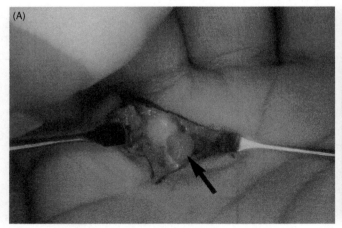
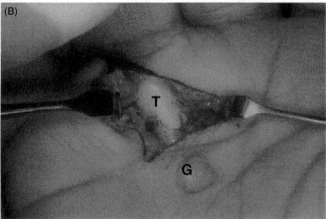

Figure 96.6. Volar flexor sheath ganglion. (A) patient presented with tender, rounded mass in distal palm. Operative finding is ganglion of the flexor tendon sheath (arrow). (B) Appearance after ganglion excision. T, tendon and tendon sheath; G, ganglion (excised).

accomplished through an angular incision for adequate exposure, identification, and mobilization of the digital neurovascular bundles. The ganglion is traced down and excised with a surrounding margin of tendon sheath (Figures 96.7). After hemostasis is obtained, skin closure is done and a simple dressing applied. Early postoperative motion is encouraged.

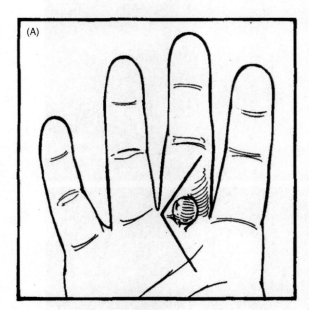

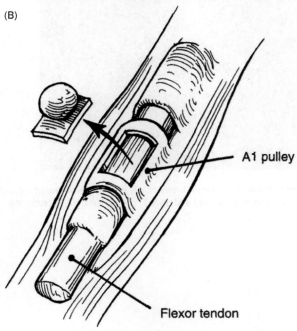

A1 pulley

Flexor tendon

Figure 96.7. Surgical technique for volar flexor tendon sheath ganglion excision. (A) Usual incision to expose flexor tendon sheath ganglion. (B) Ganglion is traced down and excised with surrounding margin of tendon sheath.

MUCOUS CYST

Nonsurgical treatments of mucous cysts have limited success and high recurrence rates, and definitive treatment is surgical excision. Exposure is done through a curved incision, and involved skin that cannot be separated from the underlying cyst is excised (Figure 96.8). The mucous cyst is mobilized and traced down to the joint. Care is taken to avoid injury to the nail matrix and extensor tendon. The cystic stalk is usually identified at the interval between the central extensor tendon and collateral ligaments (Figure 96.9). The lesion is excised and the joint is exposed. Bone spurs or osteophytes are leveled with a small rongeur. Simple closure of skin is preferred, but a rotation flap is used if there is a significant skin defect. The DIP joint is splinted for 1 week.

COMPLICATIONS

Nail plate deformities can occur if the germinal matrix is injured. Extensor lag and DIP joint instability are also possible if the extensor tendon and collateral ligaments are not protected intraoperatively.

POSTOPERATIVE CARE

A simple dressing is applied to protect the wound and to absorb drainage. The dressing is replaced or reduced by about the fourth postoperative day. A short arm splint may be used for one week, sutures are removed in 10 days, and then scar massage is encouraged. Early motion is encouraged, and hand therapy is continued until a full range of motion has been achieved.

ARTHROSCOPIC PROCEDURES

Indications for arthroscopic ganglionectomy are identical to open procedures. Enthusiasm for arthroscopic ganglionectomy rests on the potential advantages of faster recovery, decreased postoperative pain, early return to function, lower recurrence rate, and improved appearance.[28–35] Regardless, there is no evidence to suggest superiority of the arthroscopic approach, and recurrence rates of dorsal ganglion excision are comparable to the open approach. Using an open technique for ganglion cyst removal avoids the unnecessary cost of an arthroscopic approach.

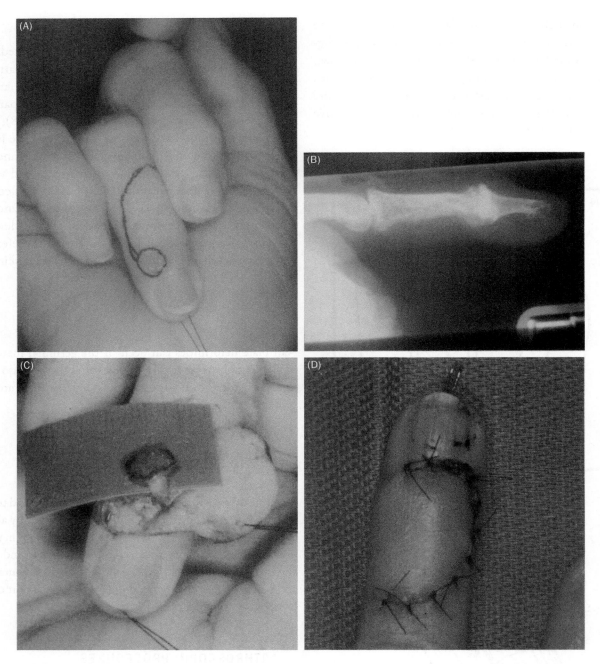

Figure 96.8. Mucous cyst. (A) Proposed surgical incision for exploration of mucous cyst with overlying skin involvement. (B) Radiograph shows associated distal interphalangeal (DIP) joint degenerative arthritis. (C) Ganglion (with adherent overlying skin) excised and traced down to joint. (D) Rotation flap closure and percutaneous longitudinal pinning of DIP joint.

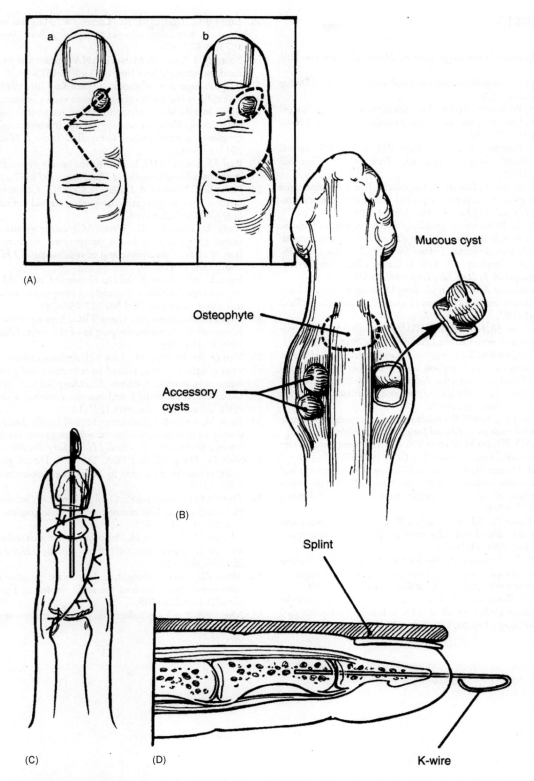

Figure 96.9. Mucous cyst excision. (A) Cyst without skin involvement and incision (a); cyst with skin involvement (b). Gently curved incision, including elliptic excision of adherent skin. (B) Cyst is mobilized, traced down to distal interphalangeal (DIP) joint, and excised with portion of joint capsule. All accessory cysts and hypertrophied synovial tissue are removed. (C) Bone spurs are leveled with small rongeur. (D) Simple closure and K-wire keep the joint in neutral position. A dorsal splint provides further finger protection.

REFERENCES

1. Evans G. *Operative Plastic Surgery*, 1st ed. New York: McGraw-Hill, 2000.
2. Thornburg LE. Ganglions of the hand and wrist. *J Am Acad Orthop Surg* 1999;7:231–238.
3. Angelides A, Wallace P. The dorsal ganglia of the wrist: its pathogenesis, gross and microscopic anatomy, and surgical treatment. *J Hand Surg Am* 1976;1:228–235.
4. Wolfe SW, Pederson WC, Hotchkiss RN, Kozin SH. *Green's Operative Hand Surgery*, 6th ed. New York: Churchill Livingston, 2010.
5. Dias JJ, Dhukaram V, Kumar P. The natural history of untreated dorsal wrist ganglia and patient reported outcome 6 years after intervention. *J Hand Surg Eur Vol* 2007;32:502–508.
6. Dias J, Buch K. Palmar wrist ganglion: does intervention improve outcome? A prospective study of the natural history and patient-reported treatment outcomes. *J Hand Surg (Br)* 2003;28:172–176.
7. Westbrook AP, Stephen AB, Oni J, Davis TRC. Ganglia: the patient's perception. *J Hand Surg (Br)* 2000;25:566–567.
8. Peters F, Vranceanu AM, Elbon M, Ring D. Ganglions of the hand and wrist: determinants of treatment choice. *J Hand Surg (Eur)*. 2012;38:151–157.
9. Head L, Gencarelli JR, Allen M, Boyd KU. Wrist ganglion treatment: systematic review and meta-analysis. *J Hand Surg Am* 2015;40:546–553.
10. Grant J, Ruff M, Janz BA. Wrist ganglions. *J Hand Surg* 2011;36:510–512.
11. Nahra M, Bucchieri JS. Ganglion cysts and other tumor related conditions of the hand and wrist. *Hand Clin* 2004;20:249–260.
12. Chung KC. *Operative Techniques: Hand and Wrist Surgery*, 2nd ed. Philadelphia, PA: Saunders, 2012.
13. Steinberg BD, Kleinman WB. Occult scapholunate ganglion: a cause of dorsal radial wrist pain. *J Hand Surg (Am)* 1999;24:225–231.
14. Greendyke SD, Wilson M, Shepier TR. Anterior wrist ganglia from the scaphotrapezial joint. *J Hand Surg (Am)* 1992;17:487–490.
15. Korkmaz M, Ozturk H, Senarslan DA, Erdogan Y. Aspiration and methylprednisolone injection to the cavity with IV cannula needle in the treatment of volar wrist ganglia: new technique. *Pakistan J Med Sci* 2013;29:5–8.
16. Rocchi L, Canal A, Pelaez J, Fanfani F, Catalano F. Results and complications in dorsal and volar wrist ganglia arthroscopic resection. *Hand Surg* 2006;11:21–26.
17. Fernandes CH, Miranda CD, Dos Santos JP, Faloppa F. A systematic review of complications and recurrence rate of arthroscopic resection of volar wrist ganglion. *Hand Surg* 2014;19:475–480.
18. Kobayashi N, Koshino T, Nakazawa A, Saito T. Neuropathy of motor branch of median or ulnar nerve induced by midpalm ganglion. *J Hand Surg (Am)* 2001;26:474–477.
19. Eaton RG, Dobranski AI, Littler JW. Marginal osteophyte excision in treatment of mucous cysts. *J Bone Joint Surg (Am)* 1973;55:570–574.
20. Naam NH, Carr SB, Massoud AHA. Intraneural ganglions of the hand and wrist. *J Hand Surg* 2015;40(8):1625–1630.
21. Burge P. Aspiration of ganglia. *J Hand Surg (Br)* 1993;8:409–410.
22. Khan PS, Hayat H. Surgical excision versus aspiration combined with intralesional triamcinolone acetonide injection plus wrist immobilization therapy in the treatment of dorsal wrist ganglion: a randomized controlled trial. *J Hand Microsurg* 2011;3:55–57.
23. Paul AS, Sochart DH. Improving the results of ganglion aspiration by the use of hyaluronidase. *J Hand Surg (Br)* 1997;22:219–221.
24. Varley GW, Needoff M, Davis TR, Clay NR. Conservative management of wrist ganglia: aspiration versus steroid infiltration. *J Hand Surg (Br)* 1997;22:636–637.
25. Kang L, Akelman E, Weiss AC. Arthroscopic versus open dorsal ganglion excision: a prospective, randomized comparison of rates of recurrence and of residual pain. *J Hand Surg Am* 2002;33:471–475.
26. Jagers M, Akkerhuis O, Van Der Heijden M, Brink P. Hyaluronidase versus surgical excision of ganglia: a prospective, randomized clinical trial. *J Hand Surg (Br)* 2002;27:256–258.
27. Stephen AB, Lyons AR, Davis TRC. A prospective study of two conservative treatments for ganglia of the wrist. *J Hand Surg (Br)* 1999;24:104–105.
28. Kim JP, Seo JB, Park HG, Park YH. Arthroscopic excision of dorsal wrist ganglion: factors related to recurrence and postoperative residual pain. *Arthrosc J Arthrosc Relat Surg* 2013;29:1019–1024.
29. Osterman AL, Raphael J. Arthroscopic resection of dorsal ganglion of the wrist. *Hand Clin* 1995;11:7–12.
30. Rizzo M, Berger RA, Steinmann SP, Bishop AT. Arthroscopic resection in the management of dorsal wrist ganglions: results with a minimum 2-year follow-up period. *J Hand Surg Am* 2004;29:59–62.
31. Shih JT, Hung ST, Lee HM, Tan CM. Dorsal ganglion of the wrist: results of treatment by arthroscopic resection. *Hand Surg* 2002;7:1–5.
32. Yamamoto M, Kurimoto S, Okui N, Tatebe M, Shinohara T, Hirata H. Sonography-guided arthroscopy for wrist ganglion. *J Hand Surg Am* 2012;37: 411–1415.
33. Edwards SG, Johansen JA. Prospective outcomes and associations of wrist ganglion cysts resected arthroscopically. *J Hand Surg Am* Mar 2009;34:395–400.
34. Ahsan ZS, Yao J. Arthroscopic dorsal wrist ganglion excision with color-aided visualization of the stalk: minimum 1-year follow-up. *Hand* 2014;9:205–208.
35. Ahsan ZS, Yao J. Complications of wrist arthroscopy. *Arthroscopy* 2012;28:855–859.

97.

PALMAR FASCIECTOMY AND FASCIOTOMY FOR DUPUYTREN DISEASE

Shepard P. Johnson and Kevin C. Chung

INTRODUCTION

Dupuytren disease is a benign connective tissue disorder of the palmar and digital fascia that may lead to profound contracture deformities and poor hand function. This condition was first described by Felix Platter in 1614, and named after Baron Guillaume Dupuytren, a French surgeon, after he described its defining characteristics and treatment in 1831.[1-4] Traditionally, the management of Dupuytren disease has included observation, fasciotomy, and fasciectomy, but needle aponeurotomy and collagenase injections have gained interest as nonsurgical alternatives.[5,6] Despite the advent of less invasive interventions, open partial fasciectomy remains the most common treatment performed.[7,8]

ASSESSMENT OF THE DEFECT

EPIDEMIOLOGY

Dupuytren disease has a genetically inherited tendency with up to 25–50% of patients reporting a family history.[1] Males are more commonly affected than females, in a 5:1 ratio, and the onset of disease peaks between 40 and 60 years.[1-4,9] Females generally present a decade later and with a more benign disease course.[1-4,9] Although observed in all ethnic groups, the highest prevalence of Dupuytren disease is among northern European populations, at 2–42%.[10] Conditions associated with Dupuytren disease include alcohol abuse, hepatic diseases, diabetes mellitus, tobacco use, chronic pulmonary diseases, tuberculosis, malignancy (paraneoplastic manifestation), human immunodeficiency virus, and epilepsy.[1-3]

HISTOPATHOLOGY

Dupuytren disease is a fibroproliferative process that results in the abnormal deposition of collagen and the transformation of palmodigital fascial structures into diseased cords. Three stages have been described in this pathologic process: (1) the proliferative phase, when fibroblast proliferate and aggregate into nodules; (2) the involution phase, characterized by myofibroblast differentiation, nodular thickening, and progressive contracture; and (3) the residual phase, marked by diffuse fibrotic thickening and type I collagen.[2,11-12] The resultant collagen produced is similar to that found in granulation tissue or hypertrophic scars.[1]

ANATOMY

To understand the pathophysiology of Dupuytren disease, a grasp of the normal palmodigital fascial elements is paramount (Figure 97.1). The palmar fascia consists of the deep fascia (which covers the interosseous muscles) and the superficial fascia (or palmar aponeurosis), but only the latter is involved in Dupuytren disease.[13-18] The principal structure affected are the pretendinous bands, which are longitudinal fibers of the palmar aponeurosis that course distally and bifurcate at the metacarpophalangeal (MCP) joints to contribute to the spiral bands.[1,2,14-18] The natatory ligament, or distal transverse fibers, can also be affected by Dupuytren disease. The natatory ligament courses superficial to the pretendinous bands and passes within the digital web.[2,13-18]

Digital fascia involved in Dupuytren disease include the spiral band, lateral digital sheath, Grayson ligament, and retrovascular band. The spiral bands wrap around the neurovascular bundle and contribute to the lateral digital sheath, which also receives fibers from the natatory ligament.[14-18] The Grayson ligament is a transverse fibrous

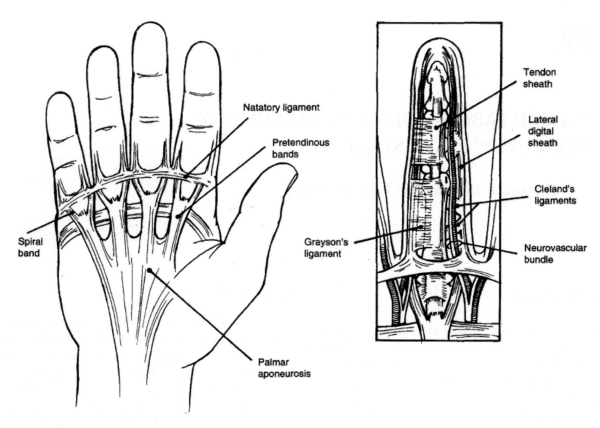

Figure 97.1. Normal palmar and digital fascia.

structure that passes from the tendon sheath to the skin and lies volar to the neurovascular bundle. Its dorsal counterpart, the Cleland ligament, is rarely involved in Dupuytren disease.[1] The retrovascular bands are longitudinally oriented fibers that are deep (dorsal) to the neurovascular bundle.[1–3,14–18]

PATHOPHYSIOLOGY

By convention, first proposed by Luck, normal fascial elements are referred to as *bands* and diseased fascia as *cords*.[11] In Dupuytren disease, joint and soft tissue contractures are a consequence of progressive shortening of these cords (Figure 97.2, Table 97.1).[17,18] For example, the pretendinous cord attaches to the palmar aponeurosis proximally and to the central band distally. Shortening of this cord results in MCP joint contractures. However, proximal interphalangeal (PIP) joint contractures are secondary to changes in a number of cords, including the central, spiral, natatory, lateral, and retrovascular cords.[1–3,15–20] Important for surgeons to consider is that the spiral cord may also displace the neurovascular bundle centrally, proximally, and superficially.[3,15–20] (Figure 97.3).

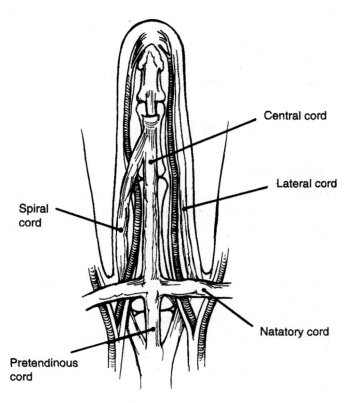

Figure 97.2. Diseased fascia in Dupuytren disease.

TABLE 97.1 NORMAL AND DISEASED PALMAR DIGITAL FASCIAL BANDS IN DUPUYTREN DISEASE

Normal bands	Diseased cords	Clinical significance
Palmar cords		
Pretendinous band	**Pretendinous cord**	MCP joint contracture
Vertical septa of Legeau and Juvara	**Vertical cord**	May contribute to associated stenosing tenosynovitis
Palmodigital cords		
Pretendinous band, spiral band, lateral digital sheath, and Grayson's ligament	**Spiral cord**	Displacement of the neurovascular bundle centrally, proximally, and superficially
Natatory ligament (distal transverse fibers)	**Natatory cord**	Digit abduction contractures and PIP flexion contractures
Digital and thumb cords		
Central fibrofatty tissue	**Central cord**	PIP joint contractures
Lateral digital sheet of Gosset	**Lateral cord**	PIP and DIP joint contractures
Grayson's ligament	**Contributes to central, spiral, and lateral cords**	
Cleland's ligament	**Contributes to spiral and lateral cords**	
Retrovascular band	**Retrovascular cord**	PIP and DIP joint contractures
Distal commissural ligament of Grapow	**Distal commissural cord**	First-web adduction contracture
Abductor digiti minimi tendon	**Abductor digiti minimi cord**	DIP joint contracture

DIP, dorsal interphalangeal; MCP, metacarpophalangeal; PIP, proximal interphalangeal.

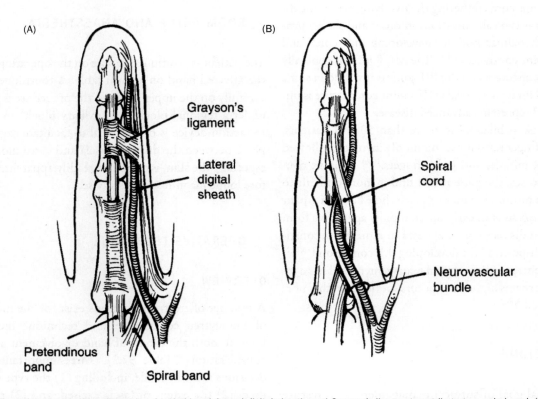

Figure 97.3. (A) Normal anatomy; pretendinous band, spiral band, lateral digital sheath, and Grayson's ligament contribute to a spiral cord. (B) Spiral cord with displacement of neurovascular bundle superficial and medial.

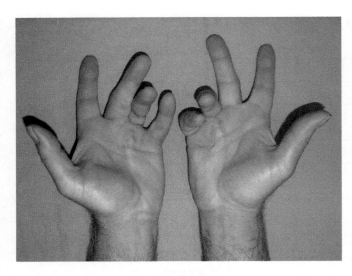

Figure 97.4. Bilateral Dupuytren disease affecting the ulnar-sided digits with nodules present in the distal palms and pitting in the right hand distal palmar crease.

CLINICAL PRESENTATION

Dupuytren disease is diagnosed based on a thorough history and clinical examination. Patients commonly present with one or more firm, painless, small nodules within the palm or at the base of the finger (Figure 97.4).[19] Pitting at the distal palmar crease is pathognomonic of Dupuytren disease, precedes nodules, and is caused by superficial fibers of pretendinous cords tethering the overlying skin.[2] The disease process is typically insidious in onset and slowly progressive, with palmar nodules developing into cords and leading to joint contracture.[1,3,8] The MCP joint is generally the first joint affected, and the PIP joint is involved in some cases. Dorsal interphalangeal (DIP) joint contracture is uncommon and represents advanced disease.

The disease is bilateral in more than 50% of patients, and the ring finger ray is most commonly involved, followed by the small, middle, and index fingers.[19,20] As joint contracture increases, the patient will find it more difficult to perform fine motor activities or place their hand in a pant pocket. A *diathesis* is an early-onset, rapidly aggressive form of Dupuytren disease, which appears to represent a constitutional predisposition for developing this condition.[1-3,19,20] Diathesis requires earlier surgical management and has a recurrence rate that is higher and occurs sooner than that normally observed.[3,19,20]

INDICATIONS

The principal goal of surgical management is to restore function by eliminating joint contracture and restoring range of motion. Although enzymatic fasciotomy with collagenase clostridium histolyticum has gained interest, long-term outcomes are not well reported and surgery remains the standard treatment for progressive Dupuytren disease.[5-7] The presence of an MCP joint flexion contracture of more than 30 degrees and/or any PIP joint contracture in conjunction with functional impairment or compromise to the digital neurovascular bundle is an indication for surgical removal of the diseased fascia.[1-3,20-26]

CONTRAINDICATIONS

There are few absolute contraindications to the surgical management of Dupuytren disease. In patients with multiple medical problems, the anesthetic risk can be minimized with the use of regional anesthesia. Conditions that may result in bleeding (e.g., coagulopathy) or poor wound healing (e.g., malnutrition) increase the risk of a poor functional and aesthetic result. Neurologic or cognitive deficits that prevent the patient from cooperating and participating in postoperative therapy may result in a less successful surgical outcome.

ROOM SETUP AND ANAESTHESIA

The patient is positioned supine on the operating table with the affected hand on an arm table. A tourniquet is placed carefully on the upper arm and the procedure is performed under a regional block (e.g., axillary block). A *lead hand* retraction device is often useful to facilitate exposure. The plane between the diseased fascia and surrounding tissues, especially the skin, is often not readily apparent, and therefore loupe magnification is advised.

OPERATIVE TECHNIQUE

OVERVIEW

A number of treatment options exist for the management of Dupuytren contracture, and technique must be tailored to both the extent of hand involvement and patient considerations (Table 97.2). Three important operative decisions must be made, including (1) the type of incision used, (2) the extent of fascia excised, and (3) the type of wound closure.

TABLE 97.2 SURGICAL CONSIDERATIONS FOR MANAGEMENT OF DUPUYTREN DISEASE INCLUDE PLACEMENT OF INCISIONS, EXTENT OF FASCIAL EXCISION, AND TYPE OF WOUND CLOSURE

Incisions		Operation	Wound closure
Palm	*Digit*		
Longitudinal +/− Z-plasties at flexion creases Bruner Transverse	Longitudinal +/− Z-plasties at flexion creases Bruner V-Y incisions Transverse	Fasciotomy Partial fasciectomy Total Fasciectomy Dermofasciectomy	Open Split thickness skin grafting Full thickness skin grafting Primary closure

Patient Markings and Incisions

Fasciotomy of an offending cord can be approached through a longitudinal incision over the pathological cord. Conversely, regional fasciectomy, or removal of fascia, requires greater exposure and more extensive incisions for adequate visualization. Suitable approaches include transverse incisions, Bruner-type zigzag incisions, midline longitudinal incision with Z-plasties, and multiple Y-V advancement flaps (Figure 97.5). Transverse incisions at the flexor creases reduce the risk of scar contracture, but the limited exposure increases the risk of incomplete fasciectomy or injury to neurovascular structures and lacks

the ability to provide skin lengthening. A classic Bruner incision avoids the potential for contracture of a longitudinal incision, but it does not permit skin lengthening and there is a risk of ischemia of the skin flaps. Skoog advocated the use of longitudinal incisions over the diseased cords with Z-plasties to improve exposure of diseased elements in the lateral portion of the digit, permit skin lengthening, and avoid a longitudinal scar (Figure 97.6).[27]

Extent of Excision

Historically, McIndie and Beare advocated a radical fasciectomy to include both the diseased and uninvolved

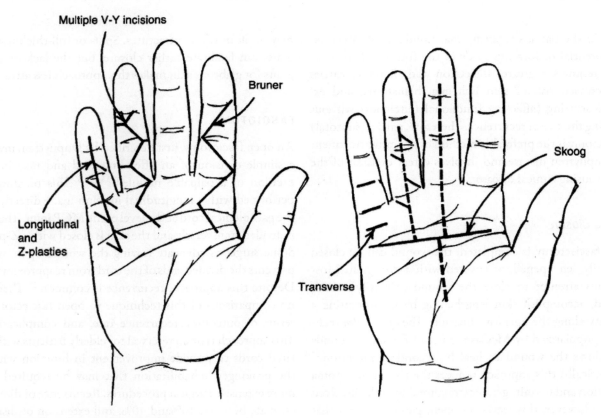

Figure 97.5. Incision options for partial fasciectomy.

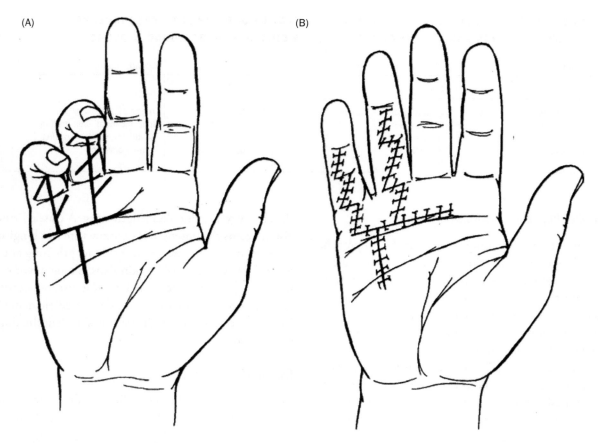

Figure 97.6. Skoog technique. (A) Preoperative markings, and (B) final skin closure following transposition of Z-plasty flaps at finger creases.

fascia in the palm, suggesting that nondiseased fascia has the potential of forming cords in the future.[28] This operation requires a greater dissection and therefore carries an increased risk of skin ischemia, hematoma, and excessive scarring (affecting functional outcomes) without lowering the rate of recurrence. Therefore, partial (subtotal) fasciectomy is the preferable method of operative treatment for Dupuytren disease and involves direct excision of the fascia causing clinical disease.

Wound Closure

After fasciectomy is completed, the wound can be closed primarily, left opened, or covered with a skin graft. Most surgeons attempt to close the wound primarily and, if needed, accomplish skin lengthening by incorporating a Z-plasty along the operative incision. The *open palm* technique popularized by McCash is useful for small wounds and allows the wound to heal by secondary intention.[29] Theoretically, this approach reduces the risk of hematoma formation and permits greater straightening of the involved digits. However, this leaves an open, painful wound that prolongs healing, limits participation in rehabilitation, and

may result in scar contractures. Split- or full-thickness skin grafts can facilitate earlier closure, but the lack of donor grafts for glabrous skin makes this approach less attractive.

FASCIOTOMY

An open fasciotomy, first described by Dupuytren, involves a simple division of an offending cord and may include excision of a palpable nodule.[1–3,8,15–16] This technique is performed with a longitudinal incision made directly over the pathological cord at the level of the MCP joint. The cord is divided transversely and the skin is closed with a Z-plasty. Some surgeons advocate leaving the wound open, which prevents the divided ends of the cord from reapproximating. Despite this approach, recurrence is common.[14] There are no comparisons of this technique to open fasciectomy in terms of outcomes, recurrence rate, and complications.[8] This approach is often reserved for elderly patients with isolated cords to provide improvement in function without the prolonged rehabilitation that may be required with more extensive surgical procedures. Recurrence of disease is estimate between 10% and 40%, and extension of diseased between 10% and 30%.[14,26]

PARTIAL FASCIECTOMY

The following is our preferred technique for partial fasciectomy for MCP and PIP joint contractures due to Dupuytren disease. The critical steps in this procedure include (1) the skin incision, (2) raising skin flaps to provide adequate exposure, (3) identifying and protecting the neurovascular bundle, (4) exposing and resecting diseased fascia (central and lateral components), and (5) closing the wound. The operation is carried out with sharp dissection using fresh no. 15 blades to minimize scar tissue formation.

The diseased fascia is marked with an incision directly over the length of the cord on the palm and volar finger (Figure 97.7). The longitudinal incision should extend from the proximal portion of the diseased cord to the PIP joint, where it terminates in a V-incision. The V-incision provides better exposure and allows easier identification of the neurovascular bundle, which is superficial at this level. We also routinely use a transverse incision at the distal

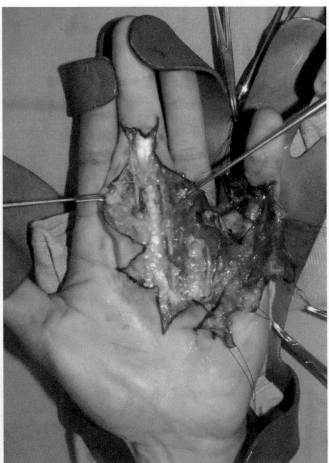

Figure 97.8. Skin flaps are raised and retracted with sutures, exposing the diseased cords.

palmar crease to elevate skin flaps that provide greater exposure. Dissecting in areas immediately proximal to the web spaces (bordered by the transverse palmar and longitudinal incisions) is avoided because it harbors the perforating vessels that supply the skin flaps.

After marking, all incisions are made and skin flaps are raised using meticulous dissection to avoid buttonholing, thinning, and compromising the viability of the skin. Sutures are placed to retract the skin and expose the diseased cord (Figure 97.8). Attention is then concentrated on the digit, and formal dissection is initiated at the level of the PIP joint where the digital neurovascular bundle is superficially located. Blunt dissection with scissors is used to mobilize the neurovascular bundle away from the diseased fascia. Surgeons must be cognizant that a diseased spiral cord may displace the neurovascular bundle medially. After both medial and lateral neurovascular bundles are identified, the central cord is dissected starting distally at the PIP joint and working proximally toward the pretendinous cord in the palm. Careful dissection is continued—while maintaining

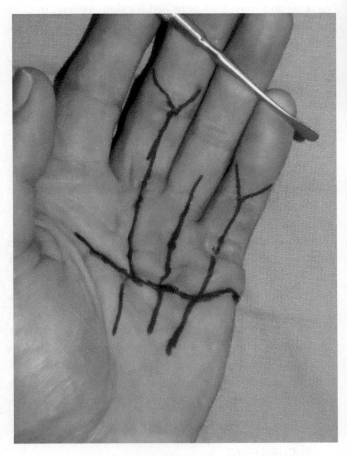

Figure 97.7. Incision markings over pretendinous cords extending onto the volar aspect of the digits. V-shaped incisions at the proximal interphalangeal (PIP) joint provide greater exposure to allow identification of the neurovascular bundle at this level. A transverse palmar incision connects the longitudinal incisions.

visualization of the neurovascular bundles at all times—to separate the cord from normal tissue and skin.

After the central diseased fascia is isolated from healthy tissue, the lateral elements can be addressed. If a spiral cord exists, the neurovascular bundle is dissected to the point where it is crosses anterior to the spiral cord. The spiral cord is then divided at this location. Excision begins with the proximal, divided end of the lateral component of the spiral cord in conjunction with excision of the lateral cord. Following removal of the spiral and lateral cords, the fascia deep to the neurovascular bundle should be examined for the presence of a retrovascular cord. Dissection of the pretendinous cord is then completed and transected proximally in the palm. Throughout the surgical procedure, emphasis should be placed on protecting the neurovascular bundle and on performing a complete dissection of the diseased fascia (Figure 97.9).

The adequacy of fascial excision is confirmed if the PIP joint digit can be straightened. If the PIP joint remains contracted, incising the A3 pulley, retracting the flexor tendon, and incising the proximal volar plate may fully release the PIP joint. We then perform a volar capsulotomy with 60-degree Z-plasty incisions at the level of the MCP finger creases. Z-plasties also improve exposure of diseased fascial elements laterally in the finger and may be performed

earlier to facilitate an adequate dissection. The tourniquet is taken down to ensure that the finger is clinically well perfused (e.g., pink), and hemostasis is achieved with a combination of pressure and electrocautery. The fingertip should be carefully inspected in full extension because straightening of a severely contracted finger may lead to vascular impairment and digital ischemia. Additionally, when closing the flaps, care must be taken to not to strangulate the neurovascular bundle at the base of the finger. Primary closure of the skin is performed loosely with a 4-0 or 5-0 monofilament nylon suture.

OTHER TECHNIQUES

Dermofasciectomy, described by Hueston, is a radical operative approach that involves removing both the diseased cord and the overlying skin.[30] This technique is useful in the treatment of recurrent disease or with Dupuytren disease with severe cutaneous involvement, which can be observed with diathesis. However, in most instances, the skin can be separated from the diseased fascia. Furthermore, this technique exposes tendons and provides a poor bed for skin grafting. In cases of severe, long-term contracture, amputation might be entertained for a fixed, severe flexion contracture in elderly patients. Other alternatives include a wedge osteotomy of the distal proximal phalanx or arthrodesis of an affected joint.

POSTOPERATIVE CARE

The hand is placed in a bulky dressing and splinted for 10 days. A volar splint is used to maintain the hand and digits in a functional position. Care should be taken to avoid overextension of interphalangeal joints, which may result in ischemia of the fingertip. Strict hand elevation is encouraged to minimize pain and to prevent edema and hematoma, both of which can compromise subsequent mobilization. Sutures are removed in 14 days. A comprehensive hand therapy program is initiated to assist the patient in edema management, mobilization, strengthening, and scar therapy. Scar massage exercises are a critical component of preventing scar tissue formation during the postoperative recovery period. Additionally, a volar resting hand splint in a functional position is used for 6 months to prevent fist clenching at nighttime.

RECURRENCE

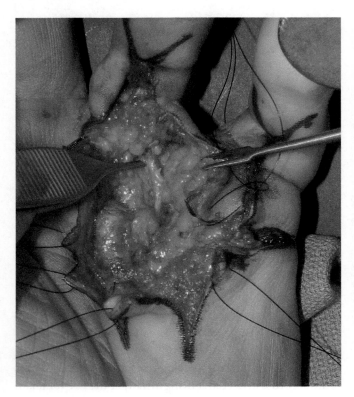

Figure 97.9. The pretendinous cord of the long finger is cut and Adson forceps shows the preserved neurovascular bundle.

Recurrence rates after partial fasciectomy are widely reported, but are approximately 20% for both MCP and PIP joint contractures.[14,25] Recurrence may be secondary to incomplete removal of the diseased fascia or shortening of the periarticular structures in long-standing disease.[1-3,8,15-21] Management of recurrent disease is often difficult because the surgeon is dealing with a combination of diseased fascia and scar tissue. Because the anatomy is distorted, the risk of injury to the neurovascular bundle is greater, and care must be taken to identify and preserve this structure early in repeat dissections. In repeat operations, incision of the fibrous flexor tendon, release of the check-rein ligaments, and release of the accessory collateral ligaments and volar plate can be performed.[1]

COMPLICATIONS

The most common early complication is hematoma formation (0–13%) and can lead to skin loss, infection, edema, delayed healing, and long-term fibrosis.[31,32] This complication is most frequently encountered after radical excisions involving a total fasciectomy because the dissection is more extensive. Skin tearing or necrosis is another common early complication and is usually a result of overly thinned flaps.[32] Infection is uncommon (less than 3%), and no evidence exists to support preoperative antibiotics to prevent surgical site infections after fasciectomy.[8,33]

Damage to the neurovascular bundle can result in nerve division, neurapraxia, or digital artery injury. Neurapraxia (<10%) may occur from traction or injury to the neurovascular bundle during dissection, but paresthesias are often self-limiting.[34] Necrosis of the fingertip may occur from direct injury of the digital artery (<2%) or overly aggressive straightening of digits that have been significantly contracted for a prolonged period.[8,32,34] Vasospasm can be managed with warm compresses or calcium channel blockers, but injury to bilateral digital arteries may require microsurgical revascularization.[8] Other long-term problems include scarring, stiffness, and complex regional pain syndrome (CRPS).[31-34]

CAVEATS

To avoid complications and recurrence, important principles should be followed in all operative cases. The appropriate incision, extent of fasciectomy, and approach to wound closure should be selected to minimize soft tissue damage, completely excise diseased fascia, and prevent skin

contractures. When raising skin flaps, care must be taken to avoid excessive manipulation, thinning, or buttonholing of the skin. During the operation, sharp dissection with a no. 15 blade scalpel is preferred to minimize scarring, but blunt dissection using scissors is an important surgical technique near the neurovascular bundle. This is critical when a spiral cord is encounter as the neurovascular bundle will be displaced medial and superficial to its normal anatomic position.

REFERENCES

1. Evans G. *Operative Plastic Surgery*, 1st ed. New York: McGraw-Hill, 2000.
2. Neligan PC. *Plastic Surgery*, 3rd ed. Philadelphia, PA: Saunders, 2012.
3. Shaw RB, Chong A, Zhang A, Hentz VR et al. Dupuytren disease: History, diagnosis, and treatment. *Plast Reconstr Surg* 2007;120:44e–54e.
4. Ross, D. C. Epidemiology of Dupuytren disease. *Hand Clin* 1999;15:53–62.
5. Badalamente, M. A., Hurst, L. C., and Hentz, V. R. Collagen as a clinical target: Nonoperative treatment of Dupuytren disease. *J. Hand Surg (Am)* 2002;27:788.
6. Hurst LC, Badalamente MA, Hentz VR et al. Injectable collagenase clostridium histolyticum for Dupuytren contracture. *N Engl J Med* 2009;361(10):968–979.
7. Chen NC, Srinivasan C, Shauver MJ, Chung KC. A systematic review of outcomes of fasciotomy, aponeurotomy, and collagenase treatments for Dupuytren contracture. *Hand* 2011;6:250–255.
8. Desai SS, Hentz VR. The treatment of Dupuytren disease. *J Hand Surg* 2011;36A:936–942.
9. Wilbrand S, Ekbom A, Gerdin B. The sex ratio and rate of reoperation for Dupuytren contracture in men and women. *J Hand Surg (Br.)* 1999;24:456.
10. Ling RS. The genetic factor in Dupuytren disease. *J Bone Joint Surg (Br)* 1963;45:709–718.
11. Luck JV. Dupuytren contracture. A new concept of the pathogenesis correlated with the surgical management. *J Bone J Surg* 1959;40:635–664.
12. Kloen P. New insights in the development of Dupuytren contracture: A review. *Br J Plast Surg* 1999;52:629–635.
13. Bojsen-Moller F, Schmidt L. The palmar aponeurosis and the central spaces of the hand. *J Anat* 1974;117:55–68.
14. Cheung K, Walley KC, Rozental TD. Management of complications of Dupuytren Contracture. *Hand Clin* 2015;31:345–354.
15. Bhandari M. *Evidence-Based Orthopedics*. Oxford: Wiley-Blackwell, 2012.
16. Wolfe SW, Pederson WC, Hotchkiss RN, Kozin SH. *Green's Operative Hand Surgery*, 6th ed. New York: Churchill Livingston, 2010.
17. Strickland JW, Leibovic SJ. Anatomy and pathogenesis of the digital cords and nodules. *Hand Clin* 1991;7:645.
18. Rayan GM. Palmar fascial complex anatomy and pathology in Dupuytren disease. *Hand Clin* 1999;15:73.
19. Rayan GM. Clinical presentation and types of Dupuytren disease. *Hand Clin* 1999;15:87.
20. Swartz WM, Lalonde DH. Dupuytren disease. *Plast Reconstr Surg* 2008;121(4):1–10.
21. Chung KC. *Operative Techniques: Hand and Wrist Surgery*, 2nd ed. Philadelphia, PA: Saunders, 2012.
22. Makela EA, Jaroma H, Harju A. Dupuytren contracture: the long-term results after day surgery. *J Hand Surg (Br)* 1991;16:272–274.

23. Becker GW, Davis TR. The outcome of surgical treatments for primary Dupuytren disease—a systematic review. *J Hand Surg Eur* 2010;35:623–626.

24. Roush TF, Stren PJ. Results following surgery for recurrent Dupuytren disease. *J Hand Surg* 2000;25(2):291–296.

25. van Rijssen AL, ter Linden HT, Werker PM. Five-year results of a randomized clinical trial on treatment in Dupuytren disease: percutaneous needle fasciotomy versus limited fasciectomy. *Plast Reconstr Surg* 2012;129(2):469–477.

26. Citron N, Hearnden A. Skin tension in the aetiology of Dupuytren disease;a prospective trial. *J Hand Surg* 2003;28B:528–530.

27. Skoog T. The transverse elements of the palmar aponeurosis in Dupuytren contracture. *Scand J Plast Reconstr Surg* 1967;1:51.

28. McIndoe A, Beare R. The surgical management of Dupuytren contracture. *Am J Surg* 1958;95:197.203.

29. McCash C. The open palm technique in Dupuytren contracture. *Br J Plast Surg* 1964;17:271.

30. Hueston T. Limited fasciectomy for Dupuytren contracture. *Plast Reconstr Surg* 1961;27:569–584.

31. Denkler K. Surgical complications associated with fasciectomy for Dupuytren disease: a 20-year review of the English Literature. *Eplasty* 2010;10:e15.

32. Boyer MI, Gelberman RH. Complications of the operative treatment of Dupuytren disease. *Hand Clin* 1999;15(1):161–166.

33. Aydin N, Uraloglu M, Yilmaz Burhanoglu AD, Sensoz O. A prospective trial on the use of antibiotics in hand surgery. *Plast Reconstr Surg* 2010;126:1617–1623.

34. Bulstrode NW, Jemec B, Smith PJ. The complications of Dupuytren contracture surgery. *J Hand Surg* 2005;30(5):1021–1025.

98.

ENDOSCOPIC CARPAL TUNNEL RELEASE

Antony Hazel and Neil F. Jones

INTRODUCTION

Conventional open carpal tunnel release surgery is one of most successful procedures in hand surgery and has been demonstrated to be an effective treatment for carpal tunnel syndrome. A known sequelae in some individuals who undergo the procedure is "pillar" pain. In an effort to avoid this condition and help people return to work more quickly, the endoscopic technique was developed. Rather than an outside-in approach to the transverse carpal ligament, this new technique incises the ligament inside-out in order to avoid the soft tissue of the palm. The techniques of endoscopic carpal tunnel release is reviewed herein.

ANATOMY

The carpal tunnel consists of the transverse carpal ligament, which spans from the hamate and triquetrum to the scaphoid and trapezium. Contents of the tunnel consist of the median nerve, flexor pollicis longus, and the four flexor digitorum superficialis and the four flexor digitorum profundus tendons. The median nerve lies directly beneath the antebrachial fascia and lies superficial to the flexor tendons in the carpal tunnel. The motor branch of the median nerve usually has a distal and radial branch point but variability does exist.[1] Common variations of the branch point of the motor nerve include an extraligamentous take-off point, where the motor branch separates distal to the transverse carpal ligament. The second most common variation is subligamentous, where the branch point occurs within the carpal tunnel. A worrisome variation is a transligamentous take-off point, where the motor branch pierces the transverse carpal ligament.

Kaplan's cardinal line, a line drawn across the palm at the level of the distal border of the fully abducted thumb, marks the level of superficial palmar arch. Some patients may have a persistent median artery that usually regresses in the second embryonic month.[1] The artery may have a superficial course within the carpal tunnel that puts it at risk during surgery.

OPERATIVE TECHNIQUE

The following technique is standard for the one-incision endoscopic carpal tunnel release developed by John Agee (Microaire, Charlottesville, VA).[2]

ANESTHESIA

Surgery can be performed under general, regional, or local anesthesia. Whichever mode of anesthesia is used, it is imperative that the patient does not move during the procedure as instrumentation is positioned close to the median nerve and sudden movements may cause injury. Local anesthesia may disrupt the tissues planes and make the approach difficult. Incorrect identification of tissue planes can lead to misplacement of instrumentation and an unsuccessful procedure. For this reason, it may be better to perform the procedure under regional or general anesthesia once the proper experience has been gained.

LANDMARKS

Important landmarks to identify prior to starting the procedure include the pisiform, hook of hamate, flexor carpi radialis (FCR), flexor carpi ulnaris (FCU), and palmaris longus tendons (Figure 98.1). A line may be drawn from

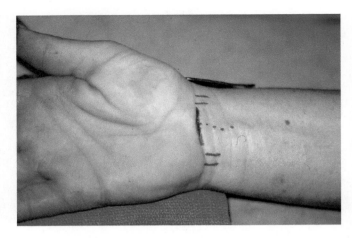

Figure 98.1. Transverse incision in the distal wrist crease between the flexor carpi radialis (FCR) and flexor carpi ulnaris (FCU) tendons.

the midpoint of the wrist flexion crease incision to the base of the proximal phalanx of the ring finger which represents the ring finger axis line. The hook of the hamate represents the ulnar-most extent of the carpal tunnel, and the endoscope should travel toward the ring finger and not be positioned ulnar to the hook of hamate in order to avoid entering Guyon's canal. Kaplan's cardinal line should mark the distal extent of the procedure because passing distal to this line may injure the superficial palmar arch or the common digital nerve to the middle-ring fingers.

TECHNIQUE

Some surgeons utilize the distal wrist crease; however, for ease of instrumentation, a transverse incision is made along the proximal wrist crease between the FCU and FCR tendons. It is important not to cut too deeply as the palmar cutaneous branch of the median nerve is at risk with this incision. There are usually one to two superficial veins that need to be cauterized. The antebrachial fascia is then identified. Using a scalpel, a distally based U-shaped flap is created and then elevated using tenotomy scissors. A synovial elevator is inserted into the carpal canal in line with the axis of the ring finger radial to the hook of the hamate. The synovial elevator should have a slight dorsal trajectory to avoid being superficial to the transverse carpal ligament and is used to scrape off or clear any synovium from the undersurface of the transverse carpal ligament, which feels like rubbing a washboard.

While holding the wrist in about 30 degrees of extension, a small and a large dilator are used to create a path for the endoscope–blade assembly. With each successive pass of the dilators, the "washboard" effect should be felt. The tip of the dilator can be palpated in the palm as it emerges

from the carpal tunnel distal to the transverse carpal ligament. The distance between the transverse incision at the wrist crease and the distal end of the transverse carpal ligament is usually 4 cm. The endoscope–blade assembly is then introduced into the carpal tunnel with the wrist in 30 degrees of extension (Figure 98.2A,B), and a clear view of the transverse carpal ligament should be seen (Figure 98.3A,B). The apparatus should be against the hook of the hamate and be pointing toward the base of the ring finger. The distal end of the transverse carpal ligament is visualized by balloting the palm with the surgeon's left thumb. The blade should not be deployed beyond the transverse carpal ligament to avoid injury to the common digital nerve to the middle-ring finger.

The blade is deployed to incise the transverse carpal ligament just proximal to where the surgeon judges the distal margin to be. This allows better visualization of the exact position of the distal margin. The distal margin of the transverse carpal ligament is now incised (Figure 98.4A, B) and the ligament released from distal to proximal. The synovial elevator is reinserted to feel whether the ligament has been completely transected. If fibrous septa are felt within the palmaris brevis muscle, another pass is performed with the blade deployed. When a complete release has been achieved, the two cut edges of the transverse carpal ligament will retract radial and ulnar to the blade-camera assembly and can be visualized by rotating the endoscope slightly (Figure 98.5).

After complete release of the transverse carpal ligament, the light from the endoscope will show through the skin of the palm. The flap of antebrachial fascia is excised, and the antebrachial fascia proximal to the incision is released by a pushing motion of the tenotomy scissors. The incision is closed with 5-0 chromic catgut sutures to the subcutaneous fat and a 4-0 Prolene subcuticular suture to approximate the skin. Steri-Strips are applied, and the incision infiltrated with 0.5% Marcaine for postoperative anesthesia.

TECHNICAL CONSIDERATIONS

When performing an endoscopic carpal tunnel release, it is important to check the apparatus to ensure that the blade deploys properly prior to beginning the surgery. Also, if the view through the endoscope is obscured by exuberant synovium, this should be cleared using the synovial elevator. Fogging of the camera is sometimes a problem. If there is any concern that the ligament cannot be seen clearly, the procedure should be abandoned and an open carpal tunnel release should be performed.

Identifying the topographical landmarks and placing the initial incision in the appropriate location are keys to ensuring the carpal canal is instrumented rather than

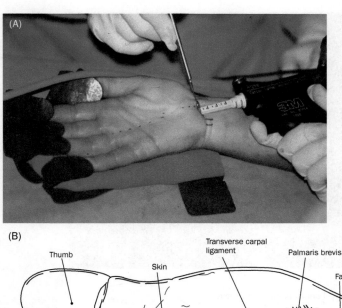

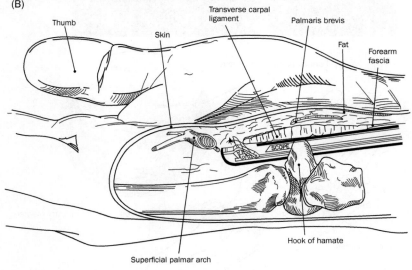

Figure 98.2. (A) The endoscope assembly is introduced into the carpal tunnel with the wrist in about 30 degrees of extension. (B) Cross-sectional depiction of endoscope within carpal tunnel. The endoscope is in close proximity to the superficial palmar arch and the communicating branch of the ulnar nerve.

Guyon's canal. With each successive introduction of an instrument, aim should be directed at the ring finger and should pass radial to the hook of the hamate.

Perfect visualization is required to perform this surgery. The synovial elevator may be used to help clear synovium off the undersurface of the transverse carpal ligament. Extending the wrist and abducting the thumb will place additional tension on the transverse carpal ligament, which may improve the view. The surgeon may also find it helpful to use the opposite thumb to palpate the palm to create counterpressure to the camera-knife assembly.

POSTOPERATIVE MANAGEMENT

Some hand surgeons do not immobilize the wrist after endoscopic carpal tunnel release and simply place the patient's hand and wrist into a soft dressing. We prefer to immobilize the wrist in 20 degrees of extension in a plaster of Paris splint which is removed 7–10 days postoperatively when the subcuticular suture is removed. The incision is then Steri-Stripped, and the patient can begin active range of motion exercises of the wrist after soaks in warm water. The patient can use a padded glove to protect the incision for another 2–3 weeks and massage the incision with hand cream to speed up softening. Hand therapy is usually never necessary. We advise patients not to use their operated hand for repetitive computing for 6 weeks.

OUTCOMES

RESULTS

The theoretical advantage of endoscopic carpal tunnel release is that with a small incision away from the palm

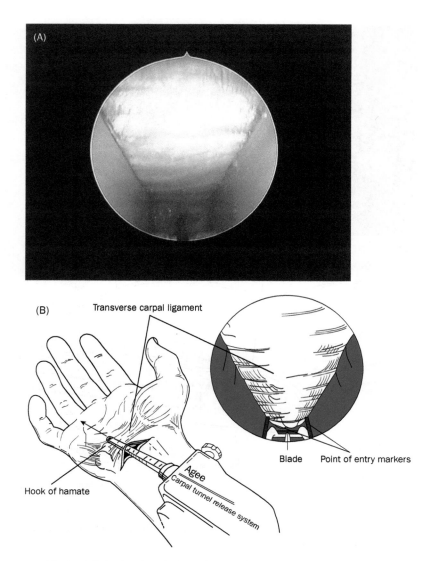

Figure 98.3. (A) Intact transverse carpal ligament. This view through the endoscope should be obtained prior to incising the ligament. If excess synovium is present, it must be cleaned off prior to proceeding. (B) Endoscope within the carpal tunnel directed toward the ring finger. The transition between the fat pad and transverse carpal ligament must be clearly visualized to avoid injury. The point of entry markers help to identify where the blade will deploy.

of the hand, patients will have a shorter recovery and faster return to work. One study performed in Denmark randomized patients to a traditional open, mini-open, or endoscopic carpal tunnel release.[3] Sick leave was shortest (7 days) in patients undergoing the endoscopic procedure compared with 16 days for patients undergoing the mini-incision procedure versus 20 days for conventional open carpal tunnel release. There were no significant differences between the treatment groups with respect to postoperative pain and resolution of paraesthesias. The incidence of "pillar" pain was also similar among the three treatment groups.

A Japanese study compared endoscopic carpal tunnel release in octogenarians with patients aged 60 years or younger. There were no complications in either group nor

were there reoperations. All patients had improvement in nocturnal pain and paresthesias. There was no difference in electrophysiological improvement between the two groups. Octogenarians did not have as good a recovery of Semmes-Weinstein filament testing, but did have better improvement of outcomes scores.[4] In a similar study of patients over the age of 65 undergoing endoscopic carpal tunnel release, all patients had resolution of their preoperative pain by the 6-month follow-up and 94% had resolution of night symptoms.[5]

COMPLICATIONS

A recent meta-analysis summarized the complications of endoscopic carpal tunnel release in randomized controlled

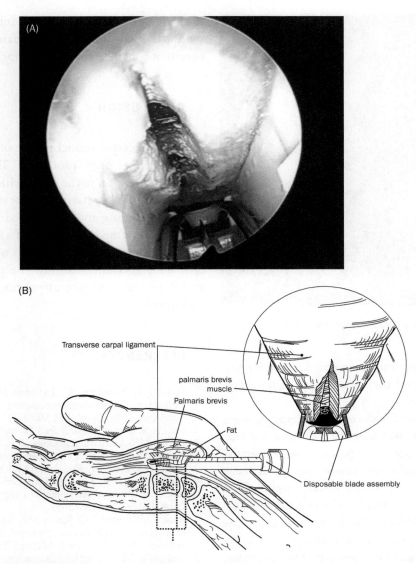

(A)

(B)

Transverse carpal ligament

palmaris brevis muscle

Palmaris brevis

Fat

Disposable blade assembly

Figure 98.4. (A) Partially incised transverse carpal ligament with the proximal portion still intact, in cross-section. (B). When the transverse carpal ligament is incised, the palmaris brevis and palmar fascia becomes visible.

trials. Early studies had reported high complication rates of up to 35%, but, more recently, complication rates have been similar to open carpal tunnel release.[6] Complications include common digital nerve injury (especially the common digital nerve to the middle-ring fingers); transient nerve symptoms consisting of neurapraxia, paresthesias and numbness; complex regional pain syndrome; wound infections; hypertrophic scarring; and tenderness over the incision ("pillar pain").

CAVEATS

Ensure that the instruments are introduced into the carpal tunnel and not Guyon's canal by feeling the "washboard"

undersurface of the transverse carpal tunnel ligament as well as a slight ulnar-to-radial "swerve" as the instrument glides around the hook of the hamate.

The axis of the planned course of the endoscope is marked from the midpoint of the incision in the distal wrist crease toward the base of the ring fingers. This means that the handle of the endoscope is positioned over the radial border of the distal forearm. Surgeons have a tendency to orient their hand and the handle of the endoscope along the long axis of the forearm, which places the tip of the endoscope more radially and could potentially result in injury to the motor branch of the median nerve.

The rectangular opening at the tip of the endoscope should be kept firmly applied to the undersurface of the transverse carpal ligament to avoid a flexor tendon or the

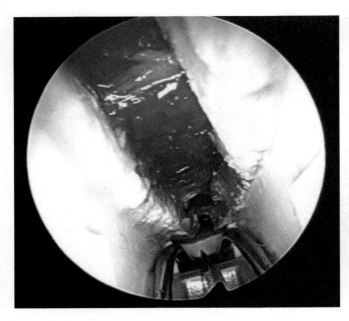

Figure 98.5. Complete release of the transverse carpal ligament.

median nerve insinuating itself between the anterior surface of the endoscope and the undersurface of the transverse carpal tunnel ligament.

If the transverse striations of the transverse carpal ligament are obscured by synovium, withdraw the endoscope and reintroduce the synovial elevator to scrape away any proliferative synovium from the undersurface of the transverse carpal ligament.

Do not immediately incise the distal margin of the transverse carpal ligament; instead, incise 1–2 mm proximal to this for approximately 5 mm. In this way, the transverse carpal ligament tends to gap open so that it is much easier to precisely define the exact distal margin of the transverse carpal ligament, which can then be incised.

If the surgeon has any concern that the transverse carpal ligament cannot be clearly visualized, it is prudent to abandon the endoscopic procedure and perform a conventional open carpal tunnel release. Unfortunately, this necessitates an inverted T-shaped incision.

CONCLUSION

Endoscopic carpal tunnel release offers an alternative to the traditional open procedure. The procedure avoids placing an incision in the palm, which is sometimes associated with scar hypersensitivity or wound complications. By understanding anatomical landmarks, the procedure may be performed safely, but if there is any difficulty in obtaining proper visualization or if there is any concern with aberrant anatomy, the procedure should be abandoned and an open carpal tunnel release should be performed.

REFERENCES

1. Presazzi A, Bortolotto C, Zacchino M, Madonia L, Draghi F. Carpal tunnel: normal anatomy, anatomical variants and ultrasound technique. *J Ultrasound* 2011 Mar;14(1):40–46.
2. Microaire. *Carpal Tunnel Release System Surgeon Training Manual.*
3. Larsen MB, Sørensen AI, Crone KL, Weis T, Boeckstyns ME. Carpal tunnel release: a randomized comparison of three surgical methods. *J Hand Surg Eur Vol* 2013 Jul;38(6):646–650.
4. Hattori Y, Doi K, Koide S, Sakamoto S. Endoscopic release for severe carpal tunnel syndrome in octogenarians. *J Hand Surg Am* 2014 Dec;39(12):2448–2453.
5. Beck JD, Wingert NC, Rutter MR, Irgit KS, Tang X, Klena JC. Clinical outcomes of endoscopic carpal tunnel release in patients 65 and over. *J Hand Surg Am* 2013 Aug;38(8):1524–1529.
6. Vasiliadis HS, Nikolakopoulou A, Shrier I, Lunn MP, Brassington R, Scholten RJ, Salanti G. Endoscopic and open release similarly safe for the treatment of carpal tunnel syndrome. A systematic review and meta-analysis. *PLoS One* 2015 Dec 16;10(12):e0143683.

99.

INFECTIONS

Scott D. Oates

Infections of the hand can lead to significant morbidity, including stiffness, scarring, and amputation. With the advent of antibiotic therapy and the development of specific surgical techniques aimed at different types of infections, the sequelae have been reduced. Nevertheless, significant morbidity still occurs as a result of delayed diagnosis or inadequate surgical treatment applied to these common problems. This chapter illustrates the most common surgical approaches to hand infections that are not amenable or responsive to drug therapy.[1-8]

ASSESSMENT OF THE DEFECT

Most infections brought to the attention of the hand surgeon have already progressed beyond the point where antibiotics alone will cure the problem. The anatomy of the hand lends itself to early confinement of infections into several closed spaces inaccessible to systemic antibiotics. The initial treatment of most hand infections is with empiric antibiotics unless certain cardinal signs are present. Elevation and splinting of the hand may also help avert progression of symptoms and should be initiated early in treatment. If the infection fails to show improvement after 24–36 hours of antibiotic therapy, surgery is indicated. Antibiotic choice is empiric initially, then guided by cultures of the wound or blood. The most common isolated organism is *Staphylococcus aureus,* followed by *Streptococcus* species.

TYPES OF INFECTIONS

FINGERTIP INFECTIONS

Paronychia

Paronychia is the term applied to infections around the nail. Classic paronychia involves an infection along the paronychial fold on one side of the nail; pain, erythema, and swelling are present immediately adjacent to the nail. This infection can extend to the eponychial area or, sometimes, all the way around the nail base, producing the so-called *run-around abscess*. Hangnails, biting of nails, or nail manipulation during manicures commonly cause these infections. The organism responsible is usually *S. aureus*. Early treatment with oral antibiotics and hot finger soaks with warm salt solutions can resolve the infection if instituted early, but surgical decompression is often necessary.

CHRONIC PARONYCHIA

Chronic paronychia occurs as the result of a recurrent fungal infection, usually *Candida albicans,* of the proximal nail fold. Recurrent infection and obstruction of the nail fold is the precipitating factor. Middle-aged women, especially those who often have their hands immersed, and diabetic patients are more commonly affected. Eliminating exposure to moist environments and use of antifungal agents and topical corticosteroids may be effective.

FELON

Felon is a subcutaneous abscess of the distal pulp of the finger. It is contained by the multiple trabeculae present in the pulp, producing a characteristic tension, swelling, and throbbing pain. A history of recent penetrating trauma can sometimes be elicited but is not always recalled. If untreated, local tissue necrosis, sinus tract formation, osteomyelitis of the distal phalanx, or, rarely, tenosynovitis may result. The most common organism is *S. aureus*. As with paronychia, early cellulitis of the pulp may be treated with antibiotics and soaks, but, once formed, a true felon requires surgical drainage.

HERPETIC WHITLOW

Herpetic whitlow is a viral infection of the fingertip caused by herpes simplex virus. It is often seen in medical or dental healthcare workers. It is characterized by pain, erythema, and small, coalescing vesicles, making differentiation from paronychia or felon sometimes difficult. The vesicles are usually filled with clear, nonpurulent fluid. Once recognized, expectant treatment results in resolution of symptoms in 3–4 weeks. One should always consider whitlow in the differential diagnosis of finger infections because operative intervention is contraindicated and can lead to bacterial superinfection, producing potential additional morbidity to the finger.

PALMAR DEEP SPACE INFECTIONS

Web Space Abscess ("Collar Button")

A "collar button" infection involves the distal palm and web space. It begins as a superficial infection in the palmar skin near the web space. In the palm, the skin is tightly adherent to the palmar fascia. This makes lateral extension of subcutaneous abscesses more difficult. As a result, the abscess develops an hourglass configuration by extending dorsally through a defect in the palmar fascia near the transverse metacarpal ligament. Pain and swelling of this region, as well as abduction of the adjacent fingers, aids in diagnosis. The swelling may be more prominent on the dorsal aspect, but the volar component cannot be overlooked.

MIDPALMAR AND THENAR INFECTIONS

Anatomy. Two potential spaces exist for abscess formation in the palm. The first is the midpalmar space. It is deep to the flexor tendons of the middle, ring, and small fingers and bounded dorsally by the interossei and metacarpals. Radially, it is bounded by the midpalmar or oblique septum. This septum originates from the volar aspect of the third metacarpal and extends to the palmar fascia. Ulnarly, the midpalmar space is defined by the fascia of the hypothenar muscles.

The thenar space is radial to the oblique septum and volar to the adductor pollicis muscle. It is deep to the flexors of the index finger and extends to the lateral edge of the adductor pollicis. An additional space, the hypothenar space, is described, but isolated infection here is extremely rare (Figure 99.1).

Midpalmar space infections. Midpalmar space infections most often result from penetrating trauma to the palm.

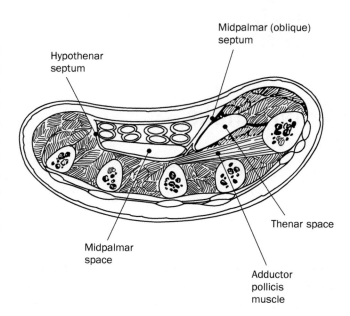

Figure 99.1. Potential midpalmar spaces.

They can also occur from a ruptured flexor tenosynovitis of the middle or ring fingers. Tenosynovitis of the small finger tracks proximally through the ulnar bursa. Pain and swelling develop volarly over the space, and there is swelling dorsally, as well as a loss of the normal concavity of the palm, a key sign to this infection.

Thenar space infections. Thenar space infections most commonly result from penetrating trauma or ruptured tenosynovitis of the thumb or index finger. Patients present with pain and swelling of the first web space. The thumb is characteristically abducted and painful to move.

FLEXOR TENOSYNOVITIS

Purulent flexor sheath infection is one of the most feared hand infections because of the potential for the development of adhesions and tendon necrosis. Usually these infections result from penetrating injuries and affect the ring, middle, and index fingers. The most common organism is *S. aureus*. Kanavel described the four classic findings of pyogenic flexor tenosynovitis: (1) flexed position of the finger, (2) symmetric enlargement of the finger, (3) tenderness over the tendon sheath, and (4) severe pain on passive extension of the finger. Patients whose disease is recognized early (within 24–48 hours) may be treated with parenteral antibiotics, splinting, elevation, and close observation. If symptoms are not resolved within 24 hours, operative intervention is indicated.

INDICATIONS

All procedures should be carried out in the operating room, with the exception of uncomplicated fingertip infections, which may be amenable to drainage under local anesthesia in the office setting. The surgical principles described here, which are generally applicable to hand surgery, are also important when draining hand abscesses. Incisions should be placed to avoid injury to underlying nerves, arteries, and tendons. Flexion creases should be crossed at angles of 45 degrees or less to prevent flexion contractures. Incisions should parallel flexion creases in the palm wherever possible. Straight incisions should be used only at the midlateral or midaxial positions of the fingers or over the dorsum of the hand. Incisions should be placed along the ulnar side of the index, middle, and ring fingers or the radial side of the thumb and small finger, when possible. Tourniquets are recommended, but forced exsanguination is contraindicated. Simple elevation should serve to exsanguinate the hand adequately in the presence of infection. Sufficient fluid for culture and Gram's stains should be obtained.

CONTRAINDICATIONS

Concurrent life-threatening conditions unrelated to the infection are a contraindication to surgery. Even then, simple drainage may be attempted at the bedside with more definitive treatment later. Systemic sepsis, although rare, should not preclude surgical treatment of these infections if they appear to be the causative factor.

ROOM SETUP

General anesthesia is preferred, although axillary or wrist blocks may be appropriate in some patients with more limited infections. Bier block anesthesia is contraindicated because of the need for forced exsanguination of the extremity. An upper arm tourniquet is used to obtain a bloodless field. A hand instrument set and hand table are used. The bed is turned 90 degrees, with the hand table in the middle of the room to allow the surgeon and an assistant to sit on opposite sides. Loupe magnification (2.5×) is recommended for dissection of vital structures. Pulsed irrigation devices are used to cleanse the involved areas after initial drainage and taking of cultures. Both normal saline and antibiotic irrigation are used for deep infections.

OPERATIVE TECHNIQUE

PARONYCHIA

The most common approach involves removal of the proximal one-fourth to one-third of the nail on the infected side. This can be done under digital block anesthesia using a Freer elevator or other flat-edged instrument to elevate the eponychial fold from the nail. The abscess cavity is entered bluntly, lateral to the proximal edge of the nail, and the nail is carefully separated from the bed using the Freer or a small clamp. The proximal part of the nail is then removed using sharp scissors and the cavity irrigated.

If an incision is required, it is made along the paronychial fold, directed away from the nailbed and germinal matrix. Additional incisions may be necessary for more extensive (i.e., run-around) abscesses (Figure 99.2). The minimal number of incisions should be used to allow access to the nail proximally and to adequately drain the abscess.

CHRONIC PARONYCHIA

If surgical treatment is required, marsupialization of the eponychial fold, as described by Keyser and Eaton, may be effective. Under digital block with tourniquet control, a crescent-shaped wedge of skin and subcutaneous tissue just proximal to the eponychial fold is removed down to, but not including, the germinal matrix (Figure 99.3). A sterile dressing is placed over the wound and changed in 48–72 hours. The matrix is thus completely exteriorized and the wound is allowed to close secondarily with dressing changes. Nail improvement after healing is slow, and residual nail deformity may still occur.

FELON

A number of different approaches for draining felons have been described. The most commonly used are the unilateral longitudinal and volar longitudinal incisions: these are described in detail. Digital block anesthesia may be used, and the procedure can be performed at the bedside, in the office, or in the emergency department.

The unilateral longitudinal incision is made along the ulnar side of the index, middle, or ring fingers or the radial side of the thumb or small finger. It begins 5 mm distal to the distal interphalangeal (DIP) joint crease and continues to just beyond the lateral end of the nail without extending onto the pulp. It should be kept high at the midaxial line of the distal phalanx, maintaining the volar pulp tissue as a unit. The dissection is carried down to the bone and the abscess

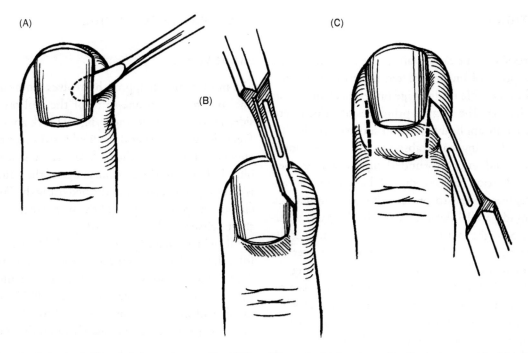

Figure 99.2. Incisions for drainage of different degrees of paronychia. (A) Use of Freer elevator to enter cavity of typical paronychia. (B) Incision used for more extensive infection. (C) Incisions used for "run around" abscess.

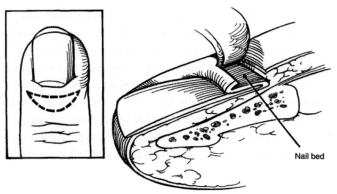

Figure 99.3. Eponychial marsupialization for chronic paronychia.

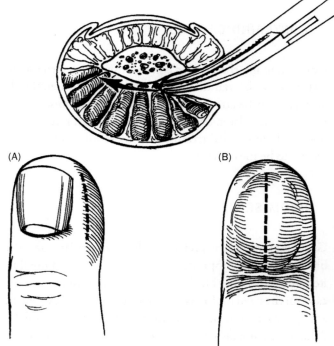

Figure 99.4. Recommended incisions for drainage of felon. (A) Unilateral longitudinal incision. (B) Volar longitudinal incision.

is entered just volar to the distal phalanx. Spreading with a clamp breaks up the fibrous septae for complete drainage.

The volar longitudinal incision is made over the point of maximal tenderness on the volar pad and extended proximally to the DIP joint crease, but not across it. Again, the fibrous septae are broken up using a clamp. Proximal probing should be minimized to avoid extension into the flexor sheath. Sinus tracts, if present, are excised with a small ellipse of skin (Figure 99.4).

Other incisions include the fish-mouth, which encompasses the entire end of the fingertip. This approach is universally condemned because of the risk of slough of the pulp, late instability of the pulp, and tender scar. Some authors recommend the J, or hockeystick, incision, but the

extension of the incision over the distal fingertip is not necessary to achieve adequate drainage of most felons and may result in a painful scar. The volar transverse incision is useful in removing sinus tracts and can achieve adequate drainage

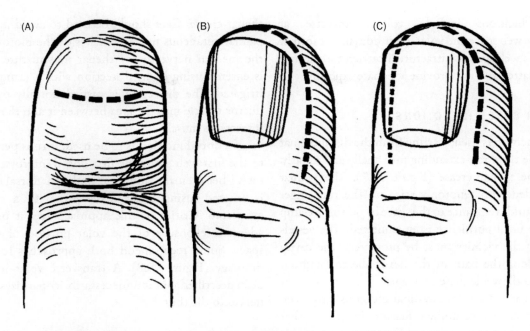

Figure 99.5. Incisions to be avoided for felon drainage. (A) Volar transverse incision. (B) Hockey stick incision. (C) Fish-mouth incision.

of the abscess but creates increased risk to the digital nerves (Figure 99.5).

WEB SPACE ABSCESS

Typically, this infection requires both dorsal and volar incisions for adequate drainage. Both curved and zigzag incisions have been described for the volar side. They extend from just proximal to the web to just distal to the midpalmar crease. The subcutaneous tissues are divided bluntly using a clamp until purulence is found. The cavity is then enlarged by dividing the adjacent palmar fascia with scissors. Dorsally, a straight longitudinal incision is made about 1.5 cm in length between the metacarpal heads (Figure 99.6). Broad communication between the two sides is developed bluntly.

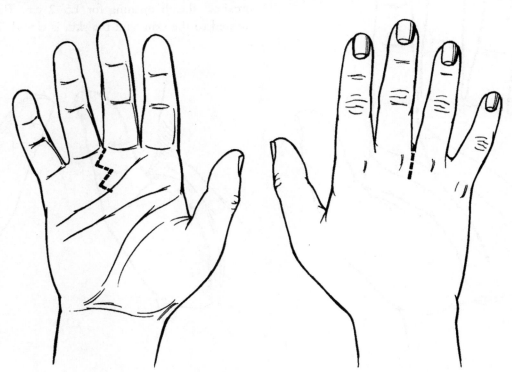

Figure 99.6. Volar and dorsal incisions for drainage of web space abscess.

Alternative incisions include volar transverse at the edge of the web space and volar longitudinal. The former may result in a web space contracture if carried too far into the web; the latter may not provide adequate exposure.

MIDPALMAR SPACE INFECTIONS

An oblique incision is used, starting from the distal palmar crease over the third ray, extending proximally and ulnarly, paralleling the thenar crease (Figure 99.7). The palmar fascia is divided with tenotomy scissors. The ring-finger flexor sheath guides entrance to the space by passing a clamp to either side until purulence is encountered. The vessels and nerves in the vicinity must be protected. The cavity is enlarged along the path of the flexor sheath (without violating it) to allow adequate drainage.

Transverse and distal longitudinal incisions have been described, as well as a combined incision, but they either limit exposure or are more extensive than necessary.

THENAR SPACE INFECTIONS

Both dorsal and volar approaches have been described. The volar incision should be made close to and parallel to the thenar crease. Care should be used to avoid injury to the palmar cutaneous nerve branches or the motor branch of the median nerve to the thenar musculature. The space is entered using blunt dissection with a clamp and then irrigated. The dissection is carried dorsally over the adductor muscle into the area between it and the first dorsal interosseus muscle.

If a dorsal incision is to be used, it runs perpendicular to the first web along the first dorsal interosseus. The interval between the adductor and first dorsal interosseus is entered, using blunt dissection with a clamp, and evacuated. Critics of this approach feel it provides inadequate exposure of the volar portion of the thenar space. Some recommend both approaches for adequate drainage (Figure 99.8). A transverse volar incision has been described, but it unnecessarily jeopardizes the digital nerves to the thumb.

FLEXOR TENOSYNOVITIS

Most authors recommend closed tendon sheath irrigation to treat this condition. An incision is made in the distal palm over the proximal end of the sheath. The sheath is opened proximal to the Al pulley. An additional incision is made on the midaxial line of the finger across the DIP joint crease. The sheath is accessed dorsal to the neurovascular bundles and excised distal to the A4 pulley. A large bore intravenous catheter (14- or 16-gauge) is inserted in the proximal sheath opening for 1.5–2 cm. The catheter is sutured to the skin, and the skin is closed. The sheath is

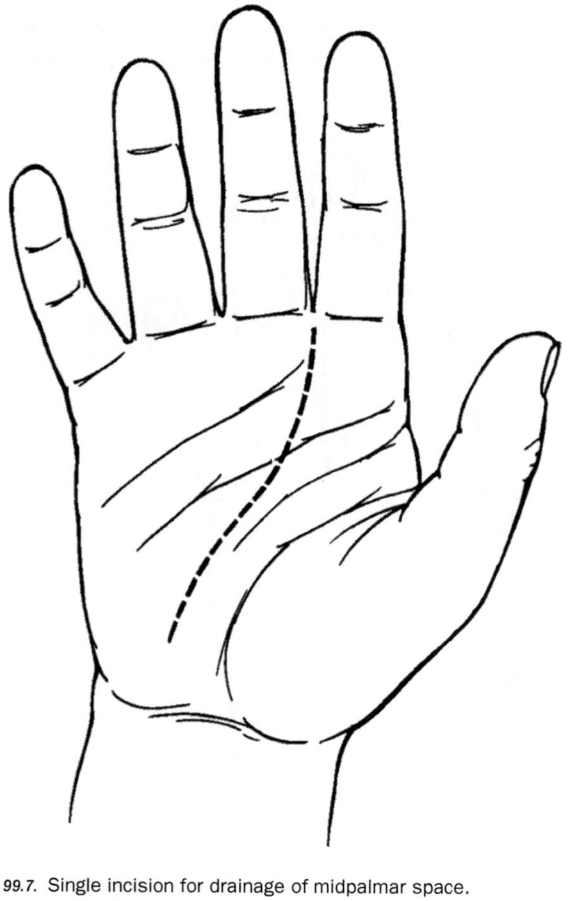

Figure 99.7. Single incision for drainage of midpalmar space.

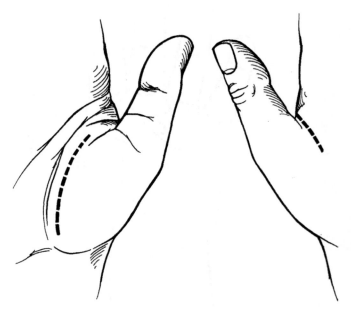

Figure 99.8. Volar and dorsal approaches for drainage of thenar space abscess.

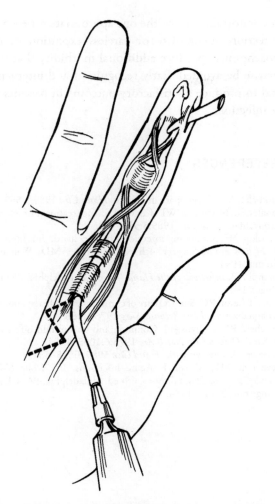

Figure 99.9. Closed tendon sheath irrigation for flexor tenosynovitis.

then copiously irrigated with antibiotic solution or saline. A small wick is placed in the distal wound, and the skin is closed loosely around it (Figure 99.9). The system is flushed again to check for patency and adequacy of drainage before leaving the operating room.

POSTOPERATIVE CARE

Aftercare for most infections involves open packing of wounds or closed irrigation systems for 24–48 hours. Once the signs of infection begin to abate, the irrigation catheters or wicks are removed. Warm soaks with one-quarter-strength Dakin's solution or saline can then commence for 20 minutes every 4 hours to dissolve fibrin and crusts. Dressing changes, using normal saline or one-fourth to half-strength Dakin's solution are used two to three times a day until wounds close secondarily. Hydrotherapy may be beneficial for several days early in the postoperative period.

PARONYCHIA

The cavity is packed for 48–72 hours with a .25-inch gauze wick. The packing is removed and warm soaks are begun. Stenting of the germinal nail fold is necessary, if the entire proximal nail is removed.

FELON

Regardless of the approach used, once adequate drainage is achieved, the cavity is packed for 48–72 hours with a gauze wick. After wick removal, soaks are begun, and the wound is allowed to close secondarily. Alternative postoperative techniques include the use of zinc oxide to prevent premature closure of the wound or continuous irrigation of the cavity using catheters in the hospitalized patient.

WEB SPACE ABSCESS

The space is packed with gauze from both sides, which is removed in 48–72 hours. Dressing changes or hydrotherapy can then commence. An alternative postoperative regimen includes irrigation with a catheter placed volarly into the wound and sewn in place on the palm. Dorsal drainage is aided by use of a Penrose drain. The catheter is irrigated with normal saline intermittently or with a continuous drip at 20–30 mL/hr for 48 hours. After removal of drains and wicks, motion is encouraged as soon as tolerated.

MIDPALMAR SPACE INFECTIONS

The space is packed or drained with a Penrose drain for 48 hours, and then dressings or hydrotherapy are begun. Alternatively, a closed irrigation system may be used postoperatively. This allows for loose primary closure of the wound and more rapid healing.

THENAR SPACE INFECTIONS

After irrigation, wicks or Penrose drains are placed into one or both incisions and left for 48 hours. Dressing changes, hydrotherapy, or a combination of both is initiated. Closed irrigation of the space may be used postoperatively with loose approximation of the wounds to allow primary healing.

FLEXOR TENOSYNOVITIS

The hand is splinted and elevated. The catheter is hooked to an intravenous pump and irrigated at 20–30 mL/hr with antibiotic or saline solution. After 48 hours, the dressing is taken down and the finger is evaluated; if signs of infection have resolved, the catheters are removed. Dressing changes or hydrotherapy can commence immediately. The wounds are allowed to close secondarily.

REHABILITATION

Most patients have rapid resolution of pain and swelling after adequate drainage of the abscess and commencement of antibiotic therapy. Motion is encouraged as soon as drains and wicks are removed, and it is tolerated by the patient. Frequent early follow-up is necessary to ensure adequate return of motion. Prolonged or chronic infections may produce enough stiffness to require formal occupational therapy referral.

CAVEATS

There are several surgical approaches for nearly all the infections described herein that can be used to achieve a successful outcome. Each surgeon should choose the most comfortable one or the one appropriate for each type of infection. Incomplete or careless execution of these approaches may produce additional morbidity that might otherwise be avoided. Early recognition and intervention is vital to produce a satisfactory outcome in patients with these infections.

REFERENCES

1. Burkhalter WE. Deep space infections. *Hand Clin* 1989;5:553–559.
2. Canales FL. Newmeyer WL, Kilgore ES. The treatment of felons and paronychias. *Hand Clin* 1989;5:515–523.
3. Crandon JH. Common infections of the hand. In: Jupiter JB, ed. *Flynn's Hand Surgery*. 4th ed. Baltimore, MD: Williams & Wilkins, 1991.
4. Kanavel AB. *Infections of the Hand*. 7th ed. Philadelphia, PA: Lea & Febiger, 1943.
5. Keyser J, Eaton RG. Surgical cure of chronic paronychia by eponychial marsupialization. *Plast Reconstr Surg* 1976;58:66.
6. Linscheid RL. Dobyns JH. Common and uncommon infections of the hand. *Orthop Clin North Am* 1975;6:1063–1104.
7. Neviaser RJ. Tenosynovitis. *Hand Clin* 1989;5:525–531.
8. Stevanovic MV, Sharpe F. Acute infections. In: Wolfe SW, ed. *Green's Operative Hand Surgery*. 6th ed. Philadelphia, PA: Churchill Livingstone, 2011; 41–84.

100.

COMPRESSION NEUROPATHIES OF THE UPPER EXTREMITY

CARPAL TUNNEL SYNDROME, CUBITAL TUNNEL SYNDROME,
AND RADIAL TUNNEL SYNDROME

Wendy Kar Yee Ng

INTRODUCTION

Compression neuropathies of the upper extremity are common, and these conditions can be symptomatically debilitating for patients. The single most common site of nerve compression of each of the three major peripheral nerves of the upper extremity is described here, noting that nerve compression can still occur at various sites from the neck proximally to the hand distally for all of the described nerves herein (Figure 100.1).

For all upper extremity compression neuropathies, the patient's age, handedness, and occupation are recorded as in any encounter for a clinical hand problem. Knowledge of prior trauma, including previous fractures, lacerations, and upper extremity surgery provides the clinician with clues as to causal factors in the patient's symptomatology. As with any medical visit, the patient's concomitant medical conditions should be noted because many systemic medical problems can contribute to symptoms of compression neuropathy. The use of blood thinners is a relative contraindication to surgery, and patients should be evaluated for bridging of anticoagulants if possible for surgical release. In addition, nonsurgical treatments such as steroid injection may cause hyperglycemia; thus, patients with diabetes mellitus should be counselled regarding this risk. Sensation, range of motion, strength, and comparisons to the contralateral extremity are documented. Electrophysiologic studies are used as an adjunct when the patient's symptoms and signs are not entirely classic.

CARPAL TUNNEL SYNDROME

Carpal tunnel syndrome is the most common upper extremity neuropathy caused by to compression of the median nerve at the wrist. Its prevalence in the general population is 0.3%, usually occurring in patients 30–50 years of age. Patients will often complain of numbness and tingling in the thumb, index, long fingers, and the radial side of the ring finger; of pain that wakes them at night; and, finally, difficulty with fine motor tasks such as turning keys or opening doors and jars.[1]

Potential causes of carpal tunnel syndrome include

- Idiopathic causes
- Repeated stress, increased pressure within carpal tunnel
- Work-related, with positioning/vibration
- Trauma
- Mass/lesions
- Tenosynovitis
- Hypothyroidism
- Rheumatoid arthritis
- Diabetes
- Pregnancy
- Renal failure; dialysis-associated amyloid deposits
- Systemic inflammatory disorders

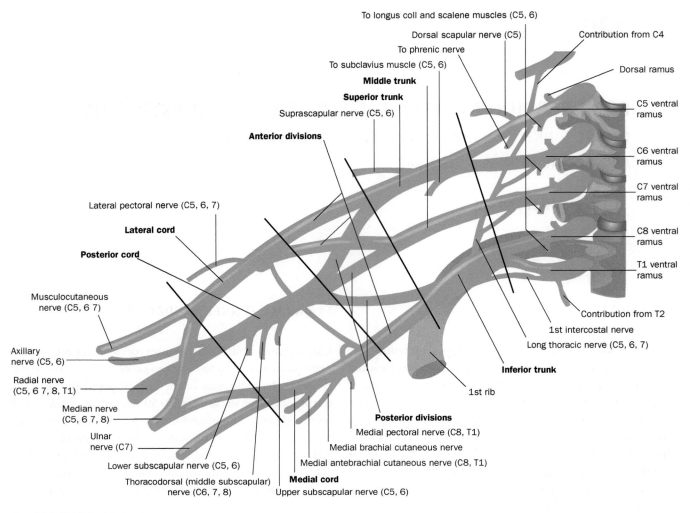

Figure 100.1. The brachial plexus.

To longus coll and scalene muscles (C5, 6)

Dorsal scapular nerve (C5)

To phrenic nerve

To subclavius muscle (C5, 6)

Middle trunk

Superior trunk

Suprascapular nerve (C5, 6)

Anterior divisions

Lateral pectoral nerve (C5, 6, 7)

Lateral cord

Posterior cord

Musculocutaneous nerve (C5, 6 7)

Axillary nerve (C5, 6)

Radial nerve (C5, 6 7, 8, T1)

Median nerve (C5, 6 7, 8)

Ulnar nerve (C7)

Lower subscapular nerve (C5, 6)

Thoracodorsal (middle subscapular) nerve (C6, 7, 8)

Medial cord

Upper subscapular nerve (C5, 6)

Posterior divisions

Medial pectoral nerve (C8, T1)

Medial brachial cutaneous nerve

Medial antebrachial cutaneous nerve (C8, T1)

Inferior trunk

1st rib

Long thoracic nerve (C5, 6, 7)

1st intercostal nerve

Contribution from T2

T1 ventral ramus

C8 ventral ramus

C7 ventral ramus

C6 ventral ramus

C5 ventral ramus

Dorsal ramus

Contribution from C4

- Sarcoid/amyloidosis

- Acromegaly

RELEVANT ANATOMY

The median nerve arises from the medial and lateral cords of the brachial plexus, derived from C6–C8 and T1 nerve roots. It runs through the carpal tunnel alongside the flexor tendons of the fingers and thumb. The flexor retinaculum comprises the roof of the carpal tunnel, reaching from the hamate and triquetrum to the scaphoid and the trapezium. Distally, the recurrent motor branch of the median nerve branches to innervate the abductor pollicis brevis muscle, the superficial head of the flexor pollicis brevis muscle, and the opponens pollicis muscle before giving off sensory branches to the radial-sided fingers of the hand and thumb (Figure 100.2).[2]

Kaplan's line refers to a line projected from the first web space of the thumb in extension to the pisiform bone in the

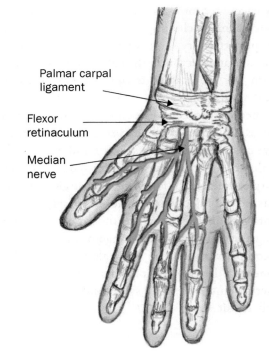

Palmar carpal ligament

Flexor retinaculum

Median nerve

Figure 100.2. Anatomy of the median nerve.

proximal palm. This is the usual distal extent of an incision for open operative carpal tunnel release. A line drawn from the radial border of the long finger intersects with Kaplan's line at the usual location that the recurrent motor branch of the median nerve innervates the thenar muscles.

PHYSICAL EXAMINATION

Provocative signs include direct pressure over the median nerve (Durkan's sign) or indirectly increasing pressure over the carpal tunnel (Phalen's sign). Most sources recommend holding such pressure for up to a minute to allow adequate time for symptoms to be elicited. A positive Tinel's sign over the carpal tunnel, decreased sensation to pinwheel or light touch over the median nerve distribution, decreased sensation to vibration with a tuning fork, and wasting of the thenar eminence may be found (Figure 100.3). The abductor pollicis brevis is tested by asking the patient to lay his or her hands flat on a table with the palms up, and then to point the thumbs toward the sky; the clinician then documents the strength of the muscle against resistance.

Vibration is a threshold test that evaluates fast-adapting sensory fibres. In comparison, measurement of two point discrimination is an innervations density test, often normal in carpal tunnel syndrome and decreased in nerve injuries; it is a test only described for glabrous skin. Whereas static two-point discrimination evaluates slowly adapting fibers, moving two-point discrimination evaluates fast-adapting fibres. Two-point discrimination correlates to axonal density, so abnormalities may not show up until later, when there is actual axonal loss. Since two-point discrimination is altered usually only with severe nerve compression, determining this for the patient preoperatively can be helpful in counseling patients and families regarding prognosis for expected recovery, although specific predictions may be challenging without preoperative nerve conduction studies.[3]

INDICATIONS

Patients should routinely be asked about concomitant back and neck pain, as symptoms of extremity neuropathies can also occur with disc herniation or spinal stenosis. Initial conservative management recommended to patients is splinting of the wrist in a neutral position at night. Care should be taken to rule out other sites of median nerve compression, such as pronator syndrome. Inflammatory tendinopathies often co-exist with carpal tunnel syndrome; patients should routinely be asked about symptoms of trigger finger as well. Nonsurgical management for carpal tunnel injection includes neutral wrist splinting and oral

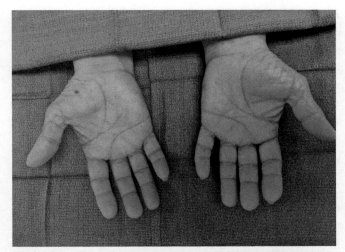
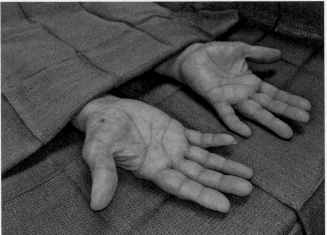
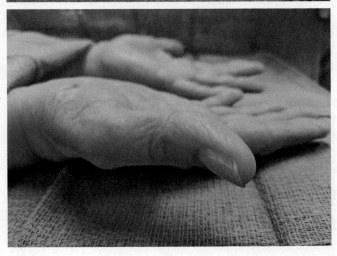

Figure 100.3. Wasting of the thenar eminence of the right hand compared to the left hand.

anti-inflammatory medications. Patients may also opt for steroid injection.

The presence of fibrillations and sharp waves on needle electromyography indicates denervation of sampled muscles. These patients should be offered surgery because conservative management will neither reverse nor halt the progression of permanent nerve damage. However, electrodiagnostic studies can be normal in early nerve compression because latency and conduction velocity only reflect the healthiest remaining myelinated nerve fibers. A nerve conduction study is not necessary in patients with classic symptoms and signs of carpal tunnel syndrome.[4]

TECHNIQUE OF STEROID INJECTION

Steroid injection can include 1% lidocaine with/without epinephrine and triamcinolone acetonide (Kenalog10). A 2 mL mixture of 1 mL of lidocaine and 1 mL of Kenalog is placed in a 5 mL syringe with a 25- or 27-gauge needle. In the clinic setting, the patient is asked to lay his or her hand flat on a table. To identify the palmaris longus for landmarking, the patient is asked to actively touch the thumb to the small finger tip and then to relax the hand flat again. Ethyl chloride is sprayed on the skin to minimize the pain of a needle poke after the area just radial to the palmaris longus and a few millimeters distal to the wrist crease is cleansed with an alcohol swab. The needle is inserted, aiming obliquely toward the third web space of the hand, through skin and the transverse carpal ligament. The patient is asked if any electric shocks are felt; if so, the needle must be readjusted so that the injection is not infiltrated directly into the nerve itself. After injection and removal of the needle, the patient is asked to actively open and close the hand several times to allow the injection to bathe the median nerve. Patients must be reminded that they may or may not see improvement of symptoms for up to 2 weeks after injection, because the effect is not immediate (Figures 100.4, 100.5, and 100.6).

ROOM SETUP

The procedure may be done in a clinic office with appropriate lighting or in a minor procedure room in an ambulatory setting, which is both more economical and more efficient than when performed in a main operating room.[5] The patient may lie supine on a stretcher or on an operating room table. A table with adjustable height to match the level of the bed, such as a tray table, can be rolled up beside the stretcher, and the patient extends the operative extremity onto the tray table over padding for the duration of the procedure. Alternatively, for an operating room table, a simple arm board abducted to 90 degrees is adequate for the operative extremity.

PREOPERATIVE PREPARATION

For operative treatment, the incision line of approximately 3–4 cm is marked preoperatively between the thenar and hypothenar eminences, in line with the third digital webspace, stopping the proximal extent of the incision at 1 cm distal to the wrist crease to minimize the risk of postoperative pillar pain.

An appropriately sized nonsterile tourniquet is placed on the upper forearm over soft padding, and the extremity is exsanguinated with an Esmarch bandage prior to tourniquet insufflation. While many surgeons do not operate on bilateral extremities for carpal tunnel release simultaneously due to concern for patients' abilities to perform self-care following surgery, this concern has not proved valid in the literature to date.[6]

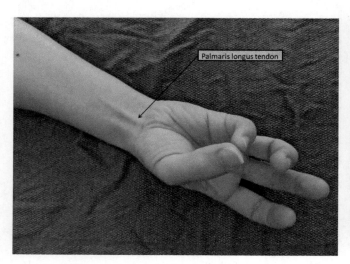

Figure 100.4. Landmarking for carpal tunnel injection. To identify the palmaris longus for landmarking, the patient is asked to actively touch the thumb to the small finger tip and then to relax the hand flat again.

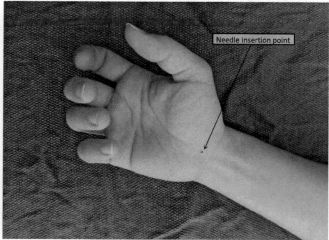

Figure 100.5. Needle insertion point for injection into the carpal tunnel. Ethyl chloride is sprayed to the skin to minimize the pain of a needle poke, after the area just radial to the palmaris longus and a few millimeters distal to the wrist crease is cleansed with an alcohol swab.

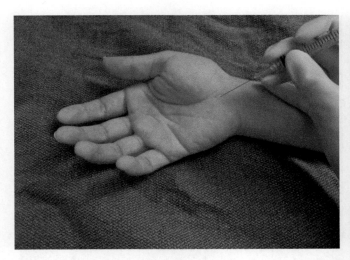

Figure 100.6. Trajectory of needle insertion into the carpal tunnel. The needle is inserted, aiming obliquely towards the 3rd web space of the hand, through skin and the transverse carpal ligament.

SURGICAL PROCEDURE

The procedure can be done under wide-awake local anesthesia only. The patient lies supine on an operating room bed with the arm abducted onto an arm board, with the hand fully supinated. After cleaning the site with an alcohol swab, 1% lidocaine with epinephrine buffered with sodium bicarbonate 8.4% is infiltrated subcutaneously to bathe the median nerve at the wrist, as well as along the proposed incision line. Time is given for the local anesthetic to take effect while sterile preparation of the upper extremity is performed (Figure 100.7).

Povidone is used for sterile preparation, and field sterility is achieved with towels. A no. 15 blade scalpel is used to incise the skin. Small tenotomy scissors are used to spread the subcutaneous tissue until the palmar fascia is visualized. This is divided with the no. 15 blade scalpel under tension, which can be achieved with a small self-retainer, such as an Alm retractor. The transverse carpal ligament is divided with a pushing motion with the no. 15 blade scalpel to avoid harm to the median nerve while the surgeon remains cognizant of potential anatomic variations of branching of the recurrent motor branch of the median nerve (Figure 100.8). Blunt-ended tenotomy scissors, or Metzenbaum scissors, are used to free the nerve from the surrounding tissue up to the level of the distal palmar fat pad; proximally, the scissors are slid under direct visualization, using a small Ragnell retractor to lift proximal skin and to divide the distal forearm antebrachial fascia by a few centimeters. If this is difficult or if resistance is encountered, the skin incision may be extended proximally, taking care to use a zig-zag incision to avoid wrist crease scar contracture, for better

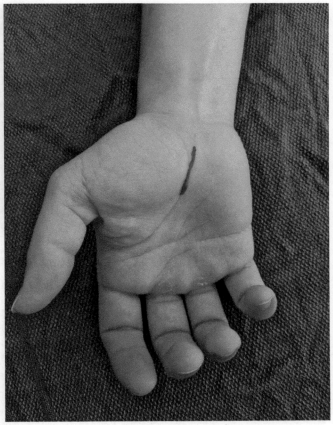

Figure 100.7. Carpal tunnel release marking. The incision line of approximately 3 to 4 cm is marked between the thenar and hypothenar eminences, in line with the 3rd digital webspace, stopping the proximal extent of the incision at 1 cm distal to the wrist crease.

visualization. A formal neurolysis is not required in primary carpal tunnel release. The tourniquet is let down and hemostasis is achieved with monopolar cautery to the skin edges if needed, but not near the median nerve itself. Skin closure is completed with simple interrupted 4-0 nylon sutures. A soft dressing such as gauze wrap (Kling) over a nonstick Xeroform or other nonadherent dressing is adequate.

The option of endoscopic carpal tunnel release is described in another chapter.

POSTOPERATIVE CARE

The patient is instructed to mobilize all fingers and the thumb immediately to allow for tendon and nerve gliding, as well as to keep the hand elevated on a few pillows when sleeping at night to decrease postoperative swelling. If a sling is offered to the patient, the patient should be reminded to take the hand out of the sling multiple times a day to ensure that the shoulder and elbow do not get stiff. Restoration of range of movement is emphasized. The patient is allowed to

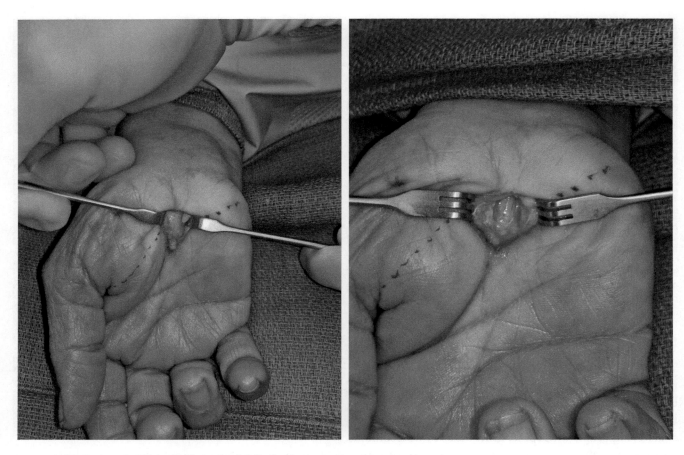

Figure 100.8. Appearance of median nerve immediately following decompression of the carpal tunnel.

remove the dressing, wash and dry the hand, and cover the incision with a new dry dressing after 2 days.

The sutures are removed 10–14 days postoperatively, and the patient may elect to wear a resting splint in a neutral position for up to 1 month postoperatively for comfort. Over the subsequent weeks following surgery, activity is gradually increased as tolerated, and patients return to full normal activities by 3 months postoperatively.

CUBITAL TUNNEL SYNDROME

Cubital tunnel syndrome refers to compression of the ulnar nerve at the elbow. Elbow flexion reduces the area of the cubital tunnel, but causes of cubital tunnel syndrome can also include the presence of anomalous muscles or nerve subluxation or sequelae after elbow trauma. It is the second most common compression neuropathy after carpal tunnel syndrome. Patients report numbness in the small finger and the ulnar half of the ring finger and hand weakness. Late symptoms include intrinsic muscle wasting and even clawing.[7,8]

RELEVANT ANATOMY

The ulnar nerve branches from the medial cord of the brachial plexus, coming from the C8 and T1 roots. It is thought that the ulnar nerve becomes susceptible to compression due to its superficial position at the elbow, while elbow flexion confers repeated tension and traction on the nerve itself (Figure 100.9).

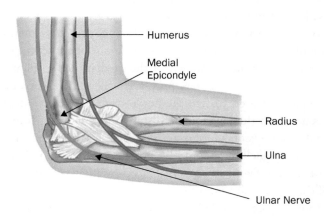

Figure 100.9. Anatomy of the ulnar nerve at the elbow.

Classic sites of compression of the ulnar nerve in the elbow include

- Arcade of Struthers (a band of deep brachial fascia that attaches to the intermuscular septum and covers the ulnar nerve approximately 8 cm proximal to the medial epicondyle)
- Medial head of triceps
- Medial intermuscular septum
- Medial epicondyle
- Cubital tunnel/Osborne's ligament (roof of the cubital tunnel)
- Anconeus epitrochlearis
- Arcuate ligament (of Osborne; in the forearm, tendinous leading edge of flexor carpi ulnaris)
- Deep flexor-pronator aponeurosis

PHYSICAL EXAMINATION

The clinician should assess for subluxation of the ulnar nerve, presence of a Tinel's sign, and perform a flexion compression test at the elbow. In the hand, ulnar intrinsic weakness and atrophy, as well as changes in two-point discrimination, should be noted (Figure 100.10).

INDICATIONS

As with other upper extremity compression neuropathies, patients are routinely asked about concomitant back and

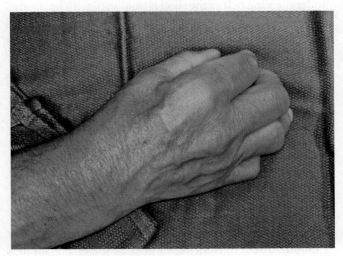

Figure 100.10. Wasting of the intrinsic muscles of the hand, including significant wasting of the first dorsal interosseous muscle.

neck pain suggestive of disc herniation or spinal stenosis. Motor neuron diseases or amyotrophic lateral sclerosis should be ruled out if motor findings are more severe than sensory findings. Nerve conduction studies are useful as electrodiagnostic investigations can reveal reduced conduction velocity. A reduction in speeds of 30% compared to normal conduction velocity values suggests that operative intervention is warranted for cubital tunnel syndrome. However, electrodiagnostic studies are not mandatory when provocative clinical testing alone clearly confirms the diagnosis.[9]

Nonsurgical management includes avoidance of overhead weight-lifting (triceps stress), avoidance of pressure to the ulnar nerve (avoid leaning on the elbow), and aiming to keep the elbows in extension or at least 45 degrees of extension. A nocturnal splint consisting of a pillow taped around the elbow prevents patients from flexing their elbows when sleeping. Most patients with mild cubital tunnel syndrome respond well to conservative management.[10]

ROOM SETUP

The procedure is performed in an operating room. The patient may remain in a stretcher or otherwise be transferred to an operating room table with a hand table set up. For operative time efficiency, it can be preferable for a patient to simply be wheeled into the operating room on a stretcher, and for the patient to remain in the same stretcher for induction and the duration of the procedure. This avoids multiple transfers of the patient from bed to bed. The surgeon ensures that the patient is at the edge of the stretcher so that, with the stretcher arm rail down after anesthetic induction, the upper extremity may easily be abducted onto a padded tray table that is locked into position beside the stretcher.

SURGICAL PROCEDURE

An incision is marked measuring 8 cm in length, extending proximally to the arm and distally to the medial forearm, centered between the olecranon and medial epicondyle (Figure 100.11).

Surgical options include various procedures ranging from simple ulnar nerve decompression alone, to medial epicondylectomy, to intramuscular or submuscular or subfascial transposition of the nerve, to endoscopic release. Most surgeons agree that in situ decompression is useful only for mild or intermittent symptoms with a nonsubluxating ulnar nerve and for patients with normal bony anatomy and no pain around the medial epicondyle.

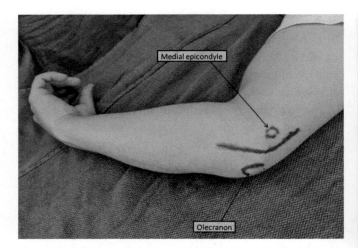

Figure 100.11. Cubital tunnel marking. An incision is marked measuring 8 cm in length extending proximally to the arm and distally to the medial forearm, centered between the olecranon and medial epicondyle.

Endoscopic cubital tunnel release is only acceptable for primary ulnar nerve decompression; if there is any difficulty visualizing the nerve, the procedure must be abandoned and the surgeon should proceed with open decompression. Meanwhile, submuscular transposition is generally preferred for thin patients and reoperative cases. Medial epicondylectomy may be useful for posttraumatic cases with bony deformity.

The ideal operation for this condition is controversial.[5,8,11,12] Since it is theoretically ideal to correct the cause of compression—including whether subluxation is a factor—the surgical option described herein is to perform an in situ decompression, evaluate intraoperatively for subluxation, and perform a transposition of the nerve if subluxation is identified under direct visualization.

Regional anesthesia is used. The patient is positioned supine on an operating room table, with the arm abducted onto an arm table. The surgeon sits between the abducted arm and the patient's body. A sterile tourniquet is applied to the upper arm over padding after the entire upper extremity has been sterilely prepared and draped. Landmarks include the olecranon and the medial epicondyle. This is where the ulnar nerve is most easily found.

An incision is made between these landmarks, extending proximally and distally by about 4 cm. Care is taken to identify and protect branches of the medial antebrachial cutaneous nerve. The ulnar nerve is identified and freed from the FCU fascia distally (Figure 100.12). Blunt finger dissection can help with proximal release.

With the ulnar nerve released, the elbow is flexed and extended while the nerve is observed for subluxation with positional changes. If no further points of compression are

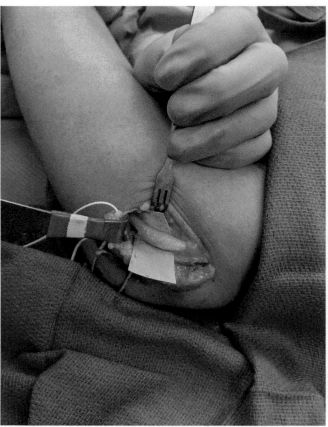

Figure 100.12. Appearance of the ulnar nerve immediately after cubital tunnel decompression.

identified with the nerve in motion, the wound is simply closed. If subluxation is observed, a fascial sling is elevated for anterior nerve transposition. Fascial flaps are elevated from the flexor-pronator origin in a stair-step fashion to create a lengthened fascial sling, and the nerve is tucked under the sling before the sling is fashioned with horizontal mattress 4-0 Monocryl sutures. Again, the nerve is checked to ensure adequate release and avoidance of kinking under the fascial sling.

For closure, a series of 3-0 Vicryl deep dermal sutures is applied, followed by either a subcuticular 4-0 Monocryl or otherwise 4-0 nylon simple interrupted sutures to the skin. Dressings include Xeroform, folded gauze, a soft dressing, and an Ace wrap. No splint is necessary.

POSTOPERATIVE CARE

Range of motion is begun immediately postoperatively, and patients are instructed to lift no more than 5 pounds at 1 month. Strength is increased gradually, and at 3 months postoperatively there are no restrictions.

RADIAL TUNNEL SYNDROME

Radial tunnel syndrome is compression of the radial nerve in the proximal forearm, where it passes under the lateral intermuscular septum. Radial tunnel syndrome and posterior interosseous nerve entrapment are often used interchangeably because they both have the same points of compression. The difference, however, is that motor dysfunction is not a hallmark of radial tunnel syndrome, whereas posterior interosseous nerve entrapment is always associated with motor weakness.[13]

RELEVANT ANATOMY

The radial nerve is derived from the posterior cord of the brachial plexus as the axillary nerve separates and arises from nerve roots C5–C8 and T1. The radial tunnel is 5 cm in length, extending from the level of the radiocapitellar joint, extending distally past the proximal edge of the supinator. The lateral boundaries are the brachioradialis (BR), the extensor carpi radialis longus (ECRL), and the extensor carpi radialis brevis (ECRB). The medial border is the biceps tendon and brachialis. The floor is the capsule of the radiocapitellar joint.

The posterior interosseous nerve, which arises as the radial nerve continues distally, innervates the ECRB, supinator, extensor carpi ulnaris (ECU), extensor digitorum (EDC), extensor indicus proprius (EIP), extensor digiti quinti (EDQ), abductor pollicis longus (AbPL), extensor pollicis longus (EPL), and extensor pollicis brevis (EPB); there is no sensory component because the superficial radial nerve has branched (Figure 100.13).[8]

Classic sites of compression in radial tunnel syndrome include:

- Tendinous margin of ECRB

- Adhesions at head of radius

- Vascular leash of Henry (radial recurrent arterial fan)

- Arcade of Frohse (proximal fibrous edge of supinator)

- Others: lateral head of triceps, superficial fibrous bands attached to the radiocapitellar joint, fascial border at *distal* edge of supinator; all locations of compression are aggravated by elbow extension and extension of long finger against resistance.

PHYSICAL EXAMINATION

Since the ECRL is innervated by the radial nerve before the branching of the posterior interosseous nerve, the wrist will tend to deviate radially in wrist extension. Due to the location of tenderness, it may be challenging to differentiate radial tunnel syndrome from lateral epicondylitis, but specific findings that can help in diagnosis have been well described in the literature. In general, tenderness in posterior interosseous nerve

PIN compression Syndrome – Sites of compression

Recurrent radial artery

1. Fibrous tissue anterior to radiocapitellar joint

5. ECRB medio-proximal edge (not shown)

Posterior interossous nerve

Superficial branch of radial nerve

Supinator

Brachioradialis

Radial nerve

Brachialis

Radial head under fat pad

2. Vascular leash of Henry

Radial artery

Pronator teres

4. Distal edge of supinator

3. Arcade of Frohse

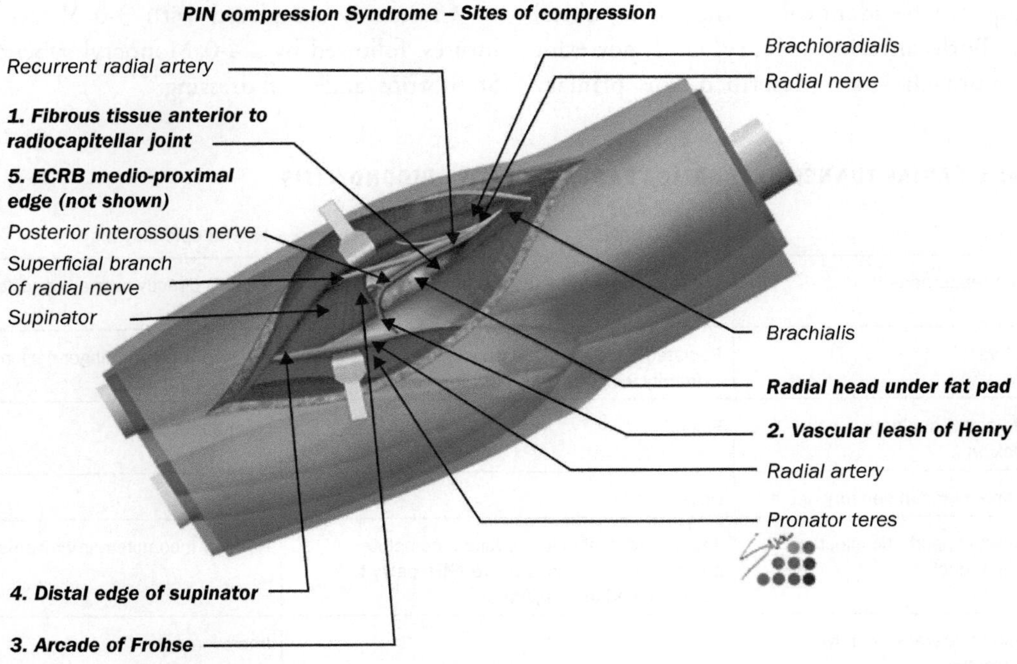

Figure 100.13. Radial tunnel syndrome compression sites.

compression is located more distally than that of lateral epicondylitis.

To perform the "middle finger test," the clinician asks the patient to extend the elbow and fingers. The clinician presses on the dorsum of the proximal phalanx of the middle finger. The test is positive if this produces pain at the edge of ECRB in the proximal forearm. However, it is still possible for this test to be positive in lateral epicondylitis.

Differentiating factors between radial tunnel syndrome and lateral epicondylitis are shown in Table 100.1.

INDICATIONS

Radial tunnel syndrome is diagnosed clinically. The clinician places pressure over the radial nerve over the forearm between the BR and the ECRB muscles and assesses for pain compared to the contralateral forearm. While it is important to differentiate radial tunnel syndrome from lateral epicondylitis, electrodiagnostic studies are not always helpful in the diagnosis aside from ruling out other conditions. Imaging such as magnetic resonance imaging (MRI) or ultrasound may rule out compressive masses, such as a lipoma or ganglion. Nonoperative care is very general, including anti-inflammatories, rest, and avoidance of provocative activities. While there is no specific conservative treatment option for radial tunnel syndrome, physiotherapy for nerve gliding may still be helpful.

SURGICAL PROCEDURE

The room setup can be identical to that of a cubital tunnel release. Both anterior (Henry) and posterior (Thompson) approaches are described for primary procedures (Figure 100.14).[13–15] The procedure can be performed under a regional block.

The patient lies supine on an operating room table with the arm abducted onto an arm board, with the forearm supinated. A tourniquet is placed on the upper arm over padding. The entire upper extremity is prepared and draped in a sterile fashion. A curvilinear incision is made on the skin over the expected interval between the brachioradialis and the brachialis in the distal arm (anterior approach, particularly for recurrent cases); if only forearm decompression is required, a straight-line incision can be made at the border of the brachioradialis and flexor-pronator muscles (posterior approach).[7] Care is taken to identify and protect branches of the lateral antebrachial cutaneous nerve. A self-retainer can help with retraction and visualization. The brachioradialis is retracted radially, so that the radial nerve can be identified along with its division at the supinator. The posterior interosseous nerve is followed distally as it goes deep to the supinator, and the fascia of the supinator is freed proximally and distally; there is no need to divide muscle itself. If needed, a portion of the fascia of the supinator can be excised, leaving the muscle intact. The surgeon should run a finger along the course of the nerve to determine that it is free; if there are any additional tendinous proximal bands of compression, the incision is extended proximally to the distal arm for further release.

Care is taken to clip off vessels in the vascular leash of Henry to further free the nerve from constricting vasculature.

Closure is completed with 3-0 Vicryl deep dermal sutures, followed by a 4-0 Monocryl subcuticular suture, Steri-Strips, and a soft dressing.

TABLE 100.1 RADIAL TUNNEL SYNDROME VERSUS LATERAL EPICONDYLITIS

	Radial tunnel	Lateral epicondylitis
Maximum tenderness	Mobile wad; deep, lateral forearm pain often at night; pain is more distal	Usually directly over epicondyle
Aggravators	Resisted middle finger extension with all upper extremity joints kept in full extension	Passive wrist and finger flexion with straight elbow
Resisted active supination with elbow flexion	Painful	Not painful
Paresthesia of radial sensory nerve	Occasionally	None
Response to anesthetic injection into radial tunnel	Improvement, should produce a complete posterior interosseous nerve (PIN) palsy to confirm location of injection	None or incomplete improvement
Response to lateral epicondyle steroid injection	None	Improvement

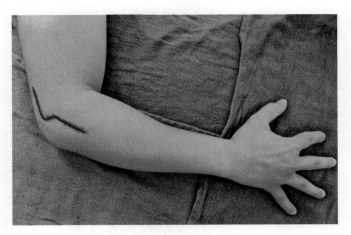

Figure 100.14. A curvilinear incision is made on the skin over the expected interval between the brachioradialis and the brachialis in the distal arm (anterior approach, particularly for recurrent cases).

POSTOPERATIVE CARE

The patient may begin range of motion immediately. The patient should lift no more than 5 pounds for the first month after surgery, but strength can be gradually increased until there are no more restrictions at 3 months postoperatively.

CAVEATS

For all compression neuropathies, the surgeon must remind the patient that operative release may not offer complete symptomatic relief, particularly if the patient has concomitant other sites of compression, such as in the neck. In addition, patients must be warned that operative release may actually aggravate other previously unnoticed symptoms, such as basal joint carpometacarpal joint arthritis pain. For example, long-standing carpal tunnel syndrome results in thumb numbness, masking osteoarthritic pain. With recovery of sensation after operative release, a patient will begin to experience arthritic thumb pain that was preexisting but previously unnoticed by the patient.

CONCLUSION

While carpal tunnel and cubital tunnel syndrome are quite common, radial tunnel syndrome is rarer. Regardless, careful preoperative assessment is critical in accurate diagnosis, and, where indicated, electrodiagnostic studies can be valuable. Various surgical approaches and procedures have been described.

REFERENCES

1. Keith MW, Masear V, Amadio PC. Treatment of carpal tunnel syndrome. *J Am Acad Orthop Surg* 2009;17:397–405.
2. Beasley RW. *Beasley's Surgery of the Hand*. New York: Thieme Medical Publishers, 2003.
3. Fowler JR, Munsch M, Huang Y, et al. Pre-operative electrodiagnostic testing predicts time to resolution of symptoms after carpal tunnel release. *J Hand Surg (Eur Vol)* 2016;41E(2):137–142.
4. Zyluk A, Szlosser Z. The results of carpal tunnel release for carpal tunnel syndrome diagnosed on clinical grounds, with or without electrophysiological investigations: a randomized study. *J Hand Surg (Eur Vol)* 2013;38(1):44–49.
5. Tang DT, Barbour JR, Davide KM, et al. Nerve entrapment: update. *Plast Reconstr Surg* 2015;135:199e–215e.
6. Osei DA, Calfee RP, Stepan JG, et al. Simultaneous bilateral or unilateral carpal tunnel release? *J Bone Joint Surg* 2014;96:889–896.
7. Duncan S. *Reoperative Hand Surgery*. New York: Springer, 2012.
8. Green DP. *Green's Operative Hand Surgery*. Philadelphia, PA: Churchill Livingstone, 2011.
9. Greenwald D, Blum LC, Adams D, et al. Effective surgical treatment of cubital tunnel syndrome based on provocative clinical testing without electrodiagnostics. *Plast Reconstr Surg* 2006;117: 87e–91e.
10. Plancher KD. *MasterCases Hand and Wrist Surgery*. New York: Thieme Medical Publishers, 2004.
11. Gaspar MP, Kane PM, Putthiwara D, et al. Predicting revision following in situ ulnar nerve decompression for patients with idiopathic cubital tunnel syndrome. *J Hand Surg Am* 2016;41(3): 427–435.
12. Matzon JL, Kutsky KF, Hoffler E, et al. Risk factors for ulnar nerve instability resulting in transposition in patients with cubital tunnel syndrome. *J Hand Surg Am* 2016;41(2):180–183.
13. Naam NH, Nemani S. Radial tunnel syndrome. *Orthop Clin N Am* 2012;43:529–536.
14. Maniker A. *Operative Exposures in Peripheral Nerve Surgery*. New York: Thieme Medical Publishers.
15. Sarris IK, Papadimitriou NG, Sotereanos DG. Radial tunnel syndrome. *Techn Hand Upper Extremity Surg* 2002;6(4):209–212.

101.

TENDON TRANSFERS IN UPPER EXTREMITY RECONSTRUCTION

Vincent G. Laurence and Gregory Rafijah

Tendon transfers have been in use since the late nineteenth century, an innovative therapy initially developed to help deal with the widespread debilitation brought on by the polio epidemics.[1] Fundamental concepts still observed today, including the need to balance antagonistic muscles, select a donor muscle with appropriate power for the function desired, and to get the patient participating in early motion rehabilitation following repair to prevent problems with adhesions were advanced before the turn of the twentieth century.[2] With the traumatic injuries of the upper extremity wrought by the trench warfare of World War I, hand surgeons continued to innovate and improve, and many of the transfers pioneered nearly a century ago are still being used today.

Today, in an era of microvascular coaptation of nerves, nerve transfers, vascularized nerve grafts, and free functional muscle transfers, tendon transfers still have a vital role to play, particularly in cases of late presentations of nerve palsies. All of these techniques within the repertoire of the reconstructive hand surgeon aim to restore function where it has been lost, whether due to trauma, disease (rheumatoid arthritis, poliomyelitis, leprosy), ischemia (stroke, compartment syndrome), or congenital absence of a muscle. For the sake of brevity, we will focus on one of the most common sets of transfers, those for a high radial nerve palsy.

GENERAL PRINCIPLES

From nearly the inception of the transfer of tendons to restore function, a number of general principles have been recognized. These include the principle of using one tendon for one function; creating as straight a line of tension as possible for a transferred tendon; ensuring mobile, supple joints, free of contracture, prior to any transfer;

ensuring a good gliding bed for the transferred tendon, free of adhesions and scar tissue; and, establishing normal tension.[2] In 1922, the Army surgeon C. L. Starr published "Army Experience with Tendon Transference," which added the need for a donor tendon to have adequate excursion for the needed function and the need to preserve wrist tenodesis.[3] Beginning in the 1970s, Paul Brand brought a new level of rigor to the field with his demonstration that "the mass or volume of a muscle is proportional to its work capacity, and the fiber length of a muscle is proportional to its potential excursion." Building on this work, Richard Lieber and Jan Fridén, among others, developed the concept of muscle architecture as a basis for optimizing the selection of donor tendons.[4–6] Although new tendon transfer–related research continues to be published, our modern repertoire of tendon transfers was essentially fully formed by the 1990s.

INDICATIONS AND TIMING

Tendon transfers are used most commonly for late reconstruction of peripheral nerve injuries, usually traumatic in nature. Other indications include more proximal neurological injuries or insults, such as those to the brachial plexus or central nervous system (e.g., cerebral palsy), traumatic absence of a muscle or tendon (e.g., from an avulsion injury), and neuromuscular conditions such as the aforementioned poliomyelitis, leprosy, and the mechanical sequelae of untreated rheumatoid arthritis. Finally, a failed attempt at repair of a peripheral nerve, or the elapse of a period of time deemed adequate for return of function, given the distance of injury from the nonfunctioning muscle (at a rate of 1 mm/day or ~1 inch/month), should warrant consideration of a tendon transfer.[7]

Timing of tendon transfers, however, remains a controversial topic. Although conventionally it was advised that "the patient should have a static condition that will not improve spontaneously,"[2,4] others now advocate for performing tendon transfers at the time of nerve repair or grafting, especially in situations with significant concomitant soft tissue injury in which spontaneous recovery is deemed unlikely.[8]

We will look now at some of the most common transfers for the most common nerve palsy.

TENDON TRANSFERS FOR HIGH RADIAL NERVE PALSY

Upper extremity peripheral nerve injuries outnumber lower extremity peripheral nerve injuries, and, in the upper extremity, peripheral nerve injuries are more common in the arm (often resulting from humeral fractures lacerating the radial nerve) than in the forearm.[9] For this reason, a high radial nerve palsy is among the most common of peripheral nerve injuries encountered. These injuries result in an extension deficit at the wrist, at the index through little finger metacarpal phalangeal (MCP) joints, and at the thumb, with loss of radial abduction of the thumb as well. The sensory deficit incurred with a radial nerve palsy, because it is dorsal and therefore not required for fine motor tasks or to control grasp, is less morbid than that associated with either a median or an ulnar nerve palsy.

Over the years, dozens of tendon transfers have been described for radial nerve palsy, but three distinct sets of transfers have emerged as dominant: the flexor carpi radialis (FCR) set, the flexor carpi ulnaris (FCU) set, and the Boyes superficialis (flexor digitorum superficialis, or FDS) set.[10] All three use the relatively redundant pronator teres (PT), the distal insertion of which is divided, then transferred to the extensor carpi radialis brevis (ECRB) tendons, to provide wrist extension. The FCR and the FCU sets of transfers also have in common the use of the expendable palmaris longus (PL) tendon (so long as it is present) transferred to extensor pollicis longus (EPL) to provide thumb extension and radial abduction. The only difference, then between the FCU and the FCR techniques is the use of their namesakes as transfers to the extensor digitorum communis (EDC) tendons for finger extension. The Boyes superficialis set of transfers was pioneered by Dr. Joseph Boyes in response to the theoretical concern that the amplitude of excursion of the wrist flexors is inadequate (classically described as 30 mm) for the function of providing finger extension (50 mm in an "average" uninjured human). A recent retrospective comparison of the three sets of transfers, however, noted no significant difference in ranges of motion, subjective satisfaction with the transfers, the relative percentages of patients able to return to work, or the time from their injury to their return to work.[11] Although the FCU transfers have long been considered the classic set,[12] we prefer the FCR set of transfers because use of the FCR preserves the more powerful FCU as wrist flexor, avoids fixed radial deviation at the wrist, and permits the ulnar deviation necessary for activities such as hammering, sawing, and throwing.

OPERATIVE TECHNIQUE

The patient should be positioned supine with the extremity being operated on positioned on a hand table and the bed rotated to allow unrestricted access on both sides and at the end of the hand table. The tourniquet is applied prior to prepping and draping the patient and can be protected with a clear plastic drape. Perioperative antibiotics and anticoagulation are administered per surgeon preference.

There are many options with respect to incisions for the FCR set of transfers, but we prefer a simple hockey stick–shaped incision along the junction of the dorsal and radial aspects of the forearm (Figure 101.1), extending ulnarly at the wrist, and a short incision volarly along the wrist crease (Figure 101.2). We perform these transfers under tourniquet control, but tendon transfers can be performed without use of a tourniquet and even under local anesthesia only, making it possible to tension the transfers with the patient's cooperation.[13]

Begin the dissection by developing a flap of subcutaneous tissue along the long dorsoradial incision, taking care to protect radial sensory branches as they are encountered. Once at fascia level, incise the fascia and continue dissecting down toward the radius, just ulnar to ECRB tendon. Identify the PT

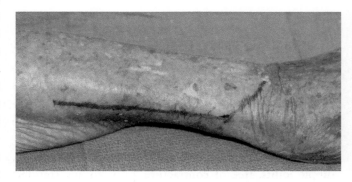

Figure 101.1 Dorsal hockey stick incision for tendon transfer.

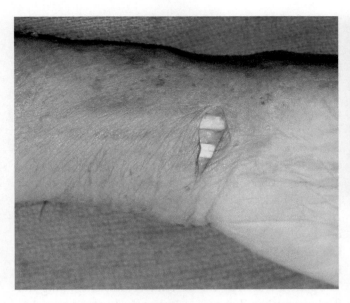

Figure 101.2 Donors dissected: Pronator teres (PT), flexor carpi radialis (FCR), and palmaris longus (PL), divided and transposed.

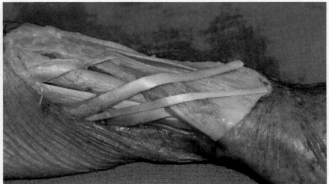

Figure 101.4 Donors dissected: Pronator teres (PT), flexor carpi radialis (FCR), and palmaris longus (PL), divided and transposed.

at its insertion on the radius and mark out a cuff of periosteum extending distally from its distal-most point (Figure 101.3). Incise the periosteum sharply, elevate off of the radius, and continue dissection as proximal as possible under direct vision.

Supinate the arm, make a transverse incision at wrist crease, and confirm the identity of PL and FCR (Figure 101.2). Take care to protect the median nerve and its palmar cutaneous branch, which is adjacent to the palmaris longus tendon. The palmaris longus tendon will not be present in approximately 15% of limbs and may require an alternate tendon transfer such as the flexor digitorum superficialis from the ring or middle finger. Divide both the FCR and PL at the flexor retinaculum, preserving as much tendon as possible, then mobilize from distal to proximal as far as is necessary to obtain a straight line of pull when transferred.

With all three donor tendons fully dissected, it is time to turn to the recipient tendons. Route all three of the donor

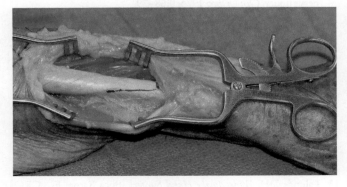

Figure 101.3 Harvest of the Pronator teres tendon with a distal cuff of periosteum.

tendons roughly into place first to assess their length with respect to where they will be sutured to their recipients (Figure 101.4). Ensure there is adequate overlap of donor and recipient before dividing any of the recipient tendons, beginning with the PL-to-EPL pair. Identify the EPL at the ulnar border of the anatomic snuffbox and follow it proximal to its musculotendinous junction. Divide it proximally enough to allow several centimeters of overlap once the PL is woven into it.

In a similar manner, identify the ECRB and confirm its identity by tugging on its tendon, looking for a nondeviated hand extension as a result of its insertion on the third metacarpal. By way of contrast, when tugged, ECRL, which inserts on the index metacarpal, will demonstrate a radial deviation. Having positively identified the ECRB, lay the PT with its periosteal extension atop it before dividing the ECRB to ensure adequate overlap with the weave. Then divide and mobilize proximal to distal. Finally, identify the four extensor digitorum communis (EDC) tendons, preserving the extensor indicis proprius (EIP), which lies ulnar to the index EDC and assessing length as before, prior to division. Then divide, mobilize, and assess for extension lag while placing equal tension on each of the tendons. If the small finger demonstrates lag, it is often because its EDC is a relatively inconsequential tendon, so you will need to add extensor digiti minimi (EDM) to the bundle of recipients. If you have full extension, however, there is no need to include the EDM. Each of the donor and recipient tendons is now ready for tensioning and weaving (Figure 101.5). Now is a good time to take down the tourniquet, obtain hemostasis, and irrigate all incisions thoroughly.

Tensioning of the transfers is critical; the goal is to provide as much function as possible (extension in this case, "opening" of the hand in order to facilitate grasp) without compromising flexion. This is done by positioning each joint in more-or-less maximal extension and placing the

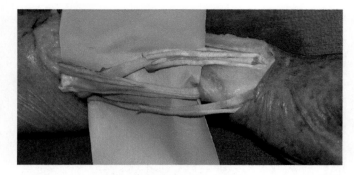

Figure 101.5 Donors and recipients laid out in place: From top to bottom, FCR to EDC, PT to ECRB, and PL to EPL

tendons you are joining under slight tension, performing the first pass of a Pulvertaft weave, but using just a single test suture. The Pulvertaft weave, which provides great strength to the tendinous connection between donor and recipient, is performed by carefully incising the recipient tendon near its proximal end with a no. 11 blade, expanding this opening as necessary with a mosquito clamp so the donor tendon will just pass through. This process is then repeated with incisions alternating in perpendicular planes every 1–2 cm, proceeding distally along the recipient, until there are 3–5 sutured junctures; any excess donor tendon may be removed or may be sutured to the recipient to strengthen the connection provided it does not create excessive bulk. In each case, after suturing the first juncture, carefully assess range of motion by passively flexing the wrist, fingers, or thumb depending on the transfer you're evaluating. If the transfer passes this test, complete the weave. If you need to adjust the tension, cut out your test suture and either increase or decrease the tension as indicated before proceeding as described earlier (Figure 101.6).

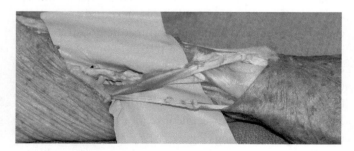

Figure 101.6 Completed transfers: Each of the donor tendons is woven through its recipient in a Pulvertaft fashion at optimal tension. Tendons are ranged gently with one test suture in place to ensure minimal lag and no flexor deficit at the wrist, then digits, then thumb. Once optimal tension has been set, then the weave is completed, with three to four points of tendon-to-tendon connection. Note that the PT to ECRB transfer is placed deep to the FCR to EDC transfer in order to create the straightest line of pull, with minimal friction between transfers.

POSTOPERATIVE CARE

Incisions are closed primarily in a single layer, using 4-0 nylon suture. Incisions are covered with a thin strip of Xeroform gauze, cotton gauze is placed in each of the web spaces, cast padding (e.g., Webril) is wrapped around the hand to the DIP joints, and a dorsal splint is applied with arm positioned in pronation, the wrist in full extension, and MCP joints fully extended, including the thumb. The extremity is immobilized for 3–4 weeks, at which point the patient is referred to occupational therapy (OT), and a dynamic finger extension splint (forearm-based, with outriggers to hold each finger and thumb in extension) is fashioned to replace the postoperative splint. This dynamic finger extension splint is maintained for another month. The patient is seen by OT for tendon transfer training and flexion exercises. The patient is then gradually advanced to unlimited activity by four months from surgery.

REFERENCES

1. Meals CG, Meals RA. Tendon versus nerve transfers in elbow, wrist, and hand reconstruction: A literature review. *Hand Clin* 2013; 29:393–400.
2. Botte MJ, Pacelli LL. "Historical aspects of tendon transfers." In *Tendon Transfers in Reconstructive Hand Surgery*, ed. Jan Friden. Routledge: Taylor & Francis, 2005.
3. Starr CL. Army experience with tendon transference. *J Bone Joint Surg* 1922; 4(1):3–21.
4. Brand PW, Beach RB, Thompson DE. Relative tension and potential excursion of muscles in the forearm and hand. *J Hand Surg (Am)* 1981; 6(3):209–219.
5. Lieber RL, Friden J. Functional and clinical significance of skeletal muscle architecture. *Muscle Nerve* 2000; 23:1647–1666.
6. Lieber RL, Jacobson MD, Fazeli BM, Abrams RA, Botte MJ. Architecture of selected muscles of the arm and forearm: Anatomy and implications for tendon transfer. *J Hand Surg* 1992; 17:787–798.
7. Sammer DM, Chung KC. Tendon transfers: Part I. Principles of transfer and transfers for radial nerve palsy. *Plast Reconstr Surg* 2009; 123:169e–177e.
8. Burkhalter WE. Early tendon transfer in upper extremity peripheral nerve injury. *Clin Orthop* 1974; 0:68–79.
9. Noble J, et al. Analysis of upper and lower extremity peripheral nerve injuries in a population of patients with multiple injuries. *J Trauma* 1998; 45(1):116–122.
10. Jones NF, Machado GR. Tendon transfers for radial, median, and ulnar nerve injuries: Current surgical techniques. *Clin Plast Surg* 2011; 38:621–642.
11. Moussavi AA, et al. Outcome of tendon transfer for radial nerve paralysis: comparison of three methods. *Indian J Orthop* 2011; 45(6): 558–562.
12. Szabo RM. Tendon transfers for radial nerve palsy. In: Van Heest A, Goldfarb CA, eds. *Tendon Transfer Surgery of the Upper Extremity: A Master Skills Publication*. Rosemont, IL: American Society for Surgery of the Hand, 2012.
13. Lalonde DH. *Wide Awake Hand Surgery*. Boca Raton, FL: CRC Press, Taylor & Francis Group, 2016.

102

METACARPAL AND PHALANGEAL FRACTURES

David T. Netscher and Kristy L. Hamilton

ASSESSMENT OF THE DEFECT

Therapeutic options for metacarpal and phalangeal fractures depend not only on fracture pattern, mechanism of injury, and location but also on associated soft tissue injuries, patient age, and occupation.

Metacarpal fractures result from crush or direct impact, such as boxer fractures, or from abduction forces, as with the thumb metacarpal. Fractures are divided into four groups: (1) head, (2) neck or subcapital, (3) shaft, and (4) base. Phalangeal fractures are commonly caused by crush injuries in the workplace and during sports secondary to direct blows to the hand. The middle finger is most commonly affected, followed by the thumb. Phalangeal fractures can be associated with injury to flexor or extensor tendons as well as the nailbed.

Nondisplaced fractures are splinted, and the hand is elevated, with motion to commence in a guarded fashion when healing permits. Displaced but stable fractures are usually managed by closed reduction and immobilization. Those that can be reduced but that demonstrate instability are treated by closed manipulation and percutaneous pinning. Open reduction and internal fixation are necessary if satisfactory closed reduction cannot be obtained or when percutaneous pinning is not possible. In the digit, open methods must be judiciously and cautiously selected because of the small dimensions of phalangeal bones and fracture fragments involved, the high technical demand of these procedures, and the potential complications, including tendon adhesion formation.

When open reduction is elected, surgical exposure is planned to allow visualization of bone fragments to gain secure fixation while minimizing devascularization and limiting adhesion-promoting soft tissue dissection. Fixation must be rigid enough to allow early active motion to minimize adhesion formation and stiffness. Avoiding hardware placement near the joint line is preferable as it can cause further joint stiffness.

Although either operative and nonoperative fracture treatment may be appropriate for isolated fractures of the hand, operative stabilization is essential for complex injuries involving combined bone and soft tissue lesions. The sequence of repair is an important component in the optimal management of these injuries and requires careful preoperative planning. Bone fixation follows debridement and is a necessary preliminary to other restorative soft tissue measures. Fixation is achieved in various ways, including internal fixation methods or external skeletal fixation, depending on existing wounds, amount of bone comminution, and the degree of contamination. Each method has its advantages and disadvantages. Bone defects created by severe comminution or bone loss are reconstructed using wire or prosthetic spacers, by the incorporation of primary autogenous bone grafts, or by external fixation. This provides the basis for achieving a stable skeletal architecture and allows the hand surgeon then to focus on the requirements of all other traumatized structures and soft tissues. Nerves and tendons are repaired early, but repair is delayed in cases of crush injury or contamination or until adequate soft tissue is in place. Early protected range-of-motion is instituted as soon as feasible to enable recovery of motion and hand function.

SURGICAL ASSESSMENT AND PREPARATION

PREOPERATIVE EVALUATION

After history-taking, the hand is examined for deformity, swelling, tenderness, ecchymosis, skin abrasions, and limitations in motion. Alignment is checked with fingers flexed into the palm (Figure 102.1). Soft tissue injury—ligaments

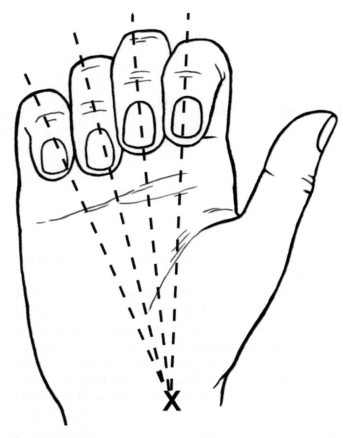

Figure 102.1. To assess malrotation of the digits, the patient flexes all digit into a fist. The digits should be parallel and point toward the scaphoid (marked by "X").

and tendons—must be differentiated from a fracture. The neurovascular integrity of the digits and hand should also be assessed. Appropriate radiographs are then obtained; these should always include three views: anteroposterior (AP), lateral, and oblique.

For metacarpal fractures, special views that are helpful include (1) the Brewerton view (Figure 102.2A,C), consisting of metacarpophalangeal (MCP) joints flexed 60 degrees with the dorsum of the fingers lying flat on the x-ray plate and tube angled 15 degrees ulnar to radial, useful for metacarpal head fractures; and (2) the Robert view (Figure 102.2B,D), consisting of true AP and lateral views of the thumb, useful for thumb metacarpal base fractures.

For phalangeal fractures, additional three-views of the affected digit focused on the proximal interphalangeal (PIP) joint should be obtained. Lateral radiographs of the interphalangeal joints may also be required in flexion and extension when indicated, such as for proximal interphalangeal fracture dislocations, as these views may reveal instability. A volar lip basilar middle phalanx fracture,

for example, may be stable in flexion, but, as the PIP joint is brought into extension, subluxation may occur.

Additional radiographic studies such as computed tomographic (CT) scanning or magnetic resonance imaging (MRI) may be needed to document and assess the extent of metaphyseal or articular fractures (Figure 102.3). They may be required for more accurate assessment of comminuted and intraarticular fractures or when the bones are crowded, which makes routine radiographs difficult to interpret (as may occur in basilar finger metacarpal fractures and fracture dislocations, more commonly seen at the fourth and fifth metacarpals).

In open fracture injuries, tetanus prophylaxis is given, a culture sample taken, and antibiotic therapy initiated.

ROOM SETUP AND INSTRUMENTATION

The base setup in the operating room is identical to that used for other hand surgery procedures. A pneumatic tourniquet and loupe magnification are recommended. Surgical instruments required are the basic hand surgery set and supplemental instruments for bone fixation. Metallic implants and devices that may be used for fixation of a fracture are listed in Tables 102.1, 102.2, 102.3, and 102.4.[1] If percutaneous fixation is planned, fluoroscopic x-ray equipment is required in the operating room. The mini C-arm is useful as it reduces risk of radiation exposure to the surgeon and the patient.

ANESTHESIA

Surgery is best performed with adequate regional (axillary or Bier block, and occasionally, wrist or digital block) or general anesthesia. Tight exsanguination with the elastic bandage may be excessively painful and preclude Bier block anesthesia.

INDICATIONS FOR SURGERY

General indications for surgical stabilization include failure to obtain and hold satisfactory closed reduction, rotational deformity, severe angulation or displacement suitable for stabilization, fractures and fracture-dislocations with unstable configuration, irreducible articular step-off, open fractures (particularly those with complex injuries of adjacent tendons, nerves, or blood vessels), fractures with comminution or bone loss, those requiring bone grafting, and fractures involving multiple digits or bones (Table 1→4).

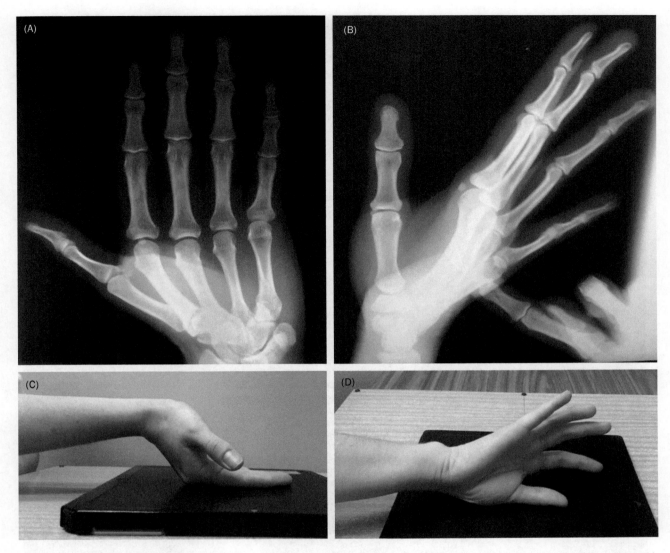

Figure 102.2. The Brewerton view is taken by flexing the metacarpophalangeal joints to create a 60-degree angle between the metacarpals and the table surface (C), while the Robert view is a true, isolated anteroposterior (AP) view of the thumb (D).

Surgery is also indicated when early mobilization is needed. Phalangeal fractures more often will fall into one of these categories and are therefore more likely to require treatment compared to metacarpal fractures, which are afforded stability by the adjacent metacarpal interconnecting ligaments.

FIXATION TECHNIQUES

The techniques for hand fracture fixation are precise and demanding. Mastering these techniques requires a thorough understanding of the procedures and their appropriate application, as well as knowledge of the many implants and devices available.[2]

KIRSCHNER WIRES

Kirschner wires, or K-wires, are 4- or 6-inch double-pointed metal wires of various diameters (i.e., 0.028, 0.035, 0.045, and 0.0625 inch). They are used after either closed reduction to secure stability or open reduction and may be used alone in different planes or as a supplement to other fixation methods. Their major disadvantage is that they lack enough stability to initiate early mobilization. They are associated with occasional but serious complications, including transfixion of tendons, pin loosening, and pin tract infection.

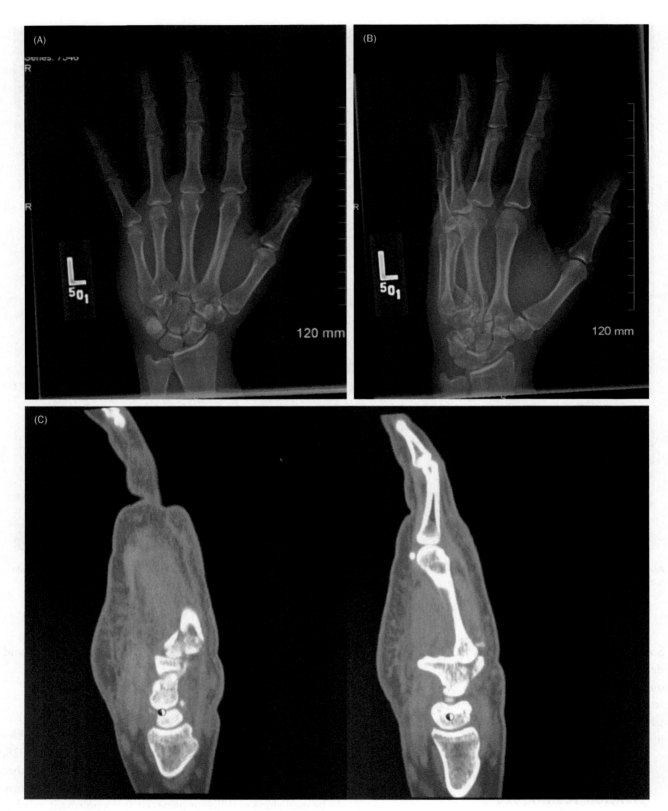

Figure 102.3. Plain films of anteroposterior (A) and oblique (B) views provide limited evaluation of this ring finger CMC fracture dislocation. Computed tomography (CT) cuts of the fourth and fifth metacarpals delineate the extent of the injury more clearly (C).

K-wires
  0.028 in.
  0.035 in.
  0.045 in.
  0.0625 in.

Intraosseus wires
  24-gauge
  26-gauge

Screws
  2.7 mm (diameter), 6–24 mm (length)
  2.0 mm (diameter), 6–20 mm (length)
  1.5 mm (diameter), 6–16 mm (length)

Plates
2.7-mm series
Quarter tubular plate
Dynamic compression plate
T-plate
Oblique L-plate

2.0- and 1.5- mm series
Straight plate
T-plate
Mini-condylar plate
Mini-H plate
2.0-mm dynamic compression plate

2.5-mm mini-external fixator

K-wires are inserted using a power-operated hand drill. The wires may be cut off at skin level with skin pulled over the sharp end, or they may protrude beyond the skin (with protection of the sharp point). The pins do not require secondary surgery for removal. They are removed with or without local anesthesia using a stout needle holder.

TABLE 102.2 BONE INSTRUMENTS

Power-operated hand drill
K-wires
  0.028 in.
  0.035 in.
  0.045 in.
  0.0625 in.
Wire cutters
Wire-bending pliers

Drill bits (assorted)
Drill guides and tap sleeves
Screwdrivers
Gauges

Plate-cutting forceps
Plate-bending pliers and bending irons

Reduction forceps
Retractors
Curettes
Rongeurs
Gouges
Bone hooks
Bone impactors
Large needle holder

The Lalonde bone clamp is particularly useful with K-wires—this specialized bone clamp includes a drill guide for the K-wire to secure fixation in the same axis as the reduction (Figure 102.4). The clamp may be used to place K-wires used in conjunction with any of the fixation methods, even if they only serve as temporary guide wires, as with percutaneous screw placement.

INTRAOSSEOUS WIRE SUTURE

Intraosseous wires are stainless steel wires passed through holes made with a power-drive drill. A 19-gauge hypodermic needle, with its hub removed, can be used as a drilled intraosseous wire passer. The wire is passed through the hollow needle bore and the needle withdrawn (Figures 102.5 and 102.6). Wires are applied in different configurations depending on the fracture type. With the Lister type A wiring technique, the intraosseous portion of the wire runs parallel to the fracture line and a single K-wire is added, passing from one cortex to another across the fracture without entering into the joint. This type of fixation is employed for shaft fractures. With Lister type B, the intraosseous wire passes perpendicular to the fracture line. Where the fragment is too small to drill, the wire can be passed through the attached ligament, hard against the bone. Other configurations include 90/90 wires and the figure-of-eight loop or tension band wire (Figure 102.7). The former is especially helpful in replantation surgery.

Intraosseous wire technique is applicable for articular fractures or for comminuted fractures with multiple small fragments. It can also be used as an adjunct to other internal fixation methods.

TENSION BAND WIRES

A tension band wire is an intraosseous wire applied in the form of a figure-of-eight loop on the convex side of the reduced fracture. It provides dynamic compression at the fracture surface (Figure 102.7). Tension band wires are indicated chiefly for avulsion fractures, for the fixation of arthrodesis, and, occasionally, for the attachment of bone grafts.

SCREW FIXATION

Screws provide high stability. Smaller screws are selected for smaller bones and smaller fragments. As a rule, a fragment should be at least three times the thread diameter of the screw to be used or there is an increased risk of shattering the fragment. Screws of 1.5 mm and 2.0 mm in diameter

TABLE 102.3 **COMMON SCREWS FOR FRACTURE FIXATION**

Device	Company	Name	Indications	Shaft diameter (mm)	Major thread diameter at tip/head (mm)	Drill size (mm)	Length (step increment; mm)	Cannulated
Headless Screw	AcuMed	Acutrak Mini	Metacarpal or IP arthrodesis	Tapered	2.8/3.1–3.6	3.1–3.6	8–26 (2)	Y
	Arthrex	Micro Compression FT	Metacarpal or IP arthrodesis	Tapered	2.8/2.8	2.0	8–14 (1), 16–30 (2)	Y
	Integra	BOLD 2.5	Metacarpal	1.8	2.5/3.3	1.9	10–30 (2)	Y
	KLS Martin	2.5 HBS 2 Mini	Metacarpal, IP arthrodesis	1.7	2.5/3.2	1.9	10–30 (1)	Y
	Medartis	2.2 SpeedTip CCS	DIP Arthrodesis, metacarpal	1.7	2.2/2.8	1.8	10–30 (1), 32–40 (2)	Y
	Synthes	HCS 1.5	DIP arthrodesis, phalanx, metacarpal	1.2	1.5/2.2	1.1	8–20 (1)	N
		HCS 2.4	Metacarpal, IP arthrodesis	2.0	2.4/3.1	2.0	9–30 (1), 32–40 (2)	Y
Headed Cannulated Screw	OsteoMed	2.0 Extremifix	Phalanx, Metacarpal	1.8	2.1/–	–	6–42 (2)	Y
		2.4 Extremifix	Phalanx, Metacarpal	1.9	2.5/–	–	6–50 (2)	Y
		3.0 Extremifix	Phalanx, Metacarpal	2.2	3.0/–	–	10–40 (2)	Y
	Stryker	Asnis micro 2.0	Phalanx, Metacarpal	1.7	2.1/–	–	8–20 (1), 22–30 (2)	Y
		Asnis micro 3.0	Phalanx, Metacarpal	2.1	3.1/–	–	8–30 (1), 32–40 (2)	Y
	Synthes	2.4 cannulated	Phalanx, Metacarpal	1.7	2.4/–	–	17–20 (1), 22–30 (2)	Y
		2.4 cannulated	Phalanx, Metacarpal	1.9	2.4/–	–	17–20 (1), 22–30 (2)	Y
		3.0 cannulated	Phalanx, Metacarpal	2.0	3.0/–	–	8–30 (1), 32–40 (2)	Y
		3.5 cannulated	Phalanx, Metacarpal	2.4	3.5/–	–	10–50 (2)	Y
	Arthrex	2.0 QuickFix cannulated	Phalanx, Metacarpal	1.7	2.0/–	–	8–30 (2)	Y
		2.4 QuickFix cannulated	Phalanx, Metacarpal	1.7	2.4/–	–	8–36 (2)	Y
		3.0 QuickFix cannulated	Phalanx, Metacarpal	2.0	3.0/–	–	10–50 (2)	Y

are generally used in the phalanges or to secure small metacarpal fragments. Screws of 2.0 mm and 2.7 mm in diameter are used for metacarpal fractures. For each screw size, an analogous set of instruments exists with drill bits, guides, countersinks, depth gauges, tap sleeves, and screwdrivers.

Self-tapping screws allow the surgeon to omit a step in the sequence of drilling, tapping, and then placing the screw, which is helpful when manipulating small fragments.

Screws used to secure two bone fragments are inserted so that the threads do not gain purchase on the proximal

TABLE 102.4 COMMON HAND SETS FOR FRACTURE FIXATION

Company	Set	Screw	Indications	Minor thread diameter (mm)	Major thread diameter (mm)	Drill size (mm)	Length (step increment; mm)
Synthes	Modular Hand	1.0 cortical	Single lag screw	0.7	1.0	0.76	6–14 (1)
		1.3 nonlocking	Phalanx	0.9	1.3	1.0	6–16 (1), 18
		1.5 nonlocking		1.1	1.5	1.1	6–16 (1), 18–24 (2)
		2.0 nonlocking		1.4	2.0	1.5	6–14 (1), 16–40 (2)
		2.4 nonlocking	Metacarpal	1.7	2.4	1.8	6–14 (1), 16–30 (2)
	LCP Compact Hand	1.5 nonlocking	Phalanx	1.1	1.5	1.1	6–16 (1), 18–24 (2)
		1.5 monoaxial locking		1.1	1.5	1.1	6–16 (1), 18–24 (2)
		2.0 nonlocking		1.4	2.0	1.5	6–14 (1), 16–40 (2)
		2.0 monoaxial locking		1.4	2.0	1.5	6–14 (1), 16–30 (2)
		2.4 nonlocking	Metacarpal	1.7	2.4	1.8	6–14 (1), 16–40 (2)
		2.4 monoaxial locking		1.8	2.4	1.8	6–14 (1), 16–30 (2)
	Mod Mini Frag LCP	2.7 nonlocking	Metacarpal	1.9	2.7	2.0	10–50 (2)
		2.7 monoaxial locking		2.1	2.7	2.0	10–50 (2)
Medartis	APTUS	1.2 nonlocking	Phalanx	0.9	1.2	1.0	4–14 (1), 16–20 (2)
		1.5 nonlocking		1.0	1.5	1.2	4–24 (1)
		1.5 variable-angle locking		1.0	1.5	1.2	4–13 (1)
		2.0 nonlocking	Proximal phalanx / metacarpal	1.3	2.0	1.6	4–24 (1)
		2.0 variable-angle locking		1.3	2.0	1.6	6–14 (1), 16–20 (2)
		2.3 nonlocking		1.6	2.3	1.9	5–24 (1), 26–34 (2)
Stryker	Profyle	1.2 nonlocking	Phalanx	1.0	1.2	1.0	4–10 (1), 12–20 (2)
		1.7 nonlocking		1.4	1.7	1.4	5–16 (1), 18–24 (2)
		2.3 nonlocking	Metacarpal	1.9	2.3	1.9	5–16 (1), 18–24 (2)
	VariAx	1.7 nonlocking	Phalanx	1.4	1.7	1.4	5–16 (1), 18–24 (2)
		1.7 variable-angle locking		1.4	1.7	1.4	5–16 (1), 18–24 (2)
		2.3 nonlocking	Metacarpal	1.9	2.3	1.9	5–16 (1), 18–24 (2)
		2.3 variable-angle locking		1.9	2.3	1.9	6, 8–16 (1), 18–26 (2)
KLS Martin	LINOS	1.2 nonlocking	Single lag screw	0.85	1.2	1.0	5–14 (1)
		1.5 nonlocking	Phalanx	1.1	1.5	1.1	6–20 (1)
		1.5 variable-angle locking		1.1	1.5	1.1	6–20 (1)
		2.0 nonlocking	Metacarpal / proximal phalanx	1.3	2.0	1.5	6–20 (1), 22–32 (2)
		2.0 variable-angle locking		1.3	2.0	1.5	6–20 (1), 22–32 (2)
		2.3 nonlocking	Metacarpal	1.7	2.3	1.8	6–20 (1), 22–32 (2)
		2.3 variable-angle locking		1.7	2.3	1.8	6–20 (1), 22–32 (2)

(continued)

TABLE 102.4 CONTINUED

Company	Set	Screw	Indications	Minor thread diameter (mm)	Major thread diameter (mm)	Drill size (mm)	Length (step increment; mm)
Biomet	ALPS	1.3 cortical	Single lag screw	1.0	1.3	1.0	8–24
		1.5 nonlocking	Phalanx	1.1	1.5	1.1	8–24
		1.5 variable-angle locking		1.1	1.5	1.1	8–24
		2.5 nonlocking	Metacarpal	2.0	2.5	2.0	8–28
		2.5 monoaxial locking		2.0	2.5	2.0	8–28
		2.5 variable-angle locking		2.0	2.5	2.0	10–28

fragment but rather glide through it to gain purchase on the distal fragment. A screw applied in this manner converts potentially disruptive, asymmetrical forces into compressive forces at the fracture line and secures the bone fragments to each other so that no movement occurs between them. This is called the *lag screw principle*, where the drill bit chosen for the proximal fragment is the same size as the screw diameter and the drill bit used distally is smaller (Figure 102.8).

Fixation with screws alone is especially applicable for displaced intraarticular fractures with large fragments, displaced periarticular fractures, and oblique and spiral fractures of shafts of the phalanges and metacarpals. In addition to these situations, screws can be used with other means of fixation, such as plates or external fixator devices.

Headless, cannulated screws are versatile, allowing for minimally invasive, percutaneous approaches to fracture fixation as well as precise screw placement in challenging scenarios, such as fixing intraarticular fragments. These

screws allow for rigid fixation while minimizing trauma to surrounding soft tissues. It may be helpful to first reduce the fracture segments with bone clamps, followed by K-wire placement. After fluoroscopic confirmation, a cannulated screw is threaded over the wire and drilled into place percutaneously without a large incision. If headless screws are unavailable, the surgeon can elect to countersink headed screws to compensate for screw projection. Benefits include stable fixation and minimal scarring with less adhesion formation secondary to the percutaneous approach.

A novel use of cannulated headless screws is to pass them distally to proximally through the joint surface in an intramedullary manner for phalangeal shaft fractures. Placement is similar to traditional percutaneous screw positioning, first with K-wire guidance, by passing the screw in a retrograde fashion (Figure 102.9). Intramedullary cannulated headless screws are useful for transverse and short oblique fractures of the phalanges and metacarpals.

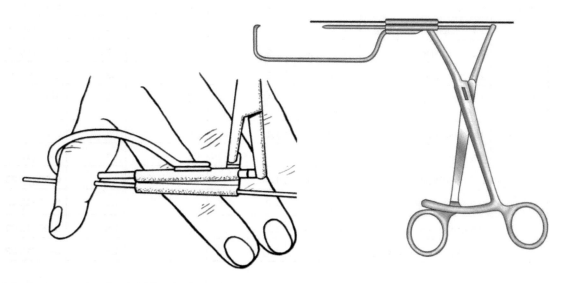

Figure 102.4. Lalonde clamps reduced and stabilize the fracture percutaneously before wires are placed.

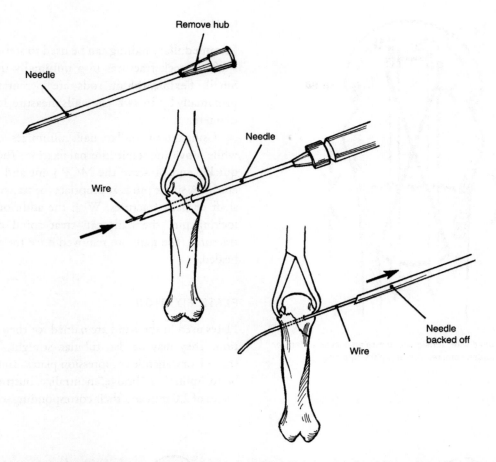

Figure 102.5. **Hypodermic needle as drilled wire passer.** 19-gauge hypodermic needle, with hub removed, can be used as drilled wire passer. Wire is passed through hollow needle bore, after which the needle is withdrawn.

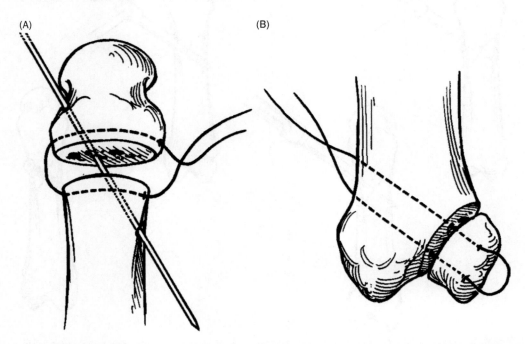

Figure 102.6. **Intraosseous wire suture.** A, Lister type A. Intraosseous portion of wire runs parallel to fracture line and single K-wire is added, passing from one cortex to another across fracture without entering joint. This fixation is used for shaft fractures. B, Lister type B. Intraosseous wire passes perpendicular to fracture line. Where the fragment is too small to drill, wire can be passed through the attached ligament, hard against bone.

NAILS

Intramedullary nailing can be used to stabilize metacarpal shaft or neck fractures in a minimally invasive fashion. Small, flexible, blunt rods are percutaneously passed proximally by an awl. The nails measure 1.1 or 1.6 mm in diameter.

Using intramedullary nails minimizes soft tissue trauma while providing stable internal fixation. They can be placed quickly and preserve the MCP joint and extensor mechanism. A single pin is appropriate for transverse metacarpal shaft or neck fractures. With the addition of a proximal locking pin, the nails can treat spiral or comminuted fractures. The nails are removed once the fracture site has healed.

PLATE FIXATION

Plates used in the hand are named for their form and function. They may be flat, tubular, straight, T-shaped or L-shaped, or dynamic compression plates. Their function may be to "splint" or "bridge," neutralize, buttress, or compress. Plates of 2.0 mm and their corresponding screws are used in

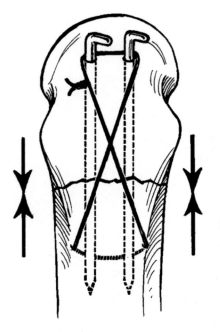

Figure 102.7. Tension band wire. Tension band wire on convex surface of reduced fracture provides compression at the fracture site.

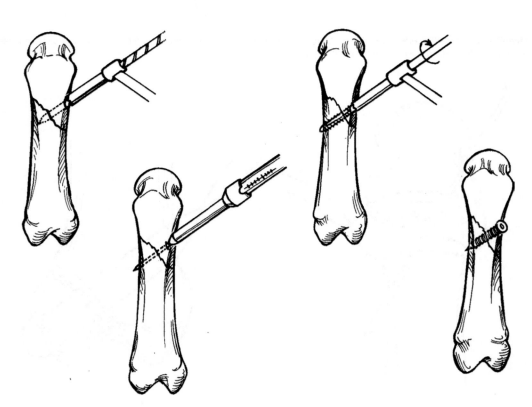

Figure 102.8. Lag screw fixation. Gliding hole is drilled in proximal fragment with bit, and smaller-diameter hole is made in distal fragment. Gliding hole is countersunk for screw head and screw length is determined with depth gauge. Hole is tapped and screw inserted.

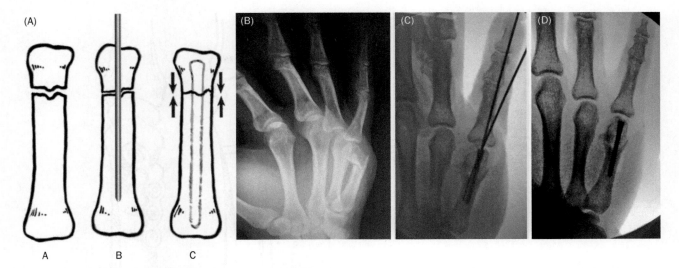

Figure 102.9 Metacarpal and phalangeal fractures may be fixed using cannulated headless screws. A K-wire is used as a guide, directed down the intramedullary canal over which the cannulated, headless compression screw is placed to reduce and fix the fracture (A). A clinical example is presented of a metacarpal fracture (B), where K-wires are used to stabilize the fracture reduction as well as act as a guide (C). The cannulated screw secures fixation (D).

the metacarpals or phalanges, and 2.7 mm plates and their corresponding screws are used for fractures in the metacarpal bones (Figure 102.10). Most fractures benefit from compression plating, which promotes healing and ensures ongoing bone-to-bone contact. Locking plates are usually implemented to bridge comminuted fractures while maintaining length. Newer plating systems have a lower profile than their earlier iterations because stronger alloys require less material to maintain the same strength. Double-row, three-dimensional plates have also been developed that allow shorter plates given the higher screw density; they boast a high load-to-failure compared to standard single-row plates. Newer plating systems are all highly polished in an attempt to limit tendon damage and tendon adhesions.[3]

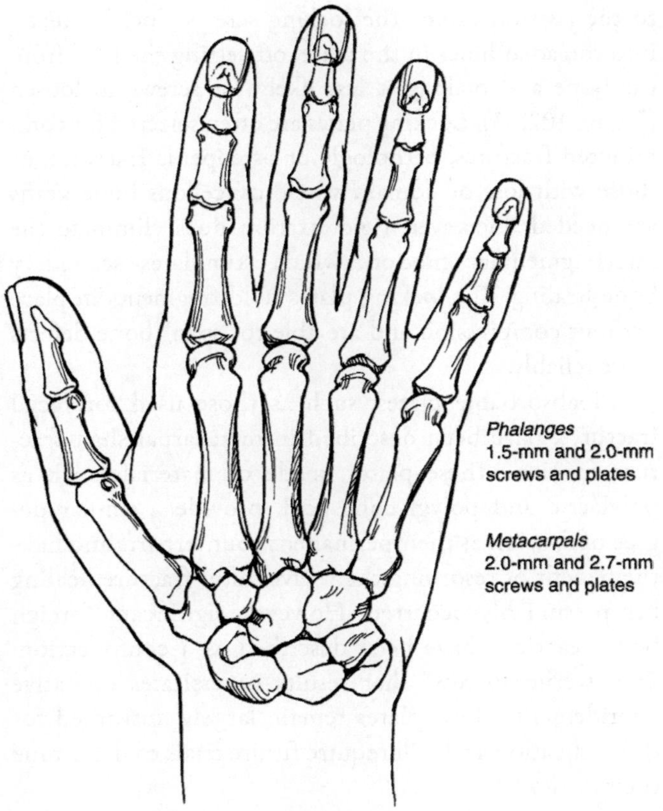

The mini-condylar plate may be useful for fractures just proximal to a phalangeal or metacarpal head (with or without a "T" component), where an ordinary plate would interfere with joint mechanics or require excessive dissection of collateral ligaments (Figure 102.11).

Nonlocking, traditional compression plates are useful. They are designed with a variable number of oval holes along the plate axis. The narrow portion of the hole is outward. Axial compression of fracture fragments using these implants is obtained by drilling a hole through the narrow portion of the hole into the bone. The screw is then engaged into the bone and tightened, causing the screw head to be forced into the wider portion of the plate hole, thus producing compression of the bone ends (Figure 102.12).

The bone and the plate share the load, and the friction between the bone ends stimulates healing.

Locking plates provide more stable fixation than conventional, nonlocking plating systems. Unlike compression plating, locking plates do not compress the plate to the cortical bone as securely, thus better preserving perfusion

Phalanges
1.5-mm and 2.0-mm
screws and plates

Metacarpals
2.0-mm and 2.7-mm
screws and plates

Figure 102.10. Guide to selection of plate and screw sizes for bones of hand.

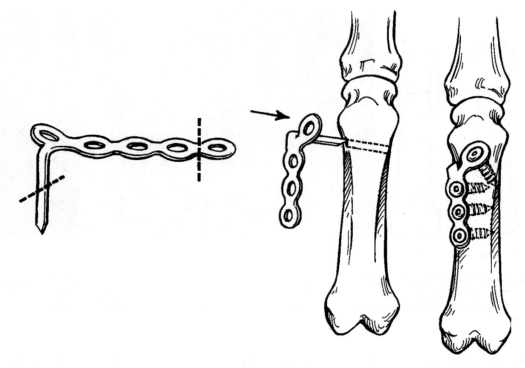

Figure 102.11. **Applying mini-condylar plate**. Length of intraosseous pin and diaphyseal part of plate must be adapted to local anatomy. They may have to be shortened with plate-cutting forceps. Transverse hole for pin is predrilled in distal fragment parallel to joint line. Pin is tentatively inserted to check and, if necessary, correct pin angle, and plate is contoured with bending pliers. Pin is inserted and distal plate screw is introduced and tightened; this screw may be lagged across fracture if desired. Finally, diaphyseal screws are introduced to produce interfragmental compression.

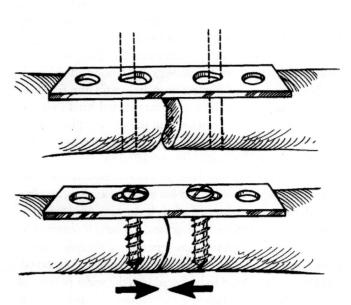

Figure 102.12. **Axial compression of fracture with dynamic compression plate**. Compression plates are designed with variable number of oval holes along plate axis. Narrow portion of hole is outward. Axial compression of fracture fragments using implants is obtained by drilling hole in narrow portion of hole into bone. Screw is then engaged and tightened, causing screw head to be forced into wider portion of plate hole, producing compression of bone ends.

to the cortical bone. The locking screws "lock" directly into threaded holes in the plate, off-setting the load from the bone and making it less likely for screws to loosen (Figure 102.13). Locking plates are often selected for comminuted fractures, pathologic or osteopenic fractures, or those with loss of domain where cancellous bone grafts are needed. However, rigid fixation does eliminate the interfragmentary motion, which stimulates secondary bone healing. The locking plates hold fragments in place without compression and are able to "span" bone defects more reliably.

Bioabsorbable plates, such as those used for facial fractures, have been described in metacarpal shaft fracture fixation. These plates, made of materials such as polylactic and polyglycolic acid, provide a similar degree of fixation as their permanent counterparts and have the benefit of resorbing themselves after fracture healing has presumably occurred. However, significant foreign body reactions have been described as a complication. The "sterile abscess" that results necessitates operative debridement. These plates remain largely unstudied for this indication and will require future trials to determine their utility.

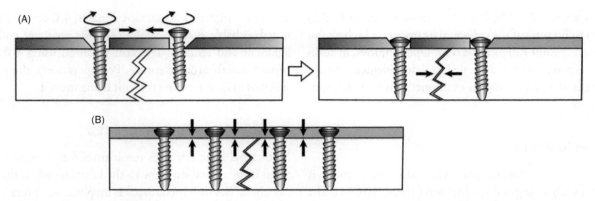

Figure 102.13 With compression plating, as the screws are tightened, they slide toward the fracture line, drawing the bone fragments together (A). With locking plating, the screws are rigidly fixed to the plate, drawing the bone fragments toward to the locking plate itself as opposed to the other fracture segments (B).

Plates are generally indicated when open reduction and fixation of metacarpal shaft fractures is required and the fracture line is not oblique enough to accommodate lag screws. If there has been bone loss, then a corticocancellous bone graft may be incorporated with the plate (and screw) fixation.

EXTERNAL SKELETAL FIXATION

External fixation for fracture repair is achieved using a number of systems. The most commonly used is the 2.5 mm mini-external fixator. The fixator has the following components:

- Pins with thread, 2.5 mm in diameter, 150 mm long

- Connecting rods, 4.0 mm in diameter, 60–200 mm long

- Swivel clamps in two sizes: 4.0/2.5 mm for use on K-wires and 4.0/4.0 mm clamp for assembling the connecting rods

- Schanz screws, 4.0 mm in diameter, with 2.7 and 3.5 mm threads for use with the 4.0 mm connecting rod

Two pins per major bone fragment, proximal and distal to the fracture site, are sufficient for most situations. The pin sites on the bone are exposed through longitudinal incisions held open with small retractors to minimize the risk of soft tissue injury. Before insertion of the pins, holes are predrilled with the 1.5 or 2.0 mm bit through the appropriate drill guide, which prevents overheating and necrosis of bone adjacent to the pin hole. The pins are inserted manually into each major bone fragment with a hand chuck. Pin holders are then applied to form the primary connection between the pins and the swivel clamps that are placed on a connecting bar to form the frame. After the correct position of the bones is secured, all the bolts on the swivel clamps are tightened. To obtain compression or distraction of the bone fragments, the bolt securing the sliding swivel clamp to the connecting bar is loosened and the wheel is turned. A single frame forms the basic frame in the hand and is sufficiently stable for most situations. Further stability can be obtained by adding a second frame, which can be triangulated or quadrangulated. Thus, a wide variety of configurations from simple to complex may be devised.

The mini-external fixator is useful in a variety of circumstances. It can be used temporarily until rigid fixation can be performed or definitively maintained until bone healing has occurred in open or complex fractures with extensive soft tissue loss, multiple fractures, and fractures complicated by bone loss.

External fixation may be dynamic or static. Dynamic external fixators have been effectively used for fracture-dislocations of the phalangeal joints in order to maintain range of motion while allowing for osseous healing. These fracture patterns are challenging and historically have had poorer outcomes.

OPERATIVE TECHNIQUES

METACARPAL HEAD FRACTURES

Head fractures may be nonarticular, intraarticular, or collateral ligament avulsion injuries. For the most part, these fractures are treated by closed methods and external immobilization. Noncomminuted fractures that have less than 25% of the articular surface involved with minimal fracture step-off (<1 mm) benefit from nonoperative management. Fractures with more extensive damage to the articular surface or with greater degrees of displacement are good candidates for operative intervention, principally with headless screws. The MCP joint is immobilized in flexion to avoid tightening of the collateral ligaments, which would permanently limit full joint flexion. Open injuries, in addition to fracture management, demand debridement of suppurative and necrotic tissue, combined with intravenous antibiotics.

Operative Technique

Exposure of the metacarpal head and MCP joint is obtained with a longitudinal incision (Figure 102.14). The MCP joint can be revealed by splitting the extensor tendon or by incising the sagittal band and retracting the tendon. The joint capsule is dissected free and opened separately. The periosteum is cut and reflected with a small periosteal elevator. If necessary, improved access may be obtained by taking down the ulnar collateral ligament. The radial collateral ligament of the fingers should generally be preserved because of the stability required in pinch motions against the thumb. (At the thumb MCP joint, in contrast, the ulnar collateral ligament is a more important stabilizing influence.) Fracture fragments are reduced using reduction forceps and fixed with K-wires, screws, or intraosseous wiring. Preference is given to the fixation technique that offers the highest stability and yet is secure enough to allow early active motion. On completion of the fixation, deep layers are closed with fine atraumatic sutures; 4-0 or 5-0 braided nonabsorbable suture may be used for repair of collateral ligament and tendon. The skin is closed using 4-0 interrupted nonabsorbable suture. Postoperatively, the joint is splinted in flexion when it is not being moved.

METACARPAL NECK FRACTURES

Metacarpal neck fractures result from direct impact, more often from an end-on blow to the knuckles when the fist is clenched. The fifth metacarpal is involved most often.

Neck fracture of the fifth metacarpal is called a boxer's fracture. Dorsal angulation and impaction are characteristic features. As a rule, minimal angulation, or angulation of less than 40 degrees, may be treated conservatively with splinting and functional exercises. Angulation of more than 40 degrees should be corrected by closed reduction, and a gutter splint or cast should be applied (Figure 102.15). Substantial residual angulation that cannot be reduced adequately with closed manipulation and stabilized, or rotational deformity that cannot be corrected, should be treated with percutaneous pin fixation or open reduction and internal fixation.

Closed reduction may be achieved using the Jahss maneuver (Figure 102.16). The affected MCP and PIP joints are flexed to 90 degrees. Dorsal force is then applied to both

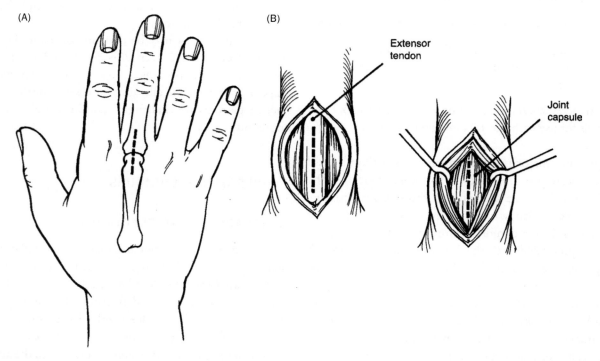

(A) (B)

Extensor tendon

Joint capsule

Figure 102.14. **Surgical approach to metacarpal head and opening of metacarpophalangeal (MCP) joint.** A, skin incision. Longitudinal incision is used for exposing MCP joint. B, deep layers. Extensor tendon is incised longitudinally, and separate longitudinal incision is made in capsule and periosteum. On completion of fixation, both structures are closed with fine atraumatic sutures.

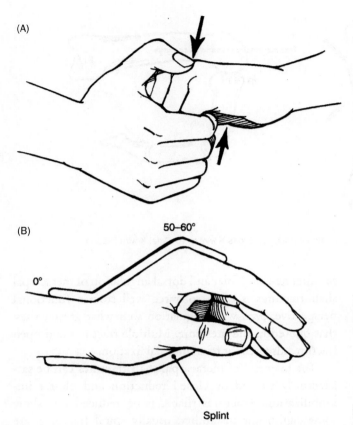

(A)

(B)

50–60°

0°

Splint

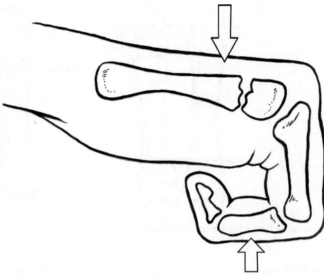

Figure 102.16. With the MCP joint flexed at 90 degrees, the collateral ligaments on the joint are tight and therefore allow for controlled maneuvering of the distal metacarpal fragment. Likewise, in this position, the deforming forces from the intrinsic muscles are relaxed, allowing for easier manipulation of the fracture fragments. In this position with the phalanges fully flexed, downward pressure is placed on the proximal fragment directly and upward pressure is placed indirectly on the distal fragment via the associated middle phalanx.

Figure 102.15. **Closed reduction method for Boxer's fracture. Anesthesia is obtained using ulnar nerve block.** Injection is made just beneath flexor carpi ulnaris tendon. Aspiration ensures that adjacent ulnar artery has not been penetrated; 3 to 5 mL of lidocaine without epinephrine is injected using 1.5-cm 25-gauge needle. Dorso-ulnar wheal is also injected to secure anesthesia of dorsal cutaneous branch of ulnar nerve. (A) closed reduction is accomplished by flexing MCP joint maximally, which relaxes deforming interosseous muscle and tightens collateral ligament, allowing proximal phalanx to exert leverage on metacarpal head. Axial traction is applied to exaggerate deformity and disimpact fragments. Metacarpal head is then pushed dorsally with flexed proximal phalanx, while downward pressure is exerted over apex of dorsally angulated fracture. (B) gutter splint or case (extending but not including the proximal interphalangeal joints of uninvolved and adjacent fingers) is applied with wrist in neutral position and MCP joints in 50 to 60 degrees of flexion. General principle of fracture splinting is to immobilize at least joint proximal to and joint immediately distal to fracture site.

the metacarpal head and the proximal phalanx to reduce the fracture. This positioning stresses the collateral ligaments of the MCP joint, improving the likelihood of successful reduction and enables stabilization of the small fragment for leveraged fracture reduction.

Operative Technique

The incisions and approach are similar to those for head fractures. A dorsal longitudinal incision and fixation with K-wires or tension band wiring are suitable (Figure 102.17)

Fixation can be achieved by placing longitudinal or oblique K-wires or by stabilizing the fracture segments to an adjacent metacarpal. Mini-condylar plates with a lower profile are available, which lend themselves to internal fixation if required for more stability. Postoperatively, a splint is applied. A removable splint is substituted and active range of motion exercises are started as soon as fracture stability allows.

The same techniques are used for angulated neck fractures of the remaining metacarpals. Open reduction is often necessary because, unlike fractures of the fifth metacarpal, considerable residual angulation cannot be compensated by motion at the carpometacarpal (CMC) joint and can cause a painful palmar mass and extensor lag. Angulation of more than 15 degrees is quoted as unacceptable for fractures of the second and third metacarpal necks, and more than 30 degrees is not acceptable for fracture of the fourth metacarpal neck, but in practice we often allow for somewhat greater angulation.

METACARPAL SHAFT FRACTURES

Shaft fractures may be transverse, oblique, spiral, or comminuted or result in segmental loss. Acute segmental bone loss

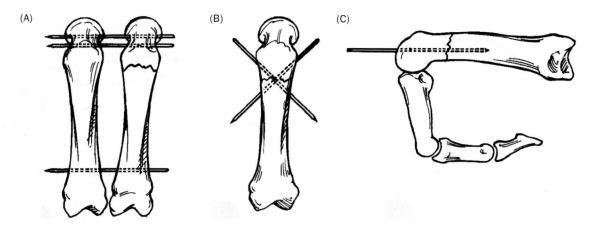

Figure 102.17 **K-wire fixation for metacarpal fractures.** (A) Transfixation to adjacent metacarpal. (B) Cross K-wires. (C) Axial K-wire fixation.

is common with open and complex injuries. These fractures are susceptible to malrotation, shortening, and angulation attributable in part to the deforming forces generated by the intrinsic muscles (Figure 102.18). Shortening by more than 1 cm results in a significant loss of intrinsic muscle contractile force, based on the Blix curve, and is an indication

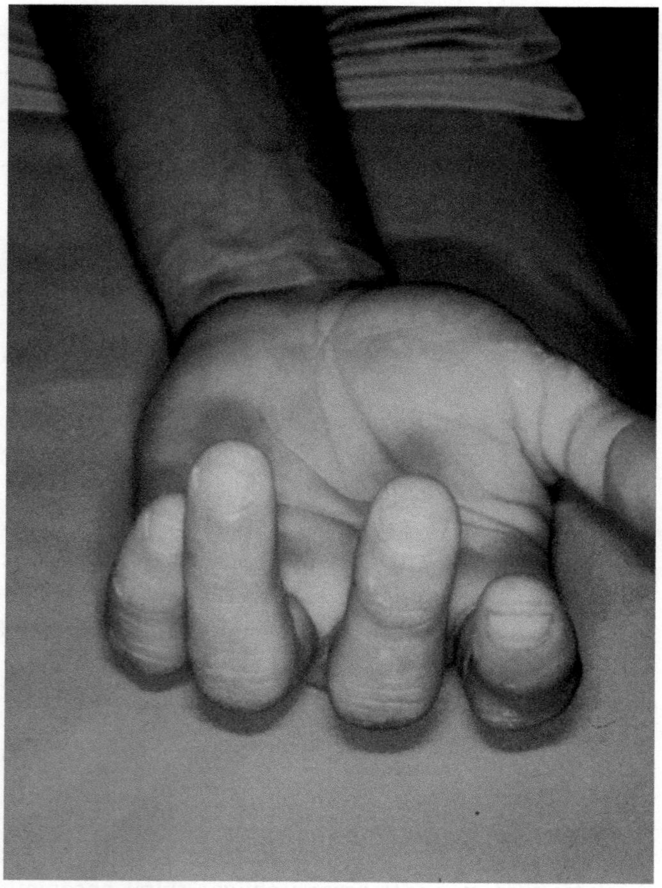

for intervention. Volar and dorsal angulation of metacarpal shaft fractures is often tolerated well from a functional perspective, even with angulation somewhat greater than that quoted in the literature. Multiple fractures and open fractures also benefit from internal fixation.

The majority of metacarpal shaft fractures can be satisfactorily treated by closed reduction and plaster immobilization. Fractures that can be reduced but show some significant instability, usually spiral fractures, are treated by closed reduction and percutaneous K-wire fixation or intramedullary nail placement. Two methods are used: (1) transfixation K-wires to the adjacent metacarpal and (2) intramedullary K-wire placement or pinning. Intramedullary fixation has gained traction recently, even with spiral, oblique, and comminuted fractures, now that devices have been developed to lock the intramedullary rod in place with pins or screws.

Displaced metacarpal shaft fractures that can be reduced closed but are unstable may be fixated percutaneously with pins or intramedullary nails. Intramedullary nails can be applied to spiral fractures and even those with rotational deformity, shortening, or a moderate amount of comminution if the nail is later secured with a locking pin. K-wires can be used in a similar fashion.

Operative Technique

Exposure is through a longitudinal incision overlying the involved bone (Figure 102.19). The extensor tendon is carefully elevated and retracted. A junctura tendinea may be divided to allow tendon retraction and later repaired. The periosteum is cut longitudinally and reflected, revealing the fracture.

The fracture is reduced with reduction forceps and fixed using K-wires, tension band wire, screws, or plates.

Figure 102.18 The ring finger is visibly malrotated in this clinical photograph, causing scissoring with the other digits.

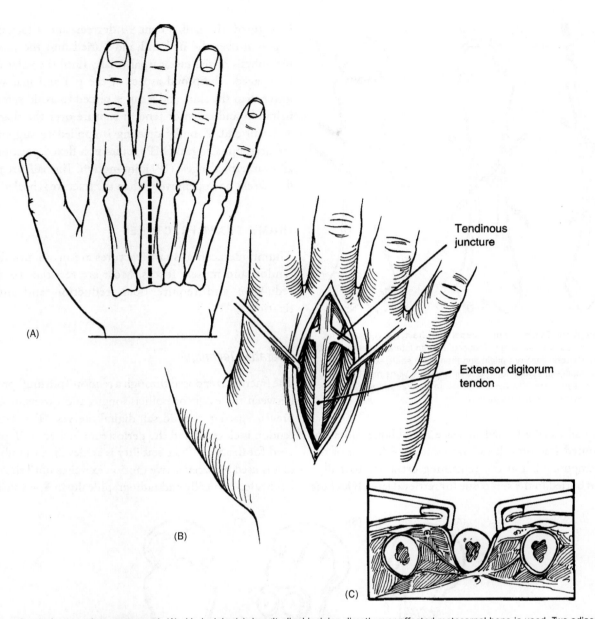

Figure 102.19 **Surgical approach to metacarpal.** (A) skin incision(s). Longitudinal incision directly over affected metacarpal bone is used. Two adjacent metacarpals may be exposed by single interosseous longitudinal incision between two metacarpals. (B) topography of superficial layers with veins and nerve fibers retracted. Extensor tendon with juntura tendonae are shown running coaxially with metacarpal bone. (C) periosteum is cut longitudinally and sparingly reflected to display fracture fragment. Fracture is reduced with reduction forceps and fixed using K-wires, tension band wire, screws, or plates, depending on nature of injury and loading of bone. Periosteum is sutured, reapproximating partially stripped interossei muscles and preventing adhesions with overlying tendon.

Transverse and short oblique fractures are best fixed with a plate, especially the more mobile second and fifth metacarpals. Long oblique or spiral fractures are fixed with K-wires or screws (Figures 102.20 and 102.21). Comminuted fractures are fixed with K-wires and, if needed, receive bone grafts. Postoperatively, a removable splint is worn and active motion exercises initiated as soon as stability is achieved.

For closed reduction percutaneous fixation, K-wires or intramedullary nails are proposed for fixation, with the latter technique subsequently described (Figure 102.22). The fracture must be easily reducible. A stab incision is made over the metacarpal base and scissors are used to bluntly dissect down to dorsal bone, avoiding injury to the overlying extensor tendons. An awl penetrates the cortex, and a 1.1 or 1.6 mm flexible, pre-bent, blunt nail is placed in the medullary canal. Under fluoroscopic guidance, the nail is passed across the fracture site and advanced into the subchondral bone of the distal fragment.

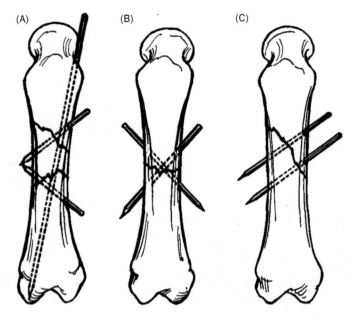

Figure 102.20. **K-wire fixation for metacarpal shaft fractures.** A, fixation for comminuted fracture. K-wire is introduced through lateral aspect of head in area of collateral ligament origin and then down shaft, so that wire does not remain within MCP joint. One or two more wires may be placed obliquely for added stability. B, crossed K-wire fixation for transverse fracture. C, fixation for oblique fracture.

The nail can be locked in place for oblique, spiral, or comminuted fractures. If not necessary, the handle of the nail is amputated, and the remaining extraosseous nail is bent and buried in the soft tissue for retrieval later. If locking

is required, the nail is bent 90 degrees, and a locking pin is passed over the nail end and buried into the proximal metaphysis of the metacarpal volarly until the volar cortex is engaged. The proud aspect of the pin and nail are cut lower than the skin, and a cap is placed to avoid soft tissue irritation and extensor tendon rupture over the sharp pin and nail end. A bulky dressing is applied to support the metacarpophalangeal (MP) joints in a flexed position and allow interphalangeal (IP) joint motion. The nail is removed 4–8 weeks postoperatively when the fracture is healed.

THUMB SHAFT FRACTURES

Thumb metacarpal shaft fractures are made unstable by tendon and muscle forces. Most are resistant to closed reduction and require open reduction and internal fixation.

Operative Technique

The fracture is exposed through a tendon-splitting approach between the extensor pollicis longus and extensor pollicis brevis, sparing the dorsal digital nerves. The extensor tendon is elevated and the periosteum incised. A T-plate is used for fixation. Once stability is achieved, a thumb spica cast is used between active motion exercises until the injury has healed clinically and radiographically in 4–6 weeks.

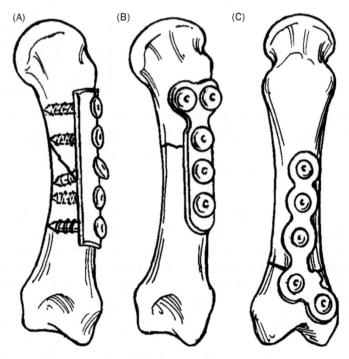

Figure 102.21. **Plate fixation for metacarpal shaft fractures.** Different plates are used, depending on fracture type. A, quarter tubular plate with interfragmental lag screw for oblique fracture. B, dorsal T-plate for distal transverse fracture. C, mini-condylar plate for fracture close to joint.

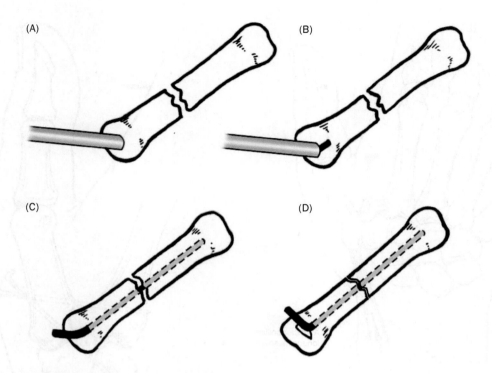

Figure 102.22 Intramedullary nailing for metacarpal neck or shaft fractures.

BASE FRACTURES

Isolated fractures of second, third, and fourth metacarpal bases are not common because of the strong support of ligaments and paucity of motion of the CMC joint. Fractures of the base of the fifth metacarpal and thumb metacarpal are more common.

Fractures of the fifth metacarpal base are frequently intraarticular and accompanied by subluxation of the CMC joint. The displacement is accentuated by the pull of extensor carpi ulnaris (Figure 102.23). These injuries are handled by closed reduction, using finger traps, distal traction, and percutaneous pinning to the adjacent intact metacarpal or carpal bones. The pins are cut off beneath the skin, and a short arm cast that leaves the MCP joints free is applied and worn for 2 weeks. Finger motion is started as soon as fracture stability allows, with pin removal at 4–8 weeks. Open reduction is required if closed reduction cannot be achieved. A dorsal incision and fixation with a mini-fragment T-plate are used.

Thumb metacarpal base fractures are extraarticular or intraarticular. Extraarticular fractures are treated similarly to other metacarpal fractures. Intraarticular fractures are more challenging and occur in two distinct patterns: Bennett fracture and Rolando fracture.

The *Bennett fracture* is a fracture-dislocation injury (Figure 102.24), characterized by a small, nondisplaced intraarticular metacarpal fragment with displacement

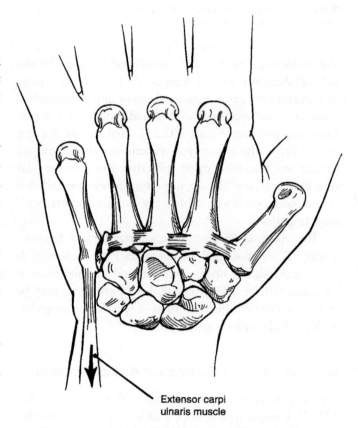

Extensor carpi
ulnaris muscle

Figure 102.23 **Fracture of base of fifth metacarpal.** Fracture of base of fifth metacarpal bone is often seen with proximal and dorsal subluxation or sometimes even complete dislocation. Deforming force is insertion of extensor carpi ulnaris tendon, which is analogous to Bennett's fracture of thumb and is sometimes called reverse Bennett's fracture. Fracture is often managed successfully by closed reduction and percutaneous pinning.

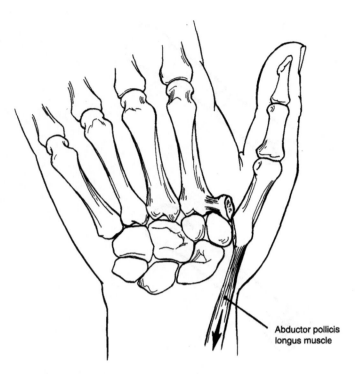

Figure 102.24. **Bennett fracture.** Bennett fracture is fracture-dislocation of thumb metacarpal. Abductor pollicis longus pulls thumb metacarpal proximally, causing it to dislocate.

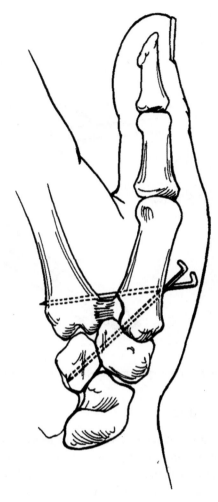

Figure 102.25. **Percutaneous K-wire fixation for Bennett's fracture.** Fracture is reduced with initial longitudinal traction on proximal and distal phalanges of thumb and countertraction on forearm. Thumb is pronated and a K-wire is drilled from first metacarpal into carpus. It is not necessary to secure small palmar- ulnar fragment. Second wire is drilled through first and second metacarpal bones. Portable intraoperative fluoroscoppy is used to assess fracture reduction and to aid in placement of K-wires.

and dislocation of the metacarpal shaft (caused by the pull of abductor pollicis longus [APL]). This fracture-dislocation requires accurate reduction and stabilization, sometimes accomplished with closed reduction and percutaneous pinning (Figure 102.25). Reduce the fracture by mobilizing the metacarpal in extension, abduction and pronation Otherwise, open reduction and internal fixation are necessary. The open method is recommended if closed reduction is not satisfactory and for fractures with large fragments.

The *Rolando fracture* is an intraarticular fracture, usually T- or Y-shaped in configuration. Treatment is individualized, but open reduction and internal fixation are often required. Fractures with comminution may be treated in a thumb spica cast for 4–6 weeks. The prognosis with marked comminution is poor.

Operative Technique (Bennett and Rolando Fracture)

The surgical approach is radiovolar (Figures 102.26 and 102.27). It begins with a "hockey stick," or L-shaped, incision (Wagner approach) with the long component centered over the metacarpal and the transverse component over the thenar eminence's proximal transverse crease. The small superficial radial nerve branches are protected. The APL is retracted. The

thenar muscles are sparingly stripped aside and the joint opened transversely. The fracture is reduced and fixed with K-wires, screws, or a small T-plate. After postoperative splinting, motion is started when fracture stability allows. A removable thumb spica splint is used between active motion exercises until the injury has healed clinically and radiographically in 4–6 weeks.

METACARPOPHALANGEAL JOINT FRACTURES

The proximal phalanx may be injured by axial loading forces or collateral ligament avulsion of a periarticular bone fragment (or by physeal injury in children). Articular fragments involving less than 20% of the joint are treated with buddy-taping for 6 weeks. Active and passive mobilization are

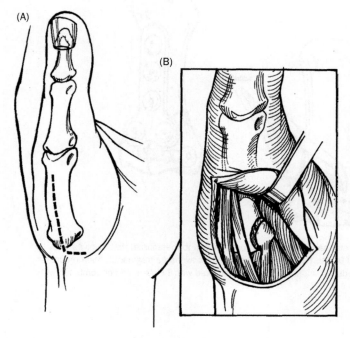

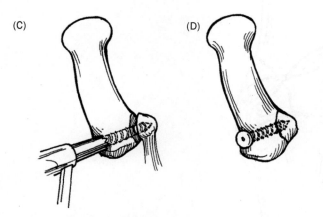

Figure 102.26. **Surgical approach for open reduction and screw fixation of Bennett fracture.** (A) skin incision with possible extensions. Incision is L-shaped with long component centered over metacarpal bone at junction of palmar skin and dorsal skin, and transverse component over proximal crease of thenar eminence. (B) thenar muscles are stripped aside and joint opened. Joint exposure is improved by elevating abductor pollicis longus tendon off its distal insertion along with joint capsular flap. (C) before reduction, gliding hole is drilled in large fragment. Fracture is reduced and held with forceps. (D) thread hole is drilled through insert sleeve, taped, and screw inserted.

encouraged. Articular involvement of more than 20% requires open reduction and internal fixation with K-wires. Comminuted fractures are reduced openly and sometimes bone-grafted.

Fractures involving the thumb proximal phalanx are usually ligamentous avulsion fractures that affect the radial or ulnar aspects of the bone and are often associated with MCP joint instability. Injuries to the ulnar collateral ligament that occur by forceful hyperextension and abduction

are "gamekeeper fractures." If nondisplaced, they are treated closed with cast immobilization. If they are significantly displaced and involve a large portion of the joint surface, open reduction and internal fixation are indicated. Extremely small fragments are fixed by 26-gauge tension-band wiring or intraosseous wiring; larger fragments are stabilized by K-wires supplemented with 26- or 28-gauge wire. Screws are reserved for large fragments that exceed three times the screw diameter. The fracture is exposed through a dorsal extensor aponeurosis-splitting incision. Postoperatively, a thumb spica cast is worn for 4 weeks (Figure 102.28).

Osteochondral metacarpal head intraarticular fractures occur from jamming injuries. They may be difficult to see on standard radiographs and Brewerton view, and a CT scan may be required. The intraarticular fragments may cause joint "locking." Headless screws enable secure fixation (Figure 102.29).

DISTAL PHALANX FRACTURE

Fractures of the distal phalanx are the most commonly encountered hand fracture (Table 102.5). The mechanism of injury is most commonly a crush injury causing a "tuft fracture," which is often accompanied by significant soft tissue damage. Treatment is wound care and protection. When debridement is necessary, the nail is preserved or replaced to help splint the soft tissues. In closed injuries with subungual hematoma, decompression may be required for pain relief; this is performed sterilely using a nail drill or fine cautery device. A subungual hematoma of greater than 50% of the nailbed was believed to indicate a significant nailbed laceration, necessitating nail removal and suture repair. Recent literature, however, suggests that this practice does not improve outcomes.

Protective splinting of the bone is required for 2–3 weeks. A foam-backed aluminum splint is applied that includes only the distal joint. Injuries with soft tissue disruption sufficient for the phalanx to lose stability require internal splinting, effected by longitudinal K-wire fixation. A technique that uses a syringe-mounted 18- or 20- gauge hypodermic needle hand-drilled into bone can be used (Figure 102.30). This technique is employed in the emergency room or office, where power equipment may not be available. Fractures that proceed to symptomatic nonunion have been effectively treated with cortical mini-screws, either in an open or percutaneous fashion. Soft tissue reconstruction helps to stabilize fracture fragments and may range from simple

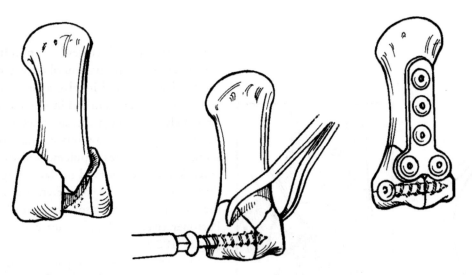

Figure 102.27. **Internal fixation of Rolando's fracture.** Rolando's fracture is T- or Y-pattern fracture at base of thumb metacarpal that involves volar lip and large dorsal lip fragment. It can be considered as type of comminuted Bennett's fracture. If fracture has two large fragments, open reduction and internal fixation are possible. L-shaped incision is used. Fracture is reduced under direct vision and fixed with T-plate alone or combined with preliminary screw fixation of joint fragment, depending on injury type.

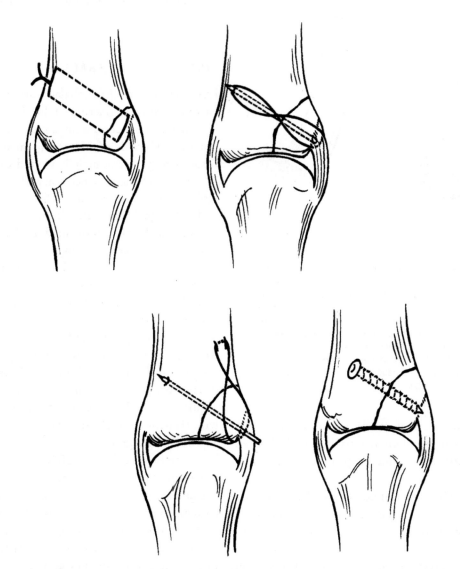

Figure 102.28. **Fixation of "game keeper's fracture".** Method depends on size of fragment. Extremely small fragments are most safely secured by 26-gauge tension band wiring, and Lister type B intraosseous wiring is suitable for larger fragments, stabilized by a 0.035-or 0.028-in K-wire, supplemented with 26-or 28-gauge wire. Screws should be reserved for large fragments that exceed three times the screw diameter in size.

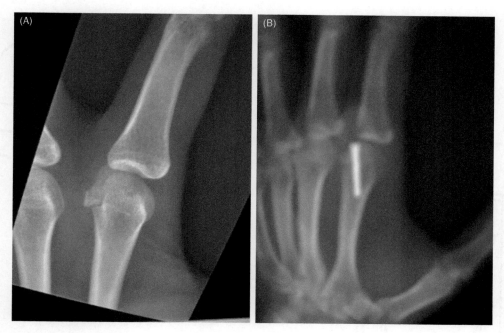

Figure 102.29. Headless screw fixation.

nail bed repair to local flaps, such as a cross-finger subcutaneous flap.

In pediatric patients, Salter I or II fractures of the distal phalanx physis in conjunction with avulsion of the proximal nail edge are called *Seymour fractures*. These are extraarticular, open fractures of distal phalanx base. They are often confused with simple mallet fingers and incorrectly splinted as sole treatment. The germinal matrix is open, interposed between the fracture fragments, leading to incomplete reduction and ultimately malunion with residual pseudo-mallet or flexion deformity.

Operative Technique

In the operating room, the nail is removed, and the open fracture is debrided and copiously irrigated. All

TABLE 102.5 CLASSIFICATION OF DISTAL PHALANGEAL FRACTURES

Distal: tuft fractures
Simple
Comminuted

Central: shaft fractures
Stable: soft tissues provide stability
Unstable: soft tissues are disrupted sufficiently for phalanx to lose stability

Proximal: articular fractures
Palmar articular
Dorsal articular (mallet fractures)
Epiphyseal separation

interposed tissue in the fracture line is completely removed. The fracture is reduced and fixed with K-wire as previously described, the nailbed repaired, and the nail fold stented.

MIDDLE AND PROXIMAL PHALANX FRACTURES

Middle and proximal phalangeal fractures that are stable and not displaced are treated nonoperatively. Stable, nondisplaced, extraarticular fractures are addressed with buddy-taping for 3–4 weeks. Less stable fractures such as spiral, oblique or comminuted fracture patterns require splinting for up to 3 weeks followed by buddy-taping, and they should be more closely monitored for instability. Displaced fractures are managed by closed reduction via axial traction and plaster immobilization with the hand placed in a gutter splint with the MCP joints flexed at 70 degrees, the PIP joints at neutral to 20 degrees, and the wrist placed in extension of 20 degrees (Figure 102.31). Hand-based splints and buddy-taping (Figure 102.32) are used once adequate healing has taken place, indicated by absence of tenderness over the fracture site. Closed reduction is achieved and maintained by maximally flexing the MCP joint to stabilize the proximal fragment and applying flexion distally. If the fracture can be reduced but shows instability, percutaneous K-wire fixation is attempted. Closed pinning works well for oblique or spiral fractures (Figure 102.33). K-wires placed obliquely address transverse or short oblique fractures and control rotation. Spiral

(A)   (B)

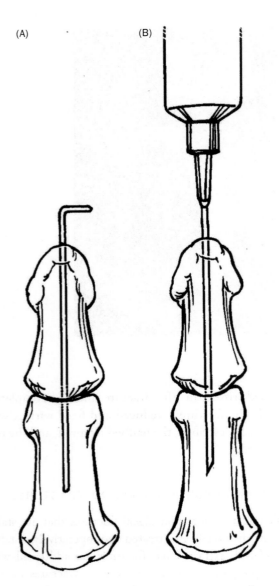

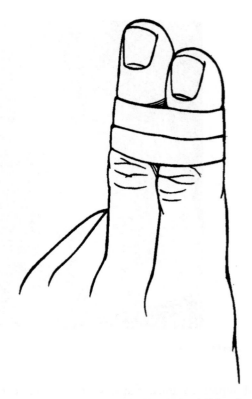

Figure 102.32. **Buddy-taping technique.** Taping of injured digit to its neighbor permits early protected motion.

Figure 102.30. **Shaft fracture of distal phalanx.** (A) stabilization of displaced shaft fracture of distal phalanx with longitudinal K-wire, which is removed at 4 weeks. (B) internal splinting can be achieved with 18- or 20-gauge hypodermic needle (on syringe) that is drilled into bone.

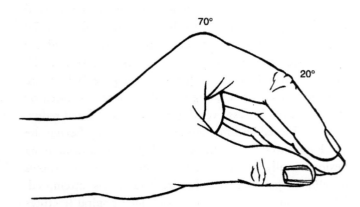

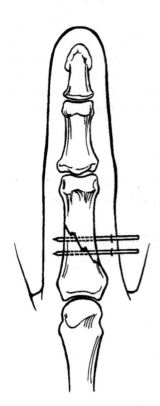

Figure 102.31. **Position of hand immobilization.** "Safe position" should be used wheneverpossible in treating phalangeal fractures. The MCP joint is flexed 70 degrees to avoid shortening of collateral ligaments, which occurs when immobilized in extension. PIP joints are held in 20 degrees of flexion to prevent contractures of involved collateral ligaments and volar plate, which occurs in flexion.

Figure 102.33. **Closed reduction and percutaneous pinning of oblique phalangeal fracture.** Fracture is reduced using longitudinal traction and compressed using tenacular clamp, while K-wires are drilled transversely across fracture.

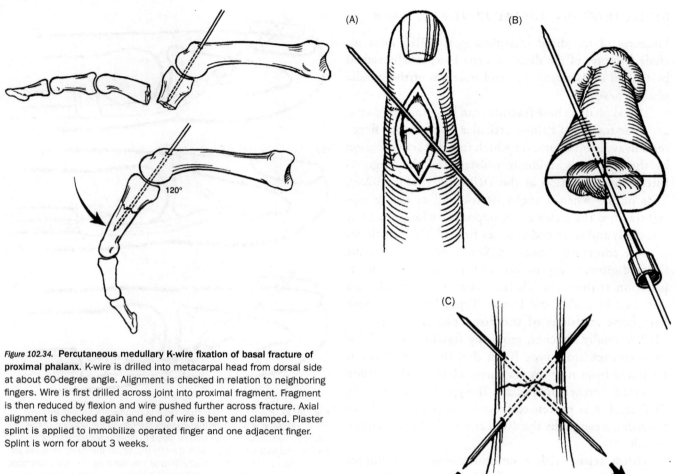

Figure 102.34. **Percutaneous medullary K-wire fixation of basal fracture of proximal phalanx.** K-wire is drilled into metacarpal head from dorsal side at about 60-degree angle. Alignment is checked in relation to neighboring fingers. Wire is first drilled across joint into proximal fragment. Fragment is then reduced by flexion and wire pushed further across fracture. Axial alignment is checked again and end of wire is bent and clamped. Plaster splint is applied to immobilize operated finger and one adjacent finger. Splint is worn for about 3 weeks.

Figure 102.35. **Open reduction with retrograde cross-pinning of transverse phalangeal fracture.** (A) "preview pin" is held over reduced fracture to help plan pin direction and angle of entry. (B) large needle may be used as drill guide to prevent pin slipping along cortex. Pins are drilled so that they are through middle of medullary canal in coronal plane. Pins are drilled through cortex and then backed up to level of fracture surface. (C) fracture is reduced and fracture ends are compressed, while two pins are drilled retrograde into other fragment.

and long oblique fractures tend toward rotational deformity and may require secure reduction with bone clamps prior to fixation with compression screws or K-wires placed at right angles to the fracture line. For basal transverse fractures of the proximal phalanx, excellent results have been obtained with a medullary K-wire inserted percutaneously across the MCP joint (Figure 102.34). Whenever possible, transfixing the extensor tendons should be avoided. Open reduction-internal fixation is required when the preceding percutaneous methods are not possible.

Operative Technique

For fractures of the middle phalanx and distal shaft of the proximal phalanx, a dorsal longitudinal incision is used. Exposure is obtained by incising between the central slip and lateral bands, avoiding injury to the central slip. The periosteum is dissected free and elevated. Fracture fragments are reduced and fixed with K-wires or screws. Transverse fractures are best fixed with K-wire, using one

of two methods: retrograde cross-pinning (Figure 102.35) or direct cross-pinning. Oblique or spiral fractures are fixed with parallel K-wires or small screws.

A longitudinal extensor tendon-splitting incision is used for fractures involving the proximal portion of the proximal phalanx. A separate longitudinal incision is made in the periosteum. Fixation is accomplished as described earlier. On completion of the fixation, deep layers are closed with fine atraumatic sutures; 4-0 or 5-0 braided nonabsorbable sutures may be used for tendons. Postoperatively, motion is started as soon as fracture stability allows.

DISTAL INTERPHALANGEAL JOINT FRACTURES

Fractures of the distal interphalangeal (DIP) joint include fractures of the distal phalanx base, usually caused by tendon avulsion injuries, and fractures of the middle phalanx head.

Distal phalanx base fractures can be palmar or dorsal articular fractures. Palmar articular fractures are flexor tendon avulsion injuries in which forceful active flexion by the patient is suddenly resisted and the finger is forced into extension at the DIP joint (Table 102.6). This occurs when a rugby or football tackler grasps tightly onto the jersey of an opponent who pulls away forcefully and is termed a "jersey finger." The ring finger is most commonly involved. With these injuries, the flexor digitorum profundus (FDP) is avulsed from its insertion at the distal phalanx base. These injuries are classified by Leddy and Packer. Types III and IV both have bone avulsions of the distal phalanx where the FDP normally attaches, requiring fixation. Type IV is distinguished from type III in that the tendon also is separated from its bony fragment, allowing the tendon to retract further proximally. In type III injuries, the FDP tendon is prevented from retracting as the bone fragment is caught by the distal end of the flexor tendon sheath.

Direct repair with a suture-over-button technique may be accomplished in the first 2 weeks after injury, although repair can be prolonged up to 4 weeks (Figure 102.36). It is important to operate within 4 weeks as tendon retraction will occur, and adequate advancement of the tendon may be impossible or result in quadriga. At this point, DIP fusion should be considered. More recently, bone anchors have been used to directly suture the tendon end to the distal phalanx. These are appropriate techniques for smaller fracture fragments. For larger fragments, treatment is open reduction and internal fixation, using the Bunnell technique for repair with additional K-wires if necessary. The repair requires

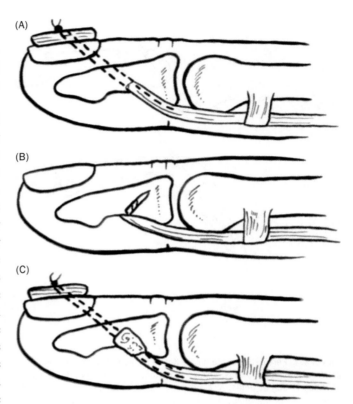

Figure 102.36. The traditional suture-over-button technique secures the tendon in place with suture that passes through to the dorsum of the digit (A). Bone anchors can also be used to directly secure the distal tendon end to the distal phalanx directly (B). When the injury includes an avulsed piece of bone that is attached to the distal tendon end, that bone fragment may also be secured to the distal phalanx using a suture-over-button technique (C).

3 weeks of protective splinting, followed by functional exercises. The pull-out wire is removed at 4–6 weeks postoperatively.

Dorsal articular fractures, or mallet fractures, are avulsion fractures of the extensor tendon insertion. They are typically caused by an axial load disrupting the terminal extensor mechanism with an associated bone fragment. Most can be treated by splinting in full

TABLE 102.6 LEDDY AND PACKER CLASSIFICATION OF FLEXOR TENDON AVULSION INJURIES

Type I: The tendon end is located in the palm with both vencula ruptured.

Type II: The tendon, along with a small bone fragment from the distal phalanx, retracts to the level of the proximal interphalangeal joint with an intact venculum.

Type III: The lesion is associated with a large bony fragment.

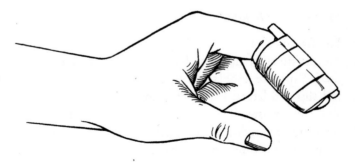

Figure 102.37. Method of splinting for mallet fracture.

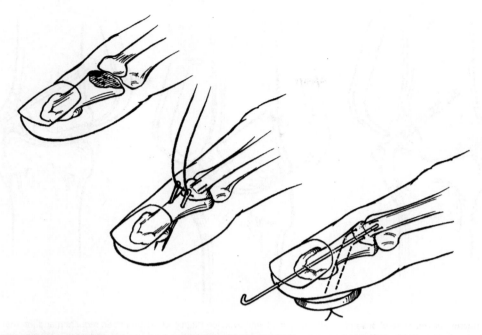

Figure 102.38. **Dorsal articular fracture (mallet fracture): repair using Bunnell pullout suture technique.** Fracture fragment is held in place with monofilament wire or monofilament nonabsorbable suture, passed through extensor tendon and palmar aspect of finger through distal phalanx. Straight needles in drill may be passed through distal phalanx to guide suture through bone. Wire or suture is tied over bolus or button underpadded with cotton. Transarticular longitudinal K-wire is used to keep joint in neutral position (K-wire protects extensor tendor at its insertion). Fingertip is checked often to avoid undue pressure from button and cotton. Wire or suture may be removed after 4 to 6 weeks by cutting one strand and pulling steadily on other.

extension for 6–8 weeks with an additional 4 weeks of night splinting (Figure 102.37). It is important to leave the PIP joint free to avoid loss of range of motion. Open reduction and internal fixation are recommended for fractures with volar subluxation and on occasion for larger fragments that involve more than 30% of the articular surface (Figure 102.38).

Occurring in torsional injuries at the DIP joint, fractures of the middle phalanx head are condylar-type fractures and can be classified as follows: Grade 1 is nondisplaced and treated by finger splinting for 3 weeks, followed by motion exercises. Grade 2 is unicondylar, displaced, and often requires open reduction and fixation with fine K-wires versus closed reduction with percutaneous pinning. The small size of fracture fragments at this level precludes the application of other internal fixation techniques, such as fixation with screws or small condyle plates. Grade 3 is bicondylar, comminuted, and usually sustained by direct trauma: it cannot be anatomically reduced and requires open reduction. This lesion may require arthrodesis or even amputation, depending on the extent of soft tissue damage.

Surgically, the DIP joint is approached dorsally through a Y- or H-shaped skin incision (Figure 102.39). The capsule is dissected free and opened to expose the joint.

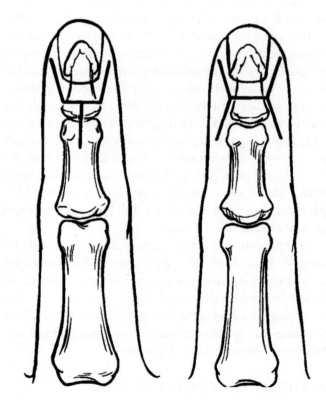

Figure 102.39. **Approach to DIP joint.** DIP joint is approached through dorsal Y- or H-shaped skin incision.

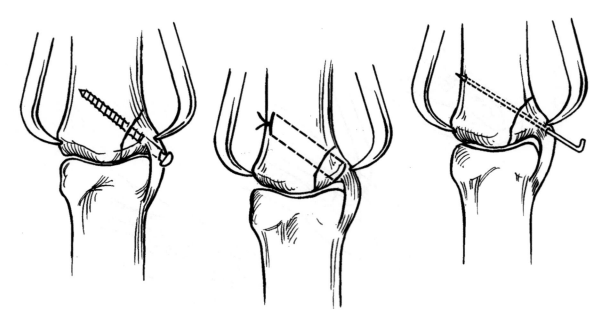

Figure 102.40. **Avulsion fracture at volar lateral base of middle phalanx.** Large avulsion fragments require open reduction and internal fixation. Small screws, Lister type B intraosseous wiring, or K-wires, often supplemented with tension band wire, can be used. This technique allows early active range of motion, which is so important in restoring functional integrity.

Operative Technique: Jersey Finger

After opening the volar skin via Bruner incisions from the PIP joint to the distal fingertip, the flexor tendon sheath is visualized. A transverse incision is made distal to the A2 pulley, and the injury is explored to find the avulsed tendon end. The Bruner incisions may be extended if the tendon has retracted proximally, or an additional incision can be made just proximal to the A1 pulley to explore the injury. The tendon is guided to its anatomic location through the flexor tendon sheath. For type III and IV injuries, the fragment may be fixated with K-wire, a mini-fragment screw, or intraosseous wire. To reattach the tendon, small holes are traditionally drilled through the bone and nail plate. After performing a Bunnell weave of the tendon end, a wire suture-passer or Keith needle is used to guide the suture ends through the drill holes, which are tied over a button on top of the nail.

The invention of bone anchors has streamlined this surgery. Instead of the suture-over-button technique, bone anchors are used to anchor permanent sutures to the desired location on the volar distal phalanx where the avulsion occurred, allowing the tendon to be secured directly to the bone. Postoperative rehabilitation is essential and may follow the Duran or Kleinert protocols.

PROXIMAL INTERPHALANGEAL JOINT FRACTURES

Fractures at the PIP joint may affect either the middle or proximal phalanx. Fractures of the middle phalanx are more common and include avulsion and intraarticular base or plateau fractures. Avulsion fractures usually occur from tension-avulsion of the bone insertion of the collateral ligament and involve the volar lateral aspect of the bone. The objectives of treatment are restoration of ligamentous and joint integrity, stability, and function. Small fragments may need no treatment or simple buddy-taping for 14–18 days, followed by motion exercises. Large fragments of more than 40% of the joint surface are managed with closed reduction. Additional stabilization with transarticular percutaneous oblique or extraarticular buttressing K-wires may be necessary. If open reduction is needed, smaller fragments are excised and the ligament repaired. Occasionally, an avulsed fragment is large enough that it can be openly reduced and secured with K-wires, often supplemented with a tension band wire, intraosseous wiring, or a small screw (Figure 102.40).

Intraarticular base or plateau fractures result from impaction rather than avulsion and are among the most difficult to treat. Outcome is often unsatisfactory and complicated by stiffness and contracture. They may involve a larger portion of the articular surface with associated joint instability and dorsal subluxation or dislocation of the middle phalanx. Goals are to reduce the PIP joint, establish early motion, and restore the anatomic joint surface. Fractures with less than 40% articular surface involvement are usually stable (Figure 102.41) and treated by a dorsal/extension block splint to keep the PIP joint

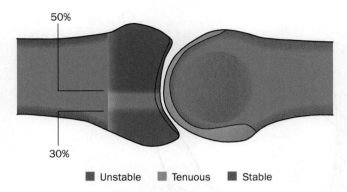

50%

30%

■ Unstable ■ Tenuous ■ Stable

Figure 102.41. PIP joint fracture stability.

in 45–60 degrees of flexion (Figure 102.42). Flexion exercises are initiated after 1 week and continued for 6 weeks, with progressive increases in the range of extension. If these fractures remain unstable, they are managed with open reduction and internal fixation using K-wire fixation with or without additional tension band wires, intraosseous wiring, or mini-fragment screw fixation. Use of mini-screws for these fractures is increasingly popular as satisfactory outcome occurs if the joint is mobilized quickly.

Base fractures with small comminuted fragments involving up to one-third of the volar articular surface may be treated by fragment excision and volar plate advancement (Figure 102.43). The joint is temporarily immobilized by pinning, followed by progressive motion using extension block splinting. Fractures with extensive comminution ("pilon" fractures) are managed with surgery confined to fragment elevation, joint realignment, and bone grafting

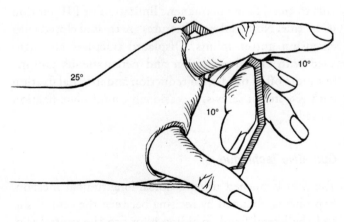

Figure 102.42 When 30% or less of the joint surface is fractured, the joint usually remains stable. Once the fracture fragment approaches 50%, the joint is unstable and requires operative fixation.

if the lesion is suitable for internal fixation or dynamic traction. The dynamic traction method has become the favored means of treating these very difficult injuries: this method combines the use of movement and traction. The motion may be either continuous or intermittent and either passive or active. The traction creates angular change at the joint and provides distal traction forces that produce several helpful effects, including reduction of articular fragments and realignment of joint surfaces, prevention of collapse of fracture fragments, prevention of contracture of joint ligaments and other periarticular structures, and enhancement of cartilage regeneration and healing. The combined results of these effects are the achievement of articular symmetry and, most important, functional recovery with excellent range of motion. Devices employing dynamic traction include the Schenck traction apparatus, the Hotchkiss device (or Compass PIP joint hinge), and the TurnKey (Hand Biomechanics Lab, Sacramento, CA) device (Figures 102.44 and 102.45). The Schenck device is of historical importance, but more modern devices are smaller, more streamlined, and easier to apply. All devices share the same concept. Dynamic traction can be constructed with K-wires across the distal proximal phalanx, proximal middle phalanx, and distal middle phalanx. With strategic placement of elastic bands to provide axial traction and K-wires for stability, the fracture fragment can be reduced and held in place while allowing active range of motion (Figure 102.46).[4]

Fractures of the PIP joint that involve the proximal phalanx are condylar fractures and can be either unicondylar or bicondylar, and either one may have displacement (Figure 102.47). Nondisplaced unicondylar fractures are inherently unstable and prone to subsequent displacement. Most are treated by percutaneous pinning to avoid displacement and allow early range of motion. When displaced, closed reduction is possible with deviation of the digit away from the fractured condyle and compression of the two condyles together by an external clamp. The fracture is then percutaneously fixed with K-wires (Figure 102.48). If a satisfactory closed reduction cannot be obtained, open reduction and internal fixation are required for definitive restoration of the articular surface. Fixation with K-wires or a 1.5 mm interfragmentary compression screw is suitable (Figure 102.49). Active range-of-motion exercises are initiated early, and the digit is protected between exercises by buddy-taping or extension PIP gutter splinting.

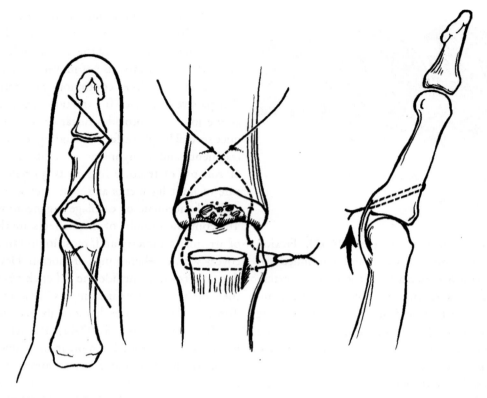

Figure 102.43. **Technique of PIP volar plate advancement.** Approach is through Brunner incision centered over PIP joint. Dorsal approach may also be used. Flexor sheath is opened from A2 to A4 pulley to allow lateral movement of tendons and thus gain exposure to volar aspect of PIP joint. Collateral ligaments that remain attached to middle phalanx are excised (major portion remaining with volar plate) and joint is maximally hyperextended, providing complete view of opposing articular surfaces. Loose bone fragments and segment attached to plate are debrided, and defect in bone is shaped into transverse groove. Plate is mobilized to advance distally into defect by means of pull-out wire suture, which spirals along lateral margins of plate and is passed through drill holes in lateral margins of defect. Holes are placed as dorsal as possible to draw plate against edge of remaining dorsal articular cartilage. Traction on sutures emerges from dorsum of middle phalanx as it is reduced concurrently with advancement of plate. K-wire is used to maintain reduced joint in 30 degrees of flexion. Immobilization is continued for 2 weeks; K-wire is then removed and active flexion started, using an extension block splint. Unrestricted active extension is allowed 4 weeks after surgery. Dynamic extension splinting is started 6 weeks after surgery, if complete extension is not possible. Swelling may persist for many months, and 6 to 8 months may be needed to regain full range of motion.

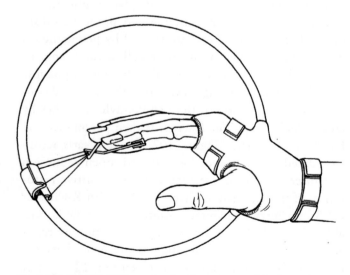

Figure 102.44. **Dynamic traction apparatus.** Apparatus consists of arcuate splint with 3-in. radius, centered on the PIP joint axis. Dynamic distal traction force is supplied by rubber band passed from one end of transosseous wire over hoop and moveable component to other end of wire.

Bicondylar fractures are less frequent but more difficult to treat. Some permanent limitation of PIP motion is the rule. Nondisplaced fractures are treated closed with extension gutter splints. Displaced fractures are managed with closed reduction and percutaneous pinning but more often need open reduction and internal fixation with K-wires or screws. Occasionally, mini-plate fixation is used.

Operative Technique

The skin is opened using a dorsal-longitudinal incision. Exposure is obtained by incising between the central slip and the lateral band, avoiding injury to the central slip. The joint capsule is dissected free and opened separately. The periosteum is cut and elevated with a small periosteal elevator. If necessary, improved access may be obtained by taking down the ulnar collateral ligament. Fracture

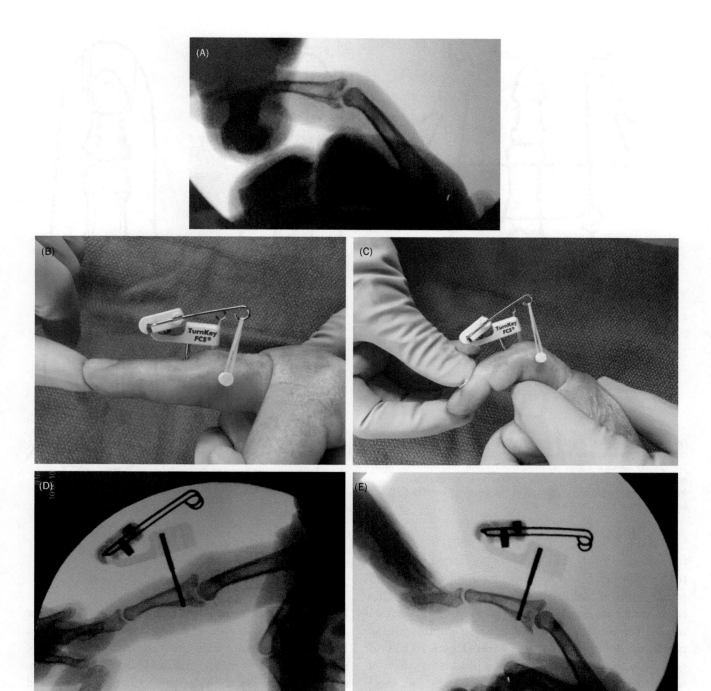

Figure 102.45. Turnkey Device.

fragments are reduced using a reduction clamp or towel clip and fixed.

COMPLEX FRACTURES

Complex fractures include multiple, segmental, and extensively comminuted fractures and fractures complicated by bone loss. Frequently, fractures occur with soft tissue damage, contusion, or loss; muscle destruction and devitalization; and injury to other deep structures, such as tendons, nerves, and blood vessels (Figure 102.50).

Complex injuries justify aggressive surgical treatment to restore anatomy, assure healing, and maximize

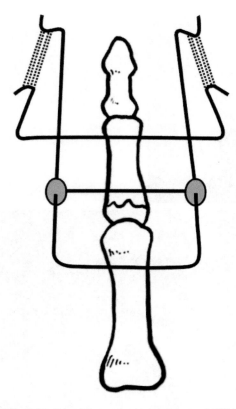

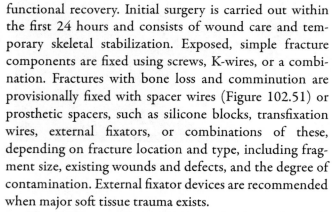

Figure 102.46 The lateral view of a proximal interphalangeal (PIP) fracture dislocation demonstrates an inherently unstable fracture pattern (A). The Turnkey device is applied allowing extension (B) and flexion (C) while holding reduction. The lateral radiographs demonstrate the fracture fragment held in appropriate reduction in extension (D) and flexion (E), allowing motion while the bone heals.

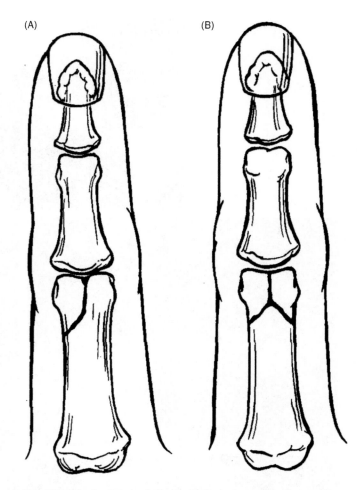

(A)   (B)

Figure 102.47 Proximal phalangeal articular fractures can be either unicondylar (A) or bicondylar (B), and either type may be displaced.

functional recovery. Initial surgery is carried out within the first 24 hours and consists of wound care and temporary skeletal stabilization. Exposed, simple fracture components are fixed using screws, K-wires, or a combination. Fractures with bone loss and comminution are provisionally fixed with spacer wires (Figure 102.51) or prosthetic spacers, such as silicone blocks, transfixation wires, external fixators, or combinations of these, depending on fracture location and type, including fragment size, existing wounds and defects, and the degree of contamination. External fixator devices are recommended when major soft tissue trauma exists.

Once adequate soft tissue coverage has been obtained, bone grafting is performed, if required. Autogenous bone grafts are necessary for restoration of bone defects, as supplementation to ensure healing of areas of comminution, and for arthrodesis in the case of an irreparable intraarticular fracture.

Operative Technique

For complex fractures involving the PIP joint, consider an external fixator made with K-wires and elastic bands. Drill the first K-wire transversely through the center of the head of the proximal phalanx. Using fluoroscopy, ensure that wire lies flush in the radio-ulnar plane and perpendicular to the longitudinal axis of the phalanx (Figure 102.52). Place the second K-wire in the same fashion through the head of the middle phalanx. Bend both ends of the first K-wire 1 cm away from the digit, at a 90-degree angle so that the ends are directed toward the second K- wire. Make a "hair-pin bend" in the first K-wire, as seen in Figure 102.51, 5–8 mm distal to the second K-wire and apply traction to the digit to engage the hair-pin bend on the second K-wire, maintaining the joint in traction. Finally, bend the ends of the second K-wire to ensure stability

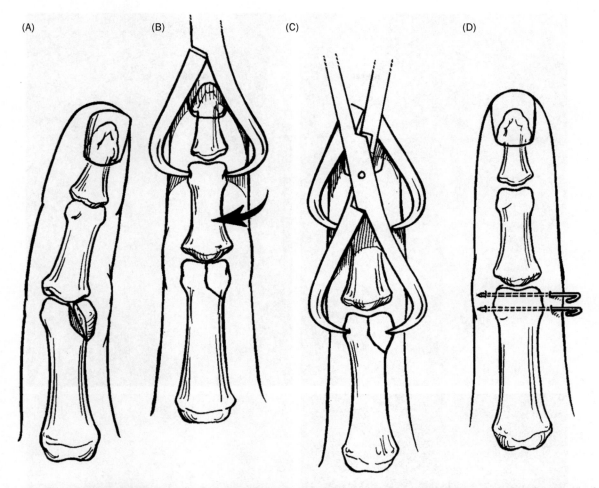

Figure 102.48. **Sequential reduction and percutaneous pin fixation of displaced unicondylar fracture of proximal phalanx.** (A) displaced unicondylar fracture results in angulation and deformity of finger at the PIP joint. (B) tenacular clamp applied transcutaneous to distal portion of middle phalanx corrects deformity and reduces fracture. (C) second tenacular clamp applied at fracture site completes and compresses reduction. (D) fracture is fixed with one or two small-gauge K-wires placed in transverse fashion. Fluoroscopic x-ray monitoring is very helpful.

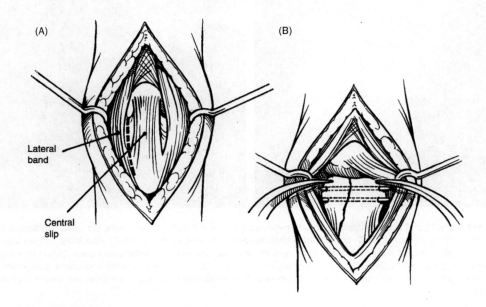

Figure 102.49. Open reduction of condylar fracture of proximal phalanx. (A) fracture is exposed betweed central slip and lateral band. Injury to central slip insertion to dorsum of base of middle phalanx must be avoided. (B) tenacular clamp is applied to reduce and hold fracture. Internal fixation is accomplished with two transverse K-wires or small screw.

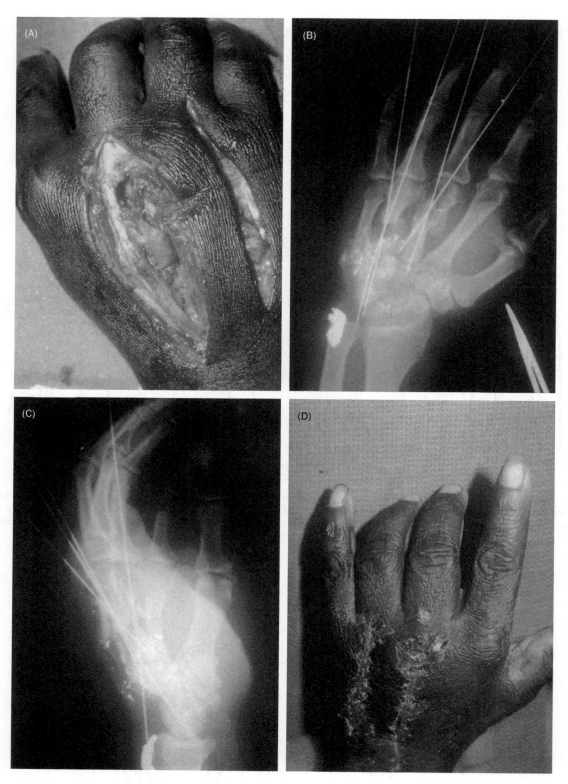

Figure 102.50. **Complex hand injury.** Open fracture of third and fourth metacarpal bones with comminution, bone loss, and shortening. (A) preliminary wound decompression and surgical cleansing. (B, C) provisional skeletal fixation performed using K-wires (D) after initial surgery, significant metacarpal shortening and extensor lag deformities of involved fingers. (E) delayed autogenous bone grafts of defects was done. Shown here are trough and peg fashioned to receive grafts. (F) bone graft in place. (G) grafts were secured with K-wires. (H, I) anteroposterior and lateral radiographs taken after bone-grafting. (J, K) 4 weeks after surgery, fractures united and K-wires removed. The patient has good range of motion and almost full functional recovery. (L, M) 2 years after surgery.

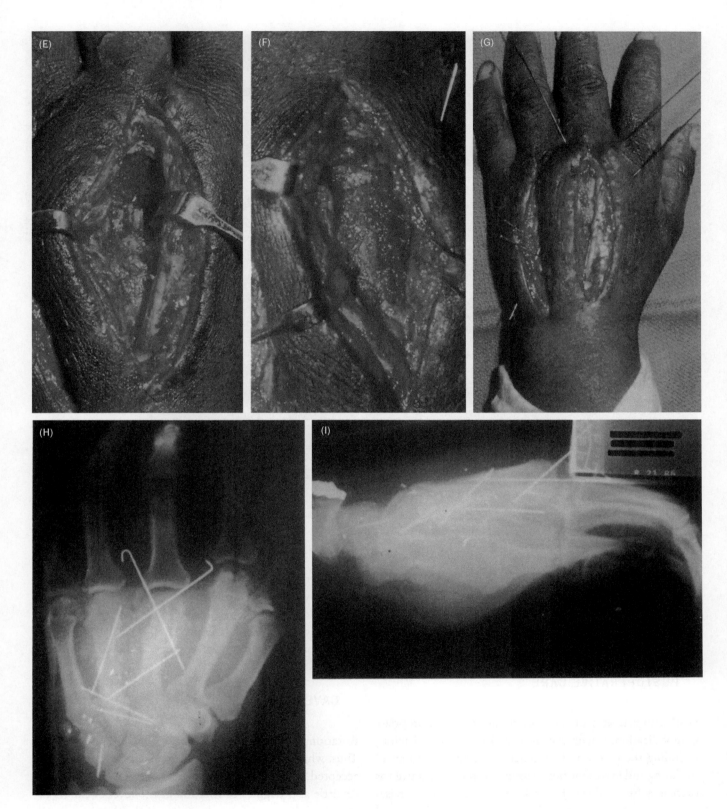

Figure 102.50. Continued

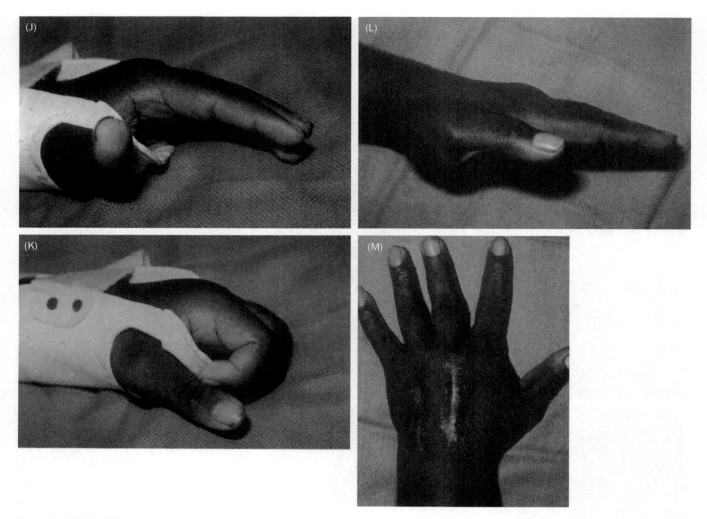

Figure 102.50. Continued

and continued engagement with the first K-wire. Confirm the joint has been distracted and range it to ensure smooth motion. Active range of motion may begin on postoperative day 1, and the external fixator may be removed in 4 weeks.

POSTOPERATIVE CARE

Postfracture treatment includes elevation and appropriate immobilization, usually for 4–6 weeks. Unaffected joints, including the elbow and shoulder, are mobilized to avoid stiffening and loss of motion. Motion exercises are started as soon as stability allows; K-wires are less stable and exercises are carried out only after about 10–14 days. Plates and screws are more secure and allow exercises to be started almost immediately. Postoperatively, the dressing is reduced or removed by the fourth day, and a removable splint is applied. Skin sutures are removed after 2 weeks. Repeat x-ray studies

are performed and follow-up films taken as needed. K-wires are removed once clinical union (i.e., absence of local pain and tenderness at the fracture site) has occurred. Generally, plates and screws are left in place unless they become palpably prominent and cause overlying soft tissue irritation.

CAVEATS

Rotational deformity will never remodel, even in children. Thus, while a certain degree of angular deformity may be accepted, rotational deformity must always be corrected. As little as 5 degrees of rotation at the level of the metacarpal results in a 1.5 cm deviation of the distal finger tip from its normal position when making a fist.

In following with the "reconstructive elevator," the best procedure that serves the purpose should be used. Noninvasive or minimally invasive measures, such as

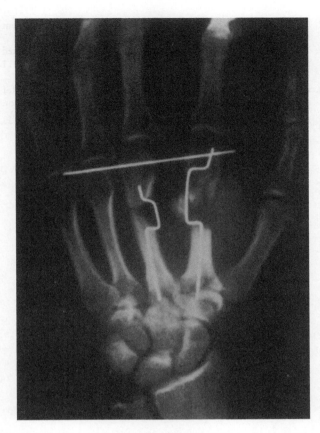

Figure 102.51. **Spacer wires.** Fractures with segmental bone loss can be provisionally fixed using spacer wires.

closed manipulation and percutaneous pinning of unstable fractures, have increasingly demonstrated excellent results that reduce the risk of postoperative sequelae of tendon adhesions, stiffness, and other soft tissue scarring. They should generally be attempted before proceeding to open reduction. However, once a clinical decision is made to open the fracture site, the most rigid fixation type should be chosen. With metacarpals, this generally implies fixation by lag screws, plates and screws, or a mini-condylar plate. While more surgical dissection may be required for plate fixation than for K-wires, the added rigidity of fixation enables early protected motion, which will help overcome stiffness and tendon adhesions.

The majority of metacarpal fractures are treated by splint immobilization. While this is considered "conservative" management, risks remain with splinting when performed incorrectly. The most frequent error is to not splint the MCP joints in sufficient flexion. Frequently, pain and swelling preclude this. Wrist block anesthesia, by abolishing pain, enables a better finger position in the splint (even when fracture manipulation is not specifically required). As swelling resolves, it may be possible to change the splint and progressively position the MCP joints in better flexion. Never leave the fingers immobilized in extension for prolonged periods. Ensuing extension contractures at the MCP joints, which may develop in a few weeks, are difficult to correct.

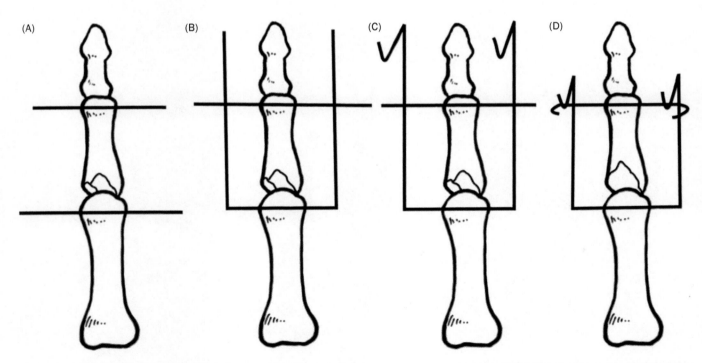

Figure 102.52. K1 is passed transversely through the distal end of the proximal phalanx, and K2 is passed through the same location on the middle phalanx of the affected finger (A). The K1 wire is bent to 90 degrees about 1 cm away from the finger surface to lie in the plane of the palm (B). The K1 wire is then bent again distal to where K1 overlaps K2 in order to be able to put the PIP joint on tension (C). The K2 wire is also bent to form a hook, allowing the PIP joint to be distracted when K1 is interfaced with K2 (D).

Additionally, poor splinting can cause pressure sores and even compartment syndrome if applied too tightly.

REFERENCES

1. Douglass N, Yao J. Nuts and bolts: dimensions of commonly utilized screws in upper extremity surgery. *J Hand Surg A* 2015 Feb;40(2):368–382.

2. Meals C, Meals R. Hand fractures: a review of current treatment strategies. *J Hand Surg A* 2013 May;38(5):1021–1031.

3. Yaffe MA, Saucedo JM, Kalainov DM. Non-locked and locked plating technology for hand fractures. *J Hand Surg A* 2011 Dec;36A:2052–2055.

4. Ruland RT et al. Use of dynamic distraction external fixation for unstable fracture-dislocations of the proximal interphalangeal joint. *J Hand Surg A* 2008 Jan;33(1):19–25.

103.

CARPAL FRACTURES AND DISLOCATIONS

Jason H. Ko, Nicholas B. Vedder, and Rahul Kasukurthi

INTRODUCTION

Carpal fractures comprise approximately 207,880 of the nearly 1.5 million hand and wrist fractures encountered in the United States annually. Most hand and forearm fractures occur in the home and are not work related. The scaphoid bone is most commonly involved, accounting for 60–85% of carpal fractures.[1,2] Prompt and accurate diagnosis and treatment are necessary to avoid long-term disability. This chapter will focus on pathophysiology, diagnosis, imaging, and treatment of carpal injuries with emphasis on scaphoid fractures and perilunate dislocations.

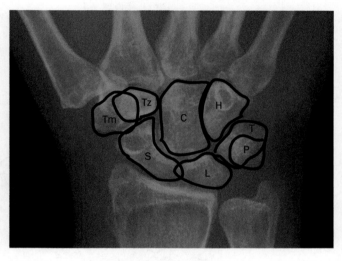

Figure 103.1. The proximal carpal row consists of the scaphoid (S), lunate (L), triquetrum (T), and pisiform (P). The distal row is formed by the trapezium (Tm), trapezoid (Tz), capitate (C), and hamate (H).

ANATOMY

The proximal carpal row consists of the scaphoid, lunate, triquetrum, and pisiform, while the distal row is formed by the trapezium, trapezoid, capitate, and hamate (Figure 103.1). The proximal row articulates with the distal radius and ulna, while the distal row, combined with the second and third metacarpals, forms the fixed unit of the hand.[3] The carpal bones have complex articulations allowing for radial and ulnar deviation, flexion, extension, pronation and supination.

LIGAMENTS

Thorough knowledge of the ligamentous anatomy of the wrist is required to understand the patterns of carpal fractures and dislocations and their treatment. Extrinsic ligaments can be palmar or dorsal and originate or insert outside the carpus. Their V-shaped configuration provides support and resists radiocarpal dislocation. Palmarly, a space between the two V-shaped bands forms an area of weakness known as the *space of Poirier*. The lunate tends to

dislocate volarly into this space during lunate dislocation. The dorsal carpal ligaments are less robust and weaker than the palmar ligaments.

Intrinsic ligaments originate and insert within the carpus. The C-shaped scapholunate (SLIL) and lunotriquetral (LTIL) interosseous ligaments provide stability to the proximal carpal row. The SLIL is strongest dorsally, while the LTIL is most robust palmarly (Figure 103.2).

KINEMATICS

The complex articulations and ligaments of the wrist dictate movement and allow for circumduction. The robust intrinsic ligaments of the distal carpal row greatly restrict interosseous movement, causing it to move as a single functional unit. No muscles arise or insert on the carpal bones, with the exception of the pisiform. The proximal carpal row,

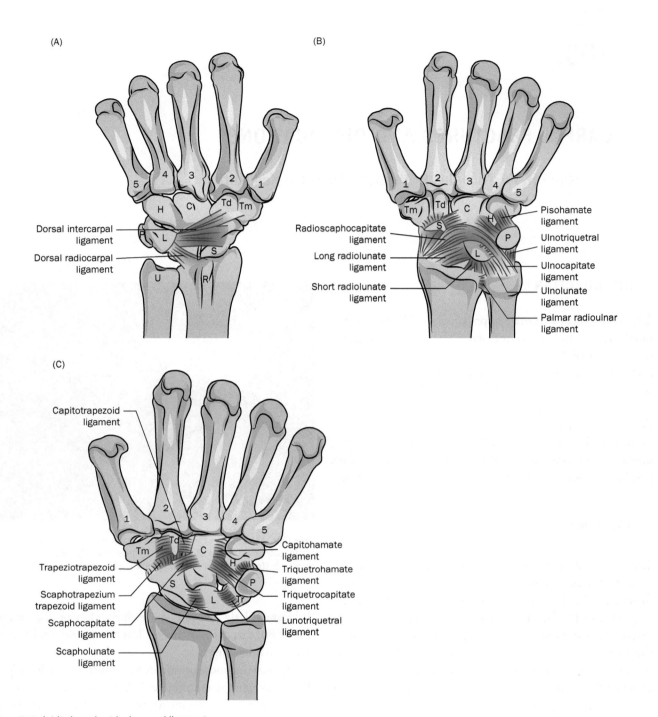

Figure 103.2. Intrinsic and extrinsic carpal ligaments.

on the other hand, does demonstrate intercarpal motion. The scaphoid flexes with radial deviation and wrist flexion, while the triquetrum extends with ulnar deviation and wrist extension. If intrinsic interosseous ligaments remain intact, the lunate moves with its adjacent carpal bone. As a result, during radial deviation, the scaphoid is flexed down by the distal carpal row, flexing the lunate and triquetrum through the SLIL. The triquetrum tends to extend during ulnar deviation, pulling the proximal carpal row into extension through the LTIL.

CARPAL INSTABILITY

Carpal instability is the result of disruption of normal intercarpal relationships by fractures or ligamentous rupture. An unstable wrist joint is characterized by symptomatic dysfunction, inability to bear loads, and abnormal kinematics during its arc of motion.[4] Carpal instability can be characterized as predynamic, dynamic, and static. A predynamic instability refers to clinical signs of ligament injury in the setting of normal x-rays. Dynamic instability occurs when stress views show intercarpal widening, but resting x-rays are normal. With static instability, abnormal carpal alignment is visible on resting x-rays.

There are several broad categories of carpal instability. Carpal instability dissociative (CID) refers to instability within a carpal row, typically as a result of SLIL or LTIL ligament injury. CID leads to abnormal rotation between the radial and ulnar aspects of the proximal carpal row. Carpal instability nondissociative (CIND) is usually caused by extrinsic ligament injury leading to disruption between the distal radius and proximal carpal row (radiocarpal) or between proximal and distal carpal rows (midcarpal instability). A carpal instability complex (CIC) pattern encompasses both CID and CIND, and requires significant ligamentous injury (e.g., perilunate dislocation). Finally, carpal instability adaptive (CIA) is the result of pathology proximal or distal to the wrist.[4–6]

DIAGNOSIS

A detailed history and physical examination of both the affected and normal wrist is necessary in order to account for normal variations that can lead to positive examination findings. Patients may present with weakness, pain, loss of motion, ecchymosis, and swelling. Radiographs should be carefully reviewed prior to aggressive physical examination maneuvers. A full neurovascular examination, including grip and pinch strength, should be performed. Specific care should be taken to rule out acute carpal tunnel syndrome. Passive and active range of motion should be documented, noting any crepitus, clunks, or clicks. Palpation of the wrist can assist in localizing the lesion. For example, pain in the anatomic snuffbox should raise suspicion of a possible scaphoid fracture.

Several provocative maneuvers are helpful in wrist injury evaluation. SLIL injury may result in a positive Watson scaphoid shift test. Volar pressure is placed over the distal scaphoid tubercle with the examiner's thumb while the wrist is moved from ulnar to radial deviation with the examiner's other hand. This resists the scaphoid's tendency to flex during radial deviation, and, in cases of SLIL disruption, the scaphoid is forced dorsally over the rim of the radius causing discomfort. Release of pressure may result in a "clunk" as the scaphoid is reduced back into its radial fossa. Examination of the unaffected wrist is important in order to rule out asymptomatic laxity.[7]

LTIL stability can be assessed using the Kleinman shear test. The examiner grasps the pisotriquetral column between his or her thumb and index finger while the wrist is moved from ulnar to radial deviation, noting any triquetral displacement. In the lunotriquetral (LT) shuck test, one hand stabilizes the lunate under the fourth extensor compartment while the thumb and index finger of the examiner's other hand applies alternating dorsal and volar pressure to the pisotriquetral column.[8] LTIL injury results in instability and discomfort during this maneuver. During the LT compression (Linscheid) test, medial to lateral pressure is applied across the LT joint. Finally, the Lichtman test assesses midcarpal instability by axially loading the hand while the wrist undergoes radial to ulnar deviation. Midcarpal instability is suspected when the proximal carpal row clunks as it rapidly extends ("catch up" clunk), a motion that usually occurs gradually in a normal wrist.[8,9]

IMAGING

Posteroanterior and lateral radiographs should be compared to the contralateral uninjured wrist. Accurate diagnosis depends on standardized views and knowledge of normal anatomic measurements on radiographs. The longitudinal axis of the radius should be in line with the third metacarpal, whereas, in a true lateral, the pisiform overlaps the distal pole of the scaphoid (Figure 103.3). If the forearm is held pronated, the pisiform will project dorsal to the distal

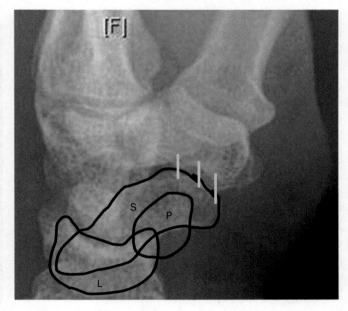

Figure 103.3. Lateral view of the wrist. The palmar border of the pisiform should fall within the middle third of the distal pole of the scaphoid. Scaphoid (S), lunate (L), pisiform (P). Yellow lines mark distal pole of scaphoid divided in thirds.

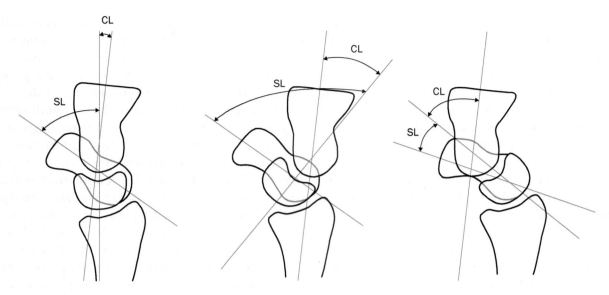

Figure 103.4. Measurement of scapholunate and capitolunate angles.

pole of scaphoid, while a supinated forearm results in a volarly projected pisiform.[10]

The lateral radiograph is useful for assessing intercarpal relationships through various angles. The scaphoid axis is formed by drawing a line tangent to its two volar convexities, while the lunate axis is perpendicular to a line joining its two distal convexities. The intersection of these axes forms the scapholunate angle, normally measuring between 30 and 60 degrees. Measurements outside these normal values suggest intercalated segment instability. The term "intercalated segment" refers to the proximal carpal row because it has no direct musculotendinous insertions. With SLIL disruption, the lunate tends to tilt dorsally while the scaphoid flexes volarly, resulting in an increased scapholunate angle. This is referred to as dorsal intercalated segment instability (DISI). On the posteroanterior view, the scaphoid appears flexed and foreshortened, resulting in a "cortical ring sign." On the other hand, a scapholunate angle of less than 30 degrees can occur with LTIL tears, causing volar tilt of the lunate and volar intercalated segment instability (VISI). The capitolunate angle normally measures less than 30 degrees and is measured by drawing intersecting lines between the lunate axis and the long axis of the capitate.[11] In a DISI or VISI deformity, the capitolunate angle exceeds ±30 degrees as the lunate tilts as part of the intercalated segment (Figure 103.4).

A disruption of the normal smooth contour of Gilula's lines suggests carpal pathology.[12] Gilula described three lines formed by the proximal and distal articular surfaces of the proximal carpal row, as well as the proximal articular surface of the distal carpal row (Figure 103.5).

SCAPHOLUNATE DISSOCIATION

Scapholunate dissociation (SLD) is the result of axial loading on a dorsiflexed, ulnarly deviated wrist. Radial and ulnar deviation generates significant stress between the scaphoid and lunate. Patients may present with discomfort and swelling distal to Lister's tubercle between the second and third extensor compartments. The Watson scaphoid shift test may be positive.[13]

Posteroanterior (PA) radiographs may demonstrate scapholunate diastasis greater than 3 mm or a cortical "ring

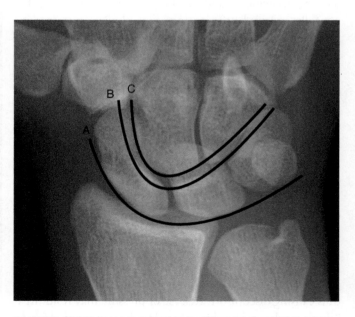

Figure 103.5. Gilula's lines are defined by the (A) proximal and (B) distal articular surfaces of the proximal carpal row in addition to the (C) proximal articular surface of the distal carpal row.

sign" as the distal pole of the scaphoid rotates forward and overlaps with its longitudinal axis. On lateral x-ray, injury to the SLIL causes the scaphoid to follow its natural tendency to flex, while the lunate extends resulting in DISI. In addition, the scapholunate angle may be increased. The clenched fist view accentuates scapholunate diastasis and can uncover dynamic instability. All x-ray findings should be compared with the contralateral wrist to rule out normal variants. Magnetic resonance imaging (MRI) can be useful to examine the severity of ligament disruption.[14]

LUNOTRIQUETRAL DISSOCIATION

Lunotriquetral dissociation (LTD) can result from axial loading on a dorsiflexed, radially deviated wrist. Patients may complain of ulnar-sided wrist pain or clicking over the lunotriquetral interval. Previously discussed provocative maneuvers such as the Kleinman lunotriquetral shear, LT shuck, and Linscheid LT compression tests should be employed.

Radiographs are often normal but in some cases may demonstrate disruption of Gilula's lines or VISI deformity. LT diastasis is typically not seen. Grip views, MRI, fluoroscopy, and arthroscopy can aid in diagnosis. Treatment options include ligament repair, reconstruction using a slip of ECU, and LT arthrodesis.[15–18]

PERILUNATE AND LUNATE DISLOCATION

Accurate diagnosis and treatment is critical with perilunate dislocations (PLD) since these injuries are frequently misdiagnosed and can result in significant functional impairment. Perilunate instability is typically caused by high-energy trauma to the extended and ulnarly deviated wrist, resulting in progressive injury of structures from the radial to ulnar side of the wrist. The Mayfield classification describes this sequence of events (Figure 103.6):

- *Stage 1*: SLIL disruption or scaphoid fracture
- *Stage 2*: Capitolunate disruption or capitate fracture
- *Stage 3*: Lunotriquetral disruption or triquetral fracture
- *Stage 4*: Dislocation of the lunate from its fossa, typically volarly through the space of Poirier.[19]

Stage 4 lunate dislocations can result in acute carpal tunnel syndrome, which should be addressed emergently. In perilunate dislocations, the lunate remains seated its radial fossa while the carpus dislocates, usually dorsally.

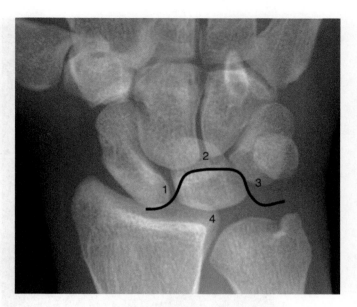

Figure 103.6. Mayfield's stages of perilunate instability. (I) Scapholunate tear, (II) space of Poirier volar capsular tear, (III) lunotriquetral tear, (IV) lunate dislocation. There is no intrinsic ligament between the capitate and lunate (Stage II).

Dislocations can be purely ligamentous in nature (lesser arc) or may interrupt ligaments with associated fractures of the radius, ulna, or carpus (greater arc injury).[20]

Patients present with diffuse hand and wrist swelling. Lateral x-rays are most useful for diagnosis and may demonstrate a spilled "tea cup" sign in lunate dislocations, while the lunate remains reduced in its radial fossa during perilunate dislocations (Figure 103.7). Reduction should be attempted in the emergency department using axial traction and wrist extension while placing volar pressure on the lunate, followed by flexion of the hand to bring the capitate over the lip of the lunate (Tavernier maneuver).

SCAPHOID FRACTURE AND NONUNION

Scaphoid fractures are typically the result of a fall on an outstretched wrist in extension and radial deviation.[1,2] The scaphoid fracture is the most commonly fractured carpal bone, and its unique anatomy and vascular supply dictates its behavior when stressed. The majority of the scaphoid's cashew-shaped surface is covered by cartilage. The scaphoid waist separates the proximal and distal poles.

Nearly 80% of the bone is supplied by dorsal scaphoid branches of the radial artery entering on the dorsal ridge and distal tubercle. This retrograde supply to the proximal pole makes it susceptible to avascular necrosis (AVN). The distal pole enjoys an anterograde blood supply from the remaining volar scaphoid branches of the

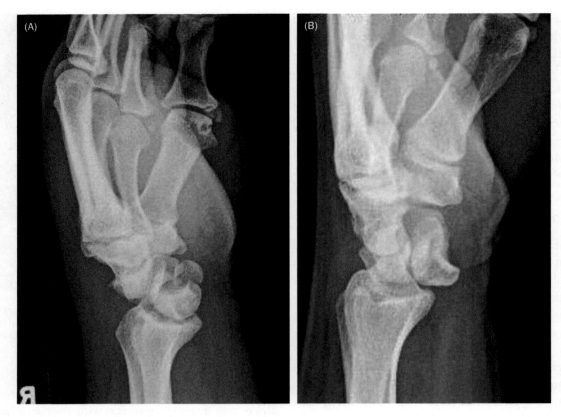

Figure 103.7. (A) Perilunate dislocation. (B) Lunate dislocation, with "spilled tea cup" sign.

radial artery entering at the level of the scaphoid tubercle. Approximately 65% of scaphoid fractures occur at the waist (Figure 103.8), 15% at the proximal pole, 10% at the distal body, and 8% at the tuberosity (a protuberance at the distal palmar aspect).[21]

The precise location of radial-sided wrist tenderness with scaphoid injury may depend on fracture location. Distal pole fractures can manifest with discomfort at the volar distal wrist crease, while proximal pole fractures may exhibit point tenderness just distal to Lister's tubercle. Waist fractures often demonstrate anatomic snuffbox tenderness.

A scaphoid view with the wrist in ulnar deviation should be obtained in addition to standard x-rays. Initial studies have a false-negative rate of approximately 25%.[22] As a result, normal x-rays in the setting of a clinical exam suggestive of scaphoid fracture should prompt immobilization in a thumb spica splint or cast, with repeat x-rays in 7–10 days. If repeat x-rays are negative but clinical suspicion remains, computed tomography (CT) or MRI should be considered. MRI has a sensitivity of approximately 97.7% and a specificity of 99.8%, while CT achieves a sensitivity of 83% and a specificity of 97%.[22]

When selecting a treatment method for scaphoid fractures, one should consider fracture chronicity, location, and stability. In general, fractures are considered unstable when any of the following are present:

- Displacement greater than 1 mm
- Scapholunate angle greater than 60 degrees
- Radiolunate or capitolunate angle greater than 15 degrees
- Fracture comminution
- Intrascaphoid angle greater than 45 degrees
- Associated ligament tear

Although some authors recommend initial immobilization of waist and proximal pole fractures with a long-arm cast for the first 4–6 weeks, followed by a short-arm cast,[23] no benefit to long-arm over short-arm thumb spica has been demonstrated to date.[24] Stable proximal pole fractures heal very slowly without operative intervention, and those treated conservatively can take up to 5 months to achieve union. Stable distal pole fractures can be immobilized in a thumb spica for at least 6 weeks.

Headless compression screws can be placed percutaneously or via an open approach. The volar approach is

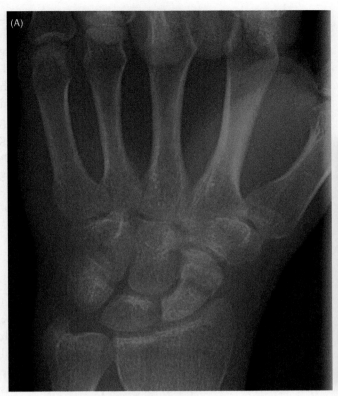

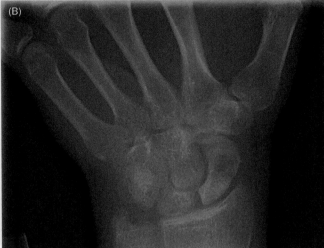

Figure 103.8. Scaphoid waist fracture.

typically reserved for distal pole fractures, while proximal pole fractures are most easily approached dorsally. Either approach can be used for waist fractures. Closed reduction and percutaneous pinning is also an option. Comminuted fractures may require primary bone grafting. Failure of nonoperative treatment should prompt consideration of open reduction and internal fixation (ORIF) with bone grafting. Patient functional status, occupation, and need to return to work should be considered with minimally displaced waist fractures. In select cases, surgical fixation of these fractures can accelerate return to activity.[25]

Scaphoid nonunion is a challenging complication caused in part by the bone's unique retrograde blood supply.[26] Prompt diagnosis, debridement of the fibrous nonunion, and corticancellous bone grafting with stable fixation are necessary to prevent long-term arthritis. Chronic nonunion ultimately leads to a sequence of arthritic changes known as *scaphoid nonunion advanced collapse* (SNAC). Initially localized to the radial scaphoid and radial styloid (Stage I), SNAC wrist then progresses to scaphocapitate arthrosis (Stage 2), and finally periscaphoid arthrosis (Stage 3).[27,28] A "humpback" deformity may be seen as the distal pole flexes and the proximal scaphoid rotates dorsally with the lunate in the setting of DISI.[29]

MRI can be a useful adjunct for diagnosis and preoperative planning.[30,31]

OPERATIVE TECHNIQUES

The patient is placed supine with the injured extremity draped and tourniqueted on a hand table. Fluoroscopic C-arm guidance is mandatory, and regional or general anesthetic may be used.

SCAPHOID OPEN REDUCTION AND INTERNAL FIXATION

When selecting an approach for scaphoid fractures, the surgeon must consider fracture location, chronicity, fixation method, and the need for bone grafting. In general, acute injuries less than 6 weeks old do not require bone grafting.

A dorsal approach is typically employed for proximal pole fractures, while a volar approach is often used in distal pole fractures, as well as in fractures with humpback deformities. Acute scaphoid waist fractures can be addressed either dorsally or volarly. Some authors advocate the volar exposure as less likely to damage the dorsal ridge vascular supply.[32]

VOLAR SCAPHOID OPEN REDUCTION AND INTERNAL FIXATION

An incision is fashioned in line with the FCR tendon proximal to the scaphoid tubercle. Distal to the tubercle, the incision angles obliquely toward the base of the thumb, over the scaphotrapezial joint. The superficial palmar branch of the radial artery can be ligated and divided, if needed, as it passes near the scaphoid tubercle. The palmar cutaneous branch of the median nerve can course near the scaphoid tubercle on the thenar eminence and should be avoided. The FCR tendon sheath is identified and incised, and the tendon itself is mobilized distally and retracted ulnarly. An oblique incision in the capsule is made from the volar rim of the radius to the tubercle distally, taking care to preserve the volar ligaments. The radioscaphocapitate ligament is divided and mobilized for scaphoid exposure, and the long radiolunate ligament may be divided proximally to provide proximal scaphoid access as needed. Distally, the thenar muscles are divided to expose the scaphotrapezial joint, while the scaphotrapezial ligament is divided in line with its fibers. Pointed reduction forceps or Kirschner wires (K-wires) can be used to joystick and reduce fracture fragments, followed by provisional fixation with a K-wire to maintain alignment. The screw guide wire is then inserted from the scaphotrapezial joint proximally with the wrist hyperextended and ulnarly deviated. A portion of the trapezium can be removed to improve the trajectory of screw placement, if needed. A dedicated depth gauge is used, and 4 mm are subtracted to determine final screw length. After drilling and tapping as needed, the headless compression screw should be inserted as orthogonal to the fracture plane as possible. The volar radioscaphocapitate and long radiolunate ligaments are repaired along with the overlying FCR tendon sheath.

DORSAL SCAPHOID OPEN REDUCTION AND INTERNAL FIXATION

For nondisplaced scaphoid waist fractures, a percutaneous or mini-open approach dorsally can be performed through a 1–2 cm longitudinal incision proximal and ulnar to Lister's tubercle. Care is taken to protect the extensor pollicis longus (EPL) tendon, and scissors are used to dissect down to the proximal pole of the scaphoid. A headless compression screw can be placed through this incision.

For displaced scaphoid fractures, a more extensive approach is required. A longitudinal dorsal skin incision is made from Lister's tubercle to approximately 4 cm distally. Taking care to protect the superficial dorsal radial sensory

nerve branches, the extensor retinaculum over the EPL tendon is incised. The interval between the third and fourth compartments is used to perform a capsulotomy, taking care to preserve vessels to the dorsal ridge of the scaphoid. A ligament-sparing capsulotomy can be performed. With the wrist flexed to expose the scaphoid, provisional fixation and guide wire insertion is performed, again subtracting 4 mm to determine final screw length. After overdrilling and screw insertion, the C-arm should be used to confirm that the implant is buried beneath subchondral bone along the central axis of the scaphoid. The capsule and third extensor compartment are closed judiciously to allow for continued EPL gliding (Figure 103.9).

SCAPHOID NONUNION

A scaphoid nonunion is defined as failure to heal within 6 months after injury, and treatment requires the use of bone grafts. Bone grafting options can include both nonvascularized and vascularized techniques. Volar distal radius autologous bone graft (Russe technique) can be used for both nondisplaced and displaced nonunions with humpback deformity by adjusting the graft shape. However, the Russe technique is contraindicated for proximal nonunions or with proximal pole AVN. In these cases, pedicled vascularized bone flaps, such as the dorsoradial 1,2 intercompartmental supraretinacular artery (1,2-ICSRA), can be used.[33] Recently, free vascularized bone flaps including the medial femoral condyle (MFC) and medial femoral trochlea (MFT) flaps have been developed. The latter flap contains a cartilage segment for lesions requiring a chondral surface.[34–38]

As implied by its name, the 1,2-ICSRA flap courses superficial to the extensor retinaculum and lies between the first and second extensor compartments. The subcutaneous tissues are dissected to identity the 1,2-ICSRA. The first and second compartments are opened at the bone graft site, and a cuff of retinaculum is preserved with the vessels overlying the bone. Small K-wires are used to perforate the perimeter of the planned bone flap site, followed by an osteotome to raise the flap. The flap is shaped to fit the previously prepared nonunion site and inset dorsally. Fixation is achieved with a headless cannulated screw. Approximately 6% of patients lack a 1,2-ICSRA, in which case a second metacarpal base flap can be used. The 1,2-ICSRA is usually used in cases without humpback deformity. In the setting of humpback deformity, a volar vascularized bone flap or a free vascularized bone flap should be used (Figure 103.10).

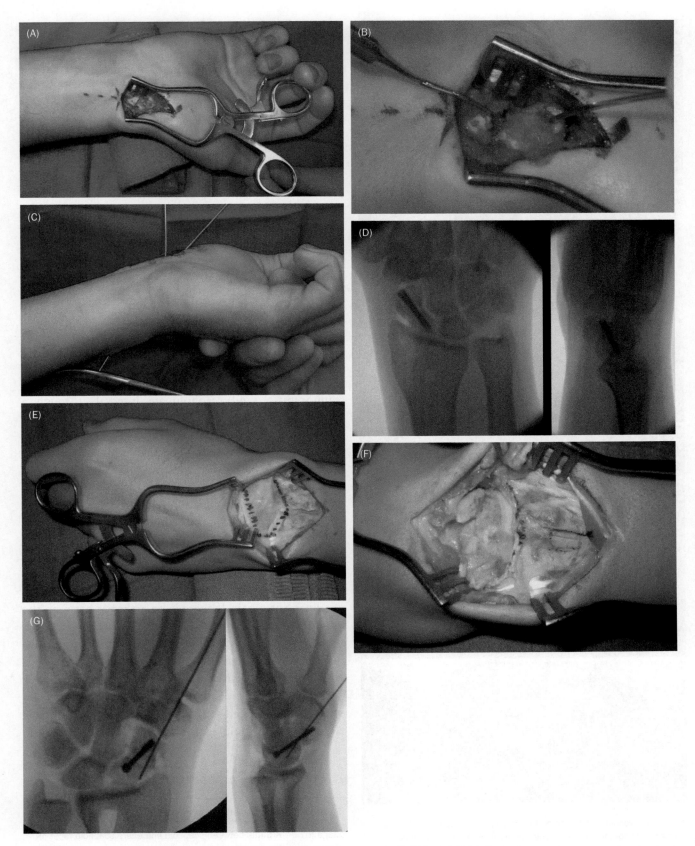

Figure 103.9. Scaphoid open reduction and internal fixation (ORIF) (A–D) Volar approach. (E–G) Dorsal approach.

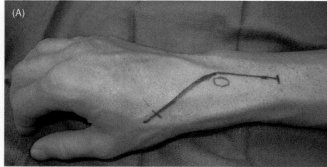

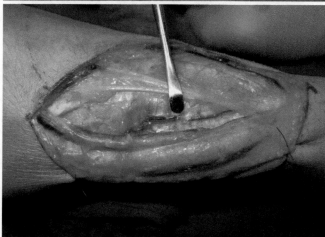

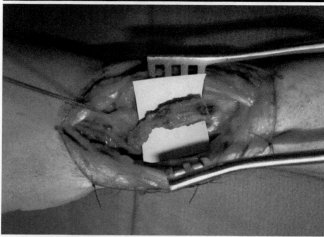

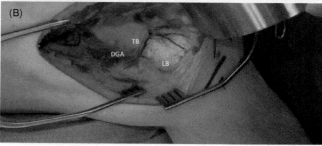

Figure 103.10. Vascularized bone grafts for scaphoid nonunion. (A) A 1,2 intercompartmental supraretinacular artery (ICSRA) demonstrating skin incision, pedicle, and raised flap. (B) Medial femoral condyle flap (MFC). Descending genicular artery (DGA), longitudinal branch (LB) and transverse branch (TB).

POSTOPERATIVE CARE OF SCAPHOID FRACTURES AND NONUNIONS

The postoperative regimen must be tailored to patient factors including age, employment, compliance, or the need to return to sports, among others. Nondisplaced scaphoid fractures treated with cast immobilization are typically followed with serial CT scans until evidence of 50% bony bridging exists. For nondisplaced scaphoid fractures treated with headless compression screws, patients can receive a removable brace and begin early active range of motion around 2 weeks postoperatively; displaced scaphoid fractures typically warrant CT at the 6-week postoperative mark or later to confirm healing prior to initiating range of motion exercises. Scaphoid nonunions usually undergo prolonged cast immobilization for 10–12 weeks, followed by CT to confirm union.

SCAPHOLUNATE DISSOCIATION TECHNIQUE

Acute complete SLIL tears are amenable to treatment via open repair with suture anchors and pinning of scaphocapitate and scapholunate intervals through a dorsal approach similar to that used for scaphoid ORIF.

Partial tears can be treated immobilized and treated nonoperatively. If this fails, arthroscopic debridement can be considered for partial tears.

Chronic scapholunate injury leads to a sequence of arthritic changes termed scapholunate advanced collapse (SLAC) (Table 103.1). The radiolunate joint is typically spared. The optimal treatment of these injuries remains controversial. Treatment is dependent on the extent of arthritic degeneration, which can be assessed via arthroscopy. Chronic SLD is typically not amenable to direct ligament repair. If there is no arthrosis between the scaphoid and lunate, soft tissue reconstruction such as a dorsal capsulodesis can be considered. Other options include bone-ligament-bone reconstruction,[39] tenodesis using FCR, or limited wrist fusion.[40-44] The Stage 1 SLAC wrist can be addressed with radial styloidectomy, while more advanced arthritis may require proximal row carpectomy, scaphoid excision with four-corner fusion,

TABLE 103.1 WATSON CLASSIFICATION

Stage I	Arthritis between scaphoid and radial styloid
Stage II	Arthritis between scaphoid and entire scaphoid facet of the radius
Stage III	Arthritis between capitate and lunate

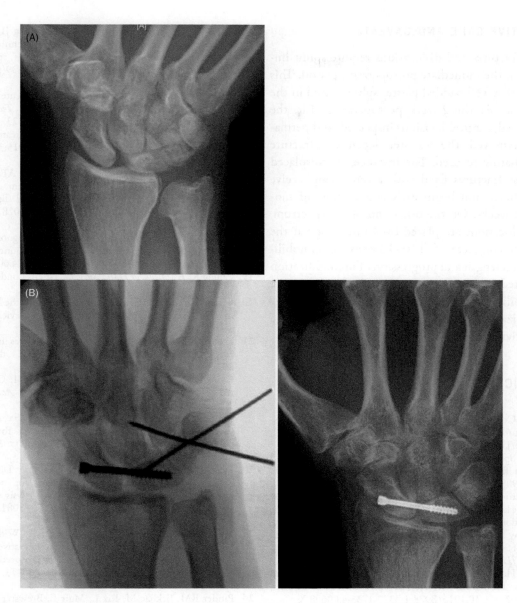

Figure 103.11. (A) Scapholunate disassociation. (B) Reduction and association of the scaphoid and lunate (RASL) procedure.

total wrist arthroplasty, or wrist fusion. The reduction and association of the scaphoid and lunate (RASL) procedure achieves fibrous union between the scaphoid and lunate by fixation with a headless compression screw and may be considered in advanced cases of SLD (Figure 103.11).[45,46] Postoperative splint and cast immobilization typically ranges from 6 to 12 weeks.

PERILUNATE DISLOCATION TECHNIQUE

Following reduction, operative fixation is achieved using a dorsal approach similar to that used for SLD. Combined dorsal and volar approaches may also be employed. Following a ligament-sparing capsulotomy, fixation of the scapholunate, scaphocapitate, and lunotriquetral intervals is performed with K-wires, and ligamentous and capsular injuries are repaired as described previously. The scaphoid is also repaired in transscaphoid perilunate injuries.[9] Salvage of proximal row carpectomy or wrist fusion may be considered in severe cases. While we typically employ a dorsal approach, severe median neuropathy or volar lunate dislocation can be addressed via an extended carpal tunnel approach, through which the space of Poirier can be repaired per surgeon preference.[47,48] A total postoperative immobilization course of 10–12 weeks is achieved with an initial plaster splint followed by cast. The K-wires are then removed in the operating room after 10–12 weeks.

POSTOPERATIVE CARE AND CAVEATS

Most carpal fractures and dislocations require splint immobilization in the immediate postoperative period. This is achieved with a well-padded plaster splint placed in the operating room. At the 2-week postoperative visit, the splint is removed, surgical incisions inspected, and permanent stitches removed. The next step depends on fracture pattern and hardware used. For instance, nondisplaced scaphoid waist fractures fixed with a screw can receive a removable brace and begin early active range of motion around 2 weeks. On the other end of the spectrum, perilunate dislocations are placed back into a cast at the 2-week mark to complete a full 10–12 weeks of immobilization. The total length and progression of immobilization must be tailored to the fracture pattern, internal fixation, and the reliability of the individual patient. Fracture specific immobilization guidelines are given in each of the preceding individual sections.

REFERENCES

1. Aitken S, Court-Brown CM. The epidemiology of sports-related fractures of the hand. *Injury* 2008;39(12):1377–1383. doi: 10.1016/j.injury.2008.04.012

2. Chung KC, Spilson SV. The frequency and epidemiology of hand and forearm fractures in the United States. *J Hand Surg Am.* 2001;26(5):908–915. doi: 10.1053/jhsu.2001.26322

3. Chang J, Valero-Cuevas F, Hentz VR, Chase RA. Anatomy and biomechanics of the hand. In: *Plastic Surgery*, 3rd ed. Amsterdam: Elsevier, 2013:1–46. doi: 10.1016/B978-1-4377-1733-4.00601-7

4. The Anatomy and Biomechanics Committee of the International Federation of Societies for Surgery of the Hand. Definition of carpal instability. *YJHSU* 1999; 24(4):866–867.

5. Chung KC, Haase SC. Fractures and dislocations of the wrist and distal radius. In: *Plastic Surgery*, 3rd ed. Amsterdam: Elsevier, 2013:161–162. doi: 10.1016/B978-1-4377-1733-4.00608-X

6. Larsen CF, Amadio PC, Gilula LA, Hodge JC. Analysis of carpal instability: I. Description of the scheme. *YJHSU* 1995;20(5): 757–764. doi: 10.1016/S0363-5023(05)80426-5

7. Watson H, Ottoni L, Pitts EC, Handal AG. Rotary subluxation of the scaphoid: a spectrum of instability. *J Hand Surg (Edinburgh)* 1993;18(1):62–64.

8. Kawamura K, Chung KC. Management of wrist injuries. *Plast Reconstr Surg* 2007;120(5):73e–89e. doi: 10.1097/01.prs.0000279385.39997.34

9. Hammert WC, Boyer MI, Bozentka DJ, Calfee RP. *ASSH Manual of Hand Surgery*. Philadelphia, PA: Lippincott Williams Wilkins, 2012.

10. Medoff RJ. Essential radiographic evaluation for distal radius fractures. *Hand Clin* 2005;21(3):279–288. doi: 10.1016/j.hcl.2005.02.008

11. Walsh JJ, Berger RA, Cooney WP. Current status of scapholunate interosseous ligament injuries. *J Am Acad Orthopaed Surg* 2002;10(1):32–42. doi: 10.5435/00124635-200201000-00006

12. Gilula LA. Carpal injuries: analytic approach and case exercises. *Am J Roentgenol* 1979;133(3):503–517. American Roentgen Ray Society. doi: 10.2214/ajr.133.3.503

13. Kuo CE, Wolfe SW. Scapholunate instability: current concepts in diagnosis and management. *J Hand Surg* 2008;33(6):998–1013. doi: 10.1016/j.jhsa.2008.04.027

14. Hsu JW, Kollitz KM, Jegapragasan M, Huang JI. Radiographic evaluation of the modified Brunelli technique versus a scapholunotriquetral transosseous tenodesis technique for scapholunate dissociation. *J Hand Surg* 2014;39(6):1041–1049. doi: 10.1016/j.jhsa.2014.03.005

15. Henry M. Arthroscopic treatment of acute scapholunate and lunotriquetral ligament injuries. *Oper Techn Orthopaed* 2003;13(1):48–55. doi: 10.1053/otor.2003.36323

16. Nicoson MC, Moran SL. Diagnosis and treatment of acute lunotriquetral ligament injuries. *Hand Clin* 2015;31(3):467–476. doi: 10.1016/j.hcl.2015.04.005

17. Shin AY, Weinstein LP, Berger RA, Bishop AT. Treatment of isolated injuries of the lunotriquetral ligament. A comparison of arthrodesis, ligament reconstruction and ligament repair. *J Bone Joint Surg (Br Vol)* 2001;83(7):1023–1028. doi: 10.1302/0301-620X.83B7.11413

18. Wagner ER, Elhassan BT, Rizzo M. Diagnosis and treatment of chronic lunotriquetral ligament injuries. *Hand Clin* 2015;31(3):477–486. doi: 10.1016/j.hcl.2015.04.006

19. Chung K. *Essentials of Hand Surgery*, 1st ed. London: JP Medical Ltd., 2015. doi: 10.5005/jp/books/12510

20. Chong AK, Tan DMK. Diagnostic imaging of the hand and wrist. In: *Plastic Surgery*, 3rd ed. Amsterdam: Elsevier, 2013:68–91. doi: 10.1016/B978-1-4377-1733-4.00603-0

21. Harris MB. Rockwood and Green's fractures in adults, fifth edition. *Arthroscopy* 2002;18(6):676–677. doi: 10.1016/S0749-8063(02)70046-7

22. Carpenter CR, Pines JM, Schuur JD, Muir M, Calfee RP, Raja AS. Adult scaphoid fracture (Kline JA, ed.). *Acad Emerg Med* 2014;21(2):101–121. doi: 10.1111/acem.12317

23. Gellman H, Caputo RJ, Carter V, Aboulafia A, McKay M. Comparison of short and long thumb-spica casts for non-displaced fractures of the carpal scaphoid. *J Bone Joint Surg (Am Vol)* 1989;71(3):354–357.

24. Doornberg JN, Buijze GA, Ham SJ, Ring D, Bhandari M, Poolman RW. Nonoperative treatment for acute scaphoid fractures: a systematic review and meta-analysis of randomized controlled trials. *J Trauma* 2011;71(4):1073–1081. doi: 10.1097/TA.0b013e318222f485

25. McQueen MM, Gelbke MK, Wakefield A, Will EM, Gaebler C. Percutaneous screw fixation versus conservative treatment for fractures of the waist of the scaphoid: a prospective randomised study. *J Bone Joint Surg (Br Vol)* 2008;90(1):66–71. Bone and Joint Journal. doi: 10.1302/0301-620X.90B1.19767

26. Pinder RM, Brkljac M, Rix L, Muir L, Brewster M. Treatment of scaphoid nonunion: a systematic review of the existing evidence. *J Hand Surg* 2015;40(9):1797–1805. doi: 10.1016/j.jhsa.2015.05.003

27. Carlsen BT, Bakri K, Al-Mufarrej FM, Moran SL. Osteoarthritis in the hand and wrist. In: *Plastic Surgery*, 3rd ed. Amsterdam: Elsevier, 2013: 411. doi: 10.1016/B978-1-4377-1733-4.00620-0

28. Shah CM, Stern PJ. Scapholunate advanced collapse (SLAC) and scaphoid nonunion advanced collapse (SNAC) wrist arthritis. *Curr Rev Musculoskeletal Med* 2013;6(1):9–17. doi: 10.1007/s12178-012-9149-4

29. Linscheid RL, Dobyns JH, Beabout JW, Bryan RS. Traumatic instability of the wrist. Diagnosis, classification, and pathomechanics. *J Bone Joint Surg (Am Vol)* 1972;54(8):1612–1632.

30. Buijze GA, Ochtman L, Ring D. Management of scaphoid nonunion. *J Hand Surg* 2012;37(5):1095–100; quiz 1101. doi: 10.1016/j.jhsa.2012.03.002

31. Moon ES, Dy CJ, Derman P, Vance MC, Carlson MG. Management of nonunion following surgical management of scaphoid fractures: current concepts. *J Am Acad Orthopaed Surg* 2013;21(9):548–557. doi: 10.5435/JAAOS-21-09-548

32. Modi CS, Nancoo T, Powers D, Ho K, Boer R, Turner SM. Operative versus nonoperative treatment of acute undisplaced and

minimally displaced scaphoid waist fractures: a systematic review. *Injury* 2009;40(3):268–273. doi: 10.1016/j.injury.2008.07.030

33. Hirche C, Heffinger C, Xiong L, Lehnhardt M, Kneser U, Bickert B, Gazyakan E. The 1,2-intercompartmental supraretinacular artery vascularized bone graft for scaphoid nonunion: management and clinical outcome. *J Hand Surg* 2014;39(3):423–429. doi: 10.1016/j.jhsa.2013.10.028

34. Iorio ML, Masden DL, Higgins JP. Cutaneous angiosome territory of the medial femoral condyle osteocutaneous flap. *YJHSU* 2012;37(5):1033–1041. doi: 10.1016/j.jhsa.2012.02.033

35. Jones DB Jr, Moran SL, Bishop AT, Shin AY. Free-vascularized medial femoral condyle bone transfer in the treatment of scaphoid nonunions. *Plast Reconstr Surg* 2010;125(4):1176–1184. doi: 10.1097/PRS.0b013e3181d1808c

36. Jones DB Jr, Rhee PC, Bishop AT, Shin AY. Free vascularized medial femoral condyle autograft for challenging upper extremity nonunions. *Hand Clin* 2012;28(4):493–501. doi: 10.1016/j.hcl.2012.08.005

37. Lin Sandeep J, Sebastin P-Y, Chung KC. Medial femoral condyle vascularized bone flap for scaphoid nonunion. In: *Operative Techniques: Hand and Wrist Surgery*. Amsterdam: Elsevier, 2012:651–659. doi: 10.1016/B978-1-4557-4024-6.00070-8

38. Capito AE, Higgins JP. Scaphoid overstuffing: the effects of the dimensions of scaphoid reconstruction on scapholunate alignment. *YJHSU* 2013;38(12):2419–2425. doi: 10.1016/j.jhsa.2013.09.035

39. Hofmeister E. Bone? Ligament? bone reconstruction for scapholunate ligament injuries. *Atlas Hand Clin* 2003;8(2):243–247. doi: 10.1016/S1082-3131(03)00051-7

40. Brunelli GA, Brunelli GR. A new surgical technique for carpal instability with scapholunate dissociation. *Surg Techn Int* 1996;5:370–374.

41. Kalb K, Blank S, van Schoonhoven J, Prommersberger K.-J. [Stabilization of the scaphoid according to Brunelli as modified by Garcia-Elias, Lluch, and Stanley for the treatment of chronic scapholunate dissociation]. *Operative Orthopadie und Traumatologie* 2009;21(4–5):429–441. Urban and Vogel. doi: 10.1007/s00064-009-1903-4

42. Links AC, Chin SH, Waitayawinyu T, Trumble TE. Scapholunate interosseous ligament reconstruction: results with a modified Brunelli technique versus four-bone weave. *J Hand Surg* 2008;33(6):850–856. doi: 10.1016/j.jhsa.2008.02.010

43. Sousa M, Aido R, Freitas D, Trigueiros M, Lemos R, Silva C. Scapholunate ligament reconstruction using a flexor carpi radialis tendon graft. *J Hand Surg* 2014;39(8):1512–1516. doi: 10.1016/j.jhsa.2014.04.031

44. Whitty LA, Moran SL. Modified Brunelli tenodesis for the treatment of scapholunate instability. In: *Fractures and Injuries of the Distal Radius and Carpus*. Amsterdam: Elsevier, 2009:481–488. doi: 10.1016/B978-1-4160-4083-5.00051-2

45. Koehler SM, Guerra SM, Kim JM, Sakamoto S, Lovy AJ, Hausman MR. Outcome of arthroscopic reduction association of the scapholunate joint. *J Hand Surg (Eur Vol)* 2016;41(1):48–55. doi: 10.1177/1753193415577335

46. Larson TB, Stern PJ. Reduction and association of the scaphoid and lunate procedure: short-term clinical and radiographic outcomes. *J Hand Surg* 2014;39(11):2168–2174. doi: 10.1016/j.jhsa.2014.07.014

47. Herzberg G, Burnier M, Marc A, Merlini L, Izem Y. The role of arthroscopy for treatment of perilunate injuries. *J Wrist Surg* 2015;4(2):101–109. doi: 10.1055/s-0035-1550344

48. Muller T, Hidalgo Diaz JJ, Pire E, Prunières G, Facca S, Liverneaux P. Treatment of acute perilunate dislocations: ORIF versus proximal row carpectomy. *Orthopaed Traumatol Surg Res* 2017;103(1):95–99. doi: 10.1016/j.otsr.2016.10.014

INDEX